Complications in
Head and Neck Surgery

Complications in Head and Neck Surgery

2nd Edition

David W. Eisele, MD, FACS

Professor and Chairman
Department of Otolaryngology—Head and Neck Surgery
University of California, San Francisco
San Francisco, California

Richard V. Smith, MD, FACS

Vice-Chair and Associate Professor
Department of Otorhinolaryngology—Head and Neck Surgery
Albert Einstein College of Medicine of Yeshiva University
Director
Head and Neck Service
Montefiore Medical Center
Bronx, New York

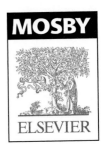

MOSBY

ELSEVIER

1600 John F. Kennedy Blvd.
Ste 1800
Philadelphia, PA 19103-2899

COMPLICATIONS IN HEAD AND NECK SURGERY, SECOND EDITION   ISBN: 978-1-4160-4220-4

Notice

Knowledge and best practice in this field are constantly changing. As new research and experience broaden our knowledge, changes in practice, treatment and drug therapy may become necessary or appropriate. Readers are advised to check the most current information provided (i) on procedures featured or (ii) by the manufacturer of each product to be administered, to verify the recommended dose or formula, the method and duration of administration, and contraindications. It is the responsibility of the practitioner, relying on their own experience and knowledge of the patient, to make diagnoses, to determine dosages and the best treatment for each individual patient, and to take all appropriate safety precautions. To the fullest extent of the law, neither the Publisher nor the Authors assume any liability for any injury and/or damage to persons or property arising out of or related to any use of the material contained in this book.

The Publisher

Previous edition copyrighted 1993

Library of Congress Cataloging-in-Publication Data
Complications in head and neck surgery / editors, David W. Eisele, Richard V. Smith. --2nd ed.
    p. ; cm.

        Includes bibliographical references and index.
        ISBN 978-1-4160-4220-4
    1. Head--Surgery--Complications. 2. Neck--Surgery--Complications. I. Eisele, David W. II. Smith, Richard V., 1962-
        [DNLM: 1. Head--Surgery. 2. Neck--Surgery. 3. Intraoperative Complications. 4. Postoperative Complications. WE 705 C73655 2009]
        RD521.C64 2009
        617.5'1059--dc22

                                                                                2008023627

Acquisitions Editor: Scott Scheidt
Editorial Assistant: Rachel Yard
Project Manager: David Saltzberg
Design Direction: Lou Forgione

Printed in the United States of America

Last digit is the print number: 9 8 7 6 5 4 3 2 1

Peter A. Adamson, MD, FRCSC, FACS
Professor
Department of Otolaryngology—Head and Neck Surgery
University of Toronto
Toronto, Ontario, Canada

Joshua S. Adler, MD
Associate Professor of Clinical Medicine
University of California, San Francisco
Director, Ambulatory Care
UCSF Medical Center
San Francisco, California

M. Jafer Ali, MD
Chief Resident
Department of Otolaryngology—Head and Neck Surgery
University of California, San Francisco
San Francisco, California

Susan K. Anderson, DO
Physician and Surgeon
Department of Otolaryngology
Ear, Nose, and Throat Specialists
Conyers, Georgia

Matthew Ashbach, MD
Chief Resident
Otorhinolaryngology—Head and Neck Surgery
Albert Einstein College of Medicine of Yeshiva University
Bronx, New York

Andrew D. Auerbach, MD, MPH
Associate Professor of Medicine in Residence
University of California, San Francisco
San Francisco, California

David Barrs, MD
Consultant and Associate Clinical Professor
Department of Otolaryngology
Mayo Clinic Arizona
Phoenix, Arizona

Amol M. Bhatki, MD
Chief Resident
Department of Otolaryngology—Head and Neck Surgery
University of California, San Francisco
San Francisco, California

Mark H. Bilsky, MD
Associate Attending
Neurosurgery
Memorial Sloan-Kettering Cancer Center
New York, New York

Jay O. Boyle, MD
Associate Professor of Otolaryngology
Weill Medical College of Cornell University
Associate Attending Surgeon
Head and Neck Service
Memorial Sloan-Kettering Cancer Center
New York, New York

Mark E. Bruley, BS, CCE
Vice President
Accident and Forensic Investigation
ECRI Institute
Plymouth Meeting, Pennsylvania

Jeffrey M. Bumpous, MD, FACS
J. Samuel Bumgardner Professor and Chief
Division of Otolaryngology—Head and Neck Surgery
University of Louisville School of Medicine
Louisville, Kentucky

C. Y. Joseph Chang, MD, FACS
Director
Texas Ear Center
Houston, Texas

Amy Y. Chen, MD, MPH, FACS
Assistant Professor
Department of Otolaryngology
Emory University
Atlanta, Georgia

Theodore Chen, MD
Southern California Permanente Medical Group
Kaiser Permanente Los Angeles Medical Center
Los Angeles, California

Douglas B. Chepeha, MD, MPH
Associate Professor and Co-director
Microvascular Program
Division of Head and Neck Surgery
Department of Otolaryngology
University of Michigan
Ann Arbor, Michigan

Steven W. Cheung, MD
Associate Professor
Department of Otolaryngology—Head and Neck Surgery
University of California, San Francisco
San Francisco, California

Michelle Ciucci, PhD, CCC-SLP
Post-Doctoral Fellow
Surgery—Division of Otolaryngology
University of Wisconsin
Madison, Wisconsin

Francisco J. Civantos, MD
Associate Professor
Co-director of Division of Head and Neck Surgery
Department of Otolaryngology
University of Miami
Miami, Florida

Kimberly P. Cockerham, MD
Associate Clinical Professor
Department of Ophthalmology
Stanford University School of Medicine
Palo Alto, California

Marc D. Coltrera, MD
Professor and Vice Chairman
Department of Otolaryngology–Head and Neck Surgery
University of Washington
Seattle, Washington

Mark S. Courey, MD
Professor
Director, Division of Laryngology
Director, UCSF Voice Center
Department of Otolaryngology—Head and Neck Surgery
University of California, San Francisco
San Francisco, California

Brian Craig, MD
Assistant Professor of Anesthesia
Medical University of South Carolina
Charleston, South Carolina

Daniel G. Deschler, MD, FACS
Associate Professor
Department of Otology and Laryngology
Harvard Medical School
Director, Division of Head and Neck Surgery
Department of Otolaryngology
Massachusetts Eye and Ear Infirmary
Director, Head and Neck Surgery Oncology
General Surgery
Massachusetts General Hospital
Boston, Massachusetts

Stephen F. Dierdorf, MD
Professor
Anesthesiology
Medical University of South Carolina
Charleston, South Carolina

Christopher F. Dowd, MD
Clinical Professor
Radiology, Neurological Surgery, Neurology and
  Anesthesia and Preoperative Care
University of California, San Francisco
San Francisco, California
The Neurovascular Medical Group
Interventional Neuroradiology Section, Department
  of Radiology
University of California, San Francisco Medical Center
San Francisco, California

David W. Eisele, MD, FACS
Professor and Chairman
Department of Otolaryngology—Head and Neck Surgery
University of California, San Francisco
San Francisco, California

Ivan H. El-Sayed, MD, FACS
Assistant Professor
Director, Otolaryngology, Minimally Invasive Skull Base
  Surgery Program
University of California San Francisco
San Francisco, California

Joseph G. Feghali, MD, FACS
Clinical Professor of Otorhinolaryngology—Head
  and Neck Surgery and Neurosurgery
Department of Otolaryngology and Neurotology
Albert Einstein College of Medicine of Yeshiva University/
  Montefiore Medical Center
Bronx, New York

Robert L. Ferris, MD, PhD, FACS
Chief, Division of Head and Neck Surgery
University of Pittsburgh Cancer Institute
Department of Otolaryngology
Pittsburgh, Pennsylvania

Rebecca E. Fraioli, MD
Department of Otolaryngology
University of Pittsburgh School of Medicine
Pittsburgh, Pennsylvania

Marvin P. Fried, MD, FACS
Professor and University Chairman
Department of Otorhinolaryngology—Head and Neck
  Surgery
Albert Einstein College of Medicine of Yeshiva University
Bronx, New York

Holger G. Gassner, MD
Division of Facial Plastic Surgery
Department of Otorhinolaryngology
University of Regensburg
Regensburg, Germany

Roberta E. Gausas, MD, FACS
Director of Oculofacial and Orbital Surgery
Associate Professor of Ophthalmology
Department of Ophthalmology
Scheie Eye Institute
Philadelphia Pennsylvania

Eric M. Genden, MD
Professor and Chairman
Department of Otolaryngology—Head and Neck Surgery
Mount Sinai School of Medicine
Director
Head and Neck Cancer Center
Mount Sinai Medical Center
New York, New York

F. Brian Gibson, MD, FACS
Clinical Assistant Professor
Department of Otolaryngology
Vanderbilt University
Nashville, Tennessee
Clinical Instructor
Department of Family Practice
Carolinas Medical Center
President
Division of Facial Plastic Surgery
Department of Otolaryngology
Charlotte Eye, Ear, Nose, and Throat Associates
Charlotte, North Carolina

M. Boyd Gillespie, MD
Associate Professor
Otolaryngology—Head and Neck Surgery
Medical University of South Carolina
Charleston, South Carolina

Andrew N. Goldberg, MD, MSCE, FACS
Professor
Director, Division of Rhinology and Sinus Surgery
Director, Outcomes Research
Department of Otolaryngology—Head and Neck Surgery
University of California, San Francisco
San Francisco, California

David P. Goldstein, MD, FRCSC
Lecturer
Department of Otolaryngology—Head and Neck Surgery
University of Toronto
Department of Otolaryngology Head and Neck Surgery
and Surgical Oncology
Princess Margaret Hospital
Toronto, Ontario
Canada

Christine G. Gourin, MD, FACS
Associate Professor
Department of Otolaryngology—Head and Neck Surgery
Johns Hopkins University
Baltimore, Maryland

Patrick J. Gullane, MD, FRCS, FACS
Professor and Chairman
Otolaryngology—Head and Neck Surgery
University of Toronto
Wharton Chair in Head and Neck Surgery
Otolaryngologist-in-Chief
University Health Network
Princess Margaret Hospital
Toronto, Ontario
Canada

Missak Haigentz, Jr., MD
Assistant Professor of Medicine
Division of Oncology
Albert Einstein College of Medicine of Yeshiva University
Montefiore Medical Center
Bronx, New York

Ronald A. Hoffman, MD
Director
The Ear Institute
New York Eye and Ear Infirmary
Professor of Otolaryngology
Albert Einstein College of Medicine of Yeshiva University
Bronx, New York

Corinne Elisabeth Horn, MD
Assistant Professor
Clinical Otolaryngology—Head and Neck Surgery
Columbia University College of Physicians and Surgeons
New York, New York

Mimi I. Hu, MD
Assistant Professor
Endocrine Neoplasia and Hormonal Disorders
University of Texas M.D. Anderson Cancer Center
Houston, Texas

Timothy E. Hullar, MD
Assistant Professor
Department of Otolaryngology—Head and Neck Surgery
Department of Anatomy and Neurobiology
Program in Audiology and Communication Sciences
Washington University School of Medicine
St. Louis, Missouri

Andrew F. Inglis, Jr., MD
Associate Professor
Pediatric Otolaryngology—Head and Neck Surgery
Children's Hospital and Regional Medical Center
University of Washington
Seattle, Washington

Jonathan C. Irish, MD, MSc, FRCS(C)
Professor
Otolaryngology—Head and Neck Surgery
University of Toronto
Chief
Surgical Oncology
University Health Network/Princess Margaret Hospital
Toronto, Ontario
Canada

Alexis H. Jackman, MD
Assistant Professor
Department of Otorhinolaryngology—Head and Neck
  Surgery
Albert Einstein College of Medicine of Yeshiva University
Bronx, New York

Adam S. Jacobson, MD
Assistant Professor
Department of Otolaryngology—Head and Neck Surgery
Beth Israel Medical Center
New York, New York

Jonas T. Johnson, MD
Professor and Chairman; The Eugene N. Myers, MD, Chair
  in Otolaryngology
Department of Otolaryngology
University of Pittsburgh School of Medicine
Pittsburgh, Pennsylvania

Haskins Kashima, MD
Professor Emeritus
Department of Otolaryngology—Head and Neck Surgery
The Johns Hopkins University School of Medicine
Baltimore, Maryland

Eric J. Kezirian, MD, MPH
Director
Division of Sleep Surgery
Assistant Professor
Department of Otolaryngology—Head and Neck Surgery
University of California, San Francisco
San Francisco, California

Nissim Khabie, MD
Medical Director
ENT SpecialtyCare of Minnesota
Minneapolis, Minnesota

David W. Kim, MD
Director
Division of Facial Plastic Surgery
Associate Professor
Department of Otolaryngology
University of California, San Francisco
San Francisco, California

Wayne M. Koch, MD
Professor of Otolaryngology—Head and Neck Surgery
Director
Division of Head and Neck Surgery
Department of Otolaryngology—Head and Neck Surgery
Johns Hopkins University
Baltimore, Maryland

Karen A. Kölln, MD
Department of Otolaryngology—Head and Neck Surgery
University of North Carolina at Chapel Hill
Chapel Hill, North Carolina

Dennis H. Kraus, MD
Attending Surgeon
Head and Neck Service
Department of Surgery
Memorial Sloan-Kettering Cancer Center
Professor
Department of Otorhinolaryngology
Cornell University Medical Center
New York, New York

Paul R. Lambert, MD
Professor and Chair
Department of Otolaryngology—Head and Neck Surgery
Medical University of South Carolina
Charleston, South Carolina

Frank R. Lin, MD
Resident
Department of Otolaryngology—Head and Neck Surgery
Johns Hopkins University
Baltimore, Maryland

Jerry Lin, MD
Assistant Professor
Department of Otorhinolaryngology
Weil Cornell Medical College
New York, New York

Jarrod Little, MD
Resident
Division of Otolaryngology
University of Louisville
Louisville, Kentucky

Errol P. Lobo, MD, PhD
Professor of Anesthesia and Perioperative Care
Chief
Vascular Anesthesia
Department of Anesthesia and Perioperative Care
University of California, San Francisco
San Francisco, California

Lawrence R. Lustig, MD
Professor
Francis A. Sooy MD Endowed Chair in Otolaryngology—
    Head and Neck Surgery
Director, Division of Otology, Neurotology, and Skull
    Base Surgery
Department of Otolaryngology—Head and Neck
    Surgery
University of California, San Francisco
San Francisco, California

Timothy M. McCulloch, MD, FACS
Professor, Department of Surgery
Chairman, Division of Otolaryngology—Head and Neck
    Surgery
University of Wisconsin
Madison, Wisconsin

Michael W. McDermott, MD, FRCSC
Professor and Vice-Chairman
Director
Patient Care Services
Co-director
Skull Base and Radiosurgery Programs
Department of Neurological Surgery
University of California, San Francisco
San Francisco, California

John T. McElveen, Jr., MD
Carolina Ear and Hearing Clinic
Raleigh, North Carolina

Laura Ellen Millender, MD
Assistant Professor
Department of Radiation Oncology
Northwestern University
Chicago, Illinois

Kris S. Moe, MD
Chief
Division of Facial Plastic Surgery
Department of Otolaryngology—Head and Neck Surgery
University of Washington School of Medicine
Seattle, Washington

Lee H. Monsein, MD
Assistant Clinical Professor
Department of Radiology
Johns Hopkins University
Baltimore, Maryland
Neuroradiologist
Radiology
Washington Hospital Center
Washington, DC

Eric J. Moore, MD
Assistant Professor/Consultant
Otorhinolaryngology
Mayo Clinic
Rochester, Minnesota

Craig S. Murakami, MD, FACS
Facial Plastic and Reconstructive Surgery
Virginia Mason Medical Center
Seattle, Washington

Andrew H. Murr, MD
Professor and Vice-Chairman
Roger Boles, MD, Endowed Chair in Otolaryngology
    Education
Director, Residency Program
Department of Otolaryngology—Head and Neck Surgery
University of California, San Francisco
San Francisco, California

James L. Netterville, MD
Professor and Director
Division of Head and Neck Surgery
Department of Otolaryngology
Vanderbilt University
Nashville, Tennessee

John K. Niparko, MD
George T. Nager Professor
Director
Division of Otology, Neurotology and Skull Base Surgery
Department of Otolaryngology—Head and Neck Surgery
The Johns Hopkins Hospital
Baltimore, Maryland

Kerry D. Olsen, MD
Professor
Otolaryngology—Head and Neck Surgery
Mayo Clinic
Rochester, Minnesota

Lisa A. Orloff, MD
Robert K. Werbe Distinguished Professor in Head and
  Neck Cancer
Director
Division of Head and Neck and Endocrine Surgery
Department of Otolaryngology—Head and Neck Surgery
University of California, San Francisco
San Francisco, California

Thomas Julian Ow, MD
Chief Resident
Otorhinolaryngology—Head and Neck Surgery
Albert Einstein College of Medicine of Yeshiva University
Montefiore Medical Center
Bronx, New York

Sanjay R. Parikh, MD, FAAP, FACS
Associate Professor
Department of Otorhinolaryngology—Head and Neck
  Surgery
Albert Einstein College of Medicine of Yeshiva University
Chief
Division of Pediatric Otorhinolaryngology
Children's Hospital at Montefiore
Bronx, New York

Shatul L. Parikh, MD
Chief Resident
Department of Otolaryngology—Head and Neck Surgery
Emory University School of Medicine
Atlanta, Georgia

Francesca Pellegrini, MD
Faculty Anesthesiologist
Department of Anesthesia
St. Anna Hospital
Ferrara, Italy

Stephen W. Perkins, MD
Clinical Associate Professor
Department of Otolaryngology—Head and Neck Surgery
Indiana University School of Medicine
Indianapolis, Indiana

Bruce A. Perler, MD, MBA
Julius H. Jacobson II Professor of Surgery
Department of Surgery
The Johns Hopkins University School of Medicine
Chief
Division of Vascular Surgery
Department of Surgery
The Johns Hopkins Hospital
Baltimore, Maryland

Karen T. Pitman, MD
Associate Professor
Department of Otolaryngology and Communicative
  Sciences
University of Mississippi Medical Center
Jackson, Mississippi

M. Anthony Pogrel, DDS, MD, FACS, FRCS
Professor and Chairman
Department of Oral and Maxillofacial Surgery
University of California, San Francisco
San Francisco, California

Elisabetta Pusceddu, MD
Resident in Anesthesia and Intensive Care
Azienda Policlinico
Università degli Studi di Caglari
Italy

Francine Rainone, DO, PhD, MS
Director of Palliative Medicine
Lourdes Hospital
Binghamton, New York

Vincent Reid, MD
Fellow
Department of Surgery
Division of Head and Neck Oncology
The Memorial Sloan-Kettering Cancer Center
New York, New York

Vicente A. Resto, MD, PhD
Assistant Professor
Department of Otolaryngology—Head and Neck Surgery
University of Texas Medical Branch
Galveston, Texas

Jennifer L. Rhodes, MD
Chief Resident
Department of Plastic Surgery
Albert Einstein College of Medicine of Yeshiva University
Montefiore Medical Center
Bronx, New York

Mark A. Richardson, MD
Dean
School of Medicine
Professor
Department of Otolaryngology—Head and Neck Surgery
Oregon Health & Science University
Portland, Oregon

David M. Saito, MD
Chief Resident
Department of Otolaryngology—Head and Neck Surgery
University of California, San Francisco
San Francisco, California

Hazem Mohammad Ali Saleh, MD
Lecturer of Otorhinolaryngology
Department of Medical Applications of Laser
National Institute of Laser Enhanced Sciences, Cairo
  University
Cairo
Egypt
Research Fellow
Otolaryngology—Head and Neck Surgery
University of California at San Francisco
San Francisco, California
Visiting Physician
Head and Neck Surgery
The Gustave Roussy Institute
Paris
France

Bradley A. Schiff, MD
Assistant Professor
Department of Otorhinolaryngology—Head and Neck
  Surgery
Albert Einstein College of Medicine of Yeshiva University
New York, New York

Brian L. Schmidt, DDS, MD, PhD
Associate Professor
Department of Oral and Maxillofacial Surgery
University of California—San Francisco
San Francisco, California

Brent A. Senior, MD, FACS, FARS
Chief
Rhinology, Allergy, and Sinus Surgery
Associate Professor, Otolaryngology—Head and Neck
  Surgery
University of North Carolina at Chapel Hill
Chapel Hill, North Carolina

Steven I. Sherman, MD
Chair and Professor
Department of Endocrine Neoplasia and Hormonal Disorders
University of Texas M. D. Anderson Cancer Center
Houston, Texas

Mark G. Shrime, MD
Clinical Fellow
Department of Otolaryngology, Head and Neck Surgery
University of Toronto
Clinical Fellow
Department of Otolaryngology, Head and Neck Surgery
Toronto General Hospital
Clinical Fellow
Department of Otolaryngology, Head and Neck Surgery
Princess Margaret Hospital
Toronto, Ontario
Canada

Richard V. Smith, MD, FACS
Vice-Chair and Associate Professor
Department of Otorhinolaryngology—Head and Neck
  Surgery
Albert Einstein College of Medicine of Yeshiva University
Director
Head and Neck Service
Montefiore Medical Center
Bronx, New York

David Alan Staffenberg, MD, DSc
Chief, Division of Plastic Surgery
Program Director, Plastic Surgery Training Program
Montefiore Medical Center
Surgical Director, Center for Craniofacial Disorders
Children's Hospital at Montefiore
Associate Professor
Clinical Plastic Surgery
Neurological Surgery and Pediatrics
Albert Einstein College of Medicine of Yeshiva University
Bronx, New York

Tracey Straker, MD, MPH
Assistant Professor of Anesthesiology
Albert Einstein College of Medicine of Yeshiva University
Attending Anesthesiologist
Montefiore Medical Center
Bronx, New York

Jonathan M. Sykes, MD, FACS
Director of Facial Plastic and Reconstructive Surgery
Professor of Otolaryngology—Head and Neck Surgery
University of California, Davis
Sacramento, California

Theodoros N. Teknos, MD
David E. and Carole Schuller Chair in Head and Neck
  Surgery
Professor, Otolaryngology—Head and Neck Surgery
Chief of the Head and Neck Cancer Program
The Arthur James Cancer Center and Richard Solove
  Research Institute
The Ohio State University Medical Center
Columbus, Ohio

David J. Terris, MD, FACS
Porubsky Distinguished Professor
Chairman, Department of Otolaryngology
Surgical Director, Medical College of Georgia Thyroid
  Center
Medical College of Georgia
Augusta, Georgia

Bradley Thedinger, MD
Neurotology
Otologic Center Inc
Kansas City, Missouri

J. Regan Thomas, MD
Lederer Professor and Chairman
Department of Otolaryngology—Head and Neck Surgery
University of Illinois, Chicago
Chicago, Illinois

Robert M. Wachter, MD
Professor and Associate Chairman
Department of Medicine
University of California, San Francisco
San Francisco, California

Rohan R. Walvekar, MD
Assistant Professor
Otolaryngology—Head and Neck Surgery
University of Pittsburgh and Veterans Affairs Medical
  Center
Pittsburgh, Pennsylvania

Brian S. Wang, MD
Resident
Department of Otolaryngology—Head and Neck Surgery
University of Texas, Houston
Houston, Texas

Steven J. Wang, MD
Assistant Professor
Department of Otolaryngology—Head and Neck Surgery
University of California, San Francisco
Chief, Otolaryngology—Head and Neck Surgery
San Francisco Veterans Affairs Medical Center
San Francisco, California

Edward Wladis, MD
Fellow, Oculofacial and Orbital Surgery
Ophthalmology
Scheie Eye Institute, University of Pennsylvania
Philadelphia, Pennsylvania

Matthew B. Zavod, MD
Staff Physician
Department of Otolaryngology—Head and Neck Surgery
Department of Facial Plastic and Reconstructive Surgery
Woodland Healthcare
Woodland, California

Mark S. Zimbler, MD
Associate Professor
Otolaryngology—Head and Neck Surgery
Albert Einstein College of Medicine of Yeshiva University
Bronx, New York
Director of Facial Plastic and Reconstructive Surgery
Department of Otolaryngology—Head and Neck Surgery
Beth Israel Medical Center
New York, New York

Christopher I. Zoumalan, MD
Chief Resident
Department of Ophthalmology
Stanford University School of Medicine
Stanford, California

Richard A. Zoumalan, MD
Resident Physician
Department of Otolaryngology—Head and Neck Surgery
New York University School of Medicine
New York, New York

Preface

This book is intended for surgeons and health care professionals at all levels of experience who are interested in the surgical management of head and neck disorders. An understanding of the potential complications that can result from the range of head and neck surgical procedures performed by surgeons of various specialties is essential to optimal patient care.

The second edition of *Complications in Head and Neck Surgery* presents a comprehensive and contemporary discussion of complications of head and neck surgical procedures. Topics are organized by anatomic region and are grouped with related procedures. Each topic is explored in depth by chapter authors from varied medical disciplines, each chosen for his or her expertise and experience. Although major surgical procedures and associated topics are emphasized, new surgical techniques and less commonly seen procedures are also covered. Some complications are discussed in more than one chapter to present different perspectives. New chapters address important contemporary issues, including patient safety and medical errors.

The avoidance, recognition, and management of complications are central to successful head and neck surgical care. Proper and prompt management prevents the complication "cascade" whereby a problem is amplified or other complications ensue. A discussion of potential risks and complications of a surgical procedure with the patient is an essential component of informed consent and risk management. It is hoped that this book will foster and facilitate increased communication between the head and neck surgeon and the patient, resulting in increased patient understanding and improved patient care, and between health care professionals, contributing to a cooperative multidisciplinary approach to care of the head and neck surgical patient.

DAVID W. EISELE, MD, FACS

RICHARD V. SMITH, MD, FACS

Contents

PART 1
General Topics

CHAPTER 1

Anesthesia Complications in Head and Neck Surgery

Errol P. Lobo, Francesca Pellegrini, and Elisabetta Pusceddu

Most surgical procedures involving the head and neck require a symbiotic relationship between the head and neck surgeon and the anesthesiologist. This is especially true for complicated surgical procedures that involve the airway, and it is also true regarding complications that occur during head and neck surgery. In critical situations in which airway compromise is anticipated, the anesthesiologist and the surgeon best appreciate the severity of the situation. This chapter focuses on some of the anesthesia complications that can occur during head and neck surgery and on how some of them may be anticipated and prevented.

The initial section of this chapter is devoted to the preoperative evaluation of the patient scheduled for head and neck surgery. Perioperative complications can often be avoided with a good presurgical workup and the optimization of existing medical conditions. This is especially true for patients with coexisting cardiovascular and pulmonary disease; these patients comprise a significant portion of the individuals who present for complicated head and neck surgery. Also included in this section is the preoperative workup of the patient with obstructive sleep apnea (OSA). As the number of people with obesity increases, there is an increase in the number of patients with OSA who present for surgery. These patients require special consideration, especially if they receive opioids as part of their anesthetic treatment.

The chapter also includes a brief discussion of the pharmacology of some of the drugs that are more commonly used for anesthesia. Most of the drugs discussed are most often used for procedures that require conscious sedation. In most facilities (particularly for office-based procedures), conscious sedation is often provided by or supervised by the surgeon. Hence, an understanding of the drugs used for conscious sedation is important. The toxicities associated with the use of some of these medications are also included. An overview of anesthetic complications that can occur during head and neck surgery and other surgical procedures is also provided. It is important to have a basic knowledge of the anesthesia complications that may require consultation from the head and neck surgeon.

The final section contains an overview of the difficult airway and discusses some techniques that can be used for tracheal intubation when a difficult airway is anticipated. Surgeries of the neck and the upper aerodigestive tract often involve patients who are difficult to manually ventilate and who also present problems for tracheal intubation. These patients merit special attention from the anesthesiologist and the head and neck surgeon. In addition, it is important for the head and neck surgeon to be aware of some of the new equipment that can be used during airway management.

PREOPERATIVE EVALUATION FOR HEAD AND NECK SURGERY

A significant percentage of complications of surgery are directly related to poor presurgical evaluation of the patient and failure to optimize medical conditions that may result in perioperative complications. Preoperative evaluation also provides information regarding any potential airway problems, including the need for additional monitoring (e.g., the use of invasive hemodynamic monitors) and the use of intraoperative transesophageal echocardiography, although the latter is not commonly used during head and neck surgery because of the operative sites involved. Also important is the disposition of the patient after surgery and the need for the patient to be monitored in an intensive care unit (ICU). The American Society of Anesthesiology has provided guidelines for categorizing the risk of patients who are undergoing surgery. These guidelines take into consideration the comorbid conditions that may be present (Box 1-1).[1-6]

In the practice of surgery today, patients with pulmonary or cardiac diseases are often referred to consultants for the assessment and perioperative management of their comorbid conditions. It is important for the surgeon to understand some of the functional and diagnostic tests that are used for the cardiac and pulmonary evaluation of patients.[7]

Basic Evaluation

The basic preoperative evaluation for most patients should include a history and physical examination. Any evidence of problems with prior surgery or anesthesia should be noted. In addition, the functional status of the patient (particularly of the elderly patient) is of major importance. Patients with a history of cardiac disease, hypertension, diabetes mellitus, pulmonary disease, or gastroesophageal reflux disease merit special consideration when general anesthesia or conscious sedation is provided. A list of the patient's medications as well as any medication allergies is also important. For head and neck surgical procedures that address disorders involving airway compromise, intubation of the trachea may be challenging. Hence, magnetic resonance imaging (MRI) or computed tomography (CT) scanning of the affected area should be performed.

For patients who are generally in good health, the basic evaluation should include a baseline laboratory evaluation that includes a complete blood count. For patients who are more than 50 years old, an electrocardiogram (EKG) is required before surgery at most institutions.

Evaluation of the Patient With Cardiac Disease

All patients who are more than 50 years old and patients with cardiac disease should receive an EKG. The preoperative EKG can provide important information about the status of the patient's cardiac and coronary circulations. Abnormal Q waves seen on the EKG suggest a previous myocardial infarction (MI). Clinical predictors of increased perioperative cardiac morbidity and mortality are listed in Box 1-2. These patients may be at increased risk for a perioperative cardiac event, and they may require further preoperative assessment, particularly if they have limitations in their exercise habits.[8–11] In fact, about 30% of MIs are silent and only detected with routine EKG; this is most notable among patients with diabetes mellitus and hypertension. In addition to the EKG, the taking of the history can provide important information regarding the patient's cardiac status.[12,13] Assessing the patient's functional status by testing his or her exercise tolerance may determine the need for a cardiac evaluation.[14] The information from cardiovascular testing may allow for the optimization of preoperative medications, and it may also provide information regarding perioperative monitoring or the need for coronary revascularization. Several tests can be used for the assessment of functional status, including the following:

1. *24-hour ambulatory EKG*: This requires the placement of a Holter monitor that records a continuous 12-lead EKG for 24 hours. This will detect arrhythmias and ischemic changes during a 24-hour period. This test will often lead to further testing, particularly if ischemic changes are noted.[15–20]

2. *Exercise stress test:* This test is essentially an exercise EKG in which a patient is asked to exercise with the EKG as well as heart rate and blood pressure monitoring. The presence of EKG signs of myocardial ischemia, patient complaints of chest pain or dyspnea, and clinical signs of left ventricular dysfunction are considered positive results. Even more important is a decrease in blood pressure in response to exercise; this may be associated with global ventricular dysfunction. Syncope during the test also signifies decreased cardiac output. A positive exercise EKG stress test should alert the anesthesiologist that the patient is at risk for ischemia at a wide range of heart rates, which may occur during surgery. These patients may require further workup and the optimization of medical management.[21–24]

3. *Thallium exercise test:* The sensitivity and specificity of the noninvasive stress test can be increased with nuclear imaging techniques. Thallium-201 (Tl-201) is a radioactive compound that mimics potassium uptake by viable myocardial cells. The sensitivity of exercise Tl-201 imaging depends on the imaging technique. Qualitative visual Tl-201 imaging has an average sensitivity of 84% and a specificity of 87% for detecting coronary artery disease, although these numbers are improved with better imaging techniques. The drawback is that patients have to remain stationary for imaging to avoid artifacts. Thallium defects are reported as normal, fixed, or reversible. Other measures of importance, particularly during stress Tl-201 imaging, are the size of defect, lung uptake, and left ventricular cavity size. A large lung uptake of isotope has been associated with myocardial ischemia that produces left ventricular dysfunction that may result in pulmonary edema. The presence of a distended left ventricular cavity on the immediate poststress image is another marker of severe coronary artery disease, presumably as a result of myocardial ischemia.

4. *Thallium imaging in patients who cannot exercise:* The use of pharmacologic agents to induce cardiac stress in patients who cannot exercise can also detect coronary artery disease. These agents can be divided into two categories: those that result in coronary artery vasodilatation (e.g., dipyridamole, adenosine) and those that increase myocardial oxygen demand (e.g., dobutamine, isoproterenol). Coronary artery vasodilators are useful for defining myocardium at risk by causing differential flows in normal coronary arteries as compared with those with a stenotic lesion. The use of dobutamine is an alternative method of increasing myocardial oxygen demand without exercise. The goal is to increase both heart rate and blood pressure.[25–30]

5. *Echocardiography:* The use of echocardiography for preoperative cardiac evaluation has increased during the last few years. Left ventricular function, pulmonary vascular pressures, and valvular competence can be evaluated. In most cases, a transthoracic approach has been used. Transesophageal echocardiography may provide a better measurement of valvular abnormalities and left ventricular function. Echocardiography can also be performed with exercise. Among patients who are unable to exercise, dobutamine has been used to mimic the stress effects of exercise. The dobutamine echocardiography examination is both sensitive and specific, and the procedure can be completed in 1 to 2 hours (as compared with angiography and thallium imaging).[31–33]

6. *Coronary angiography:* Coronary angiography has been called the gold standard for defining coronary anatomy because of its sensitivity and specificity. In addition, angiography can also assess valvular function and hemodynamic indices, including ventricular pressure and gradients across valves. In most cases, angiography is performed after a positive stress test to determine whether coronary revascularization will improve cardiac function and reduce perioperative cardiac morbidity after noncardiac surgery. One major difference between the stress tests described previously and coronary angiography is that the latter provides the clinician with anatomic—rather than functional—information. It is also an expensive test with potential complications.

Preoperative Pulmonary Evaluation

Patients scheduled for head and neck surgery may present with coexisting pulmonary disease. For patients with acute pulmonary disease who are scheduled for elective surgery, the surgery may be postponed until the pulmonary disease resolves; this is especially true for children and adults with upper respiratory tract infections. If these patients present with a history of fever and a productive cough with discolored sputum, then it is prudent to postpone elective surgery. Viral upper respiratory tract infections may adversely affect the respiratory immune system, thereby predisposing a patient who requires general anesthesia with endotracheal intubation to bacterial infections during the perioperative period.

Patients with chronic pulmonary disease may benefit from a preoperative pulmonary workup that includes an arterial blood gas determination, a chest radiograph, and pulmonary function tests (PFTs). The presence of pulmonary disease may increase perioperative morbidity and mortality (Box 1-3). Preoperative PFTs measure the severity of lung disease and the efficacy of bronchodilator therapy for improving pulmonary function, and they can predict the need for postoperative mechanical ventilation.[34–37]

The two most common patterns of abnormal breathing as determined by preoperative PFTs are obstructive and restrictive breathing patterns. Obstructive lung diseases are the most common form of pulmonary dysfunction, and they commonly afflict smokers. Asthma, emphysema, chronic bronchitis, cystic fibrosis, bronchiectasis, and bronchiolitis are all forms of obstructive lung disease. The primary characteristic of these disorders is resistance to airflow.[38–42]

Restrictive pulmonary diseases are characterized by decreased lung compliance, and lung volumes are typically reduced. Expiratory flow rates are unchanged. Restrictive pulmonary diseases include many acute and chronic intrinsic pulmonary disorders as well as extrinsic (extrapulmonary) disorders involving the pleura, the chest wall, the diaphragm, or neuromuscular function. Reduced lung compliance increases the work of breathing, which results in a characteristic rapid but shallow breathing pattern. Respiratory gas exchange is usually maintained until the disease process is advanced.

The evaluation of pulmonary function is obtained by PFTs. The evaluation of lung diffusion capacity, flow–volume loops, and nitrogen washout techniques are not discussed in this chapter. For detailed information about PFTs, refer to a textbook of pulmonary medicine or anesthesiology.

The cornerstone of the PFTs is clinical spirometry. Gas exchange can be assessed by other means, including arterial blood gas assessment. It is important for the head and neck surgeon to appreciate some of the lung volumes that are measured as part of the PFTs. The most common measurement of lung function is the vital capacity (VC). The VC is the largest volume measured, and it is measured after an individual inspires deeply and maximally to total lung capacity and then exhales completely to residual volume into a spirometer. The value of the VC depends on the position of the patient, and it is considered abnormal if the VC is less than 80% of what was predicted. In general, a VC of less than 80% of the predicted value indicates possible restrictive lung disease. A decreased VC can be associated with lung pathology, including pneumonia, atelectasis, or pulmonary fibrosis. Muscle weakness, pain, and abdominal swelling can also cause a decrease in VC.

In contrast with VC, another test has the subject exhale as forcefully and rapidly as possible after a maximum inspiratory effort, and the volume of gas exhaled is called the *forced vital capacity (FVC)*. This exhaled volume can be recorded with respect to time. The rate of airflow during this rapid, forceful exhalation indirectly reflects the flow resistance properties of the airways. If obstructive pulmonary disease is present, the FVC tends to be less than the standard VC, because the airway reaches flow limitation early, and air trapping occurs. During the measurement of FVC, the patient is instructed to take a breath to full inspiration (total lung capacity), and this is followed by an abrupt onset of exhalation and continued maximum effort throughout exhalation to residual volume. The exhalation should take at least 4 seconds, and it should not be interrupted by coughing, glottic closure, or any mechanical obstruction.

A reduction in FVC is noted in the presence of the same conditions that reduce VC. The assessment of airway obstruction is determined by the calculation of the volume exhaled during certain time intervals. Most commonly measured is the volume exhaled in the first second, called the *forced expiratory volume in 1 second (FEV1)*. The FEV_1 can be expressed as the absolute volume in liters; however, the FEV_1 provides a better perspective on the degree of airway obstruction when it is expressed as a percentage of the FVC (FEV_1/FVC). Table 1-1 shows the FVC, the FEV_1, and the FEV_1/FVC in different pulmonary disease states.

TABLE 1-1 Forced Vital Capacity and 1-Second Forced Expiratory Volume in Obstructive and Restrictive Lung Disease

Disease State	FVC	FEV_1	FEV_1/FVC
Obstructive lung disease (e.g., asthma, bronchitis)	Normal	Decreased	Decreased
Restrictive lung disease (e.g., pneumonia, pulmonary edema, pulmonary fibrosis)	Decreased	Decreased	Normal
Respiratory muscle weakness (e.g., myasthenia gravis, myopathies)	Decreased	Decreased	Normal

FEV1, 1-Second forced expiratory volumes; *FVC*, forced vital capacity.

Although the purpose of this subsection is to provide the reader with a brief overview of PFTs, it should be emphasized that obtaining PFTs for patients is done primarily to ascertain the type and severity of pulmonary disease in a patient and to determine whether postoperative care should involve recovery in an ICU. In some situations, the treatment of pulmonary disease (particularly obstructive disease) may be improved if bronchodilator treatment results in an improvement in the airway during the PFT workup.

Evaluation of the Patient With Obstructive Sleep Apnea

During the last several years, the number of patients who present for surgery with OSA has risen dramatically. In fact, OSA is a significant medical problem that affects at least 10% to 25% of the middle-aged population. OSA is more common among men than women. The most common complaints are loud snoring at night, disrupted sleep, and excessive daytime sleepiness. Over time, patients with OSA may develop significant cardiac and pulmonary problems.[43–46] Although it is clear that a significant proportion of patients who have OSA are obese with short, thick necks, some patients with OSA have a normal weight with a receding jaw. Because symptoms of OSA are exacerbated during anesthesia, both the surgeon and the anesthesiologist should be aware of potential problems when dealing with the patient with OSA. Patients who present for procedures at same-day surgery centers may require special consideration.[47–49]

Treatment for OSA in adults includes weight loss and the use of a nighttime continuous positive airway pressure (CPAP) apparatus. With CPAP, the patient wears a snugly fitting nasal mask, and positive pressure keeps the airway open during sleep. Patients with a history of OSA who present for surgery should be instructed to bring their CPAP apparatuses with them.[50–53]

Among children and some adults, the use of a CPAP mask may not be a viable treatment. Among selected younger patients, uvulopalatopharyngoplasty, which involves the removal of part of the soft palate, the uvula, and redundant pharyngeal tissues (usually including the tonsils), is an alternative therapy. Such procedures are often performed by a head and neck surgeon, so knowledge of the diagnostic criteria for OSA is important.

Diagnosis of Obstructive Sleep Apnea

The obstruction of airflow in OSA can be incomplete (hypopnea) or total (apnea). The diagnostic criterion for OSA is based on the Apnea/Hypopnea Index (AHI). The AHI is derived from the total number of apneas and hypopneas divided by the total sleep time.

Currently a normal cutoff for the AHI is between 5 and 10 per hour. The severity of OSA can be defined on the basis of the AHI as follows:

- *Mild:* AHI = 5 to 15 per hour
- *Moderate:* AHI = 15 to 30 per hour
- *Severe:* AHI = More than 30 per hour

The physical examination of patients with OSA is often unremarkable except for the presence of obesity (defined as a body mass index of more than 30 kg/m^2) and hypertension. Often the clues to the presence of OSA will come from family members who complain of loud snoring at night as well as a disrupted sleep pattern and nocturnal gasping and choking. Patients with OSA will also be observed to have excessive daytime sleepiness and fatigue.[44]

A complete physical examination of the patient with suspected OSA is of paramount importance. As for all patients who are being prepared for surgery, this should include a detailed examination of the airway. In nonobese patients with OSA, a careful evaluation of the oral cavity and the airway is also important.

Some physical features associated with OSA include the following:

- Narrowing of the lateral airway walls (this may be an independent predictor of the presence of OSA in men but not in women)
- Enlarged tonsils
- Retrognathia or micrognathia
- A prominent overbite
- Swelling of the soft palate
- A high, arched soft palate

Laboratory Diagnosis of Obstructive Sleep Apnea

Nocturnal polysomnography is the gold standard for the diagnosis of OSA. With this technique, multiple physiologic parameters are measured while the patient sleeps in a sleep laboratory. Typical parameters of a sleep study include eye movement observations (to detect rapid eye movement sleep), an electroencephalogram (to determine arousals from sleep), chest wall monitors (to document respiratory movements), nasal and oral airflow measurements, an EKG, an electromyogram (to look for limb movements that cause arousals), and oximetry (to measure oxygen saturation). Apneic events can then be documented on the basis of chest wall movement with no airflow and oxyhemoglobin desaturations.[50,54]

Perioperative care of the patient with OSA requires the careful consideration of medications that may affect the respiratory status of the patient. The use of sedative and analgesic agents will aggravate or precipitate OSA by decreasing pharyngeal tone and depressing ventilatory responses to hypoxia and hypercapnia. Limiting the amount of opioids may reduce the respiratory complications seen in patients with OSA during the postoperative period.

PHARMACOLOGY OF SOME COMMONLY USED DRUGS FOR CONSCIOUS SEDATION AND LOCAL ANESTHESIA

An understanding of the drugs used for sedation and their potential toxicities is important for the head and neck surgeon, particularly if that surgeon is to provide conscious sedation for procedures or if he or she is to supervise other health care personnel during the provision of conscious sedation. In addition to addressing the medications used for conscious sedation, this section will also review the pharmacology of local anesthetics and antiemetic medications. The use of local anesthesia for local infiltration as well as for the placement of regional nerve blocks also requires some understanding of the pharmacology of local anesthetics.

Analgesics

Opioids

Opioids mediate analgesia through a complex interaction of opioid receptors in the supraspinal central nervous system. They produce reliable analgesia, and they also provide some sedation and euphoria. There is no impairment of myocardial contractility, but sympathetically mediated vascular tone is reduced. Ventilation is depressed as a result of the elevation of the carbon dioxide threshold for respiration. Opioids given at recommended doses do not reliably produce unconsciousness. However, they may cause decreased bowel motility, biliary spasm, nausea, and pruritus. A brief review of the pharmacology of some of the more common opioids is presented later in this chapter.[55–57] For an overview of the dosing guidelines of opioids, see Table 1-2.

Morphine

Morphine has been described as the gold standard of opioid therapy. The drug can be given orally, intramuscularly, or intravenously. Morphine is relatively hydrophilic, and thus it has a slower onset with a longer clinical effect. Only a small amount of administered morphine gains access to the central nervous system, but it accumulates rapidly in the kidneys, the liver, and skeletal muscles. Morphine has several metabolites, including morphine-6-glucuronide, which causes additional analgesia,[58] and morphine-3-glucuronide, which causes adverse effects.[59]

Morphine can cause profound vasodilatation, which may be induced as a result of the effects of histamine release and a reduction of sympathetic nervous system tone. Like other opioids, addiction to morphine can occur with chronic use.[60]

Hydromorphone

Hydromorphone is opioid that binds to the μ-receptor. It is three to five times more potent than morphine orally and five to seven times as potent parenterally. Its duration of analgesic effect, at 3 to 4 hours, is similar to that of morphine. During recent years, hydromorphone has become the drug of choice for use with patient-controlled analgesia. Dosing guidelines for patient-controlled analgesia are shown in Table 1-3.

Pruritus, sedation, nausea, and vomiting occur less frequently with hydromorphone as compared with morphine. The metabolite of hydromorphone is hydromorphone-3-glucoronide. It lacks the analgesic property of the metabolite of morphine, but it possesses neuroexcitatory properties that are similar to those of morphine-3-glucuronide.

Fentanyl

Fentanyl is a potent synthetic opiate agonist that is very lipid soluble and that is commonly used in perioperative settings. Fentanyl is a phenylpiperidine derivative, and it is structurally similar to meperidine, alfentanil, and sufentanil. A 100-mcg dose of fentanyl is approximately equipotent to 10 mg of morphine. As compared with morphine or meperidine, fentanyl has a shorter duration of action and half-life.[59,61] The lipid solubility of fentanyl is the reason for its rapid onset and its shorter duration of action. This reflects faster entrance into the central nervous system as well as prompt redistribution. Elevated doses may lead to progressive saturation in adipose tissues. When this occurs, plasma concentrations do not decline promptly. Thus, pharmacodynamic effects, including ventilatory depression, may be prolonged.

Remifentanil

Remifentanil has a much more rapid onset and offset than fentanyl. With an initial dose, anesthesia may be achieved in 30 to 60 seconds; offset of the drug can occur within 5 to 10 minutes after the discontinuation of an infusion. Because remifentanil is metabolized in the blood and the skeletal muscle, it can be administered as a single dose or as an infusion. For awake tracheal intubation and airway examination, the use of remifentanil has been advocated.[62] Because of the potency of this opioid and because chest wall rigidity and rapid respiratory depression may occur with its use, remifentanil should be administered by an anesthesiologist or an anesthetist.

Meperidine

Commonly known as *Demerol,* meperidine has a tenth of the potency of morphine, a poor and variable oral absorption, and a short duration of action (2–3 hours). In low doses, it has been shown to decrease the shivering

TABLE 1-2 Dosing Guidelines of Common Opioids

Agent	Use	Route	Dose
Morphine	Premedication	IM	0.05–0.2 mg/kg
	Intraoperative anesthesia	IV	0.1–1 mg/kg
	Postoperative analgesia	IM	0.05–0.2 mg/kg
		IV	0.03–0.15 mg/kg
Meperidine	Premedication	IM	0.5–1 mg/kg
	Intraoperative anesthesia	IV	2.5–5 mg/kg
	Postoperative analgesia	IM	0.5–1 mg/kg
		IV	0.2–0.5 mg/kg
Fentanyl	Intraoperative anesthesia	IV	1–5 mcg/kg
	Postoperative analgesia	IV	0.5–1.5 mcg/kg
Sufentanil	Intraoperative anesthesia	IV	0.25–2 mcg/kg
Alfentanil	*Intraoperative anesthesia*		
	Loading dose	IV	8–100 mcg/kg
	Maintenance infusion	IV	0.5–2 mcg/kg/min
Remifentanil	*Intraoperative anesthesia*		
	Loading dose	IV	0.5–2 mcg/kg
	Maintenance infusion	IV	0.1–1 mcg/kg/min
	Postoperative analgesia/sedation	IV	0.025–0.2 mcg/kg/min

IM, Intramuscular; *IV,* intravenous.

TABLE 1-3 General Guidelines for Patient-Controlled Analgesia Orders for the Average Adult

Opioid	Bolus Dose	Lockout (min)	Infusion Rate
Morphine	1–3 mg	10–20	0–1 mg/h
Meperidine (Demerol)	10–15 mg	5–15	0–20 mg/h
Fentanyl (Sublimaze)	15–25 mcg	10–20	0–50 mcg/h
Hydromorphone (Dilaudid)	0.1–0.3 mg	10–20	0–0.5 mg/h

that is associated with rewarming after surgery and after the administration of amphotericin.

Several metabolites are excreted by the kidney and may accumulate in the presence of renal disease. Meperidine has numerous undesirable side effects, including additional anticholinergic effects and high lipophilicity, which induces drug-seeking behavior. The major metabolite, normeperidine, is a proconvul-sant that may cause seizures in patients with renal compromise.

Methadone

The use of methadone for postoperative pain management has increased during the past few years, especially for patients with chronic pain and chronic opioid usage. Methadone has an excellent bioavailability profile (60% to 95%), a high potency, and a long duration of action. Its increased use is the result of its ideal properties, which include its lack of an active metabolite, its low cost, and its activity at sites in addition to the opioid receptor. Methadone is an N-methyl-D-aspartic acid receptor antagonist, and it inhibits serotonin uptake; both of these properties provide analgesia by interfering with peripheral pain transmission. Methadone's potency as compared with that of morphine ranges from 1:1 to 1:4.

The long half-life of methadone makes it difficult to use to achieve steady-state plasma concentrations. In addition, it may accumulate when given in high doses.[63]

Complications Associated With Opioid Use

In the perioperative setting, side effects of opioid use include pruritus, nausea, respiratory depression, and delirium.[64] The latter may result in serious consequences, including death. There are multiple factors that affect the magnitude and duration of opioid-induced respiratory depression. Older patients are more sensitive to the anesthetic and respiratory-depressant effects of opioids, and, in general, they have an increased frequency of apneic episodes, periodic breathing, and upper airway obstruction after morphine use as compared with young adults. In fact, older patients develop higher plasma concentrations of opioids as compared with younger patients when the drugs are administered on a weight basis. Morphine also produces greater respiratory depression on a weight basis in neonates than in adults. In neonates and infants with incomplete blood–brain barriers, morphine easily penetrates the brain.

Complications from respiratory depression induced by opioids can lead to serious consequences, including respiratory failure and death. Box 1-4 lists some of the factors that can increase the incidence of opioid-induced

---

BOX 1-4 Factors That Increase Opioid-Induced Respiratory Depression

High dose of opioid given
Older age
Opioid naive
Opioids given with central nervous system depressants, including the following:

- Inhaled anesthetics
- Alcohol
- Barbiturates
- Benzodiazepines

Presence of renal insufficiency
Hyperventilation
Hypocapnia
Respiratory acidosis
Decreased clearance of opioids (reduction of hepatic blood flow)
Secondary peaks in plasma opioid levels (commonly seen with intrathecal morphine)
Reuptake of opioids from muscle, lung, fat, and intestine
Pain

---

respiratory depression. Special care should be taken when caring for patients who receive opioids for postoperative analgesia. Patients who receive opioids via a patient-controlled delivery system should be carefully monitored. Similar vigilance should be exercised when treating patients with a history of sleep apnea. Because access to the airway may be challenging in patients after head and neck surgery, extreme caution should be used during the postoperative period. Opioids can be titrated to effect using the patient's respiratory rate as a guide. Patients who demonstrate narcotic tolerance may require a consultation with the pain service.

The effects of narcotics may be reversed with a variety of antagonists (e.g., naloxone). Acute reversal may be accompanied by agitation, pulmonary and systemic hypertension, and pulmonary edema.[65]

Sedatives and Hypnotics

Benzodiazepines

Benzodiazepines produce anxiolysis and sedation by the facilitation of the inhibitory actions of γ-aminobutyric acid on nerve conduction in the cerebral cortex. They may be used to produce sedation or amnesia, to facilitate cooperation with care, to attenuate alcohol withdrawal syndrome, to treat seizures, and to relieve muscle spasm.

In general, benzodiazepines have no analgesic properties. They may cause transient decreases in blood pressure resulting from decreased catecholamine levels and systemic vascular resistance, but they have little effect on contractility. Respiratory depression is usually well tolerated in clinical doses, but it may be accentuated in the elderly and in those with chronic obstructive pulmonary disease. Titration to a cooperative, oriented, and tranquil state (level 2 on the Ramsey scale) is the desired effect. Patients with a history of heavy alcohol or sedative use may require considerably more drug to achieve this response. Diazepam, midazolam, and lorazepam are three of the more commonly used benzodiapines.[66,67] Recommended dosages for some of the benzodiazepines can be found in Table 1-4.

Diazepam

Diazepam has a long clinical duration as a result of the long half-life of several active metabolites. It is not water soluble, and the parenteral suspension of propylene glycol is irritating when given intravenously or intramuscularly. Because diazepam requires microsomal nonconjugative pathways for degradation and elimination, it should not be used for patients with acute hepatitis.

Midazolam

Midazolam is the most commonly used benzodiazepine in the ICU. It is water soluble with a short clinical duration and few active metabolites. Midazolam offers a

TABLE 1-4 Doses of Commonly Used Benzodiazepines

Agent	Use	Route	Dose (mg/kg)
Diazepam	Premedication	Oral	0.2–0.5
	Sedation	IV	0.04–0.2
	Induction	IV	0.3–0.6
Midazolam	Premedication	IM	0.07–0.15
	Sedation	IV	0.01–0.1
	Induction	IV	0.1–0.4
Lorazepam	Premedication	Oral	0.053
	Premedication	IM	0.03–0.05
	Sedation	IV	0.03–0.04

IM, Intramuscular; *IV,* intravenous.

more rapid onset and a greater degree of amnesia, which makes it a good choice for brief procedures such as esophagoscopy and bronchoscopy.[68]

Lorazepam

Lorazepam is another commonly used long-acting benzodiazepine. There is no pain on injection, and lorazepam has no active metabolites. This agent has become a popular choice for patients with liver disease, because its metabolism does not depend on hepatic microsomal enzymes.

Potential Problems With the Use of Benzodiazepines

Tolerance

Tolerance to benzodiazepines develops as it does with prolonged alcohol and opiate use. Withdrawal may result in a profound sympathetic autonomic response. The replacement of benzodiazepine plasma levels and transient autonomic control would be indicated for the control of withdrawal symptoms.

Effects on Respiration and Cardiovascular Function

At hypnotic doses, benzodiazepines have an effect on respiration that is comparable with that of the changes seen during natural sleep. In patients with pulmonary disease, however, even at therapeutic doses, benzodiazepines can produce significant respiratory depression. The effects of benzodiazepines appear to be dose related, and depression of the medullary respiratory center is the usual cause of death as a result of an overdose of sedative hypnotics. In patients without a history of cardiac disease, the use of benzodiazepines produces no significant ill effects. In patients with cardiovascular disease (including hypovolemic states, heart failure, and other diseases that impair cardiovascular function)

normal doses of sedative hypnotics may cause cardiovascular depression, probably as a result of actions on the medullary vasomotor centers. At toxic doses, myocardial contractility and vascular tone may both be depressed by central and peripheral effects, leading to circulatory collapse. Respiratory and cardiovascular effects are more pronounced when benzodiazepines are given intravenously.

The reversal of benzodiazepine-induced sedation has been reported with physostigmine and aminophylline. The most specific antagonist of the effects of benzodiazepines, however, is flumazenil. Flumazenil is a specific benzodiazepine receptor antagonist that provides consistent reversal of sedation within 2 minutes of intravenous administration.[69] It is a 1,4-benzodiazepine derivative with a high affinity for the benzodiazepine binding site on the γ-aminobutyric acid$_A$ receptor, and it acts as a competitive antagonist. The short half-life (0.7–1.3 hours) of flumazenil is the result of rapid hepatic clearance. Because all benzodiazepines have a longer duration of action than flumazenil, sedation commonly recurs, thus requiring repeated administration of the antagonist.

Flumazenil also has been reported to transiently reverse the somnolence of hepatic encephalopathy. Therapy with this agent should be gradual to avoid excitatory symptoms. Convulsions have been reported with flumazenil use in seizure-prone and benzodiazepine-dependent patients. The antagonism of benzodiazepine-induced respiratory depression by flumazenil is less predictable.[70]

Other Drugs of Interest That Are Used for Conscious Sedation

α_2-Agonist

The α_2-agonist dexmedetomidine is a class of sedative drug that has been approved by the U.S. Food and Drug Administration for use as a sedative and analgesic in the operating room and in the ICU. Dexmedetomidine has pharmacologic actions similar to those of clonidine except that its affinity for the α_2-receptor is eight times greater, thereby making dexmedetomidine five to ten times more potent than clonidine. During the past few years, the use of dexmedetomidine for the management of sedation and analgesia in the perioperative setting has increased significantly.[71,72] Dexmedetomidine also possesses several properties that may additionally benefit postoperative patients who have an opioid tolerance or who are sensitive to opioid-induced respiratory depression. In spontaneously breathing volunteers, intravenous dexmedetomidine caused marked sedation with only mild reductions in resting ventilation at higher doses. Head and neck surgeons will find this drug useful for conscious sedation cases, augmented sleep studies, fiber-optic intubations, and percutaneous tracheostomy placement.[73]

The drug does cause some cardiovascular instability, although this can be avoided if the drug is carefully titrated. Nevertheless, it should be appreciated that dexmedetomidine does cause some moderate reductions in blood pressure and heart rate.

Propofol

Propofol is an ultra–short-acting intravenous anesthetic agent. An anesthetist should administer the drug because of its ability to cause profound respiratory depression and apnea.[74] It is discussed here because of a desire of nonanesthesia personnel to use this drug. The soluble form of propofol, which is still undergoing evaluation, may be approved for use by nonanesthetists. Both the soluble and insoluble forms of propofol can cause unconsciousness in less than 30 seconds if given in certain doses; this is followed by awakening within 4 to 8 minutes. Propofol has potent sedative hypnotic activity, but, unlike other agents, awakening is markedly rapid from even deep sedation with minimal residual sedative effects, and the agent has good antiemetic qualities. Hepatic metabolism is rapid, but rapid redistribution also plays a role in early awakening. It has no pharmacologically active metabolites. Propofol has been shown to decrease systemic blood pressure as a result of myocardial depression and vasodilatation. When used in low doses (i.e., 10–50 mcg/kg/min) as a continuous infusion for sedation, these effects are minimal. It has no analgesic effects, but it has been shown to decrease narcotic requirements.[75]

One of the disadvantages of propofol use is that it is only slightly water soluble. It must be formulated in an oil and water emulsion of soybean oil, egg lecithin, and glycerol (this is similar to Intralipid 10%). Thus, this agent is contraindicated in patients with the potential for allergic responses to the emulsion components. Pain on injection is common, but it is often attenuated by the pretreatment of the intravenous bolus with a 20- to 40-mg lidocaine bolus before infusion. With prolonged use of propofol, blood chemistries should be assessed, because prolonged use may result in hypertriglyceridemia.

Propofol should be treated with the same degree of caution as parenteral nutrition solutions. Multiple reports of bacterial contamination as a result of manipulations of the emulsion medium demonstrate that it supports rapid bacterial growth. Recent formulations of propofol have included bacteriostatic agents (e.g., ethylenediaminetetraacetic acid, sulfites), which have made this issue less of a clinical concern. Nonetheless, clinical guidelines still limit the use of opened vials to less than 12 hours. When used as a prolonged infusion (e.g., in the ICU), the changing of the intravenous line apparatus at regular (usually 12-hour) intervals is advocated.

A soluble cousin of propofol that is marketed as Aquavan (fospropofol disodium) is currently undergoing phase III studies. The drug is described as having similar properties as propofol without the pain that can be experienced during injection. The drug has been used for conscious sedation for colonoscopies with success in several phase III studies. Aquavan does cause respiratory depression similar to propofol, and it should be used in a monitored setting.

Ketamine

Ketamine is a phencyclidine derivative (similar to lysergic acid diethylamide) that produces a dose-related, dissociative state that may be exploited as a sedative. Agitated patients may be given an intramuscular injection (3–5 mg/kg) or a titration of 10-mg intravenous boluses to produce a cataleptic state in which the eyes remain open with a slow nystagmic gaze. Amnesia is present, and analgesia is intense. Additional advantages include the maintenance of airway reflexes, cardiovascular stimulation, and bronchial relaxation. The addition of benzodiazepines may attenuate these untoward sensory effects. Examples of clinical use include conscious sedation for burn wound dressing changes and the facilitation of endotracheal intubation in the hypotensive patient.[76]

Ketamine does have several side effects in addition to cataleptic symptoms. These include increased airway secretions that may facilitate laryngospasm, particularly with the manipulation of the airway. Ketamine increases cerebral blood flow and metabolism, and, hence, it may cause an increase in intracranial pressure. The unpleasant visual or auditory illusions are perhaps the least desirable in adults, although pretreatment with benzodiazepines may prevent the occurrence of hallucinations.

Ketorolac

Ketorolac is a potent parenteral nonsteroidal analgesic without opioid-related side effects such as respiratory depression. Intramuscular doses of 60 mg are reported to be equivalent to 10 mg of morphine for up to 3 hours. Clinical dosing is performed every 8 hours. The drug appears to be most effective in situations in which swelling contributes to pain (e.g., dental, gynecologic, and orthopedic surgery). There is minimal impact on ventilation, hemodynamics, and bowel motility. Disadvantages include a limited analgesia effect beyond recommended doses and impaired platelet function. Substantial gastrointestinal mucosal breakdown may occur with use during periods as short as 1 week. The prolonged use of ketorolac can lead to renal insufficiency.[77,78]

Anticholinergics

These agents are sometimes used to produce sedation and amnesia. They also have an antisialogogue effect, and they can prevent reflex bradycardia. In fact, anticholinergics produce an increased heart rate and can be used to treat bradycardia. Atropine and scopolamine are tertiary amines that cross the lipid barrier that protects the central nervous system. Scopolamine has 10 times the potency of atropine in terms of centrally induced sedation and amnesia. Scopolamine is a popular choice as an urgent amnestic for the hemodynamically unstable or hypovolemic patient (e.g., a trauma victim). Glycopyrrolate is an anticholinergic agent that demonstrates antisialogogue activity and increases the heart rate without the undesirable central nervous system side effects, because the drug does not cross the blood–brain barrier. It is used during awake fiber-optic intubation of the trachea for its antisialogogue activity, and it can also be used during the treatment of sinus bradycardia in the operating room.

Undesirable side effects of atropine and scopolamine include toxic delirium (i.e., central cholinergic syndrome), tachycardia, the relaxation of lower esophageal sphincter tone (with the associated potential for regurgitation), mydriasis, and the potential elevation of temperature via the suppression of sweat-gland function.

Local Anesthetics

The use of local anesthetics for skin infiltration for head and neck procedures is fairly common. The use of local anesthetics may reduce the use of opioids and other kinds of anesthesia. An understanding of the pharmacology of local anesthetics is important. The primary mechanism of action of local anesthetics is by blockade of the voltage-gated sodium channels. Local anesthetics reversibly block impulse conduction along nerve axons and other excitable membranes that use sodium channels as the primary means of action potential generation. Local anesthetics bind to receptors near the intracellular end of the sodium channel and block the channel in a time- and voltage-dependent fashion.

When nerves are exposed to increasing concentrations of local anesthetic, the threshold for excitation increases. In addition, there is a slowing of impulse conduction and a decreased rate of rise of action potential. With more exposure, the action potential amplitude continues to decrease, and eventually the ability to generate an action potential is abolished.

Local anesthetics can be classified as esters or amides, depending on their structure. Ester local anesthetics are predominantly metabolized by pseudocholinesterases. Ester hydrolysis is very rapid, and the water-soluble metabolites are excreted in the urine. Two examples of ester local anesthetics are procaine and benzocaine. Both are metabolized to para-aminobenzoic acid, which has been associated with allergic reactions. Cocaine, which is an ester local anesthetic, is partially metabolized in the liver and partially excreted unchanged in the urine.

Amide local anesthetics are metabolized (N-dealkylation and hydroxylation) by microsomal P450 enzymes in the liver. Most local anesthetics that are used in the operating room belong to the amide group of local anesthetics. Included in this group are prilocaine, lidocaine, mepivacaine, ropivacaine, and bupivacaine.

Local anesthetics with a fast onset of action are generally of a lower molecular weight, and they are more lipophilic. These local anesthetics have a faster rate of interaction with the sodium channel receptor. Potency is also positively correlated with lipid solubility as long as the agent retains sufficient water solubility to diffuse to the site of action on the neuronal membrane. Local anesthetics that are more water soluble, such as lidocaine, procaine, and mepivacaine, have shorter durations of action than tetracaine, bupivacaine, and ropivacaine.

Local anesthetics have different effects on different nerve fibers. In fact, local anesthetics preferentially block small fibers, primarily because the distance over which such fibers can passively propagate an electrical impulse is shorter. In the case of myelinated nerves, at least two and preferably three successive nodes of Ranvier must be blocked by the local anesthetic to halt impulse propagation. With larger and thicker nerve fibers (e.g., motor neurons), the nodes are further apart, thus creating greater resistance to blockade. In general, myelinated nerves tend to become blocked before unmyelinated nerves of the same diameter. For this reason, the preganglionic B fibers are blocked before the smaller unmyelinated C fibers, which are involved in pain transmission, are blocked (Table 1-5).

Uses of Local Anesthesia

Anesthesia of the mucous membranes of the nasal cavity, the oral cavity, the pharynx, and the tracheobronchial tree can be produced by direct application of local anesthetics such as tetracaine (2%) or lidocaine (2%–10%). For the nasal cavity, cocaine (1%–4%) can be used; it uniquely produces vasoconstriction as well as anesthesia. The shrinking of mucous membranes decreases operative bleeding while improving surgical visualization. Comparable vasoconstriction can be achieved with other local anesthetics by the addition of a low concentration of a vasoconstrictor such as phenylephrine (0.005%). Maximal safe total dosages for topical anesthesia in a healthy 70-kg adult are 300 mg for lidocaine and 150 mg for cocaine (Table 1-6).

Many surgical procedures, particularly those procedures involving the head and neck, require local infiltration. Infiltration anesthesia is the injection of local anesthetic directly into the skin and other tissue to achieve

TABLE 1-5   Susceptibility of Different Types of Nerve Fibers to Local Anesthetics on the Basis of Size and Myelination

Fiber Type	Function	Diameter (µm)	Myelination	Conduction Velocity (m·s⁻¹)	Sensitivity to Block
Type A					
α	Proprioception, motor	12–20	Heavy	70–120	+
β	Touch, pressure	5–12	Heavy	30–70	+ +
γ	Muscle spindles	3–6	Heavy	15–10	+ +
δ	Pain, temperature	2–5	Heavy	12–30	+ + +
Type B	Preganglionic	<3	Light	2–15	+ + + +
Type C					
Dorsal root	Pain	0.4–1.2	None	0.5–2.3	+ + + +
Sympathetic	Postganglionic	0.3–1.3	None	0.7–2.3	+ + + +

TABLE 1-6   Clinical Use of Local Anesthetic Agents With Toxic Doses

Agent	Techniques	Concentrations Available	Maximum Dose (mg/kg)
Esters			
Cocaine	Topical	4%, 10%	3
Procaine	Spinal, infiltration, peripheral nerve block	2%, 10%	10
Amides			
Bupivacaine	Epidural, spinal, infiltration, peripheral nerve block	0.25%, 0.5%, 0.75%	3
Lidocaine	Epidural, spinal infiltration, peripheral nerve block, intravenous regional, topical	0.5%, 1%, 1.5%, 2%, 4%, 5%	4.5; 7 (with epinephrine)
Mepivacaine	Epidural, infiltration, peripheral nerve block	1%, 1.5%, 2%, 3%	4.5; 7 (with epinephrine)
Ropivacaine	Epidural, spinal, infiltration, peripheral nerve block	0.2%, 0.5%, 0.75%, 1%	3

anesthesia. The duration of infiltration anesthesia can be approximately doubled by the addition of epinephrine (final concentration, 1:200,000) to the injection solution; epinephrine also decreases peak concentrations of local anesthetic in blood. It is important to note that epinephrine-containing solutions should not be injected into tissues supplied by end arteries (e.g., fingers, toes, ears, nose, penis), because the resulting vasoconstriction may cause gangrene if perfusion is compromised by vasoconstriction. Epinephrine should be used with caution in those patients for whom adrenergic stimulation is undesirable. This includes patients with cardiac disease who cannot tolerate an increased heart rate or an increased blood pressure. Commonly used local anesthetics for local infiltration are lidocaine (0.5%–2%) and bupivacaine (0.125%–0.5%). The maximum suggested doses are 4.5 mg/kg for lidocaine and 2 mg/kg of bupivacaine. When epinephrine is added, the toxic doses can be increased by one third.

Commonly Used Local Anesthetics
Lidocaine

Lidocaine is the most commonly used local anesthetic in the operating room. It is the prototype amide local anesthetic. Lidocaine is absorbed rapidly after parenteral administration and from the gastrointestinal and respiratory tracts. Lidocaine is metabolized in the liver, and it has active metabolites.

The toxic side effects of lidocaine occur with increasing concentrations of the drug in the blood. With increasing doses, patients will experience drowsiness, tinnitus, dysgeusia, dizziness, and muscle twitching. With toxic doses (see Table 1-5), patients may experience seizures, coma, and respiratory depression. With further increases in toxic levels of local anesthetics, cardiac arrest can occur. Clinically significant cardiovascular depression usually occurs at the same serum levels of lidocaine that produce marked central nervous system effects. The metabolites of lidocaine—monoethylglycine xylidide and glycine xylidide—may contribute to some of the toxic side effects.

Bupivacaine

Bupivacaine belongs to the amide family, and its structure is similar to that of lidocaine. Bupivacaine is a potent agent capable of producing prolonged anesthesia. Its long duration of action plus its tendency to provide more sensory than motor block has made it a popular drug for providing prolonged analgesia during labor or during the postoperative period. Bupivacaine, like lidocaine, can be used for infiltration anesthesia.

Elevated serum levels of bupivacaine can lead to cardiac toxicity. Clinically, this manifests as severe ventricular arrhythmias and myocardial depression. Both lidocaine and bupivacaine rapidly block cardiac sodium channels during systole; however, bupivacaine dissociates much more slowly than lidocaine does during diastole. Hence, a significant fraction of the sodium channels remain blocked with bupivacaine at the end of diastole. The cardiac toxicity caused by bupivacaine may also be partially mediated centrally, because the direct injection of small quantities of bupivacaine into the medulla can produce malignant ventricular arrhythmias. The treatment of bupivacaine-induced cardiac toxicity is difficult, particularly in the presence of coexisting acidosis, hypercarbia, and hypoxemia.

Antiemetics

A significant complication of surgery and anesthesia is postoperative nausea and vomiting (PONV), which can be caused by medications such as nitrous oxide, inhaled anesthetics, and opioids, or by the procedure itself. Surgical procedures involving the ear, eye, and brain, as well as laparoscopic procedures involving the abdomen, often stimulate PONV. Moreover, procedures that involve the stretching of the peritoneal membrane may also cause PONV. Most patients who are scheduled for surgery express a profound fear of PONV. The following section contains a brief presentation of some of the current medications that can be used for the treatment of PONV.

PONV can also be treated or prevented by nonpharmacologic means, including adequate hydration (20 ml/kg) after fasting and stimulation of the P6 acupuncture point (wrist). The latter may include the application of pressure, electrical current, or injections.

Droperidol

Droperidol was the most popular antiemetic 15 years ago. In fact, the drug also has excellent sedative effects, with minimal respiratory depression. If it is administered alone, dysphoria can occur; however, in most clinical situations, it is used in combination with a narcotic or a benzodiazepine for sedation with only mild dysphoria. More recently, the U.S. Food and Drug Administration has discouraged the use of droperidol in an unmonitored setting. Droperidol can prolong the QT interval, and it has been associated with fatal cardiac arrhythmias. Nevertheless, intravenous droperidol (0.625–1.25 mg in adults, 0.05–0.075 mg/kg in children), when given intraoperatively, significantly decreases the likelihood of PONV.

Ondansetron and Dolasetron

Ondansetron and dolasetron selectively block serotonin 5-hydroxytryptamine 3 receptors with little or no effect on dopamine receptors. Unlike droperidol, these agents do not cause sedation, extrapyramidal signs, or alteration of gastrointestinal motility and lower esophageal sphincter tone. 5-Hydroxytryptamine 3 receptors are found in the chemoreceptor trigger zone of the area postrema, in the nucleus tractus solitarius, and also along the gastrointestinal tract. The most common reported side effect is headache. Dolasetron can also cause a mild prolongation of the QT interval.

INTRAOPERATIVE COMPLICATIONS RELATED TO ANESTHESIA

Although the number of complications from anesthesia has decreased with the use of standard monitoring techniques (e.g., pulse oximetry, capnography), anesthetic complications can still occur. A review of the American Society of Anesthesiologists Closed Claims Project shows that complications can arise from several sources. Complications are classified as human error, equipment error, and anesthesia mishaps unrelated to human error or equipment malfunction. Of note is that adverse respiratory events were previously more than twice as likely as adverse cardiovascular events to be associated with death or permanent brain damage. This is shown in Table 1-7.

This section discusses select perioperative complications related to anesthesia and surgery, which may be of

TABLE 1-7   Distribution of Adverse Respiratory Events in the American Society of Anesthesiologists Closed Claims Study

Event	No. of Cases	Percent of 522 Respiratory Claims
Inadequate ventilation	196	38%
Esophageal intubation	94	18%
Difficult tracheal intubation	87	17%
Inadequate inspired oxygen concentration	11	2%

From Caplan RA, Ward RJ, Posner K, et al: Unexpected cardiac arrest during spinal anesthesia: A closed claims analysis of predisposing factors. *Anesthesiology* 1988;68:5–11.

particular interest to head and neck surgeons. For a more concise discussion of the scientific and clinical basis of anesthesiology, refer to an anesthesiology textbook.[79]

Complications of Endotracheal Intubation

Cardiovascular Response to Laryngoscopy and Tracheal Intubation

Laryngoscopy together with the intubation of the trachea is a stressful process that can elicit a significant sympathetic response that can result in myocardial stress, ischemia, and even infarction. Intubation of the trachea for an elective surgical procedure requires a careful preoperative evaluation of the patient, making sure that all necessary equipment and medications are available and that the patient is carefully monitored. A knowledge of the medications—including anesthetics, muscle relaxants, and opioids—that facilitate tracheal intubation is imperative. This is because the intubation of the trachea without proper preparation and premedication can result in significant cardiovascular stress. The cardiovascular responses to laryngoscopy include hypertension, tachycardia, and dysrhythmias. In the patient without a history of cardiac disease, these responses to laryngoscopy are tolerated with limited morbidity; however, in patients with limited coronary or myocardial reserve, myocardial ischemia or failure may follow. The stress response to laryngoscopy can be blunted with various medications.[79–81]

Airway Reaction to Tracheal Intubation

Instrumentation of the airway can lead to several complications, some of which were described previously. All of these complications can occur with head and neck surgery.[82] One of the most feared complications of instrumentation of the airway is laryngospasm.[83,84] *Laryngospasm* is defined as closure of the glottis by the constriction of the intrinsic/extrinsic laryngeal muscles. It can occur in all patients, but it occurs more commonly among children and adults with reactive airway disease. Laryngospasm can completely restrict

ventilation and oxygenation, and it is therefore life threatening, particularly among patients with minimal reserve capacity and comorbid conditions. In most cases, laryngospasm persists long after the inciting stimulus has ceased. Laryngospasm can occur as a result of instrumentation of the airway and mouth. Stimuli such as a light touch to receptors on the tongue, palate, and oropharynx can precipitate laryngospasm. In addition, traction of the pelvic/abdominal viscera can also cause laryngospasm. Chemical irritation, secretions, blood, water, and vomitus may also cause laryngospasm. Both laryngospasm and bronchospasm occur more often in children, particularly after recent respiratory tract infections.

Laryngospasm can be avoided by extubating patients when they are either deeply asleep or in a fully awake state. Nevertheless, laryngospasm can occur during the extubation of an awake patient with reactive airway disease. The treatment of laryngospasm includes providing gentle positive-pressure ventilation with 100% oxygen. In some cases, the administration of intravenous lidocaine (1–1.5 mg/kg) may help, although this prolongs anesthesia. In some severe cases, if laryngospasm persists and hypoxia develops, low-dose succinylcholine (0.25–1 mg/kg) can be given to relax the laryngeal muscles and allow for controlled ventilation.[85] If the patient is an aspiration risk, then the trachea should be reintubated. It should be noted that the large negative intrathoracic pressures generated by a struggling patient during laryngospasm can result in the development of negative-pressure pulmonary edema, even in healthy young adults.[86-88]

Bronchospasm

Instrumentation of the airway can also lead to bronchospasm, which is another reflex response that occurs most commonly among asthmatic patients. In some cases, bronchospasm can be a clue to endobronchial irritation such as the end of the endotracheal tube touching the carina. Bronchospasm can also occur in lightly anesthetized patients. Intubation of the trachea increases the airway resistance.

The symptoms of intraoperative bronchospasm include wheezing, increasing peak inflation pressures (the plateau pressure should remain unchanged), decreasing exhaled tidal volumes, and a slowly rising waveform on the capnograph.[89] Because light anesthesia can cause bronchospasm, the first step in the treatment should be increasing the concentration of the volatile anesthetic agent. If the bronchospasm does not resolve after deepening the anesthetic, then other drugs should be considered.[90,91]

Bronchospasm can be treated with the administration of inhaled or intravenous β-agonists. Bronchospasm can be blunted by the prior administration of anticholinergics, steroids, inhaled $β_2$-agonists, lidocaine (topical, nerve block, or intravenous), and narcotics. Muscle relaxants may improve ventilation in extreme situations.

The following situations can also stimulate bronchospasm: obstruction of the tracheal tube from kinking, secretions, or an overinflated balloon; bronchial intubation; active expiratory efforts (straining); pulmonary edema or embolism; and pneumothorax.

Possible Injuries Occurring with Laryngoscopy and Intubation of the Trachea

In general, injury during laryngoscopy and intubation is more likely among children, women, and patients with poor dentition. Injuries are also more common among patients in whom there is a difficulty with tracheal intubation. Injuries include broken teeth, laceration and perforation of the pharynx, subluxation of the arytenoid cartilage, hoarseness, sore throat, paralysis of the vocal cords, and nerve damage. The use of certain instruments that facilitate tracheal intubation can also cause injuries. This includes perforation of the trachea, which usually occurs during difficult intubations with the use of a stylet. If subcutaneous emphysema is noted after a difficult intubation, the patient must be evaluated for mediastinitis and pneumothorax.[92,93]

Pharyngitis and Sore Throat

Intubation of the trachea even for a brief period can result in several complications. Often a head and neck surgeon may be consulted if these complications do not resolve in a timely fashion. Pharyngitis and sore throat after tracheal intubation are common. Although these symptoms are generally seen with endotracheal intubation, such symptoms are also noted in patients undergoing anesthesia by mask. In the case of the latter, the cause of pharyngitis and sore throat is attributed to the use of dry gases. This is in opposition with

tracheal intubation, where symptoms may occur from a reaction to the lubricant, the tube cuff pressure, patient motion while the tube is in place, repeated attempts at intubation, or excessive tube size. Some patients may have hoarseness, which is another postintubation problem associated with tube size. Supraglottic devices such as the laryngeal mask airway (LMA) that may be used in the delivery of general anesthesia also cause pharyngeal irritation and pharyngitis. Pharyngitis that occurs as a result of tracheal intubation usually resolves within 72 hours.[94-96] If resolution does not occur, a head and neck surgeon should be consulted.

Injuries to the Vocal Folds and the Nerves That Innervate the Vocal Folds

Laryngeal injury after short-term intubation has been reported to occur in 6.2% of patients, with the most common injury being hematoma of the vocal cords. With laryngoscopy and intubation, mucosal lacerations occur in approximately 1 in 1000 patients.

Other rare but serious complications of endotracheal intubation include vocal cord paralysis from damage to the recurrent laryngeal nerve. This nerve damage can occur as a result of the endotracheal tube cuff pressing the recurrent laryngeal nerve between the thyroid lamina and the arytenoid cartilage. Surgical procedures of the head and neck can also lead to nerve injury. It is important to note that unilateral injury causes no respiratory obstruction. Bilateral recurrent nerve injury, however, may result in respiratory distress, stridor, and significant airway obstruction. When viewed with a fiber-optic bronchoscope, both true vocal folds fail to abduct. A tracheostomy may be required during the 6-week recovery period.[97-99]

Complications of Nasal Intubation

Some procedures involving the head and neck may require a nasal intubation of the trachea. There are several complications that are associated with nasal intubation. The most common complication is epistaxis, which may occur even when vasoconstriction, a lubricated tube, and careful placement of the endotracheal tube are employed. Patients with a history of abnormal clotting or easy bruising, and those who use pharmacologic anticoagulants, are not good candidates for nasal intubation. In some cases, the inflated cuff of the endotracheal tube may tamponade the hemorrhage, if correctly positioned. Severe hemorrhage often requires consultation with a head and neck surgeon for evaluation and control.[100–102]

Another potential complication of nasal intubation is the damage of the nasal or nasopharyngeal mucosa and the creation of false passages by forcing the endotracheal tube into the nasal passages. Adenoids, polyps, and foreign bodies may be displaced, causing bleeding and even airway obstruction. Long-term nasal intubation can lead to nasal necrosis, septal perforation, ulceration of the inferior turbinate, and infection.[100,103,104]

Possible Complications That May Occur During Endotracheal Extubation

Complications from endotracheal intubation can also arise during extubation. In the operating room, extubation can be performed under deep anesthesia, provided that the patient is spontaneously breathing with adequate tidal volumes and fully recovered from neuromuscular blockade. Extubation during a light plane of anesthesia or stage II of anesthesia (i.e., a state between deep and awake) should be avoided because of the increased risk of laryngospasm. To distinguish between deep and light anesthesia, one technique is to attempt pharyngeal suctioning. If there is any reaction to suctioning such as breath holding or "bucking," this signals a light plane of anesthesia, and extubation should be postponed until the patient is awake. If there is no reaction to suctioning, this is characteristic of the patient being in a deep plane of anesthesia. Patients with reactive airway disease may have reduced wheezing, bronchospasm, or coughing if extubated under deep anesthesia.

Extubation can also be performed in an awake patient. The patient also should have neuromuscular blockade reversed. Extubation is often accompanied by increased heart rate, increased blood pressure, high central venous pressure, and an increase in intracranial and intraocular pressures. Patients who are at risk for aspiration should be extubated when awake.

Complications during extubation of the trachea can be reduced with good suctioning before extubation; this may avoid aspiration and laryngospasm after the removal of the endotracheal tube.

Other Anesthesia Complications

Aspiration of Gastric Contents During Anesthesia

The aspiration of gastric contents can occur at any time during general anesthesia or with heavy sedation. The aspiration of gastric contents, especially those with high acid concentrations, can lead to a serious aspiration pneumonitis, which can be severely debilitating or even fatal. Susceptible individuals include patients with a history of gastroesophageal reflux disease, patients who have consumed food or drink within the 6 hours before the induction of anesthesia, pregnant women, and morbidly obese patients. In high-risk patients, general anesthesia should be induced with a rapid-sequence technique and with the application of pressure to the cricoid cartilage. Cricoid pressure can help to prevent the movement of gastric contents into the lungs. The cricoid forms a complete

ring, and pressure on it can occlude the esophagus. The pressure on the cricoid cartilage required to occlude the esophagus appears to be a force of approximately 8 to 9 lb of weight. If properly applied, cricoid pressure can prevent aspiration, because the force of vomiting is blunted by the muscle relaxant. If the vocal cords are not visualized with laryngoscopy, then the mask ventilation should be instituted with cricoid pressure. The release of cricoid pressure should occur only after it is established that the trachea is intubated. Recently, the value of cricoid pressure for preventing aspiration has been disputed. Nevertheless, the use of cricoid pressure for tracheal intubation remains the standard of care for high-risk patients.

Cricoid pressure should only be applied if the patient is unconscious. The application of cricoid pressure to the awake patient is very uncomfortable and may provoke vomiting or obstruction of the airway by laryngospasm.

Malignant Hyperthermia

Malignant hyperthermia (MH) is a clinical syndrome that occurs during anesthesia with a potent volatile agent (e.g., halothane) and the depolarizing muscle relaxant succinylcholine, which produces rapidly increasing temperature and extreme acidosis. The incidence of MH is rare, ranging from 1 in 15,000 among pediatric patients to 1 in 40,000 among adult patients. Patients who are predisposed to MH have a genetic susceptibility. The earliest signs reported during anesthesia are masseter muscle rigidity, tachycardia, and hypercarbia as a result of increased carbon dioxide production. Two or more of these signs greatly increase the likelihood of MH. Fever is an inconsistent and often late sign. In the past, the mortality rate as a result of MH was about 70%; however, with the introduction of dantrolene for the treatment of MH, the incidence of mortality is now less than 5%. The common cause of death is from ventricular fibrillation from an elevated hypercarbia and acidosis.

Although the precise cellular origin of MH remains to be clearly delineated, current studies reveal that there is an uncontrolled increase in intracellular calcium in skeletal muscle. The sudden release of calcium from the sarcoplasmic reticulum removes the inhibition of troponin, which results in intense muscle contractions. Markedly enhanced and sustained adenosine triphosphatase activity results in an uncontrolled increase in aerobic and anaerobic metabolism.

MH is triggered by several anesthetic drugs, including halothane, enflurane, isoflurane, desflurane, sevoflurane, and succinylcholine. Desflurane and sevoflurane are less potent triggers, producing a more gradual onset of MH. The evaluation of the patient with MH reveals a mixed metabolic and respiratory acidosis, a marked base deficit, hyperkalemia, hypermagnesemia, and a very low mixed venous oxygen saturation. Although the serum ionized calcium concentration may initially increase, it ultimately falls to low levels. With muscle hyperactivity, patients with MH will have increased serum myoglobin, creatine kinase, lactic dehydrogenase, and aldolase levels. In fact, serum creatine kinase levels usually exceed 20,000 International Units/L.

The treatment of MH includes hyperventilation and the use of bicarbonate for the acidosis. As the patient's temperature rises, he or she needs to be cooled. Sometimes this involves dialysis with cold fluid or cardiopulmonary bypass. Hyperkalemia should be treated with insulin and glucose, and cardiac arrhythmias should be treated with antiarrhythmic medications.

A mannitol infusion as well as an infusion of furosemide should be used to establish diuresis and to prevent acute renal failure from myoglobinuria. The mainstay of therapy for an MH crisis is the immediate administration of intravenous dantrolene.

In some normal individuals, trismus-masseter spasm may occur after the administration of a depolarizing muscle relaxant (succinylcholine). *Trismus-masseter spasm* is defined as jaw muscle rigidity in association with limb muscle flaccidity. Muscle fibers from masseter and lateral pterygoid muscles contain slow tonic fibers that can respond to depolarizers with contracture. This causes a "locked-jaw" syndrome. If there is an increase in jaw muscle tone such that increased muscle tone is prolonged and tight, then there may be an increased risk of the patient developing MH.

Difficult Airway

The intubation of the trachea may prove challenging in some patients. If the manual ventilation of these patients is also difficult, then the process of securing the airway can be extremely difficult and even life threatening.[105,106] When such encounters occur, they should be recorded for future anesthetic considerations, which may require an awake placement of the endotracheal tube. Difficulty with the visualization of the vocal cords during direct laryngoscopy occurs in 1.5% to 8.5% of general anesthetics, and failed intubation occurs in 0.13% to 0.3%.

Difficult intubations are usually caused by anatomic abnormalities such as micrognathia, limited mouth opening, protruding teeth, or congenital syndromes. Other causes of difficult intubations include obesity, acromegaly, cervical spine problems, rheumatoid arthritis, and even gastric reflux.

Patients who are suspected of having difficult airways should be carefully evaluated before conventional intubation is attempted.[107] Evaluation of the head, neck, mandible, tongue, teeth, and oropharynx can help predict a potentially difficult intubation. In morbidly obese individuals, a neck circumference of more than 50 cm can predict a difficult airway. The keys to success in the intubation of the trachea in a patient with a difficult airway are having the operating room prepared with all of the necessary equipment and having a plan of action.[108-110] This should also include thorough communication between the anesthesiologist and the surgeon. The surgeon should be present and prepared to assist with intubation or, if necessary, with the establishment of a surgical airway.

Identifying Patients with Potentially Difficult-to-Manage Airways

With improvements in record keeping and patient–physician communications, the patient history should provide important information regarding the patient's airway and potential problems for securing the airway in the operating room. Knowledge of a history of difficult intubation, surgery of the head and neck, immobility of the cervical vertebrae, and radiation therapy to the airway should be basic warning signs of a potentially difficult airway. Other warning signs should include dysphagia, trauma to the head and neck, and hoarseness or stridor (Box 1-5).

Preoperative evaluation of the airway by the surgeon, either by endoscopic evaluation or with other diagnostic tools (e.g., CT scanning, MRI), may provide valuable information to the anesthesiologist, particularly if a difficult airway is involved.

Physical Examination of the Airway

In most procedures involving head and neck surgery, a detailed preoperative assessment of the airway should be performed by both the surgeon and the anesthesiologist. This is extremely helpful for determining which patients are going to be challenges for tracheal intubation. The preoperative examination should include the following:

- A detailed frontal and a profile view to assess mandibular size and mobility

---

BOX 1-5 Situations and Signs That May Help Identify the Difficult Airway

Prior difficulty with endotracheal intubation
Cervical immobility (limited or no range of motion of neck)
Hoarseness or stridor
Trauma
Prior radiation therapy
Prior surgery of the head and/or neck
Morbid obesity
Dyspnea or dyspnea on exertion
Dysphagia
Shortness of breath

- The examination and assessment of the mental–alveolar process and the mental–hyoid bone or the mental–thyroid cartilage distance
- The assessment of neck rotation and flexion–extension mobility
- An examination of the neck for evidence of masses, tracheal deviation, the size of the tracheal and cricoid cartilages, and tissue plasticity

The recognition of certain breathing patterns and phonation may also provide important clues about airway patency and potential difficulty with endotracheal intubation.

In addition, a preoperative intraoral examination should be performed and should include an assessment of tongue size, protrusive occlusion, and degree of overbite (Box 1-6). Evaluation for a potentially difficult airway can done by examining the oral cavity and assessing the structures that can be seen in a wide-open mouth. The classification of these views are shown in Figure 1-1; they are called the *Mallampati classification*. The bottom of Figure 1-1 shows the graded views of the vocal folds that are seen during laryngoscopy.

Awake Intubations and Preparation of the Patient

In patients with anticipated difficult airways, those who are unable to open their mouths, or those who have cervical spine precautions, an awake intubation is often necessary. This can be done after anesthetizing the oropharynx with a local anesthetic. The use of 2% lidocaine sprayed into the mouth and throat may cause the loss of a gag reflex and allow for awake laryngoscopy (see later discussion). In other situations, tracheal intubation via either the oral or nasal route using a fiber-optic scope should be done with the patient awake. In this latter situation, the facilitation of fiber-optic intubation may require the blockade of specific nerves (Table 1-8).

- In the oral cavity, the anterior aspect of the tongue is innervated by the lingual nerve. By contrast, the posterior third of the tongue and the oropharynx are innervated by the pharyngeal branches of the glossopharyngeal nerve and by the vagus nerve. The mucosal distribution of these nerves can be easily anesthetized by spraying the oral cavity with local anesthetic and then asking the patient to gargle and

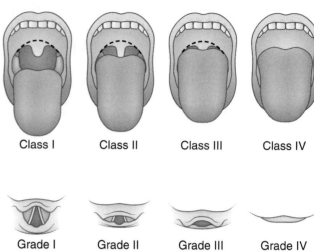

Figure 1-1. The correlation between views obtained before laryngoscopy with the naked eye and views obtained with laryngoscopy. In about 80% of class 1 oral views, a grade 1 laryngoscopic view is observed. For Mallampati class II, only the posterior vocal cords may be visualized in about 50% of cases. Class III and IV merit special attention, because the intubation of the trachea in these patients may be difficult and may merit an awake intubation. The degree of vigilance should also be increased in class III and IV patients, because manual ventilation may be a challenge.

swallow it. Alternatively, these nerves are easily blocked by the bilateral injection of 2 ml of local anesthetic into the base of the palatoglossal arch with a 25-gauge spinal needle. The inferior aspect of the larynx to the level of the vocal cords is innervated by the superior laryngeal nerve, which is a branch of the vagus nerve. This nerve can be blocked by the placement of gauze soaked in local anesthetic in the pyriform sinuses. In addition, this nerve may be blocked externally by locating the hyoid bone and injecting 3 ml of 2% lidocaine 1 cm below each greater cornu of the hyoid bone, near where the internal branch of the superior laryngeal nerves penetrates the thyrohyoid membrane.

- The recurrent laryngeal nerve innervates the mucosa below the cords. This nerve may be blocked by the transtracheal injection of local anesthetic. A transtracheal block is performed by identifying and penetrating the cricothyroid membrane while the neck is extended. After confirmation of an intratracheal position by the aspiration of air, 4 ml of 4% lidocaine is injected into the trachea at the end of expiration. A deep inhalation and cough immediately after injection distributes the anesthetic throughout the trachea.

The use of local anesthetic to block these nerves may facilitate the awake intubation of the trachea by depressing the protective cough reflex and the swallowing reflex. The patient may require sedation and amnesia. Various combinations of medications have been used with success.[111] Recently, dexmedetomidine in combination with ketamine or midazolam has been found to be effective. Most drugs that provide sedation can be used; the important consideration is to avoid oversedation.[112]

BOX 1-6 Examination of the Oral Cavity

Examination of the oral cavity can provide important information regarding potential airway difficulties. Such an examination should determine the following:

- The presence of loose, missing, or overly large teeth
- The degree of overbite or protrusive occlusion
- The size of the tongue
- The visibility and size of faucial structures
- The patency and size of the nares or the deviation of the nasal septum

TABLE 1-8 Nerves That Innervate the Oropharynx and the Area Just Above and Below the Vocal Cords

Nerves	Sensory Innervation	Motor Innervation
Superior laryngeal (internal division)	Epiglottis Base of tongue Supraglottic mucosa Thyroepiglottic joint Cricothyroid joint	None
Superior laryngeal (external division)	Anterior subglottic mucosa	Cricothyroid (adductor, tensor)
Recurrent laryngeal	Subglottic mucosa Muscle spindles Trachea	Thyroarytenoid Lateral cricoarytenoid Interarytenoid (adductors) Posterior cricoarytenoid (abductor)

In all patients with difficult airways, it is important to note that only after endotracheal placement is confirmed with the fiber-optic bronchoscope should the patient receive any anesthesia or muscle relaxant.

Devices That Address the Difficult Airway

In cases in which a difficult airway was not anticipated and patients who already may be medicated with anesthetic induction drugs and neuromuscular blockers cannot be quickly awakened, a patent airway and adequate ventilation are essential. If manual ventilation by mask is adequate, then this is not a life-threatening situation, and the patient may be ventilated until conscious; subsequently, intubation can be attempted by an alternative technique with the patient awake. In cases in which manual ventilation is difficult, even with the use of oral or nasal airways, then aggressive intervention including a surgical airway may become imperative. The LMA and the LMA Fastrach (Figure 1-2) can be used when conventional methods of tracheal intubation with a laryngoscope are unsuccessful and respiratory compromise is imminent. The LMA was introduced in 1981, and it is used extensively throughout the world for the delivery of anesthesia. It has been included in the American Society of Anesthesiologists' algorithm for the difficult airway. It requires no direct visualization of the cords, but the one drawback of this device is that it does not prevent aspiration. Hence, in a patient who is at high risk for aspiration, a small endotracheal tube (size 5.0–5.5) can be placed under fiber-optic guidance through the positioned LMA. More recently, two new laryngeal masks have been introduced: the LMA Fastrach and the LMA ProSeal (Figure 1-3; see Figure 1-2). The LMA Fastrach can be used as a regular LMA. Its main advantage is that it allows for the placement of endotracheal tubes without direct laryngoscopy (see Figure 1-2). The LMA ProSeal is very similar to the LMA but with an extra lumen for the suction of stomach and intestinal contents. It should be emphasized that none of the three types of LMA protects against the aspiration of gastrointestinal contents if the patient vomits.

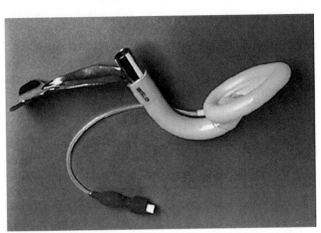

Figure 1-2. The LMA Fastrach allows for the intubation of the trachea with a laryngeal mask airway.

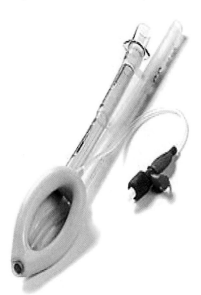

Figure 1-3. The LMA ProSeal may be the most versatile laryngeal mask airway. Its design includes a double-cuff design that allows for higher seal pressures and the ability to aspirate material from the stomach.

The esophageal–tracheal Combitube is another device that can be used in emergency situations. The Combitube is a hybrid of the traditional endotracheal tube and the old esophageal obturator airway. This device can prevent aspiration as a result of the presence of both a tracheal cuff and an esophageal cuff. The proper use of the device is important, because the Combitube has been implicated in esophageal rupture as a result of the overinflation of the esophageal cuff.

Perhaps one of the most effective tools not only for tracheal intubation but also for assessing airway pathology is the GlideScope (Saturn Biomedical Systems Inc, Burnaby, British Columbia, Canada). The GlideScope is a new video laryngoscope that can be a useful alternative to the conventional fiber-optic scope for the placement of an endotracheal tube when confronted with a difficult airway. The GlideScope has a high-resolution digital camera incorporated into the blade that displays a view of the vocal cords on a monitor. The blade is fashioned after the Macintosh blade, with a 60-degree curvature to match the anatomic alignment. The blade is made of a soft plastic material with a thickness of 18 mm. The blade also has an embedded antifogging mechanism. The GlideScope can be used with minimal treatment of the oropharynx with local anesthetic, and it is useful for both endotracheal intubation and as a diagnostic tool (Figure 1-4).

Perioperative Nerve Injuries

Nerve injuries during surgery and anesthesia can result in significant perioperative complications. These injuries usually occur as a result of patient malpositioning.

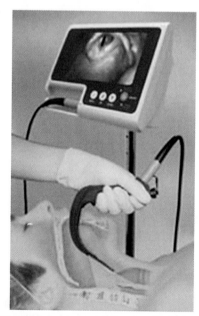

Figure 1-4. The GlideScope is a device that combines a curved laryngoscope blade attached to a fiber-optic scope that allows the user to manipulate structures in the oropharynx while visualizing the process of intubation.

The positioning of the patient on the operating table is the result of an effective compromise between what the patient undergoing surgery can tolerate from an anatomic–functional perspective and the need to provide the surgeon with suitable access. Injury to peripheral nerves in the anesthetized patient is most commonly caused by ischemia to the vasa nervorum. This occurs as a result of the stretching of the nerve and also from the compression of the nerve. Stretching a nerve can cause rupture of the epineural canal with the formation of ischemic areas in the nerve itself. The seriousness of the lesions is directly proportional to the extent of the stretching; in certain cases, it may be severe enough to cause the rupture of the nerve sheath with hernia of the nerve fibers and the formation of a pseudoneuroma. Compression of an already stretched nerve makes it extremely susceptible to injury. Compression and the subsequent ischemic injury to a nerve are usually caused by external agents (e.g., a pneumatic tourniquet, operating table accessories) as well as anatomic structures such as bones in the vicinity. In this case, the severity of the lesion is directly proportional to the duration of the insult. It is important to bear in mind that, during the intraoperative period, ischemia of the peripheral nerve may be favored by the contemporary appearance of slight hypothermia and hypotension, which reduce the flow of blood and oxygen, thereby rendering the nerve more vulnerable to ischemic insult.

Perhaps the most important thing to remember is that patients are under anesthesia and have reduced muscle tone as a result of the use of muscle relaxants. This also increases the risk of injury, because patients can be placed in unnatural positions without the ability to complain about insults and injuries.[113]

Thus it is imperative that the surgeon, the anesthesiologist, and the operating-room nursing staff cooperate when positioning the patient. During the last few years, the introduction of devices and material that may prevent perioperative positioning injuries has resulted in a reduction in the incidence of injuries. In fact, the use of intraoperative protective padding and the securing of the patient's position seem to be important factors for preventing these injuries.[114] A review of some of the potential nerve injuries is presented in Table 1-9.

Perioperative Nerve Injuries During Head and Neck Surgery

Supraorbital Nerve Injuries

Supraorbital nerve compression injuries may result from pressure applied to the face during surgery. This may occur as a result of the improper positioning of the patient or the incorrect placement of the face mask or mask straps during anesthesia. The patient may complain of periorbital numbness, and edema may be noted. Injury to this nerve presents with eye pain, forehead numbness,

TABLE 1-9 Perioperative Nerve Injuries and Potential Causes

Common Nerve Injuries in Head and Neck Surgery	Causes
Supraorbital nerve	Compression by face mask, mask straps, or endotracheal tube pressure on the nerve
Facial nerve	Compression by excessive and prolonged pressure by fingers against the mandible
Lingual nerve	Compression by endotracheal tube or laryngeal mask airway placement
Hypoglossal nerve	Compression by endotracheal and laryngeal mask airway placement
Recurrent laryngeal and superior laryngeal nerve	Compression by endotracheal tube cuff situated too high; compression by esophageal stethoscope, nasogastric tube, transesophageal echocardiogram, and laryngeal mask airway placement
Cervical vertebrae injury	Compression and disruption by excessive extension or flexion of the head, which may occur during positioning for tonsillectomy with extension of the head and neck and without support for cervical vertebrae; also seen during laryngoscopy
Brachial plexus	Stretching and compression in supine position with arm hyperabducted and head turned to the contralateral side; also occurs in supine and lateral positions with dorsal extension and lateral flexion with the head on the opposite side; also seen when patient is in lateral position and table is flexed and in a Trendelenburg position
Circumflex nerve	Pinching of nerve during Trendelenburg position with the arm in abduction against the ether screen
Radial nerve	Compression of the mid humerus by arm boards or the edge of the table; also seen with automatically cycled blood pressure cuff and injection of thiopental into a vein near the nerve
Median nerve	Compression with pronated arm off of the table; trauma during injection or cannulation of an antecubital vein
Ulnar nerve	Compression against the posterior part of the medial epicondyle of the humerus; stretching during supine or prone position when the arm is abducted between 60 and 90 degrees on an arm board; also seen with automatically cycled blood pressure cuff

and photophobia. One case involved a neuropraxic injury after the endotracheal tube was secured to the face with a Hudson harness, apparently placing pressure directly on the nerve in the forehead.

Facial Nerve Injuries

Injury to the facial nerve can result in paralysis of the muscles of the face, depending on which branches of the nerve are affected. In some individuals, an anatomic variant of the mandibular branch travels around the angle of the mandible, rendering it susceptible to compression injury at this level. Injuries to the mandibular branch have been reported after the use of the jaw lift during mask ventilation from excessive and prolonged pressure by fingers against the angles and body of the mandible. These injuries typically involve the lower face. As a result of the loss of muscle tone, chewing is difficult, the corner of the mouth sags, and the patient drools.[115]

Lingual Nerve Injuries

Palsy of the lingual nerve generally results in tongue numbness and a loss of the ability to taste. Injury to this nerve can occur from compression within the oropharynx from endotracheal tube or LMA placement. This can occur with long surgical procedures of the head and neck with the compression of the endotracheal tube against tissue. On occasion, lingual nerve injury occurs after placement of the patient in the prone position. In general, lingual nerve injury occurs as a result of pressure against the mandible and the stretching of the pterygoid muscles, which results in compression of the nerve.[116]

Hypoglossal Nerve Injuries

The hypoglossal nerve provides motor innervation to the tongue. Paralysis of this nerve results in unilateral tongue weakness, slurred speech, difficulty swallowing, and deviation to the ipsilateral side on examination. Like the lingual nerve, the hypoglossal nerve may become damaged during either endotracheal or laryngeal mask intubation, especially with the use of the LMA. In the case of the LMA, compression of the nerve between the relatively firm tube and the hyoid bone may occur.

Recurrent Laryngeal and Superior Laryngeal Nerve Injuries

Recurrent laryngeal nerve injury may result in vocal cord paralysis and hoarseness. Injury may be caused by an endotracheal tube cuff that is situated too high or by a centrally positioned esophageal stethoscope or nasogastric tube that can compress the posterior branch of the recurrent laryngeal nerve. This type of injury has also been reported after the placement of a transesophageal EKG probe followed by neck flexion. It may also occur infrequently after LMA placement.

In the subglottic larynx, an anterior branch of the recurrent laryngeal nerve enters between the cricoid and the thyroid cartilage, thus innervating the intrinsic muscles of the larynx. An inflated cuff at this location can compress the nerve between the cuff and the overlying thyroid cartilage, thereby causing injury.

Bilateral injuries present considerably more risk and often require emergency reintubation or tracheostomy. Unilateral injury to a recurrent laryngeal nerve results in the immobility of the ipsilateral vocal cord. This is associated with hoarseness that is usually noted during the immediate postoperative period. Recurrent nerve injury can be prevented by avoiding overinflation of the endotracheal tube cuff and preventing excessive endotracheal tube migration during anesthesia.

Brachial Plexus Injuries

Injuries to the brachial plexus are fairly common as a result of the malpositioning of the upper extremities, the head, and the neck during general anesthesia and operative procedures. The brachial plexus is particularly susceptible to injury. It has a long, superficial course in the axilla, and it is attached to two firm points of fixation: the vertebrae and the prevertebral fascia proximally in the neck and the axillary fascia distally in the arm.

During surgery and anesthesia, injuries to the brachial plexus from improper positioning occur as a result of the stretching and compression of the nerves. The stretching of the brachial plexus occurs especially with the patient in the supine position, during dorsal extension and lateroflexion of the head; this increases in distance between the transversal process of the vertebra and the armpit. The compression of the brachial plexus with the patient in a supine position occurs most often when the arm is abducted and the shoulder supports are positioned in the center of the trapezium muscle instead of the acromioclavicular joint. In this case, the shoulder supports may compress the plexus between the first rib and the collar bone or directly at the level of the neck triangle.

Particular attention must be paid when the patient is in the Trendelenburg position, especially when he or she is in the lithotomy position. The abduction of the arm placed on a lower level of the trunk may cause damage to the brachial plexus as a result of the stretching of the nerve.

With the patient in the prone position, brachial plexus injury can occur when the arms are abducted at 90 degrees and the elbows are bent at 90 degrees, with the hands close to the head. In the latter situation, the brachial plexus stretching usually occurs when the head is not well supported. Injuries to the brachial plexus can also occur with the patient in the lateral position when the arm is suspended on an arch, especially when the arm is in extreme abduction (i.e., more than 90 degrees of abduction).

With the patient in the lateral position, the compression of the plexus between the collar bone and the first rib may occur when the upper limb is left free to lean against the front wall of the chest and when the dependent arm and shoulder are positioned between the thorax and the table.[117–119]

Ulnar Nerve Injuries

Injuries to the ulnar nerve are also common during surgery and the postoperative period. These injuries may occur at the level of the cubital tunnel in the vicinity of the elbow, and they are characterized by numbness and tingling in the fourth and fifth digits. In addition, ulnar nerve injury may result in pain along the medial forearm and the hand, weakness of the flexor digitorum profundus muscle, and marked weakness of the muscles, namely the lumbricals and the intrinsic muscles of the hand.

The compression of the ulnar nerve may occur with the patient in the supine or prone position with the limb abducted and the hand positioned supine so that the posteromedial area of the elbow is compressed against the operating room table. More specifically, injury to the nerve occurs in the area of the olecranic groove by compression between the medial epicondyle of the humerus and the olecranus of the ulna. This is because, at this level of the elbow, the ulnar nerve can be superficial and relatively unprotected by overlying soft tissues.

In addition, perioperative injury to the ulnar nerve may occur as a result of intermittent compression by an automatically cycled blood pressure cuff, especially when the edge of the cuff is placed too far on the extremity.

Careful positioning of the patient in the operating room with appropriate padding as well as constant vigilance both in the operating room and during the postoperative period are key to avoiding injuries during surgery.

REFERENCES

1. Castellano P, Lopez-Escamez JA: American Society of Anesthesiology classification may predict severe post-tonsillectomy haemorrhage in children. *J Otolaryngol* 2003;32(5):302–307.
2. Donati A, Ruzzi M, Adrario E, et al: A new and feasible model for predicting operative risk. *Br J Anaesth* 2004;93(3):393–399.
3. Han KR, Kim HL, Pantuck AJ, et al: Use of American Society of Anesthesiologists physical status classification to assess perioperative risk in patients undergoing radical nephrectomy for renal cell carcinoma. *Urology* 2004;63(5):841–847.
4. Ragonesi M, Ivaldi C: Anaesthesiological risk assessment in young/adult and elderly dental patients. *Gerodontology* 2005;22(2):109–111.
5. Voney G, Biro P, Roos M, et al: Interrelation of peri-operative morbidity and ASA class assignment in patients undergoing gynaecological surgery. *Eur J Obstet Gynecol Reprod Biol* 2007;132(2):220–225.
6. Yilmazlar T, Guner O, Yilmazlar A: Criteria to consider when assessing the mortality risk in geriatric surgery. *Int Surg* 2006;91(2):72–76.
7. Buitelaar DR, Balm AJ, Antonini N, et al: Cardiovascular and respiratory complications after major head and neck surgery. *Head Neck* 2006;28(7):595–602.
8. Dunkelgrun M, Schouten O, Feringa HH, et al: Perioperative cardiac risk stratification and modification in abdominal aortic aneurysm repair. *Acta Chir Belg* 2006;106(4):361–366.
9. Kojima Y, Narita M: Postoperative outcome among elderly patients after general anesthesia. *Acta Anaesthesiol Scand* 2006;50(1):19–25.
10. Older P, Smith R, Hall A, French C: Preoperative cardiopulmonary risk assessment by cardiopulmonary exercise testing. *Crit Care Resusc* 2000;2(3):198–208.
11. Ozturk E, Yilmazlar T: Factors affecting the mortality risk in elderly patients undergoing surgery. *ANZ J Surg* 2007;77(3):156–159.
12. Rodanant O, Chinachoti T, Veerawatakanon T, et al: Perioperative myocardial ischemia/infarction: Study of incidents from Thai Anesthesia Incidence Study (THAI Study) of 163,403 cases. *J Med Assoc Thai* 2005;88(7 Suppl):S54–S61.
13. Rodriguez CO, Medina-Ruiz A: Evaluation of cardiovascular risks for non cardiac surgery. *Bol Asoc Med P R* 2005;97(4):296–303.
14. Sista RR, Ernst KV, Ashley EA: Perioperative cardiac risk: Pathophysiology, assessment and management. *Expert Rev Cardiovasc Ther* 2006;4(5):731–743.
15. Deedwania PC: Silent myocardial ischaemia in the elderly. *Drugs Aging* 2000;16(5):381–389.
16. Dionne MV, Kruyer WB, Snyder QC Jr: Results of Holter monitoring U.S. Air Force aircrew with ectopy on 12-lead electrocardiograms. *Aviat Space Environ Med* 2000;71(12):1190–1196.
17. Giada F, Raviele A: Diagnostic management of patients with palpitations of unknown origin. *Ital Heart J* 2004;5(8):581–586.
18. Landesberg G: Monitoring for myocardial ischemia. *Best Pract Res Clin Anaesthesiol* 2005;19(1):77–95.
19. Osman F, Gammage MD, Sheppard MC, Franklyn JA: Clinical review 142: Cardiac dysrhythmias and thyroid dysfunction: The hidden menace? *J Clin Endocrinol Metab* 2002;7(3):963–967.
20. Savelieva I, Camm AJ: Clinical relevance of silent atrial fibrillation: Prevalence, prognosis, quality of life, and management. *J Interv Card Electrophysiol* 2000;4(2):369–382.
21. Kertai MD, Boersma E, Bax JJ, et al: A meta-analysis comparing the prognostic accuracy of six diagnostic tests for predicting perioperative cardiac risk in patients undergoing major vascular surgery. *Heart* 2003;89(11):1327–1334.
22. Vinjamuri S, Jayan R: Role of myocardial perfusion imaging in risk stratification. *Nucl Med Rev Cent East Eur* 2003;6(2):147–149.
23. Passamonti E, Pirelli S: Reducing risk of cardiovascular events in noncardiac surgery. *Expert Opin Pharmacother* 2005;6(9):1507–1515.
24. Fletcher GF, Mills WC, Taylor WC: Update on exercise stress testing. *Am Fam Physician* 2006;74(10):1749–1754.
25. Romero L, de Virgilio C: Preoperative cardiac risk assessment: An updated approach. *Arch Surg* 2001;136(12):1370–1376.
26. Glance LG: Selective preoperative cardiac screening improves five-year survival in patients undergoing major vascular surgery: A cost-effectiveness analysis. *J Cardiothorac Vasc Anesth* 1999;13(3):265–271.
27. Leppo JA: Comparison of pharmacologic stress agents. *J Nucl Cardiol* 1996;3(6 Pt 2):S22–S26.
28. Johns JP, Abraham SA, Eagle KA: Dipyridamole-thallium versus dobutamine echocardiographic stress testing: A clinician's viewpoint. *Am Heart J* 1995;130(2):373–385.
29. Fleg JL: Diagnostic and prognostic value of stress testing in older persons. *J Am Geriatr Soc* 1995;43(2):190–194.
30. Hendel RC, Leppo JA: The value of perioperative clinical indexes and dipyridamole thallium scintigraphy for the prediction of myocardial infarction and cardiac death in patients undergoing vascular surgery. *J Nucl Cardiol* 1995;2(1):18–25.
31. Picano E, Pasanisi E, Venneri L, et al: Stress echocardiography. *Curr Pharm Des* 2005;11(17):2137–2149.
32. Paul B, Kasliwal RR: Dobutamine stress echocardiography—methodology, clinical applications and current perspectives. *J Assoc Physicians India* 2004;52:653–657.
33. Arruda-Olson, AM, Pellikka PA: Appropriate use of exercise testing prior to administration of drugs for treatment of erectile dysfunction. *Herz* 2003;28(4):291–297.
34. Chetta A, Tzani P, Marangio E, et al: Respiratory effects of surgery and pulmonary function testing in the preoperative evaluation. *Acta Biomed* 2006;77(2):69–74.
35. Khan MA, Hussain SF: Pre-operative pulmonary evaluation. *J Ayub Med Coll Abbottabad* 2005;17(4):82–86.
36. Smetana GW: Preoperative pulmonary evaluation: Identifying and reducing risks for pulmonary complications. *Cleve Clin J Med* 2006;73(1 Suppl):S36–S41.
37. Zollinger A, Hofer CK, Pasch T: Preoperative pulmonary evaluation: Facts and myths. *Curr Opin Anaesthesiol* 2001;14(1):59–63.
38. Smetana GW: Preoperative pulmonary assessment of the older adult. *Clin Geriatr Med* 2003;19(1):35–55.
39. Evans SE, Scanlon PD: Current practice in pulmonary function testing. *Mayo Clin Proc* 2003;78(6):758–763.
40. Gagarine A, Urschel JD, Miller JD, Bennett WF, Young JE: Preoperative and intraoperative factors predictive of length of hospital stay after pulmonary lobectomy. *Ann Thorac Cardiovasc Surg* 2003;9(4):222–225.
41. Sutherland ER, Cherniack RM: Management of chronic obstructive pulmonary disease. *N Engl J Med* 2004;350(26):2689–2697.
42. Wang JS: Pulmonary function tests in preoperative pulmonary evaluation. *Respir Med* 2004;98(7):598–605.
43. Weitzenblum E, Chaouat A: Obstructive sleep apnea syndrome and the pulmonary circulation. *Ital Heart J* 2005;6(10):795–798.
44. Van Meerhaeghe A, Moscariello A, Velkeniers B: Obstructive sleep apnoea-hypopnoea syndrome and arterial hypertension. *Acta Cardiol* 2006;61(1):95–102.
45. Dincer HE, O'Neill W: Deleterious effects of sleep-disordered breathing on the heart and vascular system. *Respiration* 2006;73(1):124–130.
46. Deane S, Thomson A: Obesity and the pulmonologist. *Arch Dis Child* 2006;91(2):188–191.
47. Coccagna G, Pollini A, Provini F: Cardiovascular disorders and obstructive sleep apnea syndrome. *Clin Exp Hypertens* 2006;28(3-4):217–224.
48. Collazo-Clavell ML, Clark MM, McAlpine DE, Jensen MD: Assessment and preparation of patients for bariatric surgery. *Mayo Clin Proc* 2006;81(10 Suppl):S11–S17.
49. Bray GA, Bellanger T: Epidemiology, trends, and morbidities of obesity and the metabolic syndrome. *Endocrine* 2006;29(1):109–117.

50. Balbani AP, Weber SA, Montovani JC: Update in obstructive sleep apnea syndrome in children. *Rev Bras Otorrinolaringol (Engl Ed)* 2005;71(1):74–80.

51. Brietzke SE, Gallagher D: The effectiveness of tonsillectomy and adenoidectomy in the treatment of pediatric obstructive sleep apnea/hypopnea syndrome: A meta-analysis. *Otolaryngol Head Neck Surg* 2006;134(6):979–984.

52. Friedman M, Vidyasagar R, Bliznikas D, Joseph N: Does severity of obstructive sleep apnea/hypopnea syndrome predict uvulopalatopharyngoplasty outcome? *Laryngoscope* 2005;115(12):2109–2113.

53. Marshall NS, Barnes M, Travier N, et al: Continuous positive airway pressure reduces daytime sleepiness in mild to moderate obstructive sleep apnoea: A meta-analysis. *Thorax* 2006;61(5):430–434.

54. Culebras A: Who should be tested in the sleep laboratory? *Rev Neurol Dis* 2004;1(3):124–132.

55. Swegle JM, Logemann C: Management of common opioid-induced adverse effects. *Am Fam Physician* 2006;74(8):1347–1354.

56. Zollner C, Stein C: Opioids. *Handb Exp Pharmacol* 2007;(177):31–63.

57. Cohen MJ, Schecter WP: Perioperative pain control: A strategy for management. *Surg Clin North Am* 2005;85(6):xi, 1243–1257.

58. van Dorp EL, Romberg R, Sarton E, Bovill JG, Dahan A: Morphine-6-glucuronide: Morphine's successor for postoperative pain relief? *Anesth Analg* 2006;102(6):1789–1797.

59. Conti G, Costa R, Pellegrini A, Craba A, Cavaliere F: Analgesia in PACU: Intravenous opioids. *Curr Drug Targets* 2005;6(7):767–771.

60. McClung CA: The molecular mechanisms of morphine addiction. *Rev Neurosci* 2006;17(4):393–402.

61. Pasero C: Fentanyl for acute pain management. *J Perianesth Nurs* 2005;20(4):279–284.

62. Battershill AJ, Keating GM: Remifentanil: A review of its analgesic and sedative use in the intensive care unit. *Drugs* 2006;66(3):365–385.

63. Lugo RA, Satterfield KL, Kern SE: Pharmacokinetics of methadone. *J Pain Palliat Care Pharmacother* 2005;19(4):13–24.

64. Fong HK, Sands LP, Leung JM: The role of postoperative analgesia in delirium and cognitive decline in elderly patients: A systematic review. *Anesth Analg* 2006;102(4):1255–1266.

65. Simons SH, Anand KJ: Pain control: Opioid dosing, population kinetics and side-effects. *Semin Fetal Neonatal Med* 2006;11(4):260–267.

66. Borchardt M: Review of the clinical pharmacology and use of the benzodiazepines. *J Perianesth Nurs* 1999;14(2):65–72.

67. Young CC, Prielipp RC: Benzodiazepines in the intensive care unit. *Crit Care Clin* 2001;17(4):843–862.

68. Nordt SP, Clark RF: Midazolam: A review of therapeutic uses and toxicity. *J Emerg Med* 1997;15(3):357–365.

69. Davis DP, Hamilton RS, Webster TH: Reversal of midazolam-induced laryngospasm with flumazenil. *Ann Emerg Med* 1998;32(2):263–265.

70. Seger DL: Flumazenil—treatment or toxin. *J Toxicol Clin Toxicol* 2004;42(2):209–216.

71. Kulkarni A, Price G, Saxena M, Skowronski G: Difficult extubation: Calming the sympathetic storm. *Anaesth Intensive Care* 2004;32(3):413–416.

72. Yildiz M, Tavlan A, Tuncer S, et al: Effect of dexmedetomidine on haemodynamic responses to laryngoscopy and intubation: Perioperative haemodynamics and anaesthetic requirements. *Drugs R D* 2006;7(1):43–52.

73. Walker J, Maccallum M, Fischer C, et al: Sedation using dexmedetomidine in pediatric burn patients. *J Burn Care Res* 2006;27(2):206–210.

74. Moos DD: Propofol. *Gastroenterol Nurs* 2006;29(2):176–178.

75. Symington L, Thakore S: A review of the use of propofol for procedural sedation in the emergency department. *Emerg Med J* 2006;23(2):89–93.

76. Bell RF, Dahl JB, Moore RA, Kalso E: Perioperative ketamine for acute postoperative pain. *Cochrane Database Syst Rev* 2006(1):CD004603.

77. Lee A, Cooper MG, Craig JC, Knight JF, Keneally JP: The effects of nonsteroidal anti-inflammatory drugs (NSAIDs) on postoperative renal function: A meta-analysis. *Anaesth Intensive Care* 1999;27(6):574–580.

78. Rocca GD, Chiarandini P, Pietropaoli P: Analgesia in PACU: Nonsteroidal anti-inflammatory drugs. *Curr Drug Targets* 2005;6(7):781–787.

79. Domino KB, Posner KL, Caplan RA, Cheney FW: Airway injury during anesthesia: A closed claims analysis. *Anesthesiology* 1999;91(6):1703–1711.

80. Bullington J, Mouton Perry SM, Rigby J, et al: The effect of advancing age on the sympathetic response to laryngoscopy and tracheal intubation. *Anesth Analg* 1989;68(5):603–608.

81. Kanaide M, Fukusaki M, Tamura S, et al: Hemodynamic and catecholamine responses during tracheal intubation using a lightwand device (Trachlight) in elderly patients with hypertension. *J Anesth* 2003;17(3):161–165.

82. Hagberg C, Georgi R, Krier C: Complications of managing the airway. *Best Pract Res Clin Anaesthesiol* 2005;19(4):641–659.

83. Hartley M, Vaughan RS: Problems associated with tracheal extubation. *Br J Anaesth* 1993;71(4):561–568.

84. Odom JL: Airway emergencies in the post anesthesia care unit. *Nurs Clin North Am* 1993;28(3):483–491.

85. Landsman IS: Mechanisms and treatment of laryngospasm. *Int Anesthesiol Clin* 1997;35(3):67–73.

86. Herrick IA, Mahendran B, Penny FJ: Postobstructive pulmonary edema following anesthesia. *J Clin Anesth* 1990;2(2):116–120.

87. Lang SA, Duncan PG, Shephard DA, Ha HC: Pulmonary oedema associated with airway obstruction. *Can J Anaesth* 1990;37(2):210–218.

88. DeVane GG: Acute postobstructive pulmonary edema. *CRNA* 1995;6(3):110–113.

89. Benumof JL: Interpretation of capnography. *AANA J* 1998;66(2):169–176.

90. Burburan SM, Xisto DG, Rocco PR: Anaesthetic management in asthma. *Minerva Anestesiol* 2007;73(6):357–365.

91. Carroll CL, Goodman DM: Endotracheal albuterol treatment of acute bronchospasm. *Am J Emerg Med* 2004;22(6):506–507.

92. Lewis RN, Swerdlow M: Hazards of endotracheal anaesthesia. *Br J Anaesth* 1964;36:504–515.

93. Dhand R, Johnson JC: Care of the chronic tracheostomy. *Respir Care* 2006;51(9):984–1004.

94. Roh JL, Lee JH: Spontaneous tracheal rupture after severe coughing in a 7-year-old boy. *Pediatrics* 2006;118(1):e224–e247.

95. Peña MT, Aujla PK, Choi SS, Zalzal GH: Acute airway distress from endotracheal intubation injury in the pediatric aerodigestive tract. *Otolaryngol Head Neck Surg* 2004;130(5):575–578.

96. Sue RD, Susanto I: Long-term complications of artificial airways. *Clin Chest Med* 2003;24(3):457–471.

97. Bielamowicz S, Stager SV: Diagnosis of unilateral recurrent laryngeal nerve paralysis: Laryngeal electromyography, subjective rating scales, acoustic and aerodynamic measures. *Laryngoscope* 2006;116(3):359–364.

98. Farrag TY, Samlan RA, Lin FR, Tufano RP: The utility of evaluating true vocal fold motion before thyroid surgery. *Laryngoscope* 2006;116(2):235–238.

99. Apfelbaum RI, Kriskovich MD, Haller JR: On the incidence, cause, and prevention of recurrent laryngeal nerve palsies during anterior cervical spine surgery. *Spine* 2000;25(22):2906–2912.

100. Zych Z, Crossley DJ: Nasotracheal intubation. *Anaesthesia* 2003;58(9):919–920.

101. Kayarkar R, Woolford TJ, Francis GA: Simple preoperative assessment to reduce the risk of traumatic epistaxis during nasotracheal intubation. *Eur J Anaesthesiol* 2002;19(9):690–691.

102. Sim WS, Chung IS, Chin JU, et al: Risk factors for epistaxis during nasotracheal intubation. *Anaesth Intensive Care* 2002;30(4):449–452.

103. Holland M, Snyder JR, Steffey EP, Heath RB: Laryngotracheal injury associated with nasotracheal intubation in the horse. *J Am Vet Med Assoc* 1986;189(11):1447–1450.

104. Onça O, Cökmez B, Aydemir S, Balcioglu T: Investigation of bacteremia following nasotracheal intubation. *Paediatr Anaesth* 2005;15(3):194–198.

105. Burkle CM, Walsh MT, Harrison BA, Curry TB, Rose SH: Airway management after failure to intubate by direct laryngoscopy: Outcomes in a large teaching hospital. *Can J Anaesth* 2005;52(6):634–640.

106. Peterson GN, Domino KB, Caplan RA, et al: Management of the difficult airway: A closed claims analysis. *Anesthesiology* 2005;103(1):33–39.

107. Pearce A: Evaluation of the airway and preparation for difficulty. *Best Pract Res Clin Anaesthesiol* 2005;19(4):559–579.

108. Berkow LC: Strategies for airway management. *Best Pract Res Clin Anaesthesiol* 2004;18(4):531–548.

109. Wheeler M: Management strategies for the difficult pediatric airway. *Middle East J Anaesthesiol* 2004;17(5):845–873.

110. Paix AD, Williamson JA, Runciman WB: Crisis management during anaesthesia: Difficult intubation. *Qual Saf Health Care* 2005;14(3):e5.

111. Oztürk T, Cakan A, Gülerçe G, et al: Sedation for fiberoptic bronchoscopy: Fewer adverse cardiovascular effects with propofol than with midazolam. *Anasthesiol Intensivmed Notfallmed Schmerzther* 2004;39(10):597–602.

112. Siobal MS, Kallet RH, Kivett VA, Tang JF: Use of dexmedetomidine to facilitate extubation in surgical intensive-care-unit patients who failed previous weaning attempts following prolonged mechanical ventilation: A pilot study. *Respir Care* 2006;51(5):492–496.

113. Cheney FW, Domino KB, Caplan RA, Posner KL: Nerve injury associated with anesthesia: A closed claims analysis. *Anesthesiology* 1999;90(4):1062–1069.

114. Hove LD, Nielsen HB, Christoffersen JK: Patient injuries in re sponse to anaesthetic procedures: Cases evaluated by the Danish Patient Insurance Association—secondary publication. *Ugeskr Laeger* 2006;168(37):3134–3136.

115. Garcia Callejo FJ, Velert Vila MM: Facial paralysis after non-otologic surgery under general anesthesia. *Acta Otorrinolaringol Esp* 1998;49(2):173–175.

116. Kadry MA, Popat MT: Lingual nerve injury after use of a cuffed oropharyngeal airway. *Eur J Anaesthesiol* 2001;18(4):264–266.

117. Winfree CJ: Peripheral nerve injury evaluation and management. *Curr Surg* 2005;62(5):469–476.

118. Winfree CJ: Iatrogenic peripheral nerve injuries. *Curr Surg* 2005;62(3):283–288.

119. Winfree CJ, Kline DG: Intraoperative positioning nerve injuries. *Surg Neurol* 2005;63(1):518.

CHAPTER 2

Nutritional Management in Head and Neck Cancer

Marc D. Coltrera

The role of nutrition in the treatment of cancer is an important, multifaceted aspect of patient care. Studies in cancer prevention have demonstrated that diet can have a significant effect on the development of different types of cancers, including head and neck carcinomas. Deficiencies of vitamins A and C along with other micronutrients such as riboflavin and zinc have been associated with the development of epithelial neoplasms in the upper aerodigestive tract.[1–5] Although diet modifications (e.g., megadoses of vitamins) have become faddish for the treatment and prevention of many types of illnesses, there is increasing evidence to support some of the popular thinking. Analogues of vitamin A have been shown to be capable of reversing early neoplastic changes in upper aerodigestive tract squamous mucosa,[6] whereas other micronutrients can directly affect immune system function with broad implications for cancer therapy.

Although the role of nutrition in the areas of cancer prevention and immunosuppression is now being examined in great detail, little is presently known that can be applied by the physician in the setting of routine clinical care. Part of the reason that nutrition's role in cancer treatment is only now coming into focus is the difficulty involved with controlling the countless, hard-to-document variables involved in clinical nutrition studies. Retrospective and epidemiologic studies dominate this literature. Still, much useful information is available, particularly regarding the links between poor nutrition and surgical complications.

There are many nutritional tests and many ideas about which ones are best in different settings. The actual application of nutritional support must deal with two practical limitations facing the typical head and neck surgeon. First, it must be recognized that the cancer patient, particularly the postsurgical patient, is a special type of patient. Many of the baseline nutritional support data and studies are based on noncancer patients and have questionable application to head and neck cancer patients. Second, ideal clinical settings—in which a team approach is recommended for all patients and which include such specialists as trained dieticians and nutritional support staff (nursing or physician)—are not always available or used. Although poor nutrition is often an issue with head and neck cancer patients, their nutritional support is often handled by their primary surgeon or physician. Many times the serious consideration

of nutritional supplementation or support first occurs postoperatively, when a feeding tube is in place. The evidence suggests that better preoperative and pretreatment assessment and nutritional support may improve the management of these cases.

This chapter outlines the areas in which nutritional support for the head and neck cancer patient may be warranted, how to evaluate the need for it, and why it might fail to make a difference for the individual patient.

CANCER-ASSOCIATED CACHEXIA: CAUSES AND EFFECTS

Protein-calorie malnutrition can be broadly characterized as acute or chronic. Acute starvation tends to result in a central pattern of protein-calorie depletion called *kwashiorkor*. Generalized cachexia is not evident, but laboratory measures of central depletion (e.g., serum albumin, total lymphocyte counts) are decreased. Chronic starvation results in a peripheral pattern of wastage referred to as *marasmus*. Body weight and anthropometric measurements of fat and muscle stores are all decreased, and the resulting body habitus is one of generalized cachexia. Head and neck cancer patients often present with a mixture of the two clinical pictures, and this requires the evaluation of both peripheral and visceral compartments to gain a true picture of the patient's nutritional status.

Tumor-related cachexia, with its attendant anorexia, losses from both fat and protein compartments, and derangements in basal energy requirements, is a well-described phenomenon among cancer patients. Approximately 40% of head and neck patients present with what is characterized as poor nutrition.[7,8] The causes can be multiple, thus complicating effective nutritional support for the cancer patient.[9] Derangements of central and peripheral control can vary depending on tumor types and individual patients.[10] Metabolic demands made by the tumor may affect the flow of nutrients to the host tissues. For example, in a study of glucose use and insulin dependency in head and neck cancer patients, Byerley and colleagues[11] demonstrated that the tumor can act as a glucose drain without evidence of altered insulin metabolism in the host. Substances made by the tumor such as tumor metabolic byproducts (e.g., lactate) can directly induce anorexia.[12,13] In addition to the tumor itself, the host response has also been implicated in tumor-associated cachexia, harming the host as well as the tumor. Cytokines such as the interleukins and interferon-γ may contribute to tumor-related cachexia.[14,15] One particularly potent cytokine, tumor necrosis factor-α, was initially independently described as a tumor-associated factor called *cachectin* because of its biologic effects on normal animals.[16–18] Further study led to the discovery that tumor necrosis factor-α and cachectin were the same protein and that the primary source was not the tumor but rather tumor-associated macrophages.

In many head and neck cancer patients, nutritional problems are compounded by excessive alcohol ingestion, mechanical obstruction, or tumor-related dysphagia, singly or in combination. In a review of more than 1000 cancer patients, Sudjiam[19] found that almost all of the patients with poor nutrition, which was defined as a loss of 12% or more of the baseline body weight, had malignant disease of the upper gastrointestinal tract. By contrast, less than 20% of the patients with adequate nutrition had malignancies that involved the upper gastrointestinal tract. The average dietary intake among the poor nutrition group was less than one half of their calculated baseline requirements. In a similar study of head and neck malignancies, Brookes[7] defined poor nutrition in terms of a general nutritional status (GNS) scoring system that is based on the percentage of weight loss and anthropometric measurements, where AMC = mid-upper arm muscle circumference; MAC = mid-upper arm circumference; TSF = triceps skin-fold thickness; P = premorbid weight; W = actual weight; and I = ideal body weight:

$$AMC = MAC - (\pi \times TSF)$$

$$AMC\% = \frac{AMC[calc] - AMC[norm]}{AMC[norm]}$$

$$P\% = \frac{P - W}{P}$$

$$I\% = \frac{I - W}{I}$$

$$AMC = \frac{P\% + I\% + AMC\%}{3}$$

Brookes found that 81.4% of his "undernourished" patients had cancers involving the oral cavity, the oropharynx, the hypopharynx, and the larynx (for further information, see Nutritional Assessment later in this chapter). Sites lacking the potential for enteral obstruction (e.g., the nasopharynx) were not found to a significant degree in the undernourished group.

In nutritionally depleted patients, surgical stress leads to further nutritional demands by creating a catabolic state.[20] Injury to tissue both from direct surgical trauma and tissue necrosis places metabolic demands on the body and can affect organ function, thereby leading to further nutritional losses.[21,22] Increased gluconeogenesis with the concomitant breakdown of fat, muscle, and visceral protein stores is the hallmark of the body's response. Infection, which is not an uncommon event in head and neck surgery, leads to further metabolic demands.

IMMUNE SYSTEM AND NUTRITION

Among the cellular components of the body, the white blood cells are some of the most metabolically active. It has long been recognized that malnutrition, particularly protein malnutrition, is associated with decreased total leukocyte counts, the decreased production of immunoglobulins, and increased infection rates.[23] Studies of cell-mediated immune response in similar malnourished populations have demonstrated reversible decreases for delayed hypersensitivity skin reactions.[24,25] Deficiencies of vitamins A, E, B_6, and folate, along with trace elements such as zinc, are associated with reduced immunocompetence.[26] More specifically, the production of lymphokines (i.e., interleukin-I) has been demonstrated to be adversely affected by malnutrition.[15] In vitro studies of vitamin-A–related molecules (e.g., beta-carotene) have demonstrated a role in stimulating effector T cells, increasing T- and B-cell proliferation in response to mitogens, enhancing natural killer cells and cytotoxic T cell activities, and increasing interleukin production.[27,28]

Although it is clear that malnutrition is related to in vitro measures of immunocompetence as well as in vivo responses to infection, it is less clear which clinical tests for malnutrition can predict a reduced immune response for the individual patient. For example, in a study of hospital patients with various degrees of malnutrition and a variety of diagnoses including neoplasm, Dowd and colleagues[29] compared historic data (e.g., weight loss), anthropometric measurements, serum proteins (e.g., albumin, transferrin), vitamins, and trace elements with measures of immunocompetence. The immune status tests included antibody-dependent cellular cytotoxicity, natural killer cell activity, and mitogen-induced lymphocyte proliferation. None of the nutritional parameters showed significant correlation with immune status, except for vitamin C levels, which correlated positively with natural killer cell activity. Low zinc and transferrin levels correlated to a lesser degree with concanavalin A mitogen stimulation of lymphocyte proliferation.

Equally hard to demonstrate is a definite improvement in immune system parameters using the standard nutritional protocols. In a study involving head and neck cancer chemotherapy patients, Picker and Bichler[30] found that demonstrable improvement in nutritional status after aggressive nutritional support did not correlate with improvement in immunologic parameters. In another study, Planas and colleagues[31] used CD4 and CD8 lymphocyte counts in an attempt to develop an immunologic assessment of parenteral nutrition efficacy. Their study showed no demonstrable improvement in lymphocyte counts after 15 days of parenteral nutritional support, which is a typical time scale for pretreatment nutritional protocols; however, they did note an improvement in mitogen-stimulated response in half of the patients. Although several studies that took place during the 1970s first noted possible trends correlating improved nutrition with improved immune status and survival,[32,33] recent reviews of the oncology literature have not found clear correlations between improved nutrition and survival other than changes in perioperative survival (see discussion later in the chapter).[34]

It must be remembered that improvement in immune parameters would not be expected to improve cancer survival statistics unless the immune system is actively responding to and is effective against the tumor. Anorexic states and nutritional intervention have direct effects on immune cell populations such as helper T cell balances.[35] A graphic example of this and nutrition's potential role is found in an experiment by Ziegler and colleagues.[36] The authors studied the effects of malnutrition in mice that were given one of two clones derived from a murine neuroblastoma cell line, C1300. The difference between the two clones was the presence (C1300-NB) or absence (TBJ-NB) of an immunogenic determinant that had been previously studied both in vitro and in vivo for its effect on host immune response. After receiving 2 weeks of either a regular diet or a protein-restricted diet, the normal and the malnourished mice received either C1300-NB or TBJ-NB. The median survival time among the mice receiving TBJ-NB was equal in both groups. By contrast, the median survival time for the Cl300-NB mice was nearly twice as long for the normal group as compared with the malnourished group. This study certainly suggests that antitumor immune response can be improved with better nutrition, but improved nutrition alone cannot be expected to improve survival. As more emphasis is being placed on the development of immunotherapies, which rely on an interaction with the patient's own immune system, nutritional support will undoubtedly become even more important.

PERIOPERATIVE MORBIDITY AND MORTALITY

Poor nutritional status and its effect on perioperative morbidity and mortality is well documented in the surgical literature. As would be expected from studies of the immune system and malnutrition, perioperative infection rates in head and neck cancer patients can be correlated with preoperative nutritional status.[37,38] The link between malnutrition and wound healing has long been recognized in nonsurgical settings (e.g., vitamin C deficiencies in sailors). The role of protein deficiencies, micronutrient deficiencies (e.g., zinc) and vitamin deficiencies (e.g., vitamins A, C, and D) has likewise been well described in surgical wounds.[39,40] It should be noted that most studies of wound healing have found that significant problems do not arise until severe malnutrition, typically involving body weight losses of more than 20%, has appeared. Many of the quantitative experiments, however, involve parameters such as the tensile strength of noninfected wound sites. As demonstrated by clinical studies, the head and neck region, with the frequent violation of mucosal and skin boundaries, coupled with the inclusion of foreign body material (e.g., reconstruction plates),[41] should be considered at higher risk for wound healing problems in the nutritionally depleted patient.

At present, the most clinically useful application of nutritional assessment is arguably in the preoperative patient. For example, in a 1984 study of head and neck patients, Goodwin and Torres[42] used a prognostic nutritional index (PNI) originally developed to assess gastrointestinal surgery patients.[43] The index is composed of serum albumin and transferrin levels, triceps skin-fold thickness (TSF), and delayed hypersensitivity reaction tests:

$$PNI~(\%~risk) = 158 - 16.6~(albumin~[g/dl])$$

$$- 0.78~(TSF~[mm]) - 0.20~(transferrin~[mg/dl])$$

$$- 5.8~(delayed~hypersensitivity~wheal~[mm])$$

Patients with a PNI of more than 40% were defined in the Goodwin and Torres study as markedly malnourished. Significant complications, including pneumonia, fistulas, and wound infections, occurred in nearly every patient in this category. Most sobering was that, within 6 months of surgery, 85% of these patients were dead.

Prospective studies using the PNI have demonstrated that preoperative nutritional support can decrease operative morbidity among those patients who are judged to be significantly malnourished.[44,45] As previously mentioned, Brookes[7] developed an analogous GNS nutritional index for assessing head and neck patients that he found to be useful. Both the PNI and the GNS scales share criteria with a more in-depth nutritional assessment that was developed by Blackburn.[46] The relative values (good to poor) for the individual laboratory tests and historic data are summarized in Table 2-1. The data and nutritional indices are discussed in more detail in the Nutritional Assessment section later in this chapter.

TABLE 2-1 General Nutritional Assessment Criteria

	Relative Assessment		
	Good	**Fair**	**Poor**
Anthropometric Data			
Weight (% ideal)	90–100	80–89	<80
Mid-upper arm circumference (cm)	29 (M)/28.9 (F)	23.0–28.9 (M)/23.0–28.8 (F)	<23 (M)/<23 (F)
Mid-upper arm muscle circumference (cm)	25 (M)/23 (F)	20.0–24.9 (M)/18.0–22.9 (F)	<20 (M)/<18 (F)
Triceps skin fold thickness (mm)	12.5 (M)/16.5 (F)	10.0–12.4 (M)/12.0–16.4 (F)	<9.9 (M)/<11.9 (F)
Laboratory Data			
Hemoglobin (g/dl)	14–17 (M)/12–15 (F)	11.0–13.9 (M)/10.0–11.9 (F)	<11 (M)/<10 (F)
Total lymphocyte count (mm^3)	<1200	800–1200	<800
Serum albumin level (g/dl)	3.5–4.5	3.0–3.4	<3
Serum transferrin level (mg/dl)	<200	150–199	<150
Creatinine-height index (%)	90–100	70–89	<70
Cell-mediated immunocompetence (mm)	<10	5–10	<5

F, Female; *M,* male.
Adapted from Bassett MR, Dobie RA: Patterns of nutritional deficiency in head and neck cancer. *Otolaryngol Head Neck Surg* 1983;91:119–125. Data originally derived from Blackburn[46] and Copeland et al.[73]

PROGNOSIS AND QUALITY OF LIFE

Although a link between poor prognosis and nutritional status is apparent, it is still not clear what overall impact improved nutritional support may have on head and neck cancer patients. The evidence certainly supports decreased surgical complications among well-nourished patients as compared with those with significant unrecompensed malnutrition. What about the effect of nutritional support and nonsurgical considerations, including tumor biology and quality-of-life issues? Once again, the multifactorial nature of nutrition studies makes it difficult to supply a clear answer to this question. Presently, no clinical studies have clearly demonstrated either improved or worsened long-term survival as a result of nutritional support during therapy. However, there have been previous as well as recent studies, both in vitro and in vivo, that suggest that improved nutrition during therapy may benefit the tumor as much as the patient.

With respect to quality of life, studies do report improvements in the sense of well-being and the overall tolerance of chemotherapy and radiation therapy.[47–52] In general, nutritional support studies report the maintenance of (rather than the improvement of) nutritional parameters during cancer therapy. By comparison, however, the ad libitum control groups tend to lose significant ground during therapy. Subjectively, nutritionally supported groups tolerate therapy protocols better, but objective improvements are harder to discern. For example, a radiation therapy study by Daly and colleagues[48] of inoperable oral cavity cancers randomized patients to oral and tube-feeding cohorts. Weight, mean mid-arm circumference, and serum albumin levels were maintained or improved in the tube-feeding group, but no improvement in overall survival was noted. In another radiation therapy study for stage III and IV head and neck cancers, Pezner and colleagues[47] found that nutritional parameters could be maintained in the tube-feeding group but that significant medical complications, failure to complete radiation therapy, and intratherapy rest periods as a result of radiation side effects were the same in both groups. The rate of complications and side effects from chemotherapy likewise appear to be unchanged by nutritional support.[34,53] Indeed, a pooled statistical analysis of parenteral nutrition support in 28 cancer treatment trials showed an apparent increase in general infection rates among patients receiving chemotherapy.[52]

Objective studies of depression and nutritional status in head and neck patients have found that the two do correlate in a manner that is independent of the tumor status.[54] When considering the number of head and neck cancer patients who undergo repeat therapy for recurrence, who are operated on for extended reconstructions, or who simply live with their untreatable disease, the potential for improving quality of life through nutritional intervention may be quite significant. For example, in a study of percutaneous endoscopic gastrostomy (PEG) for head and neck cancer patients, subjective quality of life was assessed using the Padilla quality-of-life index.[50] Evaluations were performed before, during, and after radiation therapy to compare the PEG group with an oral alimentation group. Along with the improvement or maintenance of the nutritional parameters used in the study, the authors found that the Padilla scores were maintained in the PEG group, which was in contrast with the deterioration seen in both nutritional parameters and quality-of-life indices in the oral alimentation group.

Basic issues of tumor biology make it quite probable that nutritional support for the patient also benefits the tumor cells. In some cases, improving a patient's nutrition could potentially have a negative effect on the tumor–host relationship or general outcome.[34] Edstroem and colleagues[55] studied the aneuploid cell populations of head and neck cancers in a group that was fed orally ad libitum and a group that was supplemented with nasogastric tube feedings for 6 to 8 days. They found a significant increase in the aneuploid tumor cell compartment in the group that was supplemented with nasogastric feedings. Similarly, total parenteral nutrition (TPN) has been shown to increase the hyperdiploid cells in head and neck cancers.[56] In an in vivo study of TPN and tumor metastases, Torosian and Donoway[57] looked at the effect of TPN on spontaneous pulmonary metastases from prostate carcinoma implants. The growth of both the primary tumors and the metastases were found to be increased.

Whether these tumor effects translate into significant negative outcomes for patients is more difficult to demonstrate. The only studies currently available are all retrospective. Samlowski and colleagues[58] followed 37 patients with metastatic melanoma or renal cell carcinoma who had been treated with high-dose interleukin-2 therapy. A cohort of patients had received 14 days of concurrent TPN during therapy. Although there was no difference in survival between nutrition groups, the group receiving the nutritional supplementation had a 50% reduction in complete and partial responses to therapy. Other studies, including randomized trials involving TPN, have failed to demonstrate such differences.[59]

The head and neck cancer literature is largely lacking convincing analyses of nutritional support and tumor-related outcomes. Arguably the best study to date is a secondary analysis of the Radiation Therapy Oncology Group (RTOG) trial 90-03.[60] RTOG 90-03 was a phase III prospective randomized trial with four radiation therapy arms for patients with locally advanced squamous cell carcinoma. The treatment results were published in 2000, and the secondary analysis was published in 2006.[60,61] RTOG 90-03 did not include nutritional support guidelines, and the limited information gathered simply differentiates among oral liquid supplements, enteral nutrition via feeding tube, and parenteral nutrition. As would be expected, the patients with the worst performance status and most advanced tumor stages received the greatest degree of nutritional support. As such, the secondary analysis is not without limitations requiring recursive partitioning analysis to make its point. Nonetheless, several intriguing points emerged. The patients receiving nutritional support before treatment had less weight loss and a trend toward decreased mucositis; however, a multivariate analysis found that pretreatment nutritional support was a significant, independently correlated prognostic factor for locoregional failure and decreased survival.

Considering the previously mentioned immune response experiment of Ziegler and colleagues[36] with the neuroblastoma cell line, the scenario of improved tumor nutrition coupled with an ineffective, tumor-nonspecific immune response is a potential concern for cancer patients. In order to avoid improved tumor nutrition, attempts have been made to use selective nutritional support formulations such as "selective" TPN, which adds or subtracts a nutrient needed for a tumor's growth; however, in vivo studies have not yet shown any advantages of these formulations.[62–64]

NUTRITIONAL ASSESSMENT

Patient Requirements

The calculation of baseline caloric needs, although not necessarily useful for assessing the patient's presenting clinical malnutrition, is certainly necessary for proper preoperative and postoperative supplemental support. A commonly used formula is the Harris–Benedict formula for basal energy expenditure (BEE):

Female BEE = 66.5 + (Height [cm] × 1.7) + (Weight [kg] × 9.6) − (Age [yr] × 4.7)

Male BEE = 66.0 + (Height [cm] × 5.0) + (Weight [kg] × 13.7) − (Age [yr] × 6.8)

Caloric estimates can be calculated by multiplying the BEE by factoring in activity levels (e.g., 1.3 for an ambulatory person) or by factoring in special needs, such as anabolic states. In general, practical standards for caloric needs can be estimated for maintenance states as 35 calories/kg/day and for anabolic states as

45 calories/kg/day. Protein requirements for the repletion of malnourished patients can be estimated from the following formula[65]:

$$\text{Protein (g)} = \frac{6.25 \times \text{Caloric needs}}{150}$$

The percentage of calories supplied by fat for most acute and chronic settings should be kept to less than 30% to 35% of total caloric needs. The use of "balanced" commercial tube-feeding formulations greatly simplifies the calculation of the proper dietary support required by most preoperative and postoperative head and neck cancer patients. For example, Ensure Plus (355 calories per 8-oz can) and other available nutritional supplements adhere to these general fat and protein recommendations. Blenderized diets should be similarly analyzed to ensure their adequacy.

The most practical questions facing the head and neck surgeon are probably what type of nutritional support to give and how long to administer it preoperatively. The type of nutritional support (e.g., TPN vs. enteral feedings) does not appear to be a significant factor for wound healing and other types of surgical complications.[44,66] What is significant is how effective the method was for delivering calories and protein. Ad libitum oral intake groups tend to do poorly with head and neck cancers involving lesions within the enteral canal.[52,67] Most authors favor the enteral route when the patient has an intact gastrointestinal tract. It should be recognized, however, that severely malnourished patients frequently have malabsorption syndromes as a consequence of changes in the gut. These malabsorption problems must improve before the full benefits of an enteral regimen can be realized. However, the time required to do this leads to arguments favoring TPN administration in these patients. Assuming that the method of support has been optimized, general recommendations are for 10 to 14 days of nutritional support before surgery.[68,69] Echoing this need, a 1988 study of diagnosis-related groups looked at the impact of nutritional status on head and neck surgery patients. The study found that decreased preoperative hospital time correlated with worse nutritional parameters at time of surgery and an increase in perioperative complications by a factor of 2.[70] In an era of cost containment requiring preoperative at-home management, the placement of a feeding tube or PEG at the time of the initial panendoscopy or examination is to be encouraged.

Practical Tests and Data: Nutritional Indexes

There are many laboratory tests of varying complexity and expense that can be used to assess nutritional status. Generally speaking, single-parameter assessments of nutritional status (e.g., weight loss, serum albumin) do not correlate well with clinical outcome unless the deficit is particularly severe, which means that the single-parameter test has little or no sensitivity (see Table 2-1). Also, it should be kept in mind that many of the more specific metabolic tests (e.g., creatinine–height index, nitrogen balance studies) can be affected by health considerations other than nutritional status in head and neck cancer patients. In addition, in an era of health care cost containment, nutritional tests that do not clearly have a direct impact on outcome may be viewed as "not indicated." Thus, it is especially important to use the routinely available laboratory data in the most efficacious manner and to add as few new tests as necessary.

Standard clinical information that should be available regarding all preoperative or pretherapeutic head and neck cancer patients includes the following: weight loss data, present weight, hemoglobin and hematocrit levels, total lymphocyte counts, and serum albumin level. As has been previously outlined, nutritional indexes, developed with the preoperative patient in mind, can be very useful. The indexes typically require the addition of anthropometric measurements, which can be simple to perform, and some add nonspecific immune function tests, such as the measurement of skin wheals. The routine use of a nutritional index is preferred, but even without the use of an index, certain generalizations can be made with regard to nutritional status.

Historic data are frequently used in an effort to estimate baseline nutritional deficits. Patient caloric intake can be an important way of evaluating clinical malnutrition. Ideally, caloric intake should be estimated from a detailed review of the patient's diet and compared with calculated baseline caloric needs. In practice, a history of restricted dietary intake (e.g., less than half of the premorbid historic intake) for more than 2 weeks correlates well with clinical malnutrition.

In typical cancer patient histories, weight loss is probably the most commonly noted historic measurement. It is generally understood that recent unplanned weight loss in excess of 10% of the normal baseline is a criterion for significant clinical malnutrition.[7,71] Two basic methods exist for estimating weight loss: patient recall of his or her normal weight and calculations of ideal body weight from standard population tables. At first glance, the latter may seem to be more objective than relying on patient recall. However, considering normal population variations, significant errors in estimating a baseline weight can be introduced.[72] At least one nutritional index recognizes the relative contribution of both methods of weight loss calculation.[7]

After weight, two additional anthropometric measurements that are commonly mentioned for nutritional assessment are the TSF and the MAC.[46,73] These can be assessed quickly with a minimum of equipment. The

TSF is designed to assess the fat stores of the body by measuring the subcutaneous fat layer in the arm. To produce a repeatable measurement that relates to the overall level of body fat, it is important to account for variations in fat deposition in the upper arm; therefore, the TSF is typically performed with calipers at three positions on the lateral surface, and the average measurement is then used. The MAC is an estimation of skeletal muscle mass made from a measurement at the midpoint of the upper arm. A further refinement of the MAC is the AMC, which is the value used in many applications for estimations of skeletal muscle mass. The AMC subtracts the fat contribution, as measured by the TSF, from the MAC (see Brookes' formula for the GNS and Table 2-1).

Hemoglobin and hematocrit levels are measures of a continually changing protein compartment in the body that is adversely affected by many factors, including both simple protein and caloric needs as well as vitamins and minerals (e.g., iron; see Table 2-1). Microcytic and macrocytic indices are well-known measures of folic acid and iron deficiencies that should be evaluated in every patient. Not only should the actual metabolite be supplemented, but the perceived lack of it can be used as an indicator of general needs.

White blood cells, as previously discussed, are cells with relatively high metabolic needs. It is generally thought that a total lymphocyte count below the range of 1200 to 1500/mm^3, lacking other reasons for immunosuppression, is an indicator of malnutrition (see Table 2-1). More specific tests of immune response do not appear to add significant information regarding the degree of clinical malnutrition, with the possible exception of delayed hypersensitivity skin tests, which have been incorporated into the PNI introduced by Buzby and colleagues.[43]

Serum albumin is the most commonly measured visceral protein. It is not an ideal measure of malnutrition, because it is relatively insensitive to generalized protein depletion, and its long half-life (20 days) means that it responds slowly to changes in demands and repletion therapies. Because of these and other reasons, other proteins such as transferrin, prealbumin, and serum retinol-binding protein have been used in addition to albumin. These other tests are probably more appropriate when trying to gauge acute changes (e.g., response to nutritional support), but, as a general screen for malnutrition, low albumin values (e.g., <3.4 g/dl) have been recognized as indicators of significant malnutrition, and they have been correlated with increased operative risk (250% increase in complications).[43,45] Likewise, in the same studies, low transferrin levels predict increased perioperative complications (see the PNI formula and Table 2-1).

Because single nutrition-related parameters do not correlate well with nutritional status, nutritional indexes attempt to improve the sensitivity of these tests by combining several parameters. Indexes generally recognize that both the peripheral (anthropometric testing) and the visceral protein compartments (serum laboratory testing) must be assessed to arrive at a useful value for nutritional status. Both the PNI and the more general nutritional survey of Blackburn[46] include these data. As previously discussed, the PNI assessment system has demonstrated prognostic capabilities for cancer patients, including head and neck patients. In his study of nutritional status and prognosis in the head and neck cancer patient, Brookes[7] introduced a modification of previous methods while developing a nutritional index (the GNS) for head and neck cancer patients (described previously). The GNS relies on anthropometric tests and includes both the reported weight loss and the calculated weight loss derived from the ideal weight tables. Brookes found that serum protein studies did not add materially to the GNS-derived nutritional categorization. Prospective study of head and neck cancer patients has demonstrated a potential usefulness of the GNS for prognostic assessment. For example, during follow up ranging from 18 months to 3.5 years, the group with GNS scores of less than −10% had a 13.9% survival rate as compared with a 59.5% survival for the group with GNS scores of more than −10%.

The use of one of these nutritional indexes or at least a knowledge of the relative degree of abnormality for individual tests (see Table 2-1) is highly recommended for all surgical patients and for patients receiving radiation or chemotherapy. Patients that meet criteria for significant malnutrition (e.g., PNI >40%, GNS <−20%) should be recognized and their diets supplemented accordingly. It is not as clear how lesser degrees of malnutrition affect outcome, but the routine assessment of nutrition with simple tests should lead the individual surgeon to his or her own conclusions regarding patients. Using a GNS of less than −10% as an indicator of "undernourishment" (with a GNS of <−20% being defined as significant malnourishment), as Brookes[7] did, one may argue that even minimally malnourished patients qualify for active preoperative nutritional support.

Optimization of Enteral Nutritional Support

Methods of nutritional support have been widely described and include supplemented oral intake, the nasogastric tube, the gastrostomy tube, the jejunostomy tube, and TPN. As previously discussed, all things being equal, it is generally accepted that enteral methods are preferred to parenteral ones if the gastrointestinal tract is intact. In addition, no studies comparing TPN and enteral methods, with the exception of oral groups, have demonstrated significant differences in perioperative morbidity and clinical outcome.

The use of PEG has become common for the treatment of head and neck cancer patients. The procedure is relatively simple, with few contraindications and low complication rates.[74,75] The PEG can be performed at the time of panendoscopy or as a separate procedure under local anesthesia. Briefly, the stomach is inflated, and the light from a flexible gastroscope is visualized below the costal margin. An angiocatheter is introduced into the inflated stomach by aiming at the light source, and a small tie line is passed through the angiocatheter, grasped, and pulled up through the mouth. The tie line is then used to pull the gastrostomy tube with its retention flange down to the stomach and out of a small stab incision in the abdomen. At our institution, we routinely use PEG for patients with significant nutritional deficits, for those undergoing extensive resections with or without reconstruction, and for those undergoing combined-modality therapy with wide treatment fields. In our experience, patients tolerate the PEG much better than nasogastric tubes for long-term outpatient nutritional support.

Although oral enteral nutrition groups fare relatively poorly for a variety of reasons, one area that is attracting increasing attention is the development of drugs that are capable of improving appetite in anorexic cancer patients.[76,77] Two of the more promising drugs are hydrazine sulfate and megestrol acetate.[78,79] The endocannabinoid-mediated pathways have also been found to be useful for patients with acquired immunodeficiency syndrome and cancer patients, but, for obvious reasons, there is currently no push for the use of marijuana among head and neck cancer populations. With the improvement of appetite and the encouragement of oral intake, both the general nutritional status and the quality of life of cancer patients have the potential for improvement.

REFERENCES

1. Barch DH: Esophageal cancer and microelements. *J Am Coll Nutr* 1989;8:99–107.
2. Marshall J, Graham S, Mettlin C, et al: Diet in the epidemiology of oral cancer. *Nutr Cancer* 1982;3:145–149.
3. Graham S, Mettlin C, Marshall J, et al: Dietary factors in the epidemiology of cancer of the larynx. *Am J Epidemiol* 1981;113:675–680.
4. Winn DM, Ziegler RG, Pickle LW, et al: Diet in the etiology of oral and pharyngeal cancer among women from the southern United States. *Cancer Res* 1984;44:1216–1222.
5. Shekelle RB, Lepper M, Lui S, et al: Dietary vitamin A and risk of cancer in the Western Electric study. *Lancet* 1981;2:1186–1190.
6. Lippman SM, Meyskens FL: Vitamin A derivatives in the prevention and treatment of human cancer. *J Am Coll Nutr* 1988;7:269–284.
7. Brookes GB: Nutritional status in head and neck cancer. *Otolaryngol Head Neck Surg* 1985;93:69–74.
8. Bassett MR, Dobie RA: Patterns of nutritional deficiency in head and neck cancer. *Otolaryngol Head Neck Surg* 1983;91:119–125.
9. Heber D, Byerley LO, Chi J, et al: Pathophysiology of nutrition in the adult cancer patient. *Cancer* 1986;58:1867–1873.
10. Holmes S, Dickerson JW: Malignant disease: Nutritional implications of disease and treatment. *Cancer Metastasis Rev* 1987;6:357–381.
11. Byerley LO, Heber D, Bergman RN, et al: Insulin action and metabolism in patients with head and neck cancer. *Cancer* 1991;67:2900–2906.
12. Baile CA, Zinn WM, Mayer J: Effects of lactate and other metabolites on food intake of monkeys. *Am J Physiol* 1970;219:1606–1613.
13. Richtsmeier WJ, Dauchy R, Sauer LA: In vivo nutrient uptake by head and neck cancers. *Cancer Res* 1987;47:5230–5233.
14. Langstein HN, Norton JA: Mechanisms of cancer cachexia. *Hematol Oncol Clin North Am* 1991;5:103–123.
15. Klasing KC: Nutritional aspects of leukocytic cytokines. *J Nutr* 1988;118:1436–1446.
16. Beutler B, Greenwald D, Hulmes JD, et al: Identity of tumor necrosis factor and the macrophage secreted factor cachectin. *Nature* 1985;316:552–554.
17. Beutler B, Cerami A: The biology of cachectin/TNF—a primary mediator of the host response. *Annu Rev Immunol* 1989;7:625–655.
18. Tracey KJ, Wei H, Manogue KR, et al: Cachectin/tumor necrosis factor induces cachexia, anemia, and inflammation. *J Exp Med* 1988;167:1211–1227.
19. Sudjiam AV: A hypothesis: Cancer cachexia and cachexia in cancer. *Acta Chir Scand Suppl* 1980;498:155–159.
20. Brennan MF: Metabolic response to surgery in the cancer patient. *Cancer* 1979;43:2053–2064.
21. Cerra FB: Hypermetabolism, organ failure and metabolic support. *Surgery* 1987;101:1–13.
22. Popp MB, Brennan MF: Metabolic response to trauma and infection. In Fischer JE, editor: *Surgical nutrition,* ed 1, Boston, 1983, Little, Brown, p 479.
23. Chandra S, Chandra RK: Nutrition, immune response, and outcome. *Prog Food Nutr Sci* 1986;10:1–65.
24. Fakhir S, Ahmad P, Faridi MA, et al: Cell-mediated immune responses in malnourished host. *J Trop Pediatr* 1989;35:175–178.
25. Copeland EM, MacFaden BV, Dudrick SJ: Effect of intravenous hyperalimentation on established delayed hypersensitivity in the cancer patient. *Ann Surg* 1976;184:60–64.
26. Hansen MA, Fernandes G, Good RA: Nutrition and immunity: The influence of diet on autoimmunity and the role of zinc in the immune response. *Annu Rev Nutr* 1982;2:151–177.
27. Bendich A: Carotenoids and the immune response. *J Nutr* 1989;119:112–115.
28. Bendich A, Olson JA: Biological actions of carotenoids. *FASEB J* 1989;3:1927–1932.
29. Dowd PS, Kelleher J, Walker BE, et al: Nutrition and cellular immunity in hospital patients. *Br J Nutr* 1986;55:515–527.
30. Picker H, Bichler E: Nutritional and immunological investigations in head and neck cancer patients before and after therapy. *Arch Otorhinolaryngol Suppl* 1985;242:149–153.
31. Planas M, Espanol T, Farriol M, et al: The use of immunologic parameters to assess the effectiveness of parenteral nutrition. Preliminary study. *Nutr Hosp* 1990;5:165–168.
32. Donaldson SS, Lenon RA: Alterations of nutritional status: Impact of chemotherapy and radiation therapy. *Cancer* 1979;43:2036–2052.
33. Schwartz G: Combined parenteral hyperalimentation and chemotherapy in the treatment of disseminated solid tumors. *Am J Surg* 1973;121:169–173.
34. Lipman TO: Clinical trials of nutritional support in cancer: Parenteral and enteral therapy. *Hematol Oncol Clin North Am* 1991;5:91–102.
35. Bazar KA, Joon Yun A, Lee PY: "Starve a fever and feed a cold": Feeding and anorexia may be adaptive behavioral modulators of autonomic and T helper balance. *Med Hypotheses* 2005;64:1080–1084.

36. Ziegler MM, Kirby J, McCarrick JW, et al: Neuroblastoma and nutritional support: Influence on the host-tumor relationship. *J Pediatr Surg* 1986;21:236–239.

37. Robbins KT, Favrot S, Hanna D, et al: Risk of wound infection in patients with head and neck cancer. *Head Neck* 1990;12:143–148.

38. Hussain M, Kish JA, Crane L, et al: The role of infection in the morbidity and mortality of patients with head and neck cancer undergoing multimodality therapy. *Cancer* 1991;67:716–721.

39. Knighton DR, Littooy F: Wound healing. In Paparella MM, Shumrick DA, Gluckman JL, et al, editors: *Otolaryngology*, ed 3, Philadelphia, 1991, WB Saunders, p 667.

40. Thompson WD, Ravdin IS, Frank IL: Effect of hypoproteinemia on wound disruption. *Arch Surg* 1938;36:500–508.

41. Klotch DW, Gump J, Kuhn L: Reconstruction of mandibular defects in irradiated patients. *Am J Surg* 1990;160:396–398.

42. Goodwin WJ, Torres J: The value of the prognostic nutritional index in the management of patients with advanced carcinoma of the head and neck. *Head Neck Surg* 1984;6:932–937.

43. Buzby GP, Mullen JL, Matthews DC, et al: Prognostic nutritional index in gastrointestinal surgery. *Am J Surg* 1980;139:160–167.

44. Smale BF, Mullen JL, Buzby GP, et al: The efficacy of nutritional assessment and support in cancer surgery. *Cancer* 1981;47:2375–2381.

45. Dempsey DT, Buzby GP, Mullen JL: Nutritional assessment in the seriously ill patient. *J Am Coll Nutr* 1983;2:15–22.

46. Blackburn GL: Nutritional and metabolic assessment of the hospitalized patient. *JPEN J Parenter Enteral Nutr* 1977;1:11–22.

47. Pezner RD, Archambeau JO, Lipsett JA, et al: Tube feeding enteral nutritional support in patients receiving radiation therapy for advanced head and neck cancer. *Int J Radiat Oncol Biol Phys* 1987;13:935–939.

48. Daly JM, Hearne B, Dunaj J, et al: Nutritional rehabilitation in patients with advanced head and neck cancer receiving radiation therapy. *Am J Surg* 1984;148:514–520.

49. Chencharick JD, Mossman KL: Nutritional consequences of the radiotherapy of head and neck cancer. *Cancer* 1983;51:811–815.

50. Fietkau R, Iro H, Sailer D, et al: Percutaneous endoscopically guided gastrostomy in patients with head and neck cancer. *Recent Results Cancer Res* 1991;121:269–282.

51. Holcomb GW, Ziegler MMJ: Nutrition and cancer in children. *Surg Annu* 1990;22:129–142.

52. Klein S, Simes J, Blackburn GL: Total parenteral nutrition and cancer clinical trials. *Cancer* 1986;58:1378–1386.

53. Evans WK, Nixon DW, Daly JM, et al: A randomized study of oral nutritional support versus ad lib nutritional intake during chemotherapy for advanced colorectal and non-small–cell lung cancer. *J Clin Oncol* 1987;5:113–124.

54. Westin T, Jansson A, Zenckert C, et al: Mental depression is associated with malnutrition in patients with head and neck cancer. *Arch Otolaryngol Head Neck Surg* 1988;114:1449–1453.

55. Edstroem S, Westin T, Delle U, et al: Cell cycle distribution and ornithine decarboxylase activity in head and neck cancer in response to enteral nutrition. *Eur J Cancer Clin Oncol* 1989;25:227–232.

56. Baron PL, Lawrence WJ, Chan WM, et al: Effects of parenteral nutrition on cell cycle kinetics of head and neck cancer. *Arch Surg* 1986;121:1282–1286.

57. Torosian MH, Donoway RB: Total parenteral nutrition and tumor metastasis. *Surgery* 1991;109:597–601.

58. Samlowski WE, Wiebke G, McMurray M, et al: Effects of TPN during high-dose interleukin-2 treatment for metastatic cancer. *J Immunol* 1998;21:65–74.

59. Clamon GH, Feld R, Evans WK, et al: Effects of adjuvant central IV hyperalimentation on the survival and response to treatment of patients with small cell lung cancer: A randomized trial. *Cancer Treat Rep* 1985;69:167–177.

60. Rabinovitch R, Grant B, Berkey BA, et al: Impact of nutritional support on treatment outcome in patients with locally advanced head and neck squamous cell cancer treated with definitive radiotherapy: A secondary analysis of RTOG trial 90–03. *Head Neck* 2006;28:287–296

61. Fu KK, Pajak TF, Trotti A, et al: A radiation therapy oncology group (RTOG) phase III randomized study to compare hyperfractionation and two variants of accelerated fractionation to standard fractionation radiotherapy for head and neck squamous cell carcinomas: First report of RTOG 90-03. *Int J Radiat Oncol Biol Phys* 2000;48:7–16.

62. Souba WW, Copeland EM: Hyperalimentation in cancer. *CA Cancer J Clin* 1989;39:105–114.

63. Millis RM, Diya CA, Reynolds ME, et al: Growth inhibition of subcutaneously transplanted hepatomas without cachexia by alteration of the dietary arginine-methionine balance. *Nutr Cancer* 1998;31:49–55

64. He YC, Wang YH, Cao J, et al: Effect of complex amino acid imbalance on growth of tumor in tumor-bearing rats. *World J Gastroenterol* 2003;9:2772–2775.

65. Blackburn G, Bistrian BR, Maini BS: Nutritional care of the injured and/or septic patient. *Surg Clin North Am* 1976;56:1192–1225.

66. Sako K, Lore JM, Kaufman S, et al: Parenteral hyperalimentation in surgical patients with head and neck cancer: A randomized study. *J Surg Oncol* 1981;16:391–402.

67. Hearne BE, Dunaj JM, Daly JM, et al: Enteral nutrition support in head and neck cancer: Tube vs. oral feeding during radiation therapy. *J Am Diet Assoc* 1985;85:669–674, 677.

68. Williams EF, Meguid MM: Nutritional concepts and considerations in head and neck surgery. *Head Neck* 1989;11:393–399.

69. Johnson JT: Postoperative infection. In Johns ME, editor: *Complications in otolaryngology–head and neck surgery*, Toronto, 1986, BC Decker, p 15.

70. Linn BS, Robinson DS: The possible impact of DRGs on nutritional status of patients having surgery for cancer of the head and neck. *JAMA* 1988;260:514–518.

71. Gardine RL, Kokal WA, Beatty JD, et al: Predicting the need for prolonged enteral supplementation in the patient with head and neck cancer. *Am J Surg* 1988;156:63–65.

72. Morgan DB, Path MRC, Hill GL, et al: The assessment of weight loss from a single measurement of body weight: The problems and limitations. *Am J Clin Nutr* 1980;33:2101–2105.

73. Copeland EM, Daly JM, Dudrick SJ: Nutritional concepts in the treatment of head and neck malignancies. *Head Neck Surg* 1979;1:351–363.

74. Luetzow AM, Chaffoo RA, Young H: Percutaneous gastrostomy: The Stanford experience. *Laryngoscope* 1988;98:1035–1039.

75. Wolfsen HC, Kozarek RA, Ball TJ, et al: Long-term survival in patients undergoing percutaneous endoscopic gastrostomy and jejunostomy. *Am J Gastroenterol* 1990;85:1120–1122.

76. Kulkarni SK, Kaur G: Pharmacodynamics of drug-induced weight gain. *Drugs Today (Barc)* 2001;37:559–571.

77. Yuvuzsen T, Davis MP, Walsh D, et al: Systematic review of the treatment of cancer-associated anorexia and weight loss. *J Clin Oncol* 2005;23:8500–8511.

78. Spaulding M: Recent studies of anorexia and appetite stimulation in the cancer patient. *Oncology* 1989;3:17–23.

79. Loprinzi CL, Ellison NM, Goldberg RM, et al: Alleviation of cancer anorexia and cachexia: Studies of the Mayo Clinic and the North Central Cancer Treatment Group. *Semin Oncol* 1990;17:8–12.

CHAPTER 3

Wound Healing

Bradley A. Schiff

Wound healing affects the outcome of all otolaryngologic surgeries. Understanding the mechanisms of wound healing can lead to improvements in patient care and outcome. Wound healing is a complex interactive process that involves numerous cells and a multitude of mediators. The nuances of wound healing (both when it occurs and when it fails to occur) have a significant impact on complications in otolaryngologic surgery. Many factors influence wound healing: Nutrition, radiation, aging, oxygenation, surgical techniques, and preexisting medical conditions such as diabetes or infection all play significant roles in wound healing and its complications.

BACKGROUND

Wound healing has classically been defined as having three unique phases: inflammation, proliferation, and remodeling. These three phases are, in fact, not sequential; they often occur simultaneously.

Inflammation: Postinjury to Days 4 to 6

The initial step in wound healing is hemostasis. Tissue injury results in the disruption of blood vessels and the extravasation of blood products. The injured blood vessels then vasoconstrict. The endothelium and nearby platelets activate the intrinsic part of the coagulation cascade and form a clot. Platelets both help form the hemostatic plug and secrete mediators that further wound healing. However, in the absence of hemorrhage, platelets are not essential to wound healing.[1] The resulting clot is made from a multitude of mediators, including collagen, platelets, thrombin, and fibronectin. These factors release cytokines and growth factors, which activate the inflammatory response.[2] The clot then provides a matrix for cells such as endothelial cells, fibroblasts, monocytes, and neutrophils.

After a clot has formed, the cyclooxygenase-2 enzyme in endothelial cells becomes activated and synthesizes prostaglandins, which induce vasodilation (thereby promoting cellular migration), platelet disaggregation, and leukotriene synthesis. This leads to increased vascular permeability, chemotaxis, and leukocyte adhesion.[2] The inflammatory effects of leukocytes also cause the endothelium to form gaps. These gaps allow for the extravasation of neutrophils and proteins, which cause the swelling that is very typical of inflammation.

Neutrophils are the first cells that are signaled after injury. Neutrophils help clear the wound of debris and bacteria via the release of proteolytic enzymes and reactive free oxygen radicals, which digest bacteria and nonviable tissue.[1] The extracellular matrix in unwounded tissue is protected from proteolytic enzymes by protease inhibitors. These inhibitors are not found in wounded tissue, which therefore is susceptible to degradation. If the inflammatory response is strong, it can overwhelm the protease inhibitors, thereby causing the degradation of normal tissue. Neutrophils soon undergo apoptosis and are replaced in the wound by macrophages.

Monocytes migrating toward the clot are transformed into macrophages between 48 and 96 hours after injury. The transformation of monocytes into macrophages is important for the activation of the proliferative phase of wound healing, because the activated macrophages help mediate angiogenesis. Although proper neutrophil function is not essential for wound healing to occur in noncomplicated wounds, proper monocyte–macrophage function is essential for proper wound healing to occur. Macrophage-depleted animals have been shown to have defective wound repair.[3]

Proliferative Phase: Days 4 to 14

The hallmark of the proliferative phase is the formation of granulation tissue and increased angiogenesis. Epithelialization also often occurs during this stage. Reepithelialization is the body's attempt to reestablish a protective barrier against fluid losses and bacterial invasion. It begins shortly after injury, and it is mediated by inflammatory cytokines.[2]

Fibroblasts and endothelial cells are the main cells of the proliferative phase. Endothelial cells form new capillaries, and fibroblasts migrate into the wound site and begin synthesizing collagen. The migration and function of endothelial cells and fibroblasts are mediated by the platelets and macrophages that are already in the wound. Fibroblasts already present in the injured area are also transformed into myofibroblasts, which initiate wound contraction.

Granulation tissue is found in the wound approximately 4 days after injury. New capillaries give granulation tissue its granular appearance. The newly formed extracellular matrix contributes to the formation of granulation tissue by providing scaffolding for cell migration.[4] As the extracellular matrix thickens, it forms a barrier to cell migration. Neovascularization is an essential component of the proliferative phase. The formation of new blood vessels is necessary to sustain the newly formed granulation tissue. Basic fibroblast growth factor and vascular endothelial growth factor are produced by macrophages and endothelial cells to promote angiogenesis via the migration of endothelial cells through the fragmented basement membrane to form new blood vessels.[1]

Maturation and Remodeling

This stage may be the most important with regard to long-term healing. The hallmark of this phase is the deposition of collagen into an organized network. Anything that compromises the structure of the collagen matrix will subsequently compromise the strength of the wound. Overactive collagen synthesis can result in a hypertrophic scar or keloid formation.

Fibrin, fibronectin, proteoglycans, and other proteins are synthesized next to fibroblasts. This newly formed extracellular matrix provides a framework for collagen deposition. Net collagen synthesis continues for about 1 month after wounding.[2] The initial collagen laid down is thinner than that found in uninjured skin, and it is oriented parallel to the skin instead of in the basket-weave pattern found in uninjured skin. As the initial collagen is resorbed, the new collagen deposited is thicker and organized along relaxed skin tension lines. This restructuring of collagen results in an increase in the tensile strength of the wound. At 1 week after injury, the newly formed wound is at only 3% of its final strength; at 3 weeks, the wound strength is 30% of its final strength; and, at 3 months, it is at 80% of its final strength.[5]

COMPLICATIONS AND WOUND HEALING

Wound healing is an essential component of all surgeries. The failure of wound healing leads to many head and neck complications. These failures can be caused by a breakdown in wound healing that results in a non-healing wound, or they can be caused by overactive wound healing with poor scarring and contracture that lead to functional defects. Many of the factors that negatively affect wound healing (e.g., nutrition, radiation) are covered in detail in other chapters of this book, so this chapter will attempt to focus on how specific factors impair wound healing and the resulting potential increases in complications.

OXYGENATION AND WOUND HEALING

Oxygenation plays a significant role in both wound healing and complications. There are a number of reasons why wound oxygenation is important for proper wound healing. Nonspecific immunity mediated by neutrophils depends on a high partial pressure of oxygen to form reactive oxygen species, which are the major component of the bactericidal defense against wound pathogens.[6] Oxidants produced by inflammatory cells also help initiate and direct wound healing[6] by increasing angiogenesis and collagen deposition.[7] Therefore, resistance to infection is significantly impaired by wound hypoxia, and, conversely, elevated oxygen partial pressure increases resistance to infection. Studies outside of the head and neck area have shown that supplemental perioperative oxygen can reduce the risk of wound infection in patients who are undergoing colorectal surgery.[8,9]

The tensile strength of maturing wounds is also mediated by oxygen tension. Collagen can only be exported from a cell when it aggregates into triple helixes. The enzymes that promote collagen peptides to aggregate into triple helixes are dependent on tissue oxygen tension. Therefore, the tensile strength of the wound is dependent on the tissue oxygen tension, and wound strength is adversely affected by wound hypoxia.

Although overall oxygen consumption in wounds is low, its presence in high concentrations is an essential component of a number of wound-healing processes. Unlike in muscle tissue, where oxygen delivery depends mostly on hemoglobin-bound oxygen, the driving force of oxygen diffusion in wounds is the partial pressure of oxygen. In surgical patients, the rate of wound infection is inversely proportional to subcutaneous wound tissue oxygen tension, whereas the rate of collagen deposition is directly proportional to subcutaneous wound oxygen tension.[10,11] Oxygen is also important in epithelialization, because the rate of epithelialization increases with increased oxygen in vivo.[12]

Peripheral vasoconstriction can negatively affect wound oxygenation. Subcutaneous tissue is particularly sensitive to vasoconstriction. Pain, cold, blood volume deficits, and nicotine use can all contribute to peripheral vasoconstriction. This can lead to a decrease in wound oxygenation, increased wound infection, and impaired wound healing. Many of these factors are under the control of the otolaryngologist. The prevention of hypothermia and adequate volume replacement have been shown to decrease wound infection (although not specifically in head and neck patients), and good pain control has been shown to improve subcutaneous tissue oxygen tension. Diseases such as diabetes and hypertension can affect the peripheral vasculature as well, and tight glucose control in diabetic patients is essential for proper wound healing. Although the rich vascularization of the head and neck makes the effects of tissue perfusion less drastic than in other parts of the body, the principles involved remain the same.

Smoking has also been shown to adversely affect wound healing through a variety of mechanisms. Nicotine itself can adversely affect wound healing. Nicotine impairs the proliferation of red blood cells, fibroblasts, and macrophages, all of which are essential for proper wound healing. It increases platelet adhesiveness, which can lead to microclots that cause diminished microperfusion, and it also can directly produce cutaneous vasoconstriction.[13] Carbon monoxide is produced in tobacco smoke, and it has a binding affinity for hemoglobin that is 200 times that of oxygen. As carboxyhemoglobin levels rise in the bloodstream, the oxygen disassociation curve shifts to the left, thereby preventing the dissociation of oxygen from red blood cells and decreasing oxygen diffusion into tissues.[13] Thus, tobacco smoke reduces the oxygen-carrying capacity of hemoglobin, thereby reducing the amount of oxygen that reaches the periphery.

There are direct clinical implications of smoking as well. The majority of studies involving tobacco use and its resulting complications surgical patients involve plastic and reconstructive surgery. The survival of skin flaps and skin grafts is dependent on adequate blood supply and oxygenation. The increase in vasoconstriction and the decrease in oxygen-carrying capacity and oxygen dissociation found in smokers can impair peripheral oxygenation and lead to increased flap mortality. Studies of patients undergoing face-lifts have shown that the risk of skin slough was 7.5% among smokers as compared with only 2.7% among nonsmokers.[14] A study of sacral incisions examined the wound infection rate and the wound rupture rate among smokers as compared with nonsmokers and found a statistically significant increase in both wound infections and wound ruptures among smokers as compared with nonsmokers.[15] Additionally, the same study demonstrated that 4 weeks of smoking abstinence reduced the incidence of wound infection.

Hyperbaric oxygen has been shown to improve wound healing. It does not play a significant role in preventing otolaryngologic complications, but it can play a role in managing and minimizing certain complications when they occur. The main role of hyperbaric oxygen is in the treatment of chronic wounds, and its main role in otolaryngology is in the treatment of radiation-induced tissue necrosis. Hyperbaric oxygen has been shown to improve wound healing among patients with the post-radiation complication of osteoradionecrosis.[16]

NUTRITION AND WOUND HEALING

Adequate nutrition is essential for proper wound healing, and nutrition is covered in detail in Chapter 2. Protein calorie malnutrition leads to decreased wound strength, decreased T-cell function, and decreased phagocyte, compliment, and antibody function, with resulting decreases in wound infection defenses and wound strength.[17] An important principle to remember is that nutritional requirements change during the healing process. An injury results in the need for increased energy production, which can lead to a catabolic state. Other factors such as fever, sepsis, or burn injury can greatly increase a patient's metabolic rate and nutritional needs. In addition, many head and neck cancer patients present in a malnourished state as a result of either decreased oral intake or increased metabolic rates as a result of tumor. Proteins can also be degraded in catabolic states such as sepsis or major burns. Collagen is the major protein in skin, so adequate protein intake is essential for skin healing. Preoperative nutritional support is generally recommended for patients with moderate malnutrition (10% to 20% weight loss or serum albumin <3.2 g/dl) who can wait at least 7 days before surgery.[18]

Vitamin deficiency also can contribute to poor wound healing and complications. The most famous example occurs among patients with vitamin C deficiency. Patients who develop scurvy have impaired collagen synthesis with a resulting significant impairment in wound healing. Vitamin A deficiency is also associated with poor healing. Vitamin A has been shown to stimulate epithelialization and collagen deposition. Vitamin A in high doses has been shown to reverse the poor healing associated with steroid use, diabetes, and radiation.[19–21] Zinc deficiency has been shown to impair healing, but there is no evidence that zinc supplementation accelerates healing among patients without a deficiency.

SURGICAL TECHNIQUES AND WOUND HEALING

Proper surgical technique is a key tenet of proper wound healing. Proper surgical preparation, the warming of the patient, and antibiotic prophylaxis can all help to reduce infection and, therefore, to prevent delayed wound healing. Proper tissue handling and hemostasis contribute to wound healing, and the use of proper surgical technique and planning can play a large part in reducing complications. Surgical incisions should be made with regard to blood supply to ensure skin-flap viability. The proper handling of tissue should be encouraged to minimize soft-tissue trauma. Retractors should be periodically released and flaps kept moist to encourage tissue perfusion and to prevent dryness. Proper fluid replacement and maintaining proper patient temperature help to reduce vasoconstriction and to encourage peripheral circulation. The use of monofilament sutures where possible and the use of sutures with the smallest diameter sufficient for the task will reduce inflammation. Care must be taken to ensure that sutures are not tied too tightly, which may result in ischemia. The effects of postsurgical tissue swelling must be taken into account when closing a wound.

Hematomas predispose a wound to breakdown. The prevention of hematomas is the best way to avoid the potential complications. A careful history, including patient use of over-the-counter medications such as aspirin or a history of easy bleeding or bruising, can identify patients who are at risk for hematomas. Proper surgical techniques and drain placement can also help with the prevention of hematomas. Iron is a major nutrient for bacteria, and wound infections are more likely after hematomas. Skin flaps over hematomas are also removed from potential sources of neovascularization, and they can be under more tension as well as exposed to an increased amount of free radicals, thereby increasing the chance of skin-flap necrosis.

RADIATION AND WOUND HEALING

Radiation produces both acute and delayed effects on tissue that can have a profound effect on surgical wound healing. Radiation causes acute degenerative changes in basement membranes, and it increases vascular permeability. Vascular changes may increase stasis and occlusion, thereby causing edema, thrombosis, and impaired neovascularization. The replacement of vessels with fibrous tissue may also eventually occur. The main effects of radiation are the result of impaired fibroblast function, which also leads to impaired collagen production.

The effects of radiation on wound healing are minimized beginning 6 months after irradiation. However, even if radiation is given years before surgery, it can still have a delayed effect on wound healing. Long-term effects of radiation include skin and subcutaneous tissue atrophy, with decreased wound vascularity and increased hypoxia; this results in impaired normal healing and increased odds of bacterial infection. Additionally, radiation affects surgical wound healing by altering the surgery itself. Operating in a radiated field, with the resultant increased scarring and fibrosis, is more challenging than operating in a nonirradiated field, and this may lead to an increase in complications.

Data regarding the surgical complications that are associated with radiation are scarce, but preoperative radiation has been shown to significantly impair wound healing. Wound bursting strength has been shown to be 62% of normal 1 week after only 18 gy of radiation.[22] Gorodetsky and colleagues[23] found a correlation between radiation dose and a reduction in wound strength beginning with doses as low as 8 gy. Arnold and colleagues[24] examined reconstruction using radiated tissue as compared with nonirradiated tissue and found a complication rate of 32% using tissue that had previously been irradiated as compared with only 19% using nonirradiated tissue. If a flap was placed into a previously irradiated field, the complication rate was 25% as compared with only 11.6% in tissue that was transposed into a radiation-naive field.[24]

Perhaps the most common otolaryngologic surgery in which the effects of radiation often result in poor wound healing and subsequent complications is the laryngectomy. Laryngectomies are often performed both in radiation-naive necks and previously irradiated necks. The single greatest risk factor for postsurgical laryngocutaneous fistula is previous irradiation. A meta-analysis of all studies has shown that the relative risk for pharyngocutaneous fistula after laryngectomy is 2.28 times greater among patients with previous larynx irradiation as compared with patients with a radiation-naive larynx.[25] In addition, patients with previous irradiation who developed fistulas required more time for the fistula to heal and more often required closure using a flap than patients with radiation-naive necks who developed fistulas.[25] To prevent complications while operating on radiated patients, irradiated tissue must be handled with care. Proper surgical techniques, including the proper use of drains and tension-free closure, must be used. Seromas and hematomas increase the incidence of late wound breakdown and must be avoided.

Because the initial 48 hours are the most critical for successful wound healing, postoperative radiation is often administered 3 to 4 weeks after surgery. To provide radiation therapy intraoperatively or immediately postoperatively, brachytherapy is often used in head and neck oncologic surgery. A study examining sarcoma resection with intraoperative brachytherapy implantation demonstrated wound-healing problems in 52% of patients receiving brachytherapy as compared with only 26% in patients not receiving brachytherapy.[26] Mantravadi and colleagues[27] compared complications among patients receiving radiation therapy with head and neck cancers and found that 15 of 92 patients receiving preoperative radiation therapy suffered wound dehiscence as compared with 0 of 60 patients receiving posttreatment radiation.

INFECTION AND WOUND HEALING

Infection plays a large role in wound healing. A differentiation must be made between bacterial colonization and infection. Colonization is defined as the presence of replicating organisms adherent to the wound in the absence of tissue damage, whereas infection is the presence of replicating organisms within a wound with subsequent host injury.[28] Increasingly, an intermediate stage between infection and colonization has been described as *critical colonization,* which is considered a transition state between colonization and invasive wound infection wherein the tissue may have an unhealthy appearance but there is no direct tissue invasion.[29] This transitional stage may also have impaired wound healing.

Tissue can tolerate normal skin flora up to a concentration of 10^5 bacteria per gram of tissue without being infected.[30] However, the exact concentration of bacterial contamination that leads to infection varies, depending on both the virulence of the organism and the organism's interaction with the surrounding microflora. Polymicrobial infections may lessen the bacterial load that is needed for infection via bacterial synergy between less and more virulent species. The presence of four or more species has been correlated with nonhealing wounds.[31] The species of bacteria present also plays a significant role in wound healing. Some species, such as *Pseudomonas* spp., can cause significant wound deterioration as a result of the production of tissue-destroying enzymes.

Bacteria can affect wound healing via a number of different mechanisms. Bacteria contribute to inflammation by increasing the consumption of compliment proteins, which results in decreased chemotaxis.[32] In addition, the increased production of cytotoxic enzymes and free oxygen radicals increases tissue damage. Finally, increased thrombosis and the release of vasoconstrictive metabolites increase the tissue hypoxia that promotes bacterial proliferation.[32] Bacteria also inhibit the migration of epithelium and digest dermal proteins.[33] Collagen formation is also impaired as a result of impaired fibroblast function, with resulting disorganized collagen production and cross-linking that leads to decreased wound strength and increased surgical dehiscence.[32,34] As a result of the deleterious effects of bacterial infection on surgical wound healing, proper wound preparation, antibiotic prophylaxis, and wound care are essential for preventing surgical complications.

STEROIDS AND WOUND HEALING

Steroids are known to adversely affect wound healing, but large-scale clinical articles are somewhat scarce. Steroids are often used in otolaryngologic surgery to prevent tissue edema and to limit scarring. However, their use systemically for medical reasons may have significant deleterious effects on wound healing. Steroid use has been shown to delay the appearance of inflammatory cells, fibroblasts, collagen formation, and regenerating capillary formation and to slow scar contraction and epithelial migration. Steroids suppress inflammation at the step where activated inflammatory cells consume oxygen, thereby resulting in tissue hypoxia and lactate formation.[6] Steroids also affect the maturation phase of wound repair, primarily through the impairment of fibroblasts and collagen formation.

Clinical studies of the effects of steroids in human wound healing are scarce, and most of the present knowledge of the deleterious effects of steroids comes from a few basic science articles. Studies in rat tracheas demonstrated that 1 week of corticosteroid use significantly impaired the bursting strength of rat tracheal anastomosis in a dose-dependent fashion. However, the bursting strength was not significantly reduced after a single high dose of steroids.[35]

The effects of steroids on wound healing have been shown to be partially reversed via the administration of retinoids. Retinoid administration has been shown to partially reverse the decreases in transforming growth factor β and insulin-like growth factor 1 that are associated with steroid use and to enhance hydroxyproline wound content and college deposition.[36] Steroids have also been shown to affect long-term wound healing. Steroid doses of more than 30 mg/day inhibit fibroblast activity and therefore block tissue contraction as well as scar shrinking and shortening.[37] Although the exact mechanisms of steroids' effects on wound healing are unclear and more specific clinical studies are required to fully delineate the effects of steroids on wound healing, it is important to use steroids judiciously and to be mindful of potential impaired healing when performing surgery on patients who are receiving systemic corticosteroid therapy.

AGING AND WOUND HEALING

Aging has been recognized as impairing wound healing for almost 100 years.[38] The effect of aging is thought to be more of a temporal delay rather than an actual impairment of wound healing.[39] The skin is particularly sensitive to aging. Skin changes associated with aging are both intrinsic (i.e., independent of environmental factors) and extrinsic (e.g., ultraviolet light exposure). Aging skin shows a progressive loss of function with increased vulnerability to the environment, and it also decreases homeostatic capabilities.[40] Aging has been shown to affect wound healing through a number of factors, including decreased levels of growth factors, impaired cellular proliferation and migration, and a diminishment of extracellular matrix secretions.[41]

Changes in macrophage function are also critical to age-related delays in wound healing. Keratinocytes, fibroblasts, and vascular endothelial cells all show reduced proliferation among aged animals,[42] with resultant delays in reepithelialization, collagen synthesis, and angiogenesis.[43] These changes have also been shown clinically to delay wound closure among humans.[44] Incisional wounds among patients who are more than 70 years old have been shown to have lower tensile strength than those among patients who are less than 70 years old.[45]

KELOIDS

Occasionally complications in wound healing result not from insufficient healing but rather from overly exuberant healing. Keloids and hypertrophic scars are examples of such exuberant wound healing. Keloids are distinct from hypertrophic scars. Hypertrophic scars arise within the confines of the original scar border, whereas keloids can proliferate outside of the confines of the original wound. The exact cause of keloids is uncertain, but some techniques can be used to minimize their formation. Mechanical tension has been thought to increase keloid formation, so incisions made parallel to skin tension lines can help reduce keloid formation.[46] The use of running absorbable subcuticular sutures (as opposed to interrupted cutaneous sutures) limits suture trauma to the skin and may reduce keloid formation. The treatment of keloids is addressed in detail elsewhere in this book, but it can involve steroid injection, radiation, silicon gel, pressure therapy, and numerous other treatments.

MEDICAL EFFECTS ON WOUND HEALING

Diabetes has been shown to significantly impair wound healing, and diabetic patients encounter increased complication rates as compared with their euglycemic counterparts. There are many reasons for impaired wound healing in diabetics, and the mechanisms are not fully understood. Some hypothesize that a buildup of advanced glycation end products in body tissues is responsible for the delay in wound healing.[47] Diabetics have also been shown to have a diminished early inflammatory response and delayed epithelialization.[17] Hyperglycemia itself interferes with the cellular transport of ascorbic acid into fibroblasts and leukocytes, and it decreases leukocyte chemotaxis. As a result of these facts, the strict control of glucose levels is essential for proper wound healing.[48] Diabetic patients are also prone to poor wound healing as a result of increased peripheral vascular disease and because of decreased host resistance to infection. Patients with hypertension and coronary artery disease may also present with peripheral vascular disease, and the decrease in vascularization must be considered when treating these patients.

CONCLUSION

Wound healing is an essential component of all aspects of head and neck surgery. Understanding the mechanisms of proper wound healing and the multitude of factors that can impair the wound healing process can greatly reduce and minimize complications in head and neck surgery.

REFERENCES

1. Singer AJ, Clark RA: Cutaneous wound healing. *N Engl J Med* 1999;341(10):738–746.
2. Broughton G 2nd, Janis JE, Attinger CE: The basic science of wound healing. *Plast Reconstr Surg* 2006;117(7 Suppl):12S–34S.
3. Leibovich SJ, Ross R: The role of the macrophage in wound repair: A study with hydrocortisone and antimacrophage serum. *Am J Pathol* 1975;78(1):71–100.
4. Clark RA, et al: Fibronectin and fibrin provide a provisional matrix for epidermal cell migration during wound reepithelialization. *J Invest Dermatol* 1982;79(5):264–269.
5. Irvin TT: Effects of malnutrition and hyperalimentation on wound healing. *Surg Gynecol Obstet* 1978;146(1):33–37.
6. Ueno C, Hunt TK, Hopf HW: Using physiology to improve surgical wound outcomes. *Plast Reconstr Surg* 2006;117(7 Suppl): 59S–71S.
7. Sen CK, et al: Oxidant-induced vascular endothelial growth factor expression in human keratinocytes and cutaneous wound healing. *J Biol Chem* 2002;277(36):33284–33290.
8. Belda FJ, et al: Supplemental perioperative oxygen and the risk of surgical wound infection: A randomized controlled trial. *JAMA* 2005;294(16):2035–2042.
9. Greif R, et al: Supplemental perioperative oxygen to reduce the incidence of surgical-wound infection: Outcomes Research Group. *N Engl J Med* 2000;342(3):161–167.
10. Hopf HW, et al: Wound tissue oxygen tension predicts the risk of wound infection in surgical patients. *Arch Surg* 1997;132(9): 997–1005.
11. Jonsson K, et al: Tissue oxygenation, anemia, and perfusion in relation to wound healing in surgical patients. *Ann Surg* 1991;214(5):605–613.
12. Feldmeier JJ, et al: UHMS position statement: Topical oxygen for chronic wounds. *Undersea Hyperb Med* 2005;32(3):157–168.
13. Silverstein P: Smoking and wound healing. *Am J Med* 1992;93(1A):22S–24S.
14. Rees TD, Liverett DM, Guy CL: The effect of cigarette smoking on skin-flap survival in the face lift patient. *Plast Reconstr Surg* 1984;73(6):911–915.
15. Sorensen LT, Karlsmark T, Gottrup F: Abstinence from smoking reduces incisional wound infection: A randomized controlled trial. *Ann Surg* 2003;238(1):1–5.
16. Narozny W, et al: Hyperbaric oxygen therapy in the treatment of complications of irradiation in head and neck area. *Undersea Hyperb Med* 2005;32(2):103–110.
17. Arnold M, Barbul A: Nutrition and wound healing. *Plast Reconstr Surg* 2006;117(7 Suppl):42S–58S.
18. Howard L, Ashley C: Nutrition in the perioperative patient. *Annu Rev Nutr* 2003;23:263–82.
19. Ehrlich HP, Hunt TK: Effects of cortisone and vitamin A on wound healing. *Ann Surg* 1968;167(3):324–328.
20. Levenson SM, et al: Supplemental vitamin A prevents the acute radiation-induced defect in wound healing. *Ann Surg* 1984;200(4):494–512.
21. Seifter E, et al: Impaired wound healing in streptozotocin diabetes: Prevention by supplemental vitamin A. *Ann Surg* 1981;194(1):42–50.
22. Bernstein EF, et al: Collagen gene expression and wound strength in normal and radiation-impaired wounds: A model of radiation-impaired wound healing. *J Dermatol Surg Oncol* 1993;19(6):564–570.
23. Gorodetsky R, et al: Radiation effect in mouse skin: Dose fractionation and wound healing. *Int J Radiat Oncol Biol Phys* 1990;18(5):1077–1081.
24. Arnold PG, Lovich SF, Pairolero PC: Muscle flaps in irradiated wounds: An account of 100 consecutive cases. *Plast Reconstr Surg* 1994;93(2):324–329.

25. Paydarfar JA, Birkmeyer NJ: Complications in head and neck surgery: A meta analysis of postlaryngectomy pharyngocutaneous fistula. *Arch Otolaryngol Head Neck Surg* 2006;132(1):67–72.

26. Arbeit JM, Hilaris BS, Brennan MF: Wound complications in the multimodality treatment of extremity and superficial truncal sarcomas. *J Clin Oncol* 1987;5(3):480–488.

27. Mantravadi RV, Skolnik EM, Applebaum EL: Complications of postoperative and preoperative radiation therapy in head and neck cancers: A comparative study. *Arch Otolaryngol* 1981;107(11):690–693.

28. Dow G, Browne A, Sibbald RG: Infection in chronic wounds: Controversies in diagnosis and treatment. *Ostomy Wound Manage* 1999;45(8):23-27, 29–42.

29. Edwards R, Harding KG: Bacteria and wound healing. *Curr Opin Infect Dis* 2004;17(2):91–96.

30. Robson MC: Wound infection: A failure of wound healing caused by an imbalance of bacteria. *Surg Clin North Am* 1997;77(3):637–650.

31. Bowler PG: The 10(5) bacterial growth guideline: Reassessing its clinical relevance in wound healing. *Ostomy Wound Manage* 2003;49(1):44–53.

32. Robson MC, Stenberg BD, Heggers JP: Wound healing alterations caused by infection. *Clin Plast Surg* 1990;17(3):485–492.

33. Lawrence JC: The aetiology of scars. *Burns Incl Therm Inj* 1987;13 Suppl:S3–S14.

34. Metzger Z, et al: The effect of bacterial endotoxin on the early tensile strength of healing surgical wounds. *J Endod* 2002;28(1):30–33.

35. Talas DU, et al: The effects of corticosteroids on the healing of tracheal anastomoses in a rat model. *Pharmacol Res* 2002;45(4):299–304.

36. Wicke C, et al: Effects of steroids and retinoids on wound healing. *Arch Surg* 2000;135(11):1265–1270.

37. Doughty DB: Preventing and managing surgical wound dehiscence. *Adv Skin Wound Care* 2005;18(6):319–322.

38. DuNouy P: The relation between the age of the patient, the area of the wound, and the index of cicatrisation. *J Exp Med* 1916;24:461–470.

39. Ashcroft GS, Horan MA, Ferguson MW: Aging is associated with reduced deposition of specific extracellular matrix components, an upregulation of angiogenesis, and an altered inflammatory response in a murine incisional wound healing model. *J Invest Dermatol* 1997;108(4):430–437.

40. Gilchrest BA, Garmyn M, Yaar M: Aging and photoaging affect gene expression in cultured human keratinocytes. *Arch Dermatol* 1994;130(1):82–86.

41. Gosain A, DiPietro LA: Aging and wound healing. *World J Surg* 2004;28(3):321–326.

42. Reed MJ, Ferara NS, Vernon RB: Impaired migration, integrin function, and actin cytoskeletal organization in dermal fibroblasts from a subset of aged human donors. *Mech Ageing Dev* 2001;122(11):1203–1220.

43. Swift ME, Kleinman HK, DiPietro LA: Impaired wound repair and delayed angiogenesis in aged mice. *Lab Invest* 1999;79(12):1479–1487.

44. Grove GL, Kligman AM: Age-associated changes in human epidermal cell renewal. *J Gerontol* 1983;38(2):137–142.

45. Sandblom P, Petersen P, Muren A: Determination of the tensile strength of the healing wound as a clinical test. *Acta Chir Scand* 1953;105(1-4):252–257.

46. Al-Attar A, et al: Keloid pathogenesis and treatment. *Plast Reconstr Surg* 2006;117(1):286–300.

47. Ahmed N: Advanced glycation endproducts—role in pathology of diabetic complications. *Diabetes Res Clin Pract* 2005;67(1):3–21.

48. Mann GV, Newton P: The membrane transport of ascorbic acid. *Ann N Y Acad Sci* 1975;258:243–252.

CHAPTER 4

Postoperative Infection

Rebecca E. Fraioli and Jonas T. Johnson

Wound infection is the most common nosocomial infection in surgical patients, and it accounts for significant patient morbidity, prolonged hospital stays, and increased costs.[1-3] Antibiotic prophylaxis has been established as an effective means of decreasing the incidence of postoperative wound infection, but antibiotics alone cannot fully eliminate the risk. Current research into the prevention of wound infection focuses on identifying and treating host factors and intraoperative factors that contribute to wound infection. Finally, pneumonias, blood infections, and urinary tract infections also may occur as nosocomial infections among postoperative patients.

WOUND HEALING

Wound healing begins at the time of tissue injury with the coagulation phase, in which hemostasis is achieved and growth factors and inflammatory mediators are liberated. The second phase of wound healing, the inflammatory phase, begins almost simultaneously with the coagulation phase as the cytokines released by platelet activation recruit white blood cells to the site of injury. The polymorphonuclear leukocyte (neutrophil) is the predominant cell type for the first 48 hours.

In a clean wound, macrophages take over as the predominant cell type by 72 hours after injury. Macrophages appear to be necessary for proper wound healing, because they secrete substances that recruit blood vessel growth and fibroblast replication. By contrast, neutrophils do not appear to be necessary for wound healing, and, when they are present for more than 72 hours, they may have a deleterious effect on wound healing. In a contaminated wound, neutrophil levels remain high. Neutrophil granules contain hydrolytic enzymes that cause collagen breakdown and tissue damage. Bacteria themselves also release toxic antigens that contribute to tissue breakdown. Infected wounds fail to progress to the proliferative phase, where angiogenesis and collagen formation normally occur and which is crucial for the development of a healed wound.[4,5] Whether this is the result of the continued presence of neutrophils or of the presence of the bacteria themselves, it has been demonstrated that wounds in which the bacterial colony count is greater than 10^5 organisms per gram of tissue will not heal. In addition, the presence of β-hemolytic *Streptococcus* in any concentration prevents wound healing.[5,6]

The seeding of the surgical wound with bacteria may come from both external and internal (patient) sources. Skin preparation and aseptic surgical technique are used to prevent or reduce the bacterial contamination of the wound by the external environment.[3] However, many surgical procedures of the head and neck involve entry into the upper aerodigestive tract. Estimates of the normal salivary bacterial count range from 10^8 to 10^9 colonies/ml, with more than 200 different bacterial species colonizing the tract of a single patient.[7] When postoperative wound sepsis does occur after head and neck surgery, infections are commonly polymicrobial, and cultures generally reflect the oropharyngeal flora that is present in the patient at the time of surgery.[8]

RISK FACTORS FOR POSTOPERATIVE WOUND INFECTION

Background

Three main elements contribute to the development of postoperative wound infection: (1) the degree of bacterial contamination of the operative site; (2) the functional status of the surgical patient; and (3) technical operative details. It is important to understand the role played by each of these factors when designing therapeutic interventions to correct them.

Study on the Efficacy of Nosocomial Infection Control Score

The Centers for Disease Control and Prevention (CDC) has developed a predictive measure to help estimate the risk of a particular patient developing a postoperative wound infection. The criteria, which were established and validated through multivariate analysis in a trial known as the Study on the Efficacy of Nosocomial Infection Control (SENIC), are listed in Box 4-1. The SENIC score ranges from 1 to 4, with one point given for each positive factor. The SENIC score correlates directly with the risk of wound infection[9] (Table 4-1).

Bacterial Inoculum

There is a direct correlation between the degree of bacterial inoculum contaminating the wound at the time of surgery and the incidence of postoperative wound infection. In the United States, the CDC has established a classification system that is based on the level of contamination of a wound that predicts the risk of postoperative wound infection[3,10] (Table 4-2). A class I/clean

BOX 4-1   Criteria for Determining the Study on the Efficacy of Nosocomial Infection Control Score

Abdominal surgery
Contaminated or dirty surgery (class III or IV)
Surgery duration of more than 2 hours
Poor patient functional status (i.e., more than three diagnoses at hospital discharge)

TABLE 4-1   Correlation Between the Study on the Efficacy of Nosocomial Infection Control Score and Postoperative Wound Infection

Study on the Efficacy of Nosocomial Infection Control Score	Risk of Postoperative Wound Infection[9]
0	1%
1	3.6%
2	9%
3	18%
4	27%

TABLE 4-2   Risk of Infection by Wound Category

Class	Description	Risk of Infection
I	Clean	Low (<3%–5%)
II	Clean-contaminated	Intermediate (10%–80%)
III	Contaminated	High (>80%)
IV	Dirty	Already infected

wound is one in which no infection exists preoperatively and no gross contamination occurs during surgery. For head and neck surgery, this includes any wound that does not include entry into the upper aerodigestive tract (e.g., thyroidectomy, parotidectomy, submandibular gland excision). A class II/clean-contaminated wound in head and neck surgery is one in which there is entry into the upper aerodigestive tract, but this entry is done in a controlled fashion with no gross spillage of oral or respiratory secretions (e.g., nasal septoplasty, sinus surgery, endoscopic laryngeal surgery). A class III/contaminated surgery is one in which there is either major spillage of secretions into the wound or a major break in aseptic technique (e.g., total laryngectomy, total glossectomy performed through a surgical approach in the neck). Class IV/dirty wounds are considered infected before the surgical incision is made (e.g., old traumatic wounds, wounds in which there is preexisting infection or perforated viscera, reoperation on a patient who developed a pharyngeal leak after laryngectomy).

Patient Factors

Diabetes Mellitus

Increased serum glucose levels have a deleterious effect on wound healing. Although the mechanism by which this occurs is likely multifactorial and has not been fully elucidated, many possible mechanisms may contribute. First, diabetic patients often have microvascular occlusive disease that limits tissue perfusion and oxygenation. Second, hyperglycemia causes the nonenzymatic glycosylation of proteins, thereby changing their function and solubility. Glycosylated enzymes may not function properly in wound healing: glycosylated collagen is less likely to be enzymatically degraded and thus collagen remodeling is not as efficient in the diabetic patient.[5] In turn, a nonhealing wound has a longer time period in which to be colonized by bacteria and to develop wound infection. These hypotheses have been corroborated by studies in animals and in humans that demonstrate slower rates of wound healing and higher rates of wound infection in the presence of hyperglycemia (i.e., a serum glucose level of >200 mg/dl).[1,5,11] Malone and colleagues[1] demonstrated in a regression analysis that diabetes mellitus is an independent risk factor for the development of postoperative wound infection. Although diabetes is not a modifiable risk factor, serum glucose concentration is. Preliminary studies have demonstrated a decrease in the incidence of postoperative wound infection in diabetic patients when tight serum glucose control was achieved with the use of an insulin drip.[11]

Nutritional Status

Given that alcohol and tobacco abuse are strong risk factors for the development of head and neck cancer and that nutritional deficiency is virtually omnipresent in patients who abuse alcohol, it is not surprising that a large percentage of patients who require head and neck surgery have significant nutritional deficiency at presentation. Specific nutritional deficiencies in patients with a history of alcohol abuse include adenosine triphosphate, amino acids, thiamin, magnesium, and potassium.[12] In addition to the nutritional deficiencies that result from alcoholism, many head and neck tumors directly involve the upper aerodigestive tract, which results in dysphagia and odynophagia. Finally, malignant tumors at any location may cause anorexia and cancer cachexia, which is a catabolic state in which protein and fat are burned indiscriminately. For all of these reasons, it is common for patients with head and neck cancer to present with a significant degree of weight loss at the time of their initial office evaluation.

Protein-calorie malnutrition has been clearly demonstrated to impair wound healing and immune function and to increase the likelihood of postoperative wound infection.[1] Aggressive nutritional support has been demonstrated to restore immunocompetence and to decrease the incidence of postoperative wound infection.[13,14] As little as 7 to 10 days of preoperative nutritional supplementation may decrease the incidence of postoperative complications by 10%. The greatest benefit from preoperative nutritional support is for patients who have had a weight loss of 10% or more from their ideal weight.[14]

Smoking

There are many mechanisms by which smoking impairs wound healing. Many of the substances released by cigarettes impair the delivery of oxygen to the tissues. Nicotine causes vasoconstriction, and a single cigarette may cause vasoconstriction for 90 minutes. Carbon monoxide competes with oxygen for binding to hemoglobin, and hydrogen cyanide inhibits the enzymes of oxidative metabolism.[5] Because adequate tissue oxygenation is critical for wound healing, it is not surprising that smoking impairs wound healing. Flap and full-thickness skin graft failure rates have been shown to be three times higher among one-pack-per-day and six times higher among two-pack-per-day smokers as compared with nonsmokers.[5,15] This delay in wound healing is clinically significant, and it translates into an increased rate of postoperative wound infection.

In a randomized, controlled study involving experimental wounds in human subjects, Sorensen and colleagues[16] demonstrated that smoking increases the risk of infection in small, clean wounds. Wound infection rates in this study were 12% in smokers and 2% in never smokers. Perhaps more important in terms of preoperative risk reduction is that the wound infection rate in smokers was significantly reduced when they abstained from smoking for 4 weeks before wounding occurred.[16] In another randomized, controlled study, Moller and colleagues[17] demonstrated that preoperative smoking cessation counseling and nicotine replacement therapy were able to reduce the wound-related complication rate from 23% in smoking control subjects to 4% in patients who underwent the intervention and subsequently quit or reduced their smoking by 50%.

Alcohol Abuse

Alcohol abuse is a common comorbidity of patients with head and neck cancer. Chronic alcohol abuse has been demonstrated to decrease immunity and to increase the risk of infection, including the development of postoperative wound infection.[18–20] Rantala and colleagues[21] measured 43 parameters among patients who were undergoing surgery in an attempt to correlate these factors with the development of postoperative wound infection. Of the 43 factors, only three were shown to have a statistically significant association with increased rates of wound infection: (1) contaminated or dirty surgical wounds ($P < 0.05$); (2) surgery duration of more than 2 hours ($P < 0.05$); and (3) a history of alcohol abuse ($P < 0.005$).[21] In a univariate analysis of patients undergoing surgery for head and neck cancer, Robbins and colleagues[18] demonstrated that the degree of alcohol consumption significantly correlated with the risk of postoperative wound infection, although this factor was not statistically significant in the multivariate analysis. Gallivan and Reiter[22] reviewed the outcomes of 17 consecutive patients who were treated with fibular free-flap reconstruction for mandibular defects and found that the flap survival rate of 25% among patients undergoing acute alcohol withdrawal was significantly lower than the survival rate of 85% among patients not undergoing acute alcohol withdrawal.

In a randomized, controlled trial, Tonnesen and colleagues[23] demonstrated a significant decrease in postoperative complications during the month after surgery among patients who underwent withdrawal from alcohol 1 month preoperatively as compared with patients who continued to drink during the preoperative period. Although postoperative infection was not a primary outcome measured in this study, hypoxemia and surgical stress response were significantly less in the intervention group, and immune function (measured as delayed type hypersensitivity) was significantly greater in the intervention group preoperatively, although no difference was demonstrated after surgery.[23] Unfortunately, sustaining alcohol abstinence for an entire month preoperatively may be difficult to achieve for some patients. Preventing postoperative withdrawal with intravenous ethanol and benzodiazepines may prevent symptoms of alcohol withdrawal, but as yet the potential benefit in terms of decreasing postoperative complications has not been determined. Patients with a history of chronic heavy alcohol abuse should be identified preoperatively, and their higher risk for postoperative complications should be taken into consideration when making the decision of whether to proceed with surgery.

Prior Radiation Therapy

Acute radiation therapy causes endothelial edema and lymphatic obstruction. Delayed tissue effects include interstitial fibrosis and capillary thrombosis and necrosis.[5,24] Experiments on wound healing in irradiated tissue show delays in fibroblast proliferation and collagen mRNA production. The time to achieve normal tensile strength in a wound may also be delayed by radiation therapy.[5,24] Ariyan and colleagues[25] studied the effect of wound inoculation with *Staphylococcus aureus* in rats after irradiation at one of three different doses and demonstrated a statistically significant increase in bacterial growth with an increased dose of preoperative radiation.

Despite the laboratory evidence implicating irradiation in faulty wound healing and at least one clinical study[26] demonstrating an increased risk of wound infection in irradiated patients, several other retrospective clinical studies have failed to demonstrate a correlation between preoperative irradiation and the development of postoperative wound infection.[5,24,27–29] The recent addition of chemotherapy to many treatment regimens can be expected to further inhibit wound healing and to increase the risk of infection, because chemotherapy suppresses the bone marrow production of the inflammatory cells that mediate the initial stages of wound healing.[5] With the current push toward concurrent chemotherapy and radiation therapy for organ preservation protocols, this issue may become more important, and further studies are warranted.

Technical Factors

Meticulous attention to surgical technique as well as attention to other intraoperative factors may also play important roles in attempts to decrease the rate of postoperative wound infection after surgery of the head and neck. The excessive maceration of tissues intraoperatively, excessive tension on the wound during wound closure, or inadequate suction drainage may all predispose patients to the development of wound infection.

PREVENTION OF WOUND INFECTION

The three main factors that contribute to wound infection—bacterial inoculum, host resistance to infection, and surgical technique—represent areas to target when attempting to reduce the incidence of wound infection. Early studies investigating the incidence of wound infection focused on determining the role of antibiotic prophylaxis. It is now universally accepted that 24 hours of appropriate antibiotic prophylaxis significantly decreases the rate of postoperative wound infection in clean-contaminated and contaminated surgery of the head and neck. More recent studies have focused on the management of host factors and adjustments to operative technique that also may help to reduce the incidence of wound infection. Each of the three main factors that affect the risk of wound infection may be viewed as an area for possible intervention.

Antibiotic Prophylaxis

A series of randomized controlled trials[30–32] has clearly established that antibiotic prophylaxis can significantly decrease the rate of postoperative wound infection in class II and class III surgeries of the head and neck. The role of antibiotic prophylaxis is to reduce the bacterial contamination of the wound at the time of surgery. The division of surgical procedures into clean, clean-contaminated, contaminated, and dirty wounds reflects this: the higher the degree of bacterial contamination of a wound at the time of surgery, the higher the risk of postoperative wound infection without antibiotics and, thus, the stronger the need for preoperative antibiotic prophylaxis. This risk stratification is not only a theory: clean surgical procedures of the head and neck carry a risk of less than 5% for postoperative wound infection without antibiotic prophylaxis, whereas clean-contaminated procedures carry a risk of 78% to 87% without prophylaxis. With antibiotic prophylaxis, the wound infection rate for contaminated surgery is in the range of 10%.[30,31,33,34] Velanovich,[35] in a meta-analysis of studies examining the effects of antibiotic prophylaxis in head and neck surgery, found that there was a 43.7% reduction in the incidence of postoperative wound infection when patients who received antibiotic prophylaxis were compared with patients who received placebo.

Timing and Duration of Antibiotic Prophylaxis

Preoperative antibiotic prophylaxis reduces the incidence of postoperative wound infection by decreasing the bacterial inoculum contaminating the wound at the time of surgery. Antibiotic prophylaxis is most effective when it is administered within 2 hours before the surgical incision.[36] After surgery, there should be no further contamination of the wound, and further antibiotic prophylaxis should not be necessary.[29,37] Randomized, controlled trials comparing the duration of antibiotic prophylaxis support this hypothesis.[29,38–41] Multiple studies have been performed, and prophylaxis durations of 1 day, 3 days, 5 days, and 7 days have all been studied. Overwhelmingly, the evidence is that prolonging antibiotic prophylaxis past 24 hours does not change the rate of wound infection. Infections that occur despite adequate prophylaxis are related to bacterial virulence, host factors, and operative technique.

Complications of Antibiotic Prophylaxis

In addition to adding to the cost of hospitalization, unnecessarily prolonging antibiotic prophylaxis also increases the risk of colonization and possible infection by resistant or more virulent organisms. An excellent example of this is *Clostridium difficile* colitis. In addition to increasing hospital stay duration and cost, *C. difficile* colitis has a high associated morbidity rate.[42,43] Although *C. difficile* colitis is most common after prolonged antibiotic administration, it is important to be aware that it may occur even after a short prophylactic dose of antibiotics; therefore, a high index of suspicion is necessary.[44] In addition, the irresponsible use of antibiotics in the population at large leads to the development of resistant bacterial strains. Therefore, prophylaxis should be limited to a 24-hour perioperative course of antibiotics.

Choice of Antimicrobial Agent

Bacteriology studies of postoperative wound infections after head and neck surgery have demonstrated that these infections are polymicrobial and that causative organisms are usually part of the patient's oropharyngeal flora. Gram-positive aerobic, gram-negative aerobic, and anaerobic bacteria as well as fungal species have all been cultured from postoperative wounds.[8,31,45,46] Randomized, controlled trials aimed at selecting the most appropriate antimicrobial agent have demonstrated a small but significant benefit from adding anaerobic coverage to gram-positive aerobic coverage.[47,48] This is not surprising given the high percentage of anaerobic bacteria in normal oropharyngeal flora. No further benefit was obtained by providing coverage for gram-negative aerobic bacteria.[34,46] In addition, the coverage of fungi does not appear to be necessary for antimicrobial prophylaxis. When fungi and gram-negative bacteria are recovered from wound infections they most likely represent contaminants of the wound culture.

Host Resistance

Several components of a patient's functional status that can contribute to his or her risk of developing postoperative wound infection have been discussed. Host resistance may be increased to some extent by abstinence from alcohol and tobacco, preoperative nutritional support, and the maintenance of tight control over blood glucose level.

Intraoperative Factors

Surgical Technique

Antibiotic prophylaxis will not prevent infection in a wound in which there is technical failure. In a retrospective review of 245 patients undergoing head and neck surgery, Brown and colleagues[49] attributed 59% of postoperative wound infections to a "probable flaw in surgical technique or judgment" such as tissue trauma or wound closure under tension.

Skin flaps must be designed to maintain perfusion to as much of the flap as possible. Intraoperatively, skin flaps must be kept moist. Tissues should be handled gently, and crushing or compressing tissue should be avoided. Closure should be free of tension to avoid compromising oxygen delivery to the skin flap. Exacting attention must be paid to the achievement of hemostasis before wound closure. Hematoma and seroma formation prevent skin-flap healing by forming a barrier between the skin flap and the soft tissue. Hematoma also predisposes the patient to wound infection by providing a culture medium for bacterial growth. The irrigation of the wound to remove foreign debris and the placement of suction drains to prevent seroma formation are also critical steps.

Oxygen Supplementation

It is surgical dictum that a wound must be well perfused to heal without complications. Although poor perfusion may have effects beyond those attributable to poor oxygenation, Jonsson and colleagues[50] have demonstrated in an animal model that the partial pressure of oxygen in tissue correlates with the risk of wound infection independent of tissue perfusion. These results were obtained by varying the concentration of inspired oxygen (FiO_2) while maintaining constant perfusion.[50]

In a follow-up study in humans, Hopf and colleagues[51] demonstrated that the partial pressure of oxygen in a patient's subcutaneous tissues (measured in an experimental wound in the upper extremity at a site distant to the surgical site) inversely correlates with the risk of postoperative wound infection. In fact, low subcutaneous oxygen tension was shown to correlate with an increased risk of wound infection to a more effective degree than the SENIC score.[51]

A recent double-blind, randomized study in patients undergoing colorectal surgery and receiving either 30% or 80% FiO_2 intraoperatively and for 6 hours postoperatively demonstrated an infection rate of 24.4% among patients receiving 30% FiO_2 and of 14.9% among patients receiving 80% FiO_2. Multivariate analysis of the data revealed a 54% reduction in the risk of postoperative infection in patients receiving 80% FiO_2 as compared with those receiving 30% FiO_2.[52] These results are similar to those of Grief and colleagues,[53] who demonstrated a 50% reduction in wound infection with a similar protocol.

One hypothesis for the mechanism by which hypoxia increases the risk of wound infection is that hypoxia limits the ability of neutrophils to initiate the "oxidative burst" whereby superoxide is generated. Superoxide, in turn, is largely responsible for the bacterial killing that is caused by neutrophils.[54] Hypoxia may also impair wound healing independent of the increased risk for wound infection, because the hydroxylation of proline and lysine residues is crucial for collagen cross-linking, and the hydroxylase enzyme is dependent on tissue oxygen tension.[55]

Normothermia

In a randomized, controlled trial, Kurz and colleagues[55] demonstrated that patients who underwent active intraoperative warming (mean temperature, 36.6 ± 0.5°C) had a significantly decreased risk of postoperative wound infection as compared with patients who received routine intraoperative care (mean temperature, 34.7 ± 0.5°C). Hypothermia causes vasoconstriction and decreased tissue oxygen tension, thereby increasing the patient's risk of wound infection.

Postoperative Pain Control

Pain causes an adrenergic response that may lead to vasoconstriction and subsequent tissue hypoxia. Akca and colleagues[56] demonstrated lower tissue oxygen tension among patients who were receiving placebo for pain after knee surgery than among patients receiving an intra-articular lidocaine injection. To every extent possible, patients should be maintained in a postoperative state that is comfortable and free of pain.

DIAGNOSIS OF WOUND INFECTION

Early recognition of developing wound infection and prompt institution of therapy are crucial to limiting patient and wound morbidity. Early treatment limits the exposure of tissue to salivary enzymes and bacterial toxins, both of which contribute to flap autolysis and which, if unchecked, may result in the exposure of critical structures.[57] However, it may be difficult to distinguish between postoperative wound infection and the normal inflammatory phase of wound healing. Many of the classic signs of inflammation (e.g., erythema, edema, induration) are normal sequelae of head and neck surgical procedures.[57] In addition, low-grade fever and leukocytosis (i.e., >12,500 white blood cells/mm³) are common during the immediate postoperative period, most commonly as a result of atelectasis, which limits the predictive value of these signs for the diagnosis of wound infection.

Johnson and colleagues[58] have developed a wound grading scale to aid in the accurate differentiation of infection from normal healing (Table 4-3). Wounds with erythema and induration that do not progress to draining purulent material are not felt to represent true wound infection, and the administration of therapeutic antibiotics for such a wound opens the patient to the risks of antibiotic administration that, in this situation, are felt to exceed the benefits.

TABLE 4-3 Grading System for Wound Infection

Grade 0	Normal healing
Grade 1	Erythema around suture line of <1 cm
Grade 2	1 cm–5 cm erythema
Grade 3	>5 cm erythema and induration
Grade 4	Purulent drainage either spontaneously or by incision and drainage
Grade 5	Orocutaneous fistula

TREATMENT OF WOUND INFECTION

As previously discussed, wound erythema, edema, leukocytosis, and low-grade fever are all common findings during the early postoperative period and should not be mistaken for wound infection. The presence of pus in the wound bed is the definitive sign of wound infection. When wound infection is diagnosed, treatment with appropriate antimicrobial therapy is indicated. Wound infection often implies wound breakdown and the continued soiling of the wound with oropharyngeal bacteria; therefore, antibiotics targeting the oropharyngeal flora with coverage for gram-positive aerobic bacteria and anaerobes are necessary. Unfortunately, cultures taken from closed suction drains are not useful for determining the causative organism of the wound infection. In fact, Becker[59] demonstrated that aerobic bacteria can be grown from all closed suction drain outputs and that 75% of these closed suction drain cultures grow pathogenic bacteria, even for patients without wound infection.

The maintenance of suction drainage is crucial to allow for the evacuation of purulent material and the healing of skin flaps down to the underlying soft tissue. For cases in which wound breakdown results in a salivary fistula, drains may continue to drain saliva, and they may even hold the fistulous tract open. In such cases, drains may be backed out slowly to allow the fistula to heal while maintaining drainage from the neck. For cases in which a drain is not properly positioned, has been removed prematurely, or was never placed, the operative drainage of the wound may be necessary.

QUALITY OF LIFE

Wound infection is correlated with delayed healing and longer hospital stays. An infected wound will often heal with a less cosmetically appealing scar, and it may require scar revision. Infection requiring prolonged treatment with antibiotics places the patient at increased risk of developing *C. difficile* colitis, with all its attendant risks and morbidities. When severe, wound infection and salivary fistula may require reoperation and tissue-flap reconstruction. Not only does this prolong the hospital stay, but it can also be demoralizing to the patient who was expecting a shorter hospital stay. Wound infection and breakdown in the lateral neck increases the risk of saliva draining onto the contents of the carotid sheath, with the subsequent risk of carotid artery blowout. Again, tissue-flap reconstruction may be necessary to avoid this problem. Wound infection delays healing, prolongs the hospital course, and often forces the postponement of oral feeding and the use of a voice prosthesis among patients who have undergone laryngectomy.

ECONOMIC IMPLICATIONS

Wound infection prolongs (often almost doubling) the duration of hospitalization; thus it also significantly increases perioperative costs. A 1992 study by Blair and colleagues[60] determined that the excess cost per patient from a wound infection was more than $36,000 (in 1992 dollars). A 24-hour period of prophylactic antibiotic therapy is inexpensive by comparison.

CONCLUSION

It is well established that up to 24 hours of antibiotic prophylaxis can decrease the risk of postoperative wound infection among patients undergoing clean-contaminated surgery of the head and neck. The majority of wound infections are caused by oropharyngeal flora; therefore, the antimicrobial spectrum should cover gram-positive aerobic bacteria and anaerobes. Extending the spectrum of coverage to include gram-negative bacteria and fungi is not necessary. It is important to discontinue prophylaxis after 24 hours, because no further benefit has been demonstrated from a prolonged course of antibiotics. However, the risk of antibiotic-related complications, including *C. difficile* colitis, increases with the duration of antibiotic treatment. Certain patient characteristics (e.g., diabetes mellitus, a history of alcohol abuse, smoking, poor nutritional status, prior radiation therapy) may increase a patient's risk of developing wound infection. Wound infections that occur despite appropriate antibiotic prophylaxis may be caused by errors in surgical technique. New research suggests that perioperative factors (e.g., the administration of supplemental oxygen, the maintenance of normothermia, the provision of adequate analgesia) may also decrease the risk of wound infection.

REFERENCES

1. Malone DL, Genuit T, Tracy JK, et al: Surgical site infections: Reanalysis of risk factors. *J Surg Res* 2002;103:89–95.
2. Hong J, Davis JM: Nosocomial infections and nosocomial pneumonia. *Am J Surg* 1996;172:33S–37S.
3. Mangram AJ, Horan TC, Pearson ML, et al: Guideline for Prevention of Surgical Site Infection, 1999. Centers for Disease Control and Prevention (CDC) Hospital Infection Control Practices Advisory Committee. *Am J Infect Control* 1999;27:97–134, 196.
4. Robson MC, Stenberg BD, Heggers JP: Wound healing alterations caused by infection. *Clin Plast Surg* 1990;17:485–492.
5. Broughton G 2nd, Janis JE, Attinger CE: Wound healing: An overview. *Plast Reconstr Surg* 2006;117:1e-S–32e-S.
6. Robson MC, Mannari RJ, Smith PD, et al: Maintenance of wound bacterial balance. *Am J Surg* 1999;178:399–402.
7. Bartlett JG, Gorbach SL: Anaerobic infections of the head and neck. *Otolaryngol Clin North Am* 1976;9:655–678.
8. Rubin J, Johnson JT, Wagner RL, et al: Bacteriologic analysis of wound infection following major head and neck surgery. *Arch Otolaryngol Head Neck Surg* 1988;114:969–972.
9. Haley RW, Culver DH, Morgan WM, et al: Identifying patients at high risk of surgical wound infection: A simple multivariate index of patient susceptibility and wound contamination. *Am J Epidemiol* 1985;121:206–215.
10. Garner J, Hughes J, Davis B: CDC Guideline for Prevention of Surgical Wound Infections, 1985. *Infect Control Hosp Epidemiol* 1986;7:193–200.
11. Zerr KJ, Furnary AP, Grunkemeier GL, et al: Glucose control lowers the risk of wound infection in diabetics after open heart operations. *Ann Thorac Surg* 1997;63:356–361.
12. Bertrand PC, Piquet MA, Bordier I, et al: Preoperative nutritional support at home in head and neck cancer patients: From nutritional benefits to the prevention of the alcohol withdrawal syndrome. *Curr Opin Clin Nutr Metab Care* 2002;5:435–440.
13. Johns ME: The nutrition problem in head and neck cancer. *Otolaryngol Head Neck Surg* 1980;88:691–694.
14. Copeland EM 3rd, Daly JM, Dudrick SJ: Nutritional concepts in the treatment of head and neck malignancies. *Head Neck Surg* 1979;1:350–365.
15. Goldminz D, Bennett RG: Cigarette smoking and flap and full-thickness graft necrosis. *Arch Dermatol* 1991;127:1012–1015.
16. Sorensen LT, Karlsmark T, Gottrup F: Abstinence from smoking reduces incisional wound infection: A randomized controlled trial. *Ann Surg* 2003;238:1–5.
17. Moller AM, Villebro N, Pedersen T, et al: Effect of preoperative smoking intervention on postoperative complications: A randomised clinical trial. *Lancet* 2002;359:114–117.
18. Robbins KT, Favrot S, Hanna D, et al: Risk of wound infection in patients with head and neck cancer. *Head Neck* 1990;12:143–148.
19. Tonnesen H, Kehlet H: Preoperative alcoholism and postoperative morbidity. *Br J Surg* 1999;86:869–874.
20. Tonnesen H: The alcohol patient and surgery. *Alcohol Alcohol* 1999;34:148–152.
21. Rantala A, Lehtonen OP, Niinikoski J: Alcohol abuse: A risk factor for surgical wound infections? *Am J Infect Control* 1997;25:381–386.
22. Gallivan KH, Reiter D: Acute alcohol withdrawal and free flap mandibular reconstruction outcomes. *Arch Facial Plast Surg* 2001;3:264–266.
23. Tonnesen H, Rosenberg J, Nielsen HJ, et al: Effect of preoperative abstinence on poor postoperative outcome in alcohol misusers: Randomised controlled trial. *BMJ* 1999;318:1311–1316.
24. Johnson JT, Bloomer WD: Effect of prior radiotherapy on postsurgical wound infection. *Head Neck* 1989;11:132–136.
25. Ariyan S, Kraft RL, Goldberg NH: An experimental model to determine the effects of adjuvant therapy on the incidence of postoperative wound infection: II. Evaluating preoperative chemotherapy. *Plast Reconstr Surg* 1980;65:338–345.
26. Girod DA, McCulloch TM, Tsue TT, et al: Risk factors for complications in clean contaminated head and neck surgical procedures. *Head Neck* 1995;17:7–13.
27. Soylu L, Kiroglu M, Aydogan B, et al: Pharyngocutaneous fistula following laryngectomy. *Head Neck* 1998;20:22–25.
28. Bengtson BP, Schusterman MA, Baldwin BJ, et al: Influence of prior radiotherapy on the development of postoperative complications and success of free tissue transfers in head and neck cancer reconstruction. *Am J Surg* 1993;166:326–330.
29. Johnson JT, Schuller DE, Silver F, et al: Antibiotic prophylaxis in high-risk head and neck surgery: One-day vs. five-day therapy. *Otolaryngol Head Neck Surg* 1986;95:554–557.
30. Becker GD, Parell GJ: Cefazolin prophylaxis in head and neck cancer surgery. *Ann Otol Rhinol Laryngol* 1979;88:183–186.
31. Johnson JT, Yu VL, Myers EN, et al: Efficacy of two third-generation cephalosporins in prophylaxis for head and neck surgery. *Arch Otolaryngol* 1984;110:224–227.
32. Johnson JT, Wagner RL: Infection following uncontaminated head and neck surgery. *Arch Otolaryngol Head Neck Surg* 1987;113:368–369.
33. Bumpous JM, Johnson JT: The infected wound and its management. *Otolaryngol Clin North Am* 1995;28:987–1001.

34. Johnson JT, Yu VL, Myers EN, et al: An assessment of the need for gram negative bacterial coverage in antibiotic prophylaxis for oncological head and neck surgery. *J Infect Dis* 1987;155: 331–333.

35. Velanovich V: A meta-analysis of prophylactic antibiotics in head and neck surgery. *Plast Reconstr Surg* 1991;87:429–435.

36. Classen DC, Evans RS, Pestotnik SL, et al: The timing of prophylactic administration of antibiotics and the risk of surgical-wound infection. *N Engl J Med* 1992;326:281–286.

37. Burke JF: Preventing bacterial infection by coordinating antibiotic and host activity: A time-dependent relationship. *South Med J* 1977;70 Suppl 1:24–26.

38. Wittmann DH, Schein M: Let us shorten antibiotic prophylaxis and therapy in surgery. *Am J Surg* 1996;172:26S–32S.

39. Righi M, Manfredi R, Farneti G, et al: Short-term versus long-term antimicrobial prophylaxis in oncologic head and neck surgery. *Head Neck* 1996;18:399–404.

40. Fee WE Jr, Glenn M, Handen C, et al: One day vs. two days of prophylactic antibiotics in patients undergoing major head and neck surgery. *Laryngoscope* 1984;94:612–614.

41. Mustafa E, Tahsin A: Cefotaxime prophylaxis in major non-contaminated head and neck surgery: One-day vs. seven-day therapy. *J Laryngol Otol* 1993;107:30–32.

42. Dallal RM, Harbrecht BG, Boujoukas AJ, et al: Fulminant *Clostridium difficile:* An underappreciated and increasing cause of death and complications. *Ann Surg* 2002;235:363–372.

43. Griebie M, Adams GL: *Clostridium difficile* colitis following head and neck surgery: Report of cases. *Arch Otolaryngol* 1985;111:550–553.

44. Yee J, Dixon CM, McLean AP, et al: *Clostridium difficile* disease in a department of surgery: The significance of prophylactic antibiotics. *Arch Surg* 1991;126:241–246.

45. Weber RS, Raad I, Frankenthaler R, et al: Ampicillin-sulbactam vs clindamycin in head and neck oncologic surgery: The need for gram-negative coverage. *Arch Otolaryngol Head Neck Surg* 1992;118:1159–1163.

46. Johnson JT, Yu VL: Role of aerobic gram-negative rods, anaerobes, and fungi in wound infection after head and neck surgery: Implications for antibiotic prophylaxis. *Head Neck* 1989;11:27–29.

47. Johnson JT, Kachman K, Wagner RL, et al: Comparison of ampicillin/sulbactam versus clindamycin in the prevention of infection in patients undergoing head and neck surgery. *Head Neck* 1997;19:367–371.

48. Robbins KT, Byers RM, Cole R, et al: Wound prophylaxis with metronidazole in head and neck surgical oncology. *Laryngoscope* 1988;98:803–806.

49. Brown BM, Johnson JT, Wagner RL: Etiologic factors in head and neck wound infections. *Laryngoscope* 1987;97:587–590.

50. Jonsson K, Hunt TK, Mathes SJ: Oxygen as an isolated variable influences resistance to infection. *Ann Surg* 1988;208:783–787.

51. Hopf HW, Hunt TK, West JM, et al: Wound tissue oxygen tension predicts the risk of wound infection in surgical patients. *Arch Surg* 1997;132:997–1005.

52. Belda FJ, Aguilera L, Garcia de la Asuncion J, et al: Supplemental perioperative oxygen and the risk of surgical wound infection: A randomized controlled trial. *JAMA* 2005;294:2035–2042.

53. Greif R, Akca O, Horn EP, et al: Supplemental perioperative oxygen to reduce the incidence of surgical-wound infection: Outcomes Research Group. *N Engl J Med* 2000;342:161–167.

54. Allen DB, Maguire JJ, Mahdavian M, et al: Wound hypoxia and acidosis limit neutrophil bacterial killing mechanisms. *Arch Surg* 1997;132:991–996.

55. Kurz A, Sessler DI, Lenhardt R: Perioperative normothermia to reduce the incidence of surgical-wound infection and shorten hospitalization: Study of Wound Infection and Temperature Group. *N Engl J Med* 1996;334:1209–1215.

56. Akca O, Melischek M, Scheck T, et al: Postoperative pain and subcutaneous oxygen tension. *Lancet* 1999;354:41–42.

57. Johnson JT, Weber RS: Management of postoperative head and neck wound infections. In Johnson JT, Yu VL, editors: *Infectious diseases and antimicrobial therapy of the ears, nose, and throat.* Philadelphia, 1996, WB Saunders.

58. Johnson JT, Myers EN, Thearle PB, et al: Antimicrobial prophylaxis for contaminated head and neck surgery. *Laryngoscope* 1984;94:46–51.

59. Becker GD: Ineffectiveness of closed suction drainage cultures in the prediction of bacteriologic findings in wound infections in patients undergoing contaminated head and neck cancer surgery. *Otolaryngol Head Neck Surg* 1985;93:743–747.

60. Blair EA, Johnson JT, Wagner RL, et al: Cost analysis of antibiotic prophylaxis in clean head and neck surgery. *Arch Otolaryngol Head Neck Surg* 1995;121:269–271.

CHAPTER 5

Medical Complications of Head and Neck Surgery

Joshua S. Adler and Andrew D. Auerbach

Patients undergoing major head and neck surgery, particularly those with cancer, pose a number of surgical and medical challenges. This chapter will focus on medical issues and complications that are common and preventable or that are highly problematic and therefore worthy of discussion. For each one, the scope of the problem will be addressed, the risk factors defined, and preventive strategies suggested. When no preventive therapies are available, a strategy for reducing the morbidity and mortality of the complication through early diagnosis and management will be outlined.

CARDIAC COMPLICATIONS OF HEAD AND NECK SURGERY

Scope of the Problem

Postoperative myocardial infarction, unstable angina, congestive heart failure, and ventricular arrhythmias occur in 2% to 5% of head and neck surgery patients. These conditions are associated with a 20% mortality rate and also lead to a cascade of additional complications that make them particularly important targets for preventive efforts.[1]

Risk Factors for Cardiac Complications

A number of methods to estimate risk for cardiac complications are available. Consensus-derived algorithms, such as those suggested by the American Heart Association and the American College of Cardiology,[2] approximate clinical decision making and incorporate specific recommendations. However, differences among algorithms may lead to conflicting advice, and the algorithms are complex and unwieldy.[3] Risk indexes such as the Revised Cardiac Risk Index (RCRI)[4] are derived using rigorous statistical methods and then tested on thousands of patients, but they do not automatically provide guidance regarding how to act on risk estimates themselves. Nevertheless, risk indexes are simpler to recall, and they can be used to frame an evidence-based approach to reducing risk. The RCRI appears to be superior to most other indexes[4] in terms of its test characteristics, and it is simpler to calculate (Figure 5-1). Although the RCRI criteria related to vascular surgery do not apply to head and neck surgical patients, other criteria (e.g., history of transient ischemic attack/cerebrovascular accident, insulin-dependent diabetes, coronary disease, heart failure, or renal failure) are risk factors commonly seen in the head and neck surgical population. With no RCRI risk factors, the estimated risk for perioperative cardiac complications is less than 0.5%; this risk rises to 1% with one RCRI criterion and to 4% with two criteria, and it exceeds 8% in the presence of three RCRI criteria.

Strategies to Reduce Cardiac Risk

Strategies to reduce perioperative cardiac risk as a result of coronary disease have relied on prophylactic revascularization (e.g., percutaneous transluminal angioplasty with or without stenting, coronary bypass surgery) and more recently on pharmacologic prevention with β-blockers and, potentially, statins.

Although interest in and hope for revascularization was high 5 to 10 years ago, the weight of the evidence since that time has suggested that "prophylactic" revascularization provides no benefit to patients before major surgery. A large, randomized trial of preoperative revascularization among veterans undergoing vascular surgery suggested no benefit of preoperative percutaneous transluminal coronary angioplasty or coronary artery bypass grafting. Moreover, patients who underwent revascularization had longer delays before their subsequent noncardiac surgery.[5] Revascularization with drug-eluting stents, which is a common revascularization modality, poses different problems, because drug-eluting stents require patients to remain on dual antiplatelet therapy for at least 6 months after stent placement. As a result, patients who require surgical procedures and who need to discontinue antiplatelet agents are exposed to substantial risk for the catastrophic consequences of acute stent closure. Revascularization and noninvasive stress testing should be pursued only among patients with new or unstable symptoms, among those with very high risk (three or more RCRI criteria; see Table 5-1), and among those with a history of anginal symptoms or claudication who are unable to walk.[1] This subset of patients would probably benefit from a thorough preoperative evaluation by a cardiologist, an internist, or a hospitalist before proceeding with head and neck surgery.

The evidence supporting the efficacy of the perioperative use of β-blockers for reducing perioperative cardiac complications has evolved rapidly during the last 2 years. After three strongly positive randomized trials

TABLE 5-1   Identifying Patients Who Are at Risk for Complications, Suggested Preventive Therapies, and Methods for Diagnosis and Management: A Summary

Problem	Methods to Identify At-Risk Patients	Preventive Therapies	Detection and Management
Cardiac complications	■ RCRI (see Figure 5-1) is the recommended initial screening tool. ■ AHA/ACC algorithms are also useful but more complex.	■ Use perioperative β-blockers for patients with two or more RCRI criteria, who have a history of coronary disease, or who are already taking β-blockers. ■ Prophylactic revascularization is not indicated unless the patient has new or unstable symptoms. ■ Ensure that statins are continued through surgery and that antiplatelet agents (e.g., aspirin) are restarted as soon as possible afterward.	■ In high-risk patients (those with two or more RCRI criteria), consider postoperative telemetry and troponin screening on the first postoperative day. ■ Elevations of troponin and new EKG abnormalities are indications for an urgent cardiology consultation. ■ Pulmonary edema during the first 72 hours should first be considered as a manifestation of coronary disease.
Pulmonary complications	■ Structured risk indexes exist but may be too complex for everyday use. In general, patients with poor functional status, baseline neurologic impairment, and poor functional status as a result of pulmonary disease are at the highest risk.	■ Early mobilization, positioning, and the hourly use of incentive spirometry can reduce risk. ■ Patients with exacerbations of pulmonary disease should be treated and stabilized before surgery. ■ Smoking cessation should be encouraged in all cases, but only abstinence from tobacco for more than 6 weeks reduces operative risk.	■ Monitoring patients in a step-down setting or an ICU may be indicated for patients at high risk. ■ Nebulizers and noninvasive ventilation (e.g., BiPAP) may be used in appropriate cases to improve ventilation. ■ Elevation of head of the bed to 30 degrees or more may decrease the risk for pneumonia among intubated patients.
Thromboembolism	■ Patients with cancer, those of advanced age, and those who are immobilized for more than 24 hours are at elevated risk.	■ Pneumatic compression devices and early ambulation should be the mainstays of therapy for all patients. ■ Patients with the highest risk should receive prophylactic doses of enoxaparin or unfractionated heparin.	■ The diagnosis of deep vein thrombosis and pulmonary embolism should be the same as for nonoperative patients. ■ Quantitative D-dimer testing has no role in postoperative patients. ■ Full-dose anticoagulation is required as soon as possible if thrombosis is diagnosed, and it should be continued for at least 6 months.
Bleeding disorders	■ Use the structured bleeding risk history (see Box 5-1) to identify patients who are at risk.	■ Routine screening with PT/PTT/INR and bleeding times is of no clinical value. ■ Early consultation with a hematologist is critical for patients with an abnormal bleeding history or abnormal tests.	■ Early consultation with a hematologist is critical.

Postoperative delirium	■ Risk indexes (see Figure 5-2) are useful ways to identify patients who are at highest risk.	■ Encourage family members to remain at the bedside after surgery. ■ Plans for the adequate treatment of pain and the avoidance of anticholinergics (e.g., Benadryl) may reduce risk. ■ Mainstays of delirium treatment include the removal of urinary catheters; addressing metabolic, pulmonary, and infectious problems; and discontinuing offending medications.
Alcohol withdrawal	■ The CAGE questionnaire and the directed drinking history are likely useful screening tools for all head and neck surgery patients.	■ If the patient has been abstinent for more than a week before surgery, no preventative measures are required. ■ If the patient continues drinking up to the time of surgery, starting symptom-triggered benzodiazepine therapy at the time of hospital admission is prudent. ■ The administration of multivitamins, folate, and thiamine may be of benefit. ■ Monitoring patients for signs of withdrawal (e.g., tremulousness, anxiety, tachycardia) should be a mainstay of treatment. ■ Structured symptom assessment tools (e.g., CIWA) may help diagnose patients as well as provide the basis for symptom-triggered treatment with lorazepam or diazepam.
Diabetes and hyperglycemia	■ All patients with known diabetes as well as those with fasting hyperglycemia (i.e., a blood sugar level of >150 mg/dl) anytime before or after surgery should be targeted for tight glucose control.	■ The overall goal is to maintain patients' blood glucose levels in the near-normal range (80–110 mg/dl); blood sugar levels in excess of 200 mg/dl should be avoided. ■ Preoperative management will depend on the type of agents used and the duration of NPO status before surgery. ■ Immediate postoperative care should involve restarting the outpatient regimen at the earliest possible opportunity. ■ Regular insulin sliding scale monotherapy is ineffective and should never be used. ■ Insulin infusion may be indicated for patients receiving TPN or tube feedings; other patients should be treated with a sliding scale that includes long- or intermediate-acting insulin in conjunction with short-acting insulin around mealtimes.

ACC, American College of Cardiology; AHA, American Heart Association; BiPAP, bi-level positive airway pressure; CIWA, Clinical Institute Withdrawal Assessment for Alcohol; EKG, electrocardiogram; ICU, intensive care unit; INR, international normalized ratio; NPO, nothing by mouth; PT, prothrombin time; PTT, partial thromboplastin time; RCRI, Revised Cardiac Risk Index; TPN, total parenteral nutrition.

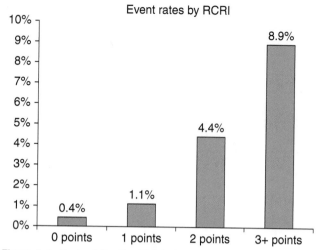

Figure 5-1. Revised Cardiac Risk Index
1. Type of surgery (1 point)
   Abdominal aortic aneurysm repair
2. History of coronary artery disease (1 point)
   History of angina, Q-waves on electrocardiogram, history of coronary bypass surgery or percutaneous coronary artery intervention, abnormal stress test, use of nitrates
3. History of congestive heart failure (CHF) (1 point)
   History of ejection fraction of less than 30%, cardiogenic pulmonary edema, paroxysmal nocturnal dyspnea, rales or clinical findings consistent with CHF on examination, chest x-ray examination consistent with CHF
4. History of cerebrovascular accident and/or transient ischemic attack (1 point)
5. History of a creatinine level of more than 2.0 mg/dl (1 point)
6. History of insulin-dependent diabetes (1 point)

were published during the mid 1990s, a subsequent series of larger randomized trials failed to demonstrate any benefit of β-blockers for reducing cardiac risks. In fact, one observational trial suggested a trend toward a higher risk of mortality when β-blockers were administered to low-risk patients.[6] As results from two large, randomized trials are collected, recent guidelines from the American Heart Association and other recommendations suggest that perioperative β-blockers should be used only for patients with documented coronary disease, and for patients who are already receiving β-blockers. Among these patients, β-blockers should be administered before surgery (optimally 3 weeks or more beforehand), titrated to a therapeutic heart rate (55–70 beats per minute) throughout hospitalization, and continued indefinitely after surgery.[1] Again, this management strategy may be facilitated through collaboration and consultation with medical specialists.

Finally, a recent body of evidence suggests that patients on statin lipid-lowering medications may have substantially lower risk for perioperative cardiac events.[6] Although these studies are preliminary, they are consistent with current knowledge of statins' effects in other settings (e.g., unstable angina). Until randomized trial data is available, it seems prudent

for surgical teams to ensure that these drugs are continued throughout the entirety of the perioperative period and after discharge.

Diagnosis and Management of Cardiac Complications

As many as 50% of clinically important postoperative cardiac events may have been detected earlier, so the diagnosis and appropriate management of cardiac complications relies on anticipating events and ensuring that patients are managed in the appropriate clinical setting. For low-risk patients (no RCRI criteria), no postoperative testing with electrocardiograms (EKGs) or troponins are required. However, patients with one RCRI criterion may benefit from screening with a 12-lead EKG the morning after surgery. Patients with two or more RCRI risk factors would likely benefit from continuous telemetry monitoring for at least 24 hours after surgery, along with a 12-lead EKG and troponin screening 6 to 10 hours after the end of surgery.

Regardless of estimated risk or monitoring strategy, elevations in troponin or new EKG abnormalities are a basis for urgent cardiology consultation, and they may prompt the initiation of antiplatelet and antithrombotic therapy (e.g., enoxaparin) if EKG and clinical factors are consistent with ST-elevation coronary events. It is important to note that any episode of postoperative congestive heart failure or pulmonary edema should be presumed to be the result of acute coronary syndromes and treated accordingly.

Risk Factors for Pulmonary Complications

A large number of studies have evaluated the risk factors for postoperative pulmonary complications (PPCs) after a variety of surgical procedures.[7,8] A small number of studies have evaluated these risks specifically among patients who are undergoing head and neck surgery.[9–11] The findings have been similar. The patient-specific factors that increase the risk of PPCs include advanced age, preexisting lung disease (especially chronic obstructive pulmonary disease [COPD]), current smoking, altered mental status, dependent functional status, American Society of Anesthesiologists class II or greater, congestive heart failure, and hypoalbuminemia. The presence of COPD is associated with an increased risk of pneumonia and respiratory failure. There is a rough correlation between the severity of the COPD and the magnitude of risk. Asthma does seem to increase the risk of perioperative bronchospasm but not of more serious pulmonary complications. Current smoking, which is common among patients who are undergoing head and neck procedures, also appears to double the risk of pneumonia. The presence of findings of congestive heart failure at the time of surgery increases the risk of PPCs nearly threefold. Morbid obesity does not appear to impart any additional risk. Patients who are totally dependent for all activities of daily living have a 2.5-fold increased risk of major pulmonary complications. Patients who are acutely confused or delirious are at increased risk for PPCs. However, the presence of chronic stable mental illness or dementia has not been found to be an independent predictor of PPCs. An American Society of Anesthesiologists class of II or greater is associated with a four- to fivefold increased risk of PPCs as compared with class I. In four studies of patients undergoing a variety of general surgical procedures, preoperative hypoalbuminemia (i.e., an albumin level of <35 g/L) is powerfully associated with pulmonary complications.

The type of procedure also appears to affect risk. Patients who undergo a major procedure for cancer that requires a tracheostomy may have a risk for postoperative pneumonia of as high as 40%. Laryngectomy, the commando procedure, and radical neck dissection seem to carry a higher risk than parotidectomy or glossectomy.[10]

Methods to Anticipate Risk Preoperatively

The primary means of assessing risk is the history and physical examination. The majority of the risk factors outlined previously in this chapter can be readily assessed during the taking of the history. A 12-lead EKG should be obtained for older patients, and those patients who have any suggestion of malnutrition should have their albumin level measured. The precise role of preoperative pulmonary function tests (PFTs) remains uncertain; however, most evidence points to selective rather than routine use. Among patients with known COPD, there is no correlation between specific PFT values and the risk of PPCs, with the exception that patients with a forced expiratory volume in 1 second of less than 500 ml or of less than 50% of the predicted value do appear to be at particularly high risk. The currently recommended approach would be to consider using preoperative PFTs for patients who are suspected of having COPD but who have not undergone prior testing or for patients with unexplained respiratory symptoms. Preoperative arterial blood gas measurement has not been shown to add appreciable value to the risk assessment and is thus not recommended.

Perioperative Strategies to Reduce Risk

Several interventions may reduce the risk of PPCs. Lung expansion maneuvers reduce atelectasis and thereby reduce the risk of postoperative pneumonia by roughly 50%.[7] Deep breathing exercises, incentive spirometry, continuous positive airway pressure, and intermittent positive pressure breathing have all been proven effective among unselected patients. No single modality has been shown to be superior in comparative trials. Deep breathing exercises and incentive spirometry are less expensive and require little or no equipment and are thus the preferred methods. Incentive spirometry must be performed for 15 minutes every 2 hours while the patient is awake to be effective. Deep breathing exercises consist of pursed lip breathing, 3-second breath holding, and coughing. Deep breathing exercise maneuvers should be done hourly while the patient is awake to ensure effectiveness.

Among patients with chronic lung disease, the preoperative optimization of pulmonary function may reduce complications, although this has not been definitively shown in clinical trials. In patients with COPD who are not at their baseline status or who may have been suboptimally controlled, a brief course of inhaled β-agonists should be used. In addition, a short course of oral corticosteroids that extends 3 to 4 days into the postoperative period has been shown to be safe and effective and to not impair wound healing. Antibiotics may be of use for patients with purulent sputum or an exacerbation of COPD symptoms before surgery. However, prophylactic antibiotics given to all patients with COPD who were undergoing major head and neck surgery did not reduce pulmonary complication rates in a single randomized trial.[8]

The value of preoperative smoking cessation is not certain. If patients can stop smoking for at least 6 weeks before surgery, there is likely a reduction in PPCs. However, for any shorter duration of abstinence, the benefits are not clear, and in at least one study there was an increased risk of PPCs.[8]

The anesthetic approach employed may also affect risk. The majority of available evidence suggests that neuraxial anesthesia is associated with a slightly lower risk of postoperative pneumonia than general anesthesia.[8] In addition, the use of postoperative epidural catheters for pain management also appears to reduce PPCs. However, the magnitude of the differences in pulmonary outcomes among various anesthetic and analgesic techniques is sufficiently small that other factors (e.g., anticoagulation, allergies, cardiac disease) have a greater influence on the decision regarding which technique to use.

Diagnosis and Management of Pulmonary Complications

The diagnosis of pulmonary complications (e.g., respiratory failure, pneumonia) of head and neck surgery is similar to that in other settings, with clinical symptoms and signs (e.g., fever, hypoxemia, leukocytosis, infiltrates by chest radiograph) being the mainstays of the diagnostic strategies. The diagnosis of ventilator-associated pneumonia is increasingly relying on mini-bronchoalveolar lavage to ascertain lower airway colonization; in both non-intubated and intubated patients, antibiotics should be used judiciously and probably for no more than 7 days to reduce the emergence of resistant organisms.

Intubated patients should have the head of the bed maintained between 30 and 45 degrees of elevation as a reasonably evidence-based approach to reducing risk for ventilator-associated pneumonia. Among patients who are at highest risk according to preoperative evaluation, the early detection of respiratory insufficiency will be helped if they receive immediate postoperative care in an intensive care unit (ICU) or a pulmonary step-down unit. In addition to expeditiously dealing with deteriorations in oxygenation and ventilation and with difficulties involving secretions, these settings are also more likely to be able to provide frequent nebulizer treatments, suctioning, or noninvasive ventilatory treatments (e.g., bi-level positive airway pressure) than typical ward settings.

THROMBOEMBOLIC COMPLICATIONS OF HEAD AND NECK SURGERY

Size of the Problem

Deep venous thrombosis (DVT) and pulmonary embolism (PE) are important causes of morbidity and mortality among surgical patients.[12] Although less common after head and neck surgery than after other forms of surgery, the consequences for the patient are often severe and include death and long-term morbidity. DVT or PE occurs in 0.1% to 0.5% of patients after head and neck surgery.[13-15] These estimates are based on case series and retrospective review studies. There are no studies that have used systematic venous thrombosis testing in all patients after head and neck surgery. Therefore, current estimates may accurately reflect the incidence of symptomatic postoperative DVT and PE, but they likely underestimate the incidence of total DVT and PE.

Risk Factors for Perioperative Deep Venous Thrombosis or Pulmonary Embolism

Several patient-specific risk factors have been identified in surgical patients. Although not specifically evaluated for head and neck surgery patients, these risk factors are likely to be relevant in any surgical population. The most important risk factors are an age of more than 40 years, cancer, a history of DVT or PE, prolonged immobilization or limb paralysis, heart failure, the use of estrogen, and known thrombophilic

states (e.g., nephrotic syndrome, myeloproliferative disorders).[12] Neck surgery may be associated with a slightly higher risk than otologic or neurotologic procedures.

Prevention of Perioperative Deep Venous Thrombosis and Pulmonary Embolism

Mechanical and pharmacologic measures have been used to prevent DVT and PE. Early ambulation to reduce the duration of immobilization is prudent for all patients after surgery, although this strategy is of unspecified clinical effectiveness. Graded compression stockings have been shown to modestly reduce the risk of DVT when used alone or in combination with pharmacologic agents. Pneumatic compression devices are effective for reducing the risk of DVT and PE, but they are often difficult for patients to tolerate and must be worn for at least 90% of the duration of immobility to be effective.[16] Low-dose unfractionated heparin and low-molecular-weight heparin (LMWH) significantly reduce the risk of perioperative DVT and PE, and they are more effective than any of the mechanical interventions.[17] There is a small but clinically significant increase in bleeding with either agent. Data regarding the effectiveness or risks of either agent specifically for head and neck surgery patients are not available.

The generally low incidence of perioperative DVT or PE in head and neck surgery patients suggests that routine prophylaxis (other than early ambulation) is not justified. In fact, no formal recommendations exist for head and neck surgery patients. Among patients with multiple risk factors who are undergoing a major procedure that is likely to result in prolonged immobilization, prophylaxis may be justified. The French Society of Anesthesiology and Intensive Care has suggested that LMWH is the prophylactic agent of choice.[16] The American College of Chest Physicians guidelines suggests using a pneumatic compression device, unfractionated heparin, or LMWH. If prophylaxis is used, it should begin within 2 hours of the completion of surgery to optimize effectiveness.[18]

Diagnosis and Management of Postoperative Deep Venous Thrombosis and Pulmonary Embolism

The diagnosis of postoperative DVT is similar to that in all other settings, with ultrasonography with Doppler being the mainstays of all diagnostic strategies to detect lower-extremity venous thromboembolism. Quantitative D-dimers are unlikely to be of clinical usefulness for postoperative patients and should be avoided for the diagnosis of DVT or PE.

Patients in whom PE is suspected should be clinically evaluated using a valid risk algorithm, with the rule suggested by Wells being one useful approach.[19] Patients with moderate to high risk for pulmonary embolism should undergo subsequent testing with either multidetector computed tomography (CT) scanning or ventilation–perfusion scintigraphy. CT scanning offers a number of advantages (e.g., speed, convenience, the provision of additional data regarding alternate diagnoses), and it is generally preferred for most patients. However, ventilation–perfusion scintigraphy should be pursued for patients with impaired renal function. Surgeons should recognize, however, that the value of a negative CT scan remains in question and that patients with a negative CT scan, no clear alternate diagnosis, and a very high clinical likelihood for PE may require pulmonary angiography to definitively rule out PE. In addition, the clinical significance of small subsegmental emboli on CT remains in doubt, although they are uniformly treated with anticoagulants.

All patients with PE or DVT should be considered for systemic, full-dose anticoagulation with either LMWH (enoxaparin 1.0 mg/kg/day) or unfractionated heparin (via weight-based nomogram). Enoxaparin is preferable, because it can be self-administered as an outpatient and because it speeds the transition to home; both enoxaparin and unfractionated heparin therapy need to be coadministered with warfarin (2.5 to 5.0 mg by mouth daily) until the patient's international normalized ratio (INR) reaches 2 to 2.5.

If patients with a proximal DVT and/or PE cannot be placed on full-dose anticoagulation because of bleeding risk, then they should be evaluated for the placement of a removable inferior vena cava filter (e.g., the Günther Tulip filter) until full-dose anticoagulation can be started. It is important to recognize that even removable inferior vena cava filter devices require patients be on lifelong anticoagulation therapy if the filter is not removed. Chances for removal are greatly increased if the filter is removed before 2 weeks have passed; after this time, the filters are often occluded with thrombus. Anticoagulation should still be started as soon as is safe after filter placement, with the goal of having the filter removed within 10 to 14 days of placement.

PERIOPERATIVE HEMATOLOGIC ISSUES

Scope of the Problem

There are three important hematologic issues to consider before surgery: (1) the presence and severity of anemia; (2) the assessment of the risk of abnormal surgical bleeding; and (3) the anticoagulated patient.

Anemia, as defined by a hematocrit (HCT) level of more than 45% for men or of more than 43% for women, is common among patients with chronic medical conditions, patients with cancer, and the elderly. A recent systematic review found that preoperative anemia was present in 25% to 50% of patients undergoing a variety of surgical procedures. Thus, a large portion of head and neck surgery patients are likely to be anemic before surgery. The severity of anemia—and, to some extent, the cause of anemia—can affect surgical outcomes. Among patients with known or suspected cardiovascular disease (especially coronary artery disease), the risks of postoperative cardiovascular complications and mortality appear to be increased when the preoperative HCT level is less than 30%. Among patients without cardiovascular disease, a preoperative HCT level of less than 25% is associated with an increased risk of complications.[20]

Certain types of anemia may be associated with increased postoperative complexity, although not necessarily with more complications. Patients with acute or chronic autoimmune hemolytic anemia may suffer a lowering of the HCT level that results from the use of perioperative medications (especially antibiotics) or from the stress of surgery itself through increasing the rate of immune-mediated red blood cell destruction. When feasible, hematologic consultation should be obtained before operating on patients with hemolytic anemia. Patients with active blood loss (e.g., from gastrointestinal bleeding) may have reductions in the HCT level that are independent of surgical blood loss, thus making the estimation of perioperative blood loss and intraoperative transfusion needs difficult. Surgery should be delayed among patients with active bleeding until the source of bleeding can be identified and treated. It is prudent for such patients to have a stable HCT level for 3 days before surgery.

Patients with stable preoperative anemia and cardiovascular risk factors may benefit from preoperative transfusion if the HCT level is less than 30%. Similarly, patients without cardiovascular disease and a preoperative HCT level of less than 25% may benefit from transfusion before surgery. This approach has not been validated in clinical trials.

ASSESSMENT OF OPERATIVE BLEEDING RISK

Scope of the Problem

Bleeding disorders are rare in a general population of patients. Because the morbidity associated with unrecognized bleeding disorders is high, the early identification of patients with bleeding problems is critical.

Risk Factors for Bleeding Disorders

The most useful approach for assessing a patient's risk for abnormal surgical bleeding is a directed bleeding history (Box 5-1). This bleeding history has been shown to be more accurate than the routine use of tests of clotting function.[21] Among patients who answer "no" to all questions in the bleeding history, the risk of abnormal surgical bleeding is very low (likely <0.5%). Despite this evidence, many hospitals and ambulatory surgery centers require preoperative tests of hemostasis (i.e., prothrombin time, partial thromboplastin time, and platelet count). The best approach is to use the directed bleeding history for all patients and to add the tests of coagulation if required.

Management and Treatment of Bleeding Disorders

For patients with an abnormal bleeding history, consultation with a hematologist or an internist before surgery is advisable.

MANAGEMENT OF THE ANTICOAGULATED PATIENT

Scope of the Problem

An increasing number of patients are taking anticoagulant medications, including patients who require surgery. Among anticoagulated patients, the risk of thrombosis varies considerably and depends almost entirely on the indication for long-term anticoagulation. Low-risk groups (e.g., patients with atrial fibrillation without prior stroke or cardiomyopathy without atrial fibrillation) have an annual thrombotic risk (without anticoagulation) of less than 4%. Moderate-risk patients (e.g., those with mechanical aortic valves) have a risk of between 4% and 7%. High-risk patients (e.g., patients with a mechanical mitral valve or with atrial fibrillation with prior stroke) have an annual risk of more than 7%.

BOX 5-1 Elements of a Directed Bleeding History

Patients who respond "yes" to one or more of these questions should be screened with prothrombin time, partial thromboplastin time, platelet count, and bleeding time:

1. Do you have frequent unprovoked nose or gum bleeding?
2. Have you had iron deficiency from heavy periods?*
3. Have you had unprovoked large bruises on your back, chest, or abdomen?
4. Have you had bleeding into a joint with mild trauma?
5. Have you previously had excessive blood loss with surgery?
6. Do you have a family history of bleeding problems?
7. Do you have kidney or liver disease?

Management and Treatment

Patients who are at low risk for thrombosis can be safely managed by withholding anticoagulant medication for the 4 to 6 days of the perioperative period. For such patients, warfarin should be stopped 4 days before surgery, and the INR value should be checked 1 day before surgery to confirm that it has decreased to less than 1.5. Warfarin should be resumed on the evening of surgery or when it is deemed safe. All other anticoagulated patients require "bridging" anticoagulation with heparin, because the risk of thrombosis when off of anticoagulation medication for 4 to 6 days is more than 1%. For most patients, LMWH is the preferred agent for bridging therapy, because it does not require intravenous or laboratory monitoring and because it can be initiated while the patient is at home (as opposed to unfractionated heparin, which requires admission).[22] LMWH is contraindicated for patients with moderate or severe renal dysfunction. These patients should be given unfractionated heparin as bridging therapy. Bridging therapy begins by discontinuing warfarin 5 days before surgery and 36 hours after the last dose of warfarin. The INR should be checked 1 day before surgery to confirm that it has decreased to less than 1.5. Bridging anticoagulation therapy should be discontinued 12 to 24 hours before surgery and resumed after hemostasis has been achieved, with warfarin restarted at the patient's usual outpatient dose at the same time. Unfractionated heparin or LMWH should be discontinued when the INR is more than 2.0.

POSTOPERATIVE DELIRIUM

Scope of the Problem

Postoperative delirium is an extraordinarily common complication of surgery that occurs in as many as 30% of patients. Although few studies have examined head and neck patients specifically, the high prevalence of risk factors for delirium (e.g., alcohol use, malnutrition) among these patients likely puts them at substantially elevated risk.[23]

Risk Factors for Delirium

A number of risk factors for delirium have been identified, many of which mirror the risks for postoperative cardiac complications. Risk indexes for postoperative delirium also exist, and they accurately identify patients for whom delirium is likely (Figure 5-2).[23]

In general, it is prudent to ask all patients whether they have ever been confused after surgery; this element of the history is highly specific and should prompt preventive measures (discussed later in this chapter).

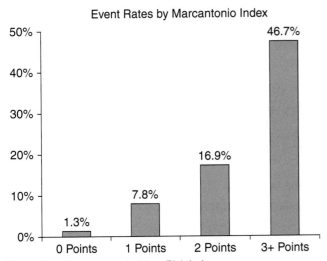

Figure 5-2. Marcantonio Delirium Risk Index
1. Type of surgery
   Aortic aneurysm surgery (2 points)
   Noncardiac thoracic surgery (1 point)
2. Age of more than 70 years (1 point)
3. Alcohol abuse (1 point)
4. Severe physical impairment (1 point)
   Unable to make bed, walk 1 block, or dress without stopping
5. Baseline dementia and/or confusion (Mini Mental State
   Examination score of <24) (1 point)
6. Abnormal sodium, potassium, or glucose level (1 point)
   A sodium level of less than 130 mmol/L or more than 150 mmol/L,
   a potassium level of less than 3 mmol/L or more than 6 mmol/L,
   a glucose level of less than 60 mg/dl or more than 300 mg/dl

For patients without a history of postoperative delirium, preoperative evaluations should assess for the presence of dementia or other cognitive disorders (e.g., sundowning, nighttime confusion) by asking both the patient and his or her family. Patients with a history of alcoholism are also at risk for postoperative delirium (see the section on alcohol withdrawal later in this chapter), as are those patients with a history of stroke and marked metabolic abnormalities (e.g., elevated blood urea nitrogen level, elevated glucose level).

Diagnosis and Management of Postoperative Delirium

Clinicians should rely on identifying patients with waxing and waning behavioral (e.g., confusion, inattention, agitation) and cognitive problems. Although families and nurses are often best able to notice that a patient is not acting normally, it is useful to ask the patient directly whether he or she feels that his or her thinking is impaired or whether he or she feels confused. The key to diagnosing delirium is to recognize its intermittent nature; acute psychoses and psychiatric disorders are rarely (if ever) a cause for postoperative delirium, thereby generally making a psychiatric consultation of low value.

The overall goal of delirium management is to reduce the duration and severity of symptoms so that patients' postoperative care (e.g., early mobilization, physical therapy, compliance with incentive spirometry) can continue apace.[24] Delirium is effectively managed through a number of fairly simple measures. First, patients should be assessed for their level of pain. Although pain medications may contribute to delirium, a growing literature suggests that the delirious patient who complains of pain should be treated with analgesics (even narcotic analgesics) first. Vaurio and colleagues[25] found that preoperative resting pain and increase in pain on the first postoperative day were independently associated with development of delirium, and that patients treated with oral narcotic medications were at decreased risk. Second, patients should be assessed and treated for other complications, such as infection, hypoxemia, hyperglycemia, or hypovolemia. Third, iatrogenic factors should be minimized, particularly the use of urinary catheters and anticholinergic medications (e.g., Benadryl, Compazine). Finally, patients' families and friends should be encouraged to remain with the patient for as much time as possible, with the goal of reorienting and reassuring the patient regularly during the immediate postoperative period.

The use of pharmacologic agents (e.g., haloperidol, benzodiazepines) and the use of restraints should be reserved only for those patients whose behavior poses a significant danger to their care (e.g., falling out of bed, wandering, pulling at surgical drains). Haloperidol (0.5–1.0 mg intramuscularly) can be used hourly until symptoms are controlled; the EKG and the QT interval should be monitored during the use of this agent. Benzodiazepines (e.g., lorazepam) should be used for patients who are agitated and whose symptoms are not controlled by haloperidol. Restraints are an option of last resort and should be removed at least once per shift to assess for skin breakdown. Furthermore, the need for restraints should be reassessed at least daily, both for the need for the restraints as well as for the careful assessment of whether pain, metabolic, infectious, and drug causes of delirium have all been addressed adequately.[24]

ALCOHOL WITHDRAWAL

Scope of the Problem

Alcoholism is among the most prevalent addictions in the United States, second only to tobacco use. As a result, withdrawal from alcohol is a very common inpatient management problem. Given the high prevalence of alcohol use among patients with head and neck cancer, an understanding of how best to manage alcohol withdrawal would seem obligatory.

Risk Factors for Alcohol Withdrawal

Given the prevalence of alcoholism in the head and neck surgery population, it would be prudent to screen all patients for current alcohol use using the standard CAGE questionnaire: Are you thinking about Cutting down? Do you get Angry when people ask about your drinking? Do you feel Guilty about your drinking? Do you ever have an Eye-opener? Answering "yes" to two or more CAGE questions is 93% sensitive and 76% specific for detecting patients with alcohol addiction problems. Patients in this category should then be screened with additional questions about the duration of their drinking, their last period of abstinence, whether or not they have had driving or work-related problems as a result of alcohol, and whether they have had withdrawal symptoms, delirium, or seizures as a result of alcohol.

Patients' peak risk for alcohol withdrawal symptoms is between 3 and 5 days after their last drink. In general, the severity and duration of withdrawal symptoms is proportional to the duration of alcohol use and the amount of alcohol consumed on a daily basis during that time period. Patients who have had delirium tremens or seizures in the past are at the highest risk.

Diagnosis and Management

Alcohol withdrawal should be suspected among all head and neck surgical patients who become acutely confused after surgery, particularly if they have a history of alcohol use. For these cases, early management should focus on the use of benzodiazepines (e.g., lorazepam, diazepam) to treat symptoms of tremulousness, tachycardia, hypertension, and anxiety using a "symptom-triggered approach." Symptom-triggered approaches are preferable to standing-dose treatment with benzodiazepines, because they allow for the rapid up-titration of benzodiazepines as part of their protocol rather than relying on the frequent rewriting of orders. A number of symptom scales are available, with the Clinical Institute Withdrawal Assessment for Alcohol being a favored guideline.[26] As the peak of withdrawal symptoms passes, most withdrawal protocols allow for an equally rapid (and symptom-triggered) reduction in benzodiazepine doses. β-Blockers and antipsychotics should never be used for the sole treatment of alcohol withdrawal, because they raise the risk for alcohol-related withdrawal seizures. Multivitamin, folic acid, and thiamine administration are indicated for all patients at the time that alcohol withdrawal is suspected.

Patients who reliably say that they have been abstinent from alcohol for more than 1 week before surgery should be monitored for withdrawal symptoms after surgery, but they do not require "prophylactic" benzodiazepine treatment. Patients who are actively drinking at the time of their surgery or who stopped less than 7 days beforehand would likely benefit from the early initiation of a symptom-triggered benzodiazepine protocol, potentially beginning as soon as the patient is admitted to the hospital.[26]

MANAGEMENT OF BLOOD SUGAR AND HYPERGYLCEMIA

Scope of the Problem

Diabetes is a comorbid illness that is ubiquitous and that is commonly perceived as a strong risk factor for postoperative complications, including infections, cardiovascular complications, and delirium. Despite the perceived strength of the evidence connecting poorer outcomes to less stringent blood sugar control, there are few data that specifically describe the degree of risk imparted to head and neck surgical patients or the goals for managing blood sugar in those patients.

Clinical Importance of Hyperglycemia

Research to date has focused primarily on fairly elevated blood sugars (e.g., >200 mg/dl) in diabetic patients, whether they are insulin dependent or not. Whether elevated blood sugar was a risk factor in itself or a marker of underlying problems (e.g., infection) has been unclear. More recent evidence suggests that this cutoff may be too high and that elevated blood sugar is of clinical importance even if the patient does not explicitly carry the diagnosis of diabetes. A randomized trial of intubated patients cared for in an ICU after cardiac surgery assigned all patients with a fasting blood glucose of 150 mg/dl or more to an insulin drip or to usual care; this trial showed a trend toward lower mortality rates and shorter lengths of stay among the insulin-treated patients.[27] Nonrandomized data, also from cardiac bypass patients, suggests that tighter glucose control (150–200 mg/dl) reduces deep sternal wound infections. Follow-up studies of tight glucose control in medical ICU patients have not definitively ascertained a clear benefit in terms of mortality or surrogate outcomes.

Diagnosis and Management of Hyperglycemia

Although several reviews have addressed the perioperative care of the diabetic patient, few have focused on the diabetic patient who is undergoing head and neck surgery.[28,29] In the light of the recent evidence described previously, many clinicians are in favor of maintaining near-normal blood sugars throughout the perioperative period.

Preoperatively, patients with noninsulin-dependent diabetes should hold or take a reduced amount of their usual oral agents on the morning of surgery. Patients with insulin-dependent diabetes should take a reduced amount of their usual morning dose of insulin while taking nothing by mouth and awaiting surgery. In both cases, the details of the management plan will depend on the time of day that the procedure will take place, the patient's diabetic regimen, and how well the patient's blood sugar is controlled at baseline.

There are no data to support use of insulin drips during or after head and neck surgery as a routine practice, although the use of insulin infusion may be indicated for diabetic patients who are receiving tube feedings or total parenteral nutrition (TPN) and who are unable to take any food by mouth. For all other patients, the use of the traditional regular insulin sliding scale should be avoided at all costs. Instead, clinicians should employ a regimen that combines once- or twice-daily intermediate-acting insulin (or once-daily Lantus insulin) with correctional short-acting insulin (aspart) at the time of meals in accordance with a sliding-scale approach. These protocols require daily attention to glucose readings and modifications to the intermediate-acting insulin or Lantus doses to reduce reliance on shorter-acting insulins. There are no data to suggest that screening finger-stick blood glucose readings should be obtained routinely from head and neck surgery patients. However, patients whose fasting blood glucose levels are elevated to more than 150 mg/dl on routine chemistries should be considered diabetic and treated accordingly.

Patients should have their outpatient regimen restarted as soon as they are eating. Patients who are receiving tube feedings or TPN after surgery (or after discharge) may require subcutaneous insulin in long-acting form (if tube feeding) or insulin added to their TPN to achieve optimal control. Metformin should not be started in patients with renal insufficiency, liver disease, or congestive heart failure, but it can be restarted among most patients who are experiencing a routine postoperative course and who are unlikely to require additional contrast studies.

REFERENCES

1. Auerbach A, Goldman L: Assessing and reducing the cardiac risk of noncardiac surgery. *Circulation* 2006;113(10):1361–1376.
2. Eagle KA, Berger PB, Calkins H, et al: ACC/AHA guideline update for perioperative cardiovascular evaluation for noncardiac surgery—executive summary: A report of the American College of Cardiology/American Heart Association Task Force on Practice Guidelines (Committee to Update the 1996 Guidelines on Perioperative Cardiovascular Evaluation for Noncardiac Surgery). *Anesth Analg* 2002;94(5):1052–1064.
3. Gordon AJ, Macpherson DS: Guideline chaos: Conflicting recommendations for preoperative cardiac assessment. *Am J Cardiol* 2003;91(11):1299–1303.
4. Lee TH, Marcantonio ER, Mangione CM, et al: Derivation and prospective validation of a simple index for prediction of cardiac risk of major noncardiac surgery. *Circulation* 1999;100(10):1043–1049.
5. McFalls EO, Ward HB, Moritz TE, et al: Coronary-artery revascularization before elective major vascular surgery. *N Engl J Med* 2004;351(27):2795–2804.
6. Lindenauer PK, Pekow P, Wang K, et al: Lipid-lowering therapy and in-hospital mortality following major noncardiac surgery. *JAMA* 2004;291(17):2092–2099.
7. Qaseem A, Snow V, Fitterman N: Risk assessment for and strategies to reduce perioperative pulmonary complications for patients undergoing noncardiothoracic surgery: A guideline from the American College of Physicians. *Ann Int Med* 2006;144(8):575–580.
8. Smetana G: Preoperative pulmonary evaluation: Identifying and reducing risks for pulmonary complications. *Cleve Clin J Med* 2006;73(Suppl 1):S36–S41.
9. Buitelaar DR, Balm AJM, Antonini N: Cardiovascular and respiratory complications after major head and neck surgery. *Head Neck* 2006;28:595–602.
10. Farwell DG, Reilly DF, Weymuller EA: Predictors of perioperative complications in head and neck patients. *Arch Otolaryngol Head Neck Surg* 2002;128:505–511.
11. Ong S, Morton RP, Kolbe J: Pulmonary complications following major head and neck surgery with tracheostomy. *Arch Otolaryngol Head Neck Surg* 2004;130:1084–1087.
12. Michota FA: Preventing venous thromboembolism in surgical patients. *Clev Clin J Med* 2006;73(Suppl 1):S88–S94.
13. Kanzaki S, Kunihiro T, Imanishi T: Two cases of pulmonary embolism after head and neck surgery. *Auris Nasus Larynx* 2004;31:313–317.
14. Moreano EH, Hutchison JL, McCulloch TM: Incidence of deep venous thrombosis and pulmonary embolism in otolaryngology-head and neck surgery. *Otolaryngol Head Neck Surg* 1998;118(6):777–784.
15. Spires JR, Byers RM, Sanchez ED: Pulmonary embolism after head and neck surgery. *South Med J* 1989;82:1111–1115.
16. Samama CM, Albaladejo P, Benhamou D: Venous thromboembolism prevention in surgery and obstetrics: Clinical practice guideline. *Eur J Anaesthiol* 2006;23(2):95–116.
17. Hirsh J, Raschke R: Heparin and low-molecular-weight heparin: The Seventh ACCP Conference on Antithrombotic and Thrombolytic Therapy. *Chest* 2004;126(Suppl 3):188S–203S.
18. Geerts WH, Pineo GF, Heit JA, et al: Prevention of venous thromboembolism: The Seventh ACCP Conference on Antithrombotic and Thrombolytic Therapy. *Chest* 2004;126(3 Suppl):338S–400S.
19. Wells PS, Anderson DR, Roger M. Derivation of a simple clinical model to categorize patients probability of pulmonary embolism: increasing the models utility with the SimpliRED D-dimer. *Thromb Haemost* 2000;83(3):416–420.
20. Shander A, Knight K, Thurer R, Adamson J, Spence R: Prevalence and outcomes of anemia in surgery: A systematic review of the literature. *Am J Med* 2004;116 Suppl A:58S–69S.
21. Baker R: Pre-operative hemostatic assessment and management. *Trans Apher Sci* 2002;27:45–53.
22. Douketis JD: Perioperative anticoagulation management in patients who are receiving oral anticoagulation therapy: A practical guide for clinicians. *Thromb Res* 2003;108:3–13.
23. Marcantonio ER, Goldman L, Mangione CM, et al: A clinical prediction rule for delirium after elective noncardiac surgery. *JAMA* 1994;271(2):134–139.
24. Marcantonio ER, Flacker JM, Wright RJ, et al: Reducing delirium after hip fracture: A randomized trial. *J Am Geriatr Soc* 2001;49(5):516–522.
25. Vaurio LE, Sands LP, Wang Y, Mullen EA, Leung JM. Postoperative delirium: the importance of pain and pain management. *Anesth Analg* 2006;102(4):1267:1273.
26. Mayo-Smith MF, Beecher LH, Fischer TL, et al: Management of alcohol withdrawal delirium: An evidence-based practice guideline. *Arch Intern Med* 2004;164(13):1405–1412.
27. van den Berghe G, Wouters P, Weekers F, et al: Intensive insulin therapy in the critically ill patients. *N Engl J Med* 2001;345(19):1359–1367.
28. Jacober SJ, Sowers JR: An update on perioperative management of diabetes. *Arch Intern Med* 1999;159(20):2405–2411.
27. Hoogwerf BJ: Perioperative management of diabetes mellitus: How should we act on the limited evidence? *Cleve Clin J Med* 2006;73(Suppl 1):S95–S99.

CHAPTER 6

Complications of Pediatric Head and Neck Surgery

Andrew F. Inglis, Jr., and Mark A. Richardson

Head and neck surgeons often care for pediatric patients. The avoidance of surgical complications in the pediatric population poses special challenges and becomes more difficult as the complexity of the pathologic condition increases. This chapter contains information about the general principles of the management of pediatric surgical patients, and it reviews the complications of specific pediatric head and neck conditions that are not covered elsewhere in this book.

GENERAL CONSIDERATIONS

Parent–Child Unit

There is an added layer of complexity in the physician–patient relationship when dealing with the pediatric population, because the physician routinely interacts with both the parent and the child. The child is often much more concerned about the details of the examination, the diagnostic workup, and the surgical intervention than with the pathologic process being treated. Additionally, the parent often has an intense emotional involvement with the child's illness. These hurdles to good medical and surgical care should be approached on two fronts. First, interactions with the child must be as gentle and playful as possible, hopefully achieving good cooperation from the patient. Second, communications with the parents should be thorough, unhurried, and often redundant. If complications do ensue as a result of any surgical procedure, having a sound relationship with the parents or caretakers is critical to the best outcome.

Anatomic Relationships and Allowances for Growth

Anatomic relationships are obviously different in the child as compared with the adult, and successful surgery will, by necessity, account for these differences. The child's facial nerve, for example, emerges from the temporal bone in a position that is higher than what is seen in the adult with regard to the attachment of the auricle to the temporal region. The facial skeleton is relatively smaller in relationship to the calvarium. The visualization of the small nasal cavities requires a microscope or a pediatric-sized endoscopic telescope. Unerupted teeth block the canine fossa approach to the maxillary antrum. The mandible may be relatively hypoplastic, which makes the visualization of the larynx

more difficult. The larynx itself is higher in the neck, which results in the alteration of surgical approaches. In the infant, the cricoid cartilage is the largest and most prominent landmark of the larynx externally, but it is also the narrowest part to the airway internally, thereby making the subglottic region especially vulnerable to endolaryngeal trauma.

Pediatric head and neck surgery, especially craniofacial surgery, should minimally interfere with future growth and development. Important growth centers are located within the nasal septum, the posterior palate, and at the skull base, and they must be maintained during surgical interventions.

Postoperative Wound Care

Suture removal may be difficult or impossible in the unsedated child; thus, absorbable sutures should be used whenever possible. Good cosmetic results can be obtained using subcuticular or intracuticular 5.0 or 6.0 fast-absorbing gut suture. Drains should be easy to care for and easily removable with minimal risk of accidental removal. For this reason, avoid using suction drains when possible. Dressings need to be practically bulletproof to survive a toddler's prying fingers. In extreme cases, arm splints will limit patient manipulation of the wound and dressings. Because infant and child skin is so fragile, areas that will require repeated taping should be protected with a layer of Tegaderm or tape, which is left in place between the skin and the tape to secure the dressing.

Anesthetic Considerations and Pain Control

Although the goals and techniques of pediatric anesthesia are in many ways similar to those of adult anesthesia, significant differences exist. With proper techniques and equipment, pediatric anesthesia can actually have lower morbidity and mortality rates than adult anesthesia. A recent review of more than 40,000 pediatric anesthetic cases revealed only one death that was partially or wholly attributable to the anesthetic.[1]

Patient age has been shown to affect the rate of anesthetic complications. Complication rates resulting from respiratory or circulatory failure have been shown to be higher among patients who are less than 1 year old (4.3 out of 1000) as compared with patients between the ages of 1 and 14 years (0.5 out of 1000).[1] This can be attributed in part to the greater precision required to maintain the infant airway and to the child's greater sensitivity to myocardial depressants. Former preterm infants of less than 44 weeks conceptual age have a higher incidence of postoperative apnea. Many pediatric anesthesiology departments require close postoperative monitoring for 12 to 24 hours for all preterm patients of less than 56 weeks postconceptual age.[2]

The patient's physical state as defined by the American Society of Anesthesiologists grading system also correlates positively with complication rates. Patients rated as grade I have a significantly lower rate of complications than patients rated in grades II to V. Complications are tripled during emergent surgery.[1]

Anesthetic complications increase if the patient has a full stomach. This is a result of the increased risk of aspiration as well as the emergent nature of these procedures. Current recommendations advise 6 hours of fasting for solids and 3 hours for clear liquids before surgery.[2] If surgery must be performed on a patient with a full stomach, preinduction treatment with antacids and ranitidine should be considered in addition to a rapid-sequence induction.

Several medical conditions that increase the risk of anesthesia are more common during childhood. Patients with asthma are at great risk for intraoperative bronchospasm and often require that steroids and bronchodilators be started before the induction of anesthesia. Bronchodilating agents such as halothane are usually employed intraoperatively.

Patients with cystic fibrosis may have difficulties with anesthesia, including bronchial and endotracheal tube plugging, atelectasis, impaired oxygenation, hypercapnia, and postoperative pneumonia caused by thick pulmonary secretions. Coagulopathies related to malabsorption are rarely present.[3] Complications can be minimized by a thorough preoperative pulmonary evaluation and an inpatient pulmonary "cleanout" consisting of vigorous chest physical therapy and intravenous (IV) antibiotics.[4]

Patients who may have sickle cell anemia require preoperative testing, and those with the disease should have hemoglobin electrophoresis performed to check their levels of hemoglobin. Patients with hemoglobin S levels of more than 30% are at increased risk of sickle cell crisis, especially in the face of hypoxia, acidosis, and dehydration; preoperative transfusion may avert these complications.[5]

Airway management before and after extubation is often a challenge among patients with craniofacial syndromes (e.g., Treacher Collins syndrome, Apert syndrome, Goldenhar syndrome, Robin sequence). The surgeon should be available to assist the anesthesiologist with securing a different airway through oral, fiber-optic nasal, or transcervical routes. A good rapport with the anesthesiologist is essential.

It is widely recognized that the preoperative anxiety and sometimes outright terror felt by patients of all ages is a major hurdle to smooth and safe anesthesia. This terror is especially common among children who are old enough to know fear but too young to be reasoned with. Measures that can reduce this response include the oral, nasal, or rectal administration of sedative narcotics and a policy that allows parents to be present during the induction of anesthesia if the patient's status warrants it.

Laryngospasm is the life-threatening reflex closure of the larynx that usually occurs during a light plane of anesthesia that is stimulated by irritation of the unsecured laryngeal airway by secretions or instrumentation. Patients with partial airway obstruction limiting the uptake of inhalational anesthetic agents are at increased risk. It occurs when blood, mucus, saliva, or stomach contents stimulate the vocal cords or when inappropriate surgical stimulation is applied to the patient or airway during procedures such as a myringotomy tube placement or laryngoscopy. It can be avoided by good airway management, the use of IV or topical lidocaine, and good communication between the surgeon and the anesthesiologist. Laryngospasm is managed with positive pressure ventilation, the deepening of the anesthetic, and, when these measures fail, the use of rapidly acting muscle relaxants before the airway is secured.

Dislodging a loose deciduous tooth during intubation is generally of little consequence as long as it is recognized and retrieved. Even hypopharyngeal or esophageal perforations occurring during intubation may be managed conservatively in neonates.[6,7] As a result of their shorter tracheas, right mainstream intubation may be more common among children, and it may be more significant as a result of a relatively smaller functional residual lung capacity. Plugging from airway secretions is more common in the smaller endotracheal tube sizes. The inadvertent administration of IV fluid volumes that would be trivial in adults can lead to fluid overload in infants and children; appropriate fluid administration devices are requisite. Similarly, blood loss in amounts that would be trivial even in young children can be significant without prompt replacement in infants and neonates.

Malignant hyperthermia (MH) is a major concern of pediatric anesthesia. MH is an autosomal-dominant genetic disorder of the skeletal muscle[8] that is triggered in susceptible persons by various agents, including inhalational anesthetics and depolarizing muscle relaxants. It is characterized by a hypermetabolic state that includes tachycardia, hyperpyrexia, hypertension, acidosis, cyanosis, and muscle rigidity.[9] It occurs more commonly among children (i.e., 1 out of 12,000) than adults (i.e., 1 out of 40,000).[10] Before the introduction of dantrolene, the mortality rate related to this condition was approximately 65%; however, with rapid recognition and appropriate intervention, the current mortality rate is near zero.[11]

Early signs of MH are tachypnea, tachycardia, tachyarrhythmias, labile blood pressure, later hyperpyrexia, and, sometimes, muscle rigidity.[11] Onset may be delayed until several hours after anesthetic administration. The treatment of MH consists of the immediate cessation of the anesthetic, the administration of dantrolene, and other supportive measures.[11]

Patients known to have MH or who have a positive family history of MH can be safely anesthetized using combinations of anesthetic agents including nitrous oxide, barbiturates, opiates, tranquilizers, and nondepolarizing muscle relaxants. Prophylactic dantrolene may not be necessary.[9] The diagnosis can be confirmed by caffeine–halothane contracture studies of biopsied vastus lateralis muscle.

The most common complication after the administration of a pediatric anesthetic is the period of confusion, disorientation, and discomfort that is called *postanesthetic excitement*. It can usually be successfully managed with a sedative or a narcotic that induces a light sleep, after which the symptoms are greatly reduced.[12]

Children and especially infants are very susceptible to hypothermia, which is often discovered in the recovery room. Prevention is the best management, and commonly employed strategies include increasing the ambient operating room temperature and using warming lights, blankets, and head and extremity wraps. Similar measures are used to correct hypothermia in the recovery room.

The aspiration of stomach contents or blood from the oral or pharyngeal operative field can occur at any stage of anesthesia, but it most commonly occurs after extubation. Awake extubation seems to lessen the incidence of aspiration. If pneumonia ensues, treatment consists of antibiotics, pulmonary toilet, oxygen therapy, and, possibly, corticosteriods.[12]

Successful postoperative pain management is crucial to achieving a favorable perception of the surgery for the patient and family. Unfortunately, some children are exquisitely sensitive to the respiratory depressant effects of narcotics, especially head and neck surgery patients, among whom there is often an underlying upper airway obstruction with altered respiratory drive. Extreme care must be used when prescribing narcotics. In a recent review of more than 40,000 pediatric anesthetic procedures, the only anesthetic death was related to narcotic overdose.[1] Patients receiving IV narcotics should be closely monitored. A range of dosages should be ordered with instructions to administer half of the recommended dose and to increase to the full dose only if necessary. In some hospitals, selected pediatric patients may use patient-controlled analgesia as directed by physicians who are experienced with its use.[2] The treatment of overdose is similar to that used for adults in that narcotic antagonists are administered and cardiorespiratory functions are supported.

Unanticipated hospital admission postoperatively is often caused by protracted nausea and vomiting. A variety of antiemetics are available, but they must be used with caution as a result of their sedative effects, especially in the outpatient setting.

In summary, pediatric anesthesia can be safe and less traumatic if allowances for the differences among infants, children, and adults are made. This is most reliably accomplished in a setting that involves experienced pediatric anesthesiologists and nurses.

SELECTED PATHOLOGIC CONDITIONS

Choanal Atresia

The congenital anomaly of choanal atresia consists of a bony, membranous, or cartilaginous plate that obstructs one or both nasal cavities just anterior to the nasopharynx. This anomaly is thought to represent a persistence of the embryonic bucconasal membrane. Hengerer and Strome[13] have written an excellent account of the embryologic aspects.

Anatomically, the nasal cavity tapers posteriorly as the vomer becomes progressively thicker, and the lateral and superior nasal walls bow medially and inferiorly. These findings are well demonstrated on an axial computed tomography (CT) scan of the nasal cavity (Figure 6-1). This broad area of narrowing has surgical implications, as will be shown.

The incidence of choanal atresia is estimated at between 1 in 5000 and 1 in 10,000 live births.[14] Unilateral cases may be slightly more common than bilateral cases. About half of the patients have other congenital anomalies. Many will have the CHARGE association, which denotes Coloboma, Heart disease, Atresia choanae, Retarded growth and development or central

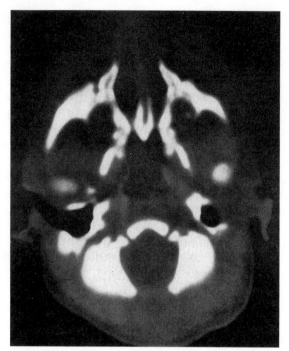

Figure 6-1. Axial computed tomography scan of the choanal atresia. Note the thickness of the atresia plate and the tapering of the nasal cavities anterior to the obstruction.

nervous system anomalies, Genital hypoplasia, and Ear anomalies or deafness.[15]

Because newborns are obligate nose breathers, bilateral choanal atresia may present as a medical emergency in the delivery room. The afflicted infant will typically struggle for breath, perhaps turn dusky, and then begin to cry with a return of normal coloration. When the patient settles down and stops crying, the cycle is repeated. A temporary airway can be secured by endotracheal intubation, the placement of an oral airway, the placement of a McGovern nipple with a large hole cut into the end, or, occasionally, by the placement of a large orogastric tube that is used as a stent to keep the oral cavity and the oropharynx open.

The various surgical approaches for repair of the atretic choanae can generally be divided in two categories: transnasal and transpalatal. There is no consensus as to which approach is best used for the newborn.

Perhaps the simplest transnasal approach is to open the nasal cavities with dilators. Urethral sounds are typically employed, with the target size generally being 14F or 16F. An opening this size will accommodate a 3-mm endotracheal tube or a Silastic stent of similar size. This technique has the limitation of being a blind procedure. Soft palate injury, septal perforation, cerebrospinal fluid leak, meningitis, and cranial nerve injury are potential complications. The risk of complications can be minimized if the dilators are carefully guided to

follow the natural curve of the floor of the nose. The progress of the dilator can to some extent be monitored by palpating the hard and soft palates during the procedure.

More precision in the creation of the nasal airway is achieved by removing the atresia plate under direct vision with the operating microscope or a nasal endoscope. Small mucosal flaps are first elevated from the atresia plate with otologic instruments, and the bony plate is removed with a drill. The preserved mucosal flaps are replaced over any exposed bone. If needed, the choanae are again kept open with stents for 6 to 8 weeks.[16]

The most aggressive transnasal approach is the sublabial transeptal approach, which is said to provide wide exposure to the nasal cavity and the choanal regions. This approach is similar to that used for transsphenoidal hypophysectomy. Mucosal flaps are raised, and the vomer is removed along with the atresia plate.[14]

The transpalatal approach involves raising a mucoperiosteal flap off of the hard palate. Bone from the posterior hard palate, the vomer, and the atresia plates is removed with a drill. The bony lateral nasal walls are widened and the mucosal flaps preserved to reline the raw bone. Stents are placed, and the palate is closed. The main advantage of the transpalatal approach is the improved exposure of the choanae and the narrowed nasal cavity anteriorly, which allows for the more aggressive removal of bone from these regions. It is technically easier to preserve the mucosal flaps. The main disadvantage to this approach is the potential sequela of the disruption of growth centers in the posterior palate; this may be associated with an increased incidence of dental occlusal abnormalities.[17] Another complication, especially in newborns, is the risk of a hemodynamically significant blood loss. There is also the possibility of postoperative deformities of the hard and soft palate, including palatal fistulas and velopharyngeal insufficiency.

The major problem with any approach to choanal atresia repair is restenosis after the removal of stents. Stahl and Jurkiewiez[18] report restenosis rates as high as 73% with the transnasal approach. However, the authors reported a 66% recurrence rate with the transpalatal approach. Restenosis rates seem to be lower when the vomer is removed, whether through a transpalatal or transnasal approach. The removal of the vomer is presumed to be safe from the standpoint of facial growth, but none of the studies performed thus far have a long enough follow-up time to give empiric assurance that this is indeed the case.

The restenosis rate after choanal atresia repair in patients with the CHARGE association seems to be much higher than in patients without it. In one series,[19] 7 of 9 CHARGE patients had restenosis as compared with 1 of 15 without the CHARGE syndrome. This was attributed to a more contracted nasopharynx and a narrowed posterior choanal region seen on the CT scans of CHARGE patients as compared with non-CHARGE patients.[20]

Accidental stent plugging with mucus is the greatest threat to the patient with stents after he or she is discharged. Home care instruction to the parents regarding the care of the nasal stents needs to be as vigorous as it is with the home tracheotomy patient. Other stent complications include dislodgment and columella ulceration.

One review suggests that restenosis of the transnasal choanal atresia repair is more likely in patients with gastroesophageal reflux disease and age younger than 10 days at initial surgery. Coexistent malformations and previous surgeries were not associated with poorer outcomes. The use of stents was associated with higher rates of restenosis.[21]

In summary, the ideal management of choanal atresia has not been established. The current management plan is to establish some form of oral airway and to obtain a preoperative CT scan to fully elucidate the nature of the choanal atresia. Atresia is repaired as soon as other major anomalies, especially cardiac anomalies, have been managed or ruled out. The initial surgery is usually a simple removal of the bony plate with a transnasal drill and the placement of stents for 6 weeks. Endoscopic or microscopic visualization is used. Stents, if they are placed, are removed in the operating room, and any granulation tissue present is removed as well. If restenosis occurs, a more aggressive procedure, including the removal of the posterior vomer, is considered. The potential for a growth abnormality caused by the removal of the vomer may be outweighed by the potential for the growth abnormality caused by chronic mouth breathing in the nasally obstructed patient.

Branchial Cleft Anomalies

First Branchial Cleft Anomalies

First branchial cleft cysts, sinuses, and fistulas are epithelial-lined tracts that probably represent duplication anomalies of the external auditory canal. The Work classification involves two categories.[22] Type I presents as a mass or sinus in the periauricular region and has a tract that runs parallel to the external auditory canal. This tract may end in a blind pouch that is separate from but at the same level as the tympanic membrane, or there may be a fistulous connection to the external auditory canal. The type II anomaly typically has a cutaneous opening around the region of the angle of the mandible. It has a thick wall that may be cartilaginous and extend up toward the external auditory canal. It usually runs adjacent and deep to the facial nerve in the parotid gland, although this relationship is not consistent. There usually is a fistulous opening in the lateral anteroinferior external auditory canal.

Both types are prone to recurrent infection with an intense local inflammatory response, and there may be discharge from the cutaneous openings. Treatment is surgical excision. The type I cysts are approached through the appropriate periauricular incisions, with the cyst dissected from the soft tissue laterally and the tract elevated from the mastoid bone medially. Cutaneous openings are excised. These cysts are usually superior to and not closely associated with the facial nerve, but anomalies of the facial nerve may be present, and facial nerve identification is advised. Facial nerve monitoring may be useful. The most likely complication is recurrence after incomplete excision; this is minimized by providing adequate exposure (sometimes including the removal of the associated mastoid bone) to ensure good visualization of the deep portions of the tract. A thorough removal of a sinus opening into the medial external auditory canal, if present, must also be accomplished.

Type II cysts can be approached through a tunnel technique or through a formal parotidectomy-style flap and facial nerve dissection. With the tunnel technique, fusiform skin incisions are made around the fistulous openings in the neck and the external auditory canal. A probe is passed through the fistula, and soft tissue is dissected from the tract by tunneling along the wall of the cyst from above and below. When the tract is freed up, it is pulled through one of the incisions. The main objection to this approach is that it is completely blind in the region of the facial nerve, and straying from the wall of the cyst in this region can result in injury to the nerve. There are advocates of this technique, however, and this approach can be considered when the tract is relatively short, superficial, thick walled, and without evidence of ongoing infection, which could lead to partial necrosis of the cyst wall.

An effective approach to the type II fistula excision is to raise a parotidectomy flap. The flap should be relatively thin, because the cyst may "tent up" the facial nerve, thereby causing it to be much more superficial than expected (Figure 6-2). A formal facial nerve dissection is performed. The dissection may be quite difficult if an intense inflammatory response is present from recurrent cyst infection. The cyst is then removed, with all branches of the facial nerve visualized and protected.

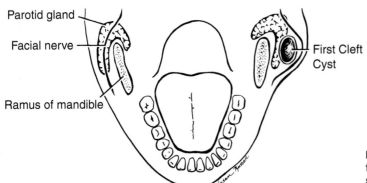

Figure 6-2. Axial view showing the normal relationship of the facial nerve to the parotid gland and the skin *(left)* and the more superficial course of the nerve when overlying a first cleft sinus.

An operating microscope should be available to be draped into the field, if necessary. Intraoperative facial nerve monitoring should be used for an additional level of safety.

If, despite all due care, the facial nerve is injured, immediate nerve repair must be undertaken. The epincurium is reapproximated with 10-0 nylon sutures in the same manner as it is for adults.

Second and Third Branchial Cleft Anomalies

Unlike the first branchial cleft anomalies, which are duplication anomalies, second and third cleft anomalies represent a failure of a normal embryonic structure to involute. These structures may be cysts, sinuses, or fistulas. Cysts present as masses between the anterior border of the sternocleidomastoid muscle and the carotid sheath. External sinuses usually open along the anterior border of the same muscle in the mid or low neck. Internal sinuses open in the tonsillar fossa or along the anterior tonsillar pillar in second cleft anomalies and in the piriform sinus in third cleft anomalies.

Treatment is excision, and complications are related to wound infection, recurrence, and injury to adjacent structures. The last two complications can be minimized with a thorough understanding of the anatomy of these anomalies.

Second cleft anomalies run lateral to the carotid sheath, then anterior to (i.e., over) the internal carotid artery (i.e., the embryologic artery of the third branchial arch) in the carotid bifurcation, lateral to the twelfth cranial nerve (i.e., embryologically derived from myotomes of the occipital somites), over the ninth cranial nerve (i.e., the nerve of the third arch), and through the constrictor muscles to the tonsillar fossa.

Third cleft anomalies are more rare than second cleft anomalies. They may begin with a sinus opening low in the neck along the anterior border of the sternocleidomastoid muscle or as a cystic swelling located similar to the second cleft anomaly. As the tract runs superiorly, it passes behind (i.e., under) the internal carotid artery (i.e., the third arch derivative), over the twelfth cranial nerve (i.e., the somite derivative), under the ninth cranial nerve (i.e., the third arch derivative), and over the superior laryngeal nerve (i.e., the nerve of the fourth branchial arch), where it penetrates the thyrohyoid membrane and enters the piriform sinus.

All of the lower cranial nerves are at risk, especially if resection is attempted in an infected surgical field. It should be noted that hypoglossal nerve paresis has been reported preoperatively as a result of inflammation from the infected cyst itself.[23] An exceedingly rare complication, death from a cerebrovascular accident as a result of carotid arteriospasm has also been reported.[24]

Thyroglossal Duct Anomalies

Thyroglossal duct anomalies represent embryologic remnants of the tract that is formed when the thyroid gland descends from its origin at the glossal foramen cecum to its usual location in the lower neck. Thyroglossal duct cysts, sinuses, and fistulas result when portions of the tract fail to involute. The most common presentation is of a midline neck mass at or below the level of the hyoid bone. The most common serious complication after surgical excision is recurrence; this can be minimized by a thorough understanding of the anatomy of this anomaly, which provides the rationale for the Sistrunk operation.

With each thyroglossal duct, there may be a tract with potential side branches that runs cephalad toward the foramen cecum. This tract is usually not visible during surgery. The tract typically extends upward from the cyst anterior to the hyoid bone, but, in a sizable minority of patients (30%), a portion of the duct may loop dorsal to the hyoid bone (Figure 6-3) from the inferior aspect of the hyoid bone.[25] Because of the potentially complex relationship of the tract with the hyoid bone, the first principle of the Sistrunk operation is to include the resection of the midportion of the hyoid bone and the adjacent soft tissue with the excision of the cyst.[26]

Cephalad to the hyoid bone, the tract may branch out like a broom, with many accessory ducts terminating in secretory glands within the substance of the tongue.[25,27]

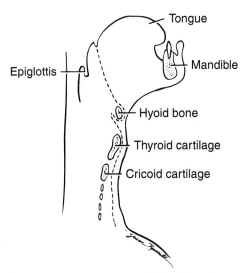

Figure 6-3. The path of the thyroglossal duct. Note the complex relationship of the hyoid bone, which necessitates the removal of the midportion of this bone to ensure the total removal of the duct.

It is considered necessary to remove all of the duct and accessory structures to prevent a recurrence. This is the basis for the second principle of the Sistrunk operation, which is that a core of tongue muscle running from the hyoid bone to the foramen cecum should be excised without attempting to visualize the tract.[26]

Several factors have been associated with higher recurrence rates. Attempted extirpation via local excision without the removal of hyoid and tongue tissue results in recurrence in about one third of cases.[28] Cysts that have undergone previous attempts at excision also have a higher rate of recurrence during subsequent operation (e.g., up to 30% in one series[27]). Recurrences tend to be secondary to incomplete excision of glandular tissue in the tongue base; this can be most effectively extirpated through the use of a heavy traction suture inserted via a spinal needle from the hyoid region through tongue base mucosa at the foramen cecum.[29] High rates of recurrence have also been associated with attempted removal when the cyst is actively infected[27,30] (e.g., as high as 24% in one series[27]). Other factors associated with recurrence include the presence of a cutaneous fistula or extensive subdermal involvement,[32] younger patient age,[30,32] and rupture of the cyst intraoperatively.[30,32] Even with a well-performed Sistrunk procedure, a recurrence rate of 4% to 7% can be expected.[30-32] Recurrences will generally show up within the first 4 months after the operation.

The prevention of recurrence is best accomplished through the generous en bloc removal of the cyst, the connective tissues between the cyst and the hyoid bone, the midportion of the hyoid bone with a small cuff of tissue both anterior and posterior to it, and a core of tissue extending from the hyoid bone to the foramen cecum through the base of the tongue. The region of the foramen cecum is best identified intraoperatively by placing a double-gloved finger through the patient's mouth and pushing the region of the junction of the anterior two thirds and posterior one third of the tongue forward through the wound.

Recurrences typically present as inflammatory masses in the neck. Treatment is wide surgical excision. Intraoperatively, one may encounter multiple pseudocysts at sites caudal to the original operative field as a result of the tendency of the inflamed cyst fluid to track along tissue planes in a dependent fashion. In addition to cleaning out palpable disease, a wider resection of the hyoid bone and base of the tongue should be undertaken.[27]

Postoperative wound infections are a more common but less serious complication. Predisposing factors include preexisting infection within the excised cyst, a large amount of dead space in the base of the tongue after excision, and potential wound contamination from the oral cavity. Most wounds should be drained externally for at least 24 hours postoperatively, and perioperative antibiotics are advised.

Hypothyroidism is a rare complication that occurs when a patient's only functioning thyroid gland is located in an ectopic position, mistaken for a thyroglossal duct cyst, and excised. This can be prevented by obtaining a preoperative technetium-99m pertechnetate scan or an ultrasound image of the thyroid gland. A review of 230 cases of presumed thyroglossal duct cyst revealed eight specimens that had ectopic thyroid or accessory thyroid tissue.[33] The majority of these patients had abnormal thyroid function tests and signs of hypothyroidism, including chronic constipation, developmental and growth delay, excessive somnolence, and weight gain despite poor feeding habits. The recommendations for preoperative workup in this study included careful questioning for signs of hypothyroidism and routine thyroid function tests; thyroid scans were reserved for patients with abnormalities found by the first two screening tests. It was pointed out that nearly all patients with palpable ectopic thyroid glands have some degree of hypothyroidism preoperatively and would benefit from thyroid replacement therapy. The impact of inadvertent total ectopic thyroidectomy is usually minimal. If one encounters a mass intraoperatively that appears to be ectopic thyroid tissue, exploration of the wound inferiorly may reveal normal thyroid tissue. If so, excision of the aberrant tissue can be completed.

Subglottic Stenosis

Infant subglottic stenosis may be acquired as a result of endotracheal intubation for respiratory distress, but more rarely it is a congenital anomaly. The infant airway is narrowest at the level of the subglottic region, and, because this region is completely encircled by the rigid cricoid cartilage, the mucosa is subject to pressure necrosis from a relatively rigid endotracheal (ET) tube. In an infant who requires endotracheal intubation, a key factor that leads to mucosal injury and subsequent subglottic stenosis from fibrous tissue or cartilaginous collapse is the size of the ET tube. Generally speaking, the smaller the ET tube, the smaller the chance of mucosal injury. The use of an ET tube that is too large may be inadvertent (e.g., when an infant undergoes urgent intubation), or it may be deliberate (e.g., when an infant has such severe respiratory compromise that a large ET tube is necessary to provide a tight seal to allow for high pressure ventilation). Other factors that may predispose an infant to increased subglottic trauma include cyanotic heart disease, repeated intubations, excessive activity in an infant who is difficult to sedate, and, possibly, oral (as opposed to nasal) intubation.[34]

Subglottic mucosal ulceration and pressure necrosis may occur even with appropriately sized ET tubes after less than 3 days of intubation.[35] During the subsequent 3 weeks, the laryngeal mucosa typically undergoes remarkable healing and reepithelialization around the ET tube; thus, subglottic stenosis is avoided in the overwhelming majority of infants and neonates.[36] No simple recommendations can be made with regard to when an intubated infant should be converted to a tracheotomy to avoid the complication of subglottic stenosis.

If a patient fails an attempted extubation from presumed subglottic swelling, reintubation with a smaller ET tube is recommended, followed by treatment with antibiotics and steroids for 2 days. The leak around the ET tube usually increases during this time period, and a second extubation is then performed. If this fails, endoscopic evaluation of the airway should be performed to assess the level and degree of injury. The accurate assessment of the lesion is probably the single most important factor that will lead to a successful operative procedure and the correction of the stenotic airway. Other laryngeal causes of airway obstruction include posterior glottic stenosis and vocal cord paralysis. Readily treatable causes include vocal cord granulations and ventricular polyps, which can be excised with the carbon dioxide laser. Airway obstruction above and below the larynx should also be ruled out.

Assuming that the obstruction is the result of subglottic stenosis, decompressing the cricoid ring is an accepted treatment for neonates and infants. The anterior cricoid split procedure, as described by Cotton and Seid,[37] has a success rate that ranges from 58% to 100% in selected populations.[37–40] The anterior cricoid split is performed through a neck incision that exposes the thyroid, cricoid, and upper tracheal cartilages. A midline incision is then made through these cartilages and through the underlying airway mucosa beginning from a point 2 mm

below the thyroid notch and extending inferiorly to include the upper two tracheal rings. The patient is then reintubated with an appropriately sized ET tube. The wound is closed loosely over a drain, and the patient remains intubated for 7 to 10 days.

Significant complications have been reported after this procedure. Intraoperatively, coordination with the anesthesiologist is vital so that the movement or changing of the delivery system for anesthetic gasses can take place in an unhurried and nonconfusing manner. The maintenance of an adequate airway during surgery becomes a shared responsibility between the surgeon and the anesthesiologist, and the details of the procedure should clearly be worked out well in advance.

Care must be taken to not disrupt the integrity of the anterior commissure, or a poor voice will result. The tip of the ET tube must be carefully positioned in the small space between the lower end of the incision and the carina. Malpositioning of the ET tube with either mainstem bronchus intubation or with the migration of the tip of the tube up to the level of the wound may result in respiratory distress.

Postoperatively, accidental extubation may result in severe respiratory distress if sufficient airway expansion has not occurred. Reintubation via the transoral or transnasal route is usually difficult, because the ET tube usually becomes misdirected through the cricoidotomy and into the tissues of the neck, which leads to further hypoventilation and pneumothorax or pneumomediastinum. In this setting, it may be best to attempt to reestablish the airway through the neck incision. The prevention of accidental extubation is preferable; this is accomplished by vigilant nursing care and the administration of appropriate sedative or relaxant agents. The advantage of sedative agents is that the patient will still breathe spontaneously if he or she is inadvertently extubated. Alternatively, relaxants greatly reduce the risk of self-extubation by the patient. Sedation without relaxation is generally preferred. Other complications include persistent tracheocutaneous fistula,[41] subcutaneous emphysema, and bleeding,[42] but these are generally not difficult to sort out or manage.

The complication of failed extubation may have several causes. The patient's pulmonary status must truly be sufficient to allow for ventilator independence. Granulation tissue or subglottic fibrosis or scarring may cause continued airway obstruction. Undetected structural problems (e.g., cricoid chondritis and collapse, posterior glottic stenosis) may also be present. Successful extubation can often be predicted by the air leak around the tube. Leaks at less than 20 cm of water pressure are predictive of good airway expansion and successful extubation, whereas leaks at more than 30 cm of water pressure are indicative of a narrow lumen and can be predictive of extubation failure.[43]

In a prospective study comparing the anterior cricoid split alone to the anterior cricoid split augmented with costal cartilage graft, three major advantages were found to augmenting the repair with rib cartilage.[44] First, reintubation after accidental extubation was less hazardous with the rib graft blocking the opening from the laryngotracheal lumen to the neck. Second, healing was faster and extubation was accomplished earlier. Finally, the overall extubation rate was improved, probably because the added cartilaginous support provided better structural expansion to the cricoid and the perichondrial surface, thereby allowing for more reliable epithelialization of the luminal surface. Obtaining adequate graft tissue, however, can be complicated by pneumothorax or other donor site morbidity. Generally, careful attention to detail when obtaining the graft will allow for the harvesting of cartilage without complications.

Assuming that the patient is successfully extubated and a tracheotomy is avoided, the main long-term complication is poor vocal quality. This may result from the original ET tube trauma to the vocal folds or from the expansion of the anterior commissure by the thyrotomy portion of the split procedure (Figure 6-4).

Lymphatic Malformations

The term *cystic hygroma* is best replaced by *lymphatic malformation*. These malformations can vary widely in their histopathologic appearance. The range includes large multiloculated cystic structures with little vascularity to capillary-like lymphatic channels with an intense

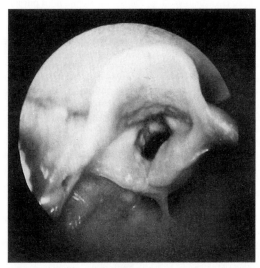

Figure 6-4. Endoscopic photograph of a patient with a poor voice result after an anterior cricoid split and a rib graft. The poor voice is the result of trauma to the vocal cords after prolonged intubation and the widening of the anterior commissure.

vascular component. Lymphatic malformations typically present as painless masses in newborns or infants, or they may arise as a result of infections of the head and neck area.

The parents must have realistic preoperative expectations regarding what can be accomplished by surgery. It should be clearly understood by both the parents and the surgeon that complications can also occur without any surgical procedures being performed. Acute bleeding into the lesion and infection can cause the rapid enlargement of the lymphatic malformation, which can cause interference with feeding and impingement of the airway. Hospital admission for IV antibiotic treatment or airway protection may be necessary.

The greatest opportunity for the successful removal of the lymphatic malformation occurs during the initial surgical procedure. An underestimation of the extent of the lesion and the need for extensive dissection are complications that can be avoided with the use of appropriate radiographic imaging techniques such as CT scanning or magnetic resonance imaging. Such imaging will allow for the accurate staging of the lymphatic malformation, appropriate operative planning, and a prognosis for recurrence.

The site of the lesion dictates the potential surgical complications. The excision of parotid lesions puts the facial nerve at risk. Suprahyoid lesions generally involve many anatomic spaces, and this leads to poor surgical cure rates. The excision of a lesion that extends to the floor of the mouth or the base of the tongue has the potential complication of altering the normal lymphatic drainage, which leads to postoperative tongue swelling with potential airway obstruction; this may result in the need for a partial glossectomy. Prolonged postoperative drainage may be required for serous fluid accumulation that occurs at the operative site.

Infection of the operative site can usually be prevented with the use of preoperative antibiotics that are continued through the early postoperative period. The nerve integrity monitor can be used in the musculature of nerves that are at risk for injury, such as the facial or spinal accessory nerves. Blood loss can be extensive as a result of the size or nature of the resection; it should be anticipated and treated with appropriate blood replacement, if necessary. Meticulous hemostasis should be obtained in conjunction with prolonged wound drainage to prevent postoperative hematoma.

The use of sclerosing agents has altered the management of macrocystic (i.e., large-chambered) lymphatic malformations. Picibanil is an experimental drug that, when injected into the cystic space of the malformation, induces scarring and collapse. It has proved useful in protocols, but repeated injections may be required, and it is accompanied by inflammation, febrile response, and tenderness in the region being treated. It cannot be used in individuals who are allergic to penicillin, because trace elements of the antibiotic are used in the preparation of picibanil.

Adenotonsillectomy

Although adenotonsillectomy is one of the most common procedures performed by otolaryngologists, it may involve significant complications. Bleeding is usually estimated to occur in 1% to 2% of cases, and it may take place late during the course of recovery. There seems to be a slightly higher incidence of bleeding among older children and adults. There is no proven association between increased bleeding and any specific technique used for tonsillectomy, but a number of studies have suggested potential associations. The coblation technique, fine-needle cautery, and cautery have been implicated as potential causes of higher bleeding rates.

Pain is a common occurrence, and it may eventually result in dehydration, with a need for readmission to the hospital for IV fluids. Control of pain can be improved with the preoperative teaching of the parents and caregivers regarding the appropriate use of narcotic and nonnarcotic analgesia. Factors associated with increased pain postoperatively are infection in the operative site and excessive trauma to the surgical site with thermal damage. Postoperative antibiotics have been recommended to diminish the likelihood of infection.

The most common indication for adenotonsillectomy is sleep-disordered breathing. Obstructive sleep apnea is one of the disorders encompassed by this term, and it may be associated with increased sensitivity to narcotics during the postoperative period. Children with severe sleep apnea (defined as a respiratory distress index of >20) should be watched carefully for signs of oversedation during the immediate postoperative period.[45] Increased caution should also be used when treating these patients with respiratory suppressants for pain control. In addition, children who are less than 3 years old are at increased risk for complications postoperatively and should be considered for brief hospital stays after surgery.

CONCLUSIONS

Pediatric patients are subject to specific types of complications as a result of their physiologic differences from adults and because of special problems associated with formative disorders. Preoperative planning and an awareness of the various issues that affect infants and children may help with the avoidance of some of the more common complications that are seen.

REFERENCES

1. Tiret L, Nivoche Y, Ha lton F, et al: Complications related to anesthesia in infants and children. *Br J Anaesth* 1988;61: 263–269.
2. Mulroy JJ, Crone RK: Anesthesia and postoperative care. *Curr Opin Pediatrics* 1990;2:545–549.
3. Komp DM, Selden RF: Coagulation abnormalities in cystic fibrosis. *Chest* 1977;58:501.
4. Morray JP, Krane EJ: Anesthesia for thoracic surgery. In Gregory GA, editor: *Pediatric anesthesia,* ed 2, New York, 1989, Churchill Livingstone.
5. Salem MR, Klowden AJ: Anesthesia for pediatric orthopedic surgery. In Gregory GA, editor: *Pediatric anesthesia,* ed 2, New York, 1989, Churchill Livingstone.
6. Krasna IH, Rosenfeld D, Benjamin BG, et al: Esophageal perforation in the neonate: An emerging problem in the newborn nursery. *J Pediatr Surg* 1987;22:784–790.
7. Blair GK, Filler RM, Theodorescu D: Neonatal pharyngoesophageal perforation mimicking esophageal atresia: Clues to diagnosis. *J Pediatr Surg* 1987;22:770–774.
8. McCarthy TV, Healy JM, Heffron JJ, et al: Localization of the malignant hyperthermia susceptibility locus to human chromosome 19q12-13.2. *Nature* 1990;343:562–564.
9. Dubrow TJ, Wackym PA, Abdul-Rasool IH, et al: Malignant hyperthermia: Experience in the prospective management of eight children. *J Pediatr Surg* 1989;24:163–166.
10. Britt BA, Endrenyl L, Peters PL, et al: Screening of malignant hyperthermia susceptible families by creating phosphokinase measurements and other clinical investigations. *Can Anaesth Soc J* 1976;23:263–284.
11. Sessler DI: Malignant hyperthermia. In Gregory GA, editor: *Pediatric anesthesia,* ed 2, New York, 1989, Churchill Livingstone.
12. Berts EK, Downes JJ: Anesthesia. In Welch KJ, Randolph JG, Ravitch MM, et al, editors: *Pediatric surgery,* ed 4, St Louis, 1986, Mosby-Year Book.
13. Hengerer AS, Strome M: Choanal atresia: New embryologic theory and its influence on surgical management. *Laryngoscope* 1982;92:913–921.
14. Krespi YP, Husain S, Levine TM, et al: Sublabial transseptal repair of choanal atresia or stenosis. *Laryngoscope* 1987;97:1402–1406.
15. Pagon RA, Graham JM, Zonana J, et al: Congenital heart disease and choanal atresia with multiple anomalies: CHARGE association. *J Pediatrics* 1981;99:223–227.
16. Stankiewiez JA: The endoscopic repair of choanal atresia. *Otolaryngol Head Neck Surg* 1990;103:931–937.
17. Freng A: Growth in width of the dental arches after partial extirpation of the midpalatal suture in man. *Scand J Plast Reconstr Surg* 1978;76:429–436.
18. Stahl RS, Jurkiewiez MJ: Congenital posterior choanal atresia. *Pediatrics* 1985;76:429–436.
19. Coniglio JU, Manzione JV, Hengerer AS: Anatomic findings and management of choanal atresia and the CHARGE association. *Ann Otol Rhinol Laryngol* 1988;97:448–453.
20. Asher BF, McGill TJ, Kaplan L, et al: Airway complications in CHARGE association. *Arch Otolaryngol Head Neck Surg* 1990;116:594–595.
21. Teissier N, Kaguelidou F, Couloigner V, François M, Van Den Abbeele T: Predictive factors for success after transnasal endoscopic treatment of choanal atresia. *Arch Otolaryngol Head Neck Surg* 2008;134(1):57–61.
22. Work WP: Newer concepts of first branchia, cleft defects. *Laryngoscope* 1972;9:1581–1587.
23. Gatot A, Tovi F, Fliss DM, et al: Branchial cleft cyst manifesting as hypoglossal nerve palsy. *Head Neck* 1991;13:249–250.
24. Osguthorpe JD, Adkins WY: Carotid arteriospasm. *Laryngoscope* 1985;95:942–944.
25. Horisawa M, Niinomi N, Ito T: Anatomical reconstruction of the thyroglossal duct. *J Pediatr Surg* 1991;26:766–769.
26. Sistrunk WE: Technique of removal of cysts and sinuses of the thyroglossal duct. *Surg Gynecol Obstet* 1928;46:109–114.

27. Hoffman MA, Schuster SR: Thyroglossal duct remnants in infants and children: Reevaluation of histopathology and methods for resection. *Ann Otol Rhinol Laryngol* 1988;97:483–486.

28. Nathanson LK, Gough IR: Surgery for thyroglossal cysts: Sistrunk's operation remains the standard. *Aust N Z J Surg* 1989;59:873–875.

29. Perkins JA, Inglis AF, Sie KC, Manning SC: Recurrent thyroglossal duct cysts: a 23-year experience and a new method for management. *Ann Otol Rhinol Laryngol* 2006;115(11):850–856.

30. Bennett KG, Organ CH Jr, Williams GR: Is the treatment for thyroglossal duct cysts too extensive? *Am J Surg* 1986;153:602–605.

31. Athow AC, Fagg NL, Drake DP: Management of thyroglossal cysts in children. *Br J Surg* 1989;76:811–814.

32. Hawkins DB, Jacobsen BE, Klatt EC: Cysts of the thyroglossal duct. *Laryngoscope* 1982;92:1254–1258.

33. Radkowski D, Arnold J, Healy GB, et al: Thyroglossal duct remnants, preoperative evaluation and management. *Arch Otolaryngol Head Neck Surg* 1991;117:1378–1381.

34. Ratner I, Whitfield J: Acquired subglottic stenosis in the very-low-birth-weight infant. *Am J Dis Child* 1983;137:40–43.

35. Hawkins DB: Pathogenesis of subglottic stenosis from endotracheal intubation. *Ann Otol Rhinol Laryngol* 1987;96:116–117.

36. Quiney RE, Gould SJ: Subglottic stenosis: A clinicopathological study. *Clin Otolaryngol* 1985;10:315–327.

37. Cotton RT, Seid AB: Management of the extubation problem in the premature child. Anterior cricoid split as an alternative to tracheotomy. *Ann Otol Rhinol Laryngol* 1980;89:508–511.

38. Anderson GJ, Tom LWC, Wemore RF, et al: The anterior cricoid split: The Children's Hospital of Philadelphia experience. *Int J Pediatr Otorhinolaryngol* 1988;16:31–38.

39. Holinger LD, Stankiewiez JA, Livingston GL: Anterior cricoid split: The Chicago experience with an alternative to tracheotomy. *Laryngoscope* 1987;97:19–24.

40. Cotton RT: Prevention and management of laryngeal stenosis in infants and children. *J Pediatr Surg* 1985;20:845–851.

41. Grundfast KM, Coffman AC, Milmoe G: Anterior cricoid split: A "simple" surgical procedure and a potentially complicated care problem. *Ann Otol Rhinol Laryngol* 1985;94:445–449.

42. Bagwell CE, Marchildon MB, Pratt LL: Anterior cricoid split for subglottic stenosis. *J Pediatr Surg* 1987;22:740–742.

43. Seid AB, Godin MS, Pransky SM, et al: The prognostic value of endotracheal tube-air leak following tracheal surgery in children. *Arch Otolaryngol Head and Neck Surg* 1991;117:880–882.

44. Richardson MA, Inglis AF: Immediate expansion of the cricoid split with costal cartilage. *Int J Pediatr Otorhinolaryngol* 1991;22:187–193.

45. Richardson MA, Freidman NR: *Clinician's guide to pediatric sleep disorders,* New York, 2007, Informa Healthcare.

CHAPTER 7

Complications of Geriatric Head and Neck Surgery

Eric M. Genden

According to the Department of Health and Human Services report on aging from 2004, persons 65 years old or older numbered 36.3 million in 2004 and represented 12.4% of the U.S. population (i.e., about 1 in every 8 Americans). By 2030, there will be about 71.5 million older persons, and they will make up 20% of the population. The elderly represent the fastest growing subpopulation in North America and Europe. As the average life expectancy increases, physicians and surgeons can expect an increasing number of geriatric patients who need special attention.[1] Undoubtedly a proportion of the elderly will present with diseases of the head and neck that will require surgical therapy. Treating this population requires an appreciation for a variety of issues specific to the elderly, including the effect of age on surgical outcomes, tumor biology, and the risks of both ablative and reconstructive surgery.

PHYSIOLOGY OF AGING

There is great debate regarding the effect of aging on physiology and the mechanisms of aging. It has been suggested that a balance between nature and nurture determine the life span of a human. *Nature* refers to the genetic control over aging, such as programmed cell death and cellular fragility. *Nurture* refers to nongenetic factors such as the environment, nutrition, and physical condition. It is the combination of these elements that are suggested to determine a person's longevity. Although some contend that age results in an inevitable decline in physiologic reserve and the ability to tolerate physical stress,[2,3] others feel that it is the comorbidities associated with advanced age that are responsible for the increased risks of surgery.[4]

Although the mechanisms of longevity remain unresolved, the process of aging has been linked to a variety of well-documented physiologic changes, including progressive declines in immune function, renal function, and endocrine function.[5] Additionally, wound healing is impaired,[6] cardiac ventricles atrophy,[7] and the vasculature becomes less compliant,[8] thereby leading to hypertension. There are also changes that occur in the pulmonary system, including a decrease in chest wall compliance[9,10] and a decline in supporting tissues in the pulmonary airways. These changes have great implications for the management of head and neck surgical patients and the potential complications of surgery among the elderly. Failure to evaluate and preoperatively manage renal, cardiac, or pulmonary failure can result in avoidable complications.

AGE-RELATED RISKS

Many of the physiologic changes associated with age do not represent a direct risk for surgical complications, assuming that the surgical team and the primary care physician work together to preoperatively optimize the patient's medical condition. However, indirectly, the physiologic changes that are characteristic of advanced age can result in a higher risk of surgical morbidity. The normal age-related decline in immunologic function, renal function, and vascular compliance may predispose elderly patients to complications of surgery if these issues are not addressed during the preoperative workup. Routine preoperative laboratory tests including the creatinine level, the blood urea nitrogen level, a complete blood cell count, a chest radiograph, and an electrocardiogram are examples of the screening evaluation that every elderly patient should undergo before surgery. The preoperative workup is the most effective method of identifying the significant problems that may predispose an elderly patient to perioperative complications. The keys to avoiding complications are a thorough workup that is aimed at evaluating the patient's comorbidities and a preoperative plan to optimize the patient's medical conditions before surgery.

The age-related decrease in vascular compliance may lead to hypertension that, if identified and managed before surgery, is not usually associated with an increased risk of complications. However, labile or recalcitrant hypertension can result in more significant complications, including stroke, aortic dissection, and myocardial infarction.[11] Therefore, the condition should be managed aggressively before surgery. Myocardial infarction is the most common cause of postoperative mortality. Thus, the preoperative management of hypertension, cardiac arrhythmia, and congestive heart failure is essential.

Deep vein thrombosis (DVT) remains a serious risk of surgery among the elderly, particularly for the bedridden patient. Although most patients are ambulatory after routine head and neck surgery, more extensive surgical procedures and flap reconstructions can delay a patient's ambulation and increase the risk of DVT. Pneumatic compression boots and subcutaneous heparin are effective for reducing the incidence of DVT after surgery, but there is no substitute for early ambulation. Elderly patients are at higher risk for heparin-related complications, so the dose must be carefully titrated. Among elderly patients with known venous stasis, the elevation of the lower extremities while the patient is in bed can also prove beneficial. Similarly, early ambulation can be very effective for preventing pulmonary complications. Atelectasis can result in a cascade of complications, including pneumonia, which is one of the leading causes of postoperative complications after surgery in the elderly. Although the use of incentive spirometry has been helpful for reducing the incidence of pulmonary complications, preoperative steroids, bronchodilators, and respiratory therapy are examples of measures that are commonly used to optimize pulmonary function. Patients that use tobacco should be discouraged from smoking for at least 2 to 3 days before surgery. Additionally, any surgical procedure that renders an elderly patient bedridden for more that 36 hours carries with it an increased risk of pulmonary complications. Early ambulation and incentive spirometry can be very effective for preventing these complications. In an effort to limit a patient's exposure, it is recommended that, if the primary care physician identifies a moderate or severe compromise in cardiac or pulmonary function, the patient should undergo a preoperative consultation with a specialist. The underlying concept is that the most effective method for managing complications among elderly patients is to avoid those complications in the first place.

PAIN MANGEMENT

Pain management deserves special attention, because it has been suggested that pain tolerance decreases with age. As a result, elderly patients will often request pain management postoperatively. However, even small doses of narcotic pain medication can result in mild side effects (e.g., nausea, vomiting, constipation) or more serious complications (e.g., decreased respiratory drive, hypotension, impaired cognition). An impaired ability to metabolize and clear narcotic analgesics can occur with age and therefore magnify both the effects and the side effects of narcotic pain medication. The liberal use of non-narcotic analgesics is recommended, and, when indicated, a carefully titrated dose of narcotic analgesics can be used to better gauge the patient's response. Pain management specialists can offer expert guidance for elderly patients.

POLYPHARMACY

The term *polypharmacy* is defined as the use of multiple drugs. This is a concern for patients of all ages, but it is particularly concerning for the elderly. Because this patient population commonly suffers from multiple comorbidities, polypharmacy is common. The consequences of polypharmacy include adverse drug reactions and drug interactions. To limit adverse reactions, a complete review of patient medications should be performed before surgery. Sedative and pain medications should be carefully reviewed and discontinued before surgery, and antihypertensive medications and bronchodilators should be reviewed. Patients taking steroids may require a supplemental dose or a "stress dose" of steroids before the induction of anesthesia. Because drug interactions can be complex, it is recommended that the operating surgeon work with the patient's primary care physician to simplify the medication list and eliminate unnecessary medications.

IMPLICATIONS OF AGING ON SURGICAL MORBIDITY

There is evidence to suggest that the geriatric population receives substandard therapy as compared with younger age groups.[12] This is largely believed to be a result of a general perception that elderly patients cannot tolerate a full course of therapy. Although biased attitudes can negatively affect a patient's prognosis, many argue that advanced age is not in itself a criterion for excluding patients from standard treatment with either radiation therapy, chemotherapy, or surgery.[13-15] There is a paucity of data to suggest that age alone is associated with a higher risk of surgical complications. However, the comorbidities associated with age may indirectly affect an elderly patient's ability to tolerate surgery and prolonged anesthesia. One recent study reviewed the American College of Surgeons National Surgical Quality Improvement Program database for patient demographics, preoperative risk factors, intraoperative risk factors, and 30-day outcomes with a focus on those aged 80 years old and older.[16] The authors reviewed 7696 surgical procedures and found that hypertension and dyspnea were the most common risk factors among members of that age group. Preoperative transfusion, emergency operation, and weight loss best predicted morbidity for those 80 years old and older. They also found that the American Society of Anesthesiologists (ASA) classification predicted mortality across all age groups. A 30-minute increment of operative duration increased the odds of mortality by 17% among patients who were more than 80 years old, and postoperative morbidity and mortality increased progressively with increasing age. Age was statistically significantly associated with cardiovascular, renal, respiratory, and wound healing complications. In contrast with several prior studies that demonstrated no relationship between advanced age and surgical morbidity,[13-15] the authors of this important study concluded that increasing age itself is an important risk factor for postoperative morbidity and mortality. It should be understood that, with the exception of this study, the majority of reports on this topic suggest that age itself is not a contraindication to surgical therapy.

As the population grows older, surgeons are more commonly faced with the dilemma of directing therapy for the elderly population, many of whom have complex medical problems. Because geriatric patients often have a higher degree of medical complexity than their younger counterparts, a comprehensive assessment may provide crucial information and help to determine the actual risk associated with therapy. There is no consensus regarding the optimal tool for assessment; however, there are several tools available, including the ASA physical status system, the Goldman Cardiac Risk Index,[17] and the Acute Physiological and Chronic Health Evaluation.[18]

An international project to help better define the general health condition of geriatric surgical candidates has been instrumental in the development of the PACE assessment tool. The PACE tool is an instrument that was generated from work at the National Institutes of Health that focused on medical decision making for the geriatric patient.[19] The PACE tool incorporates several previously described instruments that are currently used for surgical risk assessment, including the Mini Mental State Examination,[20] the Eastern Cooperative Oncology Group Performance Status,[21] the ASA Scale, and the Physiological and Operative Severity Score for enUmeration of Mortality and Morbidity (POSSUM).[22]

Results are now available from an interim analysis of 215 patients who were entered from seven recruiting centers in the United Kingdom, Italy, the Netherlands, and Japan; the authors of this landmark work conclude that the aspects of PACE that relate to psychologic well-being do not appear to be significantly associated with postoperative complications.[23] By contrast, aspects that relate to physical frailty and morbidity (i.e., Activities of Daily Living, Instrumental Activities of Daily Living) seem to best predict surgical complications.

IMPLICATIONS OF AGING ON TUMOR BIOLOGY

Cancer is a disease that disproportionately affects the elderly. The elderly have an 11-fold increased incidence of cancer as compared with their younger counterparts and a 15-fold increase of cancer-related mortality.[24,25] The impact of age on tumor formation and tumor biology is an interesting topic; however, there is little data to suggest that tumors in the elderly are more aggressive than those found in their younger counterparts. There are several theories regarding the impact of age on tumor biology. One theory suggests that tumor formation results from carcinogen exposure and an accumulation of cellular events that ultimately lead to malignant transformation. Because older patients have extended exposure to carcinogens, they are considered to be more vulnerable to the development of cancer. Other theories include an increase in oncogenic activation that has been suggested to occur with an age-related decrease in tumor-suppressor gene activity. Although these theories may account for the observed higher incidence of malignancy among the older population, it does not suggest altered biology or clinical behavior.

Advanced age has been associated with a decline in immune surveillance and the development of faulty DNA repair mechanisms.[26] Although these mechanisms are related to cellular replication, the relationship between age and malignancy remains unproven. Koch and colleagues[27] investigated biologic and epidemiologic factors associated with the development of head and neck squamous cell carcinoma. They found that individuals who developed squamous cell cancer of the head and neck after the age of 75 years demonstrated genetic changes less often than younger patients and that heavy carcinogen exposure and p53 gene mutations are present less often among elderly individuals.

IMPLICATIONS OF AGING ON NONSURGICAL THERAPY

There appears to be a considerable paradigm shift in the management of advanced head and neck cancer from primary surgical therapy to combined chemoradiation. The majority of patients with cancers of the oropharynx and the laryngopharyngeal area are now treated with combined chemoradiation. This has generated considerable debate regarding whether the elderly patients can tolerate chemoradiation therapy for a period of 2 to 3 months; however, the majority of the chemotherapy protocols do not include elderly patients in their studies. One does need to keep in mind that salvage surgery in elderly individuals may be extremely complex and that the patients may not tolerate salvage surgery. Clayman and colleagues[28] reviewed 43 patients who were 80 years old and older in a case-control study. Only 23.3% of the octogenarians were treated with adjuvant therapy, whereas 44.1% of the younger controls received adjuvant therapy. The authors found that multimodality therapy among the octogenarian population may be limited by the patient. Similarly, postoperative radiation therapy may not be well tolerated by elderly patients. The authors point out that, after major surgery, the patient and the family may refuse postoperative radiation therapy, especially if the patient had postoperative complications related to surgery. It is not uncommon for the patient and the family to refuse surgery, especially if the patient is going to be transferred to a long-term care facility or a nursing home. The authors suggest that the majority of literature regarding this topic exclusively focuses on epidemiologic aspects or on the therapeutic consequences. Psychosocial aspects are less interesting, although the psychosocial status of elderly patients has a significant impact on the course of the disease, highlighting both the predilection for less aggressive and substandard therapy among the elderly and the likely misperception that age may adversely affect disease-free survival.

IMPLICATIONS OF AGING ON SURGICAL RECONSTRUCTION

The goal of reconstruction of the head and neck is to restore speech and swallowing to as close to the preoperative state as possible. Local tissue flaps (e.g., cervicofacial advancement flaps) often provide a simple means of reconstruction. However, extensive defects often represent a reconstructive challenge, particularly among elderly patients. Because elderly patients experience a progressive age-related demyelination process[29] that may affect functional performance by decreasing sensation and muscular coordination, elderly patients tend to be more vulnerable to the functional morbidity that is associated with surgery and reconstruction. For these reasons, it is imperative to restore the native anatomy and to reestablish sensation in an effort to achieve optimal functional rehabilitation.

Although the extent of ablative surgery for head and neck malignancies is often determined by the nature of the primary lesion, the method of reconstruction is usually left to the discretion of the surgeon. Limited defects may be managed with local flaps and skin grafts, but extensive defects that are not amenable to local flap reconstruction often require either regional pedicled flaps or microvascular free tissue transfer. Regional pedicled flaps offer an efficient reconstructive alternative to free tissue transfer. However, although there are few age-specific risks, there are several age-related risks associated with regional pedicled flaps. Some authors[30] found that patients with preexisting pulmonary disease may be at higher risk for pulmonary complications, including pulmonary atelectasis and restrictive lung disease, after pectoralis flap harvest. Talmi and colleagues[31] prospectively evaluated the effects of pectoralis muscle harvest on pulmonary function and found that, although patients with normal preoperative pulmonary function performed well postoperatively, patients with severe preexisting pulmonary disorders had a decrease in forced vital capacity. However, the degree of pulmonary dysfunction is related to the size of the skin paddle, and pulmonary restriction seldom occurred when the skin paddle was less than 40 cm^2.[32]

Since the early 1990s, concern regarding the safety of free flap reconstruction for elderly patients has resulted in a number of studies examining the indications and limitations of free tissue transfer in the geriatric population. Early reports found that major complications in the elderly population after free tissue transfer occurred in those patients with "significant underlying medical problems."[33] It has been suggested that the ASA classification of patients provided a predictor of postoperative medical and surgical morbidity.[34] Shaari and colleagues[35] found that, although free tissue transfer can be performed safely in the elderly, when postoperative complications occur, they are most commonly pulmonary and cardiovascular in nature. Microvascular free flap reconstruction always generates considerable debate with regard to elderly patients, especially octogenarians. Clearly, the free flap will increase the duration of surgery by a number of hours. This occasionally may be detrimental to the patient's general health, and it may precipitate comorbid complications and cardiac problems.

Similar to the data related to ablative surgery, the safety of free tissue transfer for elderly patients appears to be related to the medical condition of the patient rather than the age of the patient. This concept also holds true for elderly patients who have been previously treated surgically or with combination medical therapy. Reece and colleagues[36] reviewed 66 elderly cancer patients who underwent tumor resection and free tissue transfer after previous radiotherapy, chemotherapy, or both and compared them with a similar group of 64 elderly patients who had not received such previous therapy. The authors found that previous cancer treatment did not predispose elderly patients to a higher rate of flap failure or wound-healing problems after reconstruction. The management of head and neck cancer in elderly patients continues to be a great challenge for the treating physician. Although family wishes need to be respected, it is important to explain the optimal treatment for controlling the cancer. Both the patient and the family should be educated. The comorbid conditions and quality of life issues need to be put in proper perspective; however, the physician should make every effort to offer the best and standard treatment, especially for patients with advanced head and neck cancer.

As surgery has been extended into the elderly population, health-related quality of life (HRQOL) has been appropriately added as a parameter to evaluate surgical success. Surgery remains of significant risk for older patients, and an estimate of the potential outcomes, including morbidity, mortality, and HRQOL, can aid in that decision. New techniques, such as laparoscopic or minimally invasive surgery, show great promise for the reduction of perioperative stress and for improved HRQOL in the elderly population.[37]

REFERENCES

1. Weiss MF, Lesnick GJ: Surgery in the elderly: Attitudes and facts. *Mt Sinai J Med* 1980;47(2):208–214.
2. Ramesh HS, et al: Optimising surgical management of elderly cancer patients. *World J Surg Oncol* 2005;3(1):17–22.
3. Audisio RA, et al: Elective surgery for gastrointestinal tumours in the elderly. *Ann Oncol* 1997;8(4):317–326.
4. Yancik R, et al: Effect of age and comorbidity in postmeno-pausal breast cancer patients aged 55 years and older. *JAMA* 2001;285(7):885–992.
5. Tsaih SW, et al: Lead, diabetes, hypertension, and renal function: The normative aging study. *Environ Health Perspect* 2004;112(11):1178–1182.
6. Rochon PA, Gurwitz JH: Drug therapy. *Lancet* 1995;346(8966): 32–36.
7. Gerstenblith G, et al: Echocardiographic assessment of a normal adult aging population. *Circulation* 1977;56(2):273–278.
8. Vaitkevicius PV, et al: Effects of age and aerobic capacity on arterial stiffness in healthy adults. *Circulation* 1993;88(4 Pt 1): 1456–1462.
9. Janssens JP, Pache JC, Nicod LP: Physiological changes in respiratory function associated with aging. *Eur Respir J* 1999;13(1):197–205.
10. Edge JR, et al: The radiographic appearances of the chest in persons of advanced age. *Br J Radiol* 1964;37:769–774.
11. Elliott WJ: Clinical features in the management of selected hyper-tensive emergencies. *Prog Cardiovasc Dis* 2006;48(5):316–325.
12. Samet J, et al: Choice of cancer therapy varies with age of patient. *JAMA* 1986;255(24):3385–3390.
13. Greimel ER, Padilla GV, Grant MM: Physical and psychosocial outcomes in cancer patients: A comparison of different age groups. *Br J Cancer* 1997;76(2):251–255.
14. Karl RC, Smith SK, Fabri PJ: Validity of major cancer operations in elderly patients. *Ann Surg Oncol* 1995;2(2):107–113.
15. Chin R, et al: Oropharyngeal cancer in the elderly. *Int J Radiat Oncol Biol Phys* 1995;32(4):1007–1016.
16. Turrentine FE, et al: Surgical risk factors, morbidity, and mortality in elderly patients. *J Am Coll Surg* 2006;203(6):865–877.
17. Goldman L, et al: Multifactorial index of cardiac risk in noncardiac surgical procedures. *N Engl J Med* 1977;297(16):845–850.
18. Knaus WA, et al: APACHE-acute physiology and chronic health evaluation: A physiologically based classification system. *Crit Care Med* 1981;9(8):591–597.
19. Balstad A, Springer P: Quantifying case management work-loads: Development of the PACE tool. *Lippincotts Case Manag* 2006;11(6):291–304.
20. Folstein MF, Folstein SE, McHugh PR: "Mini-mental state": A practical method for grading the cognitive state of patients for the clinician. *J Psychiatr Res* 1975;12(3):89–198.
21. Repetto L, et al: Comprehensive geriatric assessment adds information to Eastern Cooperative Oncology Group performance status in elderly cancer patients: An Italian Group for Geriatric Oncology Study. *J Clin Oncol* 2002;20(2):494–502.
22. Prytherch DR, et al: POSSUM and Portsmouth POSSUM for predicting mortality. Physiological and Operative Severity Score for the enUmeration of Mortality and Morbidity. *Br J Surg* 1998;85(9):1217–1220.
23. Lawrence VA, et al: Risk of pulmonary complications after elective abdominal surgery. *Chest* 1996;110(3):744–750.
24. Yancik R: Cancer burden in the aged: An epidemiologic and demographic overview. *Cancer* 1997;80(7):1273–1283.
25. Yancik R, Ries LA: Aging and cancer in America: Demographic and epidemiologic perspectives. *Hematol Oncol Clin North Am* 2000;14(1):17–23.
26. Wei Q, et al: DNA repair and aging in basal cell carcinoma: A molecular epidemiology study. *Proc Natl Acad Sci USA* 1993;90(4):1614–1618.
27. Koch WM, et al: Squamous cell carcinoma of the head and neck in the elderly. *Arch Otolaryngol Head Neck Surg* 1995;121(3): 262–265.
28. Clayman GL, et al: Surgical outcomes in head and neck cancer patients 80 years of age and older. *Head Neck* 1998;20(3): 216–223.
29. Bhattacharyya N: A matched survival analysis for squamous cell carcinoma of the head and neck in the elderly. *Laryngoscope* 2003;113(2):368–372.
30. Kowalski LP, et al: A case-control study on complications and sur-vival in elderly patients undergoing major head and neck surgery. *Am J Surg* 1994;168(5):485–490.
31. Talmi YP, et al: Pulmonary function after pectoralis major myocu-taneous flap harvest. *Laryngoscope* 2002;112(3):467–471.
32. Schuller DE, et al: Analysis of frequency of pulmonary atelectasis in patients undergoing pectoralis major musculocutaneous flap reconstruction. *Head Neck* 1994;16(1):25–29.
33. Singh B, et al: Outcome differences in younger and older patients with laryngeal cancer: A retrospective case-control study. *Am J Otolaryngol* 2000;21(2):92–97.
34. Serletti JM, et al: Factors affecting outcome in free-tissue transfer in the elderly. *Plast Reconstr Surg* 2000;106(1):66–70.
35. Shaari CM, et al: Complications of microvascular head and neck surgery in the elderly. *Arch Otolaryngol Head Neck Surg* 1998;124(4):407–411.
36. Reece GP, et al: Morbidity associated with free-tissue transfer after radiotherapy and chemotherapy in elderly cancer patients. *J Reconstr Microsurg* 1994;10(6):375–382.
37. Hornick TR: Surgical innovations: Impact on the quality of life of the older patient. *Clin Geriatr Med* 2006;22(3):499–513.

CHAPTER 8

Endocrine Complications of Head and Neck Surgery

Mimi I. Hu and Steven I. Sherman

Surgical therapy of endocrine gland dysfunction may be associated with morbidity characteristic of the underlying endocrinopathy, such as decompensated thyrotoxicosis after surgery for hyperthyroidism. Endocrine deficiency states often result from the excision of a secretory gland or from preoperative hypofunction, thereby increasing the surgical risk if not corrected. As a consequence of mass lesions or of surgery on the endocrine organs, potentially life-threatening injuries to the surrounding structures can occur. The morbidity of these endocrine complications of head and neck surgery can be minimized or avoided with appropriate preoperative assessment and anticipatory perioperative management of the surgical patient.

THYROID SURGERY

Thyroid resection for benign disease is typically reserved for patients who refuse radioactive iodine ablation, who develop severe side effects from medical therapy (especially during pregnancy), or who have very large goiters.[1] Additionally, surgery may provide relief of obstructive symptoms (e.g., dysphagia, pain, tracheal compromise causing stridor or shortness of breath), allow cosmesis, or prevent the exacerbation of severe Graves' ophthalmopathy.[2] Thyrotoxicosis caused by toxic multinodular goiter or a solitary toxic nodule is another indication for surgery, which may cure the mass lesion more effectively than iodine-131. Toxic multinodular goiters tend to have lower radioiodine uptakes, thus requiring larger doses of radioactivity to ablate the thyroid. The treatment of hyperfunctioning solitary nodules with large doses of radioiodine may lead to excessive postablative hypothyroidism.[1] Although the role of thyroidectomy for the differential diagnosis of thyroid neoplasia has declined as a result of the availability of fine-needle aspiration biopsy, surgery remains the preferred initial therapy for well-differentiated carcinoma (e.g., papillary, follicular, medullary) and for the debulking of anaplastic carcinoma. The inability to adequately exclude malignancy on clinical and cytologic grounds is an indication for the surgical excision of benign nodules or goiter.

Preoperative Evaluation

In anticipation of thyroid surgery, patients require both general medical and thyroid-specific assessment to identify and minimize their surgical and anesthetic risks.

Evaluation should focus on the cardiovascular and pulmonary systems, the medical and surgical history, and current medications. This review should also include an assessment of thyroid function, a determination of the presence of laryngeal nerve compromise or upper airway compression, and an evaluation of the potential for associated endocrine conditions (e.g., multiple endocrine neoplasia type 2 [MEN2], radiation-induced parathyroid adenoma). Selected laboratory and imaging studies can be helpful for determining these risks and for directing preoperative and intraoperative management for minimizing them.

Clinical Assessment

Most patients undergoing thyroidectomy are euthyroid. Exceptions include patients whose indication for surgery is thyrotoxicosis and those with iatrogenic hypothyroidism as a result of previous gland irradiation or antithyroid drugs. The classic signs and symptoms of thyrotoxicosis should be sought, but they may be absent in elderly patients with apathetic thyrotoxicosis. This syndrome is characterized predominantly by cardiovascular signs and symptoms, depression or lethargy, muscle weakness, or weight loss; these patients typically lack sympathomimetic symptoms. Clinical manifestations of hypothyroidism may also be subtle or absent, particularly among older patients.

Among patients undergoing surgery for known or potential thyroid malignancies, careful palpation for cervical adenopathy is essential given the frequency of cervical metastases with papillary thyroid carcinoma.[3] Clinical features suggestive of familial medullary thyroid carcinoma or MEN2 include the following: flushing, diarrhea, or pruritus with medullary thyroid carcinoma; renal stones or hypercalcemia with hyperparathyroidism; or severe or paroxysmal hypertension, palpitations, headache, or diaphoresis with pheochromocytoma. For the patient with medullary carcinoma, physical findings that may suggest MEN2B include neuromas of the tongue and of the buccal and conjunctival mucosa as well as a Marfanoid habitus.

Biochemical Assessment

When there is little clinical suspicion of hyperthyroidism or hypothyroidism, a serum thyroid-stimulating hormone (TSH) determination with a highly sensitive assay is appropriate. Third-generation TSH chemiluminometric assays with detection limits of about 0.01 milli-international units/ml can detect both a suppressed TSH typical of hyperthyroidism (even mild cases) and an elevated TSH typical of hypothyroidism.[3,4]

When hyperthyroidism is suspected or likely, serum for free thyroxine (T_4) or free triiodothyronine (T_3) and TSH should be evaluated to confirm the diagnosis, stratify perioperative risk, and monitor the response to antithyroid drug therapy. For most forms of hyperthyroidism that require surgery, the serum T_3 level is more elevated than the T_4 level. Furthermore, T_3 toxicosis can exist alone in the absence of T_4 elevations.

Primary hypothyroidism is confirmed by hypothyroxinemia (low free T_4) and an elevated serum TSH. Subclinical hypothyroidism, which is defined as an elevation of the serum TSH in the presence of a normal free T_4 concentration, occurs in approximately 4% to 8.5% of the adult U.S. population without known thyroid disease, with an increase to 20% among women who are more than 60 years old. There are insufficient data to support the association of subclinical hypothyroidism or any benefit of treatment with adverse cardiac end points (including atherosclerotic disease and cardiovascular mortality).[5] Difficulty with the diagnosis of primary hypothyroidism can arise when the TSH is not elevated in the presence of hypothyroxinemia, which occurs frequently in patients with conditions of severe nonthyroidal illness (i.e., the so-called *euthyroid sick syndrome*) as well as in those with secondary or tertiary causes of hypothyroidism. In cases of nonthyroidal illness, the abnormal binding of T_4 to serum transport proteins, the decreased peripheral conversion of T_4 to T_3, and the suppression of TSH production result in low free T_4 and T_3 levels without a compensatory TSH rise. In these patients, elevation in the T_3 resin uptake frequently reflects the plasma protein binding abnormality, and it can serve as a marker of the condition. The significance of nonthyroidal illness as a risk factor for increased perioperative morbidity is not known, and there is no clear evidence to support the need for thyroid hormone replacement.[6]

Recent guidelines for the diagnosis and management of thyroid nodules recommend an efficient strategy for laboratory testing by starting with an evaluation of the serum TSH level. If it is normal, no further testing is warranted. If the TSH level is high, the patient should be evaluated for hypothyroidism with the use of free T_4 and thyroid peroxidase antibody levels. If the TSH level is low, then the patient should be evaluated for hyperthyroidism with the use of free T_4 and T_3 levels.[3]

Imaging Studies

Radioactive isotopes of iodine and technetium can be used to evaluate the structure and function of the thyroid. In hyperthyroid patients, the fractional uptake by the thyroid of a tracer dose may help distinguish conditions in which there is gland hyperfunction (e.g., Graves' disease) from inflammatory thyroiditis or exogenous hyperthyroidism. A thyroid scan can reveal the diffuse inhomogeneous uptake typical of autoimmune thyroiditis; it can demonstrate hypofunctioning and hyperfunctioning nodules, and, when the whole body is examined; it can localize ectopic thyroid tissue and metastases from well-differentiated thyroid carcinomas. Scanning with radioactive iodine can distinguish most substernal goiters from other anterior mediastinal masses.

Ultrasound imaging of the thyroid is useful for the examination of nodules, and it is currently recommended for all patients with one or more suspected thyroid nodules.[7] It can measure lesion dimensions to evaluate the efficacy of suppression therapy, differentiate thyroidal from extrathyroidal lesions, detect nonpalpable nodules in patients exposed to ionizing radiation, guide fine-needle aspiration biopsy when a nodule is not readily accessible to unguided percutaneous biopsy, identify other intrathyroidal nodules suspicious for malignancy (i.e., hypoechogenicity, irregular margins, intranodular vascularity, microcalcifications),[8] and evaluate for the presence of metastatic cervical lymphadenopathy in cases of thyroid carcinoma.

Cross-sectional anatomic imaging of the thyroid with computed tomography (CT) scanning and magnetic resonance imaging (MRI) have limited applications. The indications for CT scanning and MRI are to assess the relationship of thyroid tissue with adjacent cervical and intrathoracic structures (e.g., carotid and jugular vessels, esophagus, lymph nodes, trachea) and to identify metastases or invasion by thyroid malignancies.

Airway Evaluation

Patients with compression or invasion of the trachea may present with cough, hemoptysis, wheezing, dyspnea, or positional stridor. With extrathoracic compression, stridor is classically inspiratory and exacerbated by increased airflow. Flow-volume determinations during spirometry identify functionally significant tracheal narrowing, distinguish intrathoracic from extrathoracic obstruction, and differentiate fixed blockages (e.g., benign goiter) from variable blockages (e.g., vocal cord paralysis, intraluminal invasion by tumor).

Associated Endocrine Conditions

Patients with a preoperative diagnosis of or a suspicion for medullary thyroid carcinoma (MTC) must be evaluated for MEN2A and MEN2B, which occur in 25% of cases.[9] A pheochromocytoma can be present in approximately 50% of patients with MEN2, and it usually occurs after the development of MTC, although it precedes the onset of MTC in 10% of cases.[10] Because of the significant perioperative risk of hypertensive crisis and cardiovascular compromise associated with pheochromocytoma, a determination of plasma metanephrine levels is necessary to rule out the disease before surgery in all patients with known medullary carcinoma.[11] When a pheochromocytoma is present, its treatment should take surgical precedence over medullary carcinoma.[9]

Hyperparathyroidism is present in approximately 20% of patients with MEN2A; it is not a component of MEN2B. Hypercalcemia and the concomitant elevation of the intact parathyroid hormone level (iPTH) are diagnostic of primary hyperparathyroidism. Its treatment should be coordinated with thyroid surgery.

Preoperative Management

Hyperthyroidism

Before the introduction of effective preoperative medical therapy, surgery in the hyperthyroid patient had a 20% to 40% mortality rate, primarily as a result of complications of decompensated thyrotoxicosis or thyroid storm (Box 8-1).[12,13] This multisystem syndrome may be precipitated by surgery or infection in inadequately treated thyrotoxic patients. Older patients, patients with intrinsic cardiopulmonary disease, and those with more severe hyperthyroxinemia are more likely to develop the syndrome. With proper medical preparation, decompensated thyrotoxicosis and perioperative mortality are now rarely reported outcomes.[14–16]

Decompensated thyrotoxicosis can be prevented by appropriate preoperative medical therapy with the goal of a euthyroid state. Several preparative regimens effectively target various points of thyroid hormone production, conversion, or action. Thionamide antithyroid drugs (methimazole [MMI], propylthiouracil [PTU], and carbimazole [not available in the United States]) are the

foundations of effective preoperative preparation, and they usually restore the patient to the euthyroid state within 1 to 3 months. These drugs inhibit thyroid hormone biosynthesis by inhibiting the intrathyroidal organification of iodine. MMI has a longer duration of action and a greater likelihood of effectiveness with a single daily dose. In the severely thyrotoxic patient, however, PTU has the advantage of partially blocking the peripheral conversion of T_4 to T_3 and, consequently, the rapid reduction of serum T_3 levels. PTU is also the preferred agent for pregnant women as a result of its lower transplacental passage and of reports of congenital cutis aplasia after fetal exposure to MMI.[17]

Pharmacologic doses of stable iodine cause a rapid decrease in the release and further synthesis of thyroid hormone. Because there is a physiologic escape from this effect, iodine administration should be initiated 10 to 14 days before elective surgery. Preoperative iodine administration can also reduce thyroid gland vascularity, thereby reducing blood loss in surgery for Graves' disease or diffuse toxic multinodular goiter.[18,19] Typically, 50 to 500 mg/day of iodide should be given in divided doses. Available forms include Lugol solution (6 mg per drop) and saturated solution of potassium iodide (50 mg per drop). Sodium iodide can be administered intravenously (IV) in a dose of 0.5 to 1.0 g/day when the oral route is not available. After therapy with iodide alone, serum T_4 and T_3 concentrations reach a nadir of approximately 50% of their initial levels within 4 to 6 days. The oral cholecystographic agent sodium ipodate, which contains iodine, not only inhibits the glandular production of thyroid hormones but also rapidly blocks the extrathyroidal conversion of T_4 to T_3. Thyrotoxicosis is ameliorated within 3 to 5 days of the oral administration of ipodate (1 g/day). As a result of the initial use of iodine as a substrate for new hormone synthesis, which can potentiate thyrotoxicosis, the administration of iodine should be delayed at least 1 hour after thionamide administration.[20]

Lithium carbonate is an alternative if patients have histories of severe allergic reactions to or side effects from previous exposure to thionamides or iodine. Lithium inhibits the release of thyroid hormone as long as it is administered without the "escape" phenomenon seen with iodine. Lithium is initiated at 300 mg by mouth every 6 hours, with titration to keep serum levels at approximately 1 mEq/L.[21]

The blockade of β-adrenergic receptors (with propranolol, metoprolol, atenolol, or esmolol) reduces the complications of thyroidectomy in hyperthyroidism. The rapid reduction of tachycardia is achieved, although complete normalization should be avoided to allow hemodynamic compensation for blood loss and possible perioperative hypotension. Propranolol in high doses has an additional

---

BOX 8-1 Clinical Presentation of Thyroid Storm

Fever
Cardiovascular effects

- Arrhythmia (sinus tachycardia, atrial fibrillation)
- Congestive heart failure
- Hypotension

Central nervous system effects

- Agitation
- Emotional lability
- Confusion
- Seizures
- Psychosis
- Coma
- Cerebrovascular accident

Gastrointestinal effects

- Abdominal pain
- Vomiting
- Diarrhea
- Jaundice

effect of inhibiting the extrathyroidal conversion of T_4 to T_3; however, this process occurs slowly over a week and does not provide significant clinical benefit.[22] Thus, longer-acting β-blockers are the preferred agents as a result of their less frequent dosing and prolonged duration of effect.[12] Additionally, β-blockers should be used with caution for patients with congestive heart failure or asthma. They should not be used alone in severely hyperthyroxinemic or older patients, because decompensated thyrotoxicosis has occurred.[23]

Combination preoperative regimens are particularly effective. Thionamides may be used until biochemical euthyroidism is achieved, with the subsequent addition of iodine to reduce glandular vascularity. Short-term therapy with a β-adrenergic receptor blocker and iodine may be similarly effective for preventing complications.

In summary, most hyperthyroid patients require aggressive preoperative treatment using a combination of prolonged antithyroid drug therapy, β-adrenergic receptor blockade, and 10 to 14 days of preoperative iodine. The goal in these patients is clinical and biochemical euthyroidism before surgery. Occasionally, young patients or those with particularly mild thyrotoxicosis may undergo surgery without additional risk if they are pretreated with a β-adrenergic receptor blocker to maintain their resting pulse rate at less than 100 beats per minute. After thyroidectomy, antithyroid medications can be discontinued and β-adrenergic receptor blockade tapered over several days. For pregnant patients, thyroidectomy can be performed after preparation with propranolol and PTU. Because compressive fetal goiters can result from prolonged in utero exposure to pharmacologic doses of iodides, these agents should be avoided in all but the severely thyrotoxic pregnant patient.

Hypothyroidism

Surgery in the hypothyroid patient is associated with increased frequencies of intraoperative hypotension and postoperative ileus, constipation, and neuropsychiatric symptoms (e.g., confusion).[24] Recently, a large prospective study of patients with subclinical and overt hypothyroidism did not demonstrate any differences in cardiovascular outcomes (coronary heart disease) or mortality (cardiovascular and all-cause deaths).[25] Overall, there is no significant increase in mortality, days of hospitalization, or days of intensive care therapy among hypothyroid surgical patients.

Nonetheless, when surgery is elective, the hypothyroid patient should ideally be made euthyroid preoperatively. L-Thyroxine is the drug of choice (1.8 mcg/kg/day), with adjustment every 4 weeks until the serum TSH concentration is normalized.[26] For older patients who have lower levothyroxine clearance rates, 50% to 75% lower initial doses are recommended to avoid symptoms of overreplacement. Because full thyroid hormone replacement can worsen myocardial ischemia in patients with coronary artery disease, it may be advisable to withhold full replacement therapy until after revascularization procedures.[27,28] When urgent surgery is required for the hypothyroid patient, lower doses of anesthetic medications may be required to avoid respiratory insufficiency and prolonged ventilatory support. The use of hypotonic IV fluids should be minimized to prevent hyponatremia. Despite equivalent rates of infection, hypothyroid patients are significantly less likely to have fever as a result of decreased thermogenesis, and they require vigilant evaluation for perioperative infection.

Perioperative Management

The perioperative course of patients undergoing thyroid surgery should typically be uneventful. Decompensated thyrotoxicosis is a rare but serious event. Hypocalcemia (with or without hypoparathyroidism) and vocal fold paralysis as a result of recurrent laryngeal nerve injury occur more commonly. Permanent hypothyroidism often follows even partial thyroidectomy; late hypothyroidism may occur in patients with Graves' disease as a result of the autoimmune destruction of the remaining thyroid tissue. Complications such as bleeding, hematoma formation, air embolism, and hypotension as a result of carotid sinus manipulation are rarely seen.

Decompensated Thyrotoxicosis

The management of decompensated thyrotoxicosis includes hemodynamic and fluid support as well as the treatment of precipitating conditions such as infection or thromboembolism. The synthesis of thyroid hormones is inhibited by PTU (200 mg by mouth or nasogastric tube every 4 to 6 hours) or MMI (20 mg by mouth or nasogastric tube every 4 hours). Although PTU may have potential additional value for its suppressive effect on the peripheral conversion of T_4 to T_3, MMI is considered the thionamide of choice by some specialists (especially if it is used in conjunction with another agent that can block peripheral thyroxine conversion) because of its longer duration of effect and its greater potency.[29] When the oral route is unavailable, methimazole (60 mg)[30] or PTU (400 mg enema or 200 mg polyethylene glycol suppository)[31] can be administered rectally. Recently, two patients with thyrotoxicosis were successfully treated with intravenous MMI.[32] To block the release of existing hormone from the thyroid gland, iodine is administered at least 1 hour after the initial dose of thionamide as a saturated solution of potassium iodide (5–8 drops every 6 hours), Lugol solution (10 drops three times daily), or ipodate or iopanoic acid (0.5–1.0 gm orally once daily). Unfortunately, ipodate and iopanoic acid are currently not available in the United States. Iodine has also been given both intravenously and rectally.[33] Therapy to reduce the effects of thyroid hormones in target organs includes the blockade of β-adrenergic receptors. Propranolol is given orally (80–120 mg every 6 hours) or intravenously (initial bolus of 0.5–1.0 mg over 10 minutes, followed by 1–3 mg over 10 minutes every few hours to titrate until the pulse is slowed to about 100 beats per minute), with careful observation for congestive heart failure or reactive airway disease.[20] Esmolol, which is a short-acting β_1-selective blocker, can be administered as a continuous intravenous infusion (bolus 0.25–0.5 mg/kg over 10 minutes, followed by continuous infusion 0.05–0.1 mg/kg/min).[34,35] Glucocorticoid therapy is effective for its ability to block the peripheral conversion of T_4 to T_3, and it should probably be given in doses equivalent to hydrocortisone 100 mg every 8 hours. The febrile patient should be rapidly cooled using cooling blankets and ice packs. Acetaminophen should be used for the medical management of fever rather than aspirin, which can displace T_4 from thyroid-binding globulin and worsen thyrotoxicosis.[20] Fluid, electrolyte, nutritional, and respiratory support are essential.

Hypocalcemia

Transient hypocalcemia after thyroidectomy is common, with reported incidences ranging from 10% to 30%. Permanent hypocalcemia as a result of hypoparathyroidism occurs in 0.4% to 2.5% of total thyroidectomy patients.[36–41] These incidence rates of hypocalcemia are highly dependent on the surgeon's level of experience with thyroid resection, the extent of surgery, and presence of hyperthyroidism. Symptoms of acute mild hypocalcemia include circumoral and distal extremity paresthesia and muscle cramps. Tetany, laryngospasm, seizures, and cardiac arrhythmias may occur with severe hypocalcemia. Chvostek's (facial twitch elicited by tapping the facial nerve) and Trousseau's (wrist flexion induced by brachial artery occlusion with a blood pressure cuff) signs, which indicate neuromuscular irritability, may develop when the serum calcium level is less than 8 mg/dl. Total serum calcium (corrected for the albumin) or ionized calcium levels can be monitored postoperatively; however, the ionized calcium level may be highly variable as a result of transient changes in the pH balance of the patient. Ionized calcium is considered to be more clinically relevant, because it is the physiologically active form of serum calcium.[42] Therapeutic decisions based on calcium levels should include the consideration of the patient's overall clinical status at the time of the blood draw and the presence of hypocalcemic signs or symptoms.

Postoperative hypoparathyroidism is the major cause of hypocalcemia in patients undergoing thyroid resection. Compromise of the vascular supply to the parathyroid glands (primarily derived from the inferior thyroid arteries, in most patients) occurs more frequently than the actual resection of the glands in procedures such as subtotal thyroidectomy.[43] More extensive procedures (e.g., total thyroidectomy, central neck dissection) are more often associated with direct physical removal as well as ischemic damage to the parathyroid glands. Although the incidence of incidental parathyroid removal during thyroidectomy ranges from 8% to 19%, there does not seem to be an increased incidence of hypocalcemia in these situations in some series.[44,45] Alternatively, the preservation of as much functional parathyroid tissue in situ as possible is the goal to minimize permanent hypoparathyroidism. When parathyroid resection is recognized intraoperatively, permanent hypoparathyroidism can be prevented by the autotransplantation of one or more glands.[46,47]

Postoperative laboratory findings consistent with hypoparathyroidism are hypocalcemia, hyperphosphatemia, metabolic alkalosis, relative hypercalciuria, and inappropriately low iPTH levels. In patients with liver disease or malnutrition, magnesium deficiency causes impaired PTH secretion and end-organ resistance to the actions of PTH; this condition should be treated if present.[48]

Thyrotoxicosis leads to accelerated bone turnover, negative calcium balance, and osteopenia.[49] As a consequence of longstanding bone demineralization leading to osteodystrophy, thyrotoxic patients have a higher rate of postoperative hypocalcemia associated with remineralization.[50,51] This process, which is known as *hungry bone syndrome,* is characterized by hypocalcemia, hypophosphatemia, hypomagnesemia, an elevated alkaline phosphatase level, and hypocalciuria.[52] With prolonged preoperative antithyroid therapy, this syndrome may be avoided, although one case has been reported to occur after successful treatment with MMI and radioactive iodine in a patient with thyrotoxicosis.[53]

For the last decade, much interest has focused on identifying biochemical parameters during the immediate postoperative period that may predict the development of hypocalcemia to help facilitate appropriate monitoring, treatment, and timely discharge. Relative change in serum calcium levels from 6 to 12 hours after surgery may be predictive of the development of significant postoperative hypocalcemia.[54] The iPTH level has been the subject of investigation as a result of the hypothesis that low levels would correlate with inadequate calcemic regulation. Prospective studies of patients undergoing thyroidectomies or cervical neck dissections have shown that postoperative iPTH levels (up to 8 hours after surgery) of less than the normal reference range are predictive of hypocalcemia in the short term.[55–59] A combination of an iPTH level of 28 pg/ml or more and a simultaneous corrected calcium level of 2.14 mmol/L or more (equivalent to 8.56 mg/dl) at 6 hours after surgery was predictive of the maintenance of normocalcemia postoperatively.[60] Although low iPTH values may correlate with the risk of hypocalcemia, this risk is not absolute; some patients who have low iPTH values but remain normocalcemic would be unnecessarily monitored or treated with the use of these criteria.

Serum calcium levels should generally be measured every 12 hours for the first 2 days after thyroid surgery. The treatment of postoperative hypocalcemia depends on the severity and expected duration of the syndrome. Emergent therapy is indicated for severe tetany, seizures, laryngospasm, or markedly prolonged electrocardiographic QT intervals. Calcium gluconate (10 ml of a 10% solution or 0.2 ml/kg for children infused IV over 10 minutes) can be employed. Continued support should include 10% calcium gluconate (1.5 ml/kg diluted in 500 ml 5% dextrose solution) administered over 6 to 12 hours, with adjustment based on serial determinations of the serum calcium level. Alkalosis should be avoided, because it increases calcium binding to plasma proteins, thereby further reducing levels of ionized calcium.

Severe hypocalcemia may require long-term calcium and vitamin D or calcitriol supplementation (Tables 8-1 and 8-2). Serum calcium levels should be maintained no higher than 9.0 mg/dl to avoid significant hypercalciuria, which can be exacerbated by the lack of PTH-mediated renal calcium resorption. Oral calcium salts (1–3 gm/day of elemental calcium) should be administered. Ergocalciferol (vitamin D_2; 50,000–100,000 international units daily) provides an inexpensive chronic therapy, but several weeks are required to accumulate therapeutic levels, because it needs to be metabolized to the active hormone calcitriol (1,25-dihydroxyvitamin D_3). Calcitriol (0.5–2.0 mcg/day) rapidly increases gastrointestinal calcium absorption and can be given acutely, although its effects may not manifest for 2 to 3 days. Treatment may be tapered after several weeks to assess the need for continued therapy.

TABLE 8-1 Oral Calcium Preparations

Calcium Preparations	Brand	Dosage	Elemental Calcium Content[†]	Vitamin D Content
Calcium acetate	PhosLo	667 mg	169 mg	None
Calcium carbonate	Generic	650 mg	260 mg	None
		667 mg	267 mg	None
		750 mg (chew)	300 mg	None
		1250 mg	500 mg	None
		1250 mg/5 ml	500 mg/5 ml	None
		1500 mg	600 mg	None
	Tums Ultra	1000 mg	400 mg	None
	Os-Cal 500	1250 mg	500 mg	None
	Os-Cal 500 + D	1250 mg	500 mg	200 IU
	Caltrate 600	1500 mg	600 mg	None
	Caltrate 600 + D	1500 mg	600 mg	200 IU
	Viactiv*	1250 mg	500 mg	100 IU
Calcium citrate	Citracal	950 mg	200 mg	None
	Citracal + D	1500 mg	315 mg	200 IU
	Citracal + D soft chews	2380 mg	500 mg	200 IU
Calcium glubionate		1.8 g/5 ml	115 mg/5 ml	None
Calcium lactate		650 mg	84.5 mg	None

*Viactiv contains 40 mcg of vitamin K.
[†]Calcium acetate = 25% elemental calcium (Ca^{++}). Calcium carbonate = 40% elemental Ca^{++}. Calcium citrate = 21% elemental Ca^{++}. Calcium glubionate = 6.5% elemental Ca^{++}. Calcium lactate = 13% elemental Ca^{++}.
IU, International units.

TABLE 8-2 Oral Vitamin D Preparations

Vitamin D Forms	Brand	Forms Available*	Half-Life	Comments
Calcitriol (1,25-dihydroxycholecalciferol)	Rocaltrol Calcijex	C: 0.25, 0.5 mcg OS: 1 mcg/ml	3–6 hours	Active form; used for renal failure and malabsorption syndromes
Calcifediol (25-hydroxycholecalciferol)	Calderol	C: 20 and 50 mcg	10–22 days	Renal conversion to calcitriol; used for liver disease
Ergocalciferol (vitamin D_2)	Calciferol Drisdol	C: 50,000 IU (1.25 mg) OS: 8000 IU/ml	Long (months)	Hepatic and renal conversion to calcitriol; derived from irradiated plant sterols; found in commercial vitamin preparations
Cholecalciferol (vitamin D_3)	Delta-D	T: 400 and 1000 IU	Long (months)	Hepatic and renal conversion to calcitriol; found in fortified food products
Dihydrotachysterol (DHT)	DHT Intensol Hytakerol	C: 0.125 mg OS: 0.2 mg/ml T: 0.125, 0.2, and 0.4 mg	8 days	Hepatic activation only; synthetic analog of vitamin D_2.

*Equivalent pharmacologic doses: ergocalciferol 50,000 IU = DHT 0.4 mg = calcifediol 50 mcg = calcitriol 1 mcg.
C, Capsules; IU, international units; OS, oral solution; T, tablets.

Patients with mild postoperative hypocalcemia may be treated with oral calcium supplementation alone. Asymptomatic patients may be observed carefully without therapy, because mild postoperative hypocalcemia may be transient and resolve spontaneously. Some investigators have shown that the empiric initiation of standard doses of oral calcium with or without calcitriol can prevent symptomatic hypocalcemia after total thyroidectomy.[61] This treatment strategy should be used with caution, because overreplacement in patients who have mild, transient hypocalcemia may lead to serious side effects, including symptomatic hypercalcemia. When calciuria exceeds 300 to 400 mg/day, a thiazide diuretic can be added to promote calcium resorption and to permit the reduction of calcium and calcitriol doses.

Postoperative Thyroid Hormone Therapy

The diagnosis of postoperative hypothyroidism is established by the presence of hypothyroxinemia and an elevated serum TSH level. Treatment is directed toward restoring the euthyroid state with levothyroxine (1.6 mcg/kg/day), with subsequent dose adjustment until the serum TSH level is normalized. Surgery for benign nodular disease, if bilateral, may leave the patient hypothyroid. If hormone deficiency does not occur, however, the indications for postoperative therapy are uncertain. There are conflicting views regarding whether routine TSH-suppressive thyroid hormone therapy prevents the recurrence of benign nodular disease, especially after surgical resection.[62] However, it may be reasonable to consider suppressive therapy if there were mass effects (e.g., airway or esophageal compromise) with the original nodular goiter.

After the diagnosis of papillary or follicular thyroid carcinoma, thyroid hormone suppression therapy is usually indicated to reduce the frequency of recurrence.[63] To suppress serum TSH levels (<0.1 milli-international units/L for persistent disease; 0.1–0.5 milli-international units/L if free of disease and at high risk for recurrence; 0.3–2.0 milli-international units/L if free of disease and at low risk for recurrence), levothyroxine (2.2 mcg/kg/day) may be initiated as empiric therapy; dose modifications are dictated by the serum TSH concentration after 4 weeks of therapy.[7] Adjunctive treatment with radioactive iodine or, less commonly, external beam radiotherapy or chemotherapy may be required for patients with one or more risk factors for cancer recurrence or death (i.e., older age; larger tumors; or evidence of soft-tissue extension, greater invasiveness, or distant metastases). To promote the uptake of radioiodine by thyroid tissue for scanning and treatment, serum TSH levels are allowed to rise maximally by withholding postoperative thyroid hormone therapy for 2 to 4 weeks and by having the patient adhere to a low-iodine diet. Levothyroxine therapy is initiated with TSH-suppressive doses after treatment with radioiodine.

After the surgical removal of a hyperfunctioning thyroid gland, thyrotoxicosis does not resolve immediately, because the circulating half-life of thyroxine is about 7 days. Because of this, agents such as β-blockers may need to continue for a few weeks after surgery. Thionamides may be discontinued sooner depending on the extent of surgical resection, because no significant thyroid tissue remains to necessitate hormone synthesis inhibition.[12] Periodic monitoring of these patients for the development of hypothyroidism or continued hyperthyroidism is required.

PARATHYROID SURGERY

Surgical parathyroidectomy is indicated for primary hyperparathyroidism complicated by end-organ dysfunction (e.g., nephrolithiasis, osteitis fibrosa cystica, symptomatic hypercalcemia). Asymptomatic primary hyperparathyroidism may also require surgical treatment if clinical or laboratory assessment suggests an increased risk for long-term complications (Box 8-2).[64] In patients with uremic secondary hyperparathyroidism complicated by parathyroid hyperplasia that has failed medical therapy, the risk of significant hypercalcemia, extraskeletal calcification, or cutaneous gangrene may necessitate the surgical reduction of the parathyroid gland mass to normalize serum calcium levels (Box 8-3).[65] Surgery also is indicated for parathyroid carcinoma, which is a rare cause of primary hyperparathyroidism that may present as an invasive neck mass or severe hypercalcemia.

Preoperative Evaluation

Clinical Assessment

Preoperative clinical assessment should be directed toward detecting manifestations of severe hypercalcemia that may complicate the perioperative course and possible features of the MEN syndromes. Hypercalcemia

---

BOX 8-2 Indications for Surgical Treatment of Asymptomatic Primary Hyperparathyroidism*

Overt signs and/or symptoms (nephrolithiasis, osteitis fibrosa cystica, neuromuscular disease)
Serum calcium concentration >1 mg/dl above the upper normal limit
24-hour urine calcium excretion >400 mg
Bone mineral density (T score) <−2.5 standard deviations from normal (at any site)
Age <50 years

*Based on the Guidelines from the 2002 National Institutes of Health Workshop.[64]

BOX 8-3 Indications for Surgical Treatment of Secondary Hyperparathyroidism[65]

Averaged intact parathyroid hormone level >85–95 pmol/L despite optimal available therapy
Averaged intact parathyroid hormone level >50 pmol/L despite optimal available therapy, in addition to the following:

- Corrected serum calcium level of >2.4 mmol/L or
- Serum phosphate level of >1.60 mmol/L or
- Calcium × phosphate product of >4 $mmol^2/L^2$ or
- Progressive loss of hip or lumbar spine bone mineral density in patients with osteoporosis receiving optimal therapy

---

may cause anorexia, nausea, vomiting, constipation, polyuria (as a result of nephrogenic diabetes insipidus), depression, obtundation, coma, and muscle weakness. Uremia associated with either secondary hyperparathyroidism or obstructive uropathy from nephrolithiasis can produce additional symptoms of central nervous system dysfunction, congestive heart failure, or coagulopathy. Hyperparathyroid bone disease may present as fractures or pain associated with focal or occasionally diffuse abnormalities of demineralization and osteomalacia. Hypertension, which may arise from abnormalities of the renin–angiotensin–aldosterone system and vascular cell dysfunction, has been associated with primary hyperparathyroidism.[66–68] Similarly, pancreatitis and peptic ulcer disease have been linked to hypercalcemia and hyperparathyroidism independent of coexistent gastrin and PTH-secreting tumors associated with MEN1 syndrome. Calcium deposition in the cornea (band keratopathy) can rarely be detected. It is distinctly unusual to palpate a parathyroid gland, except in the presence of parathyroid carcinoma or parathyroid cysts. However, none of these aforementioned processes may be present, because asymptomatic primary hyperparathyroidism (the disease that lacks classical signs and symptoms of hyperparathyroidism) is more commonly found (up to 80% of patients) than the classical disease phenotype.[69] Recent data has suggested that asymptomatic primary hyperparathyroidism may actually demonstrate other characteristic effects on the renal, skeletal, neuropsychiatric, and cardiovascular systems.

Although rare (i.e., <10% of patients), a family history of parathyroid disease should be sought.[70] In cases of MEN1, hyperparathyroidism is the most common endocrinopathy and usually the presenting manifestation of the syndrome. Hyperplasia involving all of the parathyroid glands is typical (>90% of MEN1 cases), and recurrence commonly occurs after surgery. Symptoms suggestive of tumors of the pancreas (e.g., insulinoma causing hypoglycemia, gastrinoma causing Zollinger–Ellison syndrome, VIPoma syndrome causing watery diarrhea) or of the pituitary gland (e.g., headache, acromegaly, galactorrhea, impotence, Cushing's syndrome) require careful evaluation. Diarrhea can also be a presentation of hypercalcitoninemia of the medullary thyroid carcinoma. The presence of hypertension, sweating, or headaches may indicate a pheochromocytoma of MEN2A. Familial hyperparathyroidism can occur independent of MEN syndrome in other hereditary patterns associated with recurrent cystic adenomas of the parathyroid glands or fibrous maxillary or mandibular tumors (hyperparathyroidism–jaw tumor syndrome; Table 8-3).

Primary hyperparathyroidism is most often the result of a solitary adenoma (89%) followed by multiple gland hyperplasia (6%). Rarely, primary hyperparathyroidism is the result of parathyroid carcinoma (0.7%).[71] The risk

TABLE 8-3   Hereditary Hyperparathyroidism Syndromes

Syndrome	Gene Mutation
MEN1	MEN1
MEN2A	RET
HPT-JT	HRPT2
FIHP*	HRPT2, HRPT3, MEN1

*FIHP may represent a variant of MEN1.[113]
FIHP, Familial isolated hyperparathyroidism; *HPT-JT*, hyperparathyroidism–jaw tumor; *HRPT2*, hyperparathyroidism type 2; *HRPT3*, hyperparathyroidism type 3; *MEN1*, multiple endocrine neoplasia type 1; *MEN2A*, multiple endocrine neoplasia type 2A; *RET*, rearranged during transfection.

of solitary versus multigland disease is a factor for determining the type of surgery necessary.

Biochemical Assessment

Hypercalcemia with an elevated or inappropriately unsuppressed iPTH is the hallmark of primary hyperparathyroidism. In early mild disease, hypercalcemia may be intermittent. Determination of the ionized calcium concentration removes the influence of the serum protein concentration, which can fluctuate as a result of illness, fasting, dehydration, or prolonged tourniquet application. Two-site immunometric assays specific for iPTH have been developed that are both highly sensitive and specific, with the normal range typically from 10 to 65 pg/ml. Hypophosphatemic, hyperchloremic acidosis is the result of PTH-mediated renal phosphate and bicarbonate wasting, and it can increase the fraction of ionized calcium. Urinary calcium levels are at the upper limits of normal. In addition, the 25-hydroxyvitamin D level tends to be on the lower end of the normal reference range, with high levels of 1,25-dihydroxyvitamin D reflecting the PTH activation of renal 1α-hydroxylase enzymatic activity.

When hypercalcemia is the result of disorders other than hyperparathyroidism, iPTH levels are typically low or undetectable. The differential diagnosis of hypercalcemia includes a wide variety of endocrine and nonendocrine conditions (Box 8-4). Humoral hypercalcemia of malignancy is mediated by the ectopic production of PTH-related peptide that contains critical sequence homology to PTH but that does not cross-react with antisera in the iPTH immunometric assay. In familial hypocalciuric hypercalcemia (FHH), which is an autosomal-dominant disorder with high penetrance, patients have mild hypercalcemia with normal or minimally elevated iPTH levels but decreased fractional clearance of calcium (<1%). FHH is the result of an inactivating mutation of the calcium-sensing receptor gene in parathyroid tissue.[72] Parathyroidectomy does not cure the hypercalcemia in FHH. In general, these patients have benign clinical courses, and they do not develop complications of hypercalcemia or hyperparathyroidism

BOX 8-4 Differential Diagnoses of Hypercalcemia

Hyperparathyroidism
- Primary (adenoma, hyperplasia)
- Tertiary (severe renal failure)

Malignancy associated
- Humoral hypercalcemia of malignancy (parathyroid-hormone–related peptide mediated)
- Osteolytic bone destruction
- 1,25-dihydroxyvitamin D3 mediated

Endocrinopathy
- Hyperthyroidism (thyrotoxicosis)
- Adrenal insufficiency
- Pheochromocytoma

Granulomatous disease
- Sarcoidosis
- Tuberculosis
- Fungal infection (histoplasmosis, coccidiomycosis, leptospirosis)
- Berylliosis
- Eosinophilic granuloma

Acquired immunodeficiency syndrome
Familial hypocalciuric hypercalcemia
Immobilization with Paget's disease of bone
Rhabdomyolysis
Iatrogenic
- Vitamin A or D intoxication
- Milk–alkali syndrome
- Drugs (lithium, thiazides, theophylline)
- Total parenteral nutrition

(e.g., nephrolithiasis, bone disease). Family screening with biochemical tests helps to confirm the diagnosis, because genetic testing is not routinely available.

Imaging Studies

Preoperative localization is necessary for patients who are being considered for minimally invasive parathyroidectomy. Evaluation of the neck anatomy can increase the success rates from 60% with no preoperative localization to more than 95% with localization in patients undergoing repeat surgery for recurrent or persistent hyperparathyroidism.[73,74] Alternatively, before the initial surgery for hyperparathyroidism, localization is usually not required, especially if bilateral neck exploration is planned. It is generally thought that the best way to localize a parathyroid adenoma is to find a surgeon with experience performing parathyroidectomies.[64] Experienced surgeons can identify and resect enlarged glands in more than 90% of initial surgeries for primary hyperparathyroidism.[75] By contrast, the sensitivities of imaging modalities such as ultrasound, thallium–technetium subtraction scanning, and MRI are all significantly less.[76,77] 99m-Technetium sestamibi scans, often in combination with a subtraction thyroid scan or sestamibi double phase studies, can be highly predictive for solitary adenomas (90%–100%) but less so for multiple adenomas or parathyroid hyperplasia.[78–80] Although sestamibi imaging is often obtained preoperatively, especially when considering a mediastinal parathyroid adenoma, its clinical reliability is unclear. It can be difficult to interpret in a patient with coexistent thyroid adenomas. However, it has been recommended that a combination of two noninvasive imaging tests (one of which is a sestamibi study) should be performed before parathyroidectomy for recurrent or persistent hyperparathyroidism.[81] More invasive imaging procedures, including ultrasound or CT-guided fine-needle aspiration for PTH assay or angiography (arterial or venous), should be reserved for patients who are not cured by initial surgery or for whom other imaging modalities are equivocal.

Preoperative Management

Severe preoperative hypercalcemia requires partial correction. Parathyroid crisis can be associated with acute renal insufficiency, cardiac arrhythmias, impaired mentation, and severe dehydration. Aggressive rehydration with saline, which often requires invasive hemodynamic monitoring, reverses dehydration and promotes calciuresis. Serum calcium levels can be reduced by 2 to 3 mg/dl in 24 hours with fluid hydration. The tubular reabsorption of calcium is inhibited by furosemide, which should be administered intravenously every 4 to 8 hours after the patient has been appropriately rehydrated. To decrease the bone resorption associated with PTH-mediated hypercalcemia and, consequently, to lower the serum calcium concentration, calcitonin (4–8 international units/kg subcutaneously or intramuscularly every 6–12 hours) or bisphosphonates (e.g., pamidronate, zoledronic acid) can be administered. Pamidronate (60–90 mg IV once) or zoledronic acid (4 mg IV once) have delayed onsets of action (48–72 hours) but a more sustained duration of effect (up to 2–3 weeks) than calcitonin (up to 48 hours), and they are thus the therapies of choice for PTH-mediated hypercalcemia. Additionally, repeated doses of calcitonin may lead to the development of tachyphylaxis. Osteonecrosis of the jaw is a rare complication (0.6%–9.9%) reported to occur in patients receiving chronic bisphosphonate therapy; however, most cases have been found in the context of patients with underlying malignancy (particularly breast cancer and multiple myeloma) who have received high and frequent doses of intravenous bisphosphonates for metastatic bone disease.[82,83] No patients have been reported to develop osteonecrosis of the jaw after bisphosphonate treatment for hypercalcemia. β-Adrenergic receptor blockade can prevent cardiac arrhythmias; doses of digoxin should be reduced to avoid hypercalcemia-induced toxicity. Electrolyte depletion, including potassium and magnesium, should be anticipated and avoided. When serum calcium levels are less than 11.5 mg/dl, therapy to reduce calcium concentrations is unnecessary before parathyroidectomy.

Intensive medical therapy of severe hyperparathyroidism resulting from renal failure should be attempted before parathyroid surgery. Oral phosphate restriction, the judicious use of oral calcium salts as phosphate binders, and, occasionally, intravenous calcitriol can reduce the severity of hyperparathyroidism. The presence of aluminum osteodystrophy must be ruled out, which may require an iliac crest bone biopsy to look for low turnover osteomalacia and aluminum staining. Patients with coexisting aluminum-related disease can develop a dramatic worsening of osteomalacia after parathyroidectomy, and treatment with desferoxamine chelation is required before surgical exploration.

Perioperative Management

The exacerbation of preoperative complications of hyperparathyroidism can occur after parathyroid resection. The acute worsening of renal function, metabolic acidosis, and hypomagnesemia should be anticipated and avoided by careful fluid and electrolyte management. If intra-articular calcification is present, acute flares of gout or pseudogout may occur during the postoperative period. Recurrent laryngeal nerve injury and neck hematoma can occur, although less commonly than after thyroid surgery.

Hypocalcemia is common after the successful surgical treatment of hyperparathyroidism. Transient hypoparathyroidism may occur for 12 to 48 hours until the previously suppressed normal glands resume PTH secretion. More severe and prolonged hypocalcemia can result from the reversal of hungry bone syndrome as a result of longstanding hyperparathyroidism-induced demineralization. The elevation of serum alkaline phosphatase levels preoperatively may identify patients at greater risk for this syndrome. Permanent hypoparathyroidism is rare after the resection of a parathyroid adenoma, but it is more common after the removal of multiple hyperplastic parathyroid glands. To monitor for the development of hypocalcemia, serum calcium levels should be measured every 12 hours for the first 2 days after surgery. The diagnosis and management of hypocalcemia after parathyroidectomy are similar to that after thyroidectomy (described previously). Recently a retrospective study found that preoperative treatment with bisphosphonate may prevent the occurrence of hungry bone syndrome after parathyroidectomy for primary hyperparathyroidism.[84]

Although the cure rate for primary hyperparathyroidism with either conventional bilateral neck exploration or minimally invasive parathyroidectomy has been reported to be as high as 97%, recurrence should be evaluated periodically, especially for patients with hereditary endocrine syndromes.[75]

PITUITARY SURGERY

With the increased use of imaging studies, clinically insignificant pituitary microadenomas are detected in about 10% of the normal adult population.[85] Thus, a thorough medical evaluation should be performed for endocrine, visual, or neurologic dysfunction before a patient is considered for surgical resection. The disturbance of multiple endocrine functions of the pituitary and hypothalamus as a result of the primary disease itself or as a complication of therapy requires evaluation and correction before and after surgery to minimize morbidity and mortality. Pituitary adenomas may present with hormonal deficiency, hypersecretion syndromes, and local mass effects. Other mass lesions of the sella also present with degrees of hypopituitarism, including craniopharyngioma, meningioma, glioma, germinoma, infiltrative diseases (e.g., sarcoidosis), infections, and congenital or vascular abnormalities.

Preoperative Evaluation

Endocrine dysfunction from sellar mass lesions can include any of the six major axes controlled by the pituitary gland: thyroid, adrenal cortex, gonads, lactation, somatic growth, and water balance. The significant compromise of structures adjacent to the sella (e.g., optic chiasm, cavernous sinus, third ventricle, sellar floor) may be apparent from the clinical presentation, or they may require careful radiographic imaging for detection. Medical therapy (e.g., cabergoline or bromocriptine for prolactinoma, glucocorticoids for sarcoidosis) may obviate the need for surgical intervention entirely.

Clinical Assessment

Hypothalamic or pituitary hypothyroidism (central hypothyroidism) produces symptoms identical to those of primary hypothyroidism, including cold intolerance, constipation, drowsiness, depression, and fatigue. Adrenocorticotropic hormone (ACTH) deficiency leading to cortisol insufficiency may present acutely as severe hypotension, nausea, and vomiting; however, chronic symptoms usually include weight loss, weakness, fatigue, and manifestations of hypoglycemia. The inadequate secretion of growth hormone (GH) causes growth retardation in children. In adults, nonspecific signs and symptoms of fatigue, decreased muscle mass, and depression may develop. In women, central hypogonadism as a result of deficiencies of luteinizing hormone (LH) and follicle-stimulating hormone (FSH) causes secondary amenorrhea, infertility, and menopausal symptoms of hot flashes and vaginal atrophy. In children, primary amenorrhea is often the presenting symptom. Impotence, infertility, and decreased libido result from central hypogonadism in men. Prolactin insufficiency may manifest clinically when a postpartum female is unable to lactate. Patients with central diabetes insipidus

(CDI) as a result of vasopressin (i.e., antidiuretic hormone [ADH]) deficiency complain of increased thirst, polyuria, nocturia, and light-colored ("like water") urine production. Physical signs of hypopituitarism include postural hypotension, bradycardia, hypothermia, slowed mentation, decreased secondary sexual features, and characteristic skin changes on the face (i.e., a wrinkled, doughy texture).

Cushing's disease, which is the result of a pituitary adenoma oversecreting ACTH, is characterized by features of cortisol excess, such as truncal obesity, hypertension, moon facies, dorsocervical fat pad, hirsutism, violaceous striae, hyperglycemia, proximal muscle weakness, menstrual irregularities, and mental status changes. There are no pathognomonic symptoms or physical signs that distinguish pituitary Cushing's disease caused by a corticotroph adenoma from other causes of hypercortisolism, although hyperpigmentation is usually not seen in patients with primary adrenal disease.

GH excess in adults produces the syndrome of acromegaly, which is characterized by the following: increased soft-tissue mass, particularly in the face and hands; excessive diaphoresis; arthralgia; dental malocclusion from jaw prognathism; skin tags; hypertension; carpal tunnel syndrome; and insulin resistance. GH excess before the closure of the epiphyseal plates results in gigantism. Cardiomegaly occurs commonly, although contractile dysfunction is unusual. Because marked enlargement of the tongue and prognathism result from chronic GH excess, intubation during anesthesia induction can be problematic.

Hyperprolactinemia is a common finding in patients with pituitary disease. Women typically present with galactorrhea and amenorrhea; men present with hypogonadism, gynecomastia, and, rarely, galactorrhea. Although prolactin-secreting pituitary tumors are more common, hyperprolactinemia can also result from the interruption of the hypothalamic dopaminergic inhibition of prolactin secretion by the extrinsic compression of the pituitary stalk or hypothalamic disease. Hypothyroidism can cause mild hyperprolactinemia, and clinical evidence of primary thyroid disease should be sought.[86]

Pituitary tumors that secrete gonadotropins or the common pituitary glycoprotein α-subunit typically present solely with hypopituitarism. Adenomas that secrete TSH produce hyperthyroidism and a diffuse goiter, but the ophthalmologic stigmata of Graves' disease should be lacking. In contrast with CDI, the syndrome of inappropriate ADH (SIADH), which can occur with numerous central nervous system disorders (e.g., infection, trauma, mass lesions) regardless of sellar involvement, leads to hyponatremia that presents with nausea, vomiting, headache, altered sensorium, seizure, coma, or death.

Large sellar lesions may cause symptoms as a result of mass effect. Headache is common as a result of meningeal traction. Because pituitary tumors tend to enlarge superiorly, the optic chiasm may be compressed, which leads to a loss of bitemporal and superior visual fields. When there is lateral invasion of the cavernous sinus, paresis of an ipsilateral third, fourth, or sixth cranial nerve can result. Papilledema and pallor of the optic disc can be noticed during funduscopic examination of a patient with a large pituitary or hypothalamic mass. Formal visual field testing is appropriate for patients with pituitary macroadenomas or other sellar lesions that may involve the optic chiasm.

Biochemical Assessment

Pituitary function testing before sellar surgery is done for the following reasons:

1. To diagnose the pituitary or hypothalamic disease

2. To recognize hypersecretory or hormone deficiency states that may require medical treatment before consideration for surgical intervention

3. To identify biochemical markers that can be monitored in response to therapy

The initial evaluation of the patient undergoing sellar surgery should include testing of all six pituitary endocrine axes for hormonal deficiency or overproduction (Table 8-4). If the clinical evaluation suggests the presence of a hypersecreting pituitary tumor, initial testing may include the measurement of the pituitary hormone itself (e.g., prolactin, GH, or TSH). To document clinically suspected acromegaly, hyperthyroidism from a TSH-producing adenoma, or hypercortisolism in Cushing's syndrome, testing should include the measurement of target tissue responses to the increased secretion of the pituitary hormone; increased insulin-like growth factor type I, free T_4, or urinary free cortisol levels would be detected, respectively. Unlike growth hormone, insulin-like growth factor type I production does not vary during the day or in response to food intake, stress, or exercise. Further dynamic testing demonstrating the unsuppressibility of hormone production is usually necessary to confirm the diagnosis of a hypersecretory tumor (Box 8-5).

Inadequately stimulated hormone levels will support insufficiency states. It is essential that adrenal function be evaluated before pituitary surgery given the significant risk of acute hypotension and mortality if left untreated. A low 8:00 AM serum cortisol level (when cortisol is normally at its highest peak concentration) with a low ACTH level suggests the presence of secondary (or central) adrenal insufficiency. A low-dose (1 mcg) ACTH test should be performed for all patients with possible secondary adrenal insufficiency, a sellar lesion of 1 cm or more in diameter, hyponatremia, or symptoms of adrenal insufficiency.[87] The low-dose ACTH test, however, has a high specificity but a low sensitivity for secondary adrenal insufficiency, especially if it is associated with

TABLE 8-4 Endocrine Testing in Patients with Pituitary Disease*

Pituitary Cell Type or Hormone	Deficiency State	Hypersecretory State
Corticotroph	*ACTH stimulation test (low dose)* Insulin tolerance test	24-hour urinary free cortisol Plasma ACTH Dexamethasone suppression test
Thyrotroph	*Free T_4* *TSH*	Free T_4 TSH
Somatotroph	*IGF-I (somatomedin C)* Insulin tolerance test GHRH–arginine stimulation test	IGF-I GH Glucose tolerance test
Lactotroph	Not clinically relevant	*Prolactin*
Gonadotroph	Female: *FSH, LH, estradiol* Male: *FSH, LH, testosterone*	FSH, LH α-Subunit glycoprotein
Vasopressin	*Serum sodium* Urine osmolality Plasma osmolality	Serum sodium Urine osmolality Plasma osmolality Water deprivation test

*Italicized tests should generally be obtained for all patients before sellar surgery. Other tests should be performed on the basis of clinical suspicion of underlying abnormalities.
ACTH, Adrenocorticotropic hormone; *FSH*, follicle-stimulating hormone; *GH*, growth hormone; *GHRH*, growth-hormone–releasing hormone; *IGF-I*, insulin-like growth factor type I; *LH*, luteinizing hormone; *T4*, thyroxine; *TSH*, thyroid-stimulating hormone.

BOX 8-5 Procedures for Commonly Performed Stimulation and Suppression Tests of Anterior Pituitary Gland Function

ADRENOCORTICOTROPIC HORMONE STIMULATION TEST (LOW DOSE, 1 MCG): EVALUATION FOR ADRENAL INSUFFICIENCY

Method: Administer 1 mcg of synthetic adrenocorticotropic hormone (ACTH; cosyntropin). Obtain plasma samples for cortisol at 0 (baseline) and 30 minutes.

Interpretation: ACTH stimulates the adrenal gland to secrete cortisol. ACTH deficiency causes blunted response within 2 weeks of onset. The normal peak plasma cortisol concentration is more than 18 to 20 mcg/dl.[87]

INSULIN TOLERANCE TEST: EVALUATION FOR GROWTH HORMONE DEFICIENCY OR ADRENAL INSUFFICIENCY

Method: Obtain baseline serum levels for glucose, cortisol, ACTH and growth hormone (GH). Administer 0.15 to 0.25 U/kg of insulin intravenously to achieve adequate hypoglycemia (serum glucose ≤35 mg/dl).* Obtain serum levels for glucose, cortisol, and/or GH at 30 and 45 minutes after hypoglycemia is achieved.

Interpretation: Hypoglycemia normally increases GH and ACTH secretion and thus increases cortisol production. The normal peak GH level is ≥5.1 mcg/L, and the normal peak cortisol level is ≥18 to 20 mcg/dl.[111,114]

GROWTH-HORMONE–RELEASING HORMONE (ARGININE STIMULATION TEST): EVALUATION FOR GROWTH HORMONE DEFICIENCY

Method: In a fasting state, administer arginine (0.5 g/kg, maximum 30 gm) intravenously over 30 minutes, followed by GH-releasing hormone (1 mcg/kg) via an intravenous bolus at time 0. Obtain serum GH levels at 0, 30, 60, 90 and 120 minutes.

Interpretation: The combination of arginine with GH-releasing hormone is a potent stimulus of GH secretion. The normal peak GH level is ≥4.1 mcg/L.[111,114]

DEXAMETHASONE SUPPRESSION TEST (HIGH DOSE): EVALUATION FOR THE SOURCE OF ADRENOCORTICO-TROPIC-HORMONE–DEPENDENT CUSHING'S DISEASE

Method: Obtain a baseline 8 AM serum cortisol level. Administer 8 mg of dexamethasone orally at 11 PM the same day. Obtain a serum cortisol level at 8 AM the next morning.

Interpretation: Pituitary adenomas oversecreting ACTH will respond to high doses of dexamethasone by decreasing the production of ACTH and cortisol, whereas an ectopic tumor producing ACTH typically will not respond to dexamethasone. A suppression of serum cortisol from baseline of 50% or more after dexamethasone administration suggests a pituitary source of ACTH production.[115]

GLUCOSE TOLERANCE TEST

Method: Administer 75 g of glucose with the patient in a fasting state. Collect serum for glucose testing at 0 (baseline), 30, 60, 90, and 120 minutes.

Interpretation: Hyperglycemia normally suppresses GH levels to ≤1 mcg/L. Failure to suppress or a paradoxic rise is seen in patients with acromegaly.[116†]

*A bedside automated glucose oxidase analyzer can approximate the level of hypoglycemia. Most automated glucose meters are inaccurate at low serum glucose concentrations in that they tend to underestimate the concentration, which leads to the premature termination of the insulin tolerance test.

†Current two-site immunoradiometric or chemiluminescent assays are more sensitive than the previous radioimmunoassay methods; therefore, the normal GH nadir for a glucose load may need to be adjusted to be 0.3 mcg/L.[116]

mild or recent-onset dysfunction; thus a subnormal cortisol level rules in secondary adrenal insufficiency, but a negative (i.e., normal) result does not sufficiently rule out the possibility of the diagnosis. Clinical reevaluation with further testing with an insulin tolerance test (ITT) may be needed if secondary adrenal insufficiency is still suspected.[88,89] The perioperative morbidity of untreated hypothyroidism, as already discussed, requires that thyroid gland function be evaluated. TSH levels may be normal or possibly elevated in immunoassays despite central hypothyroidism as a result of the secretion of bioinactive TSH molecules that can cross-react in these assays. Therefore hypothyroidism should be suspected in pituitary surgery patients with low or low-normal free T_4 levels.

Diseases that affect the posterior pituitary or the hypothalamus may cause CDI. The diagnosis should be suspected in patients with polyuria or hypernatremia. Urine osmolality is inappropriately low in the face of hyperosmolar plasma. *DI* is defined as the production of a large volume of dilute urine (>30 cc/kg/24 hr or >3 L/day) with a urine osmolality of less than 300 mOsm/kg. Dehydration normally leads to maximal urinary concentration by the kidney under the influence of vasopressin secretion by the posterior pituitary. Normal persons will concentrate their urine to 800 mOsm/kg or more in the setting of hyperosmolar plasma. CDI is caused by a lack of ADH secretion, and nephrogenic DI is the result of renal resistance to ADH action; however, both conditions are associated with the insufficient concentration of urine despite dehydration. If random plasma osmolality is not elevated despite polyuria, a water deprivation test followed by desmopressin (DDAVP) administration may be required to distinguish CDI from nephrogenic DI or primary polydipsia. In CDI, DDAVP administration will typically produce an increase of more than 50% in urinary osmolality. In nephrogenic DI, there will be an insufficient concentration (<50%) of urine after DDAVP injection. Primary polydipsia, which can occur commonly in patients with hypothalamic disease, may not be excluded if plasma and urinary osmolality remain dilute as a result of the impairment of the concentrating ability of the kidneys from longstanding washout of the medullary interstitial gradient and from the downregulation of ADH production with chronic water intake. The water deprivation test can begin at bedtime if basal urine output is less than 6 L/day; otherwise it should be initiated during the early morning to prevent the development of severe dehydration and complications. After weighing the patient and collecting plasma and urine for osmolality, all fluid intake (oral or intravenous) is discontinued. Hourly measurements of weight, plasma, urine osmolality, serum sodium, and urine output are performed. If the patient's weight drops more than 5% from baseline, if the plasma osmolality rises to more than 295 mOsm/kg, or if the urine osmolality fails to rise to more than 600 mOsm/kg or more than 30 mOsm/kg in successive hours, DDAVP (1 mcg subcutaneously or 10 mcg intranasally) is administered. Urine osmolality is then measured at 30 minutes, 60 minutes, and 2 hours after DDAVP is given. The test concludes after the last urine collection, and the patient may resume water intake.

Alternatively, SIADH is diagnosed when a clinically euvolemic patient has a decreased plasma osmolality (<270 mOsm/kg), an inappropriately elevated urine osmolality (>100 mOsm/kg), and an elevated urine sodium concentration (>40 mEq/L).[90] Because renal dysfunction, hypothyroidism, and adrenal insufficiency can cause hyponatremia, these disorders should be ruled out before a diagnosis of SIADH can be made.

Elevated levels of the pituitary glycoprotein hormone α-subunit are frequently seen in pituitary tumors that are otherwise described as "nonfunctioning" because of the lack of the hypersecretion of an intact hormone. The documentation of increased blood α-subunit concentration identifies a biochemical marker of the tumor, thereby allowing for the subsequent measurement of response to therapy or recurrence of disease.

Imaging Studies

MRI with gadolinium enhancement is the single best imaging procedure for most sellar masses.[91] Tumors as small as 2 to 3 mm can be resolved using this technique. Although there are characteristic features on imaging that are suggestive of pituitary adenomas, some sellar lesions cannot be determined other than with pathologic examination. Pituitary adenomas will take up gadolinium to a degree that is between that of normal pituitary (high uptake) and other central nervous system tissue (low uptake). Extrasellar extension, the compression of the optic chiasm, and the invasion of the cavernous sinus are readily detected. High-resolution CT imaging of the sella before and after intravenous contrast administration is also valuable but inferior to MRI; however, CT can detect calcifications in craniopharyngiomas and meningiomas better than MRI.

In general, invasive localization procedures are not indicated for the evaluation of pituitary lesions. The exception is in cases of ACTH-dependent forms of Cushing's syndrome, when the source of ACTH hypersecretion (pituitary or ectopic production) remains unclear. In this situation, bilateral inferior petrosal sinus sampling may be performed. Simultaneous blood specimens for ACTH obtained from each sinus and from a peripheral vein before and after corticotropin-releasing hormone stimulation will reveal a post–corticotropin-releasing hormone inferior-petrosal-sinus–to–peripheral ratio of 3 or more, with more than 95% sensitivity and specificity for Cushing's disease.[92]

Preoperative Management

Replacement therapy for ACTH and TSH deficiency should be initiated as soon as the diagnoses are established. Hydrocortisone (12 mg/m[2]/day) or cortisone acetate (25 to 37.5 mg/day) should be administered orally in divided daily doses to treat chronic secondary adrenal insufficiency. Typically, two thirds of the total dose is taken when arising in the morning and one third is taken during the late afternoon to mimic the normal circadian concentrations of serum cortisol. If the patient presents with signs and symptoms of acute adrenal crisis, therapy should be initiated emergently with saline hydration. Blood for cortisol determination should be obtained, and 100 mg of IV hydrocortisone should be administered immediately and every 6 to 8 hours thereafter. Equivalently, 4 mg of dexamethasone or 20 mg of methylprednisolone can be administered. Steroid doses should be tapered as rapidly as clinically tolerated. Unlike primary adrenal insufficiency, patients with hypopituitarism usually do not require mineralocorticoid supplementation.

When hypothyroidism is documented, treatment is initiated with levothyroxine (1.8 mcg/kg/day), with subsequent dose adjustments every 4 weeks until the free T_4 level is within the upper half of the normal range. The administration of sex hormones may be desirable to treat the symptoms of hypogonadism and to prevent long-term complications (e.g., osteoporosis). GH therapy is initiated in deficient adults if a clinical benefit is anticipated; in children, GH replacement is necessary for adequate linear growth.

Prolactinomas should first be treated medically with dopamine agonists, because these drugs are typically more effective than surgery for decreasing the size and secretion of these tumors.[93] Available dopamine agonists include cabergoline (0.25–1 mg twice weekly) and bromocriptine (2.5–15 mg/day in divided doses). Pergolide, which is approved by the U.S. Food and Drug Administration for the treatment of Parkinson's disease but not for hyperprolactinemia, effectively treated prolactinomas with the benefits of being less expensive than cabergolide and requiring only once-daily dosing.[94] Pergolide is no longer recommended for the treatment of hyperprolactinemia, however, as a result of its association with the development of valvular heart disorders.[95] Cabergoline is the preferred therapy because of its greater efficacy for decreasing the serum prolactin concentration with less gastrointestinal side effects than bromocriptine.[96,97] Because there is more evidence available to support a lack of teratogenicity, bromocriptine (rather than cabergoline) is recommended for the treatment of pregnant women. Macroprolactinomas can shrink in 70% of patients within 6 weeks, with the concomitant relief of symptoms caused by optic chiasm compression or other mass effects; however, therapy should be continued for at least 6 months to allow for maximal tumor shrinkage before determining if surgery is required.[98]

Patients with Cushing's disease are at increased perioperative risk for hyperglycemia, hypertension, fluid retention, opportunistic infection, impaired homeostasis, and poor wound healing. Preoperative therapy to diminish hypercortisolism with the goal of eucortisolemia for 4 to 6 weeks before surgery may reduce the frequency of these complications.[99] Oral inhibitors of adrenal steroidogenesis include mitotane, metyrapone, aminoglutethimide, and ketoconazole; etomidate is the only inhibitory agent given parentally.[100] Unfortunately, the use of these drugs is often limited by adverse side effects. In addition, hypoadrenalism and adrenal crisis need to be avoided by implementing replacement therapy with a glucocorticoid and a mineralocorticoid. Mitotane (4–12 g/day)—a derivative of the insecticide dichlorodiphenyltrichloroethane, which causes necrosis and atrophy of the adrenal cortex—was the first adrenolytic used. The onset of action can be up to 6 to 8 weeks, and maximal benefit occurs after 4 to 6 months of continued use. However, side effects of nausea, vomiting, diarrhea, and depression often become intolerable, causing most patients to discontinue therapy prematurely. Metyrapone (0.75–2 g/day), an 11β-hydroxylase inhibitor, prevents cortisol synthesis. Increasing ACTH in response to decreasing cortisol levels does not overcome the adrenolytic effects of metyrapone. Aminoglutethimide (0.5–6 g/day) inhibits cholesterol processing, which disrupts the production of cortisol, aldosterone, and androgens; however, the hypersecretion of ACTH in pituitary tumors can overcome the enzymatic blockade caused by aminoglutethimide.[101] The combination of metyrapone and aminoglutethimide can be used to lower the required individual dosages of each. Ketoconazole (200–1200 mg/day) is an antimycotic agent that inhibits P450-dependent enzymes involved with adrenal and gonadal steroidogenesis and that also prevents cortisol from binding to glucocorticoid receptors. Of the adrenal-blocking agents, ketoconazole is the best tolerated (despite its risks for hepatotoxicity and gynecomastia), and it can be administered orally for several weeks before surgery.

Perioperative risks in a patient with a TSH-secreting adenoma are similar to other causes of hyperthyroidism. Antithyroid drug therapy should be initiated as outlined, with biochemical and clinical euthyroidism restored before surgery, as described previously in this chapter. Patients with pituitary tumors that secrete GH, FSH, LH, or α-subunit do not require specific preoperative therapy to minimize surgical risks.

The control of chronic polyuria and hyperosmolality in patients with CDI is achieved with DDAVP (2–4 mcg/day IV or subcutaneously, 10–40 mcg/day intranasally, 0.05–1.2 mg/day orally). Initial therapy can be attempted as a single dose at bedtime to eliminate nocturia and to allow for the appropriate thirst mechanisms to compensate for daytime polyuria. If necessary, DDAVP can be given in divided doses two to three times daily. The careful monitoring of volume status and electrolytes is necessary, and iatrogenic hyponatremia should be avoided.

Fluid restriction is the cornerstone of the treatment of SIADH. Free water intake should be limited to less than 800 ml/day initially. Severe, acute hyponatremia presenting as disorientation or seizures requires aggressive therapy to reverse the manifestations of cerebral edema with the avoidance of overly rapid correction, which can lead to osmotic demyelination.[102] Patients who underwent rapid correction (i.e., a change in serum sodium concentration of >0.55 mEq/L/hr) demonstrated neurologic sequelae after the resolution of hyponatremia.[103] Symptomatic hyponatremia may be initially treated with intravenous hypertonic 3% saline (2 ml/kg/hr), with the goal of increasing serum sodium concentrations by 1 to 2 mEq/L/hr. Serum sodium should be monitored every 1 to 2 hours, and the patient's volume status should be carefully managed with furosemide diuresis. The rate of correction of the serum sodium level should be approximately 8 mEq/L/day.[104,105] When the serum sodium concentration has increased by 5% to 10%, symptoms usually abate, and more conservative therapy can be initiated. Demeclocycline (600–1200 mg/day), which is considered for the chronic treatment of hyponatremia that is not responsive to water restriction, induces renal resistance and nephrogenic diabetes insipidus. Its use arginine vasopressin (AVP) is limited by the development of nephrotoxicity, hepatotoxicity, and photosensitivity. Recently the U.S. Food and Drug Administration approved a vasopressin-receptor antagonist, conivaptan (20 mg loading dose IV then a continuous infusion of 20 mg/day for 1–3 days), for the inpatient treatment of SIADH, although it has been studied in hypervolemic states as well.[106] Other vasopressin-receptor antagonists are currently under investigation.[106,107]

Postoperative Management

Glucocorticoid therapy should be administered to all pituitary surgery patients. Initially, 100 mg of intravenous hydrocortisone should be given when the patient is transported to the operating room. This should be repeated every 6 hours, with a dose reduction of 50% every day as part of an uncomplicated recovery. Oral dosing is preferred, when possible. Glucocorticoid doses should not be reduced below those required for maintenance (hydrocortisone 12 mg/m^2/day or cortisone acetate 25–37.5 mg/day). If dexamethasone is used to minimize postoperative cerebral edema, additional steroid therapy is unnecessary; appropriate doses of hydrocortisone or cortisone acetate should be initiated when dexamethasone is discontinued. Thyroid hormone and sex hormone therapy should be continued in patients who were treated preoperatively.

Disorders of vasopressin secretion are common postoperatively, and they classically present as one of the following triphasic responses:

1. DI as a result of acute vasopressin insufficiency caused by hypophyseal neuronal shock

2. SIADH as a result of the release of vasopressin from severed and degenerating hypothalamic neurons

3. DI as a result of permanent hypothalamic neuronal loss (Figure 8-1)

Each phase can last several hours to several days, and all phases do not necessarily occur in every patient. Because significant fluctuations in serum osmolality and volume status can occur rapidly, the serum sodium concentration should be determined every 12 hours, and the patient's weight should be obtained every day. Careful monitoring of fluid intake and output are mandatory. Urine and serum osmolality should be measured when DI is suspected. With these essential monitoring steps, the development of significant DI or SIADH can be detected early and treatment instituted as described previously.

Postoperative endocrine testing is directed toward detecting new pituitary hormone deficiency states and assessing the adequacy of surgical intervention. If sufficient pituitary tissue is resected to potentially cause secondary adrenal insufficiency, the diagnosis should be established by one or more dynamic tests 4 to 6 weeks after surgery with an insulin tolerance test or a low-dose (1 mcg) ACTH stimulation test.[108] Testing done before

4 to 6 weeks is more unreliable. Although the insulin tolerance test is the established gold standard method for evaluating the hypothalamic–pituitary–adrenal axis, it is labor intensive, and it requires close patient monitoring. It is also contraindicated among patients with seizure disorders, ischemic heart disease, and cerebrovascular disease. An overnight metyrapone test was recommended in the past; however, the drug is no longer accessible, and it is available only for compassionate use from the pharmaceutical company. Additionally, a morning serum cortisol (8–9 am) drawn 7 days postoperatively may give an earlier indication of adrenal insufficiency: less than 3.6 mcg/dl is highly diagnostic of adrenal insufficiency; a level of more than 10 mcg/dl is predictive of a normal hypothalamic–pituitary–adrenal axis; and a level of 3.6 to 9 mcg/dl requires further testing with an ITT or a low-dose ACTH stimulation test.[109] Glucocorticoid therapy should be withheld 24 hours before any of these tests are performed. Thyroid (TSH and free T_4) and gonadal (FSH, LH, testosterone in males, estradiol in premenopausal females) function should be assessed at least 1 week postoperatively as well. An elevated FSH level is reassuring for normal pituitary function, because the secretion of gonadotrophins and GH typically becomes impaired before that of ACTH or TSH.[110] GH secretion can be assessed by stimulating GH with intravenous arginine alone, GH-releasing hormone plus arginine, oral levodopa, or hypoglycemia induced by ITT. Testing for GH deficiency is not necessary for patients with multiple other pituitary deficiencies ($\geq$3) documented, because there is a high correlation with GH insufficiency in these patients.[111] Any hormone with a level that was elevated preoperatively should be reevaluated at this time as well.

The majority of patients who are treated surgically for acromegaly, hyperprolactinemia, Cushing's disease, and "nonfunctioning" macroadenomas experience improvement but not long-term cure of their underlying disease. Postoperative external beam radiation or appropriate medical therapy (e.g., cabergoline for hyperprolactinemia, octreotide or pegvisomant for acromegaly) should be considered.

SURGERY FOR NONENDOCRINE DISEASE

In addition to disease or injury to the endocrine glands, metabolic problems can result from surgery or diseases involving other organs. Hypercalcemia of malignancy and cerebral salt wasting will be discussed.

Hypercalcemia is a common complication of malignant disease. The secretion of PTH-related peptide occurs particularly frequently among patients with squamous cell carcinomas, including those that involve the head, neck, lung, and esophagus. Patients present with typical symptoms of severe hypercalcemia, and they may

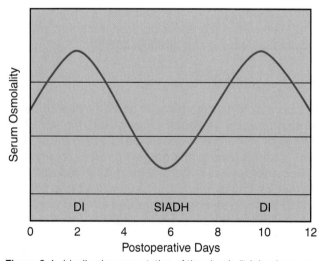

Figure 8-1. Idealized representation of the classic "triple-phase response" of water metabolism after pituitary surgery. The final phase of diabetes insipidus may be permanent. *DI,* Diabetes insipidus; *SIADH,* syndrome of inappropriate antidiuretic hormone.

be significantly dehydrated as a result of calciuresis. The diagnosis should be suspected among patients whose intact PTH levels are low in the presence of hypercalcemia, regardless of whether a malignancy has been previously diagnosed. Treatment should be directed toward the restoration of intravascular volume and the promotion of calciuresis with aggressive saline replacement. When the patient is euvolemic, furosemide diuresis can increase calcium excretion. Specific therapy to reduce bone resorption acutely includes intravenous bisphosphonate (e.g., pamidronate, zoledronic acid) or calcitonin.

Cerebral salt wasting is an uncommon syndrome of hypovolemic hyponatremia that is typically seen among elderly patients after head trauma, intracranial surgery, or subarachnoid hemorrhage. The mechanism that causes inappropriate natriuresis after cerebral injury is not known. Clinical and laboratory findings include dehydration, hypotension, severe hyponatremia, markedly elevated urinary sodium excretion (typically >200 mEq/day), and increased plasma vasopressin levels in response to hypovolemia. Thyroid, adrenal, and renal functions are normal. Treatment requires the invasive monitoring of fluid status, aggressive rehydration with isotonic saline, and, occasionally, 0.1 to 0.4 mg/day of fludrocortisone acetate to promote salt retention.[112]

REFERENCES

1. Cooper DS: Hyperthyroidism. *Lancet* 2003;362(9382):459-468.
2. Abe Y et al: Effect of subtotal thyroidectomy on natural history of ophthalmopathy in Graves' disease. *World J Surg* 1998;22(7):714–717.
3. AACE/AME Task Force on Thyroid Nodules: American Association of Clinical Endocrinologists and Associazione Medici Endocrinologi medical guidelines for clinical practice for the diagnosis and management of thyroid nodules. *Endocr Pract* 2006;12(1):63–102.
4. Baloch Z et al: Laboratory medicine practice guidelines: Laboratory support for the diagnosis and monitoring of thyroid disease. *Thyroid* 2003;13(1):3–126.
5. Surks MI et al: Subclinical thyroid disease: Scientific review and guidelines for diagnosis and management. *JAMA* 2004;291(2):228–238.
6. Stathatos N, Wartofsky L: Perioperative management of patients with hypothyroidism. *Endocrinol Metab Clin North Am* 2003;32(2):503–518.
7. Cooper DS et al: Management guidelines for patients with thyroid nodules and differentiated thyroid cancer. *Thyroid* 2006;16(2):109–142.
8. Papini E et al: Risk of malignancy in nonpalpable thyroid nodules: Predictive value of ultrasound and color-Doppler features. *J Clin Endocrinol Metab* 2002;87(5):1941–1946.
9. Quayle FJ, Moley JF: Medullary thyroid carcinoma: Including MEN 2A and MEN 2B syndromes. *J Surg Oncol* 2005;89(3):122–129.
10. Kouvaraki MA et al: RET proto oncogene: A review and update of genotype-phenotype correlations in hereditary medullary thyroid cancer and associated endocrine tumors. *Thyroid* 2005;15(6):531–544.
11. Sawka AM et al: A comparison of biochemical tests for pheochromocytoma: Measurement of fractionated plasma metanephrines compared with the combination of 24-hour urinary metanephrines and catecholamines. *J Clin Endocrinol Metab* 2003;88(2):553–558.
12. Langley RW, Burch HB: Perioperative management of the thyrotoxic patient. *Endocrinol Metab Clin North Am* 2003; 32(2):519–534.
13. Gimm O et al: An update on thyroid surgery. *Eur J Nucl Med Mol Imaging* 2002;29(Suppl 2):S447–S452.
14. Gaujoux S et al: Extensive thyroidectomy in Graves' disease. *J Am Coll Surg* 2006;202(6):868–873.
15. Sivanandan R et al: Postoperative endocrine function in patients with surgically treated thyrotoxicosis. *Head Neck* 2004;26(4):331–337.
16. Panzer C, Beazley R, Braverman L: Rapid preoperative preparation for severe hyperthyroid Graves' disease. *J Clin Endocrinol Metab* 2004;89(5):2142–2144.
17. Ferraris S et al: Malformations following methimazole exposure in utero: An open issue. *Birth Defects Res A Clin Mol Teratol* 2003;67(12):989–992.
18. Marigold JH et al: Lugol's iodine: Its effect on thyroid blood flow in patients with thyrotoxicosis. *Br J Surg* 1985;72(1):45–47.
19. Ansaldo GL et al: Doppler evaluation of intrathyroid arterial resistances during preoperative treatment with Lugol's iodide solution in patients with diffuse toxic goiter. *J Am Coll Surg* 2000;191(6):607–612.
20. Sarlis NJ, Gourgiotis L: Thyroid emergencies. *Rev Endocr Metab Disord* 2003;4(2):129–136.
21. Lazarus JH et al: Treatment of thyrotoxicosis with lithium carbonate. *Lancet* 1974;2(7890):1160–1163.
22. Geffner DL, Hershman JM: Beta-adrenergic blockade for the treatment of hyperthyroidism. *Am J Med* 1992;93(1):61–68.
23. Eriksson M et al: Propranolol does not prevent thyroid storm. *N Engl J Med* 1977;296(5):263–264.
24. Ladenson PW et al: Complications of surgery in hypothyroid patients. *Am J Med* 1984;77(2):261–266.
25. Cappola AR et al: Thyroid status, cardiovascular risk, and mortality in older adults. *JAMA* 2006;295(9):1033–1041.
26. Hennessey JV et al: L-thyroxine dosage: A reevaluation of therapy with contemporary preparations. *Ann Intern Med* 1986;105(1):11–15.
27. Ladenson PW: Recognition and management of cardiovascular disease related to thyroid dysfunction. *Am J Med* 1990;88(6): 638–641.
28. Sherman SI, Ladenson PW: Percutaneous transluminal coronary angioplasty in hypothyroidism. *Am J Med* 1991;90(3):367–370.
29. Ross DS: The medical management of Graves' disease. *Endocr Pract* 1995;1(3):193–199.
30. Nabil N, Miner DJ, Amatruda JM: Methimazole: An alternative route of administration. *J Clin Endocrinol Metab* 1982;54(1): 180–181.
31. Jongjaroenprasert W et al: Rectal administration of propylthiouracil in hyperthyroid patients: Comparison of suspension enema and suppository form. *Thyroid* 2002;12(7):627–631.
32. Hodak SP et al: Intravenous methimazole in the treatment of refractory hyperthyroidism. *Thyroid* 2006;16(7):691–695.
33. Yeung SC, Go R, Balasubramanyam A: Rectal administration of iodide and propylthiouracil in the treatment of thyroid storm. *Thyroid* 1995;5(5):403–405.
34. Brunette DD, Rothong C: Emergency department management of thyrotoxic crisis with esmolol. *Am J Emerg Med* 1991;9(3): 232–234.
35. Isley WL, Dahl S, Gibbs H: Use of esmolol in managing a thyrotoxic patient needing emergency surgery. *Am J Med* 1990;89(1):122–123.
36. Pattou F et al: Hypocalcemia following thyroid surgery: Incidence and prediction of outcome. *World J Surg* 1998; 22(7):718–724.
37. Zambudio AR et al: Prospective study of postoperative complications after total thyroidectomy for multinodular goiters by surgeons with experience in endocrine surgery. *Ann Surg* 2004;240(1):18–25.
38. Rosato L et al: Complications of total thyroidectomy: Incidence, prevention and treatment. *Chir Ital* 2002;54(5):635–642.

39. Ozbas S et al: Comparison of the complications of subtotal, near total and total thyroidectomy in the surgical management of multinodular goitre. *Endocr J* 2005;52(2):199–205.

40. Sanchez-Blanco JM et al: Influence of superspecialization in endocrine surgery on outcomes of thyroidectomy in a general surgery department. *Cir Esp* 2005;78(5):323–327.

41. Goncalves Filho J, Kowalski LP: Surgical complications after thyroid surgery performed in a cancer hospital. *Otolaryngol Head Neck Surg* 2005;132(3):490–494.

42. Ladenson JH, Lewis JW, Boyd JC: Failure of total calcium corrected for protein, albumin, and pH to correctly assess free calcium status. *J Clin Endocrinol Metab* 1978;46(6):986–993.

43. Demeester-Mirkine N et al: Hypocalcemia after thyroidectomy. *Arch Surg* 1992;127(7):854–858.

44. Sakorafas GH et al: Incidental parathyroidectomy during thyroid surgery: An underappreciated complication of thyroidectomy. *World J Surg* 2005;29(12):1539–1543.

45. Sasson AR et al: Incidental parathyroidectomy during thyroid surgery does not cause transient symptomatic hypocalcemia. *Arch Otolaryngol Head Neck Surg* 2001;127(3):304–308.

46. Palazzo FF et al: Parathyroid autotransplantation during total thyroidectomy—Does the number of glands transplanted affect outcome? *World J Surg* 2005;29(5):629–631.

47. Lo CY: Parathyroid autotransplantation during thyroidectomy. *ANZ J Surg* 2002;72(12):902–907.

48. Rude RK, Oldham SB, Singer FR: Functional hypoparathyroidism and parathyroid hormone end-organ resistance in human magnesium deficiency. *Clin Endocrinol (Oxf)* 1976;5(3):209–224.

49. Smith DA, Fraser SA, Wilson GM: Hyperthyroidism and calcium metabolism. *Clin Endocrinol Metab* 1973;2(2):333–354.

50. See AC, Soo KC: Hypocalcaemia following thyroidectomy for thyrotoxicosis. *Br J Surg* 1997;84(1):95–97.

51. Abboud B et al: Risk factors for postthyroidectomy hypocalcemia. *J Am Coll Surg* 2002;195(4):456–461.

52. de Ronde W et al: "Hungry bone" syndrome, characterized by prolonged symptomatic hypocalcemia, as a complication of the treatment for hyperthyroidism. *Ned Tijdschr Geneeskd* 2004;148(5):231–234.

53. Grieff M: The hungry bone syndrome after medical treatment of thyrotoxicosis. *Ann Intern Med* 2003;139(8):706–707.

54. Nahas ZS et al: A safe and cost-effective short hospital stay protocol to identify patients at low risk for the development of significant hypocalcemia after total thyroidectomy. *Laryngoscope* 2006;116(6):906–910.

55. Chia SH et al: Prospective study of perioperative factors predicting hypocalcemia after thyroid and parathyroid surgery. *Arch Otolaryngol Head Neck Surg* 2006;132(1):41–45.

56. Ghaheri BA et al: Perioperative parathyroid hormone levels in thyroid surgery. *Laryngoscope* 2006;116(4):518–521.

57. Lindblom P, Westerdahl J, Bergenfelz A: Low parathyroid hormone levels after thyroid surgery: A feasible predictor of hypocalcemia. *Surgery* 2002;131(5):515–520.

58. Soon PS et al: Serum intact parathyroid hormone as a predictor of hypocalcaemia after total thyroidectomy. *ANZ J Surg* 2005;75(11):977–980.

59. Lombardi CP et al: Early prediction of postthyroidectomy hypocalcemia by one single iPTH measurement. *Surgery* 2004;136(6):1236–1241.

60. Payne RJ et al: Same-day discharge after total thyroidectomy: The value of 6-hour serum parathyroid hormone and calcium levels. *Head Neck* 2005;27(1):1–7.

61. Bellantone R et al: Is routine supplementation therapy (calcium and vitamin D) useful after total thyroidectomy? *Surgery* 2002;132(6):1109–1113.

62. Mandel SJ, Brent GA, Larsen PR: Levothyroxine therapy in patients with thyroid disease. *Ann Intern Med* 1993;119(6):492–502.

63. Pujol P, et al: Degree of thyrotropin suppression as a prognostic determinant in differentiated thyroid cancer. *J Clin Endocrinol Metab* 1996;81(12):4318–4323.

64. Bilezikian JP et al: Summary statement from a workshop on asymptomatic primary hyperparathyroidism: A perspective for the 21st century. *J Bone Miner Res* 2002;17(Suppl 2):N2–N11.

65. Elder GJ: Parathyroidectomy in the calcimimetic era. *Nephrology (Carlton)* 2005;10(5):511–515.

66. Lafferty FW: Primary hyperparathyroidism. Changing clinical spectrum, prevalence of hypertension, and discriminant analysis of laboratory tests. *Arch Intern Med* 1981;141(13):1761–1766.

67. Kovacs L et al: The effect of surgical treatment on secondary hyperaldosteronism and relative hyperinsulinemia in primary hyperparathyroidism. *Eur J Endocrinol* 1998;138(5):543–547.

68. Kosch M et al: Studies on flow-mediated vasodilation and intima-media thickness of the brachial artery in patients with primary hyperparathyroidism. *Am J Hypertens* 2000;13(7):759–764.

69. Silverberg SJ, Bilezikian JP: The diagnosis and management of asymptomatic primary hyperparathyroidism. *Nat Clin Pract Endocrinol Metab* 2006;2(9):494–503.

70. Wassif WS et al: Genetic studies of a family with hereditary hyperparathyroidism-jaw tumour syndrome. *Clin Endocrinol (Oxf)* 1999;50(2):191–196.

71. Ruda JM, Hollenbeak CS, Stack BC Jr: A systematic review of the diagnosis and treatment of primary hyperparathyroidism from 1995 to 2003. *Otolaryngol Head Neck Surg* 2005;132(3):359–372.

72. Pollak MR et al: Mutations in the human Ca(2+)-sensing receptor gene cause familial hypocalciuric hypercalcemia and neonatal severe hyperparathyroidism. *Cell* 1993;75(7):1297–1303.

73. Jaskowiak N et al: A prospective trial evaluating a standard approach to reoperation for missed parathyroid adenoma. *Ann Surg* 1996;224(3):308–321.

74. Shen W et al: Reoperation for persistent or recurrent primary hyperparathyroidism. *Arch Surg* 1996;131(8):861–869.

75. Grant CS et al: Primary hyperparathyroidism surgical management since the introduction of minimally invasive parathyroidectomy: Mayo Clinic experience. *Arch Surg* 2005;140(5):472–479.

76. Thompson CT, Bowers J, Broadie TA: Preoperative ultrasound and thallium-technetium subtraction scintigraphy in localizing parathyroid lesions in patients with hyperparathyroidism. *Am Surg* 1993;59(8):509–512.

77. Yao M, Jamieson C, Blend R: Magnetic resonance imaging in preoperative localization of diseased parathyroid glands: A comparison with isotope scanning and ultrasonography. *Can J Surg* 1993;36(3):241–244.

78. Taillefer R et al: Detection and localization of parathyroid adenomas in patients with hyperparathyroidism using a single radionuclide imaging procedure with technetium-99m-sestamibi (double-phase study). *J Nucl Med* 1992;33(10):1801–1807.

79. Thule P et al: Preoperative localization of parathyroid tissue with technetium-99m sestamibi 123I subtraction scanning. *J Clin Endocrinol Metab* 1994;78(1):77–82.

80. Civelek AC et al: Prospective evaluation of delayed technetium-99m sestamibi SPECT scintigraphy for preoperative localization of primary hyperparathyroidism. *Surgery* 2002;131(2):149–157.

81. Alexander HR Jr et al: Role of preoperative localization and intraoperative localization maneuvers including intraoperative PTH assay determination for patients with persistent or recurrent hyperparathyroidism. *J Bone Miner Res* 2002;17(Suppl 2):N133–N140.

82. Bamias A et al: Osteonecrosis of the jaw in cancer after treatment with bisphosphonates: Incidence and risk factors. *J Clin Oncol* 2005;23(34):8580–8587.

83. Badros A et al: Osteonecrosis of the jaw in multiple myeloma patients: Clinical features and risk factors. *J Clin Oncol* 2006;24(6):945–952.

84. Lee IT et al: Bisphosphonate pretreatment attenuates hungry bone syndrome postoperatively in subjects with primary hyperparathyroidism. *J Bone Miner Metab* 2006;24(3):255–258.

85. Melmed S: Evaluation of pituitary masses. In DeGroot LJ, Jameson JL, editors: *Endocrinology*, ed 5, Philadelphia, 2006, Elsevier Saunders.

86. Grubb MR, Chakeres D, Malarkey WB: Patients with primary hypothyroidism presenting as prolactinomas. *Am J Med* 1987;83(4):765–769.

87. Thaler LM, Blevins LS Jr: The low dose (1-microg) adrenocorticotropin stimulation test in the evaluation of patients with

suspected central adrenal insufficiency. *J Clin Endocrinol Metab* 1998;83(8):2726–2729.

88. Dorin RI, Qualls CR, Crapo LM: Diagnosis of adrenal insufficiency. *Ann Intern Med* 2003;139(3):194–204.

89. Mayenknecht J et al: Comparison of low and high dose corticotropin stimulation tests in patients with pituitary disease. *J Clin Endocrinol Metab* 1998;83(5):1558–1562.

90. Baylis PH: The syndrome of inappropriate antidiuretic hormone secretion. *Int J Biochem Cell Biol* 2003;35(11):1495–1499.

91. Pressman B: Pituitary imaging. In Melmed S, editor: *The pituitary,* ed 2, Malden, Mass, 2002, Blackwell Science.

92. Oldfield EH et al: Petrosal sinus sampling with and without corticotropin-releasing hormone for the differential diagnosis of Cushing's syndrome. *N Engl J Med* 1991;325(13):897–905.

93. Acquati S et al: A comparative evaluation of effectiveness of medical and surgical therapy in patients with macroprolactinoma. *J Neurosurg Sci* 2001;45(2):65–69.

94. Kleinberg DL et al: Pergolide for the treatment of pituitary tumors secreting prolactin or growth hormone. *N Engl J Med* 1983;309(12):704–709.

95. Flowers CM et al: The US Food and Drug Administration's registry of patients with pergolide-associated valvular heart disease. *Mayo Clin Proc* 2003;78(6):730–731.

96. Webster J, et al: A comparison of cabergoline and bromocriptine in the treatment of hyperprolactinemic amenorrhea: Cabergoline Comparative Study Group. *N Engl J Med* 1994;331(14):904–909.

97. Sabuncu T et al: Comparison of the effects of cabergoline and bromocriptine on prolactin levels in hyperprolactinemic patients. *Intern Med* 2001;40(9):857–861.

98. Molitch ME et al: Bromocriptine as primary therapy for prolactin-secreting macroadenomas: Results of a prospective multicenter study. *J Clin Endocrinol Metab* 1985;60(4):698–705.

99. Lamberts SW, van der Lely AJ, de Herder WW: Transsphenoidal selective adenomectomy is the treatment of choice in patients with Cushing's disease: Considerations concerning preoperative medical treatment and the long-term follow-up. *J Clin Endocrinol Metab* 1995;80(11):3111–3113.

100. Drake WM et al: Emergency and prolonged use of intravenous etomidate to control hypercortisolemia in a patient with Cushing's syndrome and peritonitis. *J Clin Endocrinol Metab* 1998;83(10):3542–3544.

101. Zachmann M et al: Effect of aminoglutethimide on urinary cortisol and cortisol metabolites in adolescents with Cushing's syndrome. *Clin Endocrinol (Oxf)* 1977;7(1):63–71.

102. Sterns RH, Silver SM: Brain volume regulation in response to hypo-osmolality and its correction. *Am J Med* 2006;119 (7 Suppl 1):S12–S6.

103. Sterns RH: Severe symptomatic hyponatremia: Treatment and outcome: A study of 64 cases. *Ann Intern Med* 1987;107(5):656–664.

104. Sterns RH et al: Neurologic sequelae after treatment of severe hyponatremia: A multicenter perspective. *J Am Soc Nephrol* 1994;4(8):1522–1530.

105. Adrogue HJ: Consequences of inadequate management of hyponatremia. *Am J Nephrol* 2005;25(3):240–249.

106. Ghali JK et al: Efficacy and safety of oral conivaptan: a V1A/V2 vasopressin receptor antagonist, assessed in a randomized, placebo-controlled trial in patients with euvolemic or hypervolemic hyponatremia. *J Clin Endocrinol Metab* 2006;91(6):2145–2152.

107. Verbalis JG: AVP receptor antagonists as aquaretics: Review and assessment of clinical data. *Cleve Clin J Med* 2006;73 (Suppl 3):S24–S33.

108. Courtney CH et al: The insulin hypoglycaemia and overnight metyrapone tests in the assessment of the hypothalamic-pituitary-adrenal axis following pituitary surgery. *Clin Endocrinol (Oxf)* 2000;53(3):309–312.

109. Courtney CH et al: Comparison of one week 0900 h serum cortisol, low and standard dose synacthen tests with a 4 to 6 week insulin hypoglycaemia test after pituitary surgery in assessing HPA axis. *Clin Endocrinol (Oxf)* 2000;53(4):431–436.

110. Singer PA, Sevilla LJ: Postoperative endocrine management of pituitary tumors. *Neurosurg Clin N Am* 2003;14(1):123–138.

111. Molitch ME et al: Evaluation and treatment of adult growth hormone deficiency: An Endocrine Society Clinical Practice Guideline. *J Clin Endocrinol Metab* 2006;91(5):1621–1634.

112. Ishikawa SE et al: Hyponatremia responsive to fludrocortisone acetate in elderly patients after head injury. *Ann Intern Med* 1987;106(2):187–191.

113. Miedlich S et al: Familial isolated primary hyperparathyroidism—A multiple endocrine neoplasia type 1 variant? *Eur J Endocrinol* 2001;145(2):155–160.

114. Erturk E, Jaffe CA, Barkan AL: Evaluation of the integrity of the hypothalamic-pituitary-adrenal axis by insulin hypoglycemia test. *J Clin Endocrinol Metab* 1998;83(7):2350–2354.

115. Tyrrell JB et al: An overnight high-dose dexamethasone suppression test for rapid differential diagnosis of Cushing's syndrome. *Ann Intern Med* 1986;104(2):180–186.

116. Lim EM, Pullan P: Biochemical assessment and long-term monitoring in patients with acromegaly: Statement from a joint consensus conference of the Growth Hormone Research Society and the Pituitary Society. *Clin Biochem Rev* 2005;26(2):41–43.

CHAPTER 9

Ophthalmic and Orbital Complications of Head and Neck Surgery

Christopher I. Zoumalan, Edward Wladis, Richard A. Zoumalan, Roberta E. Gausas, and Kimberly P. Cockerham

PREOPERATIVE OPHTHALMIC ASSESSMENT

Surgery performed in the head and neck region can affect the visual system in a variety of ways. A preoperative ophthalmic assessment should be performed for all patients undergoing surgery in the regions adjacent to the orbit. Ophthalmic and orbital complications include—but are not limited to—double vision, pupillary abnormalities, and a loss of vision as a result of direct or indirect optic nerve trauma (Box 9-1).

A complete eye examination should include visual acuity, pupillary assessment, the assessment of motility in all cardinal directions with the documentation of diplopia, the quantification of globe position (with an exophthalmometer, if possible), and standard evaluations of the anterior and posterior segments of the eye. Lid laxity must be assessed with a snap test. During this test, the lower eyelid is pulled away from the globe. A normal result consists of the lid being able to be comfortably pulled less than 6 to 8 mm and then quickly snapping back into place. Intercanthal distance should also be evaluated preoperatively, and it should be half the interpupillary distance (30–35 mm). If there is any concern that optic nerve function is impaired (i.e., decreased vision, afferent pupillary defect, color vision abnormalities, or optic nerve changes), formal visual field testing should be performed. External photographs to document eyelid and globe position are helpful. If optic nerve damage is present preoperatively, red-free digital fundus photography and nerve fiber layer analysis are helpful to document the preoperative status.

Evaluation of Diplopia

The term *diplopia* refers to double vision. Cases that resolve with the coverage of one eye are usually caused by an obstruction of the visual axis of the affected eye (e.g., cataract, corneal disease). Binocular double vision may occur in a variety of postoperative settings and is the result of a misalignment of the eyes. Specifically, binocular diplopia may result from damage to the rectus muscles (either direct, as occurs with laceration, or indirect, in cases of hemorrhage, entrapment, or edema) or to the nerves that govern their actions.

Several tests may be employed to assess the alignment of a patient's eyes. When the eyes are properly aligned, shining a light directly into both eyes should result in a light reflex in a symmetric position on the cornea. Deviations (i.e., differences in light reflex position) should indicate a misalignment. Furthermore, the careful monitoring of extraocular motility may reveal deficiencies. When an inability to move an eye becomes apparent, clinicians must differentiate between restrictive and nonrestrictive causes. To perform forced duction testing, the bulbar conjunctiva should be anesthetized and grasped with a toothed forceps. This instrument can then be used to attempt to move the eye in the direction of the decreased motility. In cases of a mechanical restriction (e.g., fibrosis, edema, hemorrhage), the eye will not slide freely; cases of neuromuscular paralysis are marked by free movement.

Several of the conditions outlined in this chapter may result in double vision, and a careful analysis for the precise cause is critical to optimal management. When a rectus muscle in impinged or "hooked" by a fragment of bone, the muscle becomes entrapped, and its action becomes limited. Ischemic processes and direct injury to the muscle from surgery usually become evident immediately after surgery. Hemorrhages within the orbit can limit the range of the muscle and can act as restrictive processes. Finally, infection within the orbit merits serious consideration as a cause of diplopia; diplopia may be the hallmark of orbital cellulitis, which may result in morbidity and mortality.

After the cause of the diplopia has been determined, it should be addressed as discussed in the separate sections of this chapter.

Evaluation of Dry Eyes

A Schirmer test should be tested preoperatively to document a dry eye. In this test, a 35 mm × 5 mm filter paper strip is used to measure the amount of tears that are produced over a period of 5 minutes. The strip is placed at the junction of the middle and lateral thirds of the lower eyelid with or without the use of a preplaced ophthalmic anesthetic drop. There is considerable variability in the assessment of tear dysfunction (or dry eyes), and usually a value of less than 5 mm indicates the condition.

BOX 9-1 Ophthalmic Complications

Ocular pain

Orbital hemorrhage

Orbital emphysema

Optic nerve injury

Orbital apex syndrome

Extraocular muscle injury

Pupil abnormality

Globe displacement

Eyelid malposition

Facial nerve palsy

Nasolacrimal duct obstruction

Vision loss from therapeutic and anesthetic injections

When an anesthetic eyedrop is used, this test is thought to measure only the basic tear secretion. When an anesthetic eyedrop is not used, this test is thought to measure the basal and reflex tear secretion. There are compelling reasons to believe that the tears measured by these two different methods may not sufficiently differentiate between basic and reflex tear production.

OCULAR PAIN

Clinical Problem

Ocular pain is a frequent complication among postoperative patients. Postoperative pain can be the result of intraoperative local ocular manipulation, local soft-tissue orbital swelling, increased intraocular pressure, and corneal abrasion.

A corneal abrasion is a very common postoperative complication. Addressing corneal abrasions is important, because the patient is at a higher risk for a corneal infection (corneal ulcer) when the cornea is deepithelialized. Intraoperative corneal exposure can occur when the eyes are left open during surgery. Other causes include postoperative facial palsy, which will leave the patient with a variable amount of lagophthalmos and a poor blinking reflex, thereby placing the patient at in increased risk for corneal decompensation or abrasion. Alternatively, an abnormal position of the eyelids (e.g., ectropion of the lower eyelid as a result of orbital floor repair) can place the patient at risk for a corneal abrasion.

Medical and Surgical Management

A corneal abrasion is characterized by a sharp, stabbing, constant eye pain. The diagnosis can be made by placing a drop of fluorescein sodium solution onto the cornea. Areas of epithelial breakdown stain yellowish green when viewed by a blue light. Treatment can include patching the eye shut for 24 hours until the epithelial defect heals.

ORBITAL HEMORRHAGE

Clinical Problem

Any orbital surgery or endoscopic sinus surgery poses a risk for an orbital hemorrhage. Entry into the orbit can result in bleeding as a result of the disruption of one of the many vessels that course through the orbital fat or as a result of the laceration of even a small region of the very vascular extraocular muscles. The thin medial orbital wall (lamina papyracea) is easily perforated during sinus surgery, and the surgeon needs to be wary of the surrounding orbital anatomy. For example, orbital fat must be quickly recognized, because damage to vessels can lead to a hematoma. If there are bony defects in the orbital walls, bleeding within the sinuses can enter the orbit inadvertently. Furthermore, bucking or gagging during extubation may result in bleeding as a result of increased venous pressure. Postblepharoplasty orbital hemorrhage has also been reported, with the incidence of permanent visual loss estimated at 0.04%.[1] Although this rate is low, the potential for permanent and severe visual loss should not be ignored, and it should be specifically mentioned to the patient as a possible complication. It is speculated that there is an association between visual loss and the removal of fat at the time of blepharoplasty[2,3]; therefore meticulous attention must be paid to hemostasis and the anatomy when excising orbital fat.

Orbital hemorrhage can cause exophthalmos, dysmotility, increased intraocular pressure, and optic nerve dysfunction. Specifically, such a hemorrhage may directly compress the orbital vasculature, occlude the central retinal artery, or damage the optic nerve. Urgent consultation with an ophthalmologist (preferably one with subspecialty training in oculoplastic and orbital surgery) should be obtained.

Medical and Surgical Management

The visual acuity and intraocular pressure should be documented. If the intraocular pressure is elevated to more than 30 mm Hg, measures should be taken to lower the pressure immediately to prevent visual loss. Glaucoma eyedrops may be initiated to decrease intraocular fluid production or to increase the egress of aqueous humor. Mannitol, acetazolamide, or both are often useful as well.

If the visual acuity is decreased with subsequent elevated intraocular pressure (>30 mm Hg), an emergent canthotomy and cantholysis (i.e., the release of the lateral canthal insertion onto the orbital tubercle) should be performed at the bedside to relieve the intraorbital pressure. Specifically, after the administration of local anesthetic into the lateral canthal region, the skin and the orbicularis muscle are incised in a horizontal fashion for several millimeters with scissors. Toothed forceps are then em-

ployed to pull the lower eyelid away from the globe, and the scissors are used to "strum" the inferior crus of the lateral canthal ligament. After the ligament is identified, it is incised, and a palpable "give" is felt along the course of the eyelid as the ligament is released. Figure 9-1 effectively demonstrates this procedure. The evacuation of

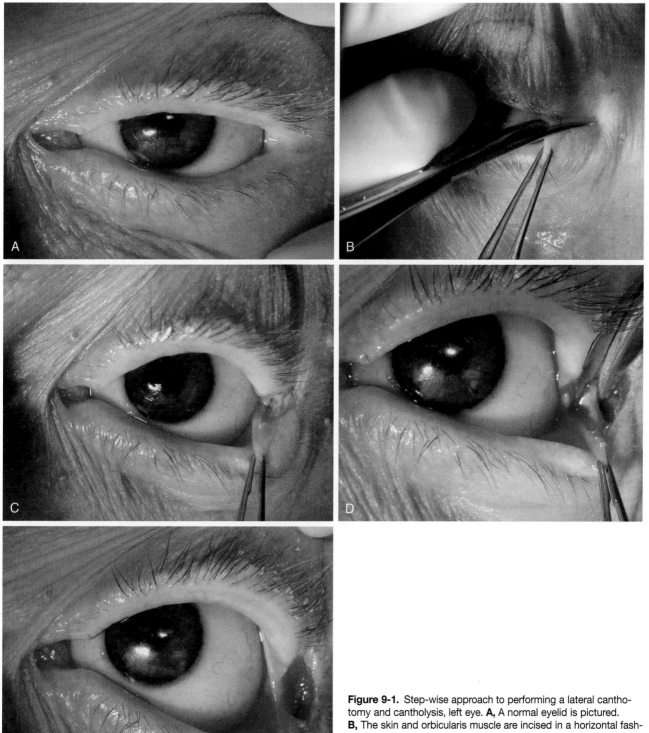

Figure 9-1. Step-wise approach to performing a lateral canthotomy and cantholysis, left eye. **A,** A normal eyelid is pictured. **B,** The skin and orbicularis muscle are incised in a horizontal fashion for several millimeters with scissors. **C,** The lower eyelid is pulled away from the globe with toothed forceps. **D and E,** Scissors are used to "strum" and incise the inferior crus of the lateral canthal ligament.

the hematoma may be necessary in some cases. Under these circumstances, scissors can be used in a spreading fashion to enter the inferotemporal orbit. The tips of the scissors should remain closed to avoid inadvertent perforation of the globe. The fibrous septae of the orbit can be opened carefully with scissors, thereby allowing for the evacuation of the hemorrhage.[4] Although the needle evacuation of a hematoma has been described,[5] this technique involves the risk of inadvertent damage to the orbital structures and globe perforation.

In cases of postoperative blepharoplasty orbital hemorrhage, treatments can also include wound incision and drainage and the cautery of active bleeders while addressing the elevated intraocular pressure, as previously mentioned. An orbital hemorrhage that is refractory to these techniques may require emergent orbital decompression. One specific technique employs a mosquito clamp, which is inserted through the inferior fornix and advanced along the medial orbital floor. Pressure is then applied to fracture the orbital floor and maxillary sinus. Although this technique theoretically risks damage to the infraorbital nerve and the inferior oblique and rectus muscles, Liu[6] reported his experience with five patients who required emergent decompression maneuvers, and he found excellent results with this approach. Of particular note is that intravenous corticosteroids can be helpful in some cases.

ORBITAL EMPHYSEMA

Clinical Problem

The most common cause of excessive air in the orbit (i.e., orbital emphysema) is sneezing or blowing the nose after trauma to the medial and/or inferior orbital bones, thus allowing for the direct entry of the air into the orbit. Any process that results in a direct communication between the orbits and a paranasal sinus can yield orbital emphysema. The air can become trapped within in the orbit and thus acts as a space-occupying mass, creating a compartment syndrome and resulting in proptosis, dysmotility, and even visual loss. Central retinal artery occlusion, direct compression of the optic nerve, and ischemia have all been implicated in the pathogenesis of vision loss related to orbital emphysema.[7]

Medical and Surgical Management

In mild cases, spontaneous resolution typically occurs within 2 weeks.[8] After fractures, patients should be cautioned against nose blowing. Despite the generally favorable prognosis, careful monitoring of visual acuity is absolutely necessary in cases of orbital emphysema. If visual acuity worsens, rapid interventions may be required to reduce the compressive effects of the air pocket. Needle decompression to deflate an air pocket

has been described,[9] although a blind needle passage into the orbit carries significant theoretic risks of damage to the orbital structures. Canthotomy and cantholysis, as previously described in this chapter, may allow for effective decompression with the return of visual function.

OPTIC NERVE INJURY

Clinical Problem

Loss of vision may be a complication of endoscopic sinus surgery or, less commonly, of the repair of facial fractures. The mechanism of action may be direct nerve injury (contusion or avulsion), retinal artery occlusion as a result of orbital edema, compression from an orbital hematoma, and central retinal vein occlusion associated with increased intraocular pressure. Whether the approach is external, internal, or endoscopic, serious visual complications involving the optic nerve injury can occur in the most routine cases. The thin medial orbital wall (lamina papyracea) may be inadvertently penetrated, with subsequent manipulation or damage to structures such as the medial rectus muscle, the trochlea, and the optic nerve. The optic nerve is very restricted in the optic canal, and small changes in volume from blood or edema can result in ischemic damage. Retinal hemorrhages have also been reported as complications of endoscopic sinus surgery.[10–14]

The optic nerve is intimately related to the ethmoid and sphenoid sinuses. Different anatomic configurations of the optic nerve can predispose the nerve to damage during functional endoscopic sinus surgery (FESS). The course of the optic nerve in relation to the posterior paranasal sinuses has been studied in computed tomography (CT) scans. The optic nerve runs adjacent to the sphenoid sinus and causes an indentation of the sinus in 12% to 15% of patients. In 6% to 8% of patients, it courses through the sphenoid sinus. In 3% of patients, the optic nerve also contacts the posterior ethmoid sinus.[15,16] One study showed that 90% of sphenoid sinuses contact the ipsilateral optic nerve, and 10% of patients have sphenoid sinuses that contact both optic nerves.[17] This anatomic variation was consistently associated with an ipsilateral clinoid process that pneumatized. In this series, protrusion into the ethmoidal air cells was not observed.[18] To reduce optic nerve damage in surgeries, preoperative CT examination of the paranasal sinuses and the optic nerves is very important for the early detection of any protrusion of the optic nerve into the sphenoid sinus or the posterior ethmoid air cells.

Lee and colleagues[19] report an unusual case of ischemic optic neuropathy (ION) in a 51-year-old man undergoing an uneventful endoscopic sinus surgery. Patient risk factors include a history of hypertension, diabetes, renal failure, and anemia. Structurally, a "disc at risk" (i.e., a small or absent cup within the optic disc) is very significant. Additionally, preoperative sildenafil has been linked to optic neuropathies. Intraoperative blood loss, hypoxia, anemia, and hypotension have been implicated in ION reported after spinal and cardiac surgery.

Bilateral ION has also been reported after bilateral radical neck dissections. In one case, histopathologic inspection demonstrated bilateral intraorbital hemorrhagic infarction without ophthalmic artery occlusion or embolization. Venous hypertension as a result of bilateral internal jugular vein ligation may contribute.[20] The aggressive correction of blood pressure and blood transfusions may be helpful.

Girotto and colleagues[21] reviewed the University of Maryland Shock Trauma experience and found that 2987 of the 29,474 patients admitted had facial fractures (10.1%) and that 1338 of these had orbital involvement (44.8%). Of the 1240 patients undergoing fracture repair, 3 had postoperative blindness. Overall, 27 patients had visual loss, and, in 18 of these patients (67%), increased orbital pressure or hemorrhage was implicated as the cause.

In another study, Girotto and colleagues[22] used cadavers to access the mechanism of optic nerve injury during elective Le Fort I osteotomy. Using a pressure transduction system, the authors demonstrated a 5-second, 10-mm Hg change in optic canal pressure during down-fracture of the maxilla. All specimens had uncontrolled propagation of fracture lines during pterygomaxillary separation that could explain the compression or optic nerve injury that is occasionally observed. In a retrospective case series of 94 patients undergoing Le Fort I osteotomy and distraction osteogenesis for craniofacial anomalies, Lo and colleagues[23] reported two cases of blindness as a result of optic nerve dysfunction. Corticosteroids were used without any visual improvement. Imaging studies were negative for hemorrhage or orbital bone abnormalities.

Medical and Surgical Management

Lamentably, there is currently no proven therapy for optic nerve injury. In their meta-analysis of traumatic optic neuropathy cases, Cook and colleagues[24] determined that patients who received some intervention (corticosteroids or surgical decompression) fared better than those who were observed. The combination of these therapies was not better than monotherapy. If a localized optic nerve sheath hematoma can be identified, surgical evacuation may improve vision.[25] The International Optic Nerve Trauma Study did not find any benefit to corticosteroid administration or optic canal decompression.[26]

In cases of postoperative ischemic optic neuropathy, the role of postoperative corticosteroids is also controversial.[19]

ORBITAL APEX SYNDROME

Clinical Problem

Orbital apex syndrome is defined as the simultaneous dysfunction of the optic nerve and the cranial nerves (manifesting with vision loss, ptosis, and a complete internal and external ophthalmoplegia) as a result of a process occurring in the region of the optic canal and the superior orbital fissure (orbital apex). It has been reported in a wide variety of procedures, usually as a result of hemorrhage, and it has also been reported after manipulation during facial fracture repair,[22] ethmoidal artery ligation for recurrent epistaxis,[27] septorhinoplasty,[28] and intranasal ethmoidectomy.[29]

Medical and Surgical Management

Because cases of orbital apex syndrome may be both devastating and irreversible, careful intraoperative manipulations must be employed. Intraorbital ligation of the ethmoidal artery should be meticulously employed under excellent visualization to avoid damage to the optic nerve.

The optimal management of orbital apex syndrome remains controversial. Although some authorities advocate observant management, the use of high-dose corticosteroids has been shown to improve vision, possibly through an antioxidant effect.[30] Surgical decompression of the optic nerve may also be beneficial.

EXTRAOCULAR MUSCLE INJURY

Clinical Problem

The orbital complications of intranasal sinus surgery have been widely described in both the ophthalmology literature and the otolaryngology literature.[13,31–41] Although the use of endoscopes and image guidance have provided some safeguards, complications still pose a significant concern, particularly with the use of mechanized instrumentation.[11,31–33,42,43] In particular, the thinness of the lamina papyracea and the proximity of the medial rectus muscle to the medial orbital wall make this muscle particularly susceptible to injury. There have been several case series that have addressed extraocular muscle damage that results in dysmotility and possible treatment strategies, and several reports exist regarding the use of botulinum toxin injections into the antagonist rectus as monotherapy.[11,31–33]

Inadvertent entry into the orbit occurs most commonly during FESS during which the ethmoid bone is removed. The muscle can be contused or avulsed, especially when power tools that quickly debride tissue are used. Even in patients without enlarged extraocular muscles, it is not unusual for the medial rectus to lie just internal to the periorbita without any significant protection from the orbital fat.

Huang and colleagues[44] retrospectively evaluated 30 cases of medial rectus injury associated with FESS. They found a wide spectrum of injury that included contusion, entrapment, and complete transection. They concluded that patients with severe muscle injury may benefit from intervention (i.e., strabismus surgery), but these patients would often have persistent limitations of ocular motility and functional impairment. Even without significant entry into the orbit, powered instrument tools can result in the attraction of the orbital contents into the tip of the cutter. In one report, a patient suffered isolated medial rectus transection, and another had

"restrictive global ophthalmoplegia."[31] Figure 9-2 depicts a patient who underwent FESS with subsequent transection of the left medial rectus muscle. Inferior rectus and inferior oblique injury are less common. In four cases reported by Rene and colleagues,[13] all patients had medial rectus injury, one had additional inferior rectus and inferior oblique injury, and two were blinded as a result of optic nerve injury.

Injury to the horizontal rectus muscles (i.e., the medial or lateral rectus muscles) can cause horizontal diplopia. Consequently, injury to the vertical rectus muscles (i.e., the superior or inferior rectus muscles) can cause vertical diplopia with some small degree of a head turn for partial or full compensation.

Patients have varying levels of tolerance to diplopia, depending the severity of the muscle palsy. For example, the total avulsion of the right medial rectus muscle will cause a severe outward deviation (exotropia) in primary gaze. By contrast, a partial right medial rectus

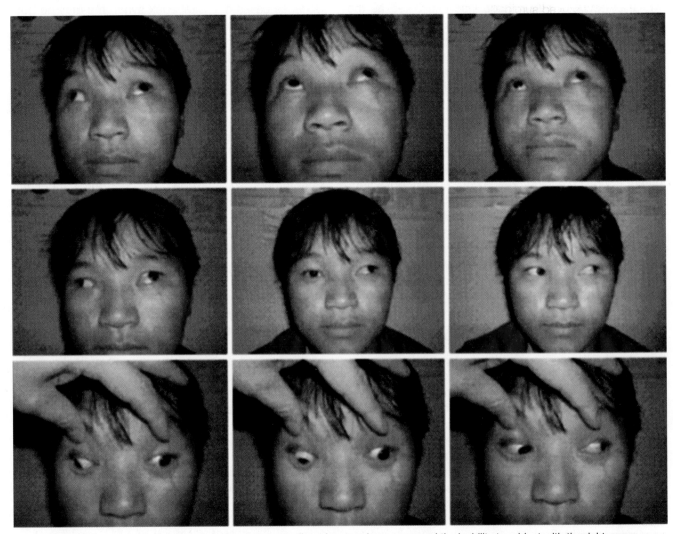

Figure 9-2. Left medial rectus palsy. Note the severe disconjugate primary gaze and the inability to adduct with the right gaze.

palsy may cause a small-angle exotropia in primary gaze that the patient may be able to compensate for by convergence for day-to-day activities. In any case, the patching of one eye can help to avoid constant diplopia while the patient is observed. Patients can alternatively be fitted into prism spectacles to help correct for the diplopia in primary gaze. It is important to note that the prism spectacles help correct the diplopia in primary gaze only and not when the patient looks in different gaze positions (e.g., right or left gaze).

Medical and Surgical Management

A formal evaluation by an ophthalmologist with a specialty in strabismus surgery is recommended if there is any suspicion of extraocular muscle injury. High-resolution CT scanning and magnetic resonance imaging help to further evaluate the nature of the injury, and surgical repair may be warranted if there is a functional remaining segment of the rectus muscles (usually >20 mm) when the patient is evaluated surgically.[33] Additionally, cases of extraocular muscle transection require early surgical intervention to identify and reappose the separated ends of the muscle. If it cannot be repaired surgically, a significant medial rectus injury is best to be initially observed for 3 to 6 months rather than repaired.[45,46] During the early postoperative period, some authorities advocate the use of systemic corticosteroids to suppress cicatrization.[47] Because trauma to the muscle often results in a myectomy, surgeons may have difficulty reanastomosing the loose ends, and they may often employ a fascial graft to enable reapproximation.[48] Options include transpositional muscle surgery with and without the use of botulinum toxin injection to inactivate the antagonist extraocular muscle.[49–51]

We have experience with a patient who had medial rectus injury from endoscopic sinus surgery who was treated successfully. The patient was a 40-year-old woman with a 2-year history of chronic sinusitis that was resistant to medical therapy who underwent bilateral CT-guided endoscopic frontal sinusotomy and ethmoidectomy. The patient noted binocular diplopia immediately upon awakening after surgery. The operative report indicated that the right lamina papyracea was extremely thinned, with bowing noted when gentle pressure was applied to the orbit. However, other than increased intraoperative bleeding, no violation of the periorbita was appreciated. CT scanning and magnetic resonance imaging obtained postoperatively revealed a defect in the medial orbital wall with an intact (although markedly attenuated) medial rectus muscle. The patient's examination was remarkable for a large outward deviation of the right eye (exotropia of 50 prism diopters in primary gaze). Forced ductions did not reveal any restriction in the excursion of the globe. The patient was treated with a series of intramuscular injections of botulinum toxin A (five injections for a total of 30 units

over 1 month). Six months after the surgical complication, the patient remained asymptomatic.

PUPIL ABNORMALITIES

Clinical Problem

During nonocular surgery performed under general anesthesia, clinicians often tape the eyelids to protect the surface of the eye to help prevent corneal abrasions. Unfortunately, this technique prevents the surgeon from observing pupillary changes that may occur intraoperatively, including an afferent pupillary defect (as a result of optic nerve damage), Horner syndrome (as a result of sympathetic denervation), or Adie pupil (as a result of damage to the ciliary ganglion or nerves).

Karkanevatos and colleagues[52] monitored pupil size and reaction during FESS in 40 patients. Miosis occurred during general anesthesia, even when nasal vasoconstriction was induced by cocaine.

In orbital surgery under general anesthesia, surgeons routinely observe the pupil intraoperatively for evidence of dilation. If the pupil enlarges in a symmetric fashion (i.e., large and round), there is a concern that the optic nerve may be ischemic.[53] If the pupil enlarges in an oval or irregular fashion, it is consistent with ischemia of the ciliary body or nerves. If the contralateral eyelid is opened, the relative response to light can be assessed: an afferent pupillary defect will go away when light stimulates the consensual light reflex.[54] By contrast, ciliary ganglion ischemic pupil changes will persist.

The determination of the cause of pupil abnormalities requires careful analysis, because several possible mechanisms may result in this disorder. *Anisocoria* refers to a difference between the size of the pupils, and this may be a normal physiologic finding in certain patients. Direct damage to the iris is another important consideration during the evaluation of nonneurologic pupillary abnormalities. Specifically, the uvea normally "plugs" scleral wounds in cases of ruptured globes, creating a "peaked" and irregularly shaped pupil. As such, pupils with this configuration should be evaluated for possible ruptures (i.e., hyphema, shallow anterior chamber, decreased vision, retinal tears or breaks, vitreous hemorrhages), particularly in cases of orbital surgery. Prior eye traumas or surgical interventions may result in tears in the iris, which create an irregular pupil. Finally, uveitis (intraocular inflammation) creates adhesions between the iris and the lens (synechiae), and it is thus characterized by pupil abnormalities. Patients will usually report histories of these problems, and they should therefore be specifically questioned about these disorders.

Horner syndrome results from damage to the sympathetic innervation to the pupil. Because the affected side becomes miotic, the anisocoria becomes worse in dark lighting, and Horner syndrome is marked by an ipsilateral ptosis. Pharmacologic testing can help to confirm and localize this diagnosis. Cocaine selectively blocks the reuptake of norepinephrine from the synaptic cleft and normally results in dilation. Because patients with Horner syndrome have reduced norepinephrine at the neuromuscular junction, the installation of 10% cocaine eyedrops will not result in dilation in these cases.

Localizing tests with 1% hydroxyamphetamine can then be used after a washout period of 24 hours. This chemical induces the release of norepinephrine from the synaptic vesicles of the third-order neuron. In cases in which the third-order neuron is intact (i.e., the defect lies in the first- or second-order neuron), the pupil should dilate in the presence of hydroxyamphetamine; the absence of such dilation indicates a postganglionic Horner syndrome. First-order neuron Horner syndrome cases are usually the result of stroke, tumor, or severe osteoarthritis. Second-order neuron cases usually result from neoplastic causes, including Pancoast tumor of the lung apex, thyroid adenoma, metastatic disease, and lymphoma. Although third-order causes are generally thought to be benign (headache syndrome, otitis media), carotid artery dissection is in the differential diagnosis. Appropriate testing for and management of these causes should be directed by such pharmacologic testing.

Conversely, damage to the parasympathetic innervation of the pupil results in mydriasis and is thus generally worse in bright light. A tonic pupil is usually characterized by blurred vision and glare. In cases of a denervation supersensitivity, dilute solutions of pilocarpine (i.e., 0.125%) eyedrops should constrict the tonic pupil considerably (without constricting a normal pupil). The therapeutic use of pilocarpine eyedrops may be necessary in these patients for both cosmetic and visual purposes.

Cases of mydriasis in the presence of ptosis suggest damage to the third cranial nerve. Pupils with this disorder should not constrict with dilute pilocarpine, but they should constrict with normal concentrations (1%). Such cases necessitate neuroimaging. Finally, mydriatic pupils that do not constrict in the presence of 1% pilocarpine are suspicious for pharmacologic dilation (i.e., the installation of atropine or mydriatic agents).

Medical and Surgical Management

If the pupillary abnormality is the result of tissue edema or a small hemorrhage, observation is indicated. The role of corticosteroids is controversial.

Surgical evacuation is indicated if there is a large hematoma compressing the ciliary ganglion or the ciliary nerves. Horner syndrome can occur in conjunction with double vision and lid ptosis if the hemorrhage involves the superior orbital fissure, the cavernous sinus, or both.

GLOBE DISPLACEMENT

Clinical Problem

Surgery of the maxilla, the orbital floor, or both after trauma or tumor removal can result in the inferior displacement of the entire eyeball (hypoglobus) or the sinking back of the eyeball into the orbit (enophthalmos).

Medical and Surgical Management

This can be a surgical challenge to repair, especially in patients with longstanding cases that are associated with intraorbital fat atrophy. Surgical options include orbital floor or, less commonly, medial wall implants to create a shelf to support the ptotic globe.

EYELID MALPOSITION

Clinical Problem

Surgery on the mid face for tumors or trauma can result in vertical scar bands or the foreshortening of the lower eyelid. This cicatrizing process most commonly results in a combination of ectropion and eyelid retraction as a result of an imbalance between protracting forces (i.e., orbicularis) and retracting forces (i.e., lower eyelid retractors, scar tissue). In severe cases, lagophthalmos (the inability to passively close the eyelids) can cause corneal breakdown and discomfort. Furthermore, ocular surface dryness often results in corneal ulceration and infection. In extreme cases, this ulceration thins the cornea, and corneal perforation may ensue. Blepharoplasties of either the upper or lower eyelid that remove too much skin, orbicularis, or both can also result in lagophthalmos.

Traditional open procedures (transconjunctival and transcutaneous) near the periorbita have up to a 5% rate of postoperative eyelid malposition complications. Complications can include lower lid retraction, lid ectropion, or entropion[55,56] (Figure 9-3). Suga and colleagues[57] reviewed 22 transconjunctival procedures for medial orbital floor fractures and found that 5 of the 22 had some evidence of lower lid retraction. Isolated cases of lower lid laceration and avulsion with lacrimal duct injury were also reported.[58] Of interest is that open procedures for isolated orbital floor repair seem to have a lower rate of incidence.

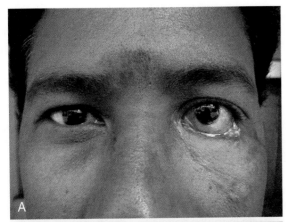

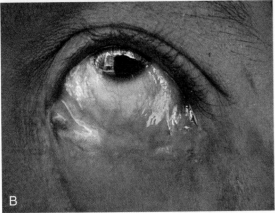

Figure 9-3. A, Postoperative cicatricial ectropion 3 months after repair of a left orbital floor and rim fracture. **B,** Severe cicatricial changes can be seen in upgaze. The patient required surgical exploration and repair, and he was found to have extensive fibrosis in the region of the plate for the rim. The hardware was removed, the cicatrix was released, and the lid was rebuilt with the use of a gelfilm spacer and a combined skin graft and Hughes flap.

Medical and Surgical Management

In mild cases, massage and time result in the resolution of the problem. Lubrication with artificial tears during the day and ointments at bedtime can be helpful during the interim. Careful monitoring of the corneal status in conjunction with an ophthalmologist is necessary to avoid excessive thinning and perforation, because these conditions represent surgical emergencies. In more severe cases of eyelid malposition, skin grafts may be necessary in conjunction with canthoplasties to horizontally tighten the lids.

FACIAL NERVE PALSY

Clinical Problem

Parotid surgery or skull-base surgery for acoustic neuromas can cause damage to the seventh nerve, which results in significant functional and aesthetic deficits. Notably, these patients may experience significant tearing and ophthalmic pain, speech disorders, impaired ability to eat and breathe, and drooling; these conditions may alter both their appearance and their self-image. Furthermore, irreversible facial paralysis may yield considerable facial asymmetry.

Because the frontalis muscle may be involved in cases of peripheral seventh nerve palsies, the involvement of the brow complex results in brow ptosis and the loss of forehead rhytids on the affected side of the face. In addition to the obvious facial asymmetry, this paralysis creates a "heavy" sensation along the eyelid, and the superior visual field may thus be compromised. Formal visual field testing can be used to quantify the amount of visual field deficit. The degree of ptosis may be assessed by manually elevating the brow to a symmetric position with the contralateral brow and measuring its descent upon release.

The loss of orbicularis oculi muscle tone results in diminished protraction in the periorbital complex, thereby causing corneal exposure. Because the upper and lower eyelids are retracted, they cannot adequately close to protect the cornea; notably, patients with seventh nerve palsies have considerable lagophthalmos. Orbicularis oculi muscle weakness may result in lower eyelid ectropion with punctual eversion. Consequently, patients may complain of pain, foreign body sensation, tearing, photophobia, and blurring in the affected eye. Eyelid position can be quantified by shining a light into the patient's eye and noting the position of the corneal light reflex. The distance from the reflex to the upper eyelid is referred to as the *upper marginal reflex distance,* and the distance to the lower eyelid is the *lower marginal reflex distance.*

Changes in the mid-face complex also affect the eyelids. Patients with facial paralysis display a descent of the malar eminence, a blunting of the nasolabial fold, and a rotation of the nasal ala.

Recent advances in acoustic neuroma resection have decreased the incidence of facial nerve injury. Preserving the facial nerve is a routine standard of care for small and intracanalicular lesions. Intraoperative monitoring of the facial nerve through various proximal-to-distal amplitude ratio and stimulus threshold devices has improved the outcomes significantly. A recent retrospective review found that 100% (8 of 8) of patients undergoing surgery for intracanalicular tumors and 95% (52 of 55) of patients with small tumors had excellent postoperative facial nerve function (i.e., House–Brackman grade 1 or 2). Medium- to large-sized acoustic neuromas were found to involve a higher incidence of facial nerve injury, with only 63% (15 of 24) of patients with medium-sized tumors maintaining a postoperative House–Brackman grade of 1 or 2. The minimum observed follow-up time in this study was 12 months.[59]

Alternatively, Samii and colleagues[60] pointed out that, among 979 cases in a retrospective study, the majority of patients that initially had facial nerve injury (i.e., House–Brackman 1–6) had a significant improvement during the course of the first postoperative year.

Of particular concern is that the nervus intermedius is equally likely to be traumatized by the surgical resection of an acoustic neuroma. Injuring the nervus intermedius, which is a component of the complex lacrimal gland secretion pattern, can often lead to dry-eye symptoms. Irving and colleagues[61] found out that a significant reduction of tears occurred in 72% of patients postoperatively and that these patients also had a variable recovery of function. This should be evaluated in postoperative patients with complaints of dry eyes with the use of a Schirmer tear film strip. The findings of dry eyes in lieu of a paralytic lower lid from facial nerve injury can significantly place the patient at a considerable risk of exposure keratopathy.

Medical and Surgical Management

Optimal care of the patient with facial paralysis depends on the reversibility of the disorder. In mild cases or reversible situations, supportive measures with topical lubricants may be sufficient. Irreversible cases generally require surgical rehabilitation. Nonetheless, the degree of corneal decompensation often dictates management. External gold weights can be applied to the pretarsal skin to assist with lid closure.[62] Moisture chambers or regular swim goggles can be worn in severe cases.

Surgical rehabilitation of the patient with irreversible facial paralysis often requires the evaluation of each complex individually. Brow ptosis can be corrected with a brow lift, and multiple approaches have been developed to address this issue. Although a direct brow lift offers the most durable solution, patients may find the risk of a facial scar unacceptable. As a result, some surgeons prefer a mid-forehead or pretricheal incision to offer elevation with minimal scarring. Endoscopic brow lifts avoid visible scars, but they may not be as durable as direct interventions.

In all cases of surgical rehabilitation of the paralyzed periorbital region, adequate corneal protection and the elimination of lagophthalmos are the desired outcomes. Although a tarsorrhaphy certainly meets these endpoints, it is marked by a cosmetically undesirable appearance, and it prevents vision in the affected eye.

Consequently, a number of other options exist to address periorbital paralysis. Lagophthalmos can be overcome with the placement of an upper eyelid gold weight (or, in cases of gold allergy, a platinum weight).

Before surgery, the adequate implant is carefully selected for the optimum size, weight, and placement within the eyelid. Such measures can help avoid the uncommon complications of gold weight implants, such as infection, extrusion, or inflammation with subsequent cicatricial entropion.[63]

Lower eyelid ectropion can be managed with a horizontal shortening procedure. Generally, a lateral tarsal strip technique is employed to this end. Specifically, a canthotomy and cantholysis are performed, and a "strip" of tarsus is shortened and reapposed to the periosteum overlying the lateral orbital rim. Optimally, this intervention results in the apposition of the punctum against the globe. Notably, the descent of mid-facial tissues may result in the residual sagging of the lower eyelids, and spacer grafts may be placed to address lower eyelid retraction.

The dynamic reanimation of the mid face involves either direct repair of the facial nerve, nerve transfer or grafting, or muscle grafting. Although these techniques are promising, their use for older patients is somewhat limited.

Alternatively, static rehabilitation techniques involve the resuspension of descended tissue through fixation to fixed structures. The standard techniques employed for cosmetic rejuvenation of the mid face (i.e., the mid-face lift) may be used for elevation. Caution should be employed in cases of facial paralysis, because the effects of gravity in the absence of natural facial animation likely require greater fixation. The fixation of the descended mid face to the orbital rim with suture anchors allows for durable elevation with the reconstitution of the nasolabial fold and the outward rotation of the nostril. Alternatively, contralateral botulinum toxin A may be applied adjunctively to restore facial symmetry and to address aberrant regeneration.

NASOLACRIMAL DUCT OBSTRUCTION

Clinical Problem

Nasolacrimal duct obstruction is a commonly reported complication with orbital surgery, endoscopic sinus surgery, maxillectomies, and rhinoplastic surgery.[64–67] Patients typically present with epiphora. Although some patients may undergo damage to the lacrimal system without symptomatic tearing, symptomatic epiphora occurs in 0.3% to 1.7% of patients after endoscopic sinus surgery.[68]

The local manipulation that occurs during paranasal sinus surgery certainly places the nasolacrimal duct at risk of transient postoperative edema and nasolacrimal duct scarring or direct injury. Anatomically, the nasolacrimal duct is variable in structure, and its paranasal location makes it susceptible to injury from intraoperative manipulation.[38,64] The areas that are most vulnerable to inadvertent surgical injury are the nasolacrimal sac, which is located just beneath the medial canthal ligament, and the ductal ostium in the inferior meatus. Interestingly enough, Meyers and Hawes[65] reviewed five case series (31 patients) involving nasolacrimal duct obstruction after nasal and sinus surgery. They showed that a significant number (21 of 31) of patients had a surgical creation of a nasoantral window as a part of their procedure. The nasolacrimal duct is certainly at risk during the placement of a nasoantral window. Serdahl and colleagues[64] also suggested that nasolacrimal duct injury can occur with a large anterior enlargement of the maxillary sinus ostium. They suggested that the ostium be limited to the thin lamellar bone of the anterior lateral wall of the middle meatus and that it not extend toward the nasolacrimal duct.

Injury to the nasolacrimal duct has also been well reported after orbital decompression for Graves' ophthalmopathy.[69,70] Seiff and Shorr[70] reported that up to 16% (14 of 90) of patients had persistent epiphora after undergoing a transantral ethmoidal orbital decompression. The epiphora presented late (an average 11–18 months postoperatively), which was suggestive of cicatricial obstruction of the nasolacrimal drainage system from surrounding scar tissue.[69,70]

Anatomically, tears are drained along the medial aspect of the eyelids through the superior and inferior punctae into the canaliculi. In the majority of patients, the two canaliculi fuse, thereby creating the common canaliculus. The system then enters into the lacrimal sac, which sits within the lacrimal fossa. The nasolacrimal duct exits from the sac into the inferior meatus, 2.5 cm posterior to the naris. Damage to the structures of this system at any point may result in the blockage of the drainage system, which results in epiphora.

Careful clinical examination can often disclose whether a blockage is present, and it may be useful for determining the location of such an obstruction. On external examination, an elevated tear meniscus along the lower eyelid suggests that tears are not adequately flowing into the drainage system. The dye disappearance test can be used to confirm blockage. With this test, fluorescein dye is instilled into the inferior fornix of both eyes, and its egress is monitored over the course of 5 minutes. If delayed dye disappearance is seen in one eye, a lacrimal system obstruction may be present.

Lacrimal system probing and irrigation are confirmatory tests. With these tests, the punctae are gently dilated, and saline is irrigated through one canaliculus. If the saline refluxes through the same punctum, a canalicular block may be present. Egress through the opposite punctum is suggestive of a more distal block (i.e., the nasolacrimal duct). Free passage into the nasal cavity and subsequently into the pharynx (i.e., the patient is able to swallow the saline) indicates that no block is present.

When performing irrigation, clinicians should be mindful of the fact that partial blockages may be present (i.e., partial reflux in the setting of some degree of free passage into the pharynx). Under such circumstances, the adjuvant use of a dacryocystogram may enable further visualization of the lacrimal drainage system. With this test, a contrast medium is injected into the canaliculus, and plain x-ray films are taken to image its flow through the system.

Medical and Surgical Management

Nasolacrimal duct obstruction is most commonly transient, although it can be permanent. In cases of rhinoplasty in which epiphora is a known complication, much of it is usually temporary and lasts 1 to 2 weeks. This has to do with local soft-tissue swelling around the lacrimal sac and the nasolacrimal duct.[67] Edema should resolve within 2 or 3 months, and scarring from chronic paranasal inflammation or direct injury to the nasolacrimal duct can cause permanent epiphora.

Epiphora that lasts longer than 2 or 3 months should prompt the evaluation of the lacrimal drainage system. Patients with nasolacrimal duct obstructions often require dacryocystorhinostomy surgery to create an artificial drainage system. For patients in which the obstruction is more proximal (i.e., at the level of the canaliculus), a conjunctivodacryocystorhinostomy should be employed to bypass the damaged system.

VISION LOSS FROM THERAPEUTIC AND ANESTHETIC INJECTIONS

The loss of vision and double vision from nasal mucosa, tonsillar fossa, sphenopalatine fossa, and scalp injections have been reported for decades.[71] Otolaryngologists commonly use corticosteroid injections for the management of inferior turbinate hypertrophy. Cases of both permanent and temporary blindness have been reported after steroid injection of the nasal turbinates, but paraffin and silicone oil emboli have also been reported.[72,73] The incidence rate of this complication 2 in patients with inferior turbinate injection of steroids is 0.006%.[74]

The mechanism of embolization is postulated to be retrograde flow from the anterior tip of the inferior turbinate through anastomosis with the anterior and posterior ethmoid arteries to the ophthalmic artery, followed by anterograde flow. Larger-particle corticosteroids (e.g., methylprednisone) are thought to present an increased risk because they can lodge in end arteries of the choroid and retinal vessels.[72,74] Transient visual loss has even been reported in patients who have been injected with triamcinolone, which is a smaller-particle corticosteroid. Numerous emboli in the retina are seen on funduscopic examination. Larger emboli can also cause severe vision loss in the absence of any visible retinal emboli; in this setting, the damage usually lies in the retrobulbar portion of the optic nerve. In such cases, a relative afferent pupillary defect in the affected eye is the only objective evidence of an injury.

Certain measures can be taken to decrease the possibility of such complications. Topical vasoconstrictors should be used along with the injections to prevent intravascular injection. When inserting the needle intranasally, the syringe should be drawn back to evaluate for any reflux of blood. Injections should be performed slowly using a small needle (i.e., 25 gauge). Additionally, the use of a small particle-based repository corticosteroid should be used.

QUALITY OF LIFE

Ophthalmic complications can certainly have a variable impact on a patient's quality of life. Quality of life can be affected in two major domains: visual function and altered appearance.

Visual Disability

Visual function can be compromised via optic nerve injury, extraocular muscle injury, chronic epiphora leading to blurry vision, or lagophthalmos causing exposure keratopathy from a facial nerve palsy. They can affect patients' ability to perform daily activities as a result of the associated diminished visual acuity, diplopia, and disturbed color perception.

A variety of pathologic changes can contribute to visual disturbance. Optic nerve injury, whether transient or permanent (as seen with orbital hemorrhages), can leave patients with deficits in vision, color perception, and contrast sensitivity. Exposure keratopathy can cause tearing, irritation, photophobia, and even blurred vision. Extraocular injury can lead to variable amounts of diplopia; some can be compensated for by patients, whereas others require monocular patch therapy, botulinum toxin A, or strabismus surgery.

Facial Disfigurement

Patients may experience psychosocial impairment related to their altered appearance. Globe displacement, strabismus, and eyelid changes (e.g., ectropion) can significantly change the way a patient perceives himself or herself and the visual impression that he or she makes on others. Visual impairment also contributes to psychosocial impairment, because patients may accomplish less at work, at home, and socially.

Pain

Patients can often have variable complications of pain. Patients with exposure keratopathy often have early corneal decompensation changes, and these can be very irritating. A corneal abrasion itself is characterized by a sharp, constant eye pain. Neither of these conditions is comforting for the patient. Often, postoperative pain from orbital surgery and endoscopic sinus surgery can leave the patient with a transient, chronic ache that may be exacerbated with eye movement.

REFERENCES

1. DeMere M, Wood T, Austin W: Eye complications with blepharoplasty or other eyelid surgery: A national survey. *Plast Reconstr Surg* 1974;53(6):634–637.
2. Jafek BW, Kreiger AE, Morledge D: Proceedings: Blindness following blepharoplasty. *Arch Otolaryngol* 1973;98(6):366–369.
3. Moser MH, DiPirro E, McCoy FJ: Sudden blindness following belpharoplasty: Report of seven cases. *Plast Reconstr Surg* 1973;51(4):364–370.
4. Burkat CN, Lemke BN: Retrobulbar hemorrhage: Inferolateral anterior orbitotomy for emergent management. *Arch Ophthalmol* 2005;123(9):1260–1262.
5. Markovits AS: Evacuation of orbital hematoma by continuous suction. *Ann Ophthalmol* 1977;9(10):1255–1258.
6. Liu D: A simplified technique of orbital decompression for severe retrobulbar hemorrhage. *Am J Ophthalmol* 1993;116(1):34–37.
7. Rubinstein A, Riddell CE, Akram I, et al: Orbital emphysema leading to blindness following routine functional endoscopic sinus surgery. *Arch Ophthalmol* 2005;123(10):1452.
8. Mohan B, Singh KP: Bilateral subcutaneous emphysema of the orbits following nose blowing. *J Laryngol Otol* 2001;115(4):319–320.
9. Hunts JH, Patrinely JR, Holds JB, et al: Orbital emphysema. Staging and acute management. *Ophthalmology* 1994;101(5):960–966.
10. Thacker NM, Velez FG, Krieger A, et al: Retinal hemorrhages as a complication of endoscopic sinus surgery. *Arch Ophthalmol* 2004;122(11):1724–1725.
11. Thacker NM, Velez FG, Demer JL, et al: Extraocular muscle damage associated with endoscopic sinus surgery: An ophthalmology perspective. *Am J Rhinol* 2005;19(4):400–405.
12. Kenawy NB, Ayou OM: Major orbital complications of endoscopic sinus surgery. *Br J Ophthalmol* 2001;85(11):1394.
13. Rene C, Rose GE, Lenthall R, et al: Major orbital complications of endoscopic sinus surgery. *Br J Ophthalmol* 2001;85(5):598–603.
14. Mafee MF, Chow JM, Meyers R: Functional endoscopic sinus surgery: Anatomy, CT screening, indications, and complications. *AJR Am J Roentgenol* 1993;160(4):735–744.
15. Chen YL, Lee LA, Lim KE: Surgical consideration to optic nerve protrusion according to sinus computed tomography. *Otolaryngol Head Neck Surg* 2006;134(3):499–505.
16. DeLano MC, Fun FY, Zinreich SJ: Relationship of the optic nerve to the posterior paranasal sinuses: A CT anatomic study. *AJNR Am J Neuroradiol* 1996;17(4):669–675.
17. Bansberg SF, Harner SG, Forbes G: Relationship of the optic nerve to the paranasal sinuses as shown by computed tomography. *Otolaryngol Head Neck Surg* 1987;96(4):331–335.

18. Dessi P, Moulin G, Castro F, et al: Protrusion of the optic nerve into the ethmoid and sphenoid sinus: Prospective study of 150 CT studies. *Neuroradiology* 1994;36(7):515–516.

19. Lee JC, Chuo PI, Hsiung MW: Ischemic optic neuropathy after endoscopic sinus surgery: A case report. *Eur Arch Otorhinolaryngol* 2003;260(8):429–431.

20. Marks SC, Jaques DA, Hirata RM, et al: Blindness following bilateral radical neck dissection. *Head Neck* 1990;12(4):342–345.

21. Girotto JA, Gamble WB, Robertson B, et al: Blindness after reduction of facial fractures. *Plast Reconstr Surg* 1998;102(6): 1821–1834.

22. Girotto JA, Davidson J, Wheatly M, et al: Blindness as a complication of Le Fort osteotomies: Role of atypical fracture patterns and distortion of the optic canal. *Plast Reconstr Surg* 1998;102(5):1409–1423.

23. Lo LJ, Hung KF, Chen YR: Blindness as a complication of Le Fort I osteotomy for maxillary distraction. *Plast Reconstr Surg* 2002;109(2):688–700.

24. Cook MW, Levin LA, Joseph MP, et al: Traumatic optic neuropathy: A meta-analysis. *Arch Otolaryngol Head Neck Surg* 1996;122(4):389–392.

25. Guy J, Sherwood M, Day AL: Surgical treatment of progressive visual loss in traumatic optic neuropathy: Report of two cases. *J Neurosurg* 1989;70(5):799–801.

26. Levin LA, Beck RW, Joseph MP, et al: The treatment of traumatic optic neuropathy: The International Optic Nerve Trauma Study. *Ophthalmology* 1999;106(7):1268–1277.

27. Yeh S, Yen MT, Foroozan R: Orbital apex syndrome after ethmoidal artery ligation for recurrent epistaxis. *Ophthal Plast Reconstr Surg* 2004;20(5):392–394.

28. Jaison SG, Bhatty SM, Chopra SK, et al: Orbital apex syndrome: A rare complication of septorhinoplasty. *Indian J Ophthalmol* 1994;42(4):213–214.

29. Vassallo P, Tranfa F, Forte R, et al: Ophthalmic complications after surgery for nasal and sinus polyposis. *Eur J Ophthalmol* 2001;11(3):218–222.

30. Eo S, Kim JY, Azari K: Temporary orbital apex syndrome after repair of orbital wall fracture. *Plast Reconstr Surg* 2005;116(5): 85e–89e.

31. Bhatti MT, Giannoni CM, Raynor E, et al: Ocular motility complications after endoscopic sinus surgery with powered cutting instruments. *Otolaryngol Head Neck Surg* 2001;125(5): 501–509.

32. Bhatti MT, Schmalfuss IM, Mancuso AA: Orbital complications of functional endoscopic sinus surgery: MR and CT findings. *Clin Radiol* 2005;60(8):894–904.

33. Thacker NM, Velez FG, Demer JL, et al: Strabismic complications following endoscopic sinus surgery: Diagnosis and surgical management. *J AAPOS* 2004;8(5):488–494.

34. Graham SM, Nerad JA: Orbital complications in endoscopic sinus surgery using powered instrumentation. *Laryngoscope* 2003;113(5):874–878.

35. Graham SM, Carter KD: Major complications of endoscopic sinus surgery: A comment. *Br J Ophthalmol* 2003;87(3):374.

36. Corey JP, Bumsted R, Panje W, et al: Orbital complications in functional endoscopic sinus surgery. *Otolaryngol Head Neck Surg* 1993;109(5):814–820.

37. Neuhaus RW: Orbital complications secondary to endoscopic sinus surgery. *Ophthalmology* 1990;97(11):1512–1518.

38. Dutton JJ: Orbital complications of paranasal sinus surgery. *Ophthal Plast Reconstr Surg* 1986;2(3):119–127.

39. Flynn JT, Mitchell KB, Fuller DG, et al: Ocular motility complications following intranasal surgery. *Arch Ophthalmol* 1979;97(3):453–458.

40. Mark LE, Kennerdell JS: Medial rectus injury from intranasal surgery. *Arch Ophthalmol* 1979;97(3):459–461.

41. Sharp HR, Crutchfield L, Rowe-Jones JM, et al: Major complications and consent prior to endoscopic sinus surgery. *Clin Otolaryngol Allied Sci* 2001;26(1):33–38.

42. Lund VJ, Wright A, Yiotakis J: Complications and medicolegal aspects of endoscopic sinus surgery. *J R Soc Med* 1997;90(8): 422–428.

43. May M, Levine HL, Mester SJ, et al: Complications of endoscopic sinus surgery: Analysis of 2108 patients—Incidence and prevention. *Laryngoscope* 1994;104(9):1080–1083.

44. Huang CM, Meyer DR, Patrinely JR, et al: Medial rectus muscle injuries associated with functional endoscopic sinus surgery: Characterization and management. *Ophthal Plast Reconstr Surg* 2003;19(1):25–37.

45. Lyon DB, Newman SA: Evidence of direct damage to extraocular muscles as a cause of diplopia following orbital trauma. *Ophthal Plast Reconstr Surg* 1989;5(2):81–91.

46. Wojno TH: The incidence of extraocular muscle and cranial nerve palsy in orbital floor blow-out fractures. *Ophthalmology* 1987;94(6):682–687.

47. Bhatti MT, Stankiewicz JA: Ophthalmic complications of endoscopic sinus surgery. *Surv Ophthalmol* 2003;48(4):389–402.

48. Trotter WL, Kaw P, Meyer DR, et al: Treatment of subtotal medial rectus myectomy complicating functional endoscopic sinus surgery. *J AAPOS* 2000;4(4):250–253.

49. Murray AD: Slipped and lost muscles and other tales of the unexpected: Philip Knapp Lecture. *J AAPOS* 1998;2(3):133–143.

50. Scott AB, Kraft SP: Botulinum toxin injection in the management of lateral rectus paresis. *Ophthalmology* 1985;92(5):676–683.

51. Osako M, Keltner JL: Botulinum A toxin (Oculinum) in ophthalmology. *Surv Ophthalmol* 1991;36(1):28–46.

52. Karkanevatos A, Lancaster JL, Osman I, et al: Pupil size and reaction during functional endoscopic sinus surgery (FESS). *Clin Otolaryngol Allied Sci* 2003;28(2):103–107.

53. Badia L, Lund VJ: Dilated pupil during endoscopic sinus surgery: What does it mean? *Am J Rhinol* 2001;15(1):31–33.

54. Zaidi FH, Moseley MJ: Use of pupil size and reaction to detect orbital trauma during and after surgery. *Clin Otolaryngol Allied Sci* 2004;29(3):288–290.

55. Zingg M, Chowdhury K, Ladrach K, et al: Treatment of 813 zygoma-lateral orbital complex fractures: New aspects. *Arch Otolaryngol Head Neck Surg* 1991;117(6):611–622.

56. Appling WD, Patrinely JR, Salzer TA: Transconjunctival approach vs subciliary skin-muscle flap approach for orbital fracture repair. *Arch Otolaryngol Head Neck Surg* 1993;119(9): 1000–1007.

57. Suga H, Sugawara Y, Uda H, et al: The transconjunctival approach for orbital bony surgery: In which cases should it be used? *J Craniofac Surg* 2004;15(3):454–457.

58. Mullins JB, Holds JB, Branham GH, et al: Complications of the transconjunctival approach: A review of 400 cases. *Arch Otolaryngol Head Neck Surg* 1997;123(4):385–388.

59. Kaylie DM, Gilbert E, Horgan MA, et al: Acoustic neuroma surgery outcomes. *Otol Neurotol* 2001;22(5):686–689.

60. Samii M, Matthies C: Management of 1000 vestibular schwannomas (acoustic neuromas): The facial nerve—Preservation and restitution of function. *Neurosurgery* 1997;40(4):684–695.

61. Irving RM, Viani L, Hardy DG, Baguley DM, et al: Nervus intermedius function after vestibular schwannoma removal: clinical features and pathophysiological mechanisms. *Laryngoscope* 1995;105(8 Pt 1):809–813.

62. Seiff SR, Boerner M, Carter SR: Treatment of facial palsies with external eyelid weights. *Am J Ophthalmol* Nov 1995;120(5): 652–657.

63. Dinces EA, Mauriello JA Jr, Kwartler JA, et al: Complications of gold weight eyelid implants for treatment of fifth and seventh nerve paralysis. *Laryngoscope* 1997;107(12 Pt 1): 1617–1622.

64. Serdahl CL, Berris CE, Chole RA: Nasolacrimal duct obstruction after endoscopic sinus surgery. *Arch Ophthalmol* 1990;108(3):391–392.

65. Meyers AD, Hawes MJ: Nasolacrimal obstruction after inferior meatus nasal antrostomy. *Arch Otolaryngol Head Neck Surg* 1991;117(2):208–211.

66. Glatt HJ, Chan AC: Lacrimal obstruction after medial maxillectomy. *Ophthalmic Surg* 1991;22(12):757–758.

67. Osguthorpe JD, Calcaterra TC: Nasolacrimal obstruction after maxillary sinus and rhinoplastic surgery. *Arch Otolaryngol* 1979;105(5):264–266.

68. Unlu HH, Goktan C, Aslan A, et al: Injury to the lacrimal apparatus after endoscopic sinus surgery: Surgical implications from active transport dacryocystography. *Otolaryngol Head Neck Surg* 2001;124(3):308–312.

69. Colvard DM, Waller RR, Neault RW, et al: Nasolacrimal duct obstruction following transantral-ethmoidal orbital decompression. *Ophthalmic Surg* 1979;10(6):25–28.

70. Seiff SR, Shorr N: Nasolacrimal drainage system obstruction after orbital decompression. *Am J Ophthalmol* 1988;106(2):204–209.

71. Hurd LM, Holden WA: A case of paraffin injection into the nose followed immediately by blindness from embolism of the central retinal artery. *Med Rec* 1903;64:53–54.

72. Byers B: Blindness secondary to steroid injections into the nasal turbinates. *Arch Ophthalmol* 1979;97(1):79–80.

73. Shin H, Lemke BN, Stevens TS, et al: Posterior ciliary-artery occlusion after subcutaneous silicone-oil injection. *Ann Ophthalmol* 1988;20(9):342–344.

74. Mabry RL: Visual loss after intranasal corticosteroid injection: Incidence, causes, and prevention. *Arch Otolaryngol* 1981;107(8):484–486.

CHAPTER 10

Neurosurgical Complications

Ivan H. El-Sayed, Hazem Mohammad Ali Saleh, and Michael W. McDermott

During the last 25 years, head and neck surgeons have worked in conjunction with neurosurgeons as part of a multidisciplinary team to treat tumors around the skull base. Several advances have occurred during this time, with improvements seen in surgical techniques, preoperative imaging, interventional radiology, image guidance, and antibiotic therapy. The advent of image guidance for skull-base surgery has provided a huge step forward in helping surgeons maintain their orientation in a small open field, particularly with respect to the bony anatomy of the skull base. Presumably surgical complications have been reduced with this enhanced anatomic information, although it would be hard to quantitate this clinically. Overall complications have dropped dramatically from the 80% complication rate reported by Ketcham[1] in 1963 in the first series of patients undergoing craniofacial resection. In a recent multi-institutional review of 433 patients undergoing craniofacial resection for anterior skull-base tumors, postoperative mortality was found to be 4.7%; the overall complication rate of 36% included wound complications (20%), central nervous system complications (16%), orbital complications (1.7%), and systemic complications (4.8%).[2] Furthermore, improvements in radiation techniques have resulted in a significant decrease in severe late toxicities for skull-base neoplasms treated with radiation therapy or radiation therapy and surgery during the past 50 years at the University of California, San Francisco (UCSF).[3]

Surgeries of the skull base can be divided into posterior fossa lesions (usually involving neurotology) and middle and anterior skull-base lesions. The history of anterior skull-base lesions has experienced a rapid succession of events during the past 40 years. The first recorded procedure was by Dandy in 1941,[4] after he transgressed into the ethmoid sinuses during a craniotomy. Klopp, Smith, and Williams performed the first planned combined sinonasal–cranial resection in 1954,[5] and they were condemned by their peers. It was not until 1963, when Ketcham reported the first series of patients treated with craniofacial resection, that the procedure began to gain acceptance[1] (Figure 10-1). Since that time, a variety of procedures have been introduced that provide access to the entire anterior and middle skull base by such surgeons as Raveh,[6] Sekhar,[7] Janecka,[8,9] Biller,[10] Catalano,[11] and Donald.[12]

Recently, endoscopic techniques have been introduced into skull-base surgery, and they are being used with increased frequency.[13–18] The minimal-access approach offered by endoscopic techniques poses new problems for the repair of the surgical defect to prevent cerebrospinal fluid (CSF) leak.[13,19] In addition, routine sinus surgery with functional endoscopic sinus surgery for benign disease can be complicated by skull-base injury with CSF leak, pneumocephalus, vessel injury, or infection. Early recognition of the problem and adequate treatment can help to reduce the chance of an adverse event for the patient.

Neurosurgical complications can be considered in terms of direct and indirect causes and grouped anatomically by the intracranial compartment affected. Direct causes include neural injury (e.g., cranial nerve, brain parenchyma) and vascular, bony, and meningeal injury, whereas indirect causes include secondary infection, intracranial hypotension, and postoperative seizures. This chapter will address complications by anatomic site, including vascular, neural, meningeal, and brain parenchymal injuries. It will also look at the consequences of indirect injury from delayed complications such as meningitis and brain abscess.

COMPLICATIONS RELATED TO VASCULAR INJURIES

Ischemic Complications

During surgeries in or near the skull base, injury to the cerebral hemispheres, brainstem, and cranial nerves may occur. Injury may occur as a result of poor blood flow or direct trauma to the brain parenchyma and its surrounding tissues or cranial nerves.[20] Preoperative assessment provides valuable information to assess the risk of injury associated with proposed procedures. Radiologic imaging and nuclear medicine studies along with a neurologic physical examination can identify patients who are at high risk of cerebrovascular accident. Intraoperative monitoring can provide real-time information about the status of the central nervous system (Table 10-1). Electromyographic neuromonitoring of the facial nerve and brainstem evoked response audiometry monitoring for the auditory nerve are standard for appropriate lateral skull-base surgeries.

Intraoperative monitoring helps the surgeon to identify brain ischemia in real time. Acute physical trauma or discrete changes in blood pressure may produce rapid or subtle neurophysiologic changes. Neurophysiologic techniques can monitor general electrical brain activity with electroencephalographic (EEG) potentials, brainstem auditory evoked potentials, somatosensory evoked

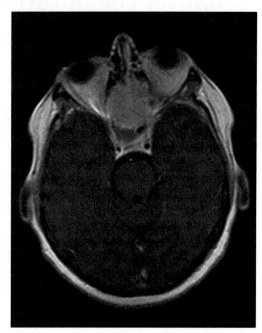

Figure 10-1. Magnetic resonance image of axial T1 with gadolinium of an anterior skull base lesion. Benign or malignant lesions can threaten important structures near the paranasal sinuses, the orbit, and the intracranial compartment. This image represents a meningioma of the skull base that produced bilateral visual loss as a result of the compression of the optic nerves.

TABLE 10-1 Commonly Employed Methods for Cranial Nerve Monitoring

Cranial Nerve	Method of Monitoring	Function Monitored
III	EMG	Inferior rectus
V	EMG	Temporalis, masseter muscles
VI	EMG	Lateral rectus
VII	EMG	Orbicularis oculi and oris
VIII	BAER	Nerve conduction cochlear nerve, brainstem, mid brain
IX	EMG	Palate via endotracheal tube electrodes
X	EMG	Vocal cords via endotracheal tube electrodes
XI	EMG	Trapezius
XII	EMG	Tongue

BAER, Brainstem auditory evoked response; *EMG,* electromyogram.

potentials, or electromyographic potentials of motor nerves. All cranial nerves, excluding the olfactory nerve, can be monitored. At UCSF, EEG potentials and somatosensory evoked potentials are monitored for evidence of ischemia during neurosurgical procedures. Electromyography is commonly used for the facial nerve, whereas brainstem evoked responses are routinely used to monitor the auditory nerve in lateral skull-base cases.[20–24]

Preoperative imaging with computed tomography (CT) scanning and magnetic resonance imaging (MRI) may suggest that the carotid artery is at risk as a result of tumor proximity during the surgical excision of tumors. If a tumor in the neck surrounds 70% of the carotid artery on an imaging study, then the carotid artery is most likely invaded with tumor. For recurrent squamous cell cancer of the head and neck, carotid resection is considered to be palliative. Adams and colleagues[9] found that 15 out of 20 patients were candidates for carotid artery resection on the basis of the balloon occlusion test. Seven patients died within the first year, 8 more died within the second year, and 2 survived for more than 2 years. Nevertheless, carotid artery resection did allow some patients valuable time to plan their affairs. Furthermore, hemorrhage occurred in only 1 patient.

Several tests exist to determine the risk of stroke if the carotid artery is resected. These tests may detect patients who are at risk of an early event; however, they do not identify the 5% to 15% of patients who are at risk of developing a delayed stroke.[20,25] The manual compression test, the balloon occlusion test with EEG monitoring, and the xenon- or CT-washout technique are three tests that are used.[20] The balloon occlusion test has replaced manual compression, because the pressure beyond the balloon can be measured during occlusion. Balloon occlusion tolerance testing can be performed preoperatively under controlled and monitored conditions along with a hypotensive challenge. If the patient can tolerate 30 minutes of occlusion under heparinization with good stump pressures measured beyond the balloon, then it can be assumed that the sacrifice of the carotid artery will be tolerated. This can be done endovascularly, and it allows time for collaterals to mature for several weeks before surgery. If the patient does not tolerate the occlusion, then he or she must be reevaluated, and the option of a high-flow carotid artery to middle cerebral vein bypass at the time of surgery must be considered.[26,27]

Transcranial Doppler ultrasonography and transcranial color duplex sonography can assess interhemispheric flow to predict the risk of stroke. The middle cerebral artery blood flow and velocity are monitored during rest and with manual compression of the ipsilateral carotid artery; the results are comparable to those of angiography.[28] The goal of each of these tests is to determine the presence of intracerebral collateral circulation of the carotid artery. Ultrasonography avoids the risks for intimal injury, air embolus, thrombus formation, and cardiac arrhythmias.[20] Manual compression of the carotid artery risks dislodging atheromatous plaques of the common carotid artery. Carotid plaques should be excluded by ultrasonography of the carotid artery at the time of compression.[20] It is suggested that, if the flow velocity in the middle cerebral artery is 90% of normal during manual compression, there is little hemodynamic risk of injury as a result of the ligation or resection of the carotid artery.[25,29]

Major Vascular Injury

Vascular injury may occur through distal injury to major vessels (e.g., the carotid artery, the vertebral artery) or by direct trauma to local vessels. During paranasal sinus surgery, transsphenoidal resections, or anterior craniofacial resections, direct injury to major vessels may occur, with devastating consequences. Trauma may cause intradural meningeal branches or subarachnoid branches of the anterior cerebral artery,[30] with resultant subdural or subarachnoid hematoma. The carotid artery is at risk of injury during endoscopic sinus surgery and during neoplasm resection via either direct trauma or traction on attached tumors. The sphenoid bone overlying the carotid artery is dehiscent in about 8% of patients.[31] Few surgeons are faced with an acute carotid artery hemorrhage during sinus surgery. Skull-base surgeons more often encounter bleeding from the cavernous sinuses and risk causing injury to the patient's carotid artery.

The management of a carotid artery tear starts immediately with the identification of the injury. Major bleeding from the cavernous sinus can often be controlled with tamponade, cautery, and packing with a hemostatic agent such as Surgicel Fibrillar (Johnson and Johnson, Somerville, NJ) or Avitene (C.R. Bard, Inc., Murray Hill, NJ). The direct compression of the cervical carotid artery may help to reduce pressures on the tear, but, ultimately, the tear must be sealed. In the event of carotid artery injury during endoscopic surgical cases, after bleeding is controlled, the patient (under the same anesthetic) is taken to the interventional radiology suite for angiography and repair. This frequently requires the sacrifice of the vessel. Less-severe injury to the carotid artery can present on a delayed basis after incomplete damage to the arterial wall at the time of surgery and then the formation of a pseudoaneurysm, with or without hemorrhage. In these cases, endovascular stenting and coiling may preserve the parent vessel and close the opening in the vessel wall. During open surgical procedures (e.g., craniofacial resection), the potential for carotid artery involvement may be anticipated on the basis of preoperative imaging. In these cases, carotid artery occlusion and bypass performed by a neurovascular surgeon may be feasible.

COMPLICATIONS RELATED TO NEURAL INJURIES: CRANIAL NERVE DYSFUNCTION

Injury to peripheral cranial nerves can result from direct trauma with procedures in the neck or as the nerves exit the skull base. Lesions of neural origin (e.g., schwannomas, paragangliomas) can intimately involve the cervical cranial nerves, thereby making resection difficult.

Carotid body tumors are often resected with a combined head and neck surgery and vascular surgery team approach in an effort to reduce complications.[32] The incidence of cranial nerve dysfunction after the surgical excision of paraganglioma ranges from 15% to 30%.[33] Twenty-four percent of excised carotid body tumors are complicated by transient paresis of the VII ramus mandibularis; 16% have cranial nerve X injury with vocal cord paralysis (reversible in three fourths of cases); and 20% have transient cranial nerve XII dysfunction. Cranial nerve injuries are more common when the tumors are larger than 4 cm.[34] Intraoperative EEG monitoring is helpful for assessing cerebral circulation if carotid artery clamping or arterial replacement becomes necessary for the resection of large tumors. Preoperative embolization significantly reduces blood loss during the resection of carotid body tumors, and many surgeons routinely embolize these tumors before resection.[35] However, some surgeons resect smaller lesions without preoperative embolization.[36,37]

Similar to carotid body tumor excisions, the resection of tumors arising from or adjacent to important nerves presents a risk of nerve injury. The affected nerve is usually the nerve of origin (most often cranial nerves IX, X, or XI), depending somewhat on the size of the tumor.[38] In the mid 1990s, Lustig and Jackler[39] reported a cranial nerve palsy rate of 30% in jugular foramen lesions, a rate of 60% with meningiomas, and a rate of 15% with schwannomas. In an updated series in 2005, Wilson and colleagues[38] reported comparable results after the excision of schwannomas of the jugular foramen.

COMPLICATIONS RELATED TO THE MENINGES

Otogenic and rhinologic CSF leaks can complicate head and neck surgery or combined surgical procedures that involve the intracranial compartment. Symptoms of CSF leak include a salty or sweet taste in the patient's throat, headaches of varying severity, constant or intermittent drainage, and headaches when assuming an upright position. The leak may increase with the Valsalva maneuver or position changes. The presence of a halo sign on tissue or a patient's clothing may also suggest a CSF leak. Beta-2 transferrin is the most specific and sensitive test for identifying CSF, because the substance is only present in the CSF, the perilymph, and the vitreous humor. A minimum of 0.5 ml of fluid is required to make the diagnosis using immunofixation electrophoresis.[40] In cases of rhinorrhea, the patient is asked to lean forward with his or her head between his or her knees for 3 to 5 minutes while catching any nasal drainage in a tube. However, a negative test does not exclude presence of CSF, and the final diagnosis should also rely on the clinical and radiologic findings.[41]

A CSF leak may be associated with acute or delayed complications such as meningitis, brain abscess, pneumocephalus, encephalocele, and, potentially, death (Figure 10-2). These complications can occur well after the onset of the leak; therefore leaks should be repaired.[41] The insertion of a lumbar subarachnoid drain for 3 to 5 days will solve the problem in up to 80% of cases. The delayed recurrence of a leak should raise the concern for the development of hydrocephalus. If the leak does not stop after 5 days of lumbar drainage, surgical repair of the dural defect should be considered. A contrast cisternogram can be performed through the lumbar drain to help localize the site of the leak. After the repair is done, the lumbar drain should remain in place for an additional 3 to 5 days, draining 15 ml to 20 ml per hour. In some cases, after attempts at direct surgical repair and repeat CSF leakage after clamping

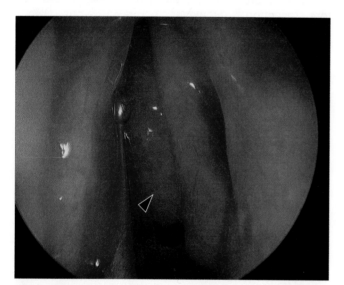

Figure 10-2. Cerebrospinal fluid leak associated with an encephalocele *(black arrowhead)* medial to the middle turbinate. The patient suffered from recurrent episodes of meningitis before being referred for management at the University of California, San Francisco. The encephalocele was resected via the transnasal endoscopic approach, and the defect was patched with a bone graft as an inlay and a mucosal overlay graft.

of the lumbar drain, a lumboperitoneal or ventriculoperitoneal shunt is necessary.

Cerebrospinal Fluid Otorrhea

Excessive CSF otorrhea can occur spontaneously, or it may result from neoplasms, infection, surgical interventions, or trauma to the temporal bone.[42–44] Temporal bone trauma can lead to acute leaks through the fracture line or to delayed leaks resulting from obstruction of the cochlear aqueduct by soft tissue or bone.[45] Spontaneous leaks can result from herniation through a defect in the tegmen or as a result of dynamic factors such as increased intracranial pressure.[42] A CSF gusher involving the cochlea can be encountered during surgery,[45] and this is often associated with developmental malformations such as cochlear hypoplasia, lateral internal auditory canal anomalies, an unusually patent cochlear aqueduct, or an enlarged vestibular aqueduct.[46,47]

Postoperative CSF leakage can occur after transtemporal skull-base surgery. Leonetti and colleagues[48] found an incidence of 4% to 8%, depending on the approach used, in a series of 589 patients. Brennan and colleagues[49] reported a 10% incidence of CSF leakage after surgery for acoustic neuroma. The authors felt the combined middle-fossa and translabyrinthine (TL) approach was associated with a high rate of CSF leakage, and they abandoned it for the retrosigmoid (RS) and TL approaches. The RS and TL approaches had similar rates of leakage. The RS approach was associated with CSF otorrhea, whereas the TL approach was associated with incisional wound leaks. In a separate study, Sanna and colleagues[50] reported a CSF leak rate of 2.8% in a series of 707 patients. Interestingly, those authors found a significantly higher rate of leakage associated with the RS approach (18.4%) as compared with the extended TL approach (1.8%). Other approaches (e.g., the extended middle fossa approach, the retrolabyrinthine approach, the transotic approach, the transcochlear approach) do not appear to be associated with a higher risk of CSF leakage. Increasing tumor size is a separate but related factor, because tumor size and location affect the selection of the surgical approach.

CSF otorrhea is initially best managed conservatively, especially in the case of a temporal bone fracture. Initial management is often with the insertion of a lumbar drain and bed rest. After acoustic neuroma surgery, Brennan and colleagues[49] found that 18% of leaks resolved without a drain and that 49% resolved with lumbar drain placement. If conservative management fails, the leak must be addressed surgically, as previously discussed.

After acoustic neuroma surgery, CSF leak usually occurs through the retrolabyrinthine cells or the apical cells.[50] Thus it is recommended that these cells be obliterated with a mastoidectomy, the meticulous removal of all of the retrolabyrinthine and apical cells, and the obliteration of the mastoid cavity using abdominal fat. Any small cells in the region of the posterior wall of the internal auditory canal should be obliterated using bone wax.[50] The common expression "wax in, wax out" is a helpful reminder to seal mastoid air cells with wax during both the exposure and the closure. Some surgeons use an endoscope to aid in the identification of cells that are capable of producing a leak but that are not directly visible. The subcutaneous tissue and the skin are sutured in a layered fashion, and a compressive wound dressing is applied for 6 to 7 days.

The most definitive method of addressing CSF leaks related to temporal bone fracture or spontaneous leaks requiring surgical intervention is through the middle fossa approach, which can be combined with a transmastoid approach.[42] Wide surgical exposure can help to identify the presence of multiple defects. The defects are then obliterated with a pedicle-based temporalis musculofascial flap and sometimes with a fat graft (Figure 10-3).

A rapid CSF leak, called a *gusher,* is encountered in approximately 1% of patients undergoing cochlear implant surgery, and it is seen with equal incidence among both children and adults. The majority of labyrinthine anomalies will be uncovered with preoperative imaging (high-resolution CT or MRI). Even after careful preoperative evaluation, unexpected CSF leaks may occur at the time of cochleostomy.[45] Furthermore, CSF gushers are not limited to patients with anatomic anomalies. Marks[51] reported three patients with CSF leak and normal cochleas, and Bhatia and colleauges[52] found that one of six patients with a CSF leak had a normal cochlea. Fahy[47] found that CSF gushers occurred in 50% of patients with enlarged vestibular aqueducts.

In the event of an intraoperative CSF gusher, intracranial pressure is lowered by placing the patient in the reverse Trendelenburg position. The anesthesiologist is instructed to administer mannitol and to lower the end-tidal carbon dioxide level to 26 to 28 mm Hg. The cochlear implant electrode is placed, and the cochleostomy is packed with fascia or periosteum.[45] Wootten and colleagues[45] recommend pressed fascia and periosteum rather than muscle, because these substances are easier to manipulate and have less tendency to atrophy than muscle. Other authors report that muscle is quite effective for controlling CSF gushers.[32] After packing, the wound is inspected to ensure that the CSF drainage is controlled. Middle-ear packing can be further reinforced with fibrin glue. A lumbar drainage is not needed, but perioperative antibiotics are recommended

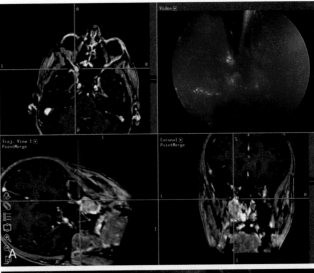

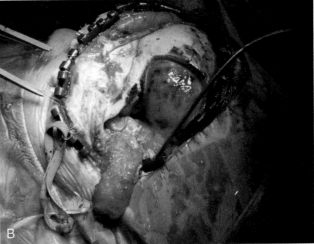

Figure 10-3. Lateral skull-base approach. **A,** Intraoperative image guidance can provide valuable assistance to the surgeon. Although knowledge of the surgical anatomy is the key to any safe surgical procedure, image-guidance technology can verify intraoperative findings. This is especially important in skull-base approaches, where the field may be bloody. In this case, an endoscope was used to allow for the safe dissection of the sphenoid wing and the inferiorly related pterygoid fossa, infratemporal fossa, and orbital apex through an orbitozygomatic approach. Image guidance verifies the dissection of the lesion medial and lateral to the optic nerve. **B,** After the completion of the resection of the lesion, the communication between the middle fossa and the nasopharynx is closed off with a temporalis myocutaneous flap, which is elevated.

as a result of a small risk of meningitis associated with cochlear implantation.[45,53]

Cerebrospinal Fluid Rhinorrhea

Similar to otologic causes, CSF rhinorrhea can result from traumatic and surgical as well as nonsurgical and nontraumatic etiologies. Nontraumatic causes include neoplasms, anomalous arachnoid granulations in the region of the olfactory groove, increased intracranial pressure, a history of radiation therapy, prior infection, the empty sella syndrome, or a congenital defect.[40] The most common surgical cause is transsphenoidal tumor surgery, with an incidence of 0.5% to 15%.[40,54–57] Open craniofacial resection and transnasal endoscopic surgery are common surgical causes as a result of the difficulty involved in closing the surgical defect. Functional endoscopic sinus surgery can also result in CSF leak caused by trauma to the anterior skull base through direct penetration or transmitted injury by the manipulation of the septum or the middle turbinate. The rate of leak in endoscopic sinus surgery is reported to be between 0.5 to 3%.[40] It is assumed that the use of image guidance during surgery will reduce the incidence of this complication.

CSF leak caused by trauma or fracture most commonly occurs in the cribriform plate as a result of the presence of thick bone positioned adjacent to extremely thin bone, with overlying and tightly adherent dura.[58] Although the cribriform plate is the more likely site of CSF leak, it is actually a thick plate of bone and relatively resistant to perforation. During sinus surgery, the thin fovea ethmoidalis is more susceptible to a penetrating injury with resultant intracranial complication. Furthermore, the height of the fovea ethmoidalis is variable with relation to the cribriform plate, and it is often assessed using the Keros classification system before surgery.[59] Three Keros types describe the height of the olfactory fossa: type I is 1 mm to 3 mm deep, type II is 4 mm to 7 mm deep, and type 3 is 8 mm to 16 mm deep. The weakest part of the anterior skull base is where the anterior ethmoidal artery leaves the ethmoid to enter the olfactory fossa.[60] This area is medial to the middle turbinate, and it offers the least resistance to intracranial perforation. It should be evaluated preoperatively on thin-sectioned, bone-windowed, axial, and coronal CT scans (Figure 10-4).

CSF fistulae can occur with all techniques of ethmoidectomy, frontal sinus surgery, and sphenoidotomy. During ethmoidectomy, the dura may be incised anywhere from the anterior ethmoid to the sphenoid sinus. CSF leaks have been associated with an approximately 10% per year risk of meningitis.[41] When leakage lasts for more than 7 days after trauma, the rate has been reported to be as high as 88%.[61] Risk factors for postoperative CSF leak include an inexperienced surgeon, ill-defined anatomic landmarks as a result of excessive bleeding, space-occupying lesions, prior surgery, and anatomic variations. Furthermore, it has been suggested that the administration of general anesthesia (rather than local anesthesia) may influence CSF fistula formation, because the patient cannot provide feedback when undue pain is experienced.[41]

After skull-base resection, the optimal technique of surgical closure is a matter of debate. Some surgeons believe that a three-layer closure or rigid fixation is

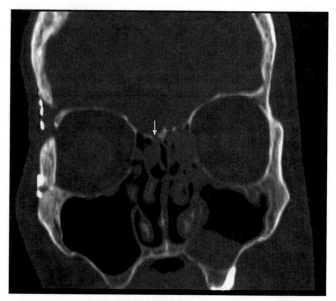

Figure 10-4. High-resolution coronal computed tomography scan of the ethmoid sinuses. The cerebrospinal fluid leak site is identified at the junction of the middle turbinate with the skull base. The patient had a history of transnasal endoscopic transsphenoidal pituitary surgery. A computed tomographic cisternogram was negative as a result of the intermittent nature of the leak. The leak occurred in the cribriform plate as a result of transmitted forces from the manipulation of the middle turbinate inferiorly. The leak was confirmed intraoperatively and successfully closed with a vascularized middle turbinate flap.

necessary for large defects of the anterior skull base. However, large defects are poorly defined in the literature. Many authors fear that so-called "brain sag" will occur or that the wound may break down. Three-layer closures include a fascial closure of the dura, a rigid layer of bone or metal mesh, and a vascularized pericranial flap.[62] However, not all surgeons use this approach.[63] At UCSF, a two-layer closure is routinely used, with a fascial or alloplastic graft used to close the dura and a pericranial flap for craniofacial resections involving the resection of bilateral ethmoids, the cribriform, and most of the planum sphenoidale. An issue can arise if the entire planum is removed without leaving a bony ledge for the pericranial flap. In these cases, the pericranial flap is sutured directly to the dural closure, or, if it is long enough, it is placed into the back of the sphenoid sinus. Lesions with supraorbital involvement are often managed with rigid material (e.g., titanium mesh) to prevent brain pulsations on the orbit. Defects including an orbital exenteration are an indication for vascularized free tissue to seal the cranial defect and provide support.

The repair of CSF leaks of the anterior cranial fossa and paranasal sinuses is approached in a similar way as the repair of otogenic leaks. Initial conservative management may include bed rest, decreasing CSF intracranial pressure with hyperosmotic agents, and possibly the placement of a lumbar drain. The use of the lumbar drain is controversial because of its potential for over-drainage and the creation of tension pneumocephalus. If the nasal cavity is sufficiently packed, however, the risk of pneumocephalus is reduced. It is rare to require a tracheostomy to divert the airway for persistent pneumocephalus, but this option should always be considered in difficult situations. If the leak persists after 3 to 7 days of drainage, then surgical intervention is generally pursued.

Dohlman performed the first extracranial repair of a CSF leak in 1948. The transnasal endoscopic closure of CSF leaks, which was first described by Wigand in 1981, created a paradigm shift in the management of CSF rhinorrhea.[64] Advantages of the endoscopic approach as compared with open craniotomy include the potential preservation of smell, a shorter hospital stay, no external scarring, no brain retraction, and less risk of bleeding, postoperative seizures, and infection. When a leak is identified during endoscopic sinus surgery, the management of a CSF leak in the initial setting is the least morbid approach, and it is successful in 95% of cases.[64] A review of an institutional skull-base series at UCSF revealed a CSF leak rate of 13%.[65] At UCSF, depending on the site of leak, endoscopic closure is attempted even after open craniofacial resection as a result of the high success rate and minimal morbidity of this approach. Leaks that are not amenable to endoscopic closure include those that originate from the posterior frontal sinus wall. Some authors indicate that defects larger than 5 cm are not amenable to endoscopic closure; however, the advances made in transnasal endoscopic tumor resection are bringing this into question. Large surgical defects may be filled with adipose grafts and covered with a pedicled vascularized

septal or turbinate flap, but the long-term stability of these grafts has not yet been reported (Figure 10-5). Transnasal endoscopic repair is now considered the treatment of choice for most anterior cranial and sphenoid CSF leaks.[66]

Powered microdebriders are widely used for endoscopic sinus surgery and also for the resection of tumors. Schnipper and Spiegel[41] raise the issue of whether powered microdebriders increase the chance of serious complications. Along with the added ease of dissection with these instruments comes a higher risk of inadvertent injury when shavers are used along the skull base or near delicate structures such as the lamina papyracea or in the sphenoid sinus. The effective cutting ability in combination with suction allows for tissues such as fat, muscle, nerves, and vessels to be pulled into the operative field before they are identified. This situation can occur with bony dehiscences of the orbital wall, anatomic variations, unrecognized low-lying skull base, or excessive bleeding. After an unintended defect is created, a powered microdebrider may result in a larger defect than nonpowered instruments would.[41] Alternatively, during endoscopic skull-base tumor resections, it is the author's experience (IE) that powered debriders may offer an advantage for visualization, because they concurrently cut and clear the bloody operative field with a single instrument during tumor debulking. This can potentially cut down on dissection time during the portions of the surgery with the most active bleeding. Despite the large surgical experience with microdebriders, there are few reports regarding associated complications. Berenholz and colleagues[30] reported a case of CSF leak and subarachnoid hemorrhage that they attributed to the use of the powered shaver along the skull base.

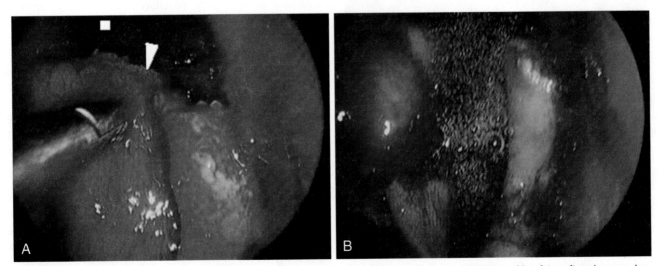

Figure 10-5. Closure of a transnasal endoscopic anterior skull-base resection for an esthesioneuroblastoma with a fat graft and a vascularized septal flap. The brain parenchyma is lined with a graft (e.g., AlloDerm (LifeCell), DuraGen). A fat graft is then placed, and the edge of the septal flap *(white arrowhead)* is brought up to the level of the frontal sinus ostia *(white block)* and lined up over the fat graft. The septal flap vascularizes the fat graft to improve healing.

Image-guidance technology may help reduce errors in endoscopic sinus surgery. Fried and colleagues[67] found that image-guidance technology appeared to be useful for endoscopic sinus surgery. In their series, patients having image-guided surgery had a lower CSF leak rate (0% vs. 2.2%), a lower overall complication rate, and required less revision procedures as compared with patients having the surgery without image guidance. Interestingly, the addition of image guidance was also associated with increased blood loss and operative time.

Pneumocephalus

Pneumocephalus may occur with a CSF leak or independently after trauma or surgical intervention (Figure 10-6). The clinical presentation of air in the intracranial space ranges from being asymptomatic to causing headaches to obtundation. Patients may develop the pathognomonic symptom, known as *bruit hydroaerique,* which is described by the patient as a splashing sound within the cranium that occurs with movement of the head. Occasionally this sound is audible to the examining physician as well. Other symptoms include dizziness, visual alterations, confusion, and personality changes.

Physical examination may identify CSF rhinorrhea, meningismus, seizures, altered mental state, and hemiparesis.[41]

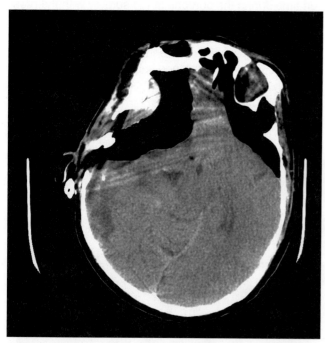

Figure 10-6. Postoperative pneumocephalus. A computed tomography scan without contrast shows bilateral subdural air after extensive combined subtotal maxillectomy and infratemporal fossa resection with orbital exenteration and the dissection of the intracranial compartment almost to vertex. Reconstruction was performed with a rectus abdominal free-tissue transfer. The treatment of the pneumocephalus included supine positioning, high levels of inspired oxygen, and surgical reexploration with a fat-graft obliteration of the communication with the nasal cavity.

In addition, there may be crepitus of the skin over the forehead. With progression to tension pneumocephalus, more extensive neural deficits and obtundation appear.

The mechanism of the intracranial entry of air is not straightforward. Because intracranial pressure is normally greater than the atmospheric pressure, this pressure differential should prevent air from entering the cranium. It is therefore hypothesized that some change must occur in the physiologic conditions that allows pneumocephalus to develop.[41] Two generally accepted theories are the ball–valve mechanism and the inverted-bottle mechanism. Air may be forced through the cranial opening for a variety of reasons and then become trapped as a result of increased intracranial pressure in a ball–valve effect. Increases in nasopharyngeal pressure (e.g., nose blowing, sneezing, coughing, mask ventilation, difficult respirations) could drive air intracranially. With the inverted-bottle mechanism, negative intracranial pressure develops as the CSF drains out of a dural tear, and air is pulled in to relieve the negative intracranial pressure.[68] Intraoperatively, nitrous oxide anesthesia is known to cause increased intracranial pressure in the presence of intracranial air and a closed cranium[69]; the increased intracranial pressure resolves rapidly after the discontinuation of the nitrous anesthesia.[41]

Pneumocephalus may also develop after craniofacial resection with the creation of large surgical defects. Some surgeons will routinely perform airway diversion with prolonged endotracheal intubation or tracheotomy on patients undergoing craniofacial resection to prevent this complication by decreasing expiratory pressure and coughing postoperatively. Routine airway diversion, however, is not considered necessary for most skull-base procedures,[70] and it may actually mask neurologic complications if a patient is kept intubated and sedated after surgery. At UCSF, barring other factors, patients are routinely extubated within 24 hours of surgery without undue consequences.

The diagnosis of pneumocephalus is made with the identification of air pockets on a brain CT scan. Patients are monitored with routine neurologic examinations in the intensive care unit setting for signs of meningitis or neurologic deterioration. The neurosurgery department is consulted to aid in the management of the patient.[41]

Tension pneumocephalus demands immediate treatment. Decompression of the air may be achieved with the inhalation of 100% oxygen, but needle aspiration of the space can be a life-saving maneuver. It is thought that inspiring 100% oxygen creates a favorable diffusion gradient to siphon off nitrogen from the aerocele and to decrease intracranial pressure.[41] Lumbar puncture or drainage in the setting of tension pneumocephalus is contraindicated because of the presence of increased intracranial pressure. Furthermore, a lumbar drain may allow more air to enter or it may allow for the rapid expansion of the intracranial air already present as a result of its higher compliance as compared with the surrounding soft tissue and fluid.[68] Closure of the intracranial defect may occur with conservative management, or it may require surgical repair. Conservative management involves keeping the patient's head elevated while he or she is on bed rest to reduce intracranial pressure as well as the placement of a subarachnoid drain. Surgical management may require an open surgical approach or an endoscopic approach. The first operative repair of tension pneumocephalus was described by Dandy[4] in 1926 using a bifrontal craniotomy,[71] which is still applicable today.[72] Some surgeons use an external ethmoidal approach[73] or, more recently, an endoscopic approach.[74]

COMPLICATIONS RELATED TO BRAIN PARENCHYMA

Hemorrhage and Direct Injury

Direct brain injury can result from surgical manipulation or from indirect vascular compromise caused by bleeding or the occlusion of important vessels. Surgery at the lowest point in the nasal cavity can lead to injury in the skull base by forces transmitted along the middle turbinate or septum. The insertion of the middle turbinate leads to a thin bone in the fovea ethmoidalis that is susceptible to fracture. With a Keros type III skull base, the central skull base is depressed, leaving a thin layer of bone along the lateral wall of the olfactory groove as it rises to meet the fovea ethmoidalis. Furthermore, the skull base generally slopes inferiorly from anterior to posterior. The anterior and posterior ethmoid arteries traverse generally within the bone of the skull base, but they may be exposed by bony dehiscences. At the posterior border of the dissection—which is the focus of tumors that involve the clivus, the nasopharynx, and the pituitary—lie important vascular structures. The cavernous sinus lies adjacent to the lateral sphenoid walls, and these are connected via the intercavernous sinus, which travels along the posterior wall of the sphenoid sinus anterior to the pituitary gland. The carotid artery traverses the posterior sphenoid wall, which can occasionally be dehiscent. Trauma along the anterior cranial fossa can lead to the intradural bleeding of the meningeal branches or the subarachnoid branches of the anterior cerebral artery. Intracranial bleeding in the setting of endoscopic approaches is complicated by limited exposure that prevents the immediate control of bleeding. Trauma to the cribriform plate can injure the anterior cerebral artery and its feeding vessels, which lie in close proximity.[41] The spasm of these vessels can lead to significant central nervous system morbidity and even death. Direct injury of the brain

parenchyma through the cribriform plate may cause a frontal lobe syndrome that involves loss of memory, forgetfulness, and behavior changes. Significant unexpected hemorrhage during surgery along the skull base may indicate cranial penetration.[41] Both major vessel injury and brain trauma require emergency craniotomy for direct neurosurgical intervention. Major vascular injury is managed as described earlier in this chapter. Subdural or subarachnoid hematoma should be evaluated by a neurosurgeon for surgical drainage. Subarachnoid hemorrhage is managed expectantly, with the understanding that there is then a risk for the development of cerebral vasospasm, hydrocephalus, or both.

Significant morbidity and mortality can arise from intracranial hemorrhage after surgery for acoustic neuroma, and this usually occurs during the first 24 hours after surgery. Progressing symptoms are caused by the compressive force at the cerebellopontine angle by a subdural hemorrhage or parenchymal cerebellar hemorrhage with subsequent brainstem and cerebellar edema. An unrecognized hematoma can progress to coma. Immediate decompression of the hematoma with the opening of the wound and the removal of the fat graft in the intensive care unit may be necessary. Delays for CT scanning may not be warranted. The immediate recognition and management of this complication may avoid subsequent devastating complications. By contrast, intraventricular hemorrhages require the placement of an external ventricular drain and possibly a CSF shunt after the acute blood products have cleared. Despite the significant, devastating complications of an intraparenchymal bleed, it is often not feasible to operate on this condition when the hematoma is within the pons or the middle cerebellar peduncle.[50]

At the time of initial tumor resection, meticulous hemostasis should be achieved and tested with a Valsalva maneuver. Continuous suction and irrigation for 10 minutes is performed while the arterial blood pressure is raised. The patient should be extubated and awakened as feasible after the surgery to obtain a baseline neurologic examination. The patient is monitored 24 to 48 hours postoperatively with continuous neurologic examinations. The deterioration of the patient's level of consciousness is the most reliable clinical parameter for recognizing the appearance of a cerebellopontine angle hematoma.[50]

DELAYED INFECTIOUS COMPLICATIONS

Meningitis

Meningitis can complicate any procedure that connects with the subarachnoid space. When postoperative CSF leaks occur, meningitis is one of the most common intracranial complications of sinus surgery. Infections spread via direct extension through a dural tear, along perivascular and vascular channels, or through the septal lymphatics that lead to the perineural spaces of the olfactory fibers.[41] Patients may develop headache, fever, photophobia, and nuchal rigidity. Other symptoms include nausea, vomiting, cranial nerve palsy, seizures, and behavioral changes such as mental status change, confusion, lethargy, and inattentiveness. The most common pathogen is *Streptococcus pneumoniae*[75] followed by gram-negative bacilli (excluding *Haemophilus influenzae*), *Neisseria meningitidis,* and other streptococcal organisms. *Staphylococcus aureus* and *Listeria monocytogenes* are pathogens in 7% to 8% of cases.[76]

A CT scan is indicated before the performance of a lumbar puncture to rule out another condition that may mimic infection, such as subacute subdural or chronic subdural hematoma. Intravenous contrast is necessary to identify an abscess by the presence of a rim-enhancing lesion. When meningitis is present without a brain abscess, the CT scan and T1- and T2-weighted MRI images are usually normal. However, MRI with gadolinium should demonstrate diffuse dural and leptomeningeal enhancement.

Empiric antimicrobial therapy is initiated for patients with suspected meningitis while the workup ensues. Patients are treated with antibiotics that are capable of crossing the blood–brain barrier (e.g., vancomycin) or with a third-generation cephalosporin and metronidazole. A lumbar puncture is performed, evaluated for the presence of inflammatory cells and organisms, and sent for culture and sensitivity. If the Gram stain of the CSF is negative, the choice of empiric therapy is guided by the knowledge of the frequency of pathogens for community-acquired versus nosocomial meningitis.

A recent U.S. Food and Drug Administration study revealed an increase in the number of reported cases of cochlear-implant–related meningitis.[53] In these cases, the pathogens were noted to be *S. pneumoniae, H. influenzae, Escherichia coli, Streptococcus viridans*, and other staphylococcal organisms. Clinical studies have shown that meningitis that occurs after cochlear implantation is more common than previously thought. Although the rate of this complication is still extremely low, every effort should be made to minimize the risk. It is recommended that patients be up to date with their vaccinations, including the *H. influenzae* type B vaccine. Half of the cases were associated with the implant positioner, which may have created a larger cochleostomy. One third of infections occurred at the time of implantation, which suggests perioperative contamination; thus the use of an antimicrobial in the carrying medium is suggested for cochlear implantation.[77] However, many

cases were delayed in onset for months to years. In these cases, it is suspected that otitis media played a role. It is not believed to be beneficial for patients who have the positioner in place to have it removed.[78]

Intracranial Infection and Abscess

Brain abscess may result from the spread from a contiguous infected structure, from a distant focus of infection, or from the integrity of the barrier surrounding the central nervous system being disrupted.[79] Fortunately, intracranial abscesses are a rare complication of paranasal sinus and skull-base surgery. For surgeries of neoplasms along the skull base, infections of the wound or the osteoplastic flap can lead to subsequent intracranial infection after craniofacial approaches. Likewise, prolonged sinusitis in the nasal cavity can lead to wound breakdown and infection along the anterior cranial fossa. In association with a CSF leak, the intracranial compartment may be breached by microorganisms, which can lead to abscess formation (Figure 10-7). During frontal craniotomy, the bone flap is devascularized and replaced with rigid fixation. The addition of preoperative or postoperative radiation therapy further reduces the vascularization of both the skin flap and the bone flap, thereby increasing the possibility of the necrosis of either. When a subcranial approach as described by Raveh[80] is used, many surgeons will wrap the frontal bone with the pericranial flap and the skull base with devascularized fascia. In these cases, the nonvascularized grafts usually heal along the skull base, with the formation of a CSF leak or abscess.

Brain abscesses often develop from the contiguous spread of infection of the paranasal sinuses, the middle ear, and the mastoid or from odontogenic infections. They may be subdural, epidural, or intraparenchymal. Pott's puffy tumor represents an indolent, circumscribed abscess.[41] The infection originates in the frontal sinus and causes a progressive osteomyelitis of the bone. Untreated, the infection may eventually form an anterior subperiosteal pericranial abscess, a periorbital abscess, or an epidural abscess.[81] Infections of the sinuses may spread intracranially via thrombophlebitis of the emissary veins, as a result of septic emboli, through the valveless diploic veins, or directly through preformed or traumatically created skull-base defects. Recent reports have found that the proportion of brain abscesses that result from neurosurgery for traumatic, benign, and neoplastic disease ranges from 19% to 37%.[79,82] This relative increase in the proportion of surgery-related abscesses may reflect the improved treatment of primary infections such as otitis media.

Intracerebral abscesses most often involve the frontal and frontoparietal lobes.[81] The infection usually begins as a local area of cerebritis that evolves into a collection

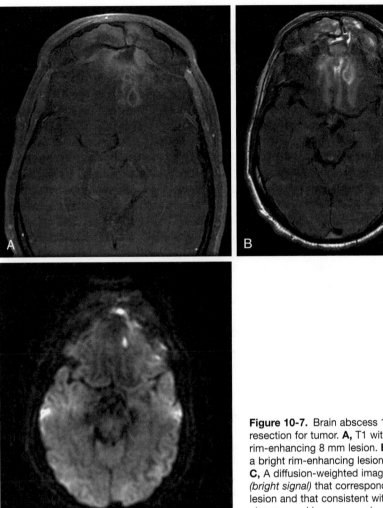

Figure 10-7. Brain abscess 12 months after craniofacial resection for tumor. **A,** T1 with gadolinium reveals a rim-enhancing 8 mm lesion. **B,** Flair sequence reveals a bright rim-enhancing lesion in the left inferior frontal lobe. **C,** A diffusion-weighted image reveals reduced diffusion *(bright signal)* that corresponds with the rim-enhancing lesion and that consistent with infection or intraparenchymal abscess and less concerning for recurrent neoplasm. Obvious pus was found intraoperatively.

of pus.[81] The fluid becomes surrounded by a well-vascularized fibrotic capsule.[81] Untreated, the abscess will progress with increased intracranial pressure, and it may eventually rupture into the ventricles, causing generalized purulent meningitis. Death may then ensue. Mortality from brain abscess is currently reported to be about 10%.[81] Nearly 80% of patients recover fully, with minimal incapacity.[81] The disease course may last days to months. The abscess may remain dormant for weeks until the capsule ruptures.[83]

In a series of 49 patients, common symptoms of brain abscess included confusion (50%) and headache (50%). Less-common symptoms included nausea, focal neurologic symptoms, fever, grand mal seizures, malaise, dysphasia, wound discharge, imbalance, focal seizure, neck stiffness, and photophobia.[79] A CT scan with intravenous contrast is necessary to identify a brain abscess. Among patients who have undergone skull-base tumor resection, the radiologic images can be difficult to interpret, and a diffusion-weighted MRI

may help to distinguish an abscess from a recurrent tumor. Serial CT scans are useful to follow the lesion throughout the course of treatment. A lumbar puncture should be avoided as a result of the risk of increased intracranial pressure and brain herniation. Stereotactic aspiration of the abscess may be necessary to reduce the mass effect and to identify the organism for appropriately directed antibiotic therapy.

Streptococcus organisms (especially *Streptococcus milleri*) appear to the most common pathogens. Other common pathogens include *S. aureus, Bacteroides spp., Proteus spp.,* and *Klebsiella spp.*[79] Antibiotic therapy includes agents that are able to penetrate the blood–brain barrier. Penicillin, trimethoprim, chloramphenicol, and metronidazole are commonly used, but antibiotic selection is most often guided by cultures and sensitivities obtained from drainage or from the needle aspiration of the abscess. Cefotaxime is an extended-spectrum cephalosporin that has a spectrum of antibiotic therapy comparable with chloramphenicol and a lower incidence of adverse reactions. Cefotaxime and metronidazole offer broad coverage of sinonasal organisms.[84] Intravenous antibiotic treatment is administered for 4 to 8 weeks. In addition, intravenous or oral corticosteroids are administered, and patients are also given anticonvulsant medications.

An attempt should be made to drain the abscess via needle aspiration of the purulent material. The primary site of infection should be drained in cases of sinusitis or of odontogenic or otologic origins. After skull-base procedures, the operative wound should be inspected. Nasal cavity defects should be cleaned of contaminated debris or packing, and the craniotomy site should be inspected for the potential infection of the bone flap. For unstable, comatose, or moribund patients, an open neurosurgical procedure may be necessary. The surgical excision of a well-encapsulated abscess or simple drainage may be attempted. In cases of increased intracranial pressure, a ventricular cannula may be placed, and continued drainage may be required. Intrathecal antibiotics may be injected through the ventricular cannula.[85]

CONCLUSION

Neurosurgical complications of head and neck surgery and skull-base surgery are not infrequent. Successful outcomes depend on prompt recognition and appropriate management. Complications related to vascular, nerve, dural, and brain injury require a multidisciplinary approach. Those involved with the care of these patients postoperatively should be aware of the potential complications of each specific surgical procedure. The prompt and appropriate management of both medical and surgical complications can yield satisfactory outcomes for most patients.

REFERENCES

1. Ketcham AS, Wilkins RH, Vanburen JM, Smith RR: A Combined Intracranial Facial Approach to the Paranasal Sinuses. *Am J Surg* 1963;106:698–703.
2. Ganly I, Patel SG, Singh B, et al: Complications of craniofacial resection for malignant tumors of the skull base: report of an International Collaborative Study. *Head Neck* 2005;27(6):445–451.
3. Chen AM, Daly ME, Bucci MK, et al: Carcinomas of the paranasal sinuses and nasal cavity treated with radiotherapy at a single institution over five decades: Are we making improvement? *Int J Radiat Oncol Biol Phys* 2007.
4. Dandy WE: Orbital tumor: results following the transcranial operative attack. New York: Oskar Piest, 1941.
5. Smith RR, Klopp, CT, Williams, JM: Surgical treatment of cancer of the frontal sinus and adjacent areas. *Cancer* 1954;7:991–994.
6. Raveh J, Laehach, K, Speiser, M, et al: The subcranial approach for fronto-orbital and anterior-posterior skull base tumors. *Arch Otolaryngol Head Neck Surg* 1993;119:385–393.
7. Sekhar LN, Janecka IP, Jones NF: Subtemporal-infratemporal and basal subfrontal approach to extensive cranial base tumours. *Acta Neurochir* (Wien) 1988;92(1–4):83–92.
8. Janecka IP, Sen CN, Sekhar LN, Arriaga M: Facial translocation: a new approach to the cranial base. *Otolaryngol Head Neck Surg* 1990;103(3):413–419.
9. Sekhar LN, Janecka IP, Jones NF: Subtempoal-infratemporal and basal subfrontal approach to extensive cranial base tumours. *Acta Neurochir* (Wien) 1988;92:83.
10. Biller HF, Shugar JMA, Krespi YP: A new technique for wide field exposure of the base of skull. *Arch Otolaryngol Head Neck Surg* 1981;107:698–702.
11. Catalano PJ, Biller HF, Sachdev V: Access to the central skull base via a modified Leforte I maxillotomy approach: the palatal hinged flap. *Skull Base Surg* 1993;3:60–68.
12. Donald P, Bernstein L: Transpalatal excision of the odontoid process. *Trans Am Acad Opthal Otolaryngol* 1978;86.
13. Hadad G, Bassagasteguy L, Carrau RL, et al: A novel reconstructive technique after endoscopic expanded endonasal approaches: vascular pedicle nasoseptal flap. *Laryngoscope* 2006;116(10):1882–1886.
14. Kassam A, Carrau RL, Snyderman CH, et al: Evolution of reconstructive techniques following endoscopic expanded endonasal approaches. *Neurosurg Focus* 2005;19(1):E8.
15. Kassam A, Snyderman CH, Mintz A, et al: Expanded endonasal approach: the rostrocaudal axis. Part II. Posterior clinoids to the foramen magnum. *Neurosurg Focus* 2005;19(1):E4.
16. Kassam A, Snyderman CH, Mintz A, et al: Expanded endonasal approach: the rostrocaudal axis. Part I. Crista galli to the sella turcica. *Neurosurg Focus* 2005;19(1):E3.
17. Kassam AB, Gardner P, Snyderman C, et al: Expanded endonasal approach: fully endoscopic, completely transnasal approach to the middle third of the clivus, petrous bone, middle cranial fossa, and infratemporal fossa. *Neurosurg Focus* 2005;19(1):E6.
18. Kassam AB, Mintz AH, Gardner PA, et al: The expanded endonasal approach for an endoscopic transnasal clipping and aneurysmorrhaphy of a large vertebral artery aneurysm: technical case report. *Neurosurgery* 2006;59(1 Suppl 1):ONSE162–165; discussion ONSE162–165.
19. Kassam A, Thomas AJ, Snyderman C, et al: Fully endoscopic expanded endonasal approach treating skull base lesions in pediatric patients. *J Neurosurg* 2007;106(2 Suppl):75–86.
20. Mann WJ, Maurer J, Marangos N: Neural conservation in skull base surgery. *Otolaryngol Clin North Am* 2002;35(2):411–424, ix.
21. Levine R: Monitoring auditory evoked potentials during cerebellopontine angle tumor surgery: relative value of electrocochleography, brainstem auditory evoked potentials, and cerebellopontine angle recordings. In: Schramm J, Moller AR eds, Intraoperative neurophysiologic monitoring. Berlin: Springer-Verlag. 1991.
22. Maurer J, Pelster H, Amedee RG, Mann WJ: Intraoperative monitoring of motor cranial nerves in skull base surgery. *Skull Base Surg* 1995;5(3):169–175.
23. Slavit DH, Harner SG, Harper CM, Jr, Beatty CW: Auditory monitoring during acoustic neuroma removal. *Arch Otolaryngol Head Neck Surg* 1991;117(10):1153–1157.
24. Gacek RR, Gacek MR, Tart R: Adult spontaneous cerebrospinal fluid otorrhea: diagnosis and management. *Am J Otol* 1999;20(6):770–776.
25. Ungersbock K, Bocher-Schwarz H, Muller-Forell W, Maurer J: The preoperative assessment of stroke risk in lesions involving the internal carotid artery. *Br J Neurosurg* 1995;9(4):477–486.
26. Hadeishi H, Yasui N, Okamoto Y: Extracranial-intracranial high-flow bypass using the radial artery between the vertebral and middle cerebral arteries. Technical note. *J Neurosurg* 1996;85(5):976–979.
27. Kinugasa K, Sakurai M, Ohmoto T: Contralateral external carotid-to-middle cerebral artery graft using the saphenous vein. Case report. *J Neurosurg* 1993;78(2):290–293.
28. Hetzel A, von Reutern G, Wernz MG, et al: The carotid compression test for therapeutic occlusion of the internal carotid artery. Comparison of angiography with transcranial Doppler sonography. *Cerebrovasc Dis* 2000;10(3):194–199.
29. Maurer J, Ungersbock K, Amedee RG, et al: Transcranial Doppler ultrasound recording with compression test in patients with tumors involving the carotid arteries. *Skull Base Surg* 1993;3(1):11–15.
30. Berenholz L, Kessler A, Sarfaty S, Segal S: Subarachnoid hemorrhage: a complication of endoscopic sinus surgery using powered instrumentation. *Otolaryngol Head Neck Surg* 1999;121(5):665–667.

31. Fujii K, Chambers SM, Rhoton AL, Jr: Neurovascular relationships of the sphenoid sinus. A microsurgical study. *J Neurosurg* 1979;50(1):31–39.

32. Persky MS, Setton A, Niimi Y, et al: Combined endovascular and surgical treatment of head and neck paragangliomas—a team approach. *Head Neck* 2002;24(5):423–431.

33. Dardik A, Eisele DW, Williams GM, Perler BA: A contemporary assessment of carotid body tumor surgery. *Vasc Endovascular Surg* 2002;36(4):277–283.

34. Kasper GC, Welling RE, Wladis AR, et al: A multidisciplinary approach to carotid paragangliomas. *Vasc Endovascular Surg* 2006;40(6):467–474.

35. LaMuraglia GM, Fabian RL, Brewster DC, et al: The current surgical management of carotid body paragangliomas. J Vasc Surg 1992;15(6):1038–1044; discussion 1044–1035.

36. Biller HF, Lawson W, Som P, Rosenfeld R: Glomus vagale tumors. *Ann Otol Rhinol Laryngol* 1989;98(1 Pt 1):21–26.

37. Litle VR, Reilly LM, Ramos TK: Preoperative embolization of carotid body tumors: when is it appropriate? *Ann Vasc Surg* 1996;10(5):464–468.

38. Wilson MA, Hillman TA, Wiggins RH, Shelton C: Jugular foramen schwannomas: diagnosis, management, and outcomes. *Laryngoscope* 2005;115(8):1486–1492.

39. Lustig LR, Jackler RK: The variable relationship between the lower cranial nerves and jugular foramen tumors: implications for neural preservation. *Am J Otol* 1996;17(4):658–668.

40. Kerr JT, Chu FW, Bayles SW: Cerebrospinal fluid rhinorrhea: diagnosis and management. *Otolaryngol Clin North Am* 2005;38(4):597–611.

41. Schnipper D, Spiegel JH: Management of intracranial complications of sinus surgery. *Otolaryngol Clin North Am* 2004;37(2):453–472, ix.

42. Brown NE, Grundfast KM, Jabre A, et al: Diagnosis and management of spontaneous cerebrospinal fluid-middle ear effusion and otorrhea. *Laryngoscope* 2004;114(5):800–805.

43. Gacek RR, Leipzig B: Congenital cerebrospinal otorrhea. *Ann Otol Rhinol Laryngol* 1979;88(3 Pt 1):358–365.

44. Mackle T, Hughes J, Fenton J, Walsh RM: Spontaneous CSF otorrhea from a defect in the medial wall of the middle ear. *Otolaryngol Head Neck Surg* 2006;134(1):166–167.

45. Wootten CT, Backous DD, Haynes DS: Management of cerebrospinal fluid leakage from cochleostomy during cochlear implant surgery. *Laryngoscope* 2006;116(11):2055–2059.

46. Megerian CA, Hadlock TA: Case records of the Massachusetts General; Hospital. Weekly clinicopathological exercises. Case 40-2001. An eight-year-old boy with fever, headache, and vertigo two days after aural trauma. *N Engl J Med* 2001;345(26):1901–1907.

47. Fahy CP, Carney AS, Nikolopoulos TP, Ludman CN, Gibbin KP: Cochlear implantation in children with large vestibular aqueduct syndrome and a review of the syndrome. *Int J Pediatr Otorhinolaryngol* 2001;59(3):207–215.

48. Leonetti J, Anderson D, Marzo S, Moynihan G: Cerebrospinal fluid fistula after transtemporal skull base surgery. *Otolaryngol Head Neck Surg* 2001;124(5):511–514.

49. Brennan JW, Rowed DW, Nedzelski JM, Chen JM: Cerebrospinal fluid leak after acoustic neuroma surgery: influence of tumor size and surgical approach on incidence and response to treatment. *J Neurosurg* 2001;94(2):217–223.

50. Sanna M, Taibah A, Russo A, et al: Perioperative complications in acoustic neuroma (vestibular schwannoma) surgery. Otol Neurotol 2004;25(3):379–386.

51. Marks HW: Simple method to control a cerebrospinal fluid gusher during cochlear implant surgery. *Otol Neurotol* 2004;25(4):483–484.

52. Bhatia K, Gibbin KP, Nikolopoulos TP, O'Donoghue GM: Surgical complications and their management in a series of 300 consecutive pediatric cochlear implantations. *Otol Neurotol* 2004;25(5):730–739.

53. FDA: Public health web notification: risk of bacterial meningitis in children with cochlear implants. In: http://www.fda.gov/cdrh/safety/101007-cochlear.html; 2003.

54. Ryall RG, Peacock MK, Simpson DA: Usefulness of beta 2-transferrin assay in the detection of cerebrospinal fluid leaks following head injury. *J Neurosurg* 1992;77(5):737–739.

55. Jho HD, Carrau RL, McLaughlin MR, Somaza SC: Endoscopic transsphenoidal resection of a large chordoma in the posterior fossa. *Acta Neurochir* (Wien) 1997;139(4):343–347; discussion 347–348.

56. Roelandse FW, van der Zwart N, Didden JH, et al: Detection of CSF leakage by isoelectric focusing on polyacrylamide gel, direct immunofixation of transferrins, and silver staining. *Clin Chem* 1998;44(2):351–353.

57. Seiler RW, Mariani L: Sellar reconstruction with resorbable vicryl patches, gelatin foam, and fibrin glue in transsphenoidal surgery: a 10-year experience with 376 patients. *J Neurosurg* 2000;93(5):762–765.

58. Som ML, Kramer R: Cerebrospinal rhinorrhea pathologic findings. *Laryngoscope* 1940;50:1167.

59. Keros P: [On the practical value of differences in the level of the lamina cribrosa of the ethmoid.]. *Z Laryngol Rhinol Otol* 1962;41:809–813.

60. Mafee MF, Chow JM, Meyers R: Functional endoscopic sinus surgery: anatomy, CT screening, indications, and complications. *AJR Am J Roentgenol* 1993;160(4):735–744.

61. Mincy JE: Posttraumatic cerebrospinal fluid fistula of the frontal fossa. *J Trauma* 1966;6(5):618–622.

62. Sinha UK, Johnson TE, Crockett D, et al: Three-layer reconstruction for large defects of the anterior skull base. *Laryngoscope* 2002;112(3):424–427.

63. Fliss DM, Gil Z, Spektor S, et al: Skull base reconstruction after anterior subcranial tumor resection. *Neurosurg Focus* 2002;12(5):e10.

64. Wax MK, Ramadan HH, Ortiz O, Wetmore SJ: Contemporary management of cerebrospinal fluid rhinorrhea. *Otolaryngol Head Neck Surg* 1997;116(4):442–449.

65. Deschler DG, Gutin PH, Mamelak AN, et al: Complications of anterior skull base surgery. *Skull Base Surg* 1996;6(2):113–118.

66. Lanza DC, O'Brien DA, Kennedy DW: Endoscopic repair of cerebrospinal fluid fistulae and encephaloceles. *Laryngoscope* 1996;106(9 Pt 1):1119–1125.

67. Fried MP, Moharir VM, Shin J, et al: Comparison of endoscopic sinus surgery with and without image guidance. *Am J Rhinol* 2002;16(4):193–197.

68. Campanelli J, Odland R: Management of tension pneumocephalus caused by endoscopic sinus surgery. *Otolaryngol Head Neck Surg* 1997;116(2):247–250.

69. Artru AA: Nitrous oxide plays a direct role in the development of tension pneumocephalus intraoperatively. *Anesthesiology* 1982;57(1):59–61.

70. Gil Z, Cohen JT, Spektor S, et al: Anterior skull base surgery without prophylactic airway diversion procedures. *Otolaryngol Head Neck Surg* 2003;128(5):681–685.

71. Dandy W: Pneumocephalus. *Archives of Surgery* 1926.;12:949–982.

72. Clevens RA, Bradford CR, Wolf GT: Tension pneumocephalus after endoscopic sinus surgery. *Ann Otol Rhinol Laryngol* 1994;103(3):235–237.

73. Daly DT, Lydiatt WM, Ogren FP, Moore GF: Extracranial approaches to the repair of cerebrospinal fluid rhinorrhea. *Ear Nose Throat J* 1992;71(7):311–313.

74. Yorgason JG, Arthur AS, Orlandi RR, Apfelbaum RI: Endoscopic decompression of tension pneumosella following transsphenoidal pituitary tumor resection. *Pituitary* 2004;7(3):171–177.

75. Younis RT, Anand VK, Childress C: Sinusitis complicated by meningitis: current management. *Laryngoscope* 2001;111(8):1338–1342.

76. Durand ML, Calderwood SB, Weber DJ, et al: Acute bacterial meningitis in adults. A review of 493 episodes. *N Engl J Med* 1993;328(1):21–28.

77. Wei BP, Robins-Browne RM, Shepherd RK, et al: Protective effects of local administration of ciprofloxacin on the risk of pneumococcal meningitis after cochlear implantation. *Laryngoscope* 2006;116(12):2138–2144.

78. Reefhuis J, Honein MA, Whitney CG, et al: Risk of bacterial meningitis in children with cochlear implants. *N Engl J Med* 2003;349(5):435–445.

79. Carpenter J, Stapleton S, Holliman R: Retrospective analysis of 49 cases of brain abscess and review of the literature. *Eur J Clin Microbiol Infect Dis* 2007;26(1):1–11.

80. Raveh J, Vuillemin T, Sutter F: Subcranial management of 395 combined frontobasal-midface fractures. *Arch Otolaryngol Head Neck Surg* 1988;114(10):1114–1122.

81. McDermott C, O'Sullivan R, McMahon G: An unusual cause of headache: Pott's puffy tumour. *Eur J Emerg Med* 2007;14(3): 170–173.

82. Kao PT, Tseng HK, Liu CP, Su SC, Lee CM: Brain abscess: clinical analysis of 53 cases. *J Microbiol Immunol Infect* 2003;36(2):129–136.

83. Snell GE: Sinogenic and otogenic brain abscesses–a review of 63 cases occurring at Toronto General Hospital, 1956–75. *J Otolaryngol* 1978;7(4):289–296.

84. Weiner GM, Williams B: Prevention of intracranial problems in ear and sinus surgery: a possible role for cefotaxime. *J Laryngol Otol* 1993;107(11):1005–1007.

85. Maniglia AJ, VanBuren JM, Bruce WB, et al: Intracranial abscesses secondary to ear and paranasal sinuses infections. *Otolaryngol Head Neck Surg* 1980;88(6):670–680.

CHAPTER 11

Complications in Interventional Neuroradiology of the Head and Neck

Lee H. Monsein and Christopher F. Dowd

Vascular lesions of the head and neck are challenging therapeutic problems for the head and neck surgeon. Endovascular techniques have played a role in the management of these lesions since selective embolization of the external carotid artery was described by Djindjian and colleagues[1] in 1972. Detailed studies of the vascular anatomy, advancements in catheterization techniques, and the introduction of new embolic materials have improved the safety and effectiveness of these techniques. Nevertheless, these are potentially dangerous procedures that require highly specialized training. Before performing such a procedure, it is important to be sure that the potential benefits will outweigh the possible risks.

The reported incidence of complications related to diagnostic and interventional neuroangiography varies widely. The skill of the angiography team, the equipment, the materials, and the patient populations are variables for which it is impossible to completely control when comparing similar studies. Prospective studies have a tendency to overemphasize adverse events, whereas retrospective analyses probably tend to underestimate them. Therefore, regardless of what is reported in the literature, data regarding the complications of neuroangiography should be obtained from the institution where a particular procedure is to be done.

COMPLICATIONS OF DIAGNOSTIC NEUROANGIOGRAPHY

Complications of diagnostic cerebral angiography are defined as any related occurrence that is detrimental to the patient that occurs during the procedure or within the following 24 hours. They may be local, systemic, or neurologic in nature.[2,3]

Local complications occur in 0.6%[4] to 23.2%[5] of cases and can involve an allergic reaction to the local anesthetic, a wound infection, a hematoma, a vessel dissection, a pseudoaneurysm, fistula formation, or thrombosis. Median nerve damage can occur with brachial artery cannulation, and cervical sympathetic fiber damage can rarely occur with direct carotid artery punctures.

Systemic complications are usually related to the contrast media, and they have been found to be less frequent with nonionic contrast agents.[6] Overall they occur in 0.5%[4] to 9.4%[7] of patients. They are classified according to their severity as major and minor reactions and according to their cause as idiosyncratic or nonidiosyncratic reactions. Minor reactions include nausea, pain, visual effects, vomiting, hives, and pruritus. Major or life-threatening reactions occur in about 1 in 3000 patients and involve facial or laryngeal edema, bronchospasm, cardiac arrest, hypotension, pulmonary edema, and ventricular fibrillation. More than 95% of these patients recover with aggressive supportive therapy.

Idiosyncratic reactions are those that are thought to have an immunologic basis. They are considered to be anaphylactoid in nature, and they are not dose dependent. Symptoms vary from mild hives and pruritus to circulatory collapse. Any previous allergic history increases the risk of severe reaction about four to five times, and a previous contrast reaction increases the risk about 11 times. Nonidiosyncratic reactions are thought to represent a direct toxic effect of contrast material, and they are usually dose dependent. These include pulmonary edema, cardiac arrhythmia, hypertensive crisis in patients with pheochromocytoma, sickle cell crisis in patients with sickle cell anemia, thyroid storm in patients with hypothyroidism, and myasthenic crisis in those with myasthenia gravis.

Neurologic complications may be transient or permanent. They can be ischemic in nature as a result of an embolic or thrombotic cause from clot formation, the dislodgement of plaque, vasospasm, or vessel injury. Transient ischemic deficits can include hemiparesis, dysphasia, sensory changes, or visual disturbances, and they occur in about 4%[2] of patients undergoing cerebral angiography. Permanent ischemic complications occur in about 1% of patients. Neurologic complications that are unrelated to technical factors are less commonly thought to be the result of direct contrast chemotoxicity. Examples include global amnesia, cortical blindness, and seizures.

COMPLICATIONS OF INTERVENTIONAL NEUROANGIOGRAPHY

General Considerations

The major risks of interventional neuroangiography of the head and neck are stroke, visual loss, cranial nerve palsy, tissue necrosis, and, rarely, hemorrhage. The location, extent, and degree of the insult are dependent on the vessel and vascular territory involved. Paying attention to anatomy, technique, and materials is crucial to minimize the risk of endovascular therapy.

Anatomy

Knowledge of normal, variant, and pathologic vascular anatomy is crucial to understanding and avoiding complications that can occur during endovascular procedures. Excellent reviews have been written on this subject.[8-11]

Lasjaunias[12] popularized the term *hemodynamic equilibrium* to describe the way in which many areas of the head and neck, including the brain, are fed by a variable number of complementary intracranial and extracranial vascular supplies. In instances in which there is acquired or iatrogenic occlusion of the internal carotid or vertebral arteries or their branches, these connections may rescue cerebral perfusion. However, these same channels can provide the route by which ischemic complications can occur during an embolization procedure. Similarly, vessels that supply tumors of the head and neck may also supply the brain, the cranial nerves, and the skin.

Important potential anastomoses exist among these arteries: the internal maxillary and the internal carotid via the artery of the foramen rotundum; the middle meningeal and the ophthalmic via the recurrent meningeal, meningoophthalmic, and meningolacrimal branches; the ascending pharyngeal and the C5 portion of the internal carotid via the lacerum branches; the ascending pharyngeal and the third cervical level of the vertebral via the musculospinal branches; the ascending pharyngeal and the second and third cervical levels of the vertebral via the hypoglossal branches; and the occipital and vertebral via the first and second cervical level collaterals (Figure 11-1 and Table 11-1). In addition, a number of anatomic variations may exist (e.g., the ophthalmic artery originating directly from the middle meningeal artery).

Dangerous anastomoses may be opacified before, during, or after embolization. However, their visualization is not an absolute contraindication to embolotherapy. Certain maneuvers can be performed to protect against embolic material traversing these channels and reaching the intracranial circulation. An embolic material that

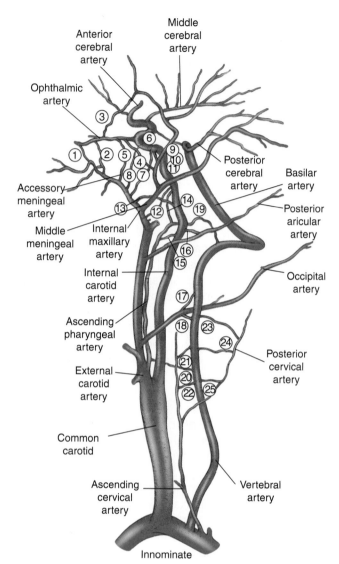

Figure 11-1. Important potential arterial anastomoses (see Table 11-1).

has physical characteristics that preclude its traversing these channels is one option, or the channels themselves may be blocked before embolization of the pathologic area. With flow control, the direction of the blood flow is stopped or reversed in an anastomosis so that embolic material does not go toward vital tissue during embolotherapy. The parent artery at or above a potentially dangerous anastomosis may be temporarily or permanently occluded to prevent the delivery of embolic material to more distant vital structures.

Caution is required when performing the embolization of vessels that may supply the cranial nerves. The transcranial nerves are supplied primarily by three branches of the internal maxillary artery: the cavernous branch of the middle meningeal artery, which supplies the Gasserian ganglion; the intracranial branches of the middle and accessory meningeal arteries, which supply the third

TABLE 11-1 Dangerous Anastomoses

Internal Carotid or Vertebral Arteries	External Carotid Artery Branches	Dangerous Connecting Artery	Figure 11-1 Legend	Course
Internal carotid artery (ophthalmic artery branches)	Internal maxillary artery	Infraorbital artery (orbital branch)	1	Inferior orbital fissure
		Sphenopalatine artery (ethmoidal anastomoses)	2	Ethmoidal canal
		Middle meningeal artery (meningoophthalmic)	3	Superior orbital fissure
		Middle meningeal artery (recurrent meningeal)	4	
		Anterior deep temporal artery (orbital branch)	5	Transmalar
Internal carotid artery siphon (inferolateral trunk)	Internal maxillary artery	Middle meningeal artery (cavernous ramus)	6	Foramen spinosum
		Accessory meningeal artery (cavernous ramus)	7	Foramen ovale
		Artery of foramen rotundum	8	Foramen rotundum
Internal carotid artery siphon (C5 portion)	Ascending pharyngeal artery	Superior pharyngeal artery (carotid branch)	9	Foramen lacerum
		Jugular artery (lateral clival branch)	10	Jugular foramen
		Hypoglossal artery (medial clival branch)	11	Hypoglossal foramen
Internal carotid artery (petrous portion)	Internal maxillary artery	Anterior tympanic artery	12	Anterior tympanic canal
		Vidian artery	13	Vidian canal
	Ascending pharyngeal artery	Superior pharyngeal artery (mandibular anastomosis)	14	Foramen lacerum
		Inferior tympanic artery	15	Jacobson's canal
	Posterior auricular or occipital arteries	Stylomastoid artery	16	Facial canal
Vertebral artery	Occipital artery	C1 anastomotic branch	17	First cervical space
		C2 anastomotic branch	18	Second cervical space
	Ascending pharyngeal artery	Hypoglossal artery (odontoid arterial arch system)	19	Third cervical space and hypoglossal foramen
		Musculospinal artery	20	Third and fourth cervical spaces

Continued

TABLE 11-1   Dangerous Anastomoses—cont'd

Internal Carotid or Vertebral Arteries	External Carotid Artery Branches	Dangerous Connecting Artery	Figure 11-1 Legend	Course
	Ascending cervical artery	C3 anastomosis	21	Third cervical space
		C4 anastomosis	22	Fourth cervical space
	Posterior cervical artery	C2 anastomosis	23	Second cervical space
		C3 anastomosis	24	Third cervical space
		C4 anastomosis	25	Fourth cervical space

Adapted from Lasjaunias P, Berenstein A: *Surgical neuroangiography, 1: Functional anatomy of the craniofacial arteries,* Berlin, 1987, Springer-Verlag.

division of the fifth cranial nerve; and the artery of the foramen rotundum, which supplies the second division of the fifth cranial nerve (and, less frequently, its first division as well as the third, fourth, and sixth cranial nerves). The intrapetrous portion of the seventh cranial nerve can be supplied by the stylomastoid artery or the petrosal branches of the middle meningeal and accessory meningeal arteries. The neuromeningeal division of the ascending pharyngeal artery supplies part of the sixth cranial nerve, the ninth though eleventh cranial nerves via the jugular branch, and the twelfth cranial nerve via the hypoglossal branch (Figure 11-2 and Table 11-2).

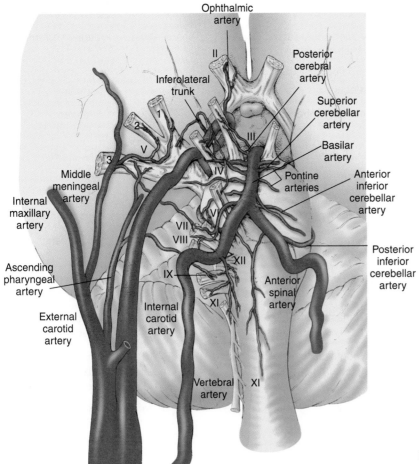

Figure 11-2. Blood supplies to the cranial nerves (see Table 11-2).

TABLE 11-2   Blood Supply of Cranial Nerves

Cranial Nerve	Location	Blood Supply
III, IV, VI, V (I)	Exiting the brainstem	Vertebral-basilar system; IV and VI have separate arteries on each side; III has arteries from each side that may arise from a common trunk
	Roof of the cavernous sinus	III and IV supplied by the marginal artery of the tentorium cerebelli
	Extradural space of the dorsum sellae	VI supplied by the jugular branch of the ascending pharyngeal artery and then by the medial branch of the lateral artery of the clivus arising from the C5 segment of the carotid siphon
	Within the cavernous sinus	III and IV by the superior branch of the inferolateral trunk; V (I) and VI supplied by other branches of the inferolateral trunk
	The superior orbital fissure	Anteromedial branch of the inferolateral trunk
V	From the brainstem to the cavernous sinus	Basilar vestige of the trigeminal artery
	The trigeminal cistern	Lateral artery of the trigeminal ganglion, cavernous branch of the middle meningeal artery, and the carotid branch of the ascending pharyngeal artery
V(II)		Artery of the foramen rotundum
V(III)		Accessory meningeal and cavernous branches of the middle meningeal arteries
VII	From the brainstem to the internal auditory canal	Vertebral–basilar system
VII, VIII	Within the internal auditory canal	Internal auditory artery from the anterior inferior cerebellar artery
VII	From the geniculate ganglion	Branch of the petrosal artery of the middle or accessory meningeal artery
IX, X	Exiting the brainstem	Vertebral artery
IX, X, XI (cranial root)	The jugular foramen	Jugular branch of the neuromeningeal trunk from the ascending pharyngeal, occipital, or anterior cervical arteries
XI (spinal root)	Exiting the brainstem	Branch of the third space and the musculospinal branch, both from the ascending pharyngeal artery
XII	Exiting the brainstem	Vertebral artery
	The hypoglossal canal	Hypoglossal branch of the neuromeningeal trunk

Adapted from Lasjaunias P, Berenstein A: *Surgical neuroangiography, 1: Functional anatomy of the craniofacial arteries,* Berlin, 1987, Springer-Verlag.

Technique

In general, an artery is considered safe for embolization if it does not supply the brain and cranial nerves directly or indirectly via dangerous anastomoses or if it supplies an area with a preexisting deficit. Successful embolization requires that the embolic material be delivered preferentially to the pathologic area and not to normal tissue. This usually requires that a catheter be positioned far enough distally in the arterial tree that it is in a vessel that only supplies pathologic tissue. When this is not possible, normal arterial territories should be protected through use of temporary occluding agents (e.g., coils) that maintain collateral supply to normal tissue. Flow control may also be implemented; this involves slowing down or reversing the flow in a normal territory with the use of an occluding catheter.

To predict whether the embolization of an extracranial vessel will lead to peripheral nervous system cranial nerve deficits, a provocative lidocaine test[13] has been recommended, although its use is controversial. A mixture of 2% lidocaine is injected into the vessel to be tested for 2 to 4 seconds. The appearance of a transient cranial nerve deficit may predict the development of a permanent one after the subsequent injection of embolic material.

Diagnostic and therapeutic angiography with local anesthetic is preferred to allow for continual neurologic testing during the procedure. This is facilitated by the use of nonionic or low-osmolality contrast agents that offer better patient tolerance than traditional ionic iodinated contrast agents. A patient must be awake enough to undergo serial neurologic examinations when lidocaine testing is used; therefore light sedation or awake monitored anesthesia should be used when possible if tolerance testing is planned. A general anesthetic can be considered for patients who are uncooperative or who cannot tolerate such an extended procedure, but this will preclude the ability to perform serial neurologic examinations and thus the use of provocative lidocaine testing.

The goal of the embolization procedure is dependent on the aggressiveness and operability of the tumor or the degree of epistaxis. In the usual case, embolization is terminated when there is a significant decrease in abnormal blush, when washout in the feeding vessel becomes stagnant, or when dangerous anastomoses become visible. Pain in the territory supplied by the embolized vessel and fever are quite common after the embolization. Other more serious complications are infrequent, and they are usually related to improper technique. These are predictable, depending on the vessels that are embolized, and they include brain infarction and transient or permanent cranial nerve palsies.

Embolic Agents

A number of agents are available for the embolization of hypervascular head and neck tumors and epistaxis (Box 11-1). Several factors determine the correct agent for a particular case. Because most of these hypervascular lesions are benign, a relatively safe agent should be chosen. In general, smaller and more permanent embolic agents are more risky.

Particles that are smaller than 100 microns as well as liquid agents have a greater tendency for aberrant migration into the vasa nervorum of the cranial nerves or through dangerous anastomoses into the intracranial circulation. Although it has been reported that meningiomas and juvenile nasopharyngeal angiofibromas rarely demonstrate arteriovenous shunting,[14] this phenomenon has been encountered quite frequently

---

BOX 11-1 Modern Embolic Agents

PARTICULATE AGENTS: ABSORBABLE

- Gelfoam* powder (Pfizer, NY, NY)
- Gelfoam* particles
- Microfibrillar collagen (Avitene [Davol, Cranston, RI])
- Autologous clot
- Dura mater

PARTICULATE AGENTS: NONABSORBABLE

- Polyvinyl alcohol
- Acrylic microspheres
- Detachable balloons
- Coils

LIQUID AGENTS: NONABSORBABLE

- N-butyl cyanoacrylate
- Ethibloc (Ethnor Laboratories/Ethicon, Norderstedt, Germany) (outside of the United States)
- Silicone

LIQUID AGENTS: CYTOTOXIC

- Ethanol 95%
- Chemotherapeutic agents
- Sodium tetradecyl sulfate
- Doxycycline

*Gelatin.

---

in patients with paragangliomas. In addition, we have injected radioactive macroaggregated microspheres (the majority measuring between 60–100 microns) into the feeders of some of these tumors before resection, resulting in significant shunting to the lungs. However, the embolic agent should be small enough to be delivered through a microcatheter and to reach the interstices of the tumor. For these reasons, particles of at least 150 microns are recommended for the presurgical embolization of most of these tumors.

Particulate and absorbable embolic agents are preferable to decrease the severity and longevity of potential ischemic complications. However, liquid and nonabsorbable agents are indicated when the pathology warrants a more aggressive approach. Liquid adhesive agents (e.g., cyanoacrylate glue) are used for permanent vascular occlusion (e.g., arteriovenous malformations) and are technically more difficult to use. Ethanol is used for permanent arterial embolization and as a sclerosing agent. Ethanol penetrates small vascular territories well, it is toxic to endothelial cells, and it causes the rapid occlusion of small arteries. As such, great care is needed to avoid the inadvertent ethanol embolization of nontarget arteries.

Specific Disease Processes

Meningiomas

Meningiomas are benign and potentially curable lesions. They can be locally invasive, however, particularly in the skull base region, and they have a propensity to recur if they are not totally removed. They usually grow slowly and evoke minimal symptoms; therefore any treatment, including embolotherapy, must be of limited risk.

The major determinant of the recurrence of meningiomas is the completeness of surgical resection. This is influenced by tumor vascularity, size, and location and the involvement of major dural venous or arterial structures. Tumor vascularity is most amenable to alteration before surgery. For this reason, as early as 1973, Manelfe and colleagues[15] and a number of subsequent investigators[16–24] recommended endovascular embolization before surgical resection or for palliation in inoperable cases. Surgery after embolization offers several advantages as compared with surgery with the ligation of arterial feeders. First, access may be gained to surgically unapproachable vessels, and the contralateral blood supply may be controlled without a bilateral surgical approach. In addition, the delivery of emboli directly into the vascular bed of the tumor results in a greater degree of ischemia and necrosis that can result in less blood loss, less mass effect, and less time in the operating room.

The indications for the preoperative embolization of a meningioma are determined by the tumor's size, location, and arterial supply. Large, highly vascular tumors of the skull base and the middle cranial fossa, in which the arterial supply is difficult to reach before surgical removal, can benefit the most from preoperative embolization. Unfortunately, however, the feeding arteries of skull-base lesions are often too small to catheterize. The objectives of the preoperative embolization of meningiomas are to facilitate surgical excision by decreasing blood loss and to lessen the chance of recurrence by causing necrosis at the site of dural attachment.

In addition to determining the feasibility and safe routes of embolization, angiography of a meningioma can provide other potentially important information. Tumor vascularity and the site of dural attachment; arterial and venous displacement, encasement, and anatomy; and the adequacy of collateral blood supply can be demonstrated by angiography. The difficulty of surgical resection can sometimes be predicted by the angiographic demonstration of arterial or venous encasement. Drainage through cortical veins may suggest cortical infiltration and portend a poor surgical cleavage plane. Supply by the superficial temporal artery or drainage through the diploic and superficial scalp veins may indicate bone or extracranial soft-tissue involvement. Lesions that can simulate the appearance of a meningioma (e.g., a giant carotid aneurysm of the sella) can be excluded.

In most cases, the middle meningeal artery is the primary blood supply to the meningioma. During embolization, it is important to be distal to the stylomastoid foramen or to the origin of the recurrent meningeal artery to minimize facial nerve damage.

In a large series of meningioma embolizations, temporary neurologic deficits were reported in 2.7% of 185 patients.[25] Permanent neurologic deficits occurred in 1.6%, which included blindness in two patients and hemiparesis and aphasia in one. There was no mortality. There have been rare reports of peritumoral, intratumoral, and subarachnoid hemorrhage after the embolization of meningiomas.[26,27]

Paragangliomas

Paragangliomas are a fascinating and diverse group of tumors that, although relatively rare, have generated significant multidisciplinary interest. They are usually benign, but they can be multicentric in 10% of cases and malignant in 3% to 18% of cases, and they can exhibit neurosecretory activity in 1%. Because of their complex vascular supply and their relation to vital structures, paragangliomas can present difficult therapeutic challenges. The mortality and morbidity rates associated with surgical resection have been reported to be as high as 33% and 50%, respectively. Since Hekster and colleagues[28] first described the preoperative embolization of paragangliomas, a number of investigators have demonstrated its benefits.[12,25,29–36] By limiting blood loss, preoperative embolization can significantly improve intraoperative surgical conditions. Definitive cures have also been reported with embolization alone.[37]

The primary vessel to be embolized with paragangliomas is the ascending pharyngeal artery. It is important to be sure that a minimum of the embolic material reaches the posterior neuromeningeal trunk to prevent injury to cranial nerves IX to XII.

Histopathologically, embolization has been shown to cause cell damage (which can be irreversible and related to ischemia), necrosis, and fibrotic transformation. Minor complications (e.g., pain, fever) can occur in up to 80% of patients. Rare fatalities have been reported as a result of uncontrollable fluctuations in blood pressure after the embolization of secretory active tumors.[38]

Juvenile Nasopharyngeal Angiofibroma

Juvenile nasopharyngeal angiofibromas (JNAs) are rare tumors that occur almost exclusively among adolescent males. They are benign, locally invasive tumors with a strong tendency to recur. Surgical resection, when possible, is considered the treatment of choice. JNAs are highly vascular lesions that are difficult to remove, and hemorrhagic fatalities have been reported. The preoperative embolization of JNAs, which was first described by Roberson and colleagues[39] in 1972, can significantly reduce the volume of blood loss.[40–46] Blood loss without embolization can reach volumes of more than 2000 ml.

JNAs are usually fed by distal branches of the internal maxillary artery. Embolization should be terminated when there is no significant residual tumor blush to prevent the delivery of embolic material to normal dental and mucosal tissues.

The largest reported series of preoperative embolization included 58 patients with JNA. No mortality and no permanent morbidity were reported.[43] There was one case of transient hemiparesis that occurred in association with the temporary balloon occlusion of the carotid artery.

Epistaxis

Epistaxis can be caused by venous, arterial, or arteriolized venous bleeding. If venous bleeding does not stop spontaneously, it can usually be controlled effectively by compression or anterior nasal packing. Arterial bleeding constitutes a medical emergency, and more aggressive therapy may require posterior nasal packing, the ligation of the maxillary or ethmoid arteries, or the embolization of the internal maxillary arterial feeders,[41,42,47-56] which was initially described by Sokoloff and colleagues.[57] In idiopathic epistaxis, particulate embolization of the distal internal maxillary and/or facial arteries can be effective for reducing or eliminating bleeding by saturating the bleeding nasal mucosa with embolic material. Embolic coils should not be used in patients with nontraumatic epistaxis, because coil embolization will simply produce proximal artery occlusion without the intended effect of mucosal devascularization. The technical issues involved in the embolization of epistaxis caused by external carotid trauma are different, because the embolic material (usually coils) must be placed at or across the injury site. Posttraumatic aneurysms of the petrous[58] or cavernous[59,60] portion of the internal carotid artery (ICA) may be permanently occluded by balloons or by coils in some cases of massive epistaxis.[61]

The control of epistaxis with embolization can be very successful.[62] Riche and colleagues[53] reported the immediate postembolization cessation of bleeding in 53 of 54 patients and no further bleeding in 29 of 42 patients at 3 months to 6 years of follow up. Three major complications occurred in their series: transient hemiplegia with dysphasia, facial nerve palsy, and hemiplegia.

Temporary and Permanent Carotid Artery Occlusion

The permanent occlusion of the ICA infrequently becomes necessary for the treatment of certain skull-base lesions.[63] Nishioka[64] demonstrated that the occlusion of the common carotid artery or the ICA in patients with intracranial aneurysms carries a 30% risk of ischemia of the ipsilateral cerebral hemisphere. In 21% of these cases, the onset of neurologic deficits is delayed for more than 48 hours after occlusion. The risk of carotid occlusion in a patient with a head and neck malignancy is thought to be similar. Inadequate collateral circulation and thromboembolism are thought to be the two causes of ischemic complications.[65]

Although intraoperative means have been advocated to assess a patient's tolerance of permanent carotid artery occlusion, preoperative testing is preferred to identify those patients who will have inadequate collateral circulation after this alteration in cerebral blood flow. As early as 1910, Matas[66] recommended a temporary occlusion test to predict a patient's tolerance for carotid occlusion.

The ICA may be temporarily occluded by a balloon catheter,[65,67-76] which is more effective and reproducible than digital compression[66,77,79] and less invasive than a ligature or clamp.[81-86] Gradual occlusion with ligatures or clamps has not been shown to be superior to abrupt occlusion with a balloon catheter.[82,87,88]

In addition to clinical examination with or without provocative hypotension, several methods of assessing the adequacy of collateral circulation during the occlusion test have been recommended. Angiography,[89] electroencephalography,[90-96] somatosensory evoked potentials,[97] and the intra-arterial measurement of stump pressures[86,96,98-101] have been used.

Cerebral blood flow assessment with xenon 133 and external probes[96,100,102,103] or stable xenon with computed tomography (CT) scanning[71-73] improves the sensitivity of test occlusions and gives quantitative information. However, the equipment required for cerebral blood flow determinations with these techniques is not widely available, and there has been some concern about the effect of xenon on the cerebral blood flow.[104] External probe measurements with xenon 133 are easily performed in the angiography suite and offer reproducible quantitative measurements, but they provide no information about regional perfusion. Stable xenon with CT gives regional information but is cumbersome and requires the transfer of the patient to another room with a carotid catheter in place. Recently, technetium-99m hexamethylpropyleneamine oxime single-photon emission computed tomography[76,79] and transcranial doppler[105] have also been recommended. These techniques are commonly available and easily used, and they offer quantitative information.

Up to 15% of patients with negative clinical test occlusions develop ischemic complications after permanent occlusion of the ICA.[73] In the experience of the authors, approximately 5% of patients who had negative clinical test occlusions of the carotid artery developed ischemic complications after permanent occlusion. Although no complications related to the test occlusion procedure itself have been experienced by the authors, others have reported up to a 4% complication rate that included carotid dissection, aphasia, and temporary neurologic deficit.[106]

Emergency Carotid Bleeding (Carotid Blowout Syndrome)

Life-threatening hemorrhage can occur either from the presence of a malignant tumor around the carotid artery or from a skull-base or paranasal sinus iatrogenic misadventure. When bleeding from the internal carotid artery is suspected, one should consider urgent intubation for airway protection (if needed) followed by radiographic investigation with both CT/CT angiography and catheter angiography. Angiography of both the internal and external carotid arteries is performed to localize the bleeding site. If an internal carotid source is confirmed in the acutely bleeding patient, it is usually prudent to consider intentional and controlled ICA occlusion to eliminate the bleeding source. One performs a carotid balloon test occlusion (as described previously) to determine patient tolerance using the neurologic examination (in the awake patient), the angiographic evidence of collaterals, and the collateral pressure measurements of the ICA. If adequate collaterals are demonstrated by these radiographic and clinical criteria, one can undertake permanent carotid occlusion using detachable balloons or embolic fibered microcoils placed at the bleeding site.[107] The posttreatment management of these patients is just as crucial as proper embolization technique, because hypotension, anemia, and patient overactivity can overwhelm the ability of collaterals to adequately perfuse the hemisphere ipsilateral to the carotid occlusion. When a patient does not tolerate carotid test occlusion, one can consider emergent external-to-internal carotid artery surgical bypass or the use of a stent[108] to cover the affected segment of ICA while preserving flow to the ipsilateral hemisphere. Generally the direct coil embolization of an acute carotid pseudoaneurysm with the preservation of the parent ICA is not advocated, because the lack of mural support for the embolic coils could permit the migration of coils though the pseudoaneurysm and thus risk rehemorrhage.[109] Such a therapy is more feasible in a subacute or chronic setting, because fibrous tissue may have formed around the pseudoaneurysm, thereby providing a structural platform for the coils. The major drawback of the use of covered stents is thrombogenicity, because long-term patency rates are suboptimal. The emergent carotid bleeding scenario represents an extreme management dilemma: treatment with carotid occlusion or stents involves the risk of ipsilateral hemisphere stroke, whereas inadequate therapy could result in exsanguination.

Vascular Birthmarks

Vascular birthmarks are a potentially confusing constellation of lesions. They may appear to be similar morphologically, yet they may behave quite differently. Physician understanding of this topic has been hindered by unclear or outdated nomenclature. In 1982, Mulliken and Glowacki[110] devised an effective classification scheme based on clinical behavior and cellular characteristics. The vast majority of cutaneous vascular anomalies may be sorted into two main categories: hemangiomas and vascular malformations.[111]

Hemangiomas

Hemangiomas represent benign neoplasms of blood-vessel origin. Clinically they demonstrate proliferation during the first year of life and involution thereafter. Their appearance via magnetic resonance imaging is characteristic, demonstrating a well-defined soft-tissue mass with an internal salt-and-pepper inhomogeneity that represents intratumoral vascularity. Treatment usually consists of observation, because these lesions involute (unless vital structures are compromised, thereby necessitating more aggressive medical management [e.g., steroids, α-interferon] or surgery). Transarterial embolization is not a commonly applied therapy for hemangiomas. However, there are two related tumors that demonstrate a similar appearance but that behave more aggressively: kaposiform hemangioendotheliomas and tufted angiomas.[112] These tumors can produce severe thrombocytopenia from platelet trapping (Kasabach–Merritt phenomenon). Transarterial embolization (usually with particulate agents) can devascularize these tumors, and it also limits thrombocytopenia.[113] As with all tumors, the inadvertent embolization of nontarget arteries is the primary risk of the procedure. This can be a particular challenge in the ill infant.

Vascular Malformations

Vascular malformations represent malformed blood vessel elements, not neoplasms. Clinically, they grow commensurate with the patient's own growth, without phases of proliferation and involution. Vascular malformations are subdivided by the affected vascular element into arteriovenous, venous, lymphatic, and capillary malformations, each of which has characteristic presentation, behavior, and imaging characteristics. Many vascular malformations are comprised of a combination of these subtypes. Endovascular therapy may provide definitive or adjunctive therapy.

Head and neck arteriovenous malformations can present as painful pulsatile masses or with worrisome bleeding. Transarterial embolization can be curative (rarely), palliative, or adjunctive to surgery. Among embolic agents, ethanol has become popular because of its efficacy.[114] However, ethanol's potential risks are significant and include skin necrosis, cranial nerve damage, and cardiopulmonary collapse.[115] Great care and experience are necessary when considering the use of ethanol in this setting.

Venous and lymphatic malformations (also called *low-flow vascular malformations*) are not treated by transarterial routes. The direct puncture of the lesion with sclerotherapy can be a useful technique for controlling mass effect and pain in these lesions.[116] Agents that are used to treat venous malformations include ethanol and sodium tetradecyl sulfate. Agents that are used to treat lymphatic malformations include ethanol and doxycycline. Clinical trials of the agent OK-432 are underway for the treatment of lymphatic malformations,[117] but its use is not yet approved in the United States. Complications of sclerotherapy include skin necrosis, infection, cranial neuropathy, and cardiopulmonary collapse. Posttreatment swelling is expected, but patient discomfort is often less than would be expected for the degree of swelling.

QUALITY OF LIFE

In considering endovascular treatment options for lesions involving the head and neck, the guiding concept of *primum non nocere* (first do no harm)[118] should be thoroughly considered as a result of the potential significant therapeutic risks of endovascular therapy. Although the preoperative embolization of a jugulotympanic paraganglioma will provide a clear benefit to the surgeon in terms of the ease of the resection and the limitation of intraoperative blood loss, a permanent lower cranial neuropathy caused by endovascular injury that results in swallowing problems, dysarthria, and aspiration represents a poor therapeutic tradeoff. During the past several decades, rapid technologic developments in microcatheters and embolic materials in combination with the increasing experience of the interventional neuroradiologist have permitted the adoption of safe and effective embolization techniques for the treatment of head and neck vascular lesions, thereby allowing for more facile surgical resection and improved patient outcomes.[119]

ACKNOWLEDGMENTS

The authors wish to thank Jacqueline Chazaly for collecting the case material and Gerard M. Debrun, MD, for his initial review of the manuscript.

REFERENCES

1. Djindjian R, Cophignon J, Theron J, et al: L'embolisation en neuroradiologie: Technique et indications a propos de 30 cas. *Nouv Press Med* 1972;1:2153–2158.
2. Hankey JH, Warlow CP, Sellar RJ: Cerebral angiographic risk in mild cerebrovascular disease. *Stroke* 1990;21:209–222.
3. Waugh JR, Sacharias N: Arteriographic complications in the DSA era. *Radiology* 1992;182:243–246.
4. Kerber CW, Cromwell LD, Drayer BP, et al: Cerebral ischaemia, I. Current angiographic techniques, complications, and safety. *Am J Roentgenol* 1978;130:1097–1103.
5. Olivecrona H: Complications of cerebral angiography. *Neuroradiology* 1977;14:175.
6. Katayama H, Yamaguchi K, Kozuka T, et al: Adverse reactions to ionic and nonionic contrast media: A report from the Japanese Committee on the Safety of Contrast Media. *Radiology* 1990;175:6616–6618.
7. Reilly LM, Ehrenfeld WK, Stoney RJ: Carotid digital subtraction angiography: The comparative roles of intra-arterial and intravenous imaging. *Surgery* 1984;96:909-917.
8. Lasjaunias P, Berenstein A: *Surgical neuroangiography. 1: Functional anatomy of the craniofacial arteries,* Berlin, 1987, Springer-Verlag.
9. Newton TH, Potts DG, editors: *Radiology of the skull and brain: Angiography: Arteries,* vol 2, book 2, Great Neck, NY, 1974, MediBooks.
10. Osborn AG: *Introduction to cerebral angiography,* Hagerstown, Maryland, 1980, Harper and Row.
11. Russel EJ: Functional angiography of the head and neck. *Am J Neuroradiol* 1986;7:927–936.
12. Lasjaunias P: *Craniofacial and upper cervical arteries: Functional, clinical, and angiographic aspects.* Baltimore, 1981, Williams and Wilkins.
13. Horton JA, Kerber CW: Lidocaine injection into external carotid branches: Provocative test to preserve cranial nerve function in therapeutic embolization. 1986;7:105–108.
14. Wickbom I: Tumor circulation. In Newton TH, Pots DG, editors: *Radiology of the skull and brain: angiography,* vol 2, book 4, Great Neck, NY, 1974, MediBooks.
15. Manelfe C, Guiraud B, David J, et al: Embolisation par catheterisme des meningiomes intracraniens. *Rev Neurol (Paris)* 1973;128:339–351.
16. Manelfe C, Lasjaunias, Ruscalleda J: Preoperative embolization of intracranial meningiomas. *AJNR Am J Neuroradiol* 1986;7:963–972.
17. Lasjaunias P, Berenstein A: Dural and bony tumors: II: Meningiomas. In *Surgical neuroangiography: Endovascular treatment of craniofacial lesions,* vol 2, Berlin, 1987, Springer-Verlag.
18. Del Favero G: Preoperative embolization of intracranial meningiomas. *Radiol Med (Torino)* 1984;70:113–117.
19. Hieshima GB, Everhart FR, Mehringer CM, et al: Preoperative embolization of meningiomas. *Surg Neurol* 1980;14:119–127.
20. Richter HP, Schachenmayr W: Preoperative embolization of intracranial meningiomas. *Neurosurgery* 1983;13:261–268.
21. Teasdale E, Patterson J, McLellan D, et al: Subselective preoperative embolization for meningiomas. *J Neurosurg* 1984;60:506–511.
22. Pandya S, Nagpal R: External carotid embolization—a useful prior adjunct to excision of convexity cerebral meningiomas. *Neurol India* 1976;24:182.
23. Rutka J, Muller Pj, Chui M: Preoperative gelfoam embolization of supratentorial meningiomas. *Can J Surg* 1985;28:441–443.
24. Fagioli L, Mavilla L, Nuzzo G, et al: Preoperative embolization of brain meningiomas. *Acta Neurochir (Wien)* 1981;57:307.
25. Lasjaunias P, Berenstein A: Temporal and cervical tumors. In *Surgical neuroangiography: Endovascular treatment of craniofacial lesions,* ed 2, Berlin, 1987, Springer-Verlag.
26. Hayashi T, Shojima K, Utsunomiya H, et al: Subarachnoid hemorrhage after preoperative embolization of a cystic meningioma. *Surg Neurol* 1987;27:295–300.
27. Suyama T, Tamaki N, Fujiwara K, et al: Peritumoral and intratumoral hemorrhage after gelatin sponge embolization of malignant meningioma: Case report. *Neurosurgery* 1987;21:944–946.
28. Hekster REM, Luyendijk W, Matricalli B: Transfemoral catheter embolization: A method of treatment of glomus jugulare tumors. *Neuroradiology* 1973;5:208–214.
29. Valvanis A: Preoperative embolization of the head and neck: Indications, patient selection, goals, and precautions. *AJNR Am J Neuroradiol* 1986;7:943–952.

30. Lacour P, Doyon D, Manelfe C, et al: Treatment of chemodectomas by arterial embolization. *J Neuroradiol* 1975;2:275–287.
31. Simpson GT, Horst RK, Takahashi M: Immediate postembolization excision of glomus jugulare tumors: Advantages of new combined techniques. *Arch Otolaryngol* 1979;105:639–643.
32. Murphy TP, Brackmann DE: Effects of preoperative embolization on glomus jugulare tumors. *Laryngoscope* 1989;99:1244–1247.
33. Young NM, Russell EJ, Wiet RJ, et al: Superselective embolization of glomus jugulare tumors. *Ann Otol Rhinol Laryngol* 1988;97:613–620.
34. Smith RF, Shetty PC, Reddy DJ: Surgical treatment of carotid paragangliomas presenting unusual technical difficulties: The value of preoperative embolization. *J Vasc Surg* 1988;7:631–637.
35. Moret J, Delvert JC, Lasjaunias P: Vascular architecture of tympanojugular glomus tumors: Its application regarding therapeutic angiography. *J Neuroradiol* 1982;9:237–260.
36. Lasjaunias P, Menu Y, Bonnel D, et al: Non-chromaffin paragangliomas of the head and neck: Diagnostic and therapeutic angiography in 19 cases explored from 1977 to 1980. *J Neuroradiol* 1981;8:281–299.
37. Iaccarino V, Sodano A, Belfiore G, et al: Embolization of glomus tumors of the carotid: Temporary of definitive? *Cardiovasc Interven Radiol* 1985;8:206–210.
38. Pandya SK, Nagpal RD, Desai AP, et al: Death following external carotid artery embolization for a functioning glomus jugulare chemodectoma. *J Neurosurg* 1978;48:1030–1034.
39. Roberson GH, Biller H, Sessions DG, et al: Presurgical internal maxillary artery embolization in juvenile angiofibroma. *Laryngoscope* 1972;82:1524–1532.
40. Lasjaunias P, Berenstein A: Nasopharyngeal tumors: Juvenile angiofibromas (JAF), I. In *Surgical neuroangiography: Endovascular treatment of craniofacial lesions,* vol 2, Berlin, 1987, Springer-Verlag.
41. Lasjaunias P, Picard L, Manelfe C, et al: Angiofibroma of the nasopharynx: A review of 53 cases treated by embolisation: The role of pretherapeutic angiography: Pathological hypotheses. *J Neuroradiol* 1980;7:73–95.
42. Davis KR: Embolization of epistaxis and juvenile nasopharyngeal angiofibromas. *AJNR Am J Neuroradiol* 1986;7:953–962.
43. Garcia-Cervignon E, Bien S, Rufenacht D, et al: Pre-operative embolization of naso-pharyngeal angiogfibromas: Report of 58 cases. *Neuroradiology* 1988;30:556–560.
44. Palmer FJ: Preoperative embolisation in the management of juvenile nasopharyngeal angiofibroma. *Australasian Radiol* 1989;33:348–350.
45. Roberson GH, Price AC, Davis JM, et al: Therapeutic embolization of juvenile angiofibroma. *AJR Am J Roentgenol* 1979;133:657–663.
46. Pletcher JD, Dedo HH, Newton TH, et al: Selective embolization of juvenile angiofibromas of the nasopharynx. *Ann Otol Rhinol Laryngol* 1975;84:740–746.
47. Lasjaunias P, Marsot-Duppuch K, Doyon D: The radio-anatomical basis of arterial embolization for epistaxis. *J Neuroradiol* 1979;6:45–53.
48. Parnes LS, Heeneman H, Vinuela F: Percutaneous embolization for control of nasal blood circulation. *Laryngoscope* 1987;97:1312–1315.
49. Strutz J, Schumacher M: Uncontrollable epistaxis. *Arch Otolaryngol Head Neck Surg* 1990;116:697–699.
50. Merland JJ, Melki JP, Chiras J, et al: Place of embolization in the treatment of severe epistaxis. *Laryngoscope* 1980;90:1694–1704.
51. Roberson GH, Reardon EJ: Angiography and embolization of the internal maxillary artery for posterior epistaxis. *Arch Otolaryngol* 1979;105:333–337.
52. Hicks JN, Vitek G: Transarterial embolization to control posterior epistaxis. *Laryngoscope* 1989;99:1027–1029.
53. Riche MC, Chiras J, Melki JP, et al: The role of embolisation in the treatment of severe epistaxis. *J Neuroradiol* 1979;6:207–220.
54. Van Wyck LG, Vinuela F, Heeneman H: Therapeutic embolization for severe epistaxis. *J Otolaryngol* 1982;11:271–274.

55. Solomons NB, Blumgart R: Severe late-onset epistaxis following le Fort I osteotomy: Angiographic localization and embolization. *J Laryngol Otol* 1988;102:260–263.
56. Breda SD, Choi IS, Persky MS, et al: Embolization in the treatment of epistaxis after failure of internal maxillary artery ligation. *Laryngoscope* 1989;99:809–813.
57. Sokoloff J, Wickbom I, McDonald D, et al: Therapeutic percutaneous embolization in intractable epistaxis. *Radiology* 1974;111:285–287.
58. Willinsky R, Lasjaunias P, Pruvost P, et al: Petrous internal carotid aneurysm causing epistaxis: Balloon embolization with preservation of the parent vessel. *Neuroradiology* 1987;29:570–572.
59. Simpson RK, Harper RL, Bryan RN: Emergency balloon occlusion for massive epistaxis due to traumatic carotid-cavernous aneurysm. *J Neurosurg* 1988;68:142–144.
60. Gelbert F, Reizine D, Stecken J, et al: Severe epistaxis by rupture of the internal carotid artery into the sphenoidal sinus: Endovascular treatment. *J Neuroradiol* 1986;13:163–171.
61. Chen D, Concus AP, Halbach VV, et al: Epistaxis originating from traumatic pseudoaneurysm of the internal carotid artery: Diagnosis and endovascular therapy. *Laryngoscope* 1998;108(3):326–331.
62. Gurney TA, Dowd CF, Murr AH: Embolization for the treatment of idiopathic posterior epistaxis. *Am J Rhinol* 2004;18:335–339.
63. Hibbert J: The compromised carotid artery. In Cummings CW, Frederickson JM, Harker LA, et al, editors: *Otolaryngology—head and neck surgery: Update I,* St Louis, 1989, Mosby.
64. Nishioka H: Report on the cooperative study of intracranial aneurysms and subarachnoid hemorrhage, section VIII, part 1: Results of the treatment of intracranial aneurysms by occlusion of the carotid artery in the neck. *J Neurosurg* 1966;24:660–682.
65. Fox AJ, Vinuela F, Pelz DM, et al: Use of detachable balloons for proximal artery occlusion in the treatment of unclippable cerebral aneurysms. *J Neurosurg* 1987;66:40–46.
66. Matas R: Testing the efficiency of the collateral circulation as a preliminary to the occlusion of the great surgical arteries. *Ann Surg* 1911;53:1–43.
67. Berenstein A, Ransohoff J, Kupersmith M, et al: Transvascular treatment of giant aneurysms of the cavernous carotid and vertebral arteries: Functional investigation and embolization. *Surg Neurol* 1984;21:3–12.
68. Raymond J, Thron J: Intracavernous aneurysms: Treatment by proximal balloon occlusion of the internal carotid artery. *AJNR Am J Neuroradiol* 1986;7:1087–1092.
69. Debrun G, Fox A, Drake F, et al: Giant unclippable aneurysms: treatment with detachable balloons. *AJNR Am J Neuroradiol* 1981;2:167–173.
70. Serbinenko FA: Balloon catheterization and occlusion of major cerebral vessels. *J Neurosurg* 1974;41:125-145.
71. Erba SM, Horton JA, Latchaw RE, et al: Balloon test occlusion of the internal carotid artery with stable xenon/CT cerebral blood flow imaging. *AJNR Am J Neuroradiol* 1988;9:533–538.
72. De Fries EJ, Sekhar LN, Horton JA, et al: A new method of to predict safe resection of the internal carotid artery. *Laryngoscope* 1990;100:85–88.
73. Johnson DW, Stringer WA, Marks MP, et al: Stable xenon CT cerebral blood flow imaging: Rationale for and role in clinical decision making. *AJNR Am J Neuroradiol* 1991;12:201–213.
74. Potts DG: Balloon test occlusion of the internal carotid artery with stable xenon/CT cerebral blood flow imaging. *Invest Radiol* 1989;24:578–579.
75. Braun IF, Battey PM, Fulenwider T, et al: Transcatheter carotid occlusion: An alternative to the surgical treatment of cervical carotid aneurysms. *J Vasc Surg* 1986;4:299–302.
76. Monsein LH, Jeffery OJ, van Heerden BB, et al: Assessing adequacy of collateral circulation during balloon test occlusion of the internal carotid artery with 99mTc-HMPAO SPECT. *AJNR Am J Neuroradiol* 1991;12:1045–1051.
77. Webster JE, Gurdjian ES: Carotid artery compression as employed both in the past and in the present. *J Neurosurg* 1958;15:372–383.

78. Toole JF, Bevilacqua JE: The carotid compression test: Evaluation of the diagnostic reliability and prognostic significance. *Neurology* 1963;13:601–606.

79. Matsuda H, Higashi S, Asli IN, et al: Evaluation of cerebral collateral circulation by technetium-99m HM-PAO brain SPECT during Matas test: Report of three cases. *J Nucl Med* 1988;29:1724–1729.

80. McKissock W, Richardson A, Walsh L: Posterior communicating aneurysms: A controlled trial of the conservative and surgical treatment of ruptured aneurysms of the internal carotid artery at or near the point of origin of the posterior communicating artery. *Lancet* 1960;1:1203–1206.

81. Mount LA: Results of treatment of intracranial aneurysms using the Silverstone clamp. *J Neurosurg* 1959;16:611–618.

82. Heros RC: Thromboembolic complications after combined internal carotid ligation and extra- to intracranial bypass. *Surg Neurol* 1984;21:75–79

83. Drake CG: Giant intracranial aneurysms: Experience with surgical treatment in 174 patients. *Clin Neurosurg* 1979;26:12–95.

84. Giannotta SL, McGillicuddy JE, Kindt GW: Gradual carotid artery occlusion in the treatment of inaccessible internal carotid artery aneurysm. *Neurosurgery* 1979;5:417-421.

85. Spetzler RF, Schuster H, Roski RA: Elective extracranial-intracranial arterial bypass in the treatment of inoperable giant aneurysms of the internal carotid artery. *J Neurosurg* 1980;53:22–27.

86. Odom GL, Woodhall B, Tindall GT, et al: Changes in distal intravascular pressure and size of intracranial aneurysm following common carotid ligation. *J Neurosurg* 1962;19:41–50.

87. Landolt M, Millikan CHL: Pathogenesis of cerebral infarction secondary to mechanical carotid artery occlusion. *Stroke* 1970;1:52–62.

88. Brice J, Dowsett D, Lower R: Some haemodynamic effects of carotid artery clamps. *J Neurol Neurosurg Psych* 1964;27:580.

89. Jeffreys RV, Holmes AE: Common carotid ligation for the treatment of ruptured posterior communicating aneurysms. *Neurol Neurosurg Psych* 1971;34:576–579.

90. Trojaborg W, Boysen G: Relation between EEG, regional cerebral blood flow and internal carotid artery pressure during carotid endarterectomy. *Electroencephalogr Clin Neurophysiol* 1973;34:61–69

91. Wells BA, Keats AS, Cooley DA: Increased tolerance to cerebral ischemia produced by general anesthesia during temporary carotid occlusion. *Surgery* 1963;54:216–222.

92. Perez-Borja C, Meyer JS: Electroencephalographic monitoring during reconstructive surgery of the neck vessels. *Electroencephalogr Clin Neurophysiol* 1965;18:161–169.

93. Youmans JR, Kindt GW, Mitchell OC: Extended studies of direction of flow and pressure in the internal carotid artery following common carotid ligation. *J Neurosurg* 1967;27:250–254.

94. Galbraith JG: Safeguards in carotid surgery. *Surgery* 1968;63:1010–1023.

95. Harris EJ, Brown WH, Pavy RN, et al: Continuous electroencephalographic monitoring during carotid artery endarterectomy. *Surgery* 1967;62:441–447.

96. Leech PJ, Miller JD, Fitch W, et al: Cerebral blood flow, internal carotid artery pressure, and the EEG as a guide to the safety of carotid ligation. *J Neurol Neurosurg Psych* 1974;37:854–862.

97. Momma F, Wang AD, Symon L: Effects of temporary arterial occlusion on somatosensory evoked responses in aneurysm surgery. *Surg Neurol* 1987;27:343–352.

98. Sweet WH, Bennett HS: Changes in internal carotid pressure during carotid and jugular occlusion and their clinical significance. *J Neurosurg* 1948;5:178–195.

99. Bakay L, Sweet WH: Intra-arterial pressures in the neck and brain; late changes after carotid closure: Acute measurements after vertebral closure. *J Neurosurg* 1953;10:353–359.

100. Holmes AE, James IM, Wise CC: Observations on distal intravascular pressure changes and cerebral blood flow after common carotid artery ligation in man. *J Neurol Neurosurg Psych* 1971;34:78–81.

101. Heyman A, Tindall GT, Finney WHM, et al: Measurement of retinal artery and intracarotid pressures following carotid artery occlusion with the Crutchfield clamp. *J Neurosurg* 1960;17:297–305.

102. Jennett WB, Harper AM, Gillespie FC: Measurement of regional cerebral blood-flow during carotid ligation. *Lancet* 1966;2:1162–1163.

103. Boysen G: Cerebral blood flow measurements as a safeguard during carotid endarterectomy. *Stroke* 1971;2:1–10.

104. Giller CA, Purdy P, Lindstrom WW: Effects of inhaled stable xenon on cerebral blood flow velocity. *AJNR Am J Neuroradiol* 1990;11:177–182.

105. Feaster SH, Powers A, Laws ER, et al: Transcranial doppler US as an alternative to angiography and balloon occlusion in estimating risk of carotid occlusion: Proceedings of the 76th Scientific Assembly and Annual Meeting of the Radiology Society of North America. *Radiology* 1990;177(P):281.

106. Tarr RW, Jungreis CA, Pentheny S, et al: *Complications of preoperative balloon test occlusion of the internal carotid arteries: Experience in 300 cases: Proceedings of the 29th Annual Meeting of the ASNR,* Washington, DC, June 9–14, 1991.

107. Chaloupka JC, Putman CM, Citardi MJ, et al: Endovascular therapy for the carotid blowout syndrome in head and neck surgical patients: Diagnostic and managerial considerations. *Am J Neuroradiol* 1996;17:843–852.

108. Desuter G, Hammer F, Gardiner Q, et al: Carotid stenting for impending carotid blowout: Suitable supportive care for head and neck cancer patients? *Palliat Med* 2005;19:427–429.

109. Lempert TE, Halbach VV, Higashida RT, et al: Endovascular treatment of pseudoaneurysms with electrolytically detachable coils. *Am J Neuroradiol* 1998;19(5):907–911.

110. Mulliken JB, Glowacki J: Hemangiomas and vascular malformations in infants and children: A classification based on endothelial characteristics. *Plast Reconstr Surg* 1982;69:412–422.

111. Mulliken JB, Young AE. *Vascular birthmarks: Hemangiomas and vascular malformations.* Philadelphia, 1988, WB Saunders.

112. Enjolras O, Wassef M, Mazoyer E, et al: Infants with Kasabach-Merritt syndrome do not have "true" hemangiomas. *J Pediatr* 1997;130:631–640.

113. Blei F, Karp N, Rofsky N, et al: Successful multimodal therapy for kaposiform hemangioendothelioma complicated by Kasabach-Merritt phenomenon: Case report and review of the literature. *Pediatr Hematol Oncol* 1998;15:295–305.

114. Do YS, Yakes WF, Shin SW, et al: Ethanol embolization of arteriovenous malformations: Interim results. *Radiology* 2005;235:674–682.

115. Mitchell SE, Shah AM, Schwengel D: Pulmonary artery pressure changes during ethanol embolization procedures to treat vascular malformations: Can cardiovascular collapse be predicted? *J Vasc Interv Radiol* 2006:17:253–262.

116. Berenguer B, Burrows PE, Zurakowski D, et al: Sclerotherapy of craniofacial venous malformations: complications and results. *Plast Reconstr Surg* 1999;104:1–11.

117. Rautio R, Keski-Nisula L, Laranne J, et al: Treatment of lymphangiomas with OK-432 (Picibanil). *Cardiovasc Intervent Radiol* 2003;26:31–36.

118. Hetts S, Werne A, Hieshima GB: "…and do no harm." *Am J Neuroradiol* 1995;16:1–5.

119. Dowd CF, Halbach VV, Higashida RT, et al: Diagnostic and therapeutic angiography. In Jackler RK, Brackman DE, editors: *Textbook of neurotology,* St Louis, 1994, Mosby Year Book.

CHAPTER 12

Head and Neck Surgical Fires

Mark E. Bruley

The risk of a fire on or within a surgical patient continues to be present in modern surgery. It is especially acute during surgery of the head, neck, and upper chest if open oxygen sources are used. Unfortunately, the sensitivity of surgical, anesthesia, and operating room (OR) nursing staff members to this hazard waned after the cessation of the use of flammable anesthetic agents during the 1970s. During the last several years, the surgical community has experienced the beginnings of a resurgence in the awareness of this continuing risk as well as an understanding of the need for a surgical team approach to the prevention of surgical fires. Preventive measures have existed for decades, but they have begun to diffuse across professional boundaries and to be put into wider practice only in recent years. Aiding in this diffusion have been initiatives by a variety of health care organizations and medical professional societies.

This chapter draws together pertinent information and recommendations regarding surgical fires with respect to the head and neck surgeon. It discusses the relevant literature that addresses surgical fires, their incidence, the various responsibilities of surgical team members for surgical fire prevention in the perioperative setting, and the procedures for surgical fire extinguishment. It significantly updates the information and recommendations presented in the first edition of *Complications in Head and Neck Surgery*.[1] It is based on an updated review of the medical literature and relevant databases, on participation in the standards activities of professional societies, and on decades of experience from field investigations and collaborations with surgeons, anesthesiologists, and OR nurses.

EFFECTS OF SURGICAL FIRE ON PATIENTS AND FAMILY

It is appropriate for this chapter to succinctly address up front the adverse effects of a surgical fire on the patient. Surgical fires of the head, neck, upper chest, and airway are frequently disfiguring or disabling and can seriously affect the quality of life of a patient.[2] Every year in the United States, there are typically two or three publicized incidents on the television news or in the newspapers. Whether the patients survive or not, their families are also adversely affected.

The horror of a surgical fire can be particularly unique in that many patients having head and neck surgery are under monitored anesthesia care with local anesthesia and therefore somewhat conscious when the fire erupts.

Their recall of the surgery, the fear and smell of the fire, and the resulting pain would obviously have a moving effect on their lives. One tragic fire incident led the daughter of the burned patient to initiate a website dedicated to surgical fire prevention and education (www.surgicalfire.org).

Virtually all surgical fires are preventable. In this new era of patient safety, surgical fires are an error worthy of no less attention by our medical profession than other low-incidence yet highly notorious surgical misadventures (e.g., retained instruments, wrong site/side/patient surgery). Surgeons owe it to their patients to become more proactive with regard to the prevention of this acutely horrific complication.

LITERATURE, NEW INITIATIVES, AND INCIDENCE OF SURGICAL FIRE

There are numerous articles of recent vintage in the medical literature that present overviews of surgical fire risks along with safety considerations, precautions, and recommendations for prevention.[1,3–25] Complementing these are a number of articles and formally promulgated recommended practices and guidelines for surgical fire prevention.[12,23,26–46] Educational initiatives and the proliferation of fire drills specific to a surgical patient fire have also recently emerged.[2,14,22,48–55]

In addition, there are references that specifically deal with surgical laser safety issues and suggested practices.[28,39,42,56–64] The even more acute risks of laser-ignited fires in the airway have stimulated significant research into laser-safe airway devices, materials, and techniques during the last 15 years.[57–61,63,65–78] At the technical level, only a few articles have discussed in detail the subtleties of accidental ignition and flame propagation as they relate to head, neck, and airway surgery.[16,17,58–60,79,80]

Of special interest are the surgical fire hazards from oxygen and flammable skin preparation agents. The concerns regarding the buildup of oxygen under surgical drapes during the use of open oxygen sources on the face and those regarding the oxygen-enriched ignition and flame spread of fires in the airway have grown considerably since the early 1990s; they have stimulated research and preventive recommendations specific to these oxygen-enriched fire hazards.[8,66,67,78,79,82,91] Surgical fires from the use of alcohol and alcohol-based skin preparation agents have also been addressed in the clinical literature apart from the fire warnings that appear on the product labels of all of these flammable agents.[26,79,92,97]

It is unfortunate that a number of references in the clinical literature have presented incorrect information regarding the flammability of common fuels in the surgical setting and the appropriate actions to take to extinguish a surgical fire.[98–100] Such incorrect information can complicate constructive dialogue among medical professionals. For example, Podnos[98] sought to address these topics for the surgical community, but his article contained significant errors and became cited in subsequent literature, thus perpetuating the errors. With regard to extinguishment, the article suggested that the best course of action for staff was to get a fire extinguisher, pull the fire alarms, and evacuate the area through the emergency exits. However, these recommendations are absolutely wrong for a surgical fire involving a patient. There is no time to get a fire extinguisher (or a fire blanket) when your patient is on fire; physically removing the burning materials from the patient is the first priority (and this is typically done instinctively by the staff). Moreover, the Podnos article's bulleted guidelines for fire prevention are limited and confusing, although they probably did not originate with the authors. The guidelines listed in that article are as follows:

- "Use only appropriately protected endotracheal tubes when operating near the trachea." This vague recommendation ignores differing ignition sources. Even laser-resistant tubes will combust under certain circumstances, depending on oxygen concentration, laser wavelength, and tube materials. In addition, laser-ignition–resistant tubes are not resistant to electrosurgical ignition.
- "Use fire-retardant surgical drapes." There are no fire-retardant surgical drapes given the potential presence of oxygen-enriched atmospheres and the high energy delivery of lasers.[60] No surgical drapes are fire-retardant treated, although some disposable drapes do have a degree of ignition resistance in air.
- The fire hazards of Betadine and iodine are misrepresented, and it is suggested that both are flammable. However, only tinctures of Betadine or iodine are flammable. Standard Betadine scrub and paint are nonflammable aqueous solutions.

Surgical Fire Safety Initiatives

Hospital-Based Initiatives

At least one health system has recently heightened its clinicians' awareness of the risks of surgical fire by adding a "Surgical Fire Risk Assessment Score" to its perioperative forms for verifying the surgical site and obtaining patient identification.[53] The surgical team is required to identify and assess several fire risk potentials related to the surgery, including, for example, the use of alcohol-based skin preparation solutions and the use of open-oxygen sources on the face. This initiative has served to stimulate collaborative communication among surgical team members.

Joint Commission Initiatives

Despite scores of clinical publications regarding surgical fire prevention during the past 30 years, it was the 2003 publication by the Joint Commission (formerly the Joint Commission on Accreditation of Healthcare Organizations) of their *Sentinel Event Alert: Preventing Surgical Fires* that began to stimulate more deliberate action within the medical community to address this surgical complication.[36] The alert described the risks of surgical fires and noted the importance of surgical fire prevention and education. This alert noted the root causes of surgical fires and described risk-reduction strategies.

The Joint Commission further highlighted the issue when it announced that its National Patient Safety Goals for 2005 would include reducing the risk of surgical fires in ambulatory care and office-based surgery. This goal, which largely mirrors the recommendations in the 2003 publication, specifies education for all surgical staff regarding "how to control heat sources and manage fuels," and it requires establishing "guidelines to minimize oxygen concentrations under [surgical] drapes." This goal was retained for ambulatory care and office-based surgery for 2006, 2007, and 2008.[37] Such Joint Commission goals are used in the formal accreditation surveys of health-care facilities, and they are also intended to provide patient safety guidance for the long term for health-care institutions and providers, even after the goals have been retired as part of the formal survey process.[37]

Professional Societies

Professional societies have begun to seriously address the risks of surgical fires at their annual conferences and, in some cases, with dedicated initiatives to educate their members. In 2006, the American Society of Anesthesiologists (www.asahq.org) established its Task Force on Operating Room Fires, Practice Advisory for the Prevention and Management of Operating Room Fires. American Society of Anesthesiologists practice advisories are systematically developed reports intended to assist clinicians with the making of patient-care decisions. The draft advisory was posted for public comment on June 29, 2007, and it was adopted at the annual meeting in the fall of 2007. The advisory was then published in *Anesthesiology* in May 2008.[38] It contains an Operating Room Fires Algorithm flowchart for assessing the potential fire risks of a surgical procedure and for management in the case of signs of a fire.

The Association of peri-Operative Registered Nurses (www.aorn.org) has for many years promulgated recommended practices for electrosurgery and lasers, which are the two most common ignition sources.[27,28] With regard to surgical fire prevention educational initiatives, in 2006 the Association produced the *Fire Safety Tool Kit* to raise the awareness of OR staff members. Its CDs contain training videos, interviews with clinicians and surgical fire researchers, slide presentations, and session evaluation forms for acquiring clinical contact hours of credit.

The American College of Surgeons has included surgical fire prevention as a session topic at its annual conference on many occasions during the past several years. In 2007, the American Academy of Otolaryngology—Head and Neck Surgery (www.entnet. org) sponsored a session regarding the prevention and management of surgical fires at its annual Quality in Otolaryngology Conference. The author of this chapter was a presenter at that conference and was encouraged by the decisive planning by senior Academy members at the conference to develop formal initiatives and outreach for members. Subsequently, the Academy officially endorsed the American Society of Anesthesiologists practice parameters (see: www.entnet. org/practice/clinicalpracticeguidelines.cfm).

Other United States Initiatives

At a national level within the United States, the National Guideline Clearinghouse (www.guideline.gov) accepted the Emergency Care Research Institute's (ECRI's) January 2003 guidance article "A Clinician's Guide to Surgical Fires" as a national guideline.[12] The Clearinghouse, which was initiated by the Agency for Healthcare Research and Quality at the U.S. Department of Health and Human Services, is a comprehensive database of evidence-based clinical practice guidelines and related documents.

At the state level, Massachusetts and New York have promulgated patient safety initiatives for the prevention of surgical fires.[40,43] Even more detailed initiatives have been undertaken by the Pennsylvania Patient Safety Authority (www.psa.state.pa.us). Their publications have addressed the surgical fire risks of airway fires, electrosurgical units (ESUs) and fires, and alcohol-based surgical fires.[44,46,96]

Within the U.S. armed forces, the Army Medical Command adopted a regulation in 2003 "to provide policy and recommendations that will help ensure minimal risk of fires associated with the performance of surgical procedures in any health care setting to include, but not limited to, the following: operating room, office-based, ambulatory surgery, and intensive care unit type."[29]

Surgical Fire Incidence

No formal repository for statistics on the incidence of surgical fires exists. However, one is not needed to understand that surgical fire is a real patient safety issue. Incidents of surgical fires during the past 15 years continue to abound in the field of head and neck surgery, where the hazards of oxygen- and nitrous-oxide–enriched atmospheres are most acute.[79,83,89,101–116] Even since the demise of flammable anesthetics during the 1970s, surgical fires of all types have continued to occur with regrettable frequency. Until recently, published estimates suggested that there are at least 50 to 100 surgical fires each year out of approximately 50 million surgical procedures performed annually.[5,9,31] These estimates were from ECRI Institute's analysis of its healthcare accident investigations, problem reports received from hospitals via their 38-year-old medical device problem reporting program, their review of the FDA medical device problem report databases, and, to some extent, published medical literature. However, as with many types of medical incidents, many fires are not reported because of embarrassment, potential adverse publicity, or the fear of investigation and possible litigation, and the overall incidence was assumed to be considerably higher. There now exists firm surgical fire data (with a denominator) from the Pennsylvania Patient Safety Authority via its mandatory statewide Patient Safety Reporting System (PA-PSRS) database.

The PA-PSRS database review revealed that the chances of a surgical fire in Pennsylvania are 1 in 87,646 operations based on 36 months of data in 2004–2007.[47] That is a reported average of 28 surgical fires per year in Pennsylvania alone based on 2,424,879 surgeries per year in that state. When the Pennsylvania statistics are used to estimate the annual number of fires in the United States, the number of fires occurring nationally range from 550 to 650, depending on whether the comparison is based on annual surgical data or populating data. Of these, ECRI Institute estimates that approximately 10 to 20 are serious or disfiguring and one or two are fatal.

Data regarding ignition sources, oxygen-enriched atmospheres, and alcohol as a fuel are available.[5,9,31] As for the ignition sources, about 70% of surgical fires involve electrosurgical equipment, another 10% involve lasers, and the balance are ignited by a variety of other heat sources, including electrocautery (i.e., hot-wire cauterization) equipment, fiber-optic light sources, defibrillators, and high-speed burs, which can produce sparks. Oxygen-enriched atmospheres are reportedly involved in approximately 75% of surgical fires, whereas alcohol or alcohol-based surgical preparations are involved in about 4% of reported fires. With regard to the actual locations of the

Locations of Surgical Fires

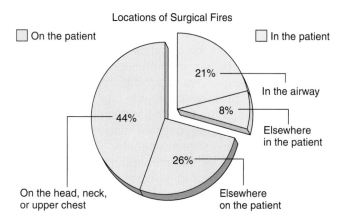

☐ On the patient   ☐ In the patient

21%

In the airway

8%

44%

Elsewhere
in the patient

26%

On the head, neck,
or upper chest

Elsewhere
on the patient

Source. The figures represented here are ECRI's estimates based on accounts of fires—including published accounts and incidents described to ECRI by involved parties—and on analyses of data in the U.S. Food and Drug Administration's medical device reporting databases.

Figure 12-1. Surgical fire data: locations on the patient. (From ECRI Institute: Surgical fires: a patient safety perspective. *Health Devices* 2006;35(2):45–66. Used with permission.)

fires on the patients, about 21% of reported fires occur in the airway; 44% occur on the head, neck, or upper chest; 26% occur elsewhere on the patient; and 8% occur elsewhere in the patient (Figure 12-1). With the abundance of high-energy surgical ignition sources, flammable surgical materials, and the potential for open-oxygen sources, the hazard of surgical fire is clearly still present.

A TEAM APPROACH TO PREVENTING SURGICAL FIRES

Understanding the Fire Triangle

A fire will occur when an ignition source, an oxidizer, and a fuel come together in the proper proportions and under the right conditions. These three basic elements of surgical fires—and of all other types of fires—constitute the traditional fire triangle (Figure 12-2). Keeping the elements of the fire triangle from coming together in ways that could lead to a fire requires that all team members be aware of the risks and that they consistently follow practices to minimize those risks.

During surgery, the three elements are typically present in a number of forms, including surgical instruments, breathing gases, and associated equipment. Consequently, each member of the surgical team is associated with and should be concerned with one or more sides of the triangle:

- Surgeons are involved mainly with ignition sources, such as ESUs, lasers, electrocautery units, and fiber-optic light sources.
- Anesthesia providers are involved mainly with oxidizers, such as oxygen, nitrous oxide (N_2O), medical compressed air, and ambient air.
- Nurses are involved mainly with fuels, such as surgical drapes and preparation agents.

Ignition Source
Surgeons—ESUs, lasers, etc.

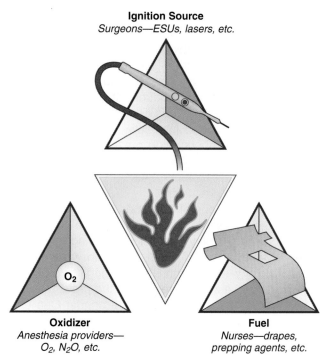

O_2

Oxidizer
Anesthesia providers—
O_2, N_2O, etc.

Fuel
Nurses—drapes,
prepping agents, etc.

Figure 12-2. The classic fire triangle and typical components. Different surgical team members are primarily involved with different sides of the triangle. *ESUs,* Electrosurgical units; *N_2O,* nitrous oxide; *O_2,* oxygen. (©2006 ECRI Institute. Used with permission.)

Of course, these areas frequently overlap. For example, tracheal tubes, breathing circuits, and masks, which are all fuels, fall within the purview of anesthesia providers during surgery. Similarly, preparations, drapes, and ointments applied by surgeons intraoperatively are also fuels, and nurses often handle ignition sources such as lasers and ESUs.

Each member of the surgical team should understand the various fire hazards presented by each side of the fire triangle and endeavor to keep the triangle's elements apart. In addition, each team member should not only understand the basics of surgical fires but also make a point of communicating information about the risks to the other team members intraoperatively or in seminars.

Later in this chapter, each of the elements of the fire triangle is discussed as it relates to the surgical setting. For each element, steps that can be taken to manage or control that side of the triangle to minimize risks are presented. The preventive recommendations that follow are summarized in the educational poster reproduced in Figure 12-3.

Controlling Ignition Sources

Ignition sources present during surgery provide the heat energy that can start a fire should the energy be directed onto or come into contact with some fuel, either in the ambient air or in an oxidizer-enriched atmosphere.

Only *You* Can Prevent Surgical Fires
Surgical Team Communication Is Essential

The applicability of these recommendations must be considered individually for each patient.

At the start of surgery:

- Enriched O_2 and N_2O atmospheres can vastly increase flammability of drapes, plastics, and hair. Be aware of possible O_2 enrichment under the drapes near the surgical site and in the fenestration, especially during head/neck surgery.
- Do not drape the patient until all flammable preps have fully dried.
- Fiberoptic light sources can start fires: Complete all cable connections before activating the source. Place the source in standby mode when disconnecting cables.
- Moisten sponges to make them ignition resistant in oropharyngeal and pulmonary surgery.

For surgery with open delivery of supplemental O_2:

- Question the need for 100% O_2 for open delivery during head/neck surgery.
- As a general policy, use air or ≤30% O_2 for open delivery to the face.
- Arrange drapes to minimize O_2 buildup underneath.
- Keep fenestration towel edges as far from the incision as possible.
- Use an incise drape to isolate head and neck incisions from O_2 and alcohol vapors.
- Coat head hair and facial hair (e.g., eyebrows, beard, moustache) within the fenestration with water-soluble surgical lubricating jelly to make it nonflammable.
- For coagulation, use bipolar electrosurgery, not monopolar electrosurgery.

During oropharyngeal surgery:

- Scavenge deep within the oropharynx with separate suction to catch leaking O_2 and N_2O.
- Soak gauze or sponges used with uncuffed tracheal tubes to minimize gas leakage into the oropharynx, and keep them wet.

When performing electrosurgery, electrocautery, or laser surgery:

- Stop supplemental O_2 (if O_2 concentration is >30%) at least one minute before and during use of the unit, if possible.
- Activate the unit only when the active tip is in view (especially if looking through a microscope or endoscope).
- Deactivate the unit before the tip leaves the surgical site.
- Place electrosurgical electrodes in a holster or another location off the patient when not in active use (i.e., when not needed within the next few moments).
- Place lasers in standby mode when not in active use. Do not place rubber catheter sleeves over electrosurgical electrodes.

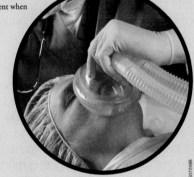

Reference: ECRI Institute. Surgical fire safety [guidance article].
Health Devices 2006 Feb;35(2):45-66.
For more information, or to purchase additional copies of this poster,
contact ECRI Institute.

ECRI Institute
The Discipline of Science. The Integrity of Independence.
5200 Butler Pike, Plymouth Meeting, PA 19462-1298, USA
▸ Telephone +1 (610) 825-6000 ▸ Fax +1 (610) 834-0240 ▸ E-mail accidents@ecri.org

Figure 12-3. Surgical fire prevention poster. (©2006 ECRI Institute. Used with permission.)

Electrosurgery

Electrosurgery is a widely used surgical technology that employs a high-frequency electric current passing through tissue to cut or cauterize that tissue. ESUs are the most common ignition source in surgical fires.[5,9] By its very nature, electrosurgery can produce a high-temperature electric arc, incandescence at the probe tip, tissue embers ejected from the surgical site (i.e., "sputtering"), a flaring flame of organic gases from desiccated tissue, or combinations thereof[117–119] (Figure 12-4). It is of note, however, that there has never been a report of a fire with bipolar electrosurgery. This is likely a result of the low power used across the forceps tips and the general lack of arcing that can occur with the tips grasping the target tissue.

Electrocautery

Electrocautery is the use of an electric current to heat a wire or scalpel blade to a high temperature. The hot wire or blade is used to cauterize tissue or vessels. In some cases, the electrocautery probe is also used to cut tissue. Unlike electrosurgery, electrocautery does not make the tissue part of the electric circuit, and no electrical arcs are generated.

Wire-type electrocautery probes have been involved in surgical fires.[15,17,31,102] With these probes, wire

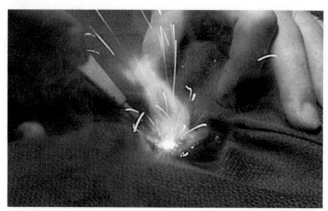

Figure 12-4. Sparks during electrosurgical cutting or coagulation in an oxygen-enriched environment are hot and can travel a distance, causing the ignition of nearby drapes or hair. (Photo by Mark E. Bruley. Used with permission.)

temperatures are typically at or above incandescence (i.e., 500°C [932°F]). Blade-style probes, by comparison, are more limited in their operating temperatures, and no incidents of surgical fires have been reported with their use.

Some hot-wire cautery units have caused fires even when they are not in use. There have been several reports of trash fires involving electrocautery pencils discarded contrary to the device's instructions. Instructions typically call for measures such as breaking off the cauterizing wire and capping the device before discarding it.[120]

Surgical Lasers

General-purpose surgical lasers are the second most frequently cited ignition source in surgical fires, but the fires that they cause are often more serious because of the methods by which the energy is delivered and applied.[5,9] No fires have been reported with ophthalmic lasers; their lower power and more precise targeting mechanisms make it unlikely that they would start a fire. Lasers use a collimated, coherent, monochromatic, directed, intense beam of electromagnetic radiation to cut, coagulate, or vaporize tissue. The wavelengths used include ultraviolet, visible, and infrared. The radiation is transmitted from the laser to the tissue through an array of mirrors, optical fibers, or waveguides. Delivered power is typically in the tens of watts, but it can be as high as 120 W in some lasers. However, the power density can be in the tens of thousands of W/cm² and can vary depending on the spot diameter. The spot diameter, in turn, can vary from a fraction of a millimeter to a few centimeters; it also varies with the distance from the laser aperture or focal point of the laser beam to the target tissue.

Fiber-Optic Light Sources

Fiber-optic light sources collect incandescent light energy and direct it into an optical fiber to illuminate specific areas during surgery. Although this is often called "cold light," these light sources can provide several hundred watts of visible, infrared, and ultraviolet light, which is enough energy to melt, scorch, or ignite materials.[10,11,121] Although some of these wavelengths can be filtered out, this power is typically focused into a fiber-optic cable of small diameter, which can deliver a power density of up to several hundred W/cm².

Defibrillators

Although rarely an ignition source during surgery, defibrillators can start a fire on the patient's chest if excess oxygen or latent alcohol vapors are present. Defibrillators use electrical energy to stimulate a patient's heart. Up to 360 J of electrical energy can be delivered through the paddles that are placed against the patient. If improper technique is used (e.g., if the paddles are applied over a bony prominence or an electrocardiograph lead), if the paddle pad is too small, if too little force is used, or if a high-impedance gel is mistakenly used, sparks can arc from the paddles to the patient. These sparks can serve as an ignition source, especially in an oxygen-enriched atmosphere or if vapors from an alcohol preparation solution are still present.[85] With oxygen present at or near the location of paddle placement, sparks can ignite body hair, including the fine sublayer of hair called *vellus,* which can then spread the fire in a flash to nearby fuels such as linens. Although most defibrillator-ignited fires have occurred in emergency or critical care settings, emergency defibrillation may be needed on a surgical patient who is receiving supplemental oxygen through an open source on the face or possibly when alcohol vapors are present on the body. As such, defibrillators are also considered a potential ignition source during surgery.

Other Surgical Ignition Sources

Other ignition sources include damaged electrosurgical cables, argon-beam coagulators, and sparks from dental and orthopedic burs.[9,122] They also include equipment failures in which an electrical component of a medical device fails, emitting smoke and sometimes flames; these are best handled by disconnecting the device from its electric power supply and removing the device from the room.

Minimizing Ignition Risks

NOTE: The applicability of the following recommendations must be considered individually for each patient.

During Electrosurgery

- Place the electrosurgical active electrode in a holster or another location off of the patient when it is not in active use (i.e., when it will not be needed within the next few moments).
- Allow the electrosurgical active electrode to be activated only by the person wielding it.

- Activate the unit only when the active electrode tip is under the surgeon's direct vision, especially if he or she is looking through a microscope or an endoscope.
- Deactivate the unit before the active electrode tip leaves the surgical site.
- If open-oxygen sources are employed, use bipolar electrosurgery whenever possible and clinically appropriate (e.g., for cauterization during head, neck, and upper-chest surgery). Bipolar electrosurgery creates little or no sparking or arcing and thus far has not been involved in the starting of any surgical fires.
- Never use insulating sleeves cut from catheters or packing material and placed over electrosurgical active electrode tips; use only active electrode tips that are manufactured with insulation. Such materials are not designed as insulators for electrosurgical currents, which are at several thousand volts and which can cause flame flare-ups in oxygen-enriched atmospheres. Figure 12-5 shows a rubber urinary catheter that had been placed over an electrosurgical pencil tip. The rubber flared during oropharyngeal surgery and ignited nearby gauze and the tracheal tube.
- Never use electrosurgery to enter the trachea.
- Never use electrosurgery in close proximity to flammable materials in oxidizer-enriched atmospheres.
- Disconnect contaminated electrosurgical active electrodes, and remove them from the surgical field.

During Laser Surgery

- Limit the laser output to the lowest clinically acceptable power density and pulse duration.
- Test fire the laser onto a safe surface (e.g., a laser firebrick) before starting the surgical procedure to ensure that the aiming and therapeutic beams are properly aligned.
- Place the laser in standby mode whenever it is not in active use.
- Activate the laser only when the tip is under the surgeon's direct vision.
- Allow the laser to be activated only by the person wielding it.
- Deactivate the laser and place it in standby mode before removing it from the surgical site.
- Use surgical devices designed to minimize laser reflectance.
- Never clamp laser fibers to drapes; clamping can break the fibers.
- When performing laser surgery through an endoscope, pass the laser fiber through the endoscope before introducing the scope into the patient. This will minimize the risk of damaging the fiber. Before inserting the scope into the patient, verify the functional integrity of the fiber.
- During lower-airway surgery, keep the laser-fiber tip in view, and make sure that it is clear of the end of the bronchoscope or the tracheal tube before laser emission.
- Use a laser backstop, if possible, to reduce the likelihood of tissue injury distal to the surgical site.
- Use appropriate laser-resistant tracheal tubes during upper-airway surgery. Follow the directions in the product literature and on the labels, which typically include information regarding the tube's laser resistance, the use of dyes in the cuff to indicate a puncture, the use of a saline fill to prevent cuff ignition, and the immediate replacement of the tube if the cuff becomes punctured.
- Place wetted gauze or sponges adjacent to the tracheal tube cuff to protect the tube from laser damage, and keep them wet.
- Wet any gauze or sponges used with uncuffed tracheal tubes to minimize the leakage of gases into the oropharynx, and keep them wet.
- Keep all moistened sponges, gauze, pledgets, and their strings moist throughout the procedure to render them ignition resistant.
- Consider the use of towels soaked in saline or sterile water around the operative site to minimize the risk of igniting the towels. Note, however, that this should be done only if it will not compromise aseptic technique during the procedure.

In General

- If possible, stop supplemental oxygen at least 1 minute before beginning the use of electrosurgery, electrocautery, or laser surgery on the head, neck, or upper chest.
- Remove unneeded foot switches so that they are not accidentally activated. (Do this only after the attached device has been placed in standby mode.)

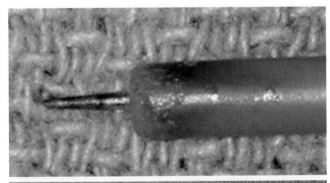

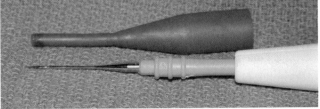

Figure 12-5. Do not cover electrosurgical probe tips with rubber catheters. The rubber can flare up and easily burn *(top photo)* in an oxygen-enriched atmosphere and ignite the tracheal tube or gauze. (Photo by Mark E. Bruley. Used with permission.)

- Dispose of electrocautery pencils properly. For example, break off the cauterizing wire and cap the pencil.
- Be aware that fiber-optic light sources can start fires. Complete all cable connections before activating the light source.
- Never place active fiber-optic cables on drapes or other flammable materials.
- Place the fiber-optic light source in standby mode or turn the light source off when disconnecting cables.

Controlling Oxidizers

Oxidizers Present in the Operating Room

Oxidizers are gases that can support combustion, such as air, oxygen, and N_2O. Oxygen at concentrations above that of ambient air is often provided to patients by means of tracheal tubes, face masks, nasal cannulas, or hyperbaric chambers. This can create oxidizer-enriched atmospheres—most often oxygen-enriched ones—that can enhance ignition and combustion.

Oxygen-Enriched Atmospheres

Oxygen-enriched atmospheres are an often-unsuspected fire risk during surgery of the airway or of the head, neck, or upper chest.[5,9,31,67] Such atmospheres are involved in the majority of reported surgical fires.[5,9] They are defined as atmospheres in which the oxygen concentration exceeds 21% by volume or the partial oxygen pressure exceeds 21.3 kPa (160 torr, 3.1 psi).

Oxygen-enriched atmospheres lower the temperature and energy at which a fuel will ignite; as the oxygen concentration increases, so typically does the risk of fire. Many materials that will not burn or sustain a flame in ambient air will do so in oxygen-enriched environments. For example, polyvinyl chloride plastic, which is a component of tracheal tubes and many other medical devices, requires 26% oxygen to maintain burning. Figure 12-6 shows a demonstration of a tracheal tube fire with flowing oxygen. In addition, fires involving oxygen-enriched atmospheres are hotter, more vigorous, and more intense than those in ambient air, and they spread more rapidly.

Nitrous Oxide

N_2O is an analgesic gas that is often mixed with oxygen and administered to surgical patients. It supports combustion by exothermally dissociating, thereby releasing heat and oxygen. Fires involving oxygen and/or N_2O mixtures (i.e., oxidizer-enriched atmospheres) can be as easily ignited and as severe as fires involving 100% oxygen.

Medical Air

Medical air is air that is produced in the facility by compressing ambient air or by combining nitrogen and oxygen in the proper proportion. Under medical gas piping system pressures of 345 to 379 kPa (i.e., 50–55 psi), medical

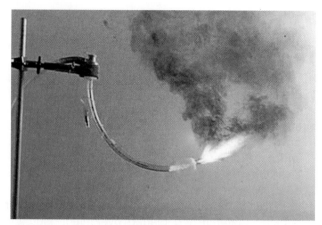

Figure 12-6. Oxygen-enriched burning of a polyvinylchloride endotracheal tube. Note the flame and smoke being emitted from the tube as well as the fire progressing inside the tube. (From ECRI Institute: Surgical fires: A patient safety perspective. *Health Devices* 2006;35(2):45–66. Used with permission.)

air is oxygen enriched in that the partial pressure of oxygen is 72 to 80 kPa (i.e., 543–597 torr, 10.5–11.5 psi). However, medical air is not oxygen enriched at ambient pressure as it is delivered to the patient.

Ambient Air

Ambient air has about 21% oxygen, 78% nitrogen, and fractional percentages of argon, carbon dioxide, and other gases. Ambient air can support the combustion of many potential fuels. In addition, some materials are flammable in atmospheres of less than 21% oxygen. For example, the red rubber used in medical equipment will ignite and burn in just 17% oxygen.

Minimizing Oxidizer Risks

NOTE: The applicability of the following recommendations must be considered individually for each patient.

During Oropharyngeal Surgery

- Use suction deep within the oropharynx to scavenge the gases from the oropharynx of an intubated patient.
- Wet any gauze or sponges used with uncuffed tracheal tubes to minimize the leakage of gases into the oropharynx, and keep them wet.
- Keep all moistened sponges, gauze, pledgets, and their strings moist throughout the procedure to render them ignition resistant.

In General

- Recognize that enriched oxygen and N_2O atmospheres can vastly increase the flammability of drapes, plastic, and hair.
- Be aware of possible oxygen- and/or N_2O-enriched atmospheres near the surgical site under the drapes and in the fenestration, especially during head, neck, and upper-chest surgery.

- Question the need for 100% oxygen for open delivery to the face when using an oxygen mask or nasal cannula during head, neck, and upper-chest surgery, for example. If possible, use air or oxygen levels at or below 30% for open delivery, consistent with patient needs.
- If possible, stop supplemental oxygen at least 1 minute before beginning the use of electrosurgery, electrocautery, or laser surgery on the head, neck, or upper chest.
- Use a pulse oximeter to monitor the patient's blood oxygen saturation, and titrate the delivery of oxygen to the patient's needs. Note that saturation readings fluctuate and that they are typically in the upper 90s, so the delivery of supplemental oxygen to maintain 100% saturation may not always be needed.
- Arrange drapes to minimize the buildup of oxygen and N_2O (e.g., from an uncuffed tracheal tube or a laryngeal mask airway) beneath the drapes.
- Use a properly applied incise drape, if possible, to help isolate head, neck, and upper-chest incisions from oxygen-enriched atmospheres and from flammable vapors beneath the drapes. The proper application of an incise drape ensures that there are no gas communication channels from the under-drape space to the surgical site.
- Dilute oxygen concentrations under drapes with medical air by placing a second cannula under the drapes near the face and providing a flow rate of at least 8 to 10 L/min. NOTE: Active gas scavenging of the space beneath the drapes during open-oxygen delivery is another possibility. This alternative may be of limited value, however, given gas-flow dynamics and the contours around the head and neck area.
- Avoid the use of N_2O during bowel surgery. (During N_2O anesthesia, the gas can diffuse into the bowel and enrich the intestinal gas mixture, thereby making it even more flammable.)

Managing Fuels

Fuels in the Operating Room

Fuels in the surgical setting encompass the following: most of the materials that come into contact with the patient or that are used on or in the patient, most of the materials that are in contact with or used by the surgical staff members, and the patient's body parts. Although the amount of fuel may in some cases be small, the potential fire from such fuels can still be injurious or deadly.

Most of the fuels discussed in this section can ignite and burn in air, but all can easily ignite and burn in oxygen-enriched atmospheres. In addition, the individual flammability characteristics of these fuels can be affected by interaction among the fuels. For example, alcohol can be absorbed into a towel, thus making the towel more flammable, or a fiber-optic light cable can penetrate a surgical drape and ignite underlying materials.

Common Operating Room Materials

Common OR materials make up the largest fuel load in the OR. Some items weigh several kilograms each. Box 12-1 lists the flammable items that are typically present

---

BOX 12-1 Fuels Commonly Encountered in Head and Neck Surgery

PATIENT

- Hair (face, scalp, body)

PREPPING AGENTS

- Degreasers (ether, acetone)
- Alcohol-based prepping agents (DuraPrep, ChloroPrep, Prevail, Hibitane)
- Alcohol (also in suture packets)
- Tinctures
- Merthiolate (thimerosal)
- Aerosol adhesives

LINENS

- Drapes (woven, nonwoven disposable, adherent)
- Gowns (reusable, nonwoven disposable)
- Masks
- Hoods and caps
- Shoe covers
- Instrument and equipment drapes and covers
- Egg-crate mattresses
- Mattresses and pillows
- Blankets

DRESSINGS

- Gauze
- Sponges
- Pledgets
- Adhesive tape (cloth, plastic, paper)

OINTMENTS

- Petrolatum (petroleum jelly)
- Tincture of benzoin (74%–80% alcohol)
- Aerosols (e.g., Aeroplast)
- White wax

EQUIPMENT/SUPPLIES

- Anesthesia components (e.g., breathing circuits, masks, airways, tracheal tubes, suction catheters)
- Flexible endoscopes
- Coverings of fiber-optic cables and wires (e.g., electrosurgical unit and electrocardiograph leads)
- Gloves
- Stethoscope tubing
- Disposable packaging materials (paper, plastic, cardboard)
- Smoke evacuator hoses
- Some instrument boxes and cabinets

on the patient or in the OR. These common materials include the following:

- Operating table mattress, sheets, blankets, pillows, and foam headrests
- Patient hair, gowns, and straps
- Staff gowns, caps, gloves, and booties
- Towels, surgical drapes, incise drapes, bandages, dressings, and sponges

Many of these materials are composed of cellulose or polymeric fibers such as rubber, nylon, polyethylene, and polypropylene. Although fire retardants are used in some of these materials, they cannot be relied on to prevent surgical fires under all conditions. It is of note that no surgical drapes are made with fire retardants. In oxygen concentrations above about 50%, the fine nap fibers on cotton surgical towels, drapes, and OR table linens can serve as a fuel that rapidly spreads a fire across the fabric surface throughout spaces of high oxygen concentration. This is a phenomenon known as *surface-fiber flame propagation.*

Alcohol and Other Volatile Organic Chemicals

Volatile organic chemicals include alcohol, acetone, and ether, which are used in liquids such as skin preparations, tinctures, and degreasers as well as some suture pack solutions and liquid wound dressings. These materials can be present during surgery in volumes from a few milliliters to about a liter. Preparation agent fires are caused by the ignition of flammable vapors at the surgical site.[92-94] Preparation solutions can wick (or be absorbed) into hair and linens, or they can pool on or under the body. If the solutions are not allowed time to fully evaporate before draping, patient-warmed vapors can diffuse throughout the space beneath the drapes and rise out of the fenestration, thereby presenting a fire hazard. Alcohol fires can be particularly difficult to detect, because they burn with a flame that can be invisible under bright surgical lights.

Body Hair

Body hair of varying density and fineness is found on all people. As with the nap on cotton fabrics, body hair—especially vellus—can easily ignite and fuel a fire that rapidly spreads across the skin in areas of high oxygen concentration (e.g., >50%). This is another example of surface-fiber flame propagation. Alternatively, in ambient air, vellus will shrivel from heat and not propagate a fire. Similarly, other types of body hair do not tend to be easily ignited in ambient air during surgery.

Intestinal Gases

Intestinal gases are composed of varying concentrations of oxygen, nitrogen, carbon dioxide, hydrogen, and methane, and this mixture that can vary widely in volume. In certain proportions, this mixture is flammable. Furthermore, during N_2O anesthesia, the gas can diffuse into the bowel and enrich the intestinal gas mixture, thereby making it even more flammable.

Tracheal Tubes

Tracheal tubes weigh a few grams and are typically made from polyvinyl chloride plastic, latex rubber, or silicone elastomer, all of which are flammable. Laser-resistant tracheal tubes often contain one or more of these materials. Although they are resistant to certain laser wavelengths, these tubes may be flammable under other conditions, such as during exposure to different laser wavelengths or other heat sources (e.g., an electrocautery pencil), or they may have flammable parts, such as the cuff or inflation tube.

The combustion of a tracheal tube, as demonstrated in Figure 12-6, delivers flames, smoke, and hot gases into the airway and lungs. Tracheal-tube fires typically produce an intraluminal fire that generates fuel and heat to produce an extraluminal free-end flame. The tracheal tube in Figure 12-7 ignited and burned severely during a tracheostomy when the surgeon cut through the tracheal rings with the flat-blade electrosurgical electrode. The patient died 2 weeks after the incident from the severe tracheal burns that were sustained.

Body Tissue

Body tissue is flammable if it has been fully desiccated by therapeutic heat, such as that from an ESU or a laser at the small target area of their application. The organic materials that remain after desiccation can ignite and become incandescent embers or flares of gas, especially if excess oxygen is present at the target tissue in the wound.

Other Fuels

Other fuels include flexible bronchoscopes, face masks, breathing systems, petroleum jelly, adhesives, surgical instrument coverings and drapes, smoke

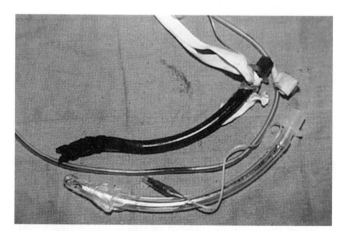

Figure 12-7. Burned tracheal tube from a fatal tracheostomy fire (shown with exemplar tube). (Photo by Mark E. Bruley. Used with permission.)

evacuator hoses, blood-pressure cuffs, and laser-fiber sheaths.

Minimizing Fuel Risks

NOTE: The applicability of the following recommendations must be considered individually for each patient.

During Preparation of the Skin

- Be aware that alcohol-based preparations are flammable.
- Avoid the pooling or wicking of flammable liquid preparations.
- Allow flammable liquid preparations to dry fully before draping; pooled or wicked liquid will take longer to dry than preparation on the skin alone.
- Keep fenestration towel edges as far from the incision as possible.

In General

- Coat hair on the head and face (including eyebrows, beards, and mustaches) within the fenestration with water-soluble surgical lubricating jelly to make the hair nonflammable.
- Be aware of the flammability of tinctures, solutions, and dressings (e.g., benzoin, phenol, collodion) used during surgery, and take steps to avoid igniting their vapors.
- Moisten sponges to make them resistant to ignition during oropharyngeal and pulmonary surgery.

HOW TO RESPOND TO A SURGICAL FIRE

Putting Out the Fire and Caring for the Patient

The initial response to a surgical fire should not be to retrieve a fire extinguisher or other fire-fighting equipment. Surgical fires can spread so rapidly that they will be out of control before an extinguisher can be used. During the past 30 years, investigators are aware of only two or three cases in which an extinguisher was needed and used in the OR for a fire that was burning on a patient.[9] An extinguisher should be employed only after other steps are taken, as described later in this chapter. The recommended actions for extinguishing a surgical fire, either on the patient or in the patient's airway, are also summarized in the poster reproduced in Figure 12-8.

For Small Fires

Small fires on the patient, such as those caused when a hot electrosurgical pencil ignites the drapes that are on a patient or when an electrocautery pencil ignites a blotting sponge, can be extinguished by patting out the fire with a gloved hand or towel. If a member of the OR staff uses a towel or sheet to smother the flames, he or she should pat out the fire in a direction away from his or her body.

For Large Fires

Large fires on or in the patient require a more comprehensive response:

- Stop the flow of oxidizers to the patient. In many fires, removing the oxidizer (i.e., oxygen and N_2O) sources (e.g., by disconnecting the breathing circuit) will cause the fire to go out or at least to lessen in intensity. Some materials burn only in oxygen-enriched atmospheres, and all materials burn more vigorously in them. Disconnection of the breathing circuit can also facilitate the rapid movement of the patient (e.g., to another OR).
- Remove the burning materials from the patient, and extinguish them. Removing the burning and burned materials is the only way to protect the patient from the heat of these materials. This applies regardless of whether the fire is burning on the patient or in the patient (e.g., as in the case of an airway fire). The heat can continue to cause thermal injury. Furthermore, should oxidizers be reintroduced to hot or molten materials, the fire may reignite. Removing these materials will allow clinicians to view all of the areas of the patient that were near the fire, thereby aiding their assessment of the injury. The burning materials should typically be removed by the surgeon and extinguished by another staff member.
- Care for the patient. The patient must be cared for swiftly. He or she is probably not breathing, may be severely bleeding, and may still be in contact with other burning materials. The anesthesia staff should restore breathing with air (never oxygen) until all possible sources of fire or of reignition are suppressed. The surgeon should deal with the patient's injuries. The nursing staff should extinguish any burning materials that are removed from or that remain on the patient.

There is some debate regarding the order in which the first two steps in this sequence should be carried out. If possible, most agree that they should be performed simultaneously; others disagree. In any case, they should both be done as close to instantaneously as possible. In the scores of fires investigated by the author, the instinctive actions of the surgical team members during a fire have resulted in these actions being performed simultaneously in almost all cases.

Note that there is no step that specifies the removal of the ignition source. In most cases, this will not be a consideration, because the surgeon almost always has the ignition source in hand and will dispose of it to deal with the fire. Because the typical ignition sources for surgical fires deactivate when they are not in use, this step generally takes care of itself.

**Emergency Procedure
Extinguishing a Surgical Fire**

Fighting Fires ON the Surgical Patient

Review before every surgical procedure.

Small fire. In the event of a small fire on the patient, immediately
    Pat out or smother the fire, or remove the burning material from the patient.
Large fire. In the event of a large fire on the patient, immediately
  1. Stop the flow of breathing gases to the patient.
  2. Remove the burning material from the patient, and have another team member
     extinguish it. If needed, use a CO_2 fire extinguisher to put out a fire on the patient.
  3. Care for the patient:
     — Resume patient ventilation.
     — Control bleeding.
     — Evacuate the patient if the room is dangerous from smoke or fire.
     — Examine the patient for injuries and treat accordingly.
  4. If the fire is not quickly controlled:
     — Notify other operating room staff and the fire department that a fire has occurred.
     — Isolate the room to contain smoke and fire.
Save involved materials and devices for later investigation.

Extinguishing Airway Fires

Review before every surgical intubation.

At the first sign of an airway or tracheal tube fire, immediately and rapidly
  1. Disconnect the breathing circuit from the tracheal tube.
  2. Remove the tracheal tube, and have another team member extinguish it. Remove cuff-
     protective devices and any segments of burned tube that may remain smoldering in the
     airway.
  3. Care for the patient:
     — Reestablish the airway, and resume ventilating with air until you are certain that
       nothing is left burning in the airway, then switch to 100% oxygen.
     — Examine the airway to determine the extent of damage, and treat the patient accordingly.
Save involved materials and devices for later investigation.

Reference: ECRI. Surgical fire safety [guidance article]. *Health Device* 2006 Feb;35(2):45–66.

5203 Butler Pilsa, Plymouth Meeting, PA 19462-1298, USA
Telephone +1(610) 825-8000 ▪ Fax + 1(610) 834–1275▪E-mail healthdevices@ecri.org

Figure 12-8. Emergency procedures for the control of surgical fires. (From ECRI Institute: Surgical fires: A patient safety perspective. *Health Devices* 2006;35(2):45–66. Used with permission.)

For Airway Fires

At the first sign of an airway or tracheal tube fire, whether during a tracheotomy or during internal tracheal and/or bronchial surgery, immediately and rapidly disconnect the breathing circuit from the tracheal tube and remove the tube. Have another team member extinguish it. Also, immediately remove cuff-protective devices and any segments of burned tube that may remain smoldering in the airway.

Care for the patient by reestablishing the airway. Resume ventilation of the patient with air until it is certain that nothing is left burning in the airway, and then switch to 100% oxygen. Using oxygen before being sure that no burning or smoldering material is present will likely reignite the fire. Examine the airway to determine the extent of damage, and treat the patient accordingly.

Other Fire-Fighting Alternatives

Use of Aqueous Solutions

Aqueous solutions such as bottled saline solution, bottled water, and tap water can be used to help put out a fire in combination with the removal of the burning materials from the patient. Some hospitals keep a saline bottle that is specially labeled "FOR FIRE" on the back table just for this purpose. However, recognize that surgical drapes are waterproof and that applied water may not penetrate to underlying burning materials.

Although basins of water or saline are also sometimes used to extinguish surgical fires, bottled solutions should be the preferred extinguishing agent. This is because some basins (e.g., suture-catch basins) may contain flammable liquids, such as alcohol. If used by mistake, these liquids could explosively increase a fire.

Use of Fire Extinguishers

Although they should not be the first choice when dealing with a surgical fire, fire extinguishers may be needed in the extremely rare instance in which a fire engulfs the patient, has migrated off the patient, or involves other materials in the OR. Surgical staff members should know why, when, and how to use fire extinguishers and other materials that can be used to put out a fire.

A 5-lb carbon dioxide fire extinguisher mounted just inside the entrance of each OR in the hospital has been recommended for many years.[9,12,15,31] In addition, it is recommended that a 20-lb dry-powder fire extinguisher be available outside of the OR but within the OR suite for use as a last resort for fighting catastrophic fires.

Fire blankets (typically wool blankets that are treated with fire retardants and that are placed over a fire to smother it) should never be located in an OR, and they should never be used for surgical patient fires.[9,31] Such blankets could trap the fire next to or under the patient, or they could displace surgical instruments, thus leading to further injury. In addition, for cases in which a fire is sustained by oxygen delivered to the patient, a fire blanket would be ineffective for extinguishing the fire; in fact, the blanket itself could burn if it is used in an oxygen-enriched atmosphere. Although fire blankets have a valid place in many industrial settings, they are not appropriate for use in the unique environment of a hospital OR.

If Evacuation of the Operating Room is Necessary

In rare cases, extreme smoke and fire conditions may force the evacuation of the specific OR in which the fire occurs. The ECRI Institute reports that it is aware of only one case in the past 35 years in which the surgical team had to evacuate the OR and temporarily leave the burning patient behind; the Institute is not aware of any incident in which the entire OR suite needed to be evacuated.[9] Nonetheless, if evacuation is necessary, the acronym *RACE* defines the actions that should take place: *R*escue, *A*lert, *C*onfine, and *E*vacuate.

Rescue

Reasonable attempts to rescue the surgical patient from the fire and the OR should be made. Several rescuers will likely be needed to deal with disconnecting the patient from any devices (e.g., an anesthesia machine, an ESU) and, possibly, to move the operating table. The rescuers should not place themselves at severe risk, although each individual will have to decide what level of risk he or she considers to be severe.

Alert

The staff members in nearby ORs should be alerted to the fire and kept informed in case they need to evacuate their patients from the area. In addition, fire alarm systems should be activated. Often, these systems call assistance from within the facility to the area of the alert; some systems also call the local fire department.

Confine

The smoke and fire should be contained in the OR by closing all of the doors. The medical gas zone (i.e., shutoff) valves for the affected OR should be shut to prevent piped gas and vacuum systems from sustaining the fire. Many facilities have automatic dampers in the air-conditioning ducts to prevent smoke migration. Some facilities have central smoke evacuator systems that are similar to vacuum systems; these should also be shut off. In addition, electric power to the involved OR should be turned off at the circuit-breaker panel; this will prevent it from sustaining electrical fires, and it will prevent an electric shock hazard for firefighters who are using water from extinguishers or hoses.

Evacuate

The incident OR and, if necessary, the surgical suite (although this is very unlikely) should be evacuated in an orderly manner to preplanned areas that are capable of handling the needs of the surgical patients.

CONCLUSION

Surgical fires present risks of serious or fatal injury to patients as well as to personnel. Surgical fires are a preventable hazard. As with other uncommon but potentially serious or fatal medical misadventures, solutions to prevent this hazard are known and published. For preventive measures to be most effective, a team approach is needed. Personnel should understand the ignition sources, fuels, and oxidizers that are present during head and neck surgery and employ the preventive measures discussed in this chapter. If a fire should occur, the emergency procedures outlined in the two boxes in Figure 12-8 should be used immediately.

REFERENCES

1. de Richemond AL, Bruley ME: Head and neck surgical fires. In Eisele DW, editor: *Complications in head and neck surgery,* St Louis, 1993, Mosby.
2. Pugliese G, Bartley JM: Home study program: Can we build a safer OR? *AORN J* 2004;79(4):764–782, 785–786.
3. Beyea SC: Preventing fires in the OR. *AORN J* 2003;78(4): 664–666.
4. Bruley ME: Frequent questions on OR fire safety. *OR Manager* 2003;19(12):17–18.
5. Bruley ME: Surgical fires: Perioperative communication is essential to prevent this rare but devastating complication. *Qual Saf Health Care* 2004;13(6):467–471.
6. Chang BW, Petty P, Manson PN: Patient fire safety in the operating room. *Plast Reconstr Surg* 1994;93(3):519–521.
7. Coulson AS, Bakhshay SA: Harmonic scalpel prevents tracheotomy fires. *Chest* 1998;114(1):349–350.
8. de Richemond AL, Bruley ME: Insidious iatrogenic oxygen-enriched atmospheres as a cause of surgical fires. In Janoff

DD, Stoltzfus JM, editors: *Flammability and sensitivity of materials in oxygen-enriched atmospheres,* vol 6, ASTM STP 1197, West Conshohocken, Penn, 1993, American Society for Testing and Materials.

9. Emergency Care Research Institute (ECRI): Surgical fire safety [guidance article]. *Health Devices* 2006; 35(2):45–66.

10. ECRI: Preventing burns and fires caused by high-powered light sources [hazard report]. *Health Devices* 2005;34(9):325–326.

11. ECRI: Endoscopic light sources and the risk of burns or fires. *Health Devices* 2004;33(4):115–116.

12. ECRI: *A clinician's guide to surgical fires: how they occur, how to prevent them, how to put them out* (website): www. guideline.gov/summary/summary.aspx?doc_id=3688&nbr=2914. Accessed April 1, 2008.

13. ECRI: Reducing the risk of fires during head and neck surgery [Eye on medical errors]. *Health Devices* 2002;31(4):125.

14. ECRI: *Only you can prevent surgical fires* [poster] (website): www.mdsr.ecri.org/static/surgical_fire_poster.pdf. Accessed April 1, 2008.

15. ECRI: The patient is on fire!: A surgical fires primer [guidance article]. *Health Devices* 1992;21(1):19–34.

16. ECRI: Fires during surgery of the head and neck area [update]. *Health Devices* 1980;9(3):82.

17. ECRI: Fires during surgery of the head and neck area [hazard report]. *Health Devices* 1979;9(2):50–52.

18. Goerig IW: Fires and explosions. *Br J Anaesth* 1995;75(5): 666–667.

19. Greco RJ: Beware of fire! *Plast Reconstr Surg* 2001;107(7): 1828–1829.

20. Macdonald AG: A brief historical review of non-anaesthetic causes of fires and explosions in the operating room. *Br J Anaesth* 1994;73(6):847–856.

21. McCranie J: Fire safety in the operating room. *Todays OR Nurse* 1994;16(1):33–37.

22. Moyer P: Operating room fires: How to prevent and minimize spread. *Todays Surg Nurse* 1998;20(6):13–17, 39–40.

23. National Fire Protection Association (NFPA): *NFPA 99: Standard for health care facilities,* Quincy, Mass, 1996, NFPA.

24. Smith TL, Smith JM: Electrosurgery in otolaryngology-head and neck surgery: Principles, advances, and complications. *Laryngoscope* 2001;111(5):769–780.

25. Wolf GL: Danger from OR fires still a serious problem. *APSF Newsl* 1999–2000;14(4):47.

26. American Society for Hospital Engineering: *NFPA accepts ASHE's amendment to NFPA 99 on alcohol based surgical prep solutions* (website): www.ashe.org/ashe/codes/nfpa/ nfpa099_proposeamend_absp.html. Accessed April 1, 2008.

27. Association of Perioperative Registered Nurses Recommended Practices Committee: Recommended practices for electrosurgery. *AORN J* 2004;79(2):432–434, 437–442, 445–450.

28. Association of Perioperative Registered Nurses Recommended Practices Committee: Recommended practices for laser safety in practice settings. *AORN J* 2004;79(4):836–838, 841–844.

29. Department of the Army—Headquarters, United States Army Medical Command. Fires associated with the performance of surgical procedures. MEDCOM Regulation No. 40–48 (website) chppm-www.apgea.army.mil/IHMSM/ms/documents/ MEDCOM%20Reg%2040-48%20Surgical%20Fires.pdf. Accessed April 1, 2008.

30. Dorsch JA, Dorsch SE: Hazards of anesthesia machines and breathing systems. In Dorsch JA, Dorsch SE, editors: *Understanding anesthesia equipment,* ed 3, Baltimore, 1994, Williams & Wilkins.

31. ECRI: A clinician's guide to surgical fires: How they occur, how to prevent them, how to put them out [guidance article]. *Health Devices* 2003;32(1):5–24.

32. ECRI: Fire blankets in the OR? [Talk to the specialist]. *Health Devices* 1999;28(11):469.

33. Ho SY, French P: Minimizing fire risk during eye surgery. *Clin Nurs Res* 2002;11(4):387–402.

34. Howard BK, Leach JL: Prevention of flash fires during facial surgery performed under local anesthesia. *Ann Otol Rhinol Laryngol* 1997;106(3):248–251.

35. Hurt TL, Schweich PJ: Do not get burned: Preventing iatrogenic fires and burns in the emergency department. *Pediatr Emerg Care* 2003;19(4):255–259.

36. Joint Commission: *Sentinel Event Alert: Preventing surgical fires* (website): www.jointcommission.org/SentinelEvents/ SentinelEventAlert/sea_29. Accessed April 7, 2008.

37. Joint Commission: *2008 National Patient Safety Goals: Ambulatory & office-based surgery programs* (website): www. jointcommission.org/PatientSafety/NationalPatientSafety-Goals/08_amb_npsgs.htm.

38. American Society of Anesthesiologists Task Force on Operating Room Fires: Practice advisory for the prevention and management of operating room fires. *Anesthesiology* 2008;108:786–801.

39. Lierz P, Heinatz A, Gustorff B, et al: Management of intratracheal fire during laser surgery. *Anesth Analg* 2002;95(2):502.

40. Massachusetts Department of Public Health: *Health care quality safety alert: Preventing operating room fires during surgery* (website) www.mass.gov/Eeohhs2/docs/dph/quality/ healthcare/hospital_alerts_or_fires.pdf. Accessed April 1, 2008.

41. Meeting JCAHO's goal on surgical fires. *OR Manager* 2004; 20(11):26–28.

42. National Fire Protection Association (NFPA): *NFPA 115: Recommended practice on laser fire protection,* Quincy, Mass, 1999, NFPA.

43. New York Department of Health—New York Patient Occurrence Reporting and Tracking System (NYPORTS): Electrosurgical burns and fire occurrences. *NYPORTS News Alert* 2003;Issue 13:1–7.

44. Pennsylvania Patient Safety Authority: Airway fires during surgery (website): www.psa.state.pa.us/psa/lib/psa/advisories/ v4n1march_2007/vol_4_no_1_mar_2007_airway_fires.pdf. Accessed April 1, 2008.

45. Pennsylvania Patient Safety Authority: Airway fires during surgery [poster] (website): www.psa.state.pa.us/psa/lib/psa/ advisories/v4n1march_2007/0307_resource_airwayfires_poster. pdf. Accessed April 1, 2008.

46. Pennsylvania Patient Safety Authority. Electrosurgical units and the risk of surgical fires (website): www.psa.state.pa.us/psa/lib/ psa/advisories/v1n3september2004/sept2004vol13_article_d_ electrosurgical_units_and_risk_of_surgical_fires.pdf. Accessed April 1, 2008.

47. Pennsylvania Patient Safety Authority: Three "never complications of surgery" are hardly that. Patient Safety Advisory 2007;4(3):82.

48. ECRI: ECRI's latest audio conference targets surgical fires: Training and communication are key, say speakers. *Health Devices* 2003;32(10):396–398.

49. ECRI: Educational videos on surgical fires [evaluation]. *Health Devices* 2003;32(1):25–38.

50. ECRI: Educational videos on surgical fires [evaluation]. *Health Devices* 2000;29(7–8):274–287.

51. Halstead MA: Fire drill in the operating room: Role playing as a learning tool. *AORN J* 1993;58(4):697–706.

52. Flowers J: Code red in the OR: Implementing an OR fire drill. *AORN J* 2004;79(4):797–805.

53. Mathias JM: Education: The best prevention for fires in the operating room. *OR Manager* 1995;11(5):30.

54. Salmon L: Fire in the OR: Prevention and preparedness [home study program]. *AORN J* 2004;80(1):42–60.

55. Smith C: Surgical fires: Learn not to burn [home study program]. *AORN J* 2004;80(1):24–40.

56. Andersen K: Safe use of lasers in the operating room: What perioperative nurses should know. *AORN J* 2004;79(1): 171–188.

57. ECRI: Laser-resistant tracheal tubes [evaluation]. *Health Devices* 1992;21(1):4–14.

58. ECRI: Do pledgets protect the tracheal tube cuff from lasers? [supplementary testing]. *Health Devices* 1992;21(1):17.

59. ECRI: Laser contact tips and tracheal tubes [supplementary testing]. *Health Devices* 1992;21(1):18.

60. ECRI: Laser ignition of surgical drapes [supplementary testing]. *Health Devices* 1992;21(1):15–16.

61. ECRI: Laser-resistant endotracheal tubes and wraps [evaluation]. *Health Devices* 1990;19(4):112–139.

62. Pashayan AG, Wolf G, Gottschalk A, et al: Upper airway management guide provided for laser airway surgery. *Anesth Patient Saf Found Newsl* 1993;8(2):13–16.

63. Sesterhenn AM, Dunne AA, Braulke D, et al: Value of endotracheal tube safety in laryngeal laser surgery. *Lasers Surg Med* 2003;32(5):384–390.

64. Waldorf HA, Leffel D, Kauvar AN, et al: The pulsed dye laser and fire: assessment of the problem and guidelines for prevention [abstract]. *Lasers Surg Med* 1995;(Suppl 7):80.

65. AlHaddad S, Brenner J: Helium and lower oxygen concentration do not prolong tracheal tube ignition time during potassium titanyl phosphate laser use. *Anesthesiology* 1994;80(4):936–938.

66. Cohen DL, Motahdi S, Wolf GL, et al: The effect of volatile anesthetics upon the flammability of endotracheal tubes [abstract]. *Anesth Analg* 1998;86(2 Suppl):S201.

67. ECRI: Fires from oxygen use during head and neck surgery [hazard report]. *Health Devices* 1995;24(4):155–157.

68. Lai HC, Juang SE, Liu TJ, et al: Fires of endotracheal tubes of three different materials during carbon dioxide laser surgery. *Acta Anaesthesiol Sin* 2002;40(1):47–51.

69. Sosis MB, Braverman B, Caldarelli DD: Evaluation of a new laser-resistant fabric and copper foil-wrapped endotracheal tube. *Laryngoscope* 1996;106(7):842–844.

70. Sosis MB, Braverman B: Prevention of cautery-induced airway fires with special endotracheal tubes. *Anesth Analg* 1993;77(4):846–847.

71. Sosis MB, Dillon FX: A comparison of CO_2 laser ignition of the Xomed, plastic, and rubber endotracheal tubes. *Anesth Analg* 1993;76(2):391–393.

72. Sosis MB, Dillon FX: CO_2 laser-resistant endotracheal tube shows no clear advantage. *Clin Laser Mon* 1993;11(8):123–124.

73. Sosis MB, Pritikin JB, Caldarelli DD: The effect of blood on laser-resistant endotracheal tube combustion. *Laryngoscope* 1994;104(7):829–831.

74. Sosis MB: Evaluation of a new laser-resistant operating room drape, eye shield, and anesthesia circuit protector. *J Clin Laser Med Surg* 1993;11(5):255–257.

75. Sosis MB: Saline soaked pledgets prevent carbon dioxide laser-induced endotracheal tube cuff ignition. *J Clin Anesth* 1995;7(5):395–397.

76. Takanashi S, Hasegawa Y, Ito A, et al: Airflow through the auxiliary line of the laser fiber prevents ignition of intra-airway fire during endoscopic laser surgery. *Lasers Surg Med* 2002;31(3):211–215.

77. Walker P, Temperley A, Thelfo S, et al: Avoidance of laser ignition of endotracheal tubes by wrapping in aluminium foil tape. *Anaesth Intensive Care* 2004;32(1):108–112.

78. Wolf GL, Sidebotham GW, Lazard JP, et al: Laser ignition of surgical drape materials in air, 50% oxygen, and 95% oxygen. *Anesthesiology* 2004;100(5):1167–1171.

79. Bruley ME, de Richemond AL: Supplemental oxygen versus latent alcohol vapors as surgical fire precursors [letter]. *Anesth Analg* 2002;95(5):1459.

80. Wolf GL, Sidebotham GW, Stern JB: Intraluminal flame spread in tracheal tubes. *Laryngoscope* 1994;104(7):874–879.

81. Mattucci KF, Militana CJ: The prevention of fire during oropharyngeal electrosurgery. *Ear Nose Throat J* 2003;82(2):107–109.

82. Barnes AM, Frantz RA: Do oxygen-enriched atmospheres exist beneath surgical drapes and contribute to fire hazard potential in the operating room? *AANA J* 2000;68(2):153–161.

83. Chou AK, Tan PH, Yang LC, et al: Carbon dioxide laser induced airway fire during larynx surgery: Case report. *Chang Gung Med J* 2001;24(6):393–398.

84. de Richemond AL, Bruley ME: Use of supplemental oxygen during surgery is not risk free [letter]. *Anesthesiology* 2000;93(2):583–584.

85. ECRI: Using external defibrillators in oxygen-enriched atmospheres can cause fires [hazard report]. *Health Devices* 2005;34(12):423–425.

86. ECRI: Responding to fires in areas of oxygen use [hazard report]. *Health Devices* 1994;23(7):306–307.

87. Galapo S, Wolf GL, Sidebotham GW, et al: Laser ignition of surgical drapes in an oxygen enriched atmosphere. *Anesthesiology* 1998;89(3A):A580.

88. Greco RJ, Gonzalez R, Johnson P, et al: Potential dangers of oxygen supplementation during facial surgery. *Plast Reconstr Surg* 1995;95(6):978–984.

89. Lai A, Ng KP: Fire during thoracic surgery. *Anaesth Intensive Care* 2001;29(3):301–303.

90. Reyes RJ, Smith AA, Mascaro JR, et al: Supplemental oxygen: Ensuring its safe delivery during facial surgery. *Plast Reconstr Surg* 1995;95(5):924–928.

91. Rodgers LA, Kulwicki A: Safety in the use of compressed air versus oxygen for the ophthalmic patient. *AANA J* 2002;70(1):41–46.

92. ECRI: Improper use of alcohol-based skin preps can cause surgical fires [hazard report]. *Health Devices* 2003;32(11):441–443.

93. ECRI: Surgical fire hazards of alcohol [Talk to the specialist]. *Health Devices* 1999;28(7):286.

94. ECRI: Fire hazard created by the misuse of DuraPrep solution [hazard report]. *Health Devices* 1998;27(11):400–402.

95. Great Britain—Medical Devices Agency: Use of spirit-based solutions during surgical procedures requiring the use of electrosurgical equipment, London, 2000, Department of Health, Safety notice no. MDA SN2000[17].

96. Pennsylvania Patient Safety Authority: Risk of fire from alcohol-based solutions (website): www.psa.state.pa.us/psa/lib/psa/advisories/v2n2june2005/vol_2-2-june-05-article_d-risk_of_fire.pdf. Accessed April 1, 2008.

97. Tooher R, Maddern GJ, Simpson J: Surgical fires and alcohol-based skin preparations. *ANZ J Surg* 2004;74(5):382–385.

98. Podnos YD, Williams RA: Fires in the operating room. *Bull Am Coll Surg* 1997;82(8):14–17.

99. Stouffer DJ: Fires in operating rooms: an unrecognized problem? *Firehouse* 1991;16:30–33.

100. Weinbaum W, Hathcock G, Whalen T, et al: Here's how to prevent laser fires in the OR. *Health Facil Mgmt* 1998;11(9):29–30.

101. Awan MS, Ahmed I: Endotracheal tube fire during tracheostomy: A case report. *Ear Nose Throat J* 2002;81(2):90–92.

102. Axelrod EH, Kusnetz AB, Rosenberg MK: Operating room fires ignited by hot wire cautery. *Anesthesiology* 1993;79(5):1123–1126.

103. Barker SJ, Polson JS: Fire in the operating room: a case report and laboratory study. *Anesth Analg* 2001;93(4):960–965.

104. Baur DA, Butler RC: Electrocautery-ignited endotracheal tube fire: Case report. *Br J Oral Maxillofac Surg* 1999;37(2):142–143.

105. Bucsi, R: Closed claim study: Fire in the operating room. *Ophthal Risk Manage Dig* 2006;16(3):7.

106. Handa KK, Bhalla AP, Arora A: Fire during the use of Nd-Yag laser. *Int J Pediatr Otorhinolaryngol* 2001;60(3):239–242.

107. Lowry RK, Noone RB: Fires and burns during plastic surgery. *Ann Plast Surg* 2001;46(1):72–76.

108. Macdonald MR, Wong A, Walker P, et al: Electrocautery-induced ignition of tonsillar packing. *J Otolaryngol* 1994;23(6):426–429.

109. Michels AM, Stott S: Explosion of tracheal tube during tracheostomy [letter]. *Anaesthesia* 1994;49(12):1104.

110. Roane KR: "I'm on fire...": Blazes sparked in surgery are on the rise. *US News World Rep* 2003;135(5):25.

111. Rogers ML, Nickalls RW, Brackenbury ET, et al: Airway fire during tracheostomy: Prevention strategies for surgeons and anaesthetists. *Ann R Coll Surg Engl* 2001;83(6):376–380.

112. Santos P, Ayuso A, Luis M, et al: Airway ignition during CO_2 laser laryngeal surgery and high frequency jet ventilation. *Eur J Anaesthesiol* 2000;17(3):204–207.

113. Scherer TA: Nd-YAG laser ignition of silicone endobronchial stents. *Chest* 2000;117(5):1449–1454.

114. Thompson JW, Colin W, Snowden T, et al: Fire in the operating room during tracheostomy. *South Med J* 1998;91(3): 243–247.

115. Varcoe RL, MacGowan KM, Cass AJ: Airway fire during tracheostomy. *ANZ J Surg* 2004;74(6):507–508.

116. Waldorf HA, Kauvar NB, Geronemus RG, et al: Remote fire with the pulsed dye laser: Risk and prevention. *J Am Acad Dermatol* 1996;34(3):503–506.

117. ECRI: Ignition of debris on active electrosurgical electrodes [hazard report]. *Health Devices* 1998;27(9-10):367–370.

118. ECRI: Selecting fire extinguishers for the operating room [Talk to the specialist]. *Health Devices* 1996;25(7):261, 263.

119. ECRI: Burns and fires from electrosurgical active electrodes [hazard report]. *Health Devices* 1993;2(8-9):421–422.

120. ECRI: Fire caused by improper disposal of electrocautery units [hazard report]. *Health Devices* 1994;23(3):98.

121. ECRI: Fiberoptic illumination systems and the risk of burns or fire during endoscopic procedures. *Health Devices* 1995; 24(11):457–459.

122. ECRI: Sparking from and ignition of damaged electrosurgical electrode cables [hazard report]. *Health Devices* 1998;27(8): 301–303.

123. Ng JM, Hartigan PM: Airway fire during tracheostomy: Should we extubate? *Anesthesiology* 2003;98(5):1303.

CHAPTER 13

Quality of Care and Patient Safety

Robert M. Wachter

During the past two decades, scores of studies have demonstrated that there are major gaps in the quality and safety of modern medical care. These gaps are particularly disconcerting to physicians, in part because their training is so rigorous and lengthy and in part because most physicians work very hard and care deeply about their work. Nevertheless, the evidence clearly demonstrates massive variations in patterns of care that are neither supported by evidence nor justified by outcomes, stunning gaps between evidence-based best practices and current practice, and staggering numbers of serious medical errors.

The recognition of these quality and safety problems has catalyzed a major transformation in medical thinking and practice, with new technologies, training models, incentive systems, regulations, and more. Even with the breathtaking changes in clinical science, diagnostics, and therapeutics, one would be hard pressed to find another area of medicine that has been transformed as completely as our approach to quality and safety during the previous decade.

This chapter begins by focusing on quality measurement and improvement and then shifts to patient safety. Although the latter is a subset of the former, there are enough differences in the approaches to measuring and improving safety that it merits a separate discussion. The chapter concludes with some observations regarding value, the nexus of safety, quality, and cost.

QUALITY

Quality of care has been defined by the Institute of Medicine (IOM) as "the degree to which health services for individuals and populations increase the likelihood of desired health outcomes and are consistent with current professional knowledge."[1] In an influential 2001 report, the IOM articulated six aims for a quality health care system (Box 13-1): patient safety, patient-centeredness, effectiveness, efficiency, timeliness, and equity.[1] These goals emphasize the fact that quality involves more than the delivery of evidence-based care.

Nevertheless, evidence-based medicine does provide much of the scientific underpinning for quality measurement and improvement. For many decades, promoted by a lack of clinical evidence and the apprenticeship model of medical training, the idiosyncratic

practice style of a senior clinician or a well-known academic medical center determined the standard of care (a tradition now sometimes called *eminence-based medicine*). Without discounting the value of experience and mature clinical judgment, the modern paradigm for determining optimal practice has changed, driven by the explosion in clinical research that occurred during the past 30 years. (The number of randomized clinical trials grew from 350 per year in 1970 to more than 15,000 per year in 2005.) This research has helped to define best practices in many areas of medicine, from preventive strategies for a healthy 64-year-old outpatient to the treatment of the patient with acute myocardial infarction and cardiogenic shock.

"Donabedian's triad," which divides quality measures into *structure* (how is care organized), *process* (what was done), and *outcomes* (what happened to the patient), represents the dominant paradigm for considering issues of quality measurement.[2] Each element of the triad has important advantages and disadvantages with regard to quality measures (Table 13-1).[3] In recent years, most widely used quality measures have been process measures, because clinical research has established a link between such processes and improved outcomes. However, for areas in which processes are less relevant and the science of case-mix adjustment is suitably advanced (e.g., cardiac bypass surgery), outcome measurement is often used. For areas in which the processes are quite complex, structural measures (e.g., the presence of intensivists in critical care units, the availability of a dedicated stroke service, the widespread implementation of computerized physician order entry) are used as proxies for quality.

Epidemiology of Quality Problems

Wennberg's pioneering studies[4] demonstrating large and clinically indefensible variations in care from one city to another were the first to hint at widespread deviations from best practices in modern medicine. More recently, McGlynn and colleagues[5] studied more than 400 measures to assess the degree to which U.S. practice comported with evidence-based guidelines. They found an average adherence to best practices of slightly more than 50%, which generated tremendous public concern about the quality of care. In most studies, adherence with evidence-based practice correlates with ultimate clinical outcomes,[6] although some studies have shown lesser amounts of correlation,[7] thus making the search for better process–outcome links and more robust case-mix adjustment methods even more pressing.

Levers for Change

For providers, patients, and policy makers, this evidence of major quality gaps has led to a recognition of structural problems that prevent the highest quality of care from being predictably delivered. These problems include the absence of incentives for quality improvement, a lack of information regarding provider or institutional performance, practicing physicians' difficulty with staying abreast of modern evidence-based medicine, and the absence of suitable system support (e.g., information technology) for quality. Each of these issues will need to be addressed if substantial progress is to be made in narrowing the gap between best practice and current practice.

The first step in quality improvement begins with quality measurement. As recently as the early 1990s, there were only a handful of generally accepted quality measures, such as whether patients with acute myocardial infarction were to receive aspirin or β-blockers. Recently, scores of such measures have been promulgated by a variety of organizations, including payers (e.g., the Centers for Medicare & Medicaid Services), accreditors (e.g., The Joint Commission on Accreditation of Healthcare Organizations), medical societies, and even organizations formed entirely for this purpose (e.g., the National Quality Forum). These measures have identified many opportunities for improvement for individual physicians, practices, and hospitals.

Given the volume of new literature published each year, no individual physician (unless practicing in a highly specialized, narrow clinical domain) can possibly remain abreast of all of the evidence-based advances in his or her field. Practice guidelines, such as those for the care of acute myocardial infarction or for prophylaxis for deep venous thrombosis, aim to synthesize evidence-based best practices into a set of summary recommendations. Although many physicians continue to harbor concerns about "cookbook medicine," there is increasing consensus that best practices should be "hard wired," if possible. The major challenges for guideline developers are the need to keep them updated as new knowledge accumulates[8] and to address the difficulties that guidelines have when patients have multiple, potentially overlapping illnesses.[9] Clinical pathways are similar to guidelines, but they attempt to codify a series of steps, usually temporally (e.g., on day one, do the following; on day two…), and they are thus are more useful for stereotypic processes such as the postoperative management of patients after hip replacement or other common surgical procedures.

TABLE 13-1 A Comparison of the Three Types of Clinical Quality Measures ("Donabedian's Triad")

Measure	Simple Definition	Advantages	Disadvantages
Structure	How was care organized?	May be highly relevant in a complex health system	• May fail to capture the quality of care provided by individual physicians • Difficult to determine the gold standard
Process	What was done?	• More easily measured and acted on than outcomes • May not require case-mix adjustment • No time lag; can be measured when care is provided • May directly reflect quality (if carefully chosen)	• A proxy for outcomes • All may not agree on gold-standard processes • May promote "cookbook" medicine, especially if physicians and health systems try to "game" their performance
Outcomes	What happened to the patient?	What is really cared about	• May take years to occur • May not reflect quality of care • Requires case-mix and other adjustments to prevent "apples-to-oranges" comparisons

Although one could argue that professionalism should be sufficient incentive to provide high-quality care, the recognition that such care often depends on a system organized to translate research into practice and to predictably deliver the right care means that it will take significant investments (i.e., providing physician education, hiring case managers or clinical pharmacists, building information systems, developing guidelines) to deliver optimal care. The traditional payment system, which compensates physicians and hospitals equally whether quality is perfect or miserable, provides no incentive to make the requisite investments. In fact, one could argue that there are financial incentives for poor quality, because both providers and hospitals often receive higher reimbursements after complications, even if they were preventable. However, this situation is changing rapidly.

Changing Environment for Quality

The recent recognition of major differences between best and current practices and of the importance of systemic change to improve quality has led to a variety of initiatives to catalyze quality improvement. Virtually all of these plans involve several steps: defining reasonable, evidence-based quality measures (i.e., capturing appropriate structures, processes, or outcomes); measuring the performance of providers or systems; and using these results to promote change. This final goal creates the greatest degree of uncertainty and experimentation.

Although one may hope that simply giving individual providers information about their own performance (perhaps as compared with either local or national benchmarks) will generate meaningful improvement, experience has shown that this strategy results in only modest change. Because of this, many payers and accrediting organizations have embraced an aggressive strategy of transparency (i.e., disseminating the results of quality measurement to key stakeholders). For example, one can now quickly obtain information about a hospital's performance with regard to simple quality measures related to the care of patients with pneumonia, acute myocardial infarction, congestive heart failure, and the prevention of surgical site infections (www.hospitalcompare.hhs.gov). In some cases, simple transparency is the main strategy, with the hope that providers will find public reporting of their quality gaps to be sufficiently concerning (or embarrassing) to motivate improvement. To date, there is little evidence that patients are using such data to make decisions about which doctor to see or hospital to attend (including a famous case in which former President Clinton received his heart surgery from a surgeon with relatively poor publicly reported outcomes). Nevertheless, studies have shown impressive improvements in some quality measures in the face of public reporting,

supporting the premise that transparency itself may generate significant change.[10]

The newest strategy is to tie payments for service to quality performance, which is also known as "pay for performance" (P4P).[11] Currently there are a number of P4P experiments that are testing whether differential payment will lead to significantly more improvement than that achieved by simple transparency. P4P also raises a host of concerns, including whether presently captured quality data are accurate, whether payments should go to best performers or those with the greatest improvements, whether existing measures adequately measure quality in patients with complex and multiorgan disease, and whether P4P will create undue focus on certain measurable practices and relative inattention to other important processes that are not being compensated.[12,13] It is not yet clear what P4P's ultimate role will be among the various strategies being used to motivate quality improvement.

Quality Improvement Strategies

Whether the motivation is professionalism, embarrassment, or economics, the next question is how to actually improve the quality of care. However, there is no simple answer. Most institutions and physicians that have been successful in this work have employed a variety of strategies. In general, most use a variation of a "plan, do, study, act" (PDSA) cycle, recognizing that quality improvement activities must be carefully planned and implemented, that their impact needs to be measured, and that the results of these activities will often be imperfect and require adjustment, after which the cycle repeats.[14]

In addition to the PDSA cycle, several other types of activities are useful. For quality improvement practices that require predictable repetition, efforts to "hard wire" the practice or to use alternative providers who focus on the activity are often beneficial. For example, the best strategy to increase the rate of pneumococcal vaccination of hospitalized patients with pneumonia will be to embed it in a standard order set (either paper-based or computerized). Having a nurse remove the patient's shoes before the doctor's entry can increase rates of diabetic foot examinations in an outpatient practice.

In some areas, however, quality improvement involves much more complex and interdependent activities. In these circumstances, bringing teams together to examine their practices and to participate in a PDSA cycle is the most likely path to success. For example, a group of cardiac surgeons in the northeastern United States participated in such an experiment in which they observed each other's practices, agreed on best practices, and measured each other's outcomes. The result was a 24% reduction in cardiac surgery mortality.[15]

PATIENT SAFETY

Introduction and Epidemiology

Although Hippocrates said "first, do no harm" more than two millennia ago and although many hospitals and departments have long hosted periodic forums to discuss errors (i.e., morbidity and mortality conferences), until recently there was little discussion of the nature of medical mistakes, investment in safety research, regulation of safety standards, or emphasis on safety improvements. In early 2000, the IOM published *To Err is Human: Building a Safer Health System.*[16] This report, which estimated that 44,000 to 98,000 Americans die each year as a result of medical mistakes (the equivalent of a jumbo jet crashing each day), generated intense public and media attention, and it set the stage for a major focus on patient safety during recent years.

The IOM death estimate, which was drawn from a review of approximately 30,000 charts in New York, Colorado, and Utah during the late 1980s and the early 1990s, was followed by studies that showed significant numbers of medication errors, fumbled handoffs within the hospital and during the discharge process, communication problems in operating rooms and intensive care units, and retained sponges. In short, everywhere one looked, one found evidence of major patient-safety issues. Added to this statistical and peer-reviewed evidence were a steady drumbeat of reports in the media of errors that appeared to be related to inadequate resident supervision or excessive on-duty hours, mistakes involving the wrong patient going to a procedure or the wrong body part being operated on, chemotherapy overdoses, mistaken mastectomies and brain surgeries, and more.

Because patients may be harmed while receiving perfect care (i.e., from an accepted complication of surgery or a medication side effect), it is important to make the distinction between adverse events and actual errors. The patient-safety literature usually defines an error as "an act or omission that leads to an unanticipated, undesirable outcome or to substantial potential for such an outcome." Alternatively, adverse events are injuries that result from medical management rather than the patient's underlying illness. This distinction is crucial: a patient who is appropriately placed on warfarin for chronic atrial fibrillation who develops a gastrointestinal bleed while his or her international normalized ratio is therapeutic is the victim of an adverse event rather than a medical error. Conversely, a similar case would represent an error if the international normalized ratio was supratherapeutic because the physician prescribed a new medication without checking for possible drug interactions.

The Modern Paradigm for Patient Safety

The traditional approach to medical errors has been to blame the provider who was at the "sharp end" of care: performing the surgery, hanging the intravenous medication, or mixing the chemotherapy. During the last decade, it has been recognized that this approach ignores the fact that most errors are committed by hardworking, well-trained individuals. Moreover, it has also been determined that such errors are unlikely to be prevented by admonishing people to be more careful or by shaming and suing them. Instead, the modern approach, known as *systems thinking,* holds that human fallibility is a universal truth and that safety depends on creating systems that anticipate errors and either prevent or catch them before they cause harm. Such an approach has been the cornerstone of safety improvements in other high-risk industries, but it has been ignored in medicine until recently.[17,18]

British psychologist James Reason's "Swiss cheese model" of accidents has been widely accepted as the dominant paradigm for system safety.[19] This model, which was drawn from innumerable accident investigations in fields such as commercial aviation and nuclear power, emphasizes that, in complex organizations, "sharp-end" errors (i.e., a single slip by an individual worker) are usually not sufficient enough to cause terrible harm by themselves. Instead, such errors must navigate multiple incomplete layers of protection (i.e., "layers of Swiss cheese") to cause catastrophic events (e.g., the crash of a space shuttle, the meltdown of a nuclear plant). Reason's model points out the need to focus less on the futile goal of trying to mint flawless human beings and more on striving to shrink the holes in the Swiss cheese and to create redundant layers of protection to decrease the probability that the holes will ever align and let an error slip through.

Ways to Improve Patient Safety

Drawing on these models, modern thinking emphasizes efforts to shore up systems to prevent or catch errors. For example, errors in routine behaviors ("slips") can best be prevented by building in redundancies and cross checks in the forms of checklists, readbacks ("let me read your order back to you"), and other standardized safety procedures (e.g., sponge counts in the operating room, signing a surgical site before an operation begins, asking a patient for his or her name before giving a medication). Recently, there has been increased emphasis on decreasing errors at the person–machine interface by using "forcing functions": engineering solutions that decrease the probability of human error.[20] The classic nonmedical example of forcing functions was when the automobile industry, responding to a rash of tragedies in which parents mistakenly backed their cars up over their children (in part because they carelessly put the car in reverse with their foot off of the brake), modified braking systems to render it impossible to place the car in reverse unless the brake pedal was being pushed. In health care, a classic forcing function was the redesign of gas nozzles and connectors to ensure that anesthesiologists could not mistakenly hook up the wrong gas (e.g., nitrogen rather than oxygen) to a patient (similar to the changes that make it impossible to fill a car that needs unleaded gas with the leaded variety). Given the ever-increasing complexity of modern medicine, building in such forcing functions (in intravenous pumps, defibrillators, mechanical ventilators, and computerized order entry systems) will be crucial to safety.

In addition to systems enhancements, there has been a growing recognition of the importance of improving communication and teamwork. Commercial pilots all participate in teamwork training exercises (called *crew resource management*) in which they drill for emergencies with other crewmembers, learning to create a culture that encourages open conversation between team members, to communicate clearly using standard and predictable language, and to use checklists and other systemic approaches to prevent errors. Although the evidence that such interventions will improve patient safety is preliminary, there is considerable enthusiasm about them in safety circles.[21] The term *culture of safety* is shorthand for an environment in which teamwork, clear communication, and openness about errors (both to other health care professionals and to patients) is the rule.

Another key patient safety principle is to learn from one's mistakes. This may take multiple forms. Safe systems have a culture in which errors are openly discussed, often in morbidity and mortality conferences or similar forums. There is a new emphasis on making sure such discussions involve the appropriate disciplines (i.e., multiple physician specialties, nursing, hospital administration) rather than single silos, that they emphasize systems thinking and solutions, that they are not overly focused on the actions of single individuals, and that they are not punitive.[22] In addition to open discussion at conferences, safe organizations build in mechanisms to hear about errors from frontline staff, often via incident-reporting systems or patient safety hotlines, and to perform detailed ("root-cause") analyses of major errors ("sentinel events") in an effort to better understand all of the layers of Swiss cheese that may require improvement.[23]

Finally, there is increasing appreciation of the importance of a well-trained, well-staffed, and well-rested workforce in the delivery of safe care. There is now evidence linking low nurse-to-patient ratios, long resident work hours, and a lack of board certification to poor patient outcomes.[24–26] Such research is catalyzing a more holistic view of patient safety and recognizing that the implementation of safer systems will not create safe patient care if the providers are overextended, poorly trained, or not adequately supervised.

Reviewing this list of potential approaches to improving safety makes clear one of the great challenges: without strong comparative evidence and in the light of the high cost of some of the interventions (e.g., improved staffing, computerized order entry, teamwork training), even institutions and departments that are highly committed to safety are sometimes unsure about how to prioritize their efforts. Prioritization is often determined by the external environment. Just as in quality improvement (in which institutions naturally focus on the practices that are measured, publicly reported, and differentially compensated), in safety institutions, physician focus first on areas that are subject to regulation (typically by The Joint Commission) and those with multiple potential benefits (e.g., computerization, which may improve both safety and efficiency).[27] Because improving culture is difficult to measure and regulate, it is an ongoing challenge to ensure that this crucial area is not perpetually shuffled to the bottom of the deck, despite its importance to safety.

VALUE: CONNECTING SAFETY AND QUALITY TO COST

Outside of health care, most purchasing decisions (e.g., cars, clothes) are based on perceptions of value, namely quality (and, where appropriate, safety) divided by cost. Health-care purchasing decisions have not traditionally been made this way, in part because of the limited ability of patients (and providers, for that matter) to make rational judgments about the quality and safety of a given provider or system and in part because health-care insurance insulated patients from the full cost of care. Much of the recent push to measure and improve quality and safety should be placed in the context of a broader effort to allow patients (or payers) to make evidence-based judgments about value, thereby catalyzing their ability to choose their providers on the basis of such judgments.[28] In this environment, it will be crucial for physicians and other health-care providers to participate in efforts to measure and improve the quality, safety, and efficiency of health care.

REFERENCES

1. Committee on Quality of Health Care in America, Institute of Medicine: *Crossing the quality chasm: A new health system for the 21st century,* Washington DC, 2001, National Academy Press.
2. Donabedian A: The quality of care. How can it be assessed? *JAMA* 1988;270:1743–1748.
3. Shojania KG, Showstack J, Wachter RM: Assessing hospital quality: A review for clinicians. *Eff Clin Pract* 2001;4:82–90.
4. Wennberg J, Gittelsohn A: Small area variations in health care delivery. *Science* 1973;182:1102–1108.
5. McGlynn EA, Asch SM, Adams J, et al: The quality of health care delivered to adults in the United States. *N Engl J Med* 2003;348:2635–2645.
6. Higashi T, Shekelle PG, Adams JL, et al: Quality of care is associated with survival in vulnerable older patients. *Ann Intern Med* 2005;143:274–281.
7. Bradley EH, Herrin J, Elbel B, et al: Hospital quality for acute myocardial infarction: Correlation among process measures and relationship with short-term mortality. *JAMA* 2006;296:72–78.
8. Shekelle PG, Ortiz E, Rhodes S, et al: Validity of the Agency for Healthcare Research and Quality clinical practice guidelines: How quickly do guidelines become outdated? *JAMA* 2001;286:1461–1467.
9. Boyd CM, Darer J, Boult C, et al: Clinical practice guidelines and quality of care for older patients with multiple comorbid diseases: Implications for pay for performance. *JAMA* 2005;294:716–724.
10. Williams SC, Schmaltz SP, Morton DJ, et al: Quality of care in U.S. hospitals as reflected by standardized measures, 2002-2004. *N Engl J Med* 2005;353:255–264.
11. Millenson ML: Pay for performance: The best worst choice. *Qual Saf Health Care* 2004;13:323–324.
12. Epstein AM: Paying for performance in the United States and abroad. *N Engl J Med* 2006;355:406–408.
13. Wachter RM: Expected and unanticipated consequences of the quality and information technology revolutions. *JAMA* 2006;205:2780–2783.
14. Langley GJ, Nolan KM, Nolan TW: *The foundation of improvement,* Silver Spring, MD, 1992, API Publishing.
15. O'Connor GT, Plume SK, Olmstead EM, et al: A regional intervention to improve the hospital mortality associated with coronary artery bypass graft surgery. *JAMA* 1996;275:841–846.
16. Kohn L, Corrigan J, Donaldson M, editors: *To err is human: Building a safer health system.* Washington DC, 2000, Committee on Quality of Health Care in America, Institute of Medicine.
17. Leape LL: Error in medicine. *JAMA* 1994;272:1851–1857.
18. Wachter RM, Shojania KG: *Internal bleeding: The truth behind America's terrifying epidemic of medical mistakes,* New York, 2004, Rugged Land.
19. Reason J: *Human error,* Cambridge, UK, 1990, Cambridge University Press.
20. Norman DA: *The design of everyday things,* New York, 2002, Basic Books.
21. Salas E, Wilson KA, Burke CS, et al: Does crew resource management training work? An update, an extension, and some critical needs. *Hum Factors* 2006;48:392–412.
22. Pierluissi E, Fischer MA, Campbell AR, et al: Discussion of medical errors in morbidity and mortality conferences. *JAMA* 2003;290:2838–2842.
23. Vincent C: Understanding and responding to adverse events. *N Engl J Med* 2003;348:1051–1056.
24. Aiken LH, Clarke SP, Sloane DM, et al: Hospital nurse staffing and patient mortality, nurse burnout, and job dissatisfaction. *JAMA* 2002;2898:1987–1993.
25. Landrigan CP, Rothschild JM, Cronin JW, et al: Effect of reducing interns' work hours on serious medical errors in intensive care units. *N Engl J Med* 2004;351:1838–1848.
26. Brennan TA, Horwitz RI, Duffy FD, et al: The role of physician specialty board certification status in the quality movement. *JAMA* 2004;292:1038–1043.
27. Wachter RM: The end of the beginning: Patient safety five years after "To err is human." *Health Aff (Millwood)* 2004;Suppl Web Exclusives:W4-534–W4-545.
28. Porter ME, Teisberg EO: *Redefining health care: Creating value-based competition on results.* Boston, 2006, Harvard Business School Press.

CHAPTER 14

Complications of Radiation Therapy

Laura Ellen Millender

Radiation therapy has a fundamental role in the definitive and adjuvant treatment of head and neck cancer. Normal tissue complications related to radiation therapy are common and determined by the region exposed, the radiation dose, and the fractionation schedule. The threshold dose beyond which one sees normal tissue injury is called *normal tissue tolerance.* Tolerance doses vary by organ, treatment volume, fraction size, and total dose.[1] Because any dose of radiation is potentially detrimental, the shielding of normal tissues is one of the more important elements for minimizing radiation-associated complications. When planning radiotherapy, it is critical to cover the appropriate target volume, to administer the necessary dose, and to respect the normal tissue tolerance within the treatment field.

Normal tissue complications of radiation therapy can be broadly divided into two groups: acute and late.[2] Acute toxicity occurs during and immediately after a course of radiation therapy. The mechanism of acute toxicity is similar to the mechanism of tumor response to radiation. Acute toxicity results from the death of rapidly dividing cells, such as the basal layers of the skin and the mucosa. The time to presentation of acute toxicity correlates with the life span of the mature functioning cells. Late effects of radiation therapy present several months to many years after treatment. Slowly proliferating tissues are more likely to manifest late damage from radiation therapy. Late toxicity is difficult to treat, but it may improve over time. The mechanisms of late toxicity are not well understood. Some believe that it is primarily a result of small-vessel ischemic disease; others propose that it is caused by the depletion of stem-cell populations.[3] Most likely it is a multifactorial process that is triggered by inflammatory cascades and compensatory responses.[4]

The severity of acute side effects and the risk of late toxicity are influenced by treatment and patient factors. The use of concurrent chemotherapy dramatically increases acute radiation toxicity.[5-7] Radiation dose escalation and altered fractionation techniques are used to improve the probability of local control, but toxicity rates are higher.[8,9] New radiation techniques (e.g., intensity-modulated radiation therapy [IMRT]) allow for the sophisticated shaping of the radiation dose distribution, and they may decrease toxicity rates. For example, lower doses given to the salivary glands improve postradiation salivary function;[10] however, a lack of homogeneity in the radiation plan may lead to unexpected acute and late toxicity in other tissues. Patient factors (e.g., cigarette smoking, a history of collagen vascular disease) have been shown to increase the risk of radiation-associated toxicity.[11,12] Because of the variability of tumor, treatment, and patient characteristics, the consent process must be individualized.

Many randomized clinical trials focus on efficacy outcomes (e.g., local and regional control) as well as disease-specific and overall survival. These end points are well understood by the oncology community, and the assessment of efficacy end points is considered to be straightforward. Toxicity and quality-of-life reporting, however, are not as well defined. Several different systems and grading scales exist for the reporting of toxicity end points.[13] Although it is important, systematic toxicity evaluation is frequently not the focus of routine follow-up visits. A recently published consensus statement recommends the routine use of the National Cancer Institute's comprehensive adverse event reporting terminology and grading system—CTCAE v3.0—as the new standard for cooperative group trials.[4] The National Cancer Institute's common toxicity criteria were established in 1983 and updated in 1998. The current version was published in 2006, and some of the toxicities relevant for the management of patients with head and neck cancer are summarized in Table 14-1.

Despite advances in imaging and treatment delivery, radiation therapy to the head and neck is a toxic treatment. With the exceptions of fatigue, nausea, and weight loss, toxicity from head and neck radiation therapy is anatomic-site specific and depends on the normal tissues included in the radiation field. What follows is a general discussion of the side effects of head and neck radiotherapy organized by tissue site.

SKIN

Skin reaction is a well-known side effect of radiation therapy. Nearly all head and neck cancer patients treated with radiation develop some level of skin toxicity. Most patients notice erythema and dryness, many patients develop dry desquamation, and some patients treated with high doses of radiation experience moist desquamation, ulceration, or even soft-tissue necrosis. Treatment factors contribute to the level of skin toxicity.

TABLE 14-1 Adverse Event Grading for Head and Neck Cancer

Toxicity	Grade 1	Grade 2	Grade 3	Grade 4
Fatigue	Mild fatigue over baseline	Moderate fatigue causing difficulty with some ADL	Severe fatigue interfering with ADL	Disabling
Weight loss	5% to <10% from baseline; intervention not indicated	10% to <20% from baseline; nutritional support indicated	≧ 20% from baseline; tube feeding or TPN indicated	—
Dermatitis	Faint erythema or dry desquamation	Moderate to brisk erythema; patchy moist desquamation, mostly confined to skin folds and creases; moderate edema	Moist desquamation other than skin folds and creases; bleeding induced by minor trauma or abrasion	Skin necrosis or ulceration of full-thickness dermis; spontaneous bleeding from involved site
Mucositis (clinical examination)	Erythema of the mucosa	Patchy ulceration or pseudomembranes	Confluent ulcerations or pseudomembranes; bleeding with minor trauma	Tissue necrosis; significant spontaneous bleeding; life-threatening consequences
Dry mouth	Symptomatic (dry or thick saliva) without significant dietary alteration; unstimulated saliva flow >0.2 ml/min	Symptomatic and significant oral intake alteration (e.g., copious water, other lubricants, diet limited to purees and/or soft, moist foods); unstimulated saliva 0.1–0.2 ml/min	Symptoms leading to an inability to adequately aliment orally; IV fluids, tube feedings, or TPN indicated; unstimulated saliva <0.1 ml/min	—
Osteonecrosis	Asymptomatic, radiographic findings only	Symptomatic and interfering with function but not interfering with ADL; minimal bone removal indicated (i.e., minor sequestrectomy)	Symptomatic and interfering with ADL; operative intervention or hyperbaric oxygen indicated	Disabling
Dysphagia	Symptomatic, able to eat regular diet	Symptomatic and altered eating/swallowing (e.g., altered dietary habits, oral supplements); IV fluids indicated <24 hrs	Symptomatic and severely altered eating/swallowing (e.g., inadequate oral caloric or fluid intake); IV fluids, tube feedings, or TPN indicated ≧24 hrs	Life-threatening consequences (e.g., obstruction, perforation)
Edema, larynx	Asymptomatic edema by examination only	Symptomatic edema, no respiratory distress	Stridor; respiratory distress; interfering with ADL	Life-threatening airway compromise; tracheotomy, intubation, or laryngectomy indicated
Hypothyroidism	Asymptomatic, intervention not indicated	Symptomatic, not interfering with ADL; thyroid replacement indicated	Symptoms interfering with ADL; hospitalization indicated	Life-threatening myxedema coma

TABLE 14-1 Adverse Event Grading for Head and Neck Cancer—cont'd

Toxicity	Grade 1	Grade 2	Grade 3	Grade 4
Myelitis	Asymptomatic, mild signs (e.g., Babinski or Lhermitte sign)	Weakness or sensory loss not interfering with ADL	Weakness or sensory loss interfering with ADL	Disabling
Cataract	Asymptomatic, detected by examination only	Symptomatic, with a moderate decrease in visual acuity (20/40 or better); decreased visual function correctable with glasses	Symptomatic, with a marked decrease in visual acuity (worse than 20/40); operative intervention indicated (e.g., cataract surgery)	—
Hearing (without monitoring program)	—	Hearing loss not requiring hearing aid or intervention (i.e., not interfering with ADL)	Hearing loss requiring hearing aid or intervention (i.e., interfering with ADL)	Profound bilateral hearing loss (>90 dB)

Selected toxicities of head and neck radiotherapy adapted from the National Cancer Institute, Cancer Therapy Evaluation Program: Common Terminology Criteria for Adverse Events v3.0 (CTCAE) (website): ctep.cancer.gov/forms/CTCAEv3.pdf. Accessed April 1, 2008.
Death due to treatment toxicity is grade 5.
ADL, Activities of daily living; *IV,* intravenous; *TPN,* total parenteral nutrition.

Low-energy x-ray beams (e.g., orthovoltage) deposit more dose in the skin than high-energy beams. The use of electron beams and normal tissue equivalent bolus also result in an increased skin dose. In some patients (e.g., those with skin cancer or the extracapsular spread of squamous cell carcinoma), treatment of the skin is intentional; therefore, a brisk skin reaction is expected and gives clinical evidence that the appropriate target volume was covered. The radiation tolerance doses for skin and other normal tissues as detailed by Emami and colleagues[1] in 1991 are listed in Table 14-2.

Acute Skin Toxicity

The skin reaction to radiation therapy is determined by skin physiology, and radiation-induced skin changes are well characterized.[2,14–17] The time to onset, the duration, and the intensity are predictable on the basis of the treatment administered (Figure 14-1). The skin is divided into two functional layers: the epidermis and the dermis. The epidermis is the target of acute radiation toxicity, whereas late toxicity results primarily from radiation-induced changes in the dermis. The epidermis is comprised of keratinizing squamous cells. These cells are continuously sloughed and then renewed by stem-cell division that occurs in the basal layer. Cells migrate from the basal layer to the surface over 12 to 48 days. Ionizing radiation therapy disrupts normal stem-cell division; therefore acute skin toxicity from radiation therapy usually manifests during the third week of treatment.

Early erythema may occur minutes to hours after a single dose of radiation. The degree of erythema depends on the fraction size. Erythema is unrecognized or minimal after 2 Gy, it is often visible after a single dose of 4 Gy, and it is readily recognizable after 8 Gy in a single fraction. This early erythema is the result of vasodilatation accompanied by skin warmth, and it generally resolves over approximately 48 hours. When standard fractionation techniques are used, persistent skin erythema resulting from inflammation is seen during the second to third week of radiation therapy. Tanning, dryness, and flaking (known as *dry desquamation*) may be seen during the fourth week of therapy. Moist desquamation occurs when the superficial cells slough more rapidly than they can be replaced. Regions of superficial ulceration, exposed dermis, and exudate present late during the course of therapy. Moist desquamation is painful, and patients with moist desquamation are at risk for superficial skin infections. The threshold dose for moist desquamation is typically 50 Gy, and the condition is most commonly seen in skin folds.

Late Skin Toxicity

The dermis contains the vascular, lymph, and connective-tissue systems that support the epidermis. The less rapidly dividing vascular endothelial cells and fibroblasts are the targets of late radiation damage.[2] The risk of late radiation toxicity rises with larger field sizes, higher total doses, and larger daily fraction sizes. Late toxicities include photosensitivity, changes in pigmentation, atrophy, fibrosis, telangiectasia, ulceration, and necrosis.[15] Late skin toxicity may present months or years after a course of radiation therapy. A history of surgery increases the risk of radiation fibrosis.

TABLE 14-2   Tolerance Doses of Normal Tissues, 5% Risk of Injury at 5 Years

Organ, End Point	One Third Total Organ Volume (Gy)	Two Thirds Total Organ Volume (Gy)	Whole Organ Volume (Gy)
Temporomandibular joint and mandible, marked limitation of joint function and pathologic fracture	65	60	60
Skin, ulceration or necrosis	70*	60†	55‡
Brain, necrosis	60	50	45
Brainstem, necrosis	60	53	50
Optic nerves and chiasm, blindness	50	50	50
Spinal cord, transverse myelitis	50§	50‖	47¶
Brachial plexus, nerve damage	62	61	60
Lens, cataract	10	10	10
Retina, blindness	45	45	45
Ear, acute/chronic otitis	30/55	30/55	30/55
Parotid, xerostomia	NR	32	32
Larynx, edema/necrosis	NR/79	45/70	45/70

Normal tissue tolerance doses adapted from Emami B, Lyman J, Brown A, et al: Tolerance of normal tissue to therapeutic irradiation. *Int J Radiat Oncol Biol Phys* 1991;21:109–122.

Tolerance dose 5% at 5 years is defined as the maximum dose limit that gives a 5% risk of a specific complication 5 years after radiation therapy. Tolerance dose 50% at 5 years are also defined but are not shown here. These data are based on standard radiation fractionation schedules without the use of concurrent chemotherapy.

*10 cc
†30 cc
‡100 cc
§5 cm
‖10 cm
¶20 cm.
NR, Not reported.

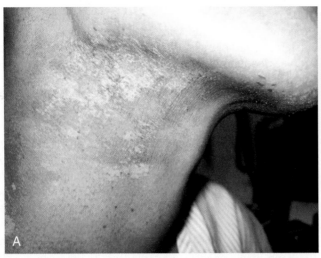 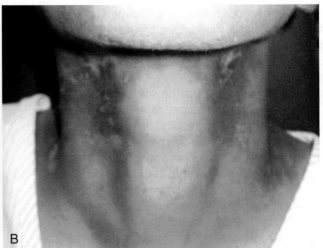

Figure 14-1. A 39-year-old man with clinical stage T1N1 poorly differentiated nasopharyngeal carcinoma. The patient was treated with intensity-modulated radiation therapy and concurrent cisplatin chemotherapy. **A,** Erythema, tanning, and dry desquamation of the skin are typically seen during the fourth to fifth week of head and neck radiotherapy. **B,** Notice the relative sparing of the skin anterior to the larynx as a result of an intentionally decreased radiation dose to this region using an intensity-modulated radiation therapy dose-painting technique.

Skin Appendages

Skin appendages such as hair follicles, sebaceous glands, and sweat glands are also sensitive to ionizing radiation.[3] Epilation occurs during the third week of treatment. The regrowth of hair is dose dependent, and it is seen approximately 3 months after the completion of radiation therapy. Areas treated with high doses may have only partial regrowth. Radiated skin is dry as a result of a loss of sebaceous glands. Sweat glands are more tolerant than sebaceous glands, and measures of electrical conductivity can be used to objectively determine levels of skin damage.

Prevention and Management

Definitive data regarding the prevention of skin reactions and the management of skin toxicity are lacking. Most institutions have protocols based on clinical experience and physician preference. Aloe vera gel is commonly recommended for the prevention of skin toxicity. Randomized studies of aloe vera have mixed results, and overall there is not good data to support its routine use.[18-21] Steroid creams and sprays decrease the symptoms of erythema, burning, and itching.[22,23] Hydrogel dressings are frequently recommended for the treatment of moist desquamation, but recent data suggest that these dressings may actually prolong skin healing time.[24] The most bothersome signs and symptoms of acute skin toxicity (e.g., moist desquamation, pain, erythema) improve during the 2 weeks after the completion of treatment. Dry desquamation may take 1 to 2 months to resolve, and tanning can persist for several months.

MUCUS MEMBRANE

The pathogenesis of radiation-induced mucositis parallels that of acute skin toxicity. When mucosal surface cells are not replaced as rapidly as they are lost, superficial ulceration occurs. Cell death triggers a severe inflammatory response, and the disturbance of the mucosal surface increases the risk of infection. The combination of ulceration, inflammation, and infection negatively affects the quality of life and leads to pain, swallowing difficulty, and weight loss. Mucositis generally presents during the third to fourth week of radiation and resolves over 4 to 6 weeks after the completion of treatment. The degree of mucositis depends on the treatment volume, the radiation dose, the fractionation schedule, and the use of neoadjuvant or concurrent chemotherapy.

Mucositis rates are substantially higher with altered fractionation schedules and with concurrent chemotherapy. The Radiation Therapy Oncology Group performed a multi-institution randomized study that evaluated four different radiation fractionation schedules. Rates of grade 3 mucositis were 25% with standard fractionation and 40% to 46% in the three arms using accelerated, hyperfractionated, and concomitant boost radiation schemes.[8] A similar French trial randomized 268 patients to standard fractionation versus a very accelerated course of radiation therapy (i.e., 63 Gy given over 22 days).[9] As expected, local control was improved by the rapid treatment schedule, but acute grade 3 mucositis rates were substantially higher at 75% in the experimental arm as compared with 23% in the standard fractionation arm. Accelerated fractionation did not result in increased late toxicity.[26]

Concurrent chemotherapy increases acute mucosal toxicity. In an Intergroup study of radiation therapy alone versus radiation with concurrent cisplatin chemotherapy, rates of grade 3 or higher mucosal toxicity were 33% with standard treatment and 45% with the addition of chemotherapy.[5] A parallel study of patients with stage III and IV oropharyngeal carcinoma compared standard radiation with the same radiation plus concurrent carboplatin and 5-fluorouracil.[6] Again, rates of mucositis were higher in the combined-modality arm, with patchy mucositis observed in 32% as compared with 57% of patients and confluent mucositis in 7% as compared with 14%. The combination of rapid fractionation and concurrent chemotherapy has been investigated. Rates of grade 3 or 4 mucositis approach 70% with these aggressive regimens.[26,27]

Management

Efforts for reducing mucositis have focused on mouthwashes and antibiotic agents. Despite multiple randomized studies, convincing evidence of any benefit with these interventions is lacking. Topical antimicrobials have been studied, with mixed results. Two randomized trials suggest that the daily use of lozenges involving a combination of polymyxin, tobramycin, and amphotericin reduces the severity of mucositis,[28,29] but another randomized study found no difference when these lozenges were compared with a placebo.[30] Chlorhexidine mouthwash and iseganan oral solution have also been studied in randomized trials, with no proven benefit for either agent.[31,32] Interestingly, a benefit of placebo mouthwash as compared with the institutional standard of care was seen in the iseganan study. Topical granulocyte macrophage colony-stimulating factor (GM-CSF) is currently under investigation for mucositis prevention.[33] The subcutaneous administration of GM-CSF for mucositis prophylaxis resulted in increased local tumor recurrence in a randomized trial; therefore the subcutaneous use of GM-CSF during radiation therapy is not recommended.[27] Amifostine, which is a pharmaceutical radioprotectant, is primarily used for the prevention of xerostomia. Some trials also suggest a benefit for rates of acute mucositis,[34,35] whereas others show no difference in mucositis rates with the concurrent use of amifostine.[36]

When the oral tongue is included in the radiation field, taste is affected. Patients complain of a loss of taste sensations during the second to third week of a conventionally fractionated course of radiation therapy. Most patients notice a gradual return of taste sensation over the several months after treatment. Decreased taste in combination with painful mucositis and dry mouth leads to significant weight loss. The author's clinical practice is to follow patient weight closely while encouraging good communication with nutrition services. Routine preradiation feeding-tube placement for healthy patients who are motivated to continue swallowing during therapy is not recommended. Percutaneous gastrostomy tubes are reasonable for the maintenance of good nutrition for elderly patients and for those patients who have lost more than 10% of their body weight during treatment.

SALIVARY GLAND

Xerostomia is a feared complication of head and neck radiation therapy. The salivary glands are sensitive to relatively low doses of radiation, and the radiation dose required for tumor control exceeds salivary-gland tolerance. A lack of saliva negatively affects the swallowing ability and increases the risk of tooth decay. Good oral hygiene can prevent serious dental complications, and saliva substitutes alleviate symptoms. The daily use of oral pilocarpine increases salivary flow in the postradiation setting,[37–39] but it does not prevent xerostomia when it is given concurrently with radiation therapy.[40] Two primary interventions are used to reduce the risk of radiation-related xerostomia: amifostine and IMRT.

Amifostine

Amifostine is a radioprotectant and a free-radical scavenger that accumulates in the salivary glands. A multinational phase III study demonstrated that intravenous amifostine given concurrently with radiation therapy reduced the incidence of grade 2 or higher xerostomia and increased the proportion of patients with meaningful salivary function. Acute xerostomia rates dropped from 78% to 51% and chronic xerostomia rates dropped from 57% to 34% with the use of amifostine. Local control and survival were not different between the two arms.[36,41] Intravenous amifostine can be difficult to tolerate, and more than 20% of patients discontinue amifostine because of its side effects, which include nausea, vomiting, hypotension, and allergic reactions. Amifostine remains efficacious as a radioprotectant when it is administered subcutaneously[35,42]; however,

discontinuation rates remain high, and rigorous comparisons of intravenous and subcutaneous routes of administration have not been performed.

Intensity-Modulated Radiation Therapy

IMRT is a radiation planning technique that permits excellent tumor coverage while shaping the radiation dose distribution to give a lower dose to the parotid glands. A single randomized study comparing IMRT with conventional radiation has been published.[10] End points of this study were quality of life and salivary function. Although dry mouth and sticky saliva were problematic for all patients, patients in the IMRT group were significantly more likely to recover salivary flow, and they had global health scores showing better physical function at 12 months after treatment. IMRT requires careful planning, and attention to the parotid dose-volume relationship is critical for the preservation of salivary function. The dose limits for the maintenance of salivary function have been well characterized. To substantially spare parotid function, the mean parotid dose must be less than 26 Gy.[43] This is a difficult treatment planning goal, because the doses required for microscopic and gross tumor control are 60 Gy and 70 Gy, respectively. Salivary gland transfer (i.e., surgically moving a submandibular gland into the submental space and out of the radiation field) is under investigation by the Radiation Therapy Oncology Group as an alternative for sparing salivary function.[44]

MANDIBLE AND TEETH

Osteoradionecrosis

Osteoradionecrosis (ORN) is defined as a nonhealing exposure of bone of at least 6 months' duration.[45] The incidence of ORN is declining, but it remains a severe complication that affects approximately 3% of patients treated with head and neck radiotherapy.[45,46] Unlike dermatitis and mucositis, ORN of the mandible is a preventable complication of radiation therapy. Preradiation dental evaluation is a key component of good multidisciplinary patient management and should be considered mandatory. It is best performed by a dentist with expertise in the management of radiation patients. The extraction of healthy teeth within the radiation field is unnecessary, but unsalvageable teeth should be removed before treatment. Meticulous oral hygiene and routine postradiation dental follow up are also important. Patients with xerostomia should be encouraged to use a fluoride supplement to prevent tooth decay as well as the subsequent need for postradiation dental extractions.

Multiple factors contribute to the risk of ORN.[45,47,48] Surgical manipulation of the mandible, including preradiation and postradiation dental extractions, increases the risk of severe complications. Patients who are edentulous at presentation are unlikely to develop ORN. Dentulous patients with teeth in poor condition are at high risk, with ORN rates of 12% to 15%.[49] The risk of ORN is higher for the mandible than the maxilla, and it is especially high for the posterior mandible. This is believed to be the result of differences in blood supply.[45] Because of the proximity of the tumor to the jaw, patients with cancer of the retromolar trigone are prone to ORN, with rates of 7% to 16% reported in single-institution retrospective studies.[50–52] Concurrent chemotherapy is another factor that contributes to late dental complications.[13] As with other normal tissue sites, total radiation dose is important. Doses of less than 60 Gy are unlikely to trigger ORN, but ORN rates of as high as 50% to 85% have been reported when the radiation dose exceeds 75 Gy.[53] Radiation technique is another consideration. With IMRT, it is possible to limit the mandibular dose, and single institutions report low ORN rates (i.e., 1 of 73 patients and 0 of 176 patients) with IMRT.[54,55] It remains to be seen if these excellent results will be maintained with longer follow up and multi-institutional experience.

Management

When it does occur, ORN can be difficult to manage. Treatment begins with conservative therapies such as antibiotic mouth rinses and oral systemic antibiotics. The removal of dental prostheses is recommended to reduce trauma to the mucosal surfaces. Because hypovascularity and hypoxia contribute to the development of ORN, hyperbaric oxygen is used for the prevention of ORN when dental extractions are required in the post-radiotherapy setting as well as for the treatment of ORN when it does occur.[56,57] Most studies of hyperbaric oxygen for the treatment of ORN show a definite or probable benefit.[58] The combination of orally administered pentoxifylline and vitamin E also promotes the healing of refractory mandibular ORN.[59] Severe ORN that does not respond to conservative management should be treated surgically.

SPEECH AND SWALLOWING

Radiation therapy is a mainstay of treatment for unresectable cancers of the head and neck. Organ preservation is an option for patients with resectable disease. The results of the Veterans Affairs Laryngeal Cancer Study Group trial support the concept that cure rates for laryngeal cancer are roughly equivalent for surgery and radiation therapy, whereas larynx preservation was possible in 64% of patients in the induction chemotherapy and radiation arm.[60] Organ preservation and the maintenance of organ function are not synonymous. Many patients experience difficulty with speech and swallowing after head and neck radiation.

Vocal Function

Vocal function after radiation therapy has been evaluated in several studies. Fung and colleagues[61] analyzed the vocal function of a group of 30 patients. Seventeen patients with nonlaryngeal tumors receiving wide-field radiation therapy that covered the primary tumor site and neck were compared with 13 patients with early glottic tumors treated with small radiation fields directed only onto the larynx. The mean larynx dose was higher in the glottic cancer patients, but voice handicap index results were significantly worse for the patients with nonlaryngeal tumors treated with wide-field radiotherapy. The authors noted that narrow-field radiation was more likely to alter the vibratory consistency of vocal-fold tissue, whereas wide-field radiation had a more pervasive influence on glottal dynamics. In another study, vocal analysis was performed on 15 patients with laryngeal or hypopharyngeal carcinoma treated with a larynx preservation protocol with radiotherapy and concurrent paclitaxel and cisplatin.[62] One patient had a normal voice after radiotherapy, four had mild dysphonia, six had moderate dysphonia, and four had severe dysphonia. Despite the fact that radiation harmed vocal function in nearly every patient, intelligible communication was possible. Voice-related quality of life (VRQOL) data was obtained for 56 patients treated in a phase II study of induction chemotherapy followed by surgery (for nonresponders) or chemoradiotherapy.[63] Organ preservation was achieved in 37 patients, and laryngectomy was performed on 19. Twelve of these 19 patients underwent early laryngectomy for poor response to induction therapy, and 7 of 19 underwent late salvage after completing chemoradiotherapy. When compared with normal subjects, VRQOL was worse for patients with an intact larynx; however, VRQOL was significantly higher for patients with an intact larynx than for laryngectomy patients.

Swallowing Dysfunction

Swallowing dysfunction is increasingly recognized as an important complication of radiation therapy. During the last several years, multiple studies of dose response with regard to swallowing function have been published.[64–67] Significant efforts are being directed toward the identification of structures that contribute to swallowing dysfunction after radiation and to the determination of whether it is possible to spare these structures with IMRT. Rates of grade 3 dysphagia are significantly higher when the structures of the pharyngoesophageal axis are not spared. In one study of two IMRT techniques, grade 3 dysphagia was 63% among patients with a midline block in the low neck field as compared with 95% among patients treated with extended-field IMRT without dose constraints on the laryngeal and pharyngeal structures.[64] In a study of long-term diet and VRQOL, a higher radiation dose delivered to the aryepiglottic folds, the false vocal cords, and the lateral pharyngeal walls correlated with a more restrictive diet.[65] The notion that a higher dose to the pharyngeal constrictor muscles and the supraglottic larynx contributes to the risk of swallowing dysfunction is supported by serial videoflouroscopy findings in a group of patients treated during a phase I study of radiotherapy and concurrent gemcitabine.[66] Laryngeal edema contributes to swallowing dysfunction, and edema rates are significantly higher when the mean larynx dose exceeds 43.5 Gy.[67]

Esophageal Stricture

Esophageal stricture formation also leads to difficulty with maintaining nutrition orally. Lee and colleagues[61] found the risk of esophageal stricture after chemoradiation to be 21%. Factors that increased the risk of stricture formation included twice-daily radiation, female sex, and hypopharyngeal primary site. Interestingly, 39 of 40 patients with strictures had percutaneous gastrostomy tubes, and the authors suggest that the use of these tubes may increase the risk of stricture as a result of the inactivity of the swallowing musculature. The dose to the proximal esophagus should be kept below 60 Gy to 65 Gy to decrease the risk of stricture.[69] When stricture does occur, it can be treated with esophageal dilation procedures.

ENDOCRINE DYSFUNCTION

Hypothyroidism

Hypothyroidism is frequent after radiation therapy to the low neck. Prospective data from the Cleveland Clinic reports hypothyroidism rates of 48% at 5 years and 67% at 8 years after treatment.[70] The median time to onset is 1.4 years, and the addition of concurrent chemotherapy does not appear to affect the risk. Nearly identical retrospective data from the University of Florida suggest that hypothyroidism rates are 42% at 5 years and 74% at 10 years after radiation therapy in a subset of patients with documented posttreatment thyroid-stimulating hormone levels.[71] The incidence of hypothyroidism is higher among patients undergoing partial thryoidectomy as a component of laryngeal or hypopharyngeal surgery,[70–72] and the presence of thyroid autoantibodies also increases the risk.[72] Because posttreatment hypothyroidism is common, routine screening during follow up is recommended.

Pituitary Dysfunction

The radiation treatment portal for advanced nasopharyngeal and paranasal sinus carcinomas commonly includes the pituitary gland and may include the hypothalamus as well. Late radiation effects on the hypothalamic–pituitary axis were summarized by Sklar and Constine.[73] Growth hormone is the hormone that is the most likely to be affected by radiotherapy. Studies of children suggest that the threshold dose for decreased secretion may be as low as 18 Gy, although the threshold dose is likely to be higher in adults. The levels of the gonadotropins, luteinizing hormone, and follicle-stimulating hormone are not likely to be impaired by doses of less than 40 Gy, but they can drop after 50 Gy of conventionally fractionated radiation therapy. Thyroid-stimulating hormone and adrenocorticotropin are the least likely hormones to be affected. The hypothalamus is more sensitive to radiation than the pituitary gland, and decreased dopaminergic tone leads to hyperprolactinemia. In a study of 31 patients with nasopharyngeal carcinoma, doses to the pituitary gland and the hypothalamus were found to be 62 Gy and 40 Gy, respectively.[74] The authors reported a 62% rate of endocrine dysfunction at 5 years. Growth hormone was the most frequently affected hormone, and it was deficient in 64% of patients. Thyroid-stimulating hormone was the least frequently affected, but it was low in 14% of the study population. Hyperprolactinemia was more common among female patients. Four patients developed hypothyroidism, but patients whose necks were also treated were more likely to develop this complication.

CAROTID ARTERY

The carotid arteries are immediately adjacent to the at-risk lymph-node regions of the head and neck. For this reason, these arteries are frequently included in the radiation field. Radiation triggers an inflammatory reaction in the vessel wall that leads to thickening of the intima media and plaque deposition,[75] and several recent studies suggest that patients treated with radiation therapy for head and neck cancer have an increased risk of carotid stenosis[76–78] and stroke.[79,80] Although carotid stenosis is usually asymptomatic, stroke can be devastating. In a group of 413 patients with squamous cell carcinoma of the head and neck, the relative risk of stroke as compared with population-based expected data was 2, and the 5-year actuarial stroke rate was 12%.[79] Dorresteijn and colleagues[80] reviewed the records of 367 patients who were less than 60 years old with diagnoses of T1 and T2 laryngeal cancer, pleomorphic adenoma, and parotid carcinoma. The median time from radiation therapy to stroke was 10.9 years, and the relative risk of stroke in irradiated patients was strikingly high at 10.

No clear relationship between radiation dose and stroke risk has been established for the range of doses that are commonly used for the treatment of head and neck cancer.[79] Increased rates of vascular disease and stroke are seen among long-term survivors of Hodgkin's lymphoma, which suggests that low doses of radiation therapy can be harmful to large vessels.[81,82] A threshold dose of 35 Gy has been suggested by one cross-sectional study.[76] The role of screening and prophylactic treatment remains to be defined by prospective trials, and the overall picture is clouded by competing risk factors such as tobacco use, hypertension, and increasing age.

CENTRAL NERVOUS SYSTEM

Spinal Cord

Temporary radiation-induced demyelination of the spinal cord results in electric-shock–like sensations of the extremities triggered by neck flexion, known as *Lhermitte syndrome*.[83] Late radiation toxicity in the central nervous system is caused by demyelination and chronic small-vessel injury.[84–86] This condition typically presents 3 months after the completion of radiation therapy, resolves spontaneously over the next 6 months, and does not predict serious late toxicity.[87] Overdose of the spinal cord results in transverse myelitis. Functionally this is equivalent to spinal-cord transection, and symptoms depend on the level of the injury. Unlike Lhermitte syndrome, transverse myelitis does not improve with time. Most radiation oncologists choose a conservative limit for the spinal cord dose (i.e., 45 Gy), although clinical evidence suggests that doses of 50 Gy should be well tolerated.[88]

Brain

Brain necrosis and cognitive decline are uncommon complications of head and neck radiotherapy. The inferior aspect of the temporal lobes is included in the conventional nasopharyngeal radiation field. In a large retrospective series from Hong Kong, the rate of temporal-lobe necrosis after definitive radiotherapy for nasopharyngeal carcinoma was 2%.[89] Higher dose per fraction and twice-daily radiation treatment were associated with an increased risk of temporal lobe damage. Symptomatic brain necrosis should be treated with oral dexamethasone, and refractory cases may require hyperbaric oxygen therapy or surgical resection. Cognitive decline has been documented after radiation to the nasopharynx and the paranasal sinuses.[90] The mechanism of cognitive decline is likely mutifactorial, with decreased neurogenesis, ischemia, and temporal lobe damage contributing to its development.[85,91]

EYE, ORBIT, AND VISUAL PATHWAY

It is not uncommon for visual structures to be immediately adjacent to tumor target volumes. When a paranasal sinus tumor invades the orbit or skull base, radiation oncologists and patients are faced with a serious dilemma: do they cover the tumor and risk a catastrophic visual complication, or do they spare the optic structures and risk local tumor recurrence? IMRT allows for the better tailoring of the radiation dose distribution as compared with conventional radiation techniques, but sophisticated radiation treatment planning cannot be expected to fully overcome the physical proximity of normal tissues and tumor targets. Exceeding tolerance doses for four separate anatomic structures—the lens, the retina, the optic nerves, and the optic chiasm—can result in vision loss after radiation therapy.

Lens

The lens is extremely sensitive to ionizing radiation. Cataract formation is seldom seen below a total fractionated radiation dose of 5 Gy,[92] but it has been reported to occur with doses as low as 4 Gy.[93] Fifty percent of patients will develop lens opacities after radiotherapy doses of 10 Gy to 12.5 Gy, but the latency period from radiation treatment to cataract formation is several years. The development of lens opacity ultimately leads to vision loss in the majority of patients, and lens-replacement surgery is the treatment of choice.[92] Because of the excellent success rates with lens-replacement surgery, radiation-induced cataract is no longer considered a severe late complication.[94]

Retinopathy and Neuropathy

Retinopathy and neuropathy cannot be remedied with surgical or medical interventions. Prevention of a catastrophic complication is key, and accurate knowledge of the dose going to these structures is necessary for the patient to give truly informed consent. Jiang and colleagues[95] published data regarding radiation injury to the visual pathway among 219 patients with cancers of the nasal cavity and the paranasal sinuses who were treated from 1969 to 1985. The study is limited by its use of conventional radiation treatment techniques and crude dose estimation methods, but, despite these limitations, the information presented remains clinically useful today. Symptomatic retinopathy occurred in 7 of 77 patients with a mean time to presentation of 11 months. Eight of ninety-eight patients developed ipsilateral blindness as a result of optic neuropathy. Only one case of optic neuropathy occurred at a dose of less than 60 Gy. Bilateral blindness as a result of optic chiasm injury was documented in 11 of 208 patients with a median time to presentation of 32 months after radiation treatment. The lowest radiation dose that resulted in bilateral blindness was 50 Gy, with a total of four cases of bilateral blindness seen at doses of less than 60 Gy.

The dose–response relationship for late retinal complications was reported by Takeda and colleagues.[94] No retinal complications were seen with doses of less than 50 Gy. In 21 eyes exposed to doses of more than 50 Gy, the probability of a severe complication was related to the amount of the retina exposed, with an increased risk of complication found when more than 50% of the retina was irradiated. Accurate radiation dose data were generated for 20 patients with advanced paranasal sinus tumors treated with three-dimensional conformal radiation therapy at a single institution.[96] The probability of any optic neuropathy at 5 years was 15%, and the probability of a severe complication was 8% at 5 years. Increasing the maximum optic-nerve dose was correlated with severe complications. Four optic nerves with severe complications received maximum doses of 64 Gy to 75.5 Gy. In this study, only one patient suffered optic chiasm damage, and that patient received a maximum chiasm dose of 59.5 Gy. Five patients with optic chiasm doses of more than 60 Gy did not have complications.

Orbit and Globe

Other visual-pathway toxicities include dry eye as a result of lacrimal gland injury, corneal ulceration, neovascular glaucoma, and retinal artery obstruction. Jiang and colleagues[95] reported corneal injury in 24 of 49 patients treated with a three-field radiation technique without any orbital shielding. The median time to corneal injury was 9 months. Orbital doses of more than 55 Gy were associated with a dramatic increase in toxicity rates, and the use of concurrent chemotherapy also predisposed patients to corneal injury. The incidence of neovascular glaucoma was 7% for eyes treated with more than 50 Gy.[94] Edema and ulcerative keratitis occurred acutely, and they usually healed with conservative management.

EAR

External and Middle Ear

Ototoxicity occurs commonly, but it has been consistently underreported. Several recent studies have explored the dose response for ototoxicity. The most comprehensive evaluation was published by Bhandare and colleagues.[97] The authors systematically reviewed ear doses and clinical outcomes for a group of 325 patients with primary tumors of the nasal cavity, the nasopharynx, and the paranasal sinuses. In total, 42% of patients experienced ototoxicity as a complication of head and neck radiotherapy. Toxicity was divided by site. Complications of the external ear (i.e., otitis externa, ulceration, cartilage necrosis, external auditory canal stenosis) were seen in 33% of patients. Chronic otitis and canal stenosis occurred in 26% and 32% of patients receiving 60 Gy to 65 Gy to the external ear. Middle-ear complications were also frequent, occurring in 29% of patients. Chronic

otitis media was seen in 60% of patients who received a middle-ear dose of more than 60 Gy. Other middle-ear complications included Eustachian tube dysfunction, tympanic membrane perforation, and transient conductive hearing loss.

Sensorineural Hearing Loss

Bhandare and colleagues[97] also reported rates of sensorineural hearing loss and noted that it occurred in 15% of patients. The risk of sensorineural hearing loss was dependent on the radiation dose. The rate of sensorineural hearing loss was 3% for inner-ear doses of less than 60.5 Gy as compared with 37% when the inner-ear dose exceeded this threshold. The median time until the development of sensorineural hearing loss was 1.8 years. Rates of sensorineural hearing loss were higher among patients who received chemotherapy. Other inner-ear complications included tinnitus, labyrinthitis, and vertigo.

Other data regarding the risk of sensorineural hearing loss suggest that the threshold dose for toxicity may be lower than reported by Bhandare and colleagues,[97] with a significantly increased risk of hearing loss seen with doses of more than 45 Gy.[98] Retrospective data from the Memorial Sloan–Kettering Cancer Center also support a lower dose threshold for hearing loss, with a significant increase in this complication seen among patients receiving more than 48 Gy.[99] Among children, hearing impairment occurs at lower dose levels, with one study suggesting a threshold dose of 32 Gy. Treatment with ototoxic chemotherapy and the presence of a cerebrospinal fluid shunt were other risk factors associated with a decline of auditory acuity in children.[100] Additional studies are needed to further clarify safe limits for the ear dose.

CONCLUSION

Radiotherapy to the head and neck is a toxic treatment. Side effects can be broadly divided into two groups: acute and late. Acute toxicity results from the death of rapidly dividing cells. Intensive regimens designed to increase local control also increase acute toxicity rates. Acute toxicity is usually self-resolving, and it should be managed conservatively. Late complications are less predictable and tend to be more difficult to manage. Close attention to the radiation dose and to volume parameters is of critical importance for the prevention of late toxicity. Despite efforts to limit the radiation dose to normal tissues, late toxicity commonly occurs. The systematic reporting of toxicity end points in cooperative group studies will lead to better understanding of the long-term consequences of head and neck radiotherapy.

REFERENCES

1. Emami B, Lyman J, Brown A, et al: Tolerance of normal tissue to therapeutic irradiation. *Int J Radiat Oncol Biol Phys* 1991;21:109–122.
2. Hall EJ: Clinical response of normal tissues. In Hall, EJ: *Radiobiology for the radiologist,* Philadelphia, 2000, Lippincott Williams & Wilkins.
3. Small W, Woloschak G: Introduction. In Small W, Woloschak GE, editors: *Radiation toxicity: A practical guide,* New York, 2006, Springer.
4. Chen Y, Trotti A, Coleman CN, et al: Adverse event reporting and developments in radiation biology after normal tissue injury: International atomic energy agency consultation. *Int J Radiat Oncol Biol Phys* 2006;64:1442–1451.
5. Adelstein DJ, Li Y, Adams GL, et al: An intergroup phase III comparison of standard radiation therapy and two schedules of concurrent chemoradiotherapy in patients with unresectable squamous cell head and neck cancer. *J Clin Oncol* 2003;21:92–98.
6. Calais G, Alfonsi M, Bardet E, et al: Randomized trial of radiation therapy versus concomitant chemotherapy and radiation therapy for advanced-stage oropharynx carcinoma. *J Natl Cancer Inst* 1999;91:2081–2086.
7. Forastiere AA, Goepfert H, Maor M, et al: Concurrent chemotherapy and radiotherapy for organ preservation in advanced laryngeal cancer. *N Engl J Med* 2003;349:2091–2098.
8. Fu KK, Pajak TF, Trotti A, et al: A Radiation Therapy Oncology Group (RTOG) phase III randomized study to compare hyperfractionation and two variants of accelerated fractionation to standard fractionation radiotherapy for head and neck squamous cell carcinomas: First report of RTOG 9003. *Int J Radiat Oncol Biol Phys* 2000;48:7–16.
9. Bourhis J, Lapeyre M, Tortochaux J, et al: Phase III randomized trial of very accelerated radiation therapy compared with conventional radiation therapy in squamous cell head and neck cancer: A GORTEC trial. *J Clin Oncol* 2006;24:2873–2878.
10. Pow EHN, Kwong DLW, McMillan AS, et al: Xerostomia and quality of life after intensity-modulated radiotherapy vs. conventional radiotherapy for early-stage nasopharyngeal carcinoma: Initial report on a randomized controlled clinical trial. *Int J Radiat Oncol Biol Phys* 2006;66:981–991.
11. Porock D, Kristjanson L: Skin reactions during radiotherapy for breast cancer: The use and impact of topical agents and dressings. *Eur J Cancer* 1999;8:143–153.
12. De Naeyer B, De Meerleer G, Breems S, et al: Collagen vascular disease and radiation therapy: A critical review. *Int J Radiat Oncol Biol Phys* 1999;44:975–980.
13. Denis F, Garaud P, Bardet E, et al: Late toxicity results of the GORTEC 94-01 randomized trial comparing radiotherapy with concomitant radiochemotherapy for advanced-stage oropharynx carcinoma: Comparison of LENT/SOMA, RTOG/EORTC, and NCI/CTC scoring systems. *Int J Radiat Oncol Biol Phys* 2003;55:93–98.
14. Archambeau JO, Pezner R, Wasserman T: Pathophysiology of irradiated skin and breast. *Int J Radiat Oncol Biol Phys* 1995;31:1171–1185.
15. Wood G, Casey L, Trotti A: Skin changes. In Small W, Woloschak GE, editors: *Radiation toxicity: A practical guide,* New York, 2006, Springer.
16. Blanco AI, Chao C: Management of radiation-induced head and neck injury. In Small W, Woloschak GE, editors: *Radiation toxicity: A practical guide,* New York, 2006, Springer.
17. White J, Joiner MC: Toxicity from radiation in breast cancer. In Small W, Woloschak GE, editors: *Radiation toxicity: A practical guide,* New York, 2006, Springer.
18. Olsen DL, Raub W, Bradley C, et al: The effect of aloe vera gel/mild soap versus mild soap alone in preventing skin reactions in patients undergoing radiation therapy. *Oncol Nurs Forum* 2001;28:543–547.
19. Heggie S, Bryant GP, Tripcony L, et al: A phase III study on the efficacy of topical aloe vera gel on irradiated breast tissue. *Cancer Nursing* 2002;25:442–451.
20. Williams MS, Burk M, Loprinzi CL, et al: Phase III double-blind evaluation of an aloe vera gel as a prophylactic agent for radiation-induced skin toxicity. *Int J Radiat Oncol Biol Phys* 1996;36:345–349.
21. Richardson J, Smith JE, McIntyre M, et al: Aloe vera for preventing radiation-induced skin reactions: A systematic literature review. *Clin Oncol* 2005;17:478–484.
22. Shukla PN, Gairola M, Mohanti BK, et al: Prophylactic beclomethasone spray to the skin during postoperative radiotherapy of carcinoma breast: A prospective randomized study. *Indian J Cancer* 2006;43:180–184.
23. Bostrom A, Lindman H, Swartling C, et al: Potent corticosteroid cream (mometasone furoate) significantly reduces acute radiation dermatitis: Results from a double-blind, randomized study. *Radiother Oncol* 2001;59:257–265.
24. Macmillan MS, Wells M, MacBride S, et al: Randomized comparison of dry dressings versus hydrogel in management of radiation-induced moist desquamation. *Int J Radiat Oncol Biol Phys* 2007;68:864–872.
25. Bourhis J, Calais G, Lapeyre M, et al: Concomitant radiochemotherapy or accelerated radiotherapy: Analysis of two randomized trials of the French head and neck cancer group (GORETC). *Semin Oncol* 2004;31:822–826.
26. Brizel DM, Albers ME, Fisher SR, et al: Hyperfractionated irradiation with or without concurrent chemotherapy for locally advanced head and neck cancer. *N Engl J Med* 1998;338:1798–1804.
27. Staar S, Rudat V, Stuetzer H, et al: Intensified hyperfractionated accelerated radiotherapy limits the additional benefit of simultaneous chemotherapy: Results of a multicentric randomized German trial in advanced head-and-neck cancer. *Int J Radiat Biol Phys* 2001;50:1161–1171.
28. Okuno SH, Foote RL, Loprinzi CL, et al: A randomized trial of a nonabsorbable antibiotic lozenge given to alleviate radiation-induced mucositis. *Cancer* 1997;79:2193–2199.
29. Symonds RP, McIlroy P, Khorrami J, et al: The reduction of radiation mucositis by selective decontamination antibiotic pastilles: A placebo-controlled double-blind trial. *Br J Cancer* 1996;74:312–317.
30. Wijers OB, Levendag PC, Harms ERE, et al: Mucositis reduction by selective elimination of oral flora in irradiated cancers of the head and neck: A placebo-controlled double-blind randomized trial. *Int J Radiat Oncol Biol Phys* 2001;50:343–352.
31. Foote RL, Loprinzi CL, Frank AR, et al: Randomized trial of a chlorhexidine mouthwash for alleviation of radiation-induced mucositis. *J Clin Oncol* 1994;12:2630–2633.
32. Trotti A, Garden A, Warde P, et al: A multinational, randomized phase III trial of iseganan HCl oral solution for reduction the severity of oral mucositis in patients receiving radiotherapy for head-and-neck malignancy. *Int J Radiat Oncol Biol Phys* 2004;58:674–681.
33. Dodd MJ, principal investigator: *Management of radiation therapy induced oral mucositis with GM-CSF mouthwash in head and neck cancer patients,* University of California, San Francisco, Committee on Human Research, Approval No: H452–26184.
34. Antonadou D, Pepelassi M, Synodinou M, et al: Prophylactic use of amifostine to prevent radiochemotherapy-induced mucositis and xerostomia in head-and-neck cancer. *Int J Radiat Oncol Biol Phys* 2002;52:739–747.
35. Koukourakis MI, Kyrias G, Kakolyris S, et al: Subcutaneous administration of amifostine during fractionated radiotherapy: A randomized phase II study. *J Clin Oncol* 2000;18:2226–2233.
36. Brizel DM, Wasserman TH, Henke M, et al: Phase III randomized trial of amifostine as a radioprotector in head and neck cancer. *J Clin Oncol* 2000;18:3339–3345.
37. Greenspan D, Daniels TE: Effectiveness of pilocarpine in post-radiation xerostomia. *Cancer* 1987;59:1123–1125.
38. Johnson JT, Ferretti GA, Nethery WJ, et al: Oral pilocarpine for post-irradiation xerostomia in patients with head and neck cancer. *N Engl J Med* 1993;329:390–395.
39. LeVeque FG, Montgomery M, Potter D, et al: A multicenter, randomized, double-blind, placebo-controlled, dose-titration

study of oral pilocarpine for treatment of radiation-induced xerostomia in head and neck cancer patients. *J Clin Oncol* 1993;11:1124–1131.

40. Warde P, O'Sullivan B, Aslanidis J, et al: A phase III placebo-controlled trial of oral pilocarpine in patients undergoing radiotherapy for head-and-neck cancer. *Int J Radiat Oncol Biol Phys* 2002;54:9–13.

41. Wasserman TH, Brizel DM, Henke M, et al: Influence of intravenous amifostine on xerostomia, tumor control, and survival after radiotherapy for head-and-neck cancer: 2-year follow-up of a prospective, randomized, phase III trial. *Int J Radiat Oncol Biol Phys* 2005;63:985–990.

42. Anne PR, Machtay M, Rosenthal DI, et al: A phase II trial of subcutaneous amifostine and radiation therapy in patients with head-and-neck cancer. *Int J Radiat Oncol Biol Phys* 2007;67:445–452.

43. Eisbruch A, Ten Haken RK, Kin HM, et al: Dose, volume, and function relationships in parotid salivary glands following conformal and intensity-modulated irradiation of head and neck cancer. *Int J Radiat Oncol Biol Phys* 1999;45:577–587.

44. Radiation Therapy Oncology Group RTOG 0244. *A phase II study of submandibular salivary gland transfer to the submental space prior to start of radiation treatment for prevention of radiation-induced xerostomia in head and neck cancer patients* (website): rtog.org/members/protocols/0244/0244.pdf. Accessed April 1, 2008.

45. Wahl MJ: Osteoradionecrosis prevention myths. *Int J Radiat Oncol Biol Phys* 2006;64:661–669.

46. Clayman L: Management of dental extractions in irradiated jaws: A protocol without hyperbaric oxygen therapy. *J Oral Maxillofac Surg* 1997;55:275–281.

47. Mendenhall WM: Mandibular osteoradionecrosis. *J Clin Oncol* 2004;22:4867–4868.

48. Engleman MA, Woloschak G, Small W: Radiation-induced skeletal injury. In Small W, Woloschak GE, editors: *Radiation toxicity: A practical guide,* New York, 2006, Springer.

49. Chang DT, Sandow PR, Morris CG, et al: Do pre-irradiation dental extractions reduce the risk of osteoradionecrosis of the mandible? *Head Neck* 2007;29:528–536.

50. Ayad T, Gelinas M, Guertin L, et al: Retromolar trigone carcinoma treatment by primary radiation therapy. *Arch Otolaryngol Head Neck Surg* 2005;131:576–582.

51. Mendenhall WM, Morris CG, Amdur RJ, et al: Retromolar trigone squamous cell carcinoma treated with radiotherapy alone or combined with surgery. *Cancer* 2005;103:2320–2325.

52. Huang CJ, Chao KSC, Tsai J, et al: Cancer of retromolar trigone: Long term radiation therapy outcome. *Head Neck* 2001;23:758–763.

53. Morrish RB, Chan E, Silverman S, et al: Osteonecrosis in patients irradiated for head and neck carcinoma. *Cancer* 1981;47:1980–1983.

54. de Arruda FF, Puri DR, Zhung J, et al: Intensity-modulated radiation therapy for the treatment of oropharyngeal carcinoma: The Memorial Sloan Kettering Cancer Center Experience. *Int J Radiat Oncol Biol Phys* 2006;64:363–373.

55. Ben-David MA, Diamante M, Radawski JD, et al: Lack of osteoradionecrosis of the mandible after intensity-modulated radiotherapy for head and neck cancer: Likely contributions of both dental care and improved dose distributions. *Int J Radiat Oncol Biol Phys* 2007;68:396–402.

56. Marx RE, Johnson RP, Kline SN: Prevention of osteoradionecrosis: A randomized prospective clinical trial of hyperbaric oxygen versus penicillin. *J Am Dent Assoc* 1985;111:49–54.

57. Bennett MH, Feldmeier J, Hampson N, et al: Hyperbaric oxygen therapy for late radiation tissue injury (review). *Cochrane Database Syst Rev* 2005;3:CD005005.

58. Feldmeir JJ, Hampson NB: A systematic review of the literature reporting the application of hyperbaric oxygen prevention and treatment of delayed radiation injuries: An evidence based approach. *Undersea Hyperb Med* 2002;29:4–30.

59. Delanian S, Depondt J, Lefaix JL: Major healing of refractory mandible osteoradionecrosis after treatment combining pentoxifylline and tocopherol: A phase II trial. *Head Neck* 2005;27:114–123.

60. Wolf GT, Hong WK, Fisher SG, et al: Induction chemotherapy plus radiation compared with surgery plus radiation in patients with advanced laryngeal cancer. *N Engl J Med* 1991;324:1685–1690.

61. Fung K, Yoo J, Leeper HA, et al: Vocal function following radiation for non-laryngeal versus laryngeal tumors for the head and neck. *Laryngoscope* 2001;111:1920–1924.

62. Carrara de Angelis E, Feher O, Barros AP, et al: Voice and swallowing in patient enrolled in a larynx preservation trial. *Arch Otolaryngol Head Neck Surg* 2003;129:733–738.

63. Fung K, Lyden TH, Lee J, et al: Voice and swallowing outcomes of an organ-preservation trial for advanced laryngeal cancer. *Int J Radiat Oncol Biol Phys* 2005;63:1395–1399.

64. Fua TF, Corry J, Milner AD, et al: Intensity-modulated radiotherapy for nasopharyngeal carcinoma: Clinical correlation of dose to the pharyngo-esophageal axis and dysphagia. *Int J Radiat Oncol Biol Phys* 2007;67:976–981.

65. Dornfeld K, Simmons JR, Karnell L, et al: Radiation doses to structures within and adjacent to the larynx are correlated with long-term diet and speech related quality of life. *Int J Radiat Oncol Biol Phys* 2007;68:750–757.

66. Eisbruch A, Schwartz M, Rasch C, et al: Dysphagia and aspiration after chemoradiotherapy for head-and-neck cancer: Which anatomic structures are affected and can they be spared with IMRT? *Int J Radiat Oncol Biol Phys* 2004;60:1425–1439.

67. Sanguineti G, Adapala P, Endrea EJ, et al: Dosimetric predictors of laryngeal edema. *Int J Radiat Oncol Biol Phys* 2007;68:741–749.

68. Lee WT, Akst LM, Adelstein DJ, et al: Risk factors for hypopharyngeal/upper esophageal stricture formation after concurrent chemoradiation. *Head Neck* 2006;28:808–812.

69. Laurell G, Kraepelien T, Mavroidis P, et al: Stricture of the proximal esophagus in head and neck carcinoma patients after radiotherapy. *Cancer* 2003;97:1693–1700.

70. Mercado G, Adelstein DJ, Saxton JP, et al: Hypothyroidism: A frequent event after radiotherapy and after radiotherapy with chemotherapy for patients with head and neck carcinoma. *Cancer* 2001;92:2892–2897.

71. Garcia-Serra A, Amdur RJ, Morris CG, et al: Thyroid function should be monitored following radiotherapy to the low neck. *Am J Clin Oncol* 2005;28:255–258.

72. Lo Glabo AM, de Bree R, Kuik DJ, et al: The prevalence of hypothyroidism after treatment for laryngeal and hypopharyngeal carcinomas: Are autoantibodies of influence? *Acta Otolaryngol* 2007;127:312–317.

73. Sklar CA, Constine LS: Chronic neuroendocrinological sequelae of radiation therapy. *Int J Radiat Oncol Biol Phys* 1995;31:1113–1121.

74. Lam KS, Tse VK, Wang C, et al: Effects of cranial irradiation on hypothalamic-pituitary function: A 5-year longitudinal study in patients with nasopharyngeal carcinoma. *Q J Med* 1991;78:165–176.

75. Abayomi OK: Neck Irradiation, carotid injury and its consequences. *Oral Oncol* 2004;40:872–878.

76. Martin JD, Buckley AR, Graeb D, et al: Carotid artery stenosis in asymptomatic patients who have received unilateral head-and-neck irradiation. *Int J Radiat Oncol Biol Phys* 2005;63:1197–1205.

77. Cheng SWK, Ting ACW, Lam LK, et al: Carotid stenosis after radiotherapy for nasopharyngeal carcinoma. *Arch Otolaryngol Head Neck Surg* 2000;126:517–521.

78. Lam WW, Leung SF, So NM, et al: Incidence of carotid stenosis in nasopharyngeal carcinoma patients after radiotherapy. *Cancer* 2001;92:2357–2363.

79. Haynes JC, Machtay M, Weber RS, et al: Relative risk of stroke in head and neck carcinoma patients treated with external cervical irradiation. *Laryngoscope* 2002;112:1883–1887.

80. Dorresteijn LDA, Kappelle AC, Boogerd W, et al: Increased risk of ischemic stroke after radiotherapy on the neck in patients younger than 60 years. *J Clin Oncol* 2002;20:282–288.

81. Hull MC, Morris CG, Pepine CJ, et al: Valvular dysfunction and carotid, subclavian, and coronary artery disease in survivors of Hodgkin lymphoma treated with radiation therapy. *JAMA* 2003;290:2831–2837.

82. Bowers DC, McNeil DE, Liu Y, et al: Stroke as a late treatment effect of Hodgkin's disease: A report from Childhood Cancer Survivor Study. *J Clin Oncol* 2005;23:6508–6515.

83. Fein DA, Marcus RB, Parsons JT, et al: Lhermitte's sign: Incidence and treatment variables influencing risk after irradiation of the cervical spinal cord. *Int J Radiat Oncol Biol Phys* 1993;25:1029–1033.

84. Sloan, AE, Arnold SM, St Clair WH, et al: Brain injury: Management and investigations. *Semin Radiat Oncol* 2003;13:309–321.

85. St Clair WH, Arnold SM, Sloan AE, et al: Spinal cord and peripheral nerve injury: Current management and investigations. *Semin Radiat Oncol* 2003;13:322–332.

86. Shaw EG, Robbins ME: The management of radiation-induced brain injury. In Small W, Woloschak GE, editors: *Radiation toxicity: A practical guide,* New York, 2006, Springer.

87. Esik O, Csere T, Stefanits K, et al: A review on radiogenic Lhermitte's sign. *Pathol Oncol Res* 2003;9:115–120.

88. Marcus RB, Million RR: The incidence of myelitis after irradiation of the cervical spinal cord. *Int J Radiat Oncol Biol Phys* 1990;19:3–8.

89. Lee AWM, Kwong DLW, Leung SF, et al: Factors affecting risk of symptomatic temporal lobe necrosis: Significance of fractional dose and treatment time. *Int J Radiat Oncol Biol Phys* 2002;53:75–85.

90. Hua MS, Chen ST, Tang LM, et al: Neuropsychological function in patients with nasopharyngeal carcinoma after radiotherapy. *Clin Exp Neuropsychol* 1998;20:684–693.

91. Abayomi OK: Pathogenesis of cognitive decline following therapeutic irradiation for head and neck tumors. *Acta Oncol* 2004;41:346–351.

92. Henk JM, Whitelocke RAF, Warrington AP, et al: Radiation dose to the lens and cataract formation. *Int J Radiat Oncol Biol Phys* 1992;25:815–820.

93. Merriam GR, Focht EF: A clinical study of radiation cataracts and the relationship to dose. *Am J Roentgenol* 1957;77:759–785.

94. Takeda A, Shigematsu N, Suzuki S, et al: Late retinal complications of radiation therapy for nasal and paranasal malignancies: Relationship between irradiated-dose area and severity. *Int J Radiat Oncol Biol Phys* 1999;44:599–605.

95. Jiang GL, Tucker SL, Guttenberger R, et al: Radiation-induced injury to the visual pathway. *Radiother Oncol* 1994;30:17–25.

96. Martel MK, Sandler HM, Cornblath WT, et al: Dose-volume complication analysis for visual pathway structures of patients with advanced paranasal sinus tumors. *Int J Radiat Oncol Biol Phys* 1997;38:273–284.

97. Bhandare N, Antonelli PJ, Morris CG, et al: Ototoxicity after radiotherapy for head and neck tumors. *Int J Radiat Oncol Biol Phys* 2007;67:469–479.

98. Pan CC, Eisbruch A, Lee JS, et al: Prospective study of inner ear radiation dose and hearing loss in head-and-neck cancer patients. *Int J Radiat Oncol Biol Phys* 2005;61:1393–1402.

99. Chen WC, Jackson A, Budnick AS, et al: Sensorineural hearing loss in combined modality treatment of nasopharyngeal carcinoma. *Cancer* 2006;106:820–829.

100. Merchant TE, Gould CJ, Xiong X, et al: Early neuro-otologic effects of three-dimensional irradiation in children with primary brain tumors. *Int J Radiat Oncol Biol Phys* 2004;58:1194–1207.

CHAPTER 15

Chemotherapy in Head and Neck Cancer

Missak Haigentz, Jr.

Since the introduction of the first chemotherapeutic agents during the 1950s, the hope of physicians involved in the care of patients with cancer has been to cure and improve the survival of patients with the use of systemic therapy. Although measures of success for meeting these goals when treating most solid tumors have been modest at best, the evolution of the multidisciplinary treatment of head and neck cancers has challenged traditional surgical oncologic principles and has become the model for organ-preserving and curative-nonsurgical therapies in clinical oncology. Furthermore, increasing knowledge of tumor and molecular biology has led to the rational development of novel and active anticancer drugs with increasingly tolerable toxicity profiles. This chapter will present an overview of chemotherapeutic and biologic therapy for head and neck cancer.

The role of chemotherapy, which was initially applied only to palliative settings, has evolved into curative management plans for patients with head and neck cancer. The roles of chemotherapy in the management of head and neck cancers are systemic disease cytoreduction, locoregional radiosensitization, or both. Challenges to achieving these end points include preserving the functional status of patients and minimizing toxicities. These conditions are often pronounced in patients with head and neck cancer, who experience considerable morbidity as a result of their disease (e.g., mucositis, dysphagia, cachexia, dyspnea). Considerable improvements in the supportive care of cancer patients have been made to ameliorate the morbidity of cancer therapy, including the use of growth-factor support (e.g., recombinant erythropoietin, granulocyte colony-stimulating factor), new antiemetics (e.g., 5-HT$_3$ antagonists, neurokinin antagonists), amifostine to prevent radiation-induced xerostomia, and ongoing research to prevent and treat mucositis. Existing supportive therapies and the development of targeted biologic therapies make increasingly aggressive, curative, nonsurgical regimens possible.

PRINCIPLES OF CHEMOTHERAPY

Clinical Settings and End Points

Before discussing the various existing therapies, it is important to define several terms used in management plans. *Neoadjuvant (induction) therapy* is treatment that is administered before a definitive locoregional therapy (e.g., surgery, radiation, chemoradiotherapy). *Adjuvant therapy* is anticancer treatment that is administered after definitive therapy, with the goal of preventing recurrence and improving survival. *Evidence of response* to therapy is generally defined as complete or partial; however, prolonged disease stability may be another measure of clinical activity in patients with incurable disease. Complete responses, which are often markers of success in clinical oncology, have been observed in laryngeal and other head and neck cancers, particularly among patients with previously untreated disease. However, only in very rare exceptions is chemotherapy alone a curative intervention for previously untreated head and neck cancer. Definitive locoregional therapy with concurrent radiation is needed to control both gross and micrometastatic locoregionally advanced disease.

Mechanism of Action and Rationale of Combination Therapy

The mechanism of chemotherapeutic activity, although varied, is generally directed toward actively dividing cancer cells. Chemotherapeutic agents are defined as *cell-cycle specific,* which means that they exert specific effects during the different phases of the cell cycle (Figure 15-1), or *nonspecific.* However, individual classes of chemotherapeutic agents have unique mechanisms of action and are associated with specific toxicity profiles. In the case of solid tumors such as those of head and neck cancer, multiple genetic defects may exist within a heterogeneous tumor population. To maximize anticancer activity and prevent drug resistance, clinical combinations of chemotherapeutic agents are frequently employed in therapeutic regimens. Ideal therapeutic combinations include active agents that have nonoverlapping toxicity profiles when each is administered according to its optimal dose and schedule. The clinical development of targeted biologic therapies in oncology offers the potential for rational combination with either chemotherapy or radiotherapy while minimizing toxicity.

Radiosensitization

The continued evolution in combinations of curative-intent chemotherapy and radiotherapy has tremendously affected the management of locally advanced head and neck cancer. Aside from the relatively independent, non-overlapping, and additive activity and toxicity profiles of

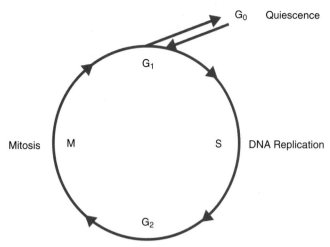

Figure 15-1. Schematic representation of the cell cycle.

the combination (i.e., local and/or regional for radiotherapy, systemic for chemotherapy), chemotherapeutic and biologic agents have been known to specifically affect tumor response to radiation. Initial studies of combined-modality therapy involved the use of induction chemotherapy before radiotherapy.[1,2] However, several randomized clinical trials involving head and neck cancer have clearly shown that the addition of chemotherapy concurrently with radiation improves locoregional control as compared with radiation alone, often enough to improve survival.[3–8] Indeed, recent large, randomized studies have supported the use of concurrent chemoradiotherapy in the postoperative adjuvant setting for patients at high risk of recurrence.[9,10] Various mechanisms for chemotherapy-induced radiosensitization (i.e., cell-cycle synchronization, hypoxia sensitization, interference with repair processes) have been proposed, but none have sufficiently explained the observed effects.[11]

Concurrent chemoradiotherapy is currently a standard treatment for the definitive management of locally advanced head and neck cancer. Although modern chemoradiotherapy regimens have made considerable advances in improving local control, distant failure appears to be increasing.[12] To address this need, several investigators are currently exploring an approach known as *sequential chemoradiotherapy,* which involves the administration of systemic doses of combination chemotherapy followed by concurrent chemoradiotherapy.[13–16] This combined approach takes advantage of the benefits of systemic disease chemosensitivity as well as radiosensitization.

Common to all such combinations, however, is the concern of additional toxicity to patients as a result not only of the added systemic toxicity of chemotherapy itself but also of the combined effect on locoregional tissues. Indeed, local tissues also appear to be radiosensitized, which results in greater mucositis, weight loss, and dysphagia. This is of particular concern in the adjuvant postoperative setting, where certain patients may indeed be overtreated. Furthermore, to accommodate the combination therapy, the toxicity of the concurrent therapy frequently requires less-than-adequate systemic drug dosing. Perhaps this challenge will be best addressed by the sequential approach, as previously described. Optimizing the chemoradiotherapy regimen and the selection of patients for appropriate therapy will be the future challenges for head and neck oncologists.

CLASSES OF CYTOTOXIC CHEMOTHERAPY

The cytotoxic chemotherapeutic agents described in this section have been commonly used for the treatment of head and neck cancers.

Platinum Analogues

The observation in 1961 that the exposure of bacteria to electromagnetic fields on platinum electrodes resulted in a profound change in their morphology led to the development of platinum complexes as anticancer therapies.[17] The platinum analogues are platinum-based compounds that work by inducing platinum-DNA adducts, which results in interstrand and intrastrand DNA cross-links; these then exert effects throughout the cell cycle. Cisplatin (i.e., *cis*-diamminedichloroplatinum), carboplatin (i.e., *cis*-diammine-cyclobutanedicarboxylatoplatinum), and oxaliplatin are members of this class of chemotherapeutic agents.

The toxicities of cisplatin are primarily myelosuppression, nausea, vomiting, peripheral neuropathy, sensorineural ototoxicity, hypokalemia, hypomagnesemia, and, renal failure, which is the most feared. The potential for severe and protracted nausea and vomiting, which occurs in almost every patient treated with cisplatin and lasts for several days after administration, has been considerably ameliorated by modern antiemetic therapies (e.g., serotonin [5-HT$_3$] receptor antagonists, neurokinin receptor antagonists, dexamethasone); approximately 70% of individuals treated with cisplatin-based chemotherapy regimens today experience no nausea or vomiting.[18,19] Aggressive hydration should be administered to prevent renal insufficiency or failure, which may become irreversible. As a result of hydration and electrolyte-replacement concerns for patients with head and neck cancer, who are already prone to dehydration as a result of disease or mucosal toxicity resulting from radiotherapy, the outpatient administration of cisplatin is challenging. Nevertheless, cisplatin is among the most active agents for the treatment of solid tumors, including those of head and neck cancer. It has systemic anticancer effects, and it also induces the potent radiosensitization of cancer cells.

Unlike cisplatin, carboplatin, which is generally associated with less nausea, vomiting, nephrotoxicity, and neurotoxicity, is easily administered in outpatient settings. Myelosuppression, nausea, and vomiting are potential toxicities. Although cisplatin is generally considered to be a more active systemic agent than carboplatin, there is no clinical evidence to support any difference in radiosensitization properties between the two drugs.

Alkylating Agents

Alkylating agents were the earliest class of chemotherapeutic agents discovered, and they remain in clinical use. Both cyclophosphamide and its isomer, ifosfamide, exert anticancer effects by alkylating DNA. In addition to causing myelosuppression, nausea, and vomiting, the urinary metabolites of these agents can induce bladder-wall irritation and cause hemorrhagic cystitis. The prevention of hemorrhagic cystitis requires adequate intravenous hydration and the administration of mesna (i.e., sodium 2-mercaptoethane sulfonate), an agent that binds and detoxifies these metabolites. Ifosfamide has been employed in aggressive combination chemotherapy regimens for head and neck cancer.

Peptides

Bleomycin is a small peptide that intercalates within DNA strands and results in single- and double-strand DNA breaks. Although bleomycin is an active agent in head and neck cancer, both the feared potential toxicity of pulmonary fibrosis and the development of other active agents for the treatment of head and neck cancer have not increased its use in modern chemotherapy regimens.

Antimetabolites

Antimetabolites interfere with the key metabolic pathways of tumor cells. These agents are thought to exert effects specific to the S-phase (i.e., the DNA synthesis phase) of the cell cycle.

5-Fluorouracil (5-FU) is a fluorinated nucleoside analogue of uracil that inhibits the thymidylate synthase enzyme, which interferes with thymine incorporation into replicating DNA. Methotrexate is an antifolate compound that inhibits the dihydrofolate reductase enzyme. Although both agents have low emetogenic potential, toxicities of these agents include myelosuppression, mucositis, and diarrhea.

Because 5-FU is commonly administered as a 24-hour continuous infusion, outpatient administration requires the placement of central venous access devices (e.g., peripherally inserted central catheter lines, port-a-caths).

Combination regimens of 5-FU with cisplatin have demonstrated high rates of clinical response in both previously untreated and recurrent disease.[20–26] The most commonly used combination regimen involves the administration of 80 mg/m^2 to 120 mg/m^2 of cisplatin on day 1 followed by a 5-day continuous infusion of 5-FU at 1000 mg/m^2/day.

Methotrexate as a single agent has considerable activity against head and neck cancer. The standard dose and schedule for palliative treatment (40–50 mg/m^2/week) is tolerable, and it is as active as cisplatin used as a single agent.[27–29] Much more aggressive doses in combination with the leucovorin rescue of myelosuppression have not been found to be more effective in randomized studies.[30]

Hydroxyurea, which is an inhibitor of ribonucleotide reductase, is an orally bioavailable agent. Although hydroxyurea has no proven systemic activity for the treatment of head and neck cancer, it is a potent radiosensitizer.[31]

Gemcitabine, which is a difluorinated analogue of deoxycytidine that is active in non–small-cell lung cancer, bladder cancer, and other malignancies, has not shown encouraging results in phase II studies of patients with head and neck cancer with recurrent disease.[32,33] Despite apparent poor systemic activity, however, it is considered a very potent radiosensitizing agent in head and neck cancer.[34]

Topoisomerase Inhibitors

Topoisomerase inhibitors inhibit DNA replication. Members of the camptothecin family, topotecan and irinotecan, are inhibitors of the topoisomerase I enzyme. Etoposide (i.e., VP-16) is an inhibitor of the topoisomerase II enzyme. Doxorubicin (Adriamycin) has antitopoisomerase II activity.

Taxanes

The taxanes are a relatively new class of anticancer agents that interfere with microtubule function. Microtubules, which are complexes of tubulin proteins, assemble (i.e., polymerize) and disassemble (i.e., depolymerize) throughout the cell cycle; these functions are critical to cell division and migration. Paclitaxel (Taxol), the first member of this class, binds to polymerized tubulin and inhibits microtubule depolymerization, resulting in cell-cycle arrest during the G2/M phase of the cell cycle (i.e., the metaphase–anaphase boundary). Docetaxel (Taxotere) has a greater affinity for tubulin than paclitaxel, and it also promotes microtubule stabilization. The taxanes are considered to be among the most active chemotherapeutic agents against head and neck cancers, with both systemic and radiosensitizing properties.[35–38] Although both agents cause minimal nausea and vomiting, they are myelosuppressive, and they can be associated with hypersensitivity reactions. Additionally, paclitaxel can induce peripheral neuropathy, which can be severe and irreversible.

ACTIVITY OF CHEMOTHERAPEUTIC AGENTS IN HEAD AND NECK CANCER

Table 15-1 presents the systemic-disease response rates of cytotoxic chemotherapies in clinical trials of individuals with recurrent or metastatic squamous cell carcinoma of the head and neck. It is important to note that the variability in response rates is associated with the extent of prior patient therapy. Of special note is that previously untreated head and neck cancer is a remarkably chemosensitive disease. However, the response rates of recurrent or metastatic head and neck cancer in

TABLE 15-1 Response Rates of Chemotherapeutic Agents in Recurrent or Metastatic Squamous Cell Carcinoma of the Head and Neck

	Response Rate (%)
Single Agents	
Methotrexate[27–30]	10–30
Cisplatin[23,24,27,39]	10–30
Carboplatin[40]	24
5-FU[23]	13
Paclitaxel[37,41]	13–40
Docetaxel[38]	32
Gemcitabine[32,33]	0–13
Vinorelbine[42,43]	7–14
Combinations	
Cisplatin + 5-FU[20–26]	27–72
Cisplatin + Paclitaxel[26–44]	26–36
Paclitaxel + Carbo[45,46]	20–30
Docetaxel + Cisplatin[47]	40
Triplets	
Pac + Ifos + Carbo[48]	59
Pac + Ifos + Cis[49]	58
Docetaxel + Cis + 5-FU[50,51]	40–44

5-FU, 5-Fluorouracil; *Carbo,* carboplatin; *Cis,* Cisplatin; *Ifos,* ifosfamide; *Pac,* paclitaxel.

patients with either distant metastases or unresectable local disease after the failure of primary radiotherapy/chemoradiotherapy are generally dismal. A critical review of the published literature for patient populations tested in clinical trials is therefore necessary.

Although combinations of chemotherapeutics are associated with greater response rates as compared with single agents, their toxicity is greater.[23] Unfortunately, no survival improvement for patients with recurrent or metastatic head and neck cancer has been demonstrated with more aggressive combinations. The role of chemotherapy in this setting is only palliative. The largest strides in this field have been in curative combinations of chemotherapy with radiotherapy.

Biologic Therapies

A growing understanding of tumor and molecular biology has led to the rational development of novel and active anticancer drugs with increasingly tolerable toxicity profiles, and several agents have shown activity in patients with head and neck cancer.

Among the most studied biologic anticancer targets has been the epidermal growth factor receptor (EGFR), a cell-surface receptor with tyrosine kinase activity involved in signal transduction pathways that relate to cell proliferation, survival, and angiogenesis. It is overexpressed in approximately 90% of head and neck cancers. This overexpression is associated with the progression of the carcinogenesis of head and neck cancer, and it is associated with a worsened prognosis, thereby making it an attractive target for the development of anticancer therapy.[52]

Although several agents targeting the EGFR are under active clinical investigation, the most studied agents have been gefitinib (i.e., ZD 1839, IRESSA), erlotinib (i.e., OSI-774, Tarceva), and cetuximab (i.e., C225, Erbitux). Both gefitinib and erlotinib are small-molecule, orally bioavailable inhibitors of the EGFR tyrosine kinase. Cetuximab is a chimeric human and mouse monoclonal antibody that tightly binds to the EGFR, thereby preventing the binding of its ligand (i.e., epidermal growth factor) and resulting in the internalization and downregulation of the receptor. The toxicity profiles of these cytostatic agents are strikingly different from those of the cytotoxic chemotherapies. The most common toxicities of these agents are the development of an acneiform skin rash and diarrhea, which are usually tolerable but can be severe. For as-yet-unknown reasons, the severity of the skin rash appears to be associated with disease response and survival for both erlotinib and gefitinib but not for cetuximab.[53–55] Cetuximab administration has rarely been associated with severe, sometimes life-threatening hypersensitivity reactions.

TABLE 15-2 Single-Agent Activity of Biologic Agents Targeting the Epidermal Growth Factor Receptor in Patients With Recurrent or Metastatic Squamous Cell Carcinoma of the Head and Neck

Single Agents	No. of Patients	Response Rate	Disease Control	Median Survival
Gefitinib (ZD 1839, Iressa)[53]	52	10.6%	53%	8.1 months
Erlotinib (OSI-774, Tarceva)[54]	115	4.5%	38%	6 months
Cetuximab (C225, Erbitux)[55]	103	12%	53%	5.9 months

Table 15-2 presents the single-agent activity of these therapies for patients with recurrent or metastatic head and neck cancer. Although clinical response rates are modest, it is important to note that they are not dissimilar to the activity of the previously mentioned cytotoxic agents in this patient population. However, the rates of disease stabilization and disease control are much higher, and they may be clinically meaningful for this incurable patient population. Furthermore, the tolerable toxicity profiles of these agents allow them to be combined safely with other chemotherapies; several such combinations are being investigated in clinical trials. Recently presented results of one randomized combination therapy have demonstrated, for the first time, a significant survival benefit associated with adding cetuximab to first-line platinum-based chemotherapy for patients with recurrent and metastatic disease.[56] There is considerable hope for integrating these relatively less toxic agents with radiotherapy regimens for the treatment of primary disease.

The first and most thoroughly studied biologic therapy combined with radiation (i.e., bioradiotherapy) to date is cetuximab, a monoclonal antibody that has high affinity for the EGFR; this combination prevents the binding of ligand to the EGFR and induces receptor downregulation. Preclinical evidence suggested the cetuximab-induced enhancement of the cytotoxic effects of radiotherapy in squamous cell carcinomas, and early clinical feasibility studies suggested that the regimen was well tolerated and active.[57] These encouraging results led to the first randomized study of bioradiotherapy in head and neck cancer, which was published in 2006.[58] A total of 424 patients with untreated, locoregionally advanced, stage III and IV head and neck cancer were randomly assigned to treatment with definitive radiotherapy or to radiotherapy with cetuximab.

Cetuximab was administered 1 week before radiotherapy as a 400 mg/m^2 intravenous loading dose, followed by weekly infusions at 250 mg/m^2 for the duration of radiotherapy. The median duration of locoregional disease control and progression-free survival was significantly greater in the cetuximab arm, and the median survival of patients was nearly doubled (i.e., 49 months vs. 29.3 months; hazard ratio (HR) = 0.74 [95% confidence interval, 0.57–0.97]; P = .03). The regimen was well tolerated; more frequently observed toxicities in the cetuximab plus radiotherapy arm included generally tolerable acneiform rash and potentially serious but uncommon infusion-related hypersensitivity reactions. The incidence of other serious (i.e., ≥grade 3) toxic events, including mucositis, did not differ significantly between the treatment arms.

Although the study has been criticized for not including a chemoradiotherapy arm and for allowing sites to select a radiotherapy regimen (i.e., once-daily fractions, twice-daily fractions, or concomitant boost), it represents the first effort to clearly demonstrate the radiosensitization of head and neck cancers induced by biologic therapies; this observation is likely to be demonstrated with other future therapies. Randomized studies comparing chemoradiotherapy with cetuximab plus radiation are warranted, and several clinical trials are investigating the incorporation of cetuximab in combination with chemoradiotherapy regimens.[59] The future of bioradiotherapy, therefore, appears to be very bright.

SUPPORTIVE CARE

The curative potential of existing therapies in head and neck cancer is limited by the morbidity that is associated with therapy. The administration of modern combination chemotherapy regimens and combinations with radiotherapy have been made possible with advances in supportive care. Although erythropoietic agents and granulocyte-colony stimulating factor use can prevent the myelosuppression associated with chemotherapy, their use in combination with radiotherapy is controversial.[60] Antiemetic therapy has additionally improved with the development of long-acting 5-HT$_3$ antagonists (e.g., palanosetron) and neurokinin antagonists (e.g., aprepitant). The prevention of radiotherapy-induced xerostomia has improved with newer radiation technologies (e.g., intensity-modulated radiation therapy) and with the use of amifostine.[61] However, mucositis and dysphagia remain common results of chemoradiotherapy, and the prevention of these toxicities has not been addressed. The use of recombinant keratinocyte growth factor to prevent mucositis is under clinical investigation, but concerns exist regarding its potential for promoting tumor growth. Improvements in supportive care for patients with this disease cannot come at a cost of sacrificing outcomes.

HOPE OF CHEMOPREVENTION

The term *chemoprevention,* which was coined by Dr. Michael Sporn in 1976, applies to therapeutic agents that are able to reverse, suppress, or prevent the development of disease.[62] Although great success in cancer chemoprevention has been documented in the adjuvant treatment of early-stage breast cancer with hormonal therapies in patients with appropriate receptor status, no such therapeutic agent has yet been found for head and neck cancer prevention. Of considerable concern is the high incidence of tumor recurrence and the development of second primary tumors, which are the leading causes of mortality among head and neck cancer patients. Although several natural and synthetic agents (e.g., α-tocopherol, beta-carotene, 13-*cis*-retinoic acid) have been studied, none have proven to consistently demonstrate effectiveness and tolerability, which are the characteristics of an ideal chemopreventive agent.[63–65] Although it is beyond the scope of this chapter to critically review these studies, the future of chemoprevention in head and neck cancer will depend on the selection of appropriate biomarkers of disease that can be targeted with specific therapies. It is hoped that ongoing studies of maintenance biologic therapies (after curative-intent treatment of primary disease) will lead to the next generation of chemoprevention research in head and neck cancer.

CONCLUSION

The development of potentially organ-preserving nonsurgical therapies in head and neck cancer has revolutionized the treatment of this disease and been a model for the nonsurgical management of other cancers. Although significant advances in care have been made, the future of head and neck cancer treatment will ultimately depend on agents and treatment plans that maximize cure while minimizing morbidity. The clinical development of biologic radiosensitizing agents and advances in supportive care are consistent with that goal. To that end, careful attention to organ functionality and quality-of-life issues is needed for all future studies of this disease. Treatment decisions and supportive care for individual patients will continue to be multidisciplinary challenges.

REFERENCES

1. Wolf GT, Hong WK, Fisher SG, et al: Department of Veterans Affairs Laryngeal Cancer Study Group: Induction chemotherapy plus radiation compared with surgery plus radiation in patients with advanced laryngeal cancer. *N Engl J Med* 1991;324: 1685–1690.
2. Lefebvre JL, Chevalier D, Luboinski B, et al: Larynx preservation in pyriform sinus cancer: Preliminary results of an European Organization for Research and Treatment of Cancer phase III trial. *J Natl Cancer Inst* 1996;88:890–899.
3. Adelstein DJ, Sharan VM, Earle AS, et al: Simultaneous versus sequential combined technique therapy for squamous cell head and neck cancer. *Cancer* 1990;65:1685–1691.
4. Merlano M, Benasso M, Corvo R, et al: Five-year update of a randomized trial of alternating radiotherapy and chemotherapy compared with radiotherapy alone in the treatment of unresectable squamous cell carcinoma of the head and neck. *J Natl Cancer Inst* 1996;88:583–589.
5. Al-Sarraf M, LeBlanc M, Giri PG, et al: Chemoradiotherapy versus radiotherapy in patients with advanced nasopharyngeal cancer: Phase III randomized Intergroup Study 0099. *J Clin Oncol* 1998;16:1310–1317.
6. Wendt TG, Grabenbauer GG, Rodel CM, et al: Simultaneous radiochemotherapy versus radiotherapy alone in advanced head and neck cancer: A randomized multicenter study. *J Clin Oncol* 1998;16:1318–1324.
7. Calais G, Alfonsi M, Bardet E, et al: Randomized trial of radiation therapy versus concomitant chemotherapy and radiation therapy for advanced-stage oropharynx carcinoma. *J Natl Cancer Inst* 1999;91:2081–2086.
8. Forastiere AA, Goepfert H, Maor M, et al: Concurrent chemotherapy and radiotherapy for organ preservation in advanced laryngeal cancer. *N Engl J Med* 2003;349:2091–2098.
9. Bernier J, Domenge C, Ozsahin M, et al: Postoperative irradiation with or without concomitant chemotherapy for locally advanced head and neck cancer. *N Engl J Med* 2004;350:1945–1952.
10. Cooper JA, Pajak TF, Forastiere AA, et al: Postoperative concurrent radiotherapy and chemotherapy for high-risk squamous cell carcinoma of the head and neck. *N Engl J Med* 2004;350: 1937–1944.
11. Fu KK, Phillips TL: Biologic rationale of combined radiotherapy and chemotherapy. *Hematol Oncol Clin North Am* 1991;5: 737–751.
12. Argiris A, Haraf DJ, Kies MS, et al: Intensive concurrent chemoradiotherapy for head and neck cancer with 5-fluorouracil- and hydroxyurea-based regimens: Reversing a pattern of failure. *Oncologist* 2003;8:350–360.
13. Kies MS, Haraf DJ, Athanasiadis I, et al: Induction chemotherapy followed by concurrent chemoradiation for advanced head and neck cancer: Improved disease control and survival. *J Clin Oncol* 1998;16:2715–2721.
14. Machtay M, Rosenthal DI, Hershock D, et al: Organ preservation therapy using induction plus concurrent chemoradiation for advanced resectable oropharyngeal carcinoma: A University of Pennsylvania Phase II Trial. *J Clin Oncol* 2002;20:3964–3971.
15. Hitt R, Lopez-Pousa A, Martinez-Trufero J, et al: Phase III study comparing cisplatin plus fluorouracil to paclitaxel, cisplatin, and fluorouracil induction chemotherapy followed by chemoradiotherapy in locally advanced head and neck cancer. *J Clin Oncol* 2005;23:8636–8645.
16. Posner MR, Hershock DM, Blajman CR, et al: cisplatin and fluorouracil alone or with docetaxel in head and neck cancer. *N Engl J Med* 2007;357:1705–1715.
17. Rosenberg B, VanCamp L., Trosko J, et al: Platinum compounds: A new class of potent antitumor agents. *Nature* 1969;222:385.
18. de Witt R, Heerstedt T, Rapoport B, et al: Addition of the oral NK1 antagonist aprepitant to standard antiemetics provides protection against nausea and vomiting during multiple cycles of cisplatin-based chemotherapy. *J Clin Oncol* 2003;21:4105–4111.
19. Hesketh PJ, Grunberg SM, Gralla RJ, et al: The oral neurokinin-1 antagonist aprepitant for the prevention of chemotherapy-induced

nausea and vomiting: A multinational, randomized, double-blind, placebo-controlled trial in patients receiving high-dose cisplatin—The Aprepitant Protocol 052 Study Group. *J Clin Oncol* 2003;21:4112–4119.

20. Al-Sarraf M: Chemotherapeutic management of head and neck cancer. *Cancer Metastasis Rev* 1987;6:181–198.

21. Kish JA, Weaver A, Jacobs J, et al: Cisplatin and 5-fluorouracil infusion in patients with recurrent and disseminated epidermoid cancer of the head and neck. *Cancer* 1984;53:1819–1824.

22. Forastiere AA, Metch B, Schuller DE, et al: Randomized comparison of cisplatin plus fluorouracil and carboplatin plus fluorouracil versus methotrexate in advanced squamous cell carcinoma of the head and neck: A Southwest Oncology Group Study. *J Clin Oncol* 1992;10:1245–1251.

23. Jacobs C, Lyman G, Velez-Garcia E, et al: A phase III randomized study comparing cisplatin and fluorouracil as single agents and in combination for advanced squamous cell carcinoma of the head and neck. *J Clin Oncol* 1992;10:257–263.

24. Clavel M, Vermorken JB, Cognetti F, et al: Randomized comparison of cisplatin, methotrexate, bleomycin and vincristine (CABO) versus cisplatin and 5-fluorouracil (CF) versus cisplatin (C) in recurrent or metastatic squamous cell carcinoma of the head and neck: A phase III study of the EORTC Head and Neck Cancer Cooperative Group. *Ann Oncol* 1994;5:521–526.

25. Schrijvers D, Johnson J, Jiminez U, et al: Phase III trial of modulation of cisplatin/fluorouracil chemotherapy by interferon alfa-2b in patients with recurrent or metastatic head and neck cancer: Head and Neck Interferon Cooperative Study Group. *J Clin Oncol* 1998;16:1054–1059.

26. Gibson MK, Li Y, Murphy B, et al: Randomized phase III evaluation of cisplatin plus fluorouracil versus cisplatin plus paclitaxel in advanced head and neck cancer (E1395): An intergroup trial of the Eastern Cooperative Oncology Group. *J Clin Oncol* 2005;23:3562–3567.

27. Hong WK, Schaefer S, Issell B, et al: A prospective randomized trial of methotrexate versus cisplatin in the treatment of recurrent squamous cell carcinoma of the head and neck. *Cancer* 1983;52:206–210.

28. Eisenberger M, Krasnow S, Ellenberg S, et al: A comparison of carboplatin plus methotrexate versus methotrexate alone in patients with recurrent and metastatic head and neck cancer. *J Clin Oncol* 1989;7:1341–1345.

29. Schornagel JH, Verweij J, de Mulder PH, et al: Randomized phase III trial of edatrexate versus methotrexate in patients with metastatic and/or recurrent squamous cell carcinoma of the head and neck: A European Organization for Research and Treatment of Cancer Head and Neck Cancer Cooperative Group Study. *J Clin Oncol* 1995;14:1649–1655.

30. Browman GP, Goodyear MD, Levine MN, et al: Modulation of the antitumor effect of methotrexate by low-dose leucovorin in squamous cell head and neck cancer: A randomized placebo-controlled clinical trial. *J Clin Oncol* 1990;8:203–208.

31. Beitler JJ, Smith RV, Owen RP, et al: Phase II trial of parenteral hydroxyurea and hyperfractionated, accelerated external beam radiation therapy in patients with advanced squamous cell carcinoma of the head and neck: Toxicity and efficacy with continuous ribonucleoside reductase inhibition. *Head Neck* 2007;29:18–25.

32. Catimel G, Vermorken JB, Clavel M, et al: A phase II study of Gemcitabine (LY188011) in patients with advanced squamous cell carcinoma of the head and neck: EORTC Early Clinical Trials Group. *Ann Oncol* 1994;5:543–547.

33. Samlowski WE, Gundacker H, Kuebler JP, et al: Evaluation of gemcitabine in patients with recurrent or metastatic squamous cell carcinoma of the head and neck: A Southwest Oncology Group phase II study. *Invest New Drugs* 2001;19:311–315.

34. Eisbruch A, Shewach DS, Bradford CR, et al: Radiation concurrent with gemcitabine for locally advanced head and neck cancer: A phase I trial and intracellular drug incorporation study. *J Clin Oncol* 2001;19:792–799.

35. Elomaa L, Joensuu H, Kulmala T, et al: Squamous cell carcinoma is highly sensitive to Taxol, a possible new radiation sensitizer. *Acta Otolaryngol (Stockh)* 1995;115:340–344.

36. Gan Y, Wientjes MG, Schuller DE, et al: Pharmacodynamics of Taxol in human head and neck tumors. *Cancer Res* 1996;56:2086–2093.

37. Forastiere AA, Shank D, Neuberg D, et al: Final report of a phase II evaluation of paclitaxel in patients with advanced squamous cell carcinomas of the head and neck: An Eastern Cooperative Group trial (PA390). *Cancer* 1998;82:2270–2274.

38. Catimel G, Verweij J, Mattijssen V, et al: Docetaxel (Taxotere): An active drug for the treatment of patients with advanced squamous cell carcinoma of the head and neck: EORTC Early Clinical Trials Group. *Ann Oncol* 1994;5:533–537.

39. Burtness B, Goldwasser MA, Flood W, et al: Phase III randomized trial of cisplatin plus placebo compared with cisplatin plus cetuximab in metastatic/recurrent head and neck cancer: An Eastern Cooperative Oncology Group study. *J Clin Oncol* 2005;23:8646–8654.

40. Al-Sarraf M, Metch B, Kish J, et al: Platinum analogs in recurrent and advanced head and neck cancer: A Southwest Oncology Group and Wayne State University Study. *Cancer Treat Rep* 1987;71:723–726.

41. Langer CJ, Li Y, Jennings T, et al: Phase II evaluation of 96-hour paclitaxel infusion in advanced (recurrent or metastatic) squamous cell carcinoma of the head and neck (E3395): A trial of the Eastern Cooperative Oncology Group. *Cancer Invest* 2004;22:823–831.

42. Saxman S, Mann B, Canfield V, et al: A phase II trial of vinorelbine in patients with recurrent or metastatic squamous cell carcinoma of the head and neck. *Am J Clin Oncol* 1998;21:398–400.

43. Degardin M, Oliveira J, Geoffrois L, et al: An EORTC-ECSG phase II study of vinorelbine in patients with recurrent and/or metastatic squamous cell carcinoma of the head and neck. *Ann Oncol* 1998;9:1103–1107.

44. Forastiere AA, Leong T, Rowinsky E, et al: Phase III comparison of high dose paclitaxel + cisplatin + granulocyte colony stimulating factor versus low dose paclitaxel + cisplatin in advanced head and neck cancer: Eastern Cooperative Oncology Group Study E1393. *J Clin Oncol* 2001;19:1088–1095.

45. Clark JI, Hofmeister C, Choudhury A, et al: Phase II evaluation of paclitaxel in combination with carboplatin in advanced head and neck carcinoma. *Cancer* 2001;92:2334–2340.

46. Pivot X, Cais L, Cupissol D, et al: Phase II trial of a paclitaxel-carboplatin combination in recurrent squamous cell carcinoma of the head and neck. *Oncology* 2001;60:66–71.

47. Glisson BS, Murphy BA, Frenette G, et al: Phase II trial of docetaxel and cisplatin combination chemotherapy in patients with squamous cell carcinoma of the head and neck. *J Clin Oncol* 2002;20:1593–1599.

48. Shin DM, Khuri FR, Glisson BS, et al: Phase II study of paclitaxel, ifosfamide, and carboplatin in patients with recurrent or metastatic head and neck squamous cell carcinoma. *Cancer* 2001;91:1316–1323.

49. Shin DM, Glisson BS, Khuri FR, et al: Phase II trial of paclitaxel, ifosfamide, and cisplatin in patients with recurrent head and neck squamous cell carcinoma. *J Clin Oncol* 1998;16:1325–1330.

50. Janinis J, Papadakou M, Xidakis E, et al: Combination chemotherapy with docetaxel, cisplatin, and 5-fluorouracil in previously treated patients with advanced/recurrent head and neck cancer: A phase II feasibility study. *Am J Clin Oncol* 2000;23:128–131.

51. Baghi M, Hambek M, Wagenblast J, et al: A phase II trial of docetaxel, cisplatin, and 5-fluorouracil in patients with recurrent squamous cell carcinoma of the head and neck (SCCHN). *Anticancer Res* 2006;26:585–590.

52. Kalyankrishna S, Grandis JR: Epidermal growth factor receptor biology in head and neck cancer. *J Clin Oncol* 2006;24:2666–2672.

53. Cohen EEW, Rosen F, Stadler WM, et al: Phase II trial of ZD1839 in recurrent or metastatic squamous cell carcinoma of the head and neck. *J Clin Oncol* 2003;21:1980–1987.

54. Soulieres D, Senzer NN, Vokes EE, et al: Multicenter phase II study of erlotinib, an oral epidermal growth factor receptor tyrosine kinase inhibitor, in patients with recurrent or metastatic squamous cell carcinoma of the head and neck. *J Clin Oncol* 2004;22:77–85.

55. Trigo J, Hitt R, Koralewski P, et al: Cetuximab monotherapy is active in patients (pts) with platinum-refractory recurrent/ metastatic squamous cell carcinoma of the head and neck (SCCHN): Results of a Phase II study. *Proc Am Soc Clin Oncol* 2004;22:5502a.

56. Vermorken J, Mesia R, Vega V, et al: Cetuximab extends survival of patients with recurrent or metastatic SCCHN when added to first line platinum based therapy—results of a randomized phase III (Extreme) study. *Proc Am Soc Clin Oncol* 2007;25:abstr 6091.

57. Huang SM, Harari PM: Anti-EGF receptor monoclonal antibody (C225) inhibits proliferation and enhances radiation sensitivity in human squamous cell carcinoma of the head and neck. *Head Neck* 1998;20:457.

58. Bonner JA, Harari PM, Giralt J, et al: Radiotherapy plus cetuximab for squamous cell carcinoma of the head and neck. *N Engl J Med* 2006;354:567–578.

59. Pfister DG, Su YB, Kraus DH, et al: Concurrent cetuximab, cisplatin, and concomitant boost radiotherapy for locoregionally advanced, squamous cell head and neck cancer: A pilot phase II study of a new combined-modality paradigm. *J Clin Oncol* 2006;24:1072–1078.

60. Henke M, Laszig R, Rube C, et al: Erythropoietin to treat head and neck cancer patients with anaemia undergoing radiotherapy: Randomised, double-blind, placebo-controlled trial. *Lancet* 2003;362:1255–1260.

61. Brizel DM, Wasserman TH, Henke M, et al: Phase III randomized trial of amifostine as a radioprotector in head and neck cancer. *J Clin Oncol* 2000;18:3339–3345.

62. Sporn MB: Approaches to prevention of epithelial cancer during the preneoplastic period. *Cancer Res* 1976;36:2699–2702.

63. Hong WK, Lippman SM, Itri LM, et al: Prevention of second primary tumors with isotretinoin in squamous-cell carcinoma of the head and neck. *N Engl J Med* 1990;323:795–801.

64. Benner SE, Pajak TF, Lippman SM, et al: Prevention of second primary tumors with isotretinoin in patients with squamous cell carcinoma of the head and neck: Long term follow up. *J Natl Cancer Inst* 1994;86:140–141.

65. Bairati I, Meyer F, Gelinas M, et al: A randomized trial of antioxidant vitamins to prevent second primary cancers in head and neck cancer patients. *J Natl Cancer Inst* 2005;97:481–488.

CHAPTER 16

Pain Management for Head and Neck Surgery

Tracey Straker

Maximized pain control includes the restoration of physical, emotional, and occupational function. The treatment regimen may include pharmacology, physiotherapy, and, when pain is refractory, interventional pain techniques.[1] The upper cervical components of the spinomesencephalic tract cells and cranial nerves V, VI, VII (nervus intermedius), IX, and X are involved in the mechanisms of acute and chronic pain from head, face, and neck structures.[2]

To format an effective pain management regimen, there must be a constant evaluation of the pain. The determination of whether pain is nociceptive or neuropathic must be recognized. *Nociceptive pain* is somatic or visceral pain, and *neuropathic pain* is a continuous dysesthesia or chronic lancinating or paroxysmal pain. Nociceptive pain is the result of actual or potential tissue damage (tumor). Somatic pain presents as aching, throbbing, or stabbing sensations, and its source is skin, muscle, or bone. Nociceptive pain is usually responsive to nonopioid analgesics. Visceral pain is usually related to internal organs and will not be discussed in this chapter.

NEUROPATHIC PAIN

Neuropathic pain has two distinctive types. The first consists of continuous dysesthesias, which are characterized by continuous burning and electrical sensations. The second type is chronic lancinating or paroxysmal pain, which is described as a sharp, stabbing, shooting, knifelike pain of sudden onset. [3]

Neuropathic pain involves peripheral or central afferent neural pathways. The terms *neuropathic, neurogenic,* and *deafferentation* have been used synonymously to describe pain associated with evidence of peripheral nerve involvement by a tumor. Patients suffering from neuropathic pain frequently respond poorly to opioids. These patients frequently respond to tricyclic antidepressants and anticonvulsants.[4] Drug therapy is the cornerstone of cancer pain management as a result of its efficacy, its rapid onset of action, and its relatively low cost. Opioids can be differentiated according to the categories of receptors that they preferentially occupy and activate. Cancer pain is an indicator for an opioid that is primarily a μ-receptor agonist. Drug therapy that follows the World Health Organization (WHO) or the treatment described by the American Pain Society is the mainstay of cancer pain management.[5,6]

The WHO has described an effective three-step ladder for the relief of cancer pain:

- Step 1—Mild to moderate pain: nonopioid ± adjuvant drug
- Step 2—Moderate to severe pain: opioid ± adjuvant drug
- Step 3—Severe pain: opioid ± adjuvant drug

Step One: Mild to Moderate Pain (Nonopioid ± Adjuvant Drug)

Drugs in this category include nonsteroidal anti-inflammatory drugs (NSAIDs) and acetaminophen. They are excellent for treating mild to moderate pain, especially when administered in a time-contingent manner. Their primary mechanism of action is the inhibition of the enzyme complex cyclooxygenase (COX). This mechanism of action results in the reduced synthesis of prostaglandins in the periphery, which is important as prostaglandins increase sensitization to nociceptors.

During the late 1990s, several COX-2–specific inhibitors were introduced that have a more limited interference with the protective effects of prostaglandins on stomach mucosa and platelet function. During the mid 2000s, several COX-2 inhibitors were removed from the market as a result of their association with myocardial infarction. Complications of COX-2 inhibitors are increased cardiovascular risks, nephrotoxicity, hepatic dysfunction, increased warfarin levels, and possible wound-healing problems.[7] A powerful nonopioid pain management agent was also removed when several of the COX-2 inhibitors were removed from the market. Subsequently, naproxen is now the NSAID of choice for outpatient chronic pain management, because it is not associated with excess cardiovascular risks. Patients with high cardiovascular and gastrointestinal risks should avoid using NSAIDs or COX-2 inhibitors. Ketorolac is administered intravenously and by mouth for short durations of acute pain. NSAIDs are especially effective for the management of bone pain and therefore play a major role in the management of cancer pain.[8]

Step Two: Moderate to Severe Pain (Opioid ± Adjuvant Drug)

The second step of the ladder requires the addition of codeine or a codeine analog of the drug. Codeine, oxycodone, and hydrocodone are commercially available, and they are used most commonly in fixed-dose combinations with acetaminophen or aspirin. These combinations limit the effective doses of codeine or oxycodone that can be used because of the toxic effects of high doses of the nonopioid drug. A preferred method is to administer the selected nonopioid drug on a time-contingent basis and to titrate the opioid dosage while administering it separately. Over-the-counter medications are a significant source of aspirin and acetaminophen in the United States. The major complications of acetaminophen and aspirin, respectively, are hepatotoxicity and gastrointestinal upset.

Acetaminophen is dangerous because of its effects on the liver, which is responsible for metabolizing drugs. When toxic levels of acetaminophen occur in the liver, the natural antioxidant defenses of the body are overwhelmed, and the liver is damaged by the buildup of dangerous free radicals. People who are taking acetaminophen should also take sufficient quantities of antioxidants to help support liver function. Complications of aspirin include gastrointestinal tract damage, altered kidney function, the inhibition of platelet function, and bleeding.[9]

Step Three: Severe Pain (Opioid ± Adjuvant Drug)

Codeine or a congener is replaced with a more effective opioid, usually morphine. Morphine, hydromorphone, and methadone are commonly used opioids. The dosage of the opioid is individualized for each patient and requires adjustment over time. Analgesic potency varies among opioids, but analgesia can be obtained with most drugs in this class. Morphine has long been considered the gold standard of opioid agents, and it is the most commonly used for the treatment of pain. Morphine has a linear dose-response curve with a broad therapeutic range. Therefore low-dose morphine may be appropriate when the pain is not advanced, and high-dose morphine may be used as the pain progresses. Controlled-release morphine is available for 8-, 12- and 24-hour dosing. Controlled-release oral opioid formulations must not be altered or damaged. Tablets should not be crushed, broken, or chewed but rather swallowed whole; otherwise large doses intended for slow absorption will be absorbed in a considerably shorter period of time, which may cause overdose and possibly death. The side effects of morphine include a decreased respiratory rate, weakness, dizziness, allergic reactions, seizures, constipation, nausea, vomiting, a decreased appetite, oliguria, a decreased sexual drive, possible unconsciousness, and addiction.[10]

Hydromorphone is a semisynthetic opioid that is more potent than morphine and that, like oxycodone, has been used as an alternative to morphine in patients with reactions or tolerance to morphine. Long-acting formulations of hydromorphone are not presently available in the United States. However, the development of controlled-release hydromorphone is currently under way for the American market. Hydromorphone in other formulations is available in the United States and has been used for the treatment of chronic pain.

Fentanyl, which is a semisynthetic opioid, is 100 times more potent than morphine. It is much more expensive than morphine and methadone. Fentanyl has been incorporated into a transdermal delivery system, an oral lollipop, and a buccal formulation. It has been released for use for the management of chronic pain requiring opioid administration. Transdermal fentanyl is effective for the treatment of both nociceptive and neuropathic pain. It is also useful for patients in whom the oral tract is no longer available for opioid delivery or who experience adverse effects to oral morphine or methadone.[11] Methadone is a potent synthetic opioid with a rapid onset of analgesia. Methadone is suitable for treating patients with severe pain, because it is inexpensive, it is well absorbed from the gastrointestinal tract, it has no active metabolites, and it is probably not affected by hepatic or renal disease. Methadone also has antagonist activity at the N-methyl-D-aspartate (NMDA) receptor. NMDA receptors are involved in neuropathic pain syndromes and the development of opioid tolerance. Side effects of methadone include difficulty breathing, hallucinations, confusion, drowsiness, dizziness, constipation, dry mouth, anorexia, and decreased sexual drive.[1]

ADJUVANT DRUGS

Adjuvant drugs are suggested at each step of the WHO three-step analgesic ladder. Adjuvant drugs are those drugs that enhance the effects of analgesics, that have independent analgesic activity in certain pain syndromes, or that lessen other symptoms that exacerbate pain. Adjuvants include tricyclic antidepressants (TCAs), anticonvulsants, and steroids.

TCAs (e.g., amitriptyline) are recommended for patients who remain depressed despite improved pain and for those patients with neuropathic pain. TCAs are also effective for patients without depression. They have been used in patients with cancer pain, they appear to have direct analgesic effects, and they may potentiate opioid analgesia in cancer pain. The mechanism of action is unclear, but it may be through blocking the reuptake of serotonin and norepinephrine at the central nervous system synapse.[12] The most common side effects of TCAs are dry mouth, blurred vision, constipation, difficult urination, tachycardia, loss of sexual drive, erectile dysfunction, weight gain, drowsiness, nausea, dizziness, and photophobia. There is a risk that antidepressant treatment may cause an increase rather than a decrease in depression. In a 2005 Public Health Advisory, the U.S. Food and Drug Administration advised that anyone taking antidepressants should be watched for an increase in suicidal thoughts and behaviors.[13]

Anticonvulsants are used for the management of chronic neuropathic pain. Carbamazepine suppresses spontaneous neuronal firing and may be effective for the management of acute neuralgic pain, particularly pain that originates from the cranial and cervical area. Carbamazepine is helpful for the management of neuralgic cancer pain, and it may be helpful for the management of acute lancinating neuralgic pain as a result of surgical trauma or nerve destruction by tumor. Carbamazepine is associated with many side effects, and it may not be tolerated. Side effects of carbamazepine include aplastic anemia, bone-marrow suppression, agranulocytosis, urticaria, Stevens–Johnson syndrome, photosensitivity, the aggravation of systemic lupus erythematosus, congestive heart failure, edema, syncope, pneumonia, leg cramps, diarrhea, diplopia, fatigue, and renal failure.[14]

Steroids have several benefits for the cancer patient. They can lower pain perception, have a sparing effect on opioid dose, improve mood, increase appetite, and lead to weight gain. Among patients with advanced disease, steroids can improve the quality of life. However, anabolic steroids can cause many unwanted side effects. Most of the side effects are dose dependent and are caused by the chemical reaction of the steroid metabolizing into other hormones. Side effects include hypertension, hypercholesterolemia, coronary artery disease, acne, hepatotoxicity, gynecomastia, temporary infertility, decreased sexual function, testicular atrophy, decreased menses, hirsutism, and phallic enlargement.[15]

NMDA receptor antagonists have been shown to possess analgesic properties in numerous patient studies involving neuropathic pain. NMDA glutamate receptor antagonists available for clinical use in the United States include ketamine, methadone, amantidine, and dextromethorphan. There are several mechanisms by which NMDA glutamate antagonists exert their antinociceptive effects. These include the prevention and possibly the reversal of central sensitization to pain, the reduction of tolerance to opioids, synergistic analgesic effects with opioids, and preemptive analgesia when given in a timely manner. NMDA receptor antagonist affinity at the phencyclidine site has been shown to modulate pain and hyperalgesia, but this is limited by an increasing dosage. Side effects include extrapyramidal symptoms, cataplexy, confusion, dizziness, gastrointestinal symptoms, hallucinations, blurred vision, ataxia, and symptoms that are consistent with narcotic side effects.[16]

Phosphodiesterase inhibitors and caffeine possess little or no analgesic activity when administered alone. Nevertheless caffeine is a widely used analgesic adjuvant that has been shown to modestly but significantly potentiate the antinociceptive effects of opiates and NSAIDs. This capacity may be related to the ability of the methylxanthines to increase circulating catecholamines, to augment the twitch response of muscles, to constrict cerebrovascular beds, and to enhance mood. Side effects include nausea, vomiting, and gastrointestinal and cardiac symptoms.[17]

Bisphosphonates have been shown to reduce pain caused by bony metastasis. The bisphosphonates pamidronate, etidronate, and clodronate have been used for the treatment of bone pain. Bisphosphonates inhibit osteoclastic activity. They may not only induce better pain control with lytic lesions of the bones, but they may also significantly slow the progression of bone metastasis, increase bone stability, and decrease hypercalcemia. Side effects of bisphosphonates include nephrotoxicity, gastrointestinal intolerance, and osteonecrosis. Reports of bisphosphonates-associated osteonecrosis of the jaw associated with pamidronate began to surface in 2003. The majority of cases have been associated with dental procedures; however, bisphosphonate osteonecrosis appears to occur spontaneously among patients who are taking these drugs. The risk of bisphosphonate osteonecrosis is much higher for cancer patients who are receiving intravenous bisphosphonate therapy.

Calcitonin is available for intranasal, intramuscular, intravenous, or subcutaneous administration. Calcitonin is postulated to reduce bone resorption and increase circulating endogenous opioids, and it acts as an endorphin-receptor agonist. Calcitonin is a polypeptide hormone that is secreted by the parafollicular cells of the thyroid gland. It enables the bones to retain more of their mass and functionality by inhibiting the bone-tissue resorbing activity of osteoclasts. Calcitonin is involved in the regulation of calcium and the decrease of bone loss and fractures. Calcitonin derived from salmon is estimated to be about 30 times more potent than the human version. Synthetic salmon calcitonin, which is identical to the natural salmon calcitonin, is available only as nasal or injectable therapy. This agent is less effective than other adjuvant medications, and it must be taken for several weeks before it becomes effective. Calcitonin is well tolerated and has minimal side effects.[18]

Consideration should be given to α-adrenergic antagonists such as clonidine for the treatment of neuropathic pain. Antispasmodics such as cyclobenzaprine can be used for spasticity and neuropathy. Cannabinoids may be used for pain relief, nausea, and vomiting.[19]

No pain management chapter would be complete without the mention of herbal alternatives. According to traditional Chinese medicine, the fundamental cause of pain is *qi* (the Chinese vital life force) stagnation, blood stagnation, or both. Effective pain relief most often requires the use of herbs that activate both *qi* and blood, thereby removing stagnation and resolving pain.

Corydalis is an herb used for the treatment of both acute and chronic neck and shoulder pain. In addition to having strong analgesic properties, it also has the ability to treat the acute and chronic changes of inflammation. White peony has demonstrated properties that relieve spasms, cramps, and pain in skeletal and smooth muscle. However, white peony pills have been associated with high levels of lead, which may accumulate in vital organs. Side effects may include headache, dullness, restlessness, irritability, poor attention span, muscle tremor, hallucinations, memory loss, weight loss, cerebral edema, paralysis, and renal toxicity.[20–22] Clinical applications include trigeminal pain, muscle spasms, and twitching in the facial region.

To date there is no reliable treatment for refractory pain from the head and neck structures. Invasive therapeutic pain regimens have been investigated, but many times the complications and side effects outweigh the benefits of the procedure. Numerous invasive techniques have been used in an attempt to treat patients with refractory head and neck pain. Therapies such as intracisternal or intraventricular injections of morphine, neurolysis of the gasserian ganglion and other cranial nerves, rhizotomy, cordotomy, and thalamotomy often provide inadequate pain relief or produce unacceptable side effects. In one study, control of pain was attempted with the injection of phenol into the cisterna magna. Eighteen percent of patients had long-lasting disabling neurologic deficits, and 71% had less severe complications. More extensive neoplastic disease that causes severe pain has been treated by performing a posterior craniotomy and sectioning the roots of cranial nerves VII, IX, and X and the sensory roots of the upper cranial nerves. Many patients cannot tolerate a major operation, and sectioning of the glossopharyngeal and vagus nerves produces paralysis of the pharyngeal and laryngeal muscles.[23]

Neurolytic procedures for the management of cancer pain have been attempted for years, but destructive nerve blocks have limited their usefulness. The destruction of the sensory component cannot be accomplished without the destruction of sympathetic and motor functions as well. Neuroablative procedures attempt to interrupt pain transmission along the neuropathway. Dorsal rhizotomy involves the interruption of the sensory nerve root. It can be completed as an open surgical procedure or with the use of a neurolytic agent. Rhizotomy of the trigeminal, glossopharyngeal, and vagus nerves has been attempted for the treatment of pain involving the head and neck areas, with variable results. Side effects of rhizotomy include sensory deficits, labial herpes, chemical meningitis, infectious meningitis, hearing deficits, dysesthesias, the loss of the corneal reflex, diplopia, blurry vision, hoarseness, vocal-cord paralysis, and dysphasia. Stereotactic radiofrequency rhizotomy should be restricted to patients with cancer pain who already have dysphagia and vocal-cord paralysis.[24]

Radiosurgical Gamma Knife treatment for trigeminal nerve involvement is the least invasive surgical option. The Gamma Knife (Elekta, Stockholm, Sweden) delivers precise, controlled beams of radiation to targeted nerves. The Gamma Knife is aimed at a target near the trigeminal nerve root where it exits the brainstem. It damages the trigeminal nerve to "short circuit" the transmission of pain signals. Benefits are the blocking of sensory pathways of pain to the trigeminal nerve distributions. Complications are the possible motor loss of musculature in the trigeminal nerve distribution.[24]

In contrast with the poor results observed with the previously mentioned therapies, the technique described by Applegren and colleagues[25] provided relatively effective analgesic therapy for select patients. The authors studied 13 patients with complex refractory pain who received continuous intracisternal or high cervical subarachnoid infusions of bupivacaine as a method of pain control for the head, face, mouth, neck, and upper extremities. For most patients, infusions of bupivacaine provided satisfactory relief, decreased systemic opioid consumption, improved nocturnal sleep patterns, and improved overall function. Associated side effects were generally dose related and included orthostatic hypotension, paresis, severe tiredness, faintness, malaise, and somnolence. The approach described by these authors can be performed at a site relatively distant from the site of pain; access to the intrathecal space is from a posterior approach at the C1 or C2 vertebral location. The authors provide an interesting and thought-provoking alternative technique for pain relief in a difficult group of patients.[25] This study is too small to garner any clinical usefulness from this technique. The most appropriate venue for collecting information would be in controlled clinical studies. The potential for serious side effects can not be ignored; the placement of a catheter next to neural tissue at high cervical levels can theoretically cause severe and irreversible nerve damage.[25]

Among the more acceptable pain management interventions is the epidural spinal cord stimulator. A catheter electrode is inserted percutaneously and provides a pain-relieving effect. Recent studies show that pain relief is achieved more in the head, the face, and the upper extremities.[26]

Spinal opioid administration can be used for long-term and end-of-life pain management. A catheter is tunneled subcutaneously and exteriorized, or an implantable drug-delivery system may be used. The implantable systems can be either intrathecal or epidural, and they feature drug reservoirs or an implanted infusion device. Opioids and low concentrations of local anesthetics may be used.[27] Complications include transient paresis, vertebral artery embolus, subdural hematoma, and spinal-cord injury.

Occipital nerve block is used to treat occipital headaches, which are sometimes the manifestation of basal-skull invasion. Myofascial pain often occurs in the area of the sternocleidomastoid and the trapezius, especially after radical neck dissection, and it can be improved with trigger-point injections of local anesthetic and steroids. Superficial cervical plexus blocks have good results for alleviating pain in postradical neck dissection syndrome, which usually occurs a few days after surgery and most commonly manifests as pain in the C2 and C3 distributions.[28]

Pain control is one of the most challenging tasks that physicians face when providing care for patients at the end of life. Despite recent advances, pain is often untreated or undertreated. Three principles should be followed when providing pain control at the end of life. First, pain can be controlled for most patients with the WHO's three-step care approach. Second, acute or escalating pain is a medical emergency that requires prompt attention; a delay in responding to this type of pain makes it more difficult to control. Third, addiction is not an issue with terminally ill patients. When pain is treated appropriately, addiction problems are rare.[29]

The initial pain assessment should include information about the location, quality, intensity, onset, duration, and frequency of pain as well as about factors that relieve or exacerbate pain. Although it is important to obtain current information about pain intensity, it is also essential to assess worst, best, and average pain intensity during a 24-hour period. Patients with terminal illnesses should be encouraged to verbalize the pain experience in their own words, and physicians should believe what the patients report.[30]

Pain syndromes can be nociceptive (somatic or visceral pain) or neuropathic (continuous dysesthesias, chronic lancinating, paroxysmal pain). Sustained-release pain medications have provided multiple therapeutic options.

Breakthrough pain can be expected to occur when a sustained-release analgesic medication becomes less effective for controlling pain. Immediate-release analgesics should be available to deal with the high incidence of breakthrough pain. Each dose of this type of medication is usually 10% to 30% of the total dose of the sustained-release analgesic. For patients who are using a significant amount of medication for breakthrough pain, the increase in the dose of sustained-release analgesic medication should reflect the total breakthrough dose taken in 24 hours.

Acute or crescendo pain occurs among patients who have good pain control but who develop an acute onset of new pain or a crescendo of established pain. This type of pain is a medical emergency, and it can be controlled with the aggressive use of an immediate-release medication every 15 minutes until the patient is comfortable. This medication should be taken in the presence of a properly trained health-care professional. After the crisis is resolved, the baseline sustained-release pain medication should be adjusted to prevent recurrence. If this type of pain persists, arrangements for more aggressive pain management regimens must be made.

Incident pain is another type of pain that patients may experience at the end of life. This pain occurs in conjunction with activities of daily living. Incident pain can be managed by giving the immediate-release medication 30 minutes before the activity is performed.

One of the most difficult challenges of providing pain management at the end of life involves changing from one medication to another, from one route of administration to another, or both. An equianalgesic dose chart can facilitate these changes. The conversions in the chart are based on studies of the effects of single doses of different pain medications, usually as compared with the effects of 10 mg of parenterally administered morphine.[31,32]

CONCLUSION

Successful pain management requires a holistic approach to the broad spectrum of problems faced by patients who are at the end of life. When providing pain management to these patients, physicians need to recognize the impact that unresolved psychosocial and spiritual issues can have on pain management. A multidiscipline hospice team can provide support for terminally ill patients.[33]

REFERENCES

1. Deng G, Cassileth BR: Principles and Practice of GI Oncology, Integrative Oncology: Complementary Therapies in Cancer Care, 2nd edition, Lippincott Williams & Wilkins, 2007.
2. Ferrante M (chair), Task Force on Pain Management: Practice guidelines for cancer pain management: A report By ASA Task Force on Pain Management, *Anesthesiology* 1996;84:256–72, 1996.
3. Miller K, Miller M, Jolly M: Challenges in pain management at the end of life. *Am Fam Phys* 2001;64(7):1227–1234.

4. Ashburn MA, Lipman AG: Management of pain in the cancer patient. *Anesth Analg* 1993;76(2):402-416.

5. World Health Organization Expert Committee, Cancer Relief and Palliative Care, Geneva, Switzerland, WHO, 1998, 1990.

6. Mitchell M, Payne R, American Pain Society: Principles of Analgesia Used in the Treatment of Acute Pain and Cancer Pain, 5th edition, Skokie, IL., IASP, 1992.

7. Schwarz SKW, McCroy C, Lindall SGE: Cox2 Inhibition for Postop Analgesia. *Anesth Analg,* 2003;96(6):1235–1236.

8. Kreuger K, Lino L, Dore R: Managing NSAID induced ulcer complications—balancing GI and CV risks. *Br Med J* 2008;67(3): 315–322.

9. Bartlett D: Life Extension: Acetaminophen and NSAID Toxicity, March 2006;30(3):281–283.

10. Veeraindar, G, Finley, R: Focus on Long Acting Opioids, Dannemiller Memorial Education Foundation, Pain Report, March 2007;(7):1–7.

11. Goulay GK, Kowalski, SP, Plummer JL: The transdermal administration of fentanyl in the treatment of postop pain. *Pain* 1989;37:193–202.

12. Majri G, Ansie D: Antidepressants in treatment of cancer pain—a survey in Italy. 1997;29:347–353.

13. Smith, M, Jaffe, J, Sejal J. Antidepressants: medications for depression: side effects, safety, and treatment guidelines, *Depression News,* January 2007, 12–20.

14. Swerdlow M: Anticonvulsant drugs and chronic pain. *Clin Neuropharmacol* 1984;7:51–82.

15. Schell HW: Adrenocorticoid therapy in far advanced cancer. Geriatrics 1972;27:131-41.

16. Hewitt DJ: The use of NMDA-receptor antagonists in the treatment of chronic pain. *Clin J Pain* 2000;16:2 (Suppl):573–579.

17. Scwynok J, Yaksh TL: Caffeine as an analgesic adjuvant: a review of pharmacology and mechanism of action. *Pharmacol Rev* 1993;45: 43–85.

18. Shoshidar HK, Lee H: Management of bone pain secondary to metastatic disease. *Cancer Control* 2005;4:153–157.

19. Hirst, RA, Lambert, DG: Pharmacology and potential therapeutic uses of cannabis. *Br J Anesth* 1998;81:77–84.

20. Ingenta Connect, Health Canada: Reactions, Warning that White Peony has High Lead Levels, Adis International. February 2006:2–21.

21. Chen J: Herbal alternatives to drugs in pain management, part II. *Acupuncture Today* 2000;1(7):45–50.

22. Kubo M, Matsoda, K: Anti-inflammatory activities of methanoic extract and alkaloidal components from corydalis tuber. *Biol Pharm Bull* 1994;17(2):262–265.

23. Carpenter, R: Refractory head and neck pain: a difficult problem and a new alternative therapy, *Anesth* 2005;6:28–32.

24. Shaw ES, Dinapoli R: Leksell Gamma Knife ® Perfexion™ Setting New Standards for Fast, Effective, Precise Radiosurgery Treatment. Int J Rad Onc May 2000;47:291–298.

25. Applegren L, Janson M: Continuous intracisternal and high cervical intrathecal bupivacaine analgesia in refractory head and neck pain. *Anesth* 1996;84(24):9–52.

26. Crul BJ, Van Dongen R: Permanent loss of cervical spinal cord function associated with the posterior approach. *Anesth Analg* 2006;102:330–331.

27. Ashburn M, Lipman A: Management of pain in cancer patient. *Anesth Analg* 1993;(76)2:402–416.

28. Ingham JM, Foley KM. Pain and the barriers to its relief at the end of life: a lesson for improving end of life health care. *Hosp J* 1998; (1-2): 89–100.

29. McCaffrey M, Pasero CL. Assessment: underlying complexities, misconceptions and practical tools: *Pain Clinical Manual*, ed. 2. St. Louis: Mosby: 1999:35–102.

30. McCaffrey M, Pasero CL. Opioid Analgesics: *Pain Clinical Manual* ed. 2. St. Louis: Mosby 1999:161–299.

31. Miettiner TT, Tiluis RS, Karppi P, Arve S: Why is the pain relief of dying patients often unsuccessful? The relatives' perspectives, *Palliat Med* 1998;12:429–435.

CHAPTER 17

Postoperative Dysphagia

Timothy M. McCulloch, Haskins Kashima, and Michelle Ciucci

The ideal treatment of head and neck malignancy continues its evolution. However, surgical management has remained a cornerstone of therapy for more than a century. The natural history of the majority of head and neck malignancies shows that they lend themselves to cure with surgical interventions. Combining the adequate resection of primary disease with the surgical management of neck nodal metastases frequently produces a long-term cure, even in patients with late-stage disease. One of the unfortunate byproducts of the resection of tissue within the aerodigestive tract and the neck is dysphagia. Dysphagia is often an unavoidable complication, because disease control and cure are paramount in treatment algorithms. Fortunately, with appropriate reconstruction and rehabilitation, patients often recover from or compensate for the swallowing disorders that result from surgical interventions. Generally the nature and severity of dysphagia are directly related to the location and extent of surgical resection and reconstruction. The goals of this chapter are to discuss the dysphagia associated with common cancer surgeries, to address some alternative treatments, and to highlight postoperative interventions that may diminish or alleviate the dysphagia. The chapter will begin with a brief discussion of the normal swallow to assist with the understanding of the complexity of the swallowing mechanism and to provide insight regarding the associated dysfunction that is seen after surgical interventions. The chapter also contains sections that discuss common surgical procedures with known dysphagia consequences, including open supraglottic laryngectomy, laser supraglottic laryngectomy, supracricoid laryngectomy, total laryngectomy, partial and total glossectomy, and neck surgical procedures. There is a complex interaction among the tissues of the head and neck region that produces a safe, efficient swallow. It is hoped that readers will gain an appreciation for this sophisticated concert of events, that they will understand how surgical interventions are likely to disrupt it, and that they will gain insight into how to manage dysphagia associated with head and neck surgery.

The twin goals of surgical resections performed for head and neck cancer are tumor eradication and functional restoration. After resections, the incidence of throat dysfunction in general and dysphagia in particular varies from report to report. The magnitude of this problem is difficult to define, because the extent and nature of the operations are variable, and dysphagia can be variously defined. Nevertheless, the restoration of normal oropharyngeal swallowing is of major concern to patients and their surgeons.

This discussion focuses on the problem of dysphagia as encountered after the supraglottic laryngectomy operation as a foundation to understand dysphagia associated with common head and neck procedures. This operation is well defined, and the principles herein described are generally applicable to and illustrative of the nature of dysphagia encountered after head and neck cancer resections. The discussion considers the following:

- The essential components for effective swallowing
- The extent of resection and the nature of reconstruction in the supraglottic laryngectomy operation
- Postoperative management, including the clinical, radiographic, and endoscopic evaluation of dysphagia
- The techniques of surgical and nonsurgical rehabilitation

NORMAL SWALLOWING

The act of swallowing (deglutition) is conventionally divided into three phases: oral, pharyngeal, and esophageal. The principal components of the swallowing action are depicted in illustrations that are based on a cineradiographic recording (Table 17-1).

The act of deglutition is a remarkable performance that completely delivers the bolus in a smooth progression from the oral phase through the pharyngeal phase to the esophageal phase, and it is described in detail elsewhere.[1] Fragmentation (the separation of the bolus) results in scattered particles that may produce symptoms as a result of misdirection into the nasopharynx or the laryngotracheal airway (e.g., cough, choke, gag, reflux) before, during, or after swallow completion.

Oral Phase

The oral phase, which consists of oral preparation and oral transport, includes the integrated functions of bolus selection, preparation, control, and delivery. A suitable bolus is selected for size (i.e., volume), texture, temperature, taste, and other characteristics; the bolus is prepared by mastication and lubrication, and it is controlled by the tongue, which supports the bolus until the appropriate instant at which it is delivered intact into the pharynx. The oral phase of swallowing is mostly voluntary, and it is subject to interruption or repetition as required.

TABLE 17-1 Summary of Normal Swallow

Swallowing Phase	Bolus	Tongue	Soft Palate	Larynx	Pharyngeal Constriction	Cricopharyngeus	
Oral	Controlled in oral cavity	Dorsum controls bolus	Resting position	Resting position	Resting	Resting	
Oral (late)	Enters oropharynx	Base assumes vertical position	Elevates to close velopharynx	Resting	Superior constriction action	Resting	
Pharyngeal	Enters hypopharynx	Strips palate and moves dorsally to close oropharynx and guides bolus	Secures velopharynx closure	Respiration inhibited, epiglottis deflects, larynx moves anterosuperiorly	Middle constrictor action	Resting	
Pharyngeal (late)	Enters pharyngo-esophageal zone	Returns to oral position	Returns to resting	Vocal folds close, epiglottis retroflexes, vestibule sheltered	Inferior constrictor action	Reflex relaxation	

Pharyngo-esophageal	Passes cricopharyngeal sphincter, enters esophagus	Returns to resting	Resting	Descends to resting and vocal folds open	Completion of inferior constrictor action	Reflex relaxation
Esophageal	Progresses down esophagus	Resting	Resting	Resting	Resting	Resting

Illustrations by Diane Robertson, AMI, Department of Radiological Sciences, The Johns Hopkins Medical Institutions, Baltimore, Md.

Pharyngeal Phase

The pharyngeal phase is controlled by a central pattern generator,[2] and it proceeds rapidly with several actions that occur virtually simultaneously but that are sequenced in a manner favorable to the effective and safe delivery of the bolus to the proximal esophagus. The pharyngeal phase typically commences with the passage of the bolus through the faucial pillars (although there is great intrapersonal and interpersonal variability), and it ends with the presentation of the bolus to the pharyngoesophageal (or cricopharyngeal) segment. The elements that constitute the pharyngeal phase of swallowing include the closure of the nasopharynx; the propulsion of the bolus by the combined actions of the posterior movement of the tongue base; and the sequential contraction of the superior, middle, and inferior constrictor muscles (the so-called *pharyngeal peristalsis*). The larynx is elevated by the action of the suprahyoid muscles, and the glottic aperture is actively closed to prevent bolus entry into the airway. Laryngeal closure results from vocal-fold adduction, and glottic sheltering is reinforced by the retroflexing epiglottis; this draws the aryepiglottic folds medially and deflects the bolus laterally. The pharyngeal phase of swallowing ends when the pharyngeal peristaltic wave reaches the cricopharyngeal segment; the synchronized relaxation of the cricopharyngeal sphincter permits the passage of the bolus into the cervical esophagus.

Esophageal Phase

The esophageal phase of swallowing begins with the entry of the bolus into and its subsequent transit through the esophagus. This is affected by a combination of gravity and peristaltic action, and it ends with the passage of the bolus through the lower esophageal sphincter into the stomach.

OPEN SUPRAGLOTTIC LARYNGECTOMY

The open supraglottic laryngectomy is less common in the modern era of cancer therapy, but it serves as an excellent framework to discuss the causes of postoperative dysphagia, which is seen in patients who have undergone many of the procedures within the region of the laryngopharynx. The supraglottic laryngectomy operation (i.e., subtotal, horizontal, and partial) is designed to excise diseased laryngeal parts with the preservation and restoration of near-normal voice and oral respiration. Its most common application is in neoplastic disease that involves the supraglottic structures (i.e., the epiglottis, the false folds, and the arytenoid and superior [roof] ventricles). The operation can also be used for the management of the acutely traumatized supraglottis and for delayed strictures that occur after infection or injury. The partial pharyngolaryngectomy operation is

an extension of the supraglottic resection for suitable lesions of the tongue base, the pyriform sinus, and the hypopharynx. The structures that remain after these resections include the true folds, one or both arytenoids, the lower thyroid ala and cricoid, the strap muscles, and the suprahyoid musculature. The objective during reconstruction and rehabilitation is the use of these remaining structures in a manner favorable to restoring throat function.

Reconstruction

Reconstruction after supraglottic resection reorganizes the remaining parts to achieve mucosal integrity, to preserve sensorimotor function, and to restore anatomic relationships. Reconstruction begins with mucosal closure of the pharynx in a manner that avoids excessive tension or mucosal redundancy, particularly over the arytenoids and the posterior larynx. The tongue base is approximated to the preserved external perichondrium at or close to the level of the true vocal folds. Precise mucosal closure over the exposed paraglottic soft tissues is not essential, and it can result in the lateralization or fixation of the vocal fold, thereby risking bolus shunting into the glottic aperture.

Favorable larynx positioning is achieved by the approximation of the strap muscles to the suprahyoid muscles (or to the hyoid, if it is preserved). The larynx remnant should be restored to a near-original level and supported in a manner that favors near-normal laryngeal elevation during the swallowing act. Favorable laryngeal placement has been achieved by wire suspension of the laryngeal remnant to the mandibular symphysis (i.e., static suspension). A beneficial procedure is to suture the digastric sling to the strap muscles below the line of the pharyngotomy closure to achieve the dynamic suspension of the larynx and to facilitate its elevation coincident with the swallow effort.

The inclusion of the cricopharyngeal myotomy as a standard part of the supraglottic laryngectomy is controversial. It is intended to facilitate bolus entry into the esophagus, and it may be particularly useful when the impairment of vocal-fold motion is anticipated as a result of arytenoid removal or vocal-fold paralysis. Reflux or regurgitation and esophageal dysfunction can be regarded as contraindications to this procedure.

Postoperative Management

Management of the postsupraglottic laryngectomy patient begins at the time of closure after resection. A leak-free pharyngotomy closure can be confirmed by instilling a mixture of methylene blue and hydrogen peroxide into the hypopharynx to facilitate the detection and closure of potential fistula sites.

Residual secretions from the hypopharynx and the trachea are aspirated while the patient remains anesthetized, and local anesthetic solution is placed into the trachea to subdue coughing spasms during the transfer of the patient from the operating table to the recovery facility. The head is supported on a pillow to prevent the risk of the hyperextension of the neck during patient transfer. The patient is instructed regarding the use of an oropharyngeal (i.e., Yankauer) suction to remove oral secretions and to minimize pooling at the pharyngotomy repair site.

At or about the third to fifth postoperative day, the patient's ability to swallow oropharyngeal secretions signals his or her preparedness to resume oral intake. When oral examination confirms the coordination, control, and strength of the tongue, jaw, and lip to manipulate and transport the bolus while protecting the airway, trials with gelatin or ice chips are used as uniformly suitable test boluses as a result of patient acceptance and minimal consequence if tracheal entry occurs. If a safe and effective swallow is noted, the diet is gradually advanced to pureed foods and then to a mechanical soft diet, with patient performance and food preferences taken into account. Contrary to usual expectations, clear liquids (water in particular) may be more difficult to swallow than thicker liquids or gels; thus advancement to tolerating liquids in the diet may lag behind that of solids.

After oral alimentation has been successfully resumed, a logical sequence of tube withdrawal begins with a gradual step down in the caliber of the tracheotomy tube until a number 4 or 5 tracheotomy tube is in place and can be occluded, initially during awake hours and later on an around-the-clock basis. The nasogastric tube is removed when the patient demonstrates an ability to meet nutrition and hydration needs orally. Tracheotomy decannulation is delayed until after the patient demonstrates success with managing oral feedings so that a safe airway is ensured. The prolonged presence of the tracheotomy aggravates laryngotracheal fixation, inhibits laryngeal elevation, and interferes with swallow recovery. However, the role of a persistent tracheotomy tube as a contributor to dysphagia remains unclear.[3]

SURGICAL REHABILITATION

The surgical approaches to the correction of dysphagia are undertaken only when difficulty persists after a full trial of rehabilitation efforts. The objectives of such surgical interventions include the following:
- The elimination of infection
- The relief of obstruction as a result of swelling or tissue redundancy
- Tissue augmentation
- The promotion of transit through the pharyngoesophageal segment by dilatation or myotomy

Surgical interventions are useful to eliminate persistent sites of infection that result in granuloma or recalcitrant soft-tissue edema. Successful swallowing has been restored after the removal of a chondronecrotic thyroid that caused episodic flare-up, inflammation, and obstructing granuloma formation. Persistent edema over the arytenoids that is attributable to mucosal redundancy may be correctable with the judicious laser vaporization of the redundant mucosa, but the possibility of underlying chondronecrosis of the arytenoid or other cartilage should be considered. These occult infection sites reveal themselves with pain or tenderness on direct palpation.

Persisting soft-tissue deficiency in the tongue base has been corrected with an inert implant. For this purpose, a Silastic testicular prosthesis of a suitable size that depends on the estimated tissue deficiency in the tongue base can be used. The prosthesis is inserted extramucosally through a skin incision in a well-healed postsupraglottic laryngectomy site. A suitable pocket is created in the tongue base, with care taken to avoid entering the hypopharyngeal lumen. The augmented tongue base, although not dynamically active, serves as the anterior buttress against which pharyngeal peristalsis can facilitate bolus advancement.

Tissue deficiency at the vocal folds can be corrected with injection thyroplasty. Tissue-volume adjustments of the vocal fold are undertaken only after an exhaustive trial of swallow rehabilitation; repeated small-volume injections are preferred, with recognition that reactive swelling may exaggerate the final result.

The elevation of the larynx during swallow is favored by the dynamic suspension of the larynx by the digastric sling. The elevation can be enhanced by the denervation or the partial division of the (infrahyoid) strap muscles. When neck dissection is performed, the suprahyoid dissection is usually omitted; this aids in the preservation of dynamic laryngeal elevation, which is an essential component of swallow recovery. Metastatic laryngeal carcinoma in the submental triangles is rare.

Delayed cricopharyngeal myotomy is only rarely successful (in the authors' experience). This additional surgical intervention may add to the scarring and fixation of the hypopharynx and larynx. If the pharyngoesophageal segment remains persistently narrowed and fails to enlarge after repeated operative dilatations and daily bougienage, the cricopharyngeal muscle can be surgically divided. In these cases, the myotomy is performed over a large-caliber bougie placed into the pharyngoesophageal segment, and the muscle is carefully divided. In certain cases in which the narrowed segment is difficult to identify with precision, a Foley catheter can be passed into the esophagus, and the myotomy is performed at the point where the narrowed segment is identified during the gradual withdrawal of the inflated balloon.

Pain accompanying dysphagia is an ominous symptom that indicates infection or tumor; tumor can be residual, or it may arise from a different site. Careful evaluation including endoscopic examination is indicated. When dysphagia persists despite all efforts in rehabilitation, the alternatives are to recommend the long-term use of a feeding tube or a completion laryngectomy. The choice is guided by the patient's wishes and general health, by an understanding of the long-term health risks of aspiration, and by the patient's trend toward recovery or debilitation.

LASER SUPRAGLOTTIC LARYNGECTOMY

Laser supraglottic laryngectomy has become an accepted alternative to the open procedures. It is purported to have the advantage of earlier recovery of aspiration-free deglutition. However, there are few studies that directly compare the techniques. The advantages of a laser technique should include less tissue resection, retained sensory fields, and no healing of neck tissues opened during the procedure. It is somewhat difficult to discern the effects of associated neck dissections, which are frequently combined with supraglottic procedures. In a comparison study by Peretti and colleagues,[4] it was found that most individuals recovered a functional swallow after either procedure. The time to recover appeared to be shorter in the laser group, with hospital discharge occurring significantly earlier. An artificial delay may be induced by the postoperative needs of an open procedure with its inherent increased risk of infection and fistula formation. After 2 years, the two groups were subjectively similar regarding their reports of aspiration (MD Anderson Dysphagia Inventory). Follow-up videofluoroscopy imaging studies identified a four-times-higher rate of silent aspiration among the open-procedure patients (80%) as compared with the laser-resection patients (21%). The early recovery and diminished aspiration may be the result of the preservation of sensory fields. Sasaki and colleagues[5] reported an earlier recovery of the glottic closure reflex in the laser-resection patients as compared with the open-supraglottic laryngectomy patients; this correlated with an earlier return to an oral diet and hospital discharge.

Although there may be evidence to support improved function as compared with open procedures, endoscopic laser excision retains a measurable risk of postoperative swallowing dysfunction. In an early experience reported by Eckel,[6] 5 of 45 patients failed to recover a safe swallow and went on to total laryngectomy. In the 1998 review conducted by Iro and colleagues,[7] of 141 consecutive patients, 6 developed postoperative aspiration pneumonia, and 12 remained tracheotomy dependent as a result

of aspiration. However, none went on to completion laryngectomy for persistent dysphagia. In this patient series, half of the group (50.4%) required unilateral or bilateral neck dissection, and a similar number (45.4%) received postoperative radiation therapy. In a similar series, Davis and colleagues[8] reported a 5% aspiration pneumonia rate and a 3% gastrostomy-tube dependency rate. It is important to recognize that these reports of "minimal" dysphagia after the successful treatment of supraglottic cancer by transoral laser resection are the experience of high-volume surgeons; they are unlikely to be reproduced by the novice.

SUPRACRICOID LARYNGECTOMY

The supracricoid laryngectomy is a technique of extended resection, but it is also a method of reconstruction designed to compensate for alterations in anatomy. This surgery requires a leap of faith by the surgeon and patient, because attempts to retain tissues beyond the described surgical method can compromise cure and interfere with the restoration of a functional voice and swallow. Hofman-Saguez[9] described this technique in the French literature circa 1950. During the later half the last century, it became an accepted procedure in much of Europe. It was finally promoted in the United States in the 1990s by Weinstein and colleagues.[10]

A nice review of the dysphagia complications that result from supracricoid laryngectomy was published by Marioni and colleagues in 2004.[11] The authors provide a summary of their own experience as well as a review of the literature, in which they highlight the lack of uniform measures to assess the true extent of posttreatment dysphagia and recognize the need to use surrogate variables to estimate swallow function (Table 17-2). The most common measures are the time to feeding-tube removal, aspiration pneumonia events, and patient questionnaires. The general themes found in this review are that most feeding tubes are removed within the first month after surgery and that approximately 90% of patients have returned to a "normal" diet within a year. This does leave a group of patients who are still aspirating or who are dependent on tube feeds and require additional care. In most cases, these patients will require completion laryngectomy.

The complications of postoperative dysphagia seem to be more commonly reported by U.S. surgeons. This increased incidence of dysphagia may be related to the use of this technique to salvage radiation therapy failures as an alternative to total laryngectomy. Laccourreye and colleagues[12] evaluated their results of supracricoid laryngectomy when it was used as a radiation therapy salvage technique and found an incidence of resulting total laryngectomy of 25%, in part as a result of recurrence and in part as a result of aspiration. Prolonged feeding-tube use, tracheotomy need, and an increased rate of

TABLE 17-2   Functional Results of Supracricoid Laryngectomy in Terms of Deglutition

Author (Year)	No. of Cases	Average NGFT Removal Time	Return to a "Normal" Oral Diet (Rate)	Remarks
Bottazzi and Ferri (1993)[a]	323	ND	60.68%	—
Naudo et al. (1997)[b]	122	22 days	91% within 12 months	SCL-CHP
De Vincentiis et al. (1998)[c]	51	15 days	79.2%	SCL-CHEP
	98	28 days	64.3%	SCL-CHP
Bussi et al. (2000)[d]	44	16 days	93.2% "good deglutition"	SCL-CHEP
Bron et al. (2000)[e]	69	22 days after CHEP	n.d.	60 SCL-CHEP
		18 days after CHP		9 SCL-CHP
Lima et al. (2001)[f]	27	43 days	97%	SCL-CHEP
Zacharek et al. (2001)[g]	10	ND	100% within 1 month	6 SCL-CHEP, 4 SCL-CHP
Present series[h]	16	21 days	90% within 12 months	14 SCL-CHEP, 2 SCL-CHP

From Marioni G, Marchese-Rafona R, Ottaviano G, et al: Supracricoid laryngectomy: Is it time to define guidelines to evaluate functional results? A review. *Am J Otolaryngol* 2004;25:98–104.
CHEP, Crico-hyoid-epiglottopexy; *CHP,* crico-hyoidopexy; *NGFT,* nasogastric feeding tube; *SCL,* supracricoid laryngectomy.
[a]Bottazzi D, Ferri T: Valutazione multicentrica dei risultati funzionali a distanza. In de Vincentiis M, editor: *Chirurgia funzionale della laringe: Stato attuale dell'arte: Relazione Ufficiale del LXXX Congresso della Societa Italiana di Otorinolaringoiatria e Chirurgia Cervico-Facciale*, 1993, Pacini Ed.
[b]Naudo P, Laccourreye O, Weinstein G, et al: Functional outcome and prognosis factors after supracricoid partial laryngectomy with cricohyoidopexy. *Ann Otol Rhinol Laryngol* 1997;106:291–296.
[c]de Vincentiis M, Minni A, Gallo A, et al: Supracricoid partial laryngectomy: Oncologic and functional results. *Head Neck* 1998;20:504–509.
[d]Bussi M, Riontino E, Cardarelli L, et al: La cricoioido-epiglottopessia: Valutazione dei risultati deglutitori su 44 casi. *Acta Otorhinolaryngol Ital* 2000;20:442–447.
[e]Bron L, Brossard E, Monnier P, et al: Supracricoid partial laryngectomy with cricohyoidoepiglottopexy for glottic and supraglottic carcinomas. *Laryngoscope* 2000;110:627–634.
[f]Lima RA, Freitas EQ, Kligerman J, et al: Supracricoid laryngectomy with CHEP: Functional results and outcome. *Otolaryngol Head Neck Surg* 2001;124:258–260.
[g]Zacharek MA, Pasha R, Meleca RJ, et al: Functional outcomes after supracricoid laryngectomy. *Laryngoscope* 2001;111:1558–1564.
[h]Marioni G, Marchese-Rafona R, Ottaviano G, et al: Supracricoid laryngectomy: Is it time to define guidelines to evaluate functional results? A review. *Am J Otolaryngol* 2004;25:98–104.

wound-healing problems are also identified with salvage patients.[13] With proper indications and good surgical technique, however, long-term successes can be expected. Laudadio and colleagues[14] evaluated 206 patients after a mean follow up of more than 5 years and found an 85% 5-year disease-free survival rate with a 97% organ-preservation rate.

It is important to note that the resection can at times include the entire epiglottis. This produces a higher rate of aspiration, because the reconstructed airway lacks the superior epiglottis, its associated sensory fields, and its mechanical advantages. The duration of swallowing problems after complete epiglottic resection repair with the tongue base and hyoid brought to the cricoid (i.e., cricohyoidopexy) is approximately twice as long as that seen with a cricohyoidoepiglottopexy.[15]

Although many patients will require completion laryngectomy to resolve aspiration issues, in some cases, abnormal pharyngoesophageal neuromuscular coordination has been identified as the primary residual problem.

Treatment with botulinum toxin into the cricopharyngeus muscle successfully restored the ability to swallow in several of these patients.[16]

TOTAL LARYNGECTOMY

Total laryngectomy was the mainstay of the treatment of laryngeal cancer for most of the last century. It was used for the treatment of stage T-2 to T-4 lesions, and it provided high levels of disease control. During the last two decades, the trend has been to make efforts to avoid the use of total laryngectomy and to instead use "organ-sparing" protocols that combine chemotherapy and radiation therapy. Although this chapter's focus is on postsurgical dysphagia, it is worthwhile to note that efforts to avoid laryngectomy may be interfering with opportunities to cure patients.[17]

Swallowing dysfunction after total laryngectomy is a commonly recognized surgical side effect, and it can be identified in up to 60% of patients.[18] Causes of dysphagia include anatomic narrowing as a result of partial pharyngectomy, postoperative inflammatory events (e.g., infection, radiation therapy, mechanical trauma for feeding tubes, dilators, voice prostheses), diverticulum, and neuromuscular causes.

Using the University of Washington Quality of Life questionnaire, version 4 (UW-QOL), Vilaseca and colleagues[19] evaluated the self-reported swallowing-related quality-of-life dysfunction in 49 total laryngectomy patients 2 years after treatment. A score of 100 indicates normal function, and a score of 0 indicates worst-possible function. The report identified that 40% of patients were not able to swallow certain foods. They reported a mean UW-QOL swallowing score of 86.67 ± 19.39. A similar result was reported by Lotempio and colleagues[20] in a study that compared the quality-of-life results of total laryngectomy and chemoradiation. They included 31 patients who received treatment with total laryngectomy and postoperative radiation therapy. In this group, 44% reported a UW-QOL score for swallowing of 100, and 6% (2 of 31) reported a score of 0.

The restoration of swallowing function depends on the identified cause. Hui and colleagues[21] looked at the relationship between residual pharyngeal mucosa and postoperative dysphagia and found no correlation in their 52 patients. The identified lower limit of tissue width was 1.5 cm, but this may have been above the threshold for causing dysphagia. The three benign dysphagia events in this study were isolated to a single bolus impaction (i.e., two events) and an inflammatory stricture (i.e., one event). Certainly the inclusion of additional mucosa when treating pharyngeal primaries does increase the incidence of postoperative dysphagia.[22]

The occasional complete pharyngeal stricture requires a reconstruction using regional flaps, free-tissue transfer, or both.[23] Figure 17-1 showed a pharyngeal reconstruction using a combination of local neck tissues and a deltopectoral flap. Incomplete strictures are often treatable with repeated dilatations.

Additional problems have been identified, including pharyngeal and tongue-base weakness and pharyngeal spasms. Few treatment options are available for pharyngeal and tongue-base weakness. Pharyngeal spasms can be addressed with botulinum toxin injections.[24] It is important to note that, after the initial recovery of swallow function after a total laryngectomy, the emergence of a new dysphagia is a common and important sign of cancer recurrence.[21]

GLOSSECTOMY

Anterior partial glossectomy is a common component of the management of tongue malignancy. Attempts to limit radiation exposure to the mandible, the salivary

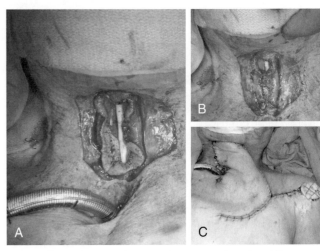

Figure 17-1. Total hypopharyngeal reconstruction. **A** and **B,** Neopharynx tube created with cervical skin flaps. **C,** Cutaneous coverage with a deltopectoral flap.

glands, and the teeth have forestalled the extensive use of combined chemotherapy and radiation therapy for the treatment of the mobile tongue. Fortunately, most individuals will compensate for anterior-tongue resections to recover swallowing function, because the anterior tongue is primarily involved with bolus manipulation rather than bolus transport. Figure 17-2 shows a hemiglossectomy reconstruction with a radial forearm free flap. Deficiencies and scar formation can interfere with dietary choice and require patients to prepare foods to simplify mastication and ease the oral phase of swallowing.

The opposite is true for the tongue base with regard to both treatment choices and swallow outcomes after resection. Resections of more than one third of the tongue base often lead to a permanent dysphagia. Swallow outcomes are related to the amount of tongue tissue that is removed.[22,25] In the modern era, the majority of tongue-base cancers are treated with chemoradiation.

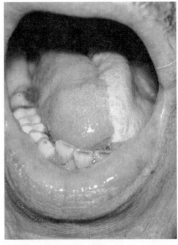

Figure 17-2. Anterior hemiglossectomy with reconstruction using a radial forearm free flap and showing near-normal oral function.

If it is required for cure, however, total glossectomy should not be avoided. Several reports have demonstrated the capacity of patients to recover functional swallowing and speech after total glossectomy when appropriate reconstruction methods are used.[26–28] Lyos and colleagues[28] looked at the MD Anderson experience with glossectomy reconstruction with a rectus abdominis flap. Their patient group included eight patients with total glossectomy and six with subtotal glossectomy. One patient required early laryngectomy to treat recurrent aspiration. Four patients died of other causes during follow up; two were alive with recurrent disease and eight were alive and free of disease at a mean survival time of 49 months. Of the 14 evaluated patients, 3 required feeding tubes for nutritional support, whereas the remaining 11 were able to eat a modified diet; none were eating a regular diet. In addition to diet modification, 8 patients received palatal augmentation prosthesis.

NECK SURGICAL PROCEDURES

Standard neck dissections are not associated with significant dysphagia. When neck dissection is required after primary radiation therapy and/or chemoradiation, there is an increased incidence of dysphagia.[29] When extensive disease requires the removal of neural tissue that is important to the swallow pattern generation, dysphagia can be expected. The vagus and pharyngeal plexus are oftentimes sacrificed or injured with surgery of the superior pharynx and with attempts to clear deeply invasive disease, skull-base disease, and vascular tumors.[30,31] Some spontaneous recovery is seen over time in many patients; however, palate weakness may require surgical repositioning,[32] and vocal-fold paralysis can be treated with medialization procedures to improve swallowing.[33] Dietary modifications are also valuable, including the restriction of thin liquids to reduce aspiration risk.[34]

EVALUATION AND MANAGEMENT OF DYSPHAGIA

Dysphagia is a common side effect of surgical interventions for head and neck cancer. Fortunately there are techniques to limit and treat associated swallowing dysfunctions. The first option is to select the appropriate surgical intervention, which will consider the preservation of life while minimizing side effects (e.g., dysphagia). However, often the appropriate surgical decision may lead to swallowing complications. In this event, postsurgical dysphagia is managed by an interdisciplinary team that includes (but is not limited to) a head and/or neck surgeon, an internal medicine specialist, a speech–language pathologist, an occupational therapist, a radiologist, a dietician, and a nursing staff member. It is paramount to consult the appropriate services when dealing with this complex patient group. If dysphagia is suspected, the most common and first step in managing the patient is to request a swallow evaluation, which is typically carried out by a speech–language pathologist. This referral will generate diet recommendations as well as follow-up diagnostics and treatment.

This assessment considers each of the anatomic elements that are relevant to the act of swallowing, including sensation and reflexes; the extent of resection (i.e., base of tongue, arytenoid, hypopharynx, pyriform sinus); adjunctive treatment (i.e., radiation therapy, chemotherapy); complications (i.e., hematoma, infection, fistula, extended need for tracheotomy); coexisting medical disorders; and mental status. The failure of safe, orderly, and effective bolus movement is recognized on the basis of three dysfunctions: (1) obstruction; (2) misdirection; and (3) bolus fragmentation.

Obstruction

Obstruction results from the failure of bolus progression caused by anatomic or functional interference. The failed passage of liquids or solids may have an abrupt or insidious onset and a swift or slow progression, and it may present with persistent or fluctuating symptoms. Symptoms often exacerbate with adjuvant therapies such as radiation. The perceived symptoms of substernal tightness and spasm can indicate esophageal spasm or stricture. Symptoms caused by pooled secretions resulting from obstruction are commonly localized to the pharyngoesophageal segment or the larynx, where a wet voice and cough–choke episodes are the result.

Misdirection

Misdirection results from bolus entry into the nasopharynx (i.e., retrograde) or into the larynx and trachea (i.e., antegrade). Misdirected bolus and oropharyngeal secretions into the larynx and trachea result from a variety of dysfunctions, such as bolus fragmentation, faulty control of the bolus, pooled secretions as a result of distal obstruction, or sensorimotor dysfunction. Cough and habitual throat clearing are symptomatic expressions of pooled secretions in the valleculae and hypopharynx resulting in overflow into the laryngeal vestibule. The entry of the bolus may provoke coughing, although these occurrences can also be asymptomatic as a result of sensory deficits. Wheezing, bronchitis, and "asthma" may result from lesser and chronic penetration and aspiration. Rhinorrhea and sneezing accompanying meals may occur with the subclinical regurgitation of the bolus into the nasopharynx or the nasal cavity.

The retrograde movement of the bolus in the esophagus is called *regurgitation,* and it may be the result of gastroesophageal reflux, an obstructing lesion, spasm, or stenosis. A bitter taste in the refluxed or regurgitated throat content indicates the return of gastric-acid–containing secretions into the hypopharynx. Asymptomatic gastroesophageal reflux is an unrecognized factor in persistent postoperative dysphagia, and a routine antireflux regimen is justified.

Bolus Fragmentation

Bolus cohesion through the aerodigestive trajectory is the hallmark of a well-executed swallow. The bolus—whether solid, liquid, or semisolid—proceeds as a compacted mass from the mouth to the stomach. Bolus fragmentation may result in a minor separation that arrives before or after the principal bolus. Premature leak into the pharynx (arriving before the larynx is actually sheltered) can produce cough or a cough–choke attack, or it can be unnoticed by the patient. Delayed bolus separation (arriving after the passage of the main bolus) pools in the oral cavity, the valleculae, or the distal hypopharynx and produces throat clearing, voluntary cough, and a wet voice. Alternatively, there may be no indication that this has occurred, and the bolus will enter the unprotected larynx after the swallow. Bolus separation as a result of a structural abnormality (e.g., retention in a cul-de-sac or diverticulum) behaves as a delayed separation. Bolus separation caused by sensory or motor dysfunction may produce symptoms that are indistinguishable from the foregoing description. In addition, bolus separation may occur when there is a regurgitation of a portion of the formed bolus; the symptoms and consequences duplicate those that result from delayed bolus separation.

Clinical Examination

The patient usually identifies the site of difficulty at the level of the hypopharynx and larynx as a result of the failure of bolus entry into the cervical esophagus with resultant aspiration. However, patients can also be asymptomatic as a result of sensory abnormalities caused by disease pathology, the primary surgery, or adjuvant therapies. The degree of postoperative dysphagia is related to the degree of pretreatment impairment and the location of the tumor.[35] The causes of dysphagia are often multiple, and they may be far removed from the site of symptoms, although this is highly correlated with the total volume that is resected.[36] Oral-phase deficiencies are often major contributing factors.[37] Physical findings that corroborate an oral site of deficiency include retained oral secretions of food particles and weakness of the tongue, the palate, or both. Indirect laryngoscopy reveals retained secretions in the hypopharynx and overflow at the laryngeal inlet. Vocal-fold mobility, the presence of mucosal redundancy, or granulation tissue is also evaluated. The presence of granulation tissues adjacent to the thyroid perichondrium may indicate subperichondrial infection or frank chondronecrosis.

Tenderness over the laryngeal remnant is strongly suggestive of subperichondrial or frank cartilaginous infection. Inspection and palpation of the neck may disclose induration of the skin and soft tissues of the neck, including the supporting musculature; swallowing effort may demonstrate a lack of laryngeal elevation.

Dynamic imaging by video or cine examination is the preferred method of radiographic study,[38] because events in oral and pharyngeal swallow occur too rapidly for visualization on fluoroscopy or spot films. This assessment is especially important because airway compromise is often asymptomatic (i.e., no coughing or choking associated with the event); laryngeal penetration or aspiration is often "silent." An imperfect oral phase of swallowing is commonly manifested by fragmentation of the contrast material, retention of contrast in the oral cavity, premature spillage or delayed arrival into the hypopharynx, and tongue pumping. A double contour of the tongue as imaged on the pharyngoesophagram indicates asymmetry that is attributable to weakness or to motion impairment as a result of fixation or paralysis.

Pharyngeal peristalsis may be absent after inflammation or neural injury that involves the constrictor muscles. Severe narrowing of the pharyngoesophageal segment may result in only small amounts of contrast entering the esophagus. It is often difficult to distinguish narrowing caused by stenosis from a failure of the sphincter to relax. A prominent cricopharyngeal "bar" on contrast radiographic examination may indicate hypertonicity or spasm of the cricopharyngeus, but it may be caused by esophageal dysfunction such as reflux, regurgitation, or dyskinesia.

Disorganized esophageal peristalsis may occur during the early postoperative period, but small amounts of contrast entering the esophagus may prohibit the satisfactory evaluation of esophageal transit. A small amount of contrast instilled into the upper esophagus by nasal catheter allows for the better evaluation of esophageal peristalsis; this includes examination for acid sensitivity, gastroesophageal reflux, or frank regurgitation of the esophageal contents into the hypopharynx.

Depending on the findings from physical and radiographic examinations, endoscopic evaluation should be performed. This examination is preferably delayed until 3 or 4 weeks into the postoperative period so that the endoscopic manipulations do not risk the disruption of the surgical closure. Examination under anesthesia includes an evaluation for the passive mobility of the laryngotracheal complex. An estimation of the pharyngoesophageal lumen caliber, particularly at the cricopharyngeus, is made, and so is a determination regarding the suitability for dilatation. The esophageal examination seeks to identify any residual secretions or food particles indicative of a failure to advance the bolus through the esophagus.

Nonsurgical Rehabilitation

On the basis of the foregoing examinations and findings, the strategy for further management is developed. In cases of infection, it is advisable to continue nasogastric feedings to permit the resolution of residual inflammation and swelling while administering appropriate antibiotics. Caloric and fluid requirements are maintained by tube feeding so that the patient's convalescence and recovery from the operation are facilitated. Nutrition and caloric demands may be increased as a result of wound healing and adjuvant therapies. Feeding via gastrostomy is preferred when a longer period of failed oral alimentation is anticipated.

Common treatment options include diet modifications, heightening sensory input, compensatory maneuvers, and exercises.[38,39] Treatment decisions are based on the detailed examination of anatomy, physiology, or both; nutrition and hydration demands; and other patient factors. Diet modifications commonly adjust food and liquid consistencies to minimize aspiration risk and to maximize efficient swallowing to meet nutrition and hydration needs. It should be noted that this may include alternatives to oral intake, including temporary and long-term tube feeding. Compensatory strategies are also based on anatomic and physiologic parameters and include the modification of postures that may alter bolus direction and flow. Finally, exercises are designed to strengthen muscles and improve the sensorimotor control of the swallowing mechanism. It should be noted that these treatment options can occur in isolation or in combination.

Evaluation and management decisions must be coordinated throughout the patient-care team. The swallowing therapist (i.e., the speech–language pathologist) is a key professional who interacts with the nurse, the dietician, the physician, the patient, and the family and who is identified as the specialist most crucial to swallow recovery.[38] The appropriate selection of bolus size and food/liquid consistency is paramount and achieved after observation as well as endoscopic and fluoroscopic evaluation. Frequent reevaluation can be important for determining the optimal form of food and liquid for ingestion as well as for determining compensatory maneuvers that can improve swallowing. Ideally, an active head and neck service should have designated speech–language pathologists with the expertise to fulfill this role.

CONCLUSION

Addressing surgery-related dysphagia requires an indepth understanding of the structural and physiologic aspects of typical swallowing and of how the surgical interventions may have altered these processes. It is necessary to consider treatment options that have a lower risk of dysphagia and, when possible, to provide appropriate patient support to maintain swallow function during and after treatment. It is imperative that this complication be discussed with patients and that the necessary support services be in place to deal appropriately with these potential postoperative sequelae.

REFERENCES

1. Logemann JA. "Anatomy and physiology of normal deglutition," in Logemann JA, editor: *Evaluation and treatment of swallowing disorders,* Austin, Tex, 1998, Pro-Ed.
2. Jean A: Brainstem control of swallowing: Localization and organization of the central pattern generator for swallowing. In Taylor A, editor: *Neurophysiology of the jaws and teeth,* London, 1990, MacMillan Press.
3. Leder SB, Joe JK, Ross DA, et al: Presence of a tracheotomy tube and aspiration status in early, postsurgical head and neck cancer patients. *Head Neck* 2005;27(9):757–761.
4. Peretti G, Piazza C, Cattaneo A, et al: Comparison of functional outcomes after endoscopic versus open-neck supraglottic laryngectomies. *Ann Otol Rhinol Laryngol* 2006;115:827–832.
5. Sasaki CT, Leder SB, Acton LM, et al: Comparison of the glottic closure reflex (GCR) in traditional "open" versus endoscopic laser supraglottic laryngectomy (ELSL). *Ann Otol Rhinol Laryngol* 2006;115:93–96.
6. Eckel HE: Endoscopic laser resection of supraglottic carcinoma. *Otolaryngol Head Neck Surg* 1997;117:681–687.
7. Iro H, Waldfahrer F, Altendorf-Hofman A, et al: Transoral laser surgery of supraglottic cancer, follow-up of 141patients. *Arch Otolaryngol Head Neck Surg* 1998;124:1245–1250.
8. Davis RK, Kriskovich MD, Galloway EB, et al: Endoscopic supraglottic laryngectomy with postoperative irradiation. *Ann Otol Rhinol Laryngol* 2004;113:132–138.
9. Hofmann-Saguez MR: Laryngectomie subtotale conservatrice. *Ann Otolaryngol* 1950;67:811–816.
10. Weinstein GS, EL-Sway MM, Ruiz C, et al: Laryngeal preservation with supracricoid partial laryngectomy results in improved quality of life when compared with total laryngectomy. *Laryngoscope* 2001;111:191–199.
11. Marioni G, Marchese-Rafona R, Ottaviano G, et al: Supracricoid laryngectomy: Is it time to define guidelines to evaluate functional results? A review. *Am J Otolaryngol* 2004;25:98–104.
12. Laccourreye O, Weinstein G, Naudo P, et al: Supracricoid partial laryngectomy after failed laryngeal radiation therapy. *Laryngoscope* 1996;106:495–498.
13. Marchese-Ragona R, Marioni G, Chiarello G, et al: Supracricoid laryngectomy with cricohyoidopexy for recurrence of early-stage glottic carcinoma after irradiation: Long-term oncological and functional results. *Acta Otoloaryngol* 2005;125:91–95.
14. Laudado P, Presutti L, O Dall'olio D, et al: Supracricoid laryngectomies: Long-term oncological and functional results. *Acta Otolaryngol* 2006;126:640–649.
15. Farrag TY, Koch WM, Cummings CW, et al: Supracricoid laryngectomy outcomes: The John Hopkins experience. *Laryngoscope* 2006;117:129–132
16. Marchese-Ragona R, De Grandis D, Restivo DA: Recovery of swallowing disorders in patients undergoing supracricoid laryngectomy with botulinum toxin therapy. *Ann Otol Rhinol Laryngol* 2003;112:258–263.
17. Hoffman HT, Porter K, Karnell LH, et al: Laryngeal cancer in the United States: Changes in demographics, patterns of care, and survival. *Laryngoscope* 2006;116(9 Pt 2 Suppl 111):1–13.
18. Braz DS, Ribas MM, Dedivitis RA, et al: Quality of life and depression in patients undergoing total and partial laryngectomy. *Clinics* 2005;60:135–142.

19. Vilaseca I, Chen AY, Backscheider AG: Long-term quality of life after total laryngectomy. *Head Neck* 2006;28:313–320.

20. Lotempio MM, Wang KH, Sadeghi A, et al: Comparison of quality of life outcomes in laryngeal cancer patients following chemoradiation v. total laryngectomy. *Otolaryngol Head Neck Surg* 2005;132:948–953.

21. Hui Y, Wei WI, Yuen PW, et al: Pharyngeal remnant after total laryngectomy and partial pharyngectomy: How much residual mucosa is sufficient? *Laryngoscope* 1996;106:490–494.

22. McConnel FMS, Duck SW, Hester TR: Hypopharyngeal stenosis. *Laryngoscope* 1984;94:1162–1164.

23. Andrews BT, McCulloch TM, Funk GF, et al: Deltopectoral flap revisited in the microvascular era: A single-institution 10-year experience. *Ann Otol Rhinol Laryngol* 2006;115(1):35–40.

24. Chao SS, Graham SM, Hoffman HT: Management of pharyngoesophageal spasm with Botox. *Otolaryngol Clin North Am* 2004;37(3):559–566.

25. Pauloski BR, Logemann JA, Rademaker AW, et al: Speech and swallowing function after oral and oropharyngeal resections: One-year follow-up. *Head Neck* 1994;16(4):313–322.

26. Brusati R, Collini M, Bozzetti A: Total glossectomy without laryngectomy. *J Maxillofac Surg* 1986;14(1):57–63.

27. Sultan MR, Coleman JJ: Oncologic and functional considerations of total glossectomy. *Am J Surg* 1989;158:297–302.

28. Lyos AT, Evans GR, Perez, D, et al: Tongue reconstruction: Outcomes with the rectus abdominis flap. *Plast Reconstr Surg* 1999;103:442–447.

29. Grabenbauer GG, Rödel C, Ernst-Stecken A, et al: Neck dissection following radiochemotherapy of advanced head and neck cancer—For selected cases only? *Radiother Oncol* 2003;66:57–63.

30. Biller HF, Lawson W, Som P, et al: Glomus vagale tumors. *Ann Otol Rhinol Laryngol* 1989;98:21–26.

31. Davidovic LB, Djukic VB, Vasic DM, et al: Diagnosis and treatment of carotid body paraganglioma: 21 years of experience at a clinical center of Serbia. *World J Surg Oncol* 2005;12:10.

32. Netterville JL, Vrabec JT: Unilateral palatal adhesion for paralysis after high vagal injury. *Arch Otolaryngol Head Neck Surg* 1994;120:218–221.

33. Fang TJ, Li HY, Tsai FC, et al: The role of glottal gap in predicting aspiration in patients with unilateral vocal paralysis. *Clin Otolaryngol* 2004;29:709–712.

34. Bhattacharyya N, Kotz T, Shapiro J: The effect of bolus consistency on dysphagia in unilateral vocal cord paralysis. *Otolaryngol Head Neck Surg* 2003;129:632–636.

35. Pauloski BR, Rademaker AW, Logemann JA, et al: Pretreatment swallowing function in patients with head and neck cancer. *Head Neck* 2000;22(5):474–482.

36. Pauloski BR, Rademaker AW, Logemann JA, et al: Surgical variables affecting swallowing in patients treated for oral/oropharyngeal cancer. *Head Neck* 2004;26(7):625–636.

37. Pauloski BR, Rademaker AW, Logemann JA, et al: Swallow function and perception of dysphagia in patients with head and neck cancer. *Head Neck* 2002;24(6):555–565.

38. Logemann JA: Swallowing disorders. *Best Pract Res Clin Gastroenterol* 2007;21(4):563–573.

39. Mittal BB, Pauloski BR, Haraf DJ, et al: Swallowing dysfunction—preventative and rehabilitation strategies in patients with head and neck cancers treated with surgery, radiotherapy, and chemotherapy: A critical review. *Int J Radiat Oncol Biol Phys* 2003;57:1219–1230.

CHAPTER 18

Palliative Medicine and End-of-Life Care

Francine Rainone

Head and neck cancer results in high rates of morbidity and mortality. Although site-specific 5-year survival rates have improved for some cancers of the head and neck, they have stayed the same or declined for others.[1] As a result, the overall 5-year survival rate remains approximately 50%. The 10-year survival rate for patients with stage III or IV head and neck cancer is no better than 23%.[2] Estimating the prognosis for an individual patient remains problematic as a result of the influence of other factors, such as comorbidities and the health-related quality of life at diagnosis.[3,4] For those who survive, persistent symptomatology after 3 years is the norm rather than the exception,[5,6] and 10-year survivors may experience a further decrease in the quality of life.[7] In light of the strong possibility that head and neck cancer will end or impair a person's life, physicians are faced with balancing the need to encourage hope without misleading patients about their prospects for the future.

As many as 98% of patients want physicians to be realistic with regard to their prognosis.[8] However, studies have repeatedly shown that physicians significantly overestimate survival.[9–15] It can be argued that giving an optimistic picture of survival provides hope for patients and their families. Alternatively, patients who expect to live longer than they actually do may die without adequate preparation, and almost everyone wants a chance to say "goodbye." In today's society, family and friends often live far apart, making it even more important to have the opportunity to plan for death rather than leaving unfinished business that negatively affects the quality of life of the patient's family and friends.

The palliative medicine approach frames the discussion of the prognosis in terms of hoping for the best and preparing for the worst. Many survivors report that they were unprepared for the long-term impact of surgery on their lives.[16] These survivors may be grateful to be alive, but they may still remain angry and unable to cope with their altered speech, taste, appearance, and so on. Physicians can play an important role in fostering good coping behaviors by frankly discussing the anticipated limitations that may result from treatment. When the prognosis likely includes death, patients report that it is still possible to support coping and to enhance hope. As one palliative medicine specialist put it, hope "is not the conviction that things will turn out well but the expectation that they will make sense, regardless of the outcome."[17]

In a recent study, patients indicated that emphasis on what is possible (including symptom control and emotional and social support), exploring realistic goals, and discussing the likely reality of day-to-day life were all ways to help them cope with a limited life expectancy.[18]

Head and neck surgeons are adept at working in multidisciplinary groups. Poor prognosis and heavy symptom burden in this population argue for the early involvement of a palliative medicine specialist as part of the standard multidisciplinary care of head and neck cancer patients. In the past, a sharp distinction was made between curable and incurable patients. Often palliative medicine specialists were not consulted until the patient was actively dying. Currently a more nuanced approach is advocated. Although there is no consensus regarding when to involve a palliative medicine specialist, all patients with stage III or higher head and neck cancer would likely benefit from a consultation. Additionally, patients with any stage of cancer who are suffering from intractable symptoms are likely to benefit from the addition of a palliative medicine specialist to the team.

QUALITY OF LIFE

Head and neck cancer and its treatment create problems in all four domains of the quality of life: (1) physical, (2) psychological, (3) social, and (4) spiritual. Often the effects overlap into more than one domain.

Physical Domain

In the physical domain, the most prevalent symptom is pain (including neck and shoulder pain). Studies have repeatedly documented the prevalence of pain in more than 80% of patients with late-stage disease.[19–22] Pain is not just unpleasant; patients with high pain scores are at increased risk for disability.[23] Other common physical symptoms include feeding disorders, speech disorders, and a loss of the senses of smell and taste.

Psychological Domain

Within the psychological domain, there remains a high rate of substance abuse, depression, anxiety, and adjustment disorders. Alcohol dependence or abuse is present in about 40% of patients.[22] Whether or not it predates the cancer diagnosis, the failure to address substance abuse can compromise recovery. Physical disfigurement and profound lifestyle changes[5] may help explain the high rates of anxiety (31%) and depression or adjustment disorder (16%–17%).[24–26]

Social Domain

Socially, patients are at high risk for becoming isolated. More than half of those working before their diagnosis become disabled either from their cancer or its treatment.[27] Feeding problems and alterations in smell and taste inhibit patients' participation in social events involving food and drink. Speech problems impair communication. Sexual problems, including problems with arousal and orgasm, are present in at least 50% of men,[28] and they persist over time.[29] Disfiguring surgery alters body image and the sense of self, and it changes the way that significant others perceive the patient, with the potential to further impair social relations.[30]

Spiritual Domain

The spiritual realm encompasses not only religious beliefs but all questions regarding meaning, purpose, and the person's place in the universe. Spiritual beliefs and practices often affect the degree to which a person is able to cope with life-threatening illness.[31] Spiritual crisis and negative religious coping behaviors impair adjustment and constitute a risk factor for mortality.[32,33]

Preventative Approach

Given the profound impact of symptoms on quality of life, a preventive approach involving routine screening is warranted. At present, the physician rating of symptoms correlates poorly with the patient rating of the impact of those symptoms on the quality of life.[34] Without such screening, the surgeon is likely to remain unaware of the need for intervention or consultation. In a recent survey, 67% of participants reported that they would like to complete a questionnaire to help them to describe their problems to their physicians as compared with 28% who said they would not.[35]

Because symptoms change over time depending on disease progression and treatment interventions, screening needs to be done at regular intervals. Several validated screening tools are available, including the European Organization for Research and Treatment of Cancer Quality of Life Questionnaire, the Functional Assessment of Cancer Therapy Head and Neck 35, and the Washington Quality of Life Questionnaire.[36]

MANAGEMENT OF COMMON SYMPTOMS

Pain is a multidimensional experience that affects the whole person. Pain has been defined as "an unpleasant sensory and emotional experience associated with actual or potential tissue damage or described in terms of such damage."[37] Galer and Dworkin[38] state that, because pain is "unpleasant," it provokes a behavioral response, and because it is "emotional," it is interpreted according to the meaning that the person experiencing it attributes to it.

The issue of meaning is particularly important for patients with life-threatening disease. The progression of cancer is accompanied by progressive disability. Progressive disability alters a patient's employment status, leisure activities, and family roles, which may erode a person's sense of identity, self-worth, and self-esteem. In this context, pain may be interpreted as meaning that disease is uncontrolled and that death is imminent. Even mild pain may trigger fears of death, disability, or the progression of disease. Providing patients with a safe environment in which to discuss the meaning of their pain is an important part of pain treatment, because pain management is unlikely to be successful without specifically addressing the emotional and behavioral responses that it elicits. Physicians, chaplains, and social workers may need to work together to ensure that relief is offered for the totality of the experience of pain.

On a physical level, pain is exhausting. It can disturb sleep, and it may exacerbate fatigue and depression, which further compromise healing and lead to greater disability. The early treatment of acute pain can prevent the development of chronic pain. The American Pain Society publishes guidelines for the management of cancer pain, including the use of radiation, chemotherapy, nerve blocks, and surgical approaches. In most situations, medical management is the first line of treatment, and it sufficiently controls 80% of pain. Another 10% to 15% of cases can be controlled with other means.[39]

Goals of Pain Management

The goals of pain management in the cancer patient are to maximize comfort and function and to prolong survival. Pain management requires a continuous cycle of assessment, intervention, and monitoring.[40] Complete assessment involves identifying the severity, quality, and timing of the pain, among other factors. The minimum acceptable assessment establishes the severity of pain by asking the patient either to rate the pain as mild, moderate, or severe or to rate it on a scale of 0 to 10, where 0 represents "no pain" and 10 represents the "worst pain imaginable." Mild pain (i.e., a rating of 1 to 3 out of 10) is usually managed with either nonpharmacologic or pharmacologic means.

Respecting patient preferences improves adherence and possibly effectiveness. Patients with mild pain who are reluctant to take medications have other options. Nonpharmacologic interventions for mild pain include distraction, heat, cold, and complementary therapies such as self-hypnosis. For some patients, counseling is helpful. Patients whose functional status remains largely intact may find that yoga or physical therapy provides relief. However, if reluctance to take medication is based on myths (e.g., the belief that opioids are invariably addicting), careful explanation and education are required.

Pharmacologic Interventions

Pharmacologic interventions for mild pain range from herbal remedies (e.g., willow bark) to acetaminophen to nonsteroidal anti-inflammatory drugs (NSAIDs). When pain is either moderate (i.e., rated 4 to 6 out of 10) or severe (i.e., rated 7 to 10 out of 10), opioids are almost always part of the treatment plan.

Moderate pain may be helped by nonpharmacologic methods, but it is rarely completely relieved by them. Medications that combine opioids with NSAIDs or acetaminophen are appropriate. Adjunctive medications (e.g., antispasmodics, antiepileptics) may be indicated in some cases.

The first-line treatment for almost all severe cancer pain is opioid medication. Relatively high doses (e.g., several grams of morphine per day) may be required to control cancer pain.

Managing the Side Effects

The higher the dose of opioids the more likely it is that the side effects will become troublesome. Patients usually do not report side effects unless they are specifically asked about them, either because they do not relate the symptom to the medication or for other reasons. Some patients endure sedation, constipation, nausea, vomiting, or pruritus because they think these effects are the price that they must pay to maintain analgesia. The following five major strategies are used to ameliorate side effects[41]:

1. Change the dose or dosing frequency.
2. Change agents.
3. Change the route of administration.
4. Add nonopioid analgesics, coanalgesics, and non-pharmaceutical methods of pain control.
5. Add an agent that counteracts a specific side effect.

Change the Dose or Dosing Frequency
The first strategy is to continue the same analgesic agent but to change the dose or the dosing frequency. A 25% decrease in opioid dose may maintain analgesic efficacy while reducing or eliminating side effects. If the decreased dose is insufficient for analgesia and the medication is short acting, give the lower dose at shorter intervals. Remember that short-acting formulas produce peaks in serum levels. Changing to long-acting formulas or to a continuous intravenous or subcutaneous infusion promotes a more constant serum level.

Change Agents
The second strategy is to change agents. Individual response to any given agent is highly variable. Often a different medication within the same class does not produce the same side effects. In other cases, known properties of medications can guide the choice of an alternative. For example, if a particular opioid produces pruritus and urticaria, it may help to change to fentanyl, which has a low potential to release histamine.

Change the Route of Administration
The third strategy is to change the route of administration. To avoid or minimize gastrointestinal side effects, try the subcutaneous, intravenous, or transdermal routes. For patients with advanced cancer, pain control may require very large doses of opioids. If effects such as sedation, nausea, or vomiting are dose related, the intraspinal route may be best, because it allows for a dramatic dose reduction (often 90%), with resultant lower levels of drugs in the brainstem, without compromising analgesia.

Add Nonopioid Analgesics, Coanalgesics, and Nonpharmaceutical Methods of Pain Control
The fourth strategy for managing opioid side effects is dose sparing by adding nonopioid analgesics, coanalgesics, and nonpharmaceutical methods of pain control. Nonopioid analgesics (e.g., acetaminophen, NSAIDs) act synergistically with opioids, and they may provide sufficient relief to permit decreased doses of opioids. Coanalgesics (e.g., caffeine) are agents that enhance analgesia and are at least partly analgesic or counteract the side effects of analgesics. Other commonly used coanalgesics include tricyclic antidepressants (TCAs), antiepileptics, and glucocorticoids. Physical, psychological, and/or complementary modalities may also provide enough pain relief to allow for a decrease in opioid dose. In this sense, they could also be said to act as coanalgesics.

Add an Agent That Counteracts a Specific Side Effect
The fifth major strategy used to manage the side effects of opioids is to add an agent that counteracts a specific side effect. Table 18-1 displays a partial list of agents that may be used to treat selected side effects of opioids.

NEUROPATHIC PAIN

Neuropathic pain is often difficult to control. It is less responsive to opioids than nociceptive pain, and it usually requires the addition of adjuvant analgesics.[42,43]

TABLE 18-1   Selected Agents for Managing Side Effects of Opioids

Nausea/Vomiting	Constipation	Pruritus	Sedation
Metoclopramide* 10 mg PO/IV q4h prn	Senna* 1–3 tablets bid or tid	Diphenhydramine* 25–50 mg PO/IV q12h	Caffeine
Prochlorperazine* 10 mg PO/IV q4h or 25 mg PR q8h	Bisacodyl 1–3 tablets bid or tid	Hydrocortisone 1% cream to affected area q6h	Dextroamphetamine 2.5–15 mg PO qd (divide doses if >5 mg)
Haloperidol 1 mg PO/IV/SC or PR bid or tid; titrate up to 20 mg if needed	Docusate 100–300 mg bid or tid	Dexamethasone 1 mg PO qd	Methylphenidate 2.5–15 mg PO qd or tid
Add meclizine if motion exacerbates symptoms	70% sorbitol or lactulose 15–60 ml bid or tid		Modafinil 100–400 mg daily is almost 5 times as expensive as methylphenidate
If severe: Transdermal scopolamines 5HT3 antagonist†	*If severe:* Sodium phosphate, magnesium citrate, or enemas		

bid, Twice daily; *IV,* intravenously; *PO,* orally; *PR,* rectally; *prn,* as needed; *qd,* daily; *q4h,* every 4 hours; *q8h, every 8 hours; q12h,* every 12 hours; *SC,* subcutaneously; *tid,* three times daily; *5HT3,* 5-hydroxytryptamine 3.
*Available in liquid form.
†Ondansetron is available in both liquid and oral transdermal forms.

Anti-Epileptic Drugs

In clinical practice, antiepileptic drugs have become the drugs of choice for lancinating pain and incident pain, and they are widely used for all types of neuropathic pain.[44,45] Gabapentin is effective and relatively well tolerated, and it has few drug–drug interactions.[46] The starting dose is between 100 mg and 300 mg given before bed. For most people, pain control is achieved at between 900 mg and 3600 mg given daily in three divided doses. Numerous other antiepileptic drugs are also used.

Tricyclic Antidepressants

Tricyclic Antidepressants (TCAs) are also commonly used to treat neuropathic pain caused by cancer.[47,48] The advantages of TCAs include their low price, their once-daily dosing, and the fact that they produce analgesia at lower doses than those required to treat depression.

The choice of agent depends on its side-effect profile, especially the agent's degree of sedation, orthostatic hypotension, weight gain, and anticholinergic action. Amitriptyline produces the greatest degree of all of these effects. Nortriptyline and desipramine are minimally sedating and anticholinergic, with only a modest effect on orthostatic hypotension and weight gain. Trazodone is as sedating as amitriptyline, without anticholinergic activity and with minimal effects on orthostasis and weight gain.[49]

Because they have class-1A (i.e., sodium-channel blocking) antiarrythmic actions, TCAs should be used with caution in patients with known arrythmias or ischemic heart disease.[50,51] As with most medications, increased doses lead to increased side effects.

Although the evidence for the practice is limited, when depression or pain is recalcitrant to treatment with TCAs or their dose must be limited because of untoward side effects, clinicians often add a selective serotonin reuptake inhibitor.[52,53] Citalopram and escitalopram do not interfere with the metabolism of TCAs, thereby making them attractive for combination therapy. Another choice is to add duloxetine, a selective serotonin and norepinephrine reuptake inhibitor for treatment of depression, diabetic peripheral neuropathy, and fibromyalgia.

Management of Plexopathies

The management of plexopathies (involving major peripheral neural plexuses) and incident pain (pain with movement) often requires interventional techniques.[54,55]

Interventional techniques include nerve blocks, the spinal administration of anesthetics and other medications, and surgical procedures. Anesthesiologists, interventional radiologists, and some general surgeons and rehabilitation specialists are trained to administer these techniques. Although there are exceptions, surgical techniques generally have relatively high morbidity rates, and they are usually used when systemic medications fail to control pain adequately and when adequate pain control requires dosing systemic medications at levels that produce unacceptable and uncontrollable side effects.

Managing Feeding Problems

Managing feeding problems (e.g., xerostomia, dysphagia, odynophagia) for the patient with head and neck cancer requires a multidisciplinary approach. Speech and swallow experts and nutritionists work with surgeons to maximize patient function. If obstruction or aspiration is intractable to pharmaceutical and non-pharmaceutical interventions, palliative tracheostomy or laryngectomy may be indicated.[56]

Managing Mucositis

Mucositis is an inevitable result of radiotherapy and a frequent result of some forms of chemotherapy. It is painful, and it may interfere with oral intake. The Cochrane Database reviewed a plethora of interventions for preventing oral mucositis and concluded the following[57]:

- Amifostine provided minimal benefit.
- Chinese medicine was beneficial for mild, moderate, and severe mucositis. Relative risk values (RR) were 0.44 (95% confidence interval [CI] 0.20 to 0.98), 0.44 (95% CI 0.33 to 0.59), and 0.16 (95% CI 0.07 to 0.35), respectively.
- Hydrolytic enzymes benefited moderate and severe mucositis, with RRs of 0.52 (95% CI 0.36 to 0.74) and 0.17 (95% CI 0.06 to 0.52), respectively
- Ice chips prevented all degrees of mucositis, with RRs of 0.64 (95% CI 0.50 to 0.82), 0.38 (95% CI 0.23 to 0.62), and 0.24 (95% CI 0.12 to 0.48).

Numerous other options are available, but there is insufficient evidence to recommend any of them.

Managing Fungating Skin Lesions

Fungating skin lesions are often malodorous as a result of the presence of anaerobic bacteria. Appropriate wound dressings, metronidazole gel with or without oral metronidazole, the use of essential oils in a bland base (e.g., A+D Ointment, Maalox, yogurt, buttermilk, topical sugar, or honey) are all effective for helping to control odor.[58] Placing cat litter in the room may also reduce odor.

PREPARATION FOR DEATH

Palliative medicine specialists are committed to ensuring that patients and their families are well prepared for what may happen during the course of illness so that there will be no surprises.[59] As the disease progresses, it is important to apprise patients and families of the likely symptoms and mechanisms of death. Hemorrhage, for example, is a very frightening complication for which advance planning can be extremely helpful. If patients elect to continue treatment, preventing hemorrhage (e.g., by maximizing nutrition and preventing constipation) should be explained.[60] If patients have forgone additional treatment, using dark-colored sheets and having dark-red or black towels at the bedside to absorb blood decreases the disturbing nature of witnessing a person bleeding.

Patients hope for a peaceful death. Many people find it comforting to know that, if suffering remains intractable, palliative sedation until death is an option. Midazolam is frequently used to induce unconsciousness during the last days of life, when symptoms such as pain, dyspnea, nausea, and agitated delirium are uncontrollable, when other options have been thoroughly explored, and when the patient, his or her family members, or both choose palliative sedation.[61]

SELF-CARE FOR SURGEONS

More than any other medical specialists, surgeons may provide life-saving interventions to patients. In addition to saving lives, head and neck cancer surgeons regularly deal with death. As with other health-care professionals, surgeons who regularly deal with patient suffering are at risk for burnout. Self-care is the best preventive and treatment strategy for burnout.[62]

People vary with regard to the specific methods that they find effective, but the basic elements of self-care plans are the same. Individual, interpersonal, and professional strategies—whether used singly or in combination—allow health-care professionals to continue caring for patients. Individual strategies involve sustained attention to the surgeon's own health needs as well as to the his or her needs for rest and rejuvenation. This attention may take the form of exercising, following a healthy diet, planning vacations and other enjoyable outings, or engaging in reflection through journaling or conversations with others. Interpersonal strategies include strengthening relationships with current family members and friends as well as expanding one's community through activism or spiritual endeavors. Professional strategies include debriefing after emotionally difficult events with colleagues or mentors and writing about these events to share experiences and insights with others. When stress interferes with regular functioning, it is often helpful to reach out to professional counselors or chaplains.

CONCLUSION

Palliative medicine specialists can assist head and neck surgeons with providing comprehensive care that is customized to reflect patient and family preferences and that maximizes the quality of life throughout the course of head and neck cancer. Head and neck surgeons should take care to prevent burnout by using effective strategies for self-care. The palliative medicine team can provide assistance with the development of self-care strategies.

REFERENCES

1. Carvalho AL, Nishimoto IN, Califano JA, et al: Trends in incidence and prognosis for head and neck cancer in the United States: A site-specific analysis of the SEER database. *Int J Cancer* 2005;114(5):806–816.
2. Zorat PL, Paccagnella A, Cavaniglia G, et al: Randomized phase III trial of neoadjuvant chemotherapy in head and neck cancer: 10-year follow-up. *J Natl Cancer Inst* 2004;96:1714–1717.
3. Piccirillo JF, Lacy PD, Basu A, et al: Development of a new head and neck cancer-specific comorbidity index. *Arch Otolaryngol Head Neck Surg* 2002;128(10):1172–1179.
4. Nordgren M, Jannert M, Boysen M, et al: Health-related quality of life in patients with pharyngeal carcinoma: A five-year follow-up. *Head Neck* 2006;28(4):339–349.
5. Abendstein H, Nordgren M, Boysen M, et al: Quality of life and head and neck cancer: A 5 year prospective study. *Laryngoscope* 2005;115(12):2183–2192.
6. Hammerlid E, Taft C: Health-related quality of life in long-term head and neck cancer survivors: A comparison with general population norms. *Br J Cancer* 2001;84(2):149–156.
7. Mehanna HM, Morton RP: Deterioration in quality of life of late (10-year) survivors of head and neck cancer. *Clin Otolaryngol* 2006;31(3):204–211.
8. Hagerty RG, Bultow PH, Ellis PM, et al: Communicating with realism and hope: Incurable cancer patients' views on the disclosure of prognosis. *J Clin Oncol* 2005;23:1278.
9. Parkes CM: Accuracy of predictions of survival in later stages of cancer. *Br Med J* 1972;2:29.
10. Evans C, McCarthy M: Prognostic uncertainty in terminal care: Can the Karnofsky index help? *Lancet* 1985;1:1204.
11. Heyse-Moore LH, Johnson-Bell VE: Can doctors accurately predict the life expectancy of patients with terminal cancer? *Palliat Med* 1987;1:165.
12. Forster LE, Lynn J: Predicting the life span for applicants to inpatient hospice. *Arch Intern Med* 1988;148:2540.
13. Maltoni M, Pirovani M, Scarpi E, et al: Prediction of survival of patients terminally ill with cancer: Results of an Italian prospective multicentric study. *Cancer* 1995;75:2613.
14. Oxenham D, Cornbleet MA: Accuracy of prediction of survival by different professional groups in a hospice. *Palliat Med* 1998;12:117.
15. Christakis NA, Lamont EB: Extent and determinants of error in doctors' prognoses in terminally ill patients: Prospective cohort study. *BMJ* 2002;320:469.
16. Newell R, Ziegler L, Stafford N, et al: The information needs of head and neck cancer patients prior to surgery. *Ann R Coll Surg Engl* 2004;86(6):407–410.
17. Creagan ET: Patient-physician communication in the cancer setting. In Berger A, Portenoy RK, Weissman DE, editors: *Principles and practice of supportive oncology*, Philadelphia, 1998, Lippincott.
18. Clayton JM, Butow PN, Arnol RM, et al: Fostering coping and nurturing hope when discussing the future with terminally ill cancer patients and their caregivers. *Cancer* 2005;103(9):1965–1975.
19. Shedd DP, Carl A, Shedd C: Problems of terminal head and neck cancer patients. *Head Neck Surg* 1980;2(6):476–482.
20. Forbes K: Palliative care in patients with cancer of the head and neck. *Clin Otolaryngol Allied Sci* 1997;22(2):117–122.
21. Ethunandan M, Rennie A, Hoffman G, et al: Quality of dying in head and neck cancer patients: A retrospective analysis of potential indicators of care. *Oral Surg Oral Med Oral Pathol Oral Radiol Endod* 2005;100(2):147–152.
22. Van Wilgen CP, Dijkstra PU, Van der Laan BF, et al: Shoulder and neck morbidity in quality of life after surgery for head and neck cancer. *Head Neck* 2004;26(10):839–844.
23. Taylor JC, Terrell JE, Ronis DL, et al: Disability in patients with head and neck cancer. *Arch Otolaryngol Head Neck Surg* 2004;30(6):764–769.
24. Vickery LE, Latchford G, Hewison J, et al: The impact of head and neck cancer and facial disfigurement on the quality of life of patients and their partners. *Head Neck* 2003;25(4):289–296.
25. Katz MR, Irish JC, Devins GM, et al: Psychosocial adjustment in head and neck cancer: The impact of disfigurement, gender and social support. *Head Neck* 2003;25(2):103–112.
26. Kugaya A, Akechi T, Okuyama T, et al: Prevalence, predictive factors, and screening for psychosocial distress in patients with newly diagnosed head and neck cancer. *Cancer* 2000;88(12):2817–2823.
27. Taylor JC: 2004. op.cit.
28. Monga U, Tan G, Ostermann HJ, et al: Sexuality in head and neck cancer patients. *Arch Phys Med Rehabil* 1997;78(3):298–304.
29. Bjordal K, Ahlner-Elmqvist M, Hammerlid E, et al: A prospective study of quality of life in head and neck cancer patients—Part II. *Longitudinal Data* 2001;111(8):1440–1452.
30. Dropkins MJ: Body image and quality of life after head and neck cancer surgery. *Cancer Pract* 1999;7(6):309–313.
31. Hinshaw DB: Spiritual issues in surgical palliative care. *Surg Clin North Am* 2005;85(2):257–272.
32. Fitchett G: Screening for spiritual risk. *Chaplaincy Today* 1999;15:2–12.
33. Pargament KI, Koenig HG, Tarakeshwar N, et al: Religious struggle as a predictor of mortality among medically ill elderly patients. *Arch Intern Med* 2001;161:1881–1885.
34. Jensen K, Bonde Jensen A, Grau C: The relationship between observer-based toxicity scoring and patient assessed symptom severity after treatment for head and neck cancer: A correlative cross sectional study of the DAHANCA toxicity scoring system and the EORTC quality of life questionnaires. *Radiother Oncol* 2006;78(3):298–305.
35. Rampling T, King H, Mais KL, et al: Quality of life measurement in the head and neck cancer radiotherapy clinic: Is it feasible and worthwhile? *Clin Oncol* 2003;15(4):205–210.
36. Mehanna HM, Morton RP: Patients' views on the utility of quality of life questionnaires in head and neck cancer: a randomized trial. *Clin Otolaryngol* 2006;31(4):310–316.
37. Merskey H: Classification of chronic pain: Description of chronic pain syndromes and definitions of pain terms. *Pain* 1979;(Suppl 3):S217.
38. Galer BS, Dworkin RH: *A clinical guide to neuropathic pain*, Minneapolis, Minn, 2000, McGraw-Hill Healthcare Information Programs.
39. Miaskowski C, Cleary J, Burney R, et al: *Guideline for the management of cancer pain in adults and children: APS clinical practice guidelines series* 2005, No. 3. Glenview, Ill, 2005.
40. Rainone F: Treating adult cancer pain in primary care. *J Am Board Fam Pract* 2004;17:S48–S56.
41. Ashburn MA, Lipman AG, Carr D, et al: *Principles of analgesia use in the treatment of acute pain and cancer pain*, ed 5, Glenview, Ill, 2003, American Pain Society.
42. Grond S, Radbruch L, Meuser T, et al: Assessment and treatment of neuropathic cancer pain following WHO guidelines. *Pain* 1999;79:15–20.
43. Cherney NI, Thaler HT, Friedlander-Klar H, et al: Opioid responsiveness of cancer pain syndromes caused by neuropathic or nociceptive mechanisms. *Neurology* 1994;44:857–861.
44. McQuay H, Carroll D, Jadad AR, et al: Anticonvulsant drugs for management of pain: A systematic review. *BMJ* 1995;311(7012):1047–1052.
45. Swerdlow M: Anticonvulsant drugs and chronic pain. *Clin Neuropharmacol* 1984;7:51–82.
46. Farrar JT, Portenoy RK: Neuropathic cancer pain: The role of adjuvant analgesics. *Oncology (Williston Park)* 2001;15(11):1435–1442, 1445; discussion 1445, 1450–1453.

47. McQuay HJ, Tramer M, Nye BA, et al: A systematic review of anti-depressants for neuropathic pain. *Pain* 1996;68(2–3):217–227.

48. Elja K, Tiina T, Pertti NJ: Amitriptyline effectively relieves neuropathic pain following treatment of breast cancer. *Pain* 1996;64(2):293–302.

49. Ventafridda V, Bonezzi C, Caraceni A, et al: Antidepressants for cancer pain and other painful syndromes with deafferentation component: Comparison of amitriptyline and trazodone. *Ital J Neurol Sci* 1987;8:579–587.

50. Hippisley-Cox J, Pringle M, Hammersley V, et al: Antidepressants as risk factor for ischemic heart disease: Case-control study in primary care. *BMJ* 2001;323(7314):666–669.

51. Cohen HW, Gibson G, Alderman MH: Excess risk of myocardial infarction in patients treated with antidepressant medications: Association with use of tricyclic agents. *Am J Med* 2000;108(1):2–8.

52. Nelson JC, Mazure C, Bowers MD, et al: *Synergistic effects of fluoxetine and desipramine: A prospective study.* Presented at the 21st meeting of the Collegium Internationale Neuro-Psychophar-macologicum Congress, Glasgow, Scotland, July 12–16, 1998.

53. Weilburg JB, Rosenbaum JF, Biederman J, et al: Fluoxetine added to non-MAOI antidepressants converts nonresponders to respond-ers: A preliminary report. *J Clin Psychiatry* 1989;50(12):447–449.

54. Marshall KA: Managing cancer pain: Basic principles and inva-sive treatments. *Mayo Clin Proc* 1996;71(5):472–477.

55. Miguel R: Interventional treatment of cancer pain: The fourth step in the World Health Organization analgesic ladder? *Cancer Control* 2000;7(2):149–156.

56. Eisele DW, Yarington CT Jr, Lindeman RC: Indications for the tracheoesophageal diversion procedure and the laryngotracheal separation procedure. *Ann Otol Rhinol Laryngol* 1988;97 (5 Pt 1):471–475.

57. Worthington HV, Clarkson JE, Eden OB: Interventions for pre-venting oral mucositis for patients with cancer receiving treat-ment. *Cochrane Database Syst Rev* 2007;(4):CD000978. DOI: 10.1002/14651858.pub3.

58. Abrahm JL: *A physician's guide to pain and symptom manage-ment in cancer patients,* Baltimore, MD, 2000, Johns Hopkins Univ. Press.

59. Shugarman LR, Lorenz K, Lynn J: End-of-life care: An agenda for policy improvement. *Clin Geriatr Med* 2005;21(1):xi, 255–272.

60. Frawley T, Bedley CM: Causes and prevention of carotid artery rupture. *Br J Nurs* 2006;14(22):1198–1202.

61. Cowan JD, Palmer TW: Practical guide to palliative sedation. *Curr Oncol* 2002;4(3):242–249.

62. Blust L: *Fast fact and concept #169: Health professional burnout: Part III* (website): http://www.eperc.mcw.edu/fastFact/ff_169.htm. Accessed April 1, 2008.

CHAPTER 19

Quality of Life in Head and Neck Cancer

Shatul L. Parikh and Amy Y. Chen

Head and neck cancer represents 5% of all cancers diagnosed annually. Although upper aerodigestive tract cancers account for a small percentage of incident cancers, the vast majority of head and neck cancers are diagnosed when the disease is in an advanced stage. Contemporary treatment consists of multimodality regimens (i.e., surgery, radiation therapy, and chemotherapy). Both the cancer and the resulting treatment can affect a patient's social functioning, including his or her ability to speak and eat.

Treatment end points for patients with cancer have historically been measured by objective tumor response, locoregional control, overall survival, and disease-free survival. For head and neck cancer, end points such as functional status and quality of life are equally important. McNeil and colleagues[1] demonstrated in their famous "fireman study" that individuals would rather die than lose their larynx to surgical resection for cancer. Within the last two decades, there has been a concerted effort by caregivers to address the loss of health and the consequences of treatment that often results in physical impairment, functional impairment, the disruption of social and family interactions, and psychological distress. These impairments have a tremendous effect on patient quality of life (QOL), and they have become increasingly important considerations in concert with previously determined cancer end points.

QUALITY OF LIFE

Quality of life is a multidimensional construct that includes physical, functional, psychological, and social well-being.[2] Other dimensions may include spirituality, sexuality, occupation functioning, treatment satisfaction, and global ratings of QOL.[3] The larger the gap that exists between the perceived reality and one's expectations, the poorer the QOL.[4] One important construct in the measurement of QOL is that patients are queried for their responses; the questionnaires are self-administered rather than completed by a health-care provider. Changes over time can occur; thus it is of utmost importance to use validated and reliable instruments that can accurately reflect the change.

Generic and disease-specific measures are available for use. Generic health questionnaires inquire into patients' general health status and are applicable to all populations. They can be completed by individuals with and without medical illnesses. These instruments provide benchmarks for comparison across diverse demographic, ethnic, and disease populations. Examples include the Nottingham Health Profile and the Short Form-36 from the Medical Outcomes Study.[5,6] Generic instruments used for patients with specific illnesses also assess general health status and each patient's individual perceptions of the functional impact of his or her illness. The Sickness Impact Profile and the Functional Assessment of Chronic Illness Therapy are both examples of these types of measures.[7,8]

Disease-specific measures are designed to assess the QOL of patients with specific disease states. A number of frequently employed instruments that are specific to head and neck cancer have been created and validated. The European Organization for Research into the Treatment of Cancer Quality of Life Questionnaire for Head and Neck Cancer is a self-administered module that assesses symptoms and side effects that are relevant for patients with head and neck cancer. The scale is sensitive to changes before and after treatment with surgery, radiation therapy, and chemotherapy.[9]

The Functional Assessment of Cancer Therapy–Head and Neck (FACT–H&N) uses the generic measurement instrument FACT, which consists of 27 questions in four domains, and adds an 11-item module that is specific to head and neck cancer.[10] The FACT–H&N is self-administered and easy to read, with clear instructions and consistent response options. The modular construction allows for comparison across cancer diagnoses while probing into issues that are specific to head and neck cancer.

A third example is the University of Washington Quality of Life Questionnaire. This is a self-administered scale that consists of 15 questions that assess nine domains in addition to overall QOL: (1) pain; (2) physical appearance; (3) activity; (4) recreation; (5) employment; (6) chewing; (7) swallowing; (8) speech; and (9) shoulder function.[11] It is a short instrument that appears to be best suited to patients undergoing surgery. There has been a recent revision that has added some issues of potential importance to patients undergoing radiation therapy, including xerostomia and dysgeusia. It has shown promising reliability, responsiveness, and validity, and it is a clinically useful tool for surgically treated patients with head and neck cancer.

Symptom-specific measures including the MD Anderson Dysphagia Inventory and the voice-related QOL measure are self-administered, validated instruments that report scores with both global and physical subscales. These tools evaluate the effects of disease and treatment on specific domains and the resulting overall effect on QOL.[12,13] In addition, the MD Anderson Dysphagia Inventory was specifically developed for use with patients with head and neck cancer.

These instruments are used throughout the course of treatment to measure changes in quality of life. Cella[14] suggests that QOL measurement take place at four points during the course of treatment and follow up:

1. Immediately before treatment

2. During treatment

3. At the end of successful treatment or at the point when the patient is considered to be nonresponsive to treatment

4. At the 6-month follow-up evaluation after time point 3

In clinical trials in which the interest may be the short- or long-term acute effects of treatment (i.e., the toxic effects of chemotherapy or radiation therapy), more frequent QOL assessment may be appropriate. Long-term assessment is also useful to determine whether the patients recover or exceed their baseline QOL.

SURGICAL TREATMENT AND QUALITY OF LIFE

Any treatment of head and neck cancer can result in disfigurement; voice loss; drooling; and difficulty with breathing, swallowing, or both.[15,16] These dysfunctions lead to psychosocial issues such as moderate to severe distress, negative self-image, and disturbed interpersonal relationships.[16] McNeil and colleagues[1] demonstrated that death was preferred over having a total laryngectomy in their fireman study. In 1991, the results of the Veterans Administration Laryngeal Cancer Study were published.[17] This study supported the use of chemotherapy and radiation therapy for patients with advanced laryngeal cancer who wished for laryngeal-conserving therapy. Several other studies followed, including the Radiation Therapy Oncology Group 91-11 and the European Organization for Research into the Treatment of Cancer, which demonstrated comparable control rates for both nonsurgical and surgical management of advanced cancer of the head and neck.

Despite the assumption that extirpative surgical resection results in greater detriments to QOL, several studies have demonstrated that the QOL is not adversely affected in the long term. Rogers and colleagues[18] classified 130 primary surgery patients into three distinct QOL groups at baseline. All groups reported diminished QOL during treatment but then recovered to baseline during the posttreatment period.

Another study by Vilaseca and colleagues[19] demonstrated that the long-term reported Short Form-12 scores of patients who had undergone laryngectomies were comparable with those of nonlaryngectomy patients with regard to the physical summary domain. In this survey of laryngectomy survivors, several commented on their questionnaires that they wished they had undergone laryngectomy earlier during the course of their disease because of their improved QOL after the procedure (in contrast with being dependent on gastrostomy or tracheostomy tubes).

The reconstruction of defects is often required after extirpative surgery. In 1987, McConnel and colleagues[20] compared three types of oral cavity reconstruction: skin grafts, hemi-tongue flaps, and autologous myocutaneous flaps. Speech and swallowing were studied in 15 surgical patients with T2 or T3 tongue and/or floor-of-mouth lesions. Additionally, end points such as speech intelligibility, articulation, tongue mobility, and oral-phase swallowing were evaluated. Tongue mobility was found to be the most significant factor in the determination of postoperative speech results. Patients with split-thickness skin grafts had the best speech and swallowing function.[20]

Komisar and colleagues[21] studied the impact of mandibular reconstruction on patients' functional status after the resection of the mandible for oropharyngeal cancer. They concluded that surgical reconstruction with reconstruction plates and screws of the lateral mandibular defects did little to improve QOL among patients with advanced oropharyngeal tumors. By contrast, Urken[22] demonstrated the functional advantages of lateral mandibular reconstruction with free-tissue transfer. In almost all functional and psychosocial categories, patients who had undergone bony reconstruction had higher scores. The average length of hospitalization was not significantly different. It was found during long-term follow up that patients who underwent bony reconstruction and eventual dental rehabilitation achieved a functional level closer to that of their predisease state as compared with the nonrepaired patients. However, this study did not address the pretreatment functional status and the impact that this may have had on posttreatment function and QOL. A prospective randomized study evaluating pretreatment QOL evaluation and its confounding effect on posttreatment QOL could address this question.

Researchers have also examined the effects of different types of neck dissections on QOL. Surgeries sparing the spinal accessory nerve have been associated with significantly less pain at comparable lengths of time aftertreatment.[23] By 12 months, however, patients who did not have spinal-accessory-nerve–sparing surgery had QOL scores that were comparable with those who did. This again demonstrates that, over the long term, surgical patients can recover to their baseline QOL and functional statuses.

NONSURGICAL TREATMENT AND QUALITY OF LIFE

Radiation therapy is not generally associated with major physical disfigurement. However, it does result in other significant long-term sequelae that affect swallowing, chewing, voice quality, loss of taste, xerostomia, esophageal stricture, osteoradionecrosis, soft-tissue fibrosis, neck contractures, facial edema, dental caries, and trismus. These complications persist after treatment and may even worsen over time. The addition of chemotherapy, which is often done for its radiation-sensitizing effects, intensifies these acute and late effects of radiation therapy.[24,25] One third of patients who receive concurrent therapy cannot complete or require modification of their treatment regimen because of the toxicity of combined treatment.

Advances in radiation therapy are judged not only by tumor-control rates but also by the impact on patients' QOL. According to a long-term follow up (7–11 years after treatment) of a randomized study, hyperfractionated radiation (2.35 Gy daily 4 days per week) was associated with similar or better QOL as compared with conventionally fractionated radiation therapy.[26] Another study compared laryngeal cancer patients receiving continuous hyperfractionated accelerated radiation therapy (CHART) with primarily stage II disease with patients with primarily stage I disease receiving conventional fractionation. Although initial QOL scores were similar across all groups, those receiving CHART showed greater improvement in QOL after 1 year despite more severe initial toxicity.[27] In a large, randomized trial of 615 patients with advanced head and neck cancer, more severe physical and emotional side effects resulted from the use of CHART as compared with conventional radiation therapy. However, symptoms appeared to be more persistent in the conventionally treated group.[28] A study comparing patients who were treated with conventional therapy and concomitant boost therapy showed no major differences in QOL but found that xerostomia was a major contributor to poorer QOL.[29]

The newest advance in radiation therapy, intensity-modulated radiation therapy (IMRT), delivers focused radiation to specific head and neck subsites in an effort to spare the salivary glands. A case-control study of head and neck cancer patients who received either standard radiotherapy or IMRT compared QOL scores and reports of xerostomia.[30] Although symptoms and QOL scores initially worsened in both groups, over time there was a significant trend toward improvement in the IMRT group that was not observed in the conventional radiation therapy group. At 12 months after treatment, xerostomia and QOL were significantly better in the IMRT group but not in those patients who received standard radiation therapy.[30]

Combined regimens with radiation therapy and chemotherapy have increasingly been used for the management of advanced head and neck cancer. Although these treatments can preserve organs (thereby minimizing the disfigurements of surgery), these regimens often result in increased toxicities that have major effects on QOL. In a longitudinal study of 64 patients with advanced head and neck cancer who were treated with therapeutic dosing concomitant with chemoradiotherapy, acute treatment toxicities were severe, with initial significant declines in virtually all QOL domains. At 1 year, general functional and physical measures had returned to baseline levels, although 30% of patients continued to report difficulties with swallowing, speech, hoarseness, and mouth pain. Pretreatment and posttreatment functional deficits were also measured at 12 months; xerostomia (6% vs. 58%), difficulty with taste (8% vs. 32%), and dysphagia (42% vs. 82%) were still issues for these patients at that time.[31]

CONCLUSION

Assumptions have arisen from studies by McNeil and colleagues[1] and others that functional deficits (e.g., speech, swallowing) result in poorer overall QOL. Although many head and neck cancer patients experience significant posttreatment functional deficits, patients often recover to their pretreatment QOL. A multidisciplinary team approach that includes social work, nutritionists, patient support groups, and psychological counseling is essential to address the functional and QOL changes that occur as a result of the cancer and its treatment, whether surgical or nonsurgical.

As more information is collected about the prevalent QOL concerns experienced by patients with head and neck cancer, clinicians can use this information to develop more comprehensive treatment plans. Although the past 5 years have shown many advances in QOL research for patients with head and neck cancer, there are still a number of continuing challenges that command attention. For example, the extent to which—and how—these data may be clinically useful for an individual patient with regard to decision making is a relatively uncharted area of investigation. Intensive efforts are not needed to encourage QOL measurements in all clinical trials. Standardizing the measurement of QOL for patients with head and neck cancer will be essential if this important construct is to be used as an end point for decision making.

REFERENCES

1. McNeil BJ, Weichselbaum R, Parker SG: Speech and survival: Tradeoffs between quality and quantity of life in laryngeal cancer. *N Engl J Med* 1981;305(17):982–987.
2. Gotay CC: Trial-related quality of life: Using quality of life assessment to distinguish among cancer therapies. *J Natl Cancer Inst Monogr* 1996;20:1–16.
3. Cella DF, Tulsky DS: Measuring quality of life today: Methodological aspects. *Oncology* 1990;4:29–38.
4. Morton RP, Davies ADM, Baker J, et al: Quality of life in treated head and neck cancer patients: A preliminary report. *Clin Otolaryngol* 1984;9:181–185.
5. Hunt SM, McEwen J, McKenna SP: Measuring health status: A new tool for clinicians and epidemiologists. *J R Coll Gen Pract* 1985;35:185–188.
6. Ware J, Sherbourne CD: The MOS 36-item short form health survey (SF-36). I: Conceptual framework and item selection. *Med Care* 1992;30:473–483.
7. Bergner M, Bobbitt RA, Carter WB, et al: The Sickness Impact Profile: Development and final revision of a health status measure. *Med Care* 1981;19:787–805.
8. Cella D: *Manual of the Functional Assessment of Chronic Illness Therapy (FACIT) scales,* Evanston, Ill, 1997, Evanston Northwestern Healthcare.
9. Bjordal K, Kaasa S: Psychometric validation of the EORTC core quality of life questionnaire: 30 item version and diagnosis-specific module for head and neck cancer patients. *Acta Oncol* 1992;31:311–321.
10. List MA, D'Antonio LL, Cella DF, et al: The Performance Status Scale for Head and Neck Cancer Patients and the Functional Assessment of Cancer Therapy–Head and Neck Scale. A study of utility and validity. *Cancer* 1996;77:2294–2301.
11. Hassan SJ, Weymuller EA Jr: Assessment of quality of life in head and neck cancer patients. *Head Neck* 1993;15:485–496.
12. Chen AY, Frankowski R, Bishop-Leone J, et al: The development and validation of a dysphagia-specific quality-of-life questionnaire for patients with head and neck cancer: The M. D. Anderson dysphagia inventory. *Arch Otolaryngol Head Neck Surg* 2001;127:870–876.
13. Hogikyan ND, Sethuraman G: Validation of an instrument to measure voice-related quality of life (V-RQOL). *J Voice* 1999;13:557–569.
14. Cella DF, Cherin EA: Quality of life during and after cancer treatment. *Compr Ther* 1988;14:69–75.
15. Dropkin MJ: Coping with disfigurement and dysfunction after head and neck cancer surgery: A conceptual framework. *Semin Oncol Nurs* 1989;5:213–219.
16. de Boer MF, Pruyn JF, van den Borne B, et al: Rehabilitation outcomes of long-term survivors treated for head and neck cancer. *Head Neck* 1995;17:503–515.
17. The Department of Veterans Affairs Laryngeal Cancer Study Group: Induction chemotherapy plus radiation compared with surgery plus radiation in patients with advanced laryngeal cancer. *N Engl J Med* 1991;324:1685–1690.
18. Rogers SN, Lowe D, Humphris G: Distinct patient groups in oral cancer: A prospective study of perceived health status following primary surgery. *Oral Oncol* 2000;36:529–538.
19. Vilaseca I, Chen AY, Backsheider A: Long-term quality of life after total laryngectomy. *Head Neck* 2006;28:313–320.
20. McConnel FMS, Teichgraeber JF, Alder RK: A comparison of three methods of oral reconstruction. *Arch Otolaryngol Head Neck Surg* 1987;113:496–500.
21. Komisar A, Warman S, Danziger E: The functional result of mandibular reconstruction. *Laryngoscope* 1990;100:364–374.
22. Urken ML, Buchbinder D, Weinberg H, et al: Functional evaluation following microvascular oromandibular reconstruction of the oral cancer patient: A comparative study of reconstructed and non-reconstructed patients. *Laryngoscope* 1991;101:935–950.
23. Terell JE, Welsh DE, Bradford CR, et al: Pain, quality of life, and spinal accessory nerve status after neck dissection. *Laryngoscope* 2000;110:620–626.
24. Fang FM, Tsai WL, Chien CY, et al: Changing quality of life in patients with advanced head and neck cancer after primary radiotherapy or chemoradiation. *Oncology* 2005;68:405–413.
25. Harrison LB, Zelefsky MJ, Pfister DG, et al: Detailed quality of life assessment in patients treated with primary radiotherapy for squamous cell cancer of the base of the tongue. *Head Neck* 1997;19:169–175.
26. Bjordal K, Frenga, Thorvik J, et al: Patient self-reported and clinician-rated quality of life in head and neck cancer patients: A cross sectional study. *Eur J Cancer* 1995;3:235–241.
27. Hammerlid E, Mercke C, Sullivan M, et al: A prospective quality of life study of patients with laryngeal carcinoma by tumor stage and different radiation therapy schedules. *Laryngoscope* 1998;108:747–759.
28. Griffiths GO, Parmar MK, Bailey AJ: Physical and psychological symptoms of quality of life in the CHART randomized trial in head and neck cancer: Short-term and long-term reported symptoms: CHART Steering Committee: Continuous hyperfractionated accelerated radiotherapy. *Br J Cancer* 1999;81:1196–1205.
29. Allal AS, Dulguerov P, Bieri S, et al: Assessment of quality of life in patients treated with accelerated radiotherapy for laryngeal and hypopharyngeal carcinomas. *Head Neck* 2000;22:288–293.
30. Jabbari S, Kim HM, Feng M, et al: Matched case-control study of quality of life and xerostomia after intensity-modulated radiotherapy or standard radiotherapy for head and neck cancer: Initial report. *Int J Radiat Oncol Biol Phys* 2005;63:725–731.
31. List MA, Siston A, Haraf D, et al: Quality of life and performance in advanced head and neck cancer patient on concomitant chemoradiotherapy: A prospective examination. *J Clin Oncol* 1999;17:1020–1028.

PART 2

Salivary Glands, Oral Cavity, and Oropharynx

CHAPTER 20

Complications of Surgery of the Salivary Glands

M. Boyd Gillespie and David W. Eisele

Surgical procedures of the major salivary glands, including the paired parotid glands, the submandibular glands, and the sublingual glands, remain technically challenging to the head and neck surgeon. Anatomic variability, the proximity of these glands to important nerves and vascular structures, structural and tissue alterations from previous surgeries, infection, radiation therapy, and diverse tumor behaviors all contribute to the challenge. A thorough understanding of the regional anatomy, the potential diagnostic studies, the disorders that affect the salivary glands, the pathologic behavior of salivary gland neoplasms, and the proper indications for surgery are necessary for the salivary gland surgeon. In addition, the surgeon must be cognizant of the potential complications and be able to differentiate them from the expected sequelae of salivary gland surgery. This chapter discusses the complications and expected sequelae of surgery of the major salivary glands. Complications of surgery of the minor salivary glands are site specific and depend on the location of the minor salivary gland lesion in the upper aerodigestive tract. The reader is therefore referred to other chapters (Chapters 23 and 27) for discussions of the site-specific complications related to surgery of the minor salivary glands.

PAROTID MASSES

A mass in the region of the parotid gland most likely represents a salivary gland neoplasm and should be considered as such until proven otherwise. Normal anatomic landmarks such as a hypertrophic masseter muscle; mandibular bony prominences, including the angle, the coronoid process, and the condylar process; and a prominent transverse process of the C1 vertebra (atlas) can be confused with a parotid neoplasm. Systemic disorders and inflammatory conditions including chronic sialadenitis can cause salivary gland enlargement. Enlarged intraparotid lymph nodes related to reactive hyperplasia or lymphadenitis, lymphoma, metastatic carcinoma from the scalp and the facial skin, or from infraclavicular primary tumors can mimic primary parotid gland neoplasms. In addition, lipoma, benign cysts, neurogenic neoplasms, and vascular or lymphatic malformations may be confused with parotid neoplasms. Chronic sialadenitis or enlarged submandibular triangle lymph nodes can mimic submandibular gland neoplasms. In addition, the submandibular gland itself may be confused with a neck mass if it descends into the neck with age as a result of the increasing laxity of the superficial musculoaponeurotic system.

DIAGNOSTIC IMAGING

Salivary gland imaging studies, including magnetic resonance imaging, computed tomography scanning, and ultrasonography, do not consistently differentiate benign from malignant tumors, and they rarely alter the therapeutic approach to salivary gland neoplasms. Therefore the routine use of imaging studies for the evaluation of salivary gland neoplasms is not always necessary. However, useful clinical information can be obtained from imaging studies performed for recurrent neoplasms, large neoplasms, suspected parapharyngeal space involvement, or the involvement of other structures that would suggest the tumor to be unresectable (e.g., the encasement of the carotid artery). In general, magnetic resonance imaging with gadolinium provides superior imaging of the parotid gland and the parapharyngeal space as compared with computed tomography scanning (Figure 20-1).

The use of F-18 fluorodeoxyglucose positron emission tomography imaging is of limited value for the routine evaluation of salivary masses, because both benign and malignant salivary tumors can demonstrate increased radiotracer uptake.[1,2] However, this type of tomography may have a role in the evaluation of large or extensive high-grade malignancies for the presence of distant metastasis before engaging in potentially morbid surgical resections with low expectations for cure.

FINE-NEEDLE ASPIRATION BIOPSY

Fine-needle aspiration biopsy (FNAB) of suspected salivary gland neoplasms is an accurate method for the proper diagnosis of a mass in the region of the major salivary glands.[3,4] The diagnostic accuracy of FNAB for salivary neoplasms is excellent. However, an experienced cytopathologist is necessary to achieve excellent results.

Because the results of FNAB rarely alter the therapeutic approach (i.e., parotidectomy) to a suspected parotid neoplasm, some surgeons do not employ FNAB routinely for parotid neoplasm evaluation. Alternatively, the information obtained by FNAB can be useful for diagnosis, preoperative patient counseling, surgical timing

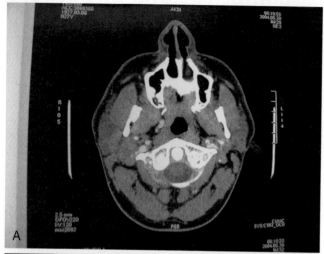

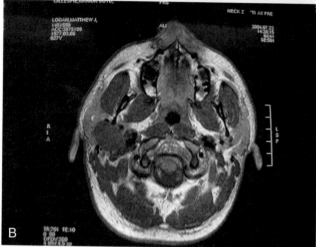

Figure 20-1. Parotid and parapharyngeal masses that are difficult to visualize with computed tomography **(A)** are often more clearly seen with magnetic resonance imaging with gadolinium **(B)**.

and planning, and prompting preoperative consultation with specialists in radiation oncology and dentistry if a malignancy is diagnosed. An FNA biopsy that is positive for malignancy affords the surgeon the opportunity to discuss with the patient before surgery the need for and potential complications of selective neck dissection and the potential need to sacrifice branches of the facial nerve. In general, the FNAB findings should contribute to rather than displace the surgeon's diagnostic impression.[5]

FNAB of salivary neoplasms is a simple and safe procedure. There have been no reports of tumor spread with this technique. Tumor seeding of a mucoepidermoid carcinoma of the parotid along a core needle (Vim-Silverman needle) tract, however, has been reported; therefore, the use of large-bore needles for aspiration or core biopsy is not recommended.[6]

Complications of FNAB of salivary masses are rare. Patients occasionally have slightly more discomfort with FNAB of a parotid mass as compared with other

head and neck sites, perhaps as a result of the extensive sensory innervation of the parotid region. Frabel and Frabel[3] reported more pain among patients with chronic sialadenitis. The injection of lidocaine before FNAB usually minimizes patient discomfort during the procedure.

Complications of FNAB of salivary masses include hemorrhage, hematoma, and ecchymosis.[7,8] FNAB is preferably performed after aspirin or anticoagulant medications have been discontinued. Firm pressure is routinely applied to the biopsy site after FNAB to prevent the rare hemorrhagic complication. If bleeding from the needle tract occurs, pressure should be applied until the hemorrhage is controlled.

Cellulitis or parotitis after salivary gland FNAB has been reported but is unusual.[4,9] Treatment consists of antibiotics with adequate streptococcal and staphylococcal coverage. Vasovagal episodes rarely occur during FNAB.[10] Patients who experience a vasovagal episode are placed in the supine position and carefully observed with the monitoring of vital signs. Such episodes are usually self-limited.

INAPPROPRIATE BIOPSY OF A PAROTID MASS

Because of their occasional superficial location, parotid neoplasms can be mistaken for skin adnexal masses, including sebaceous and dermoid cysts or superficial lymphadenopathy. This clinical confusion can result in the inappropriate biopsy of a parotid neoplasm. Incisional biopsy, excisional biopsy, or enucleation of parotid neoplasms can result in tumor recurrence, especially for pleomorphic adenoma. Such a biopsy also risks facial nerve injury (Figure 20-2) and spillage of

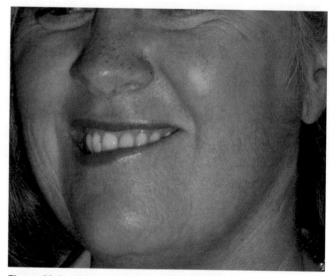

Figure 20-2. Incisional biopsy of a left parotid carcinoma with injury to the marginal mandibular branch of the facial nerve.

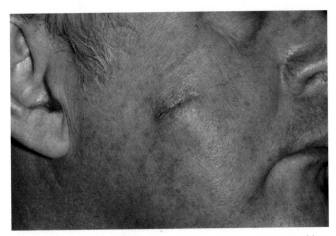

Figure 20-3. Incisional biopsy of a right parotid carcinoma resulting in a facial scar.

tumor with the possibility of tumor cell seeding of the wound. In addition, inflammation and scarring can make subsequent definitive surgery more difficult. The biopsy wound occasionally makes surgical incision planning difficult and can result in an additional facial scar (Figure 20-3).

SURGICAL INDICATIONS

The most common indications for parotidectomy are a neoplasm of the parotid gland, metastases to parotid lymph nodes, and access to structures deep to the facial nerve. In addition, parotidectomy may be a component of first branchial cleft cyst resection, the management of chronic parotid sialadenitis refractory to medical therapy, and sialolithiasis with an impacted sialolith. Rarely, parotidectomy is performed for cosmesis in cases of sialadenosis.

The generally accepted surgical approach to parotid neoplasms is to perform a parotidectomy with the identification and preservation of the facial nerve to ensure complete tumor removal with a surrounding margin of normal salivary tissue. This is particularly important for pleomorphic adenoma. Enucleation of pleomorphic adenoma results in a high incidence of recurrent tumor as compared with parotidectomy with nerve dissection (48% vs. 7%) as a result of poor tumor encapsulation with the expansion of tumor pseudopodia through the fibrous pseudocapsule.[11,12]

Because most parotid tumors are benign, parotidectomy is both diagnostic and curative for the majority (approximately 85%) of patients with parotid neoplasms. Parotidectomy is also curative for patients with small, low-grade malignancies, such as low-grade mucoepidermoid carcinoma and acinic cell carcinoma. The facial nerve is preserved, except in cases of confirmed malignancy invading the nerve. In instances of facial nerve invasion by

carcinoma, facial nerve resection is performed. Proximal and distal nerve resection margins are examined by frozen-section pathology to ensure negative margins. If nerve resection is undertaken, immediate reconstruction with a nerve graft is performed.

Indications for submandibular gland excision include submandibular gland neoplasm, chronic sialadenitis refractory to medical management, and impacted submandibular duct stones in the hilum of the gland. Many submandibular duct stones can be removed transorally by sialodochotomy or by sialendoscopy techniques.

Benign neoplasms of the submandibular gland are usually confined to the gland. Malignant submandibular neoplasms can extend beyond the gland into the surrounding tissues. Glandular excision is indicated for benign neoplasms. Surgical resection of the gland and of the contents of the submandibular triangle is usually appropriate for most malignant tumors to ensure complete tumor resection. All nerves in the submandibular triangle are preserved unless there is evidence of malignant tumor invasion. If a malignant tumor invades the surrounding tissues, the surgical resection is extended to include the involved structures with appropriate tumor-free margins.

COMPLICATIONS OF PAROTIDECTOMY

Complications of parotidectomy can be divided into early complications (including those that occur intraoperatively and during the immediate postoperative period) and late postoperative complications (Box 20-1). Each complication of parotidectomy is discussed separately. Expected sequelae of parotidectomy should be differentiated from complications and are also presented.

BOX 20-1 Complications of Parotidectomy

EARLY COMPLICATIONS

Facial nerve injury
Hemorrhage
Hematoma
Infection
External otitis
Sialocele
Seroma
Salivary fistula

LATE COMPLICATIONS

Frey syndrome
Trismus
Amputation neuroma (greater auricular nerve)
Tumor recurrence
Cosmetic deformity
Hypertrophic scar
Keloid
Earlobe malpositioning

Early Complications

Facial Nerve Injury

Facial nerve paralysis represents the major complication of parotid surgery. The risk of this complication can be minimized with proper and careful surgical techniques.

At the time of surgery, paralysis agents (except for short-acting agents such as succinylcholine at the time of anesthesia induction) should be avoided. If the local injection of epinephrine along the proposed incision is used for vasoconstriction, then the injection solution should contain no local anesthetic (e.g., lidocaine), which may cause temporary neural blockade. The facial skin flap should be carefully raised to avoid injury to the peripheral facial nerve branches beyond the anterior border of the gland. Intraoperatively, the facial nerve should be carefully identified with the aid of anatomic landmarks (Box 20-2). Wide surgical exposure is recommended to allow for the adequate visualization of these landmarks. Adequate operative exposure reduces the risk of inadvertent nerve injury during the dissection for facial nerve identification and allows for safe hemostasis if bleeding occurs during dissection near the facial nerve.

A disposable nonpulsed direct current nerve stimulator should be used judiciously for facial nerve stimulation. However, this current can damage nerves, because it is transmitted to the nerve for the duration of stimulator tip contact with the nerve.[13,14] Prolonged nerve contact with this type of stimulator may result in excessive current delivery to the nerve. Repeated nerve stimulation with such a stimulator may be responsible for temporary nerve paresis postoperatively.

Intraoperative nerve monitoring with commercially available electromyograph units can provide valuable intraoperative information regarding facial nerve identity and integrity. Such monitoring can be particularly useful for reoperation. In a retrospective review of 56 patients who received facial nerve monitoring during parotidectomy and of 61 patients who did not, a significant reduction in temporary facial paresis was observed in the monitored group as compared with the unmonitored group (44% vs. 62%); however, there was no significant difference in the rate of permanent facial paralysis.[15] Another retrospective review of 20 monitored and 33 unmonitored patients failed to demonstrate a difference in temporary paresis between the monitored (20%) and unmonitored (15%) groups.[16] A recent survey found that 60% of otolaryngologist–head and neck surgeons and 79% of frequent U.S. parotid surgeons (i.e., those who perform more than 10 parotidectomies per year) used a facial nerve monitoring system some or all of the time during parotidectomy.[17] Interestingly, surgeons who used monitoring were 21% less likely to have a history of a parotidectomy-related lawsuit.[17]

After the facial nerve is identified, it is followed peripherally. The surgeon must keep in mind the initial steep lateral course of the nerve to the mid-gland level as well as the anatomic variability of the facial nerve branches. Care must be taken to avoid nerve stretch injury during dissection, and the manipulation of the nerve during dissection should be minimized. Operating loupes or other magnification tools can be helpful for nerve branch visualization.

After the removal of the surgical specimen, the integrity of the facial nerve is determined both visually and with electrical stimulation. Nerve transection necessitates immediate microsurgical neurorrhaphy.

Temporary facial nerve paralysis involving the entire facial nerve (Figure 20-4) or one or more branches of the nerve is reported to occur in 5% to 65% of cases.[18–23]

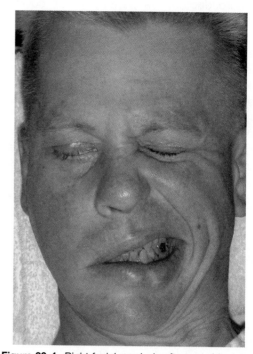

Figure 20-4. Right facial paralysis after parotidectomy.

BOX 20-2 Anatomic Landmarks for Facial Nerve Identification

1. Tragal pointer (The nerve is approximately 1-cm medial and anteroinferior to the tip of the pointer.)
2. Tympanomastoid suture (The nerve is approximately 6–8-mm medial to the suture.)
3. Digastric muscle attachment to digastric groove (The nerve is just superior to and on the same plane as the muscle attachment.)
4. Nerve within the mastoid bone
5. Retrograde dissection of the peripheral facial nerve branch

The facial nerve branch that is most at risk for temporary paralysis is the marginal mandibular branch.[19–21,23] This is thought to be the result of the high length-to-diameter ratio of this nerve branch and of the relative lack of interconnections with other branches of the facial nerve as compared with other facial nerve branches (e.g., the buccal and zygomatic branches). Paralysis of the marginal mandibular branch results in a loss of ipsilateral lower lip depressor function (Figure 20-5). Recovery from temporary facial paresis occurs within 6 months in the majority of patients.[19,20,23]

Permanent facial nerve paralysis occurs less commonly than temporary paresis. Permanent paralysis after partial parotidectomy for benign tumors is uncommon and generally reported to occur in less than 5% to 6% of cases.[19–22] A higher incidence of both temporary and permanent facial paralysis occurs with total parotidectomy as compared with superficial parotidectomy, perhaps as a result of the increased nerve manipulation that is necessary for complete gland removal.[18,20–23] In addition, permanent facial paralysis is more common with reoperation for recurrent tumors.[21,24,25] The performance of a neck dissection at the time of parotidectomy is associated with a higher incidence of permanent paralysis of the marginal mandibular branch of the facial nerve.[20] Care must be taken to protect the exposed facial nerve if parotidectomy is performed before the neck dissection. Another protective option is to perform the neck dissection before the parotidectomy.

Perzik[26] reported a 100% incidence of temporary facial paralysis with parotidectomy for chronic sialadenitis. This is not the experience of the authors, and other reports have shown no higher incidence of paralysis for parotidectomies performed for chronic inflammation than with those performed for benign neoplasms.[18,27,28]

In addition, total parotidectomy does not appear to be associated with a higher incidence of permanent paralysis than superficial parotidectomy when surgery is performed for chronic parotitis.[28]

Facial paralysis involving the orbicularis oculi muscle often results in incomplete eye closure. Conjunctivitis, keratitis, and corneal ulceration can result from eye exposure. Epiphora results from the loss of the normal pumping action of the eyelids and lower-lid laxity or ectropion (Figure 20-6). With facial paralysis involving the orbicularis oculi, eye-protection measures should be instituted immediately and should include the frequent instillation of artificial tears during the day and lubricant ophthalmic ointment and eyelid closure with tape or the application of a moisture chamber (Figure 20-7) at night. If prolonged or permanent paralysis is anticipated, upper-lid gold-weight implantation is a useful technique to provide adequate eye closure.[29] In addition, lower-lid tightening procedures may be beneficial. The patient should be questioned periodically about eye symptoms and examined for signs of eye injury. Ophthalmologic consultation should be obtained immediately if any eye complication is suspected.

The management of permanent facial paralysis is beyond the scope of this chapter. Facial reanimation procedures include nerve crossover techniques such as facial–hypoglossal anastomosis, cross-face nerve transplantation, masseter or temporalis muscle transfer, and free-tissue transfer. Brow lift, rhytidectomy, blepharoplasty, cheiloplasty, contralateral frontal neurectomy, and botulinum toxin injections to achieve forehead symmetry

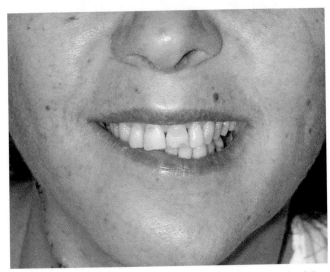

Figure 20-5. Paresis of the right marginal mandibular branch of the facial nerve. Note the lack of lip depressor function.

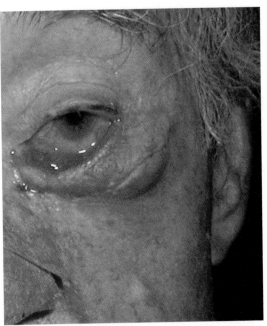

Figure 20-6. Ectropion of the lower eyelid after intentional sacrifice of the facial nerve for a malignant parotid neoplasm.

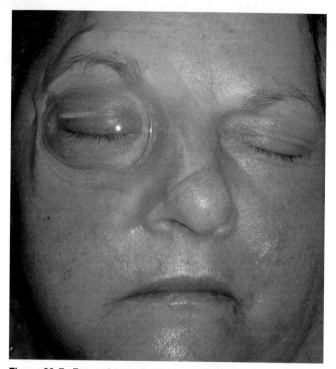

Figure 20-7. Eye-moisture chamber for nocturnal eye protection.

for frontal paralysis are some of the other reconstructive techniques that may help to improve the cosmetic deformities associated with facial paralysis.

Hemorrhage and Hematoma

Hemorrhage is an uncommon intraoperative complication. Patients should be instructed to avoid aspirin and nonsteroidal anti-inflammatory medications for several weeks before surgery. Patients taking clopidogrel and warfarin should have medical clearance to stop these medications at least 1 week before surgery. If these medications cannot be safely discontinued, then replacement with low-molecular-weight heparin therapy is recommended. Heparin can be stopped immediately before surgery and resumed after all sanguinous wound drainage has ceased. The proper identification, division, and ligation of blood vessels during surgical dissection usually prevents significant intraoperative bleeding. During total parotidectomy and the removal of the deep lobe, the internal maxillary artery and its branches are the primary vessels of concern for significant bleeding.

During the removal of tumors of the superficial lobe, the posterior facial vein, which courses deep to the facial nerve, can usually be preserved. The ligation of this vessel can contribute to the venous congestion of the gland and to increased venous bleeding from the cut surface of the gland during dissection.

Intraoperative bleeding should be controlled with careful technique using ligatures or bipolar electrocautery. Care should be taken to avoid suction or clamp compression

injury to the facial nerve during attempts at hemostasis. Unipolar electrocautery should be used with extreme care because of the risk of electrical current transmission to the facial nerve. There continues to be interest among parotid surgeons to identify surgical instruments that provide hemostasis without excessive facial nerve stimulation during parotidectomy. A retrospective review comparing 44 patients who underwent parotidectomy with the Harmonic Scalpel (Ethicon Endo-Surgery, Inc., Cincinnati, Ohio) with 41 patients who had conventional parotidectomy observed significantly less intraoperative blood loss and a reduced incidence of facial nerve paresis in the Harmonic Scalpel group.[30] Similarly, a retrospective series of 50 patients who underwent parotidectomy with the Hemostatix Scalpel (Hemostatix Medical Technologies, Bartlett, TN) were found to have significantly shorter operative times and less intraoperative blood loss as compared with patients undergoing conventional parotidectomy.[31] Another study of 77 parotidectomy patients asserted that the Hemostatix Scalpel was an independent risk factor for facial nerve paralysis. However, the larger Hemostatix #10 blade was used in this series rather than the more widely accepted #15 blade.[32]

Postoperative hematoma formation is unusual, and it is reported to occur in 3% to 7% of cases.[19,21,22] Hematoma is typically related to inadequate hemostasis or increased venous blood pressure during emergence from anesthesia. Hematoma results in wound and facial swelling (Figure 20-8), and the patient will often complain of pain. Hemorrhage may occur from the wound and drain sites. Although some minor hematomas can be

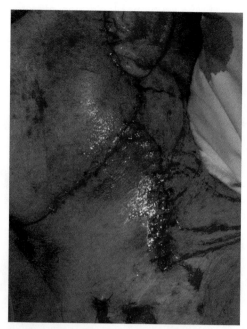

Figure 20-8. Hematoma after left parotidectomy and neck dissection. Note the swelling of the wound and bleeding from the wound and drain sites.

evacuated at the bedside, hematoma formation usually requires a return to the operating room for hematoma evacuation and wound exploration. Any identified bleeding sites are carefully controlled with ligatures or bipolar electrocautery with the identification and protection of the facial nerve.

Infection

Parotidectomy is considered a clean surgical procedure. Postoperative infection is uncommon, and it is reported to occur in less than 3% of patients.[19,22] Infection is an unusual complication of parotidectomy, probably because of the rich vascular supply to the parotid region. Infection is avoided by adherence to sterile surgical technique and the careful handling of tissues intraoperatively. Care must be taken during parotidectomy to avoid entry into the external auditory canal and to avoid oral flora contamination of the wound. Cellulitis (Figure 20-9) is treated with an intravenous antibiotic with activity against gram-positive organisms until the tissue edema and erythema begin to fade (usually 24–48 hours). This is followed by a course of oral antibiotics. Abscess formation requires incision and drainage as well as appropriate antibiotics.

Johnson and Wagner[33] examined the benefit of prophylactic antibiotics for parotidectomy for cases in which no infection existed before surgery and found no difference in infection rates with or without perioperative antibiotics. However, perioperative prophylactic antibiotics are recommended for patients who have had recent parotid gland infection or recent surgery.

External Otitis

External otitis can occur postoperatively, and it is related to blood collection in the external auditory canal intraoperatively. Blood provides an excellent medium for bacterial growth in the ear canal. External otitis can be prevented by carefully placing a petrolatum gauze pack in the ear canal at the beginning of the procedure to prevent the entry of blood (Figure 20-10). If blood enters the ear canal intraoperatively, saline irrigation and careful suctioning of the ear canal are performed at the completion of surgery. The treatment of postoperative external otitis consists of the careful removal of blood and debris from the external auditory canal and the instillation of antibiotic eardrops.

Flap Necrosis

Flap necrosis is an uncommon complication of parotidectomy.[19] Necrosis occurs most commonly in the distal tip of the inframastoid portion of the parotid flap (Figure 20-11). Proper flap design and plane of elevation, careful handling of the flap, and the avoidance of flap desiccation intraoperatively are all important factors for the prevention of this complication. Other factors that may be responsible for the development of this complication include the impairment of the flap's blood supply as a result of smoking, diabetes mellitus, or prior radiation therapy. Patients who smoke should be strongly encouraged to quit smoking several weeks before surgery to reduce the risk of skin-flap necrosis.[34,35] Venous congestion of cervicofacial rotation flaps can be reduced with the rapid institution of leech therapy for flap salvage (Figure 20-12).

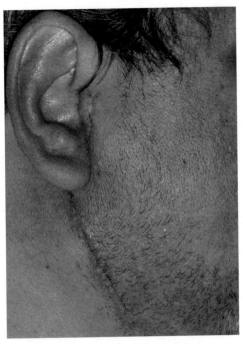

Figure 20-9. Cellulitis after parotidectomy.

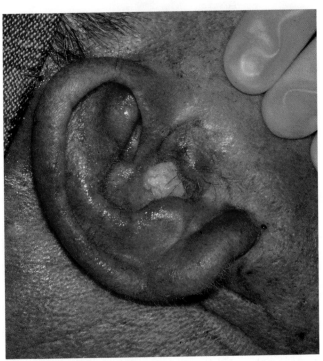

Figure 20-10. Petrolatum gauze pack placed in the external auditory canal to prevent the entry of blood.

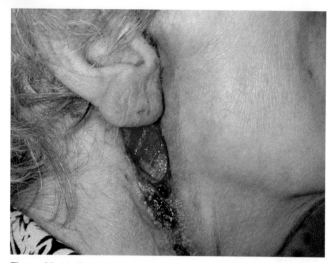

Figure 20-11. Parotid flap necrosis in a patient with diabetes mellitus.

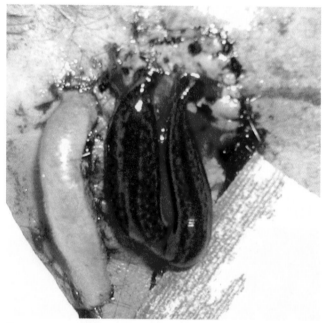

Figure 20-12. Venous congestion in a cervical facial rotation flap of a heavy smoker treated with leech therapy.

The treatment of parotid flap necrosis includes the debridement of necrotic tissue in the wound. Depending on the size of the defect, secondary wound closure, closure by secondary intention, or split-thickness skin grafting are options for wound closure.

Sialocele and Seroma

Sialocele represents a collection of saliva under the parotid flap and presents as a nontender, cystic mass (Figure 20-13, *A*). Sialocele occurs after partial parotidectomy related to salivary leakage from the cut surface of the gland remnant. This complication occurs in approximately 5% to 10% of patients after partial parotidectomy.[18,19,22]

Seroma is clinically similar to sialocele but differs in that it has lower amylase content on fluid analysis. However, such differentiation has little practical importance for the management of these two uncommon complications. Postoperative seroma is unusual if closed-suction drainage is employed until the wound drainage falls below 30 cc in a 24-hour period. However, a reduction in drain output of this degree may take several days and result in a prolonged hospital stay in patients who underwent extensive dissection or who have particularly large parotid glands. A recent randomized, controlled study found significantly less postoperative drainage volume and fewer postoperative seromas among 30 patients treated with a fibrin tissue glue to the wound bed before closure as compared with 30 patients who underwent standard closure alone.[36] The use of tissue sealants during parotidectomy may increase in the future to allow for shorter hospital stays.

The management of sialocele and seroma includes needle aspiration of the fluid collection after careful antibacterial skin preparation. Aspirated fluid is usually clear and yellow (Figure 20-13, *B*). Pressure dressings are of little value for this problem, and they are cumbersome to the patient. Patients should be counseled regarding potential reoccurrence after needle aspiration but reassured that sialoceles are rarely a chronic problem. Alternatively, the fluid collection may be observed, and fluid reabsorption will often occur spontaneously. Large, persistent fluid collections may necessitate Penrose or suction drain replacement.

Salivary Fistula

Salivary fistula is manifested by salivary drainage from the wound (Figure 20-14). It is an uncommon complication of subtotal parotidectomy, occurring in less than 3% of cases.[18,21] Salivary fistulas are generally self-limited and usually close spontaneously with local care within several weeks. A fistula will rarely persist for months or chronically. The skin surrounding a chronic fistula is often excoriated and scarred as a result of the irritative effect of saliva.[37]

A chronic salivary fistula usually requires additional treatment to effect closure. Completion total parotidectomy is curative for chronic salivary fistula but involves the risk of facial nerve injury.[38] Anticholinergic medications have been reported to have a beneficial effect on the reduction of salivary flow with resultant fistula resolution.[39,40] Transdermal scopolamine may have a similar effect on salivary flow reduction.[41] Tympanic neurectomy, which interrupts the parasympathetic innervation to the parotid gland, has also been advocated as a successful method for the closure of chronic salivary fistulas.[37,42] Recent reports have shown benefit with the use of botulinum toxin for salivary fistula.[43,44] Ultrasonography is useful for

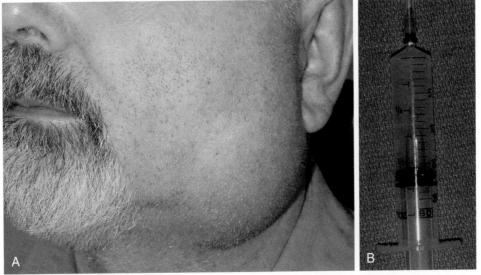

Figure 20-13. **A,** Sialocele after partial parotidectomy. **B,** Needle aspirate of sialocele fluid.

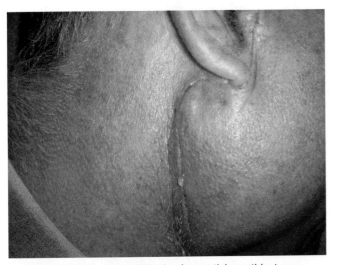

Figure 20-14. Salivary fistula after partial parotidectomy.

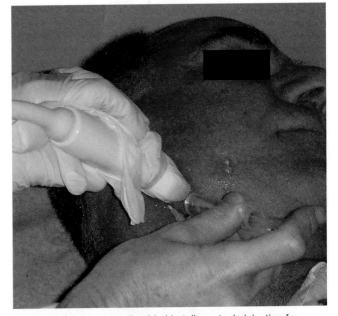

Figure 20-15. Ultrasound-guided botulinum toxin injection for postparotidectomy salivary fistula.

proper injection into the remaining parotid gland parenchyma (Figure 20-15).

Late Complications

Frey Syndrome

Frey syndrome (gustatory sweating, auriculotemporal syndrome) is a relatively common late complication of parotidectomy. This complication is thought to occur in relation to the aberrant regeneration of the postganglionic secretomotor parasympathetic nerve fibers, which are carried in the auriculotemporal nerve from the otic ganglion to the parotid to the severed postganglionic sympathetic fibers that supply the sweat glands of the skin (Figure 20-16). As a result, sweating, dermal flush, or both occur in the distribution of the auriculotemporal nerve during salivary stimulation.

The Minor starch–iodine test will objectively demonstrate the area affected by Frey syndrome.[45] An iodine solution consisting of 3 g of iodine, 20 g of castor oil, and 200 ml of absolute alcohol is applied to the skin of the face and neck. After the solution dries, the face is dusted with starch powder. The patient is given a sialogogue such as lemon candy. In areas of sweating, the starch and iodine react, producing a dark-blue discoloration (Figure 20-17). An alternative simple method for the objective assessment of Frey syndrome is to apply one ply of a two-ply tissue to the patient's face after the patient has been given a sialogogue. The tissue will adhere to areas of perspiration (Figure 20-18).

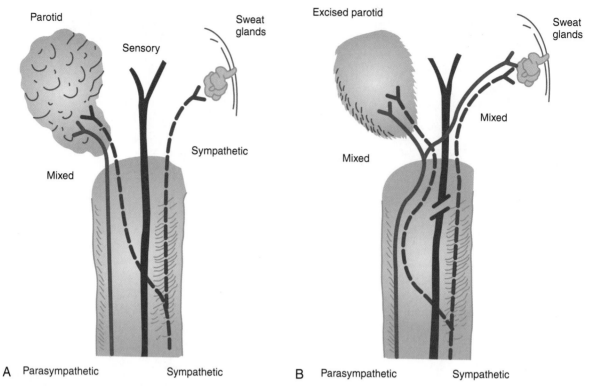

Figure 20-16. Proposed aberrant regeneration mechanism of Frey syndrome. **A,** Normal parotid gland and sweat gland parasympathetic and sympathetic innervation. **B,** Aberrant regeneration of severed parotid postganglionic parasympathetic nerve fibers to severed sweat gland postganglionic sympathetic fibers.

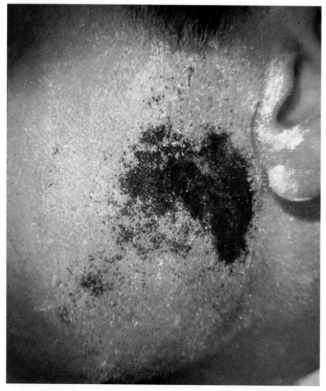

Figure 20-17. Minor starch–iodine test for Frey syndrome. Discoloration occurs in the affected area after gustatory stimulation.

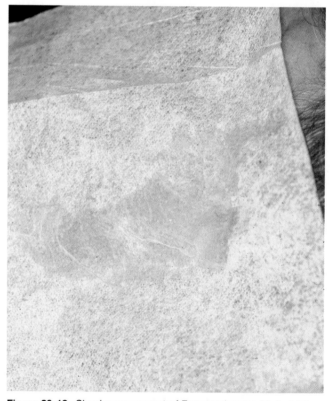

Figure 20-18. Simple assessment of Frey syndrome with facial tissue. The affected area is demarcated by the wet area on the tissue.

The reported incidence of Frey syndrome after parotidectomy varies greatly depending on how closely patients are questioned and examined for the condition. The incidence of objectively documented Frey syndrome by the Minor starch–iodine test approaches 95% to 100%.[46–53] Reports indicate incidences of patient awareness of this problem of between 20% and 65%.[18,19,46–49] Symptomatic Frey syndrome, however, occurs in only approximately 10% to 15% of patients.[18,46,50] Symptoms usually develop after a latent period of many months to a year or more after surgery.[18,51] The delayed development of symptoms of up to 8.5 years after surgery has been reported.[49]

Frey syndrome may be preventable by the elevation of a thick skin flap at the time of parotid exposure. Singleton and Cassisi[52] reported only a 2.6% incidence of this complication with thick-flap elevation as compared with a 12.5% incidence with a thinner flap. The use of a sternocleidomastoid muscle flap for the prevention of Frey syndrome has been shown to be ineffective.[53,54] Other reports have examined the use of barriers placed at the time of parotidectomy to prevent Frey syndrome. Various biologic barriers placed between the parotid bed and the skin, including lyophilized dura, polyglactin 910-polydioxane, and expanded polytetrafluoroethylene, may reduce the incidence of Frey syndrome, but they have not been widely accepted as a result of an observed increase in postoperative seroma and salivary fistula with their use.[55] Acellular dermis has also been reported to significantly reduce the incidence of Frey syndrome while improving postoperative facial contour. However, an increased rate of postoperative seroma formation has also been noted with its use.[56,57]

After they understand the condition, many patients choose to tolerate the symptoms of Frey syndrome and do not opt for treatment.[19,21] Some patients benefit from the daily or twice-daily application of antiperspirants to the affected area.[49,58] Treatment with anticholinergic medications is based on the fact that the postganglionic sympathetic innervation to the sweat gland is cholinergic rather than adrenergic. However, systemic anticholinergic medications are associated with a high incidence of side effects such as dry mouth and blurred vision, which are usually undesirable.

Topical 1% or 2% glycopyrrolate applied to the affected area of gustatory sweating has been shown in double-blind studies to be an effective treatment with a low incidence of side effects.[49,59] The relief of symptoms lasts for several days after the application of topical glycopyrrolate. This medication is not available commercially as a topical preparation; therefore a lotion or cream must be made specially by a pharmacist. Contraindications to the use of this medication include glaucoma, pyloric obstruction, and prostate hypertrophy.

Currently a common and effective method for the management of Frey syndrome is botulinum toxin injections. The recommended administration of botulinum toxin A for Frey syndrome is 2.5 IU/0.1 ml injected subcutaneously into each 1.0 cm^2 of affected area, with total dosages ranging from 80 IU to 100 IU.[60,61] The majority of patients treated with botulinum toxin A will have an objective return of gustatory sweating by starch iodine testing by 18 months after the injection; however, subjective symptoms are usually reported to be less severe.[60–62] Patients with a symptomatic recurrence of Frey syndrome often benefit from repeat injections.[61]

The surgical correction of Frey syndrome includes fascial graft interposition between an elevated skin flap and the gland.[63,64] This technique has been shown to have long-term benefit for some patients, but there have been few reports of this procedure.[63] Extreme care must be taken to avoid facial nerve injury during skin-flap elevation with this approach. As a result of the efficacy of the nonsurgical management of Frey syndrome, surgical management is presently an uncommon remedy.

Gustatory rhinorrhea has occasionally been reported after parotidectomy.[65–67] Patients complain of ipsilateral rhinorrhea with eating. A proposed pathway for this symptom is the regeneration of damaged preganglionic parasympathetic fibers in the lesser superficial petrosal nerve through the greater superficial petrosal nerve to the Vidian nerve, the sphenopalatine ganglion, and the long sphenopalatine nerve, which supplies the nasal mucous glands.[65]

Trismus

Trismus occurs rarely after parotidectomy, and, if it occurs, it is usually mild and transient (Figure 20-19). Trismus is most likely related to masseter inflammation

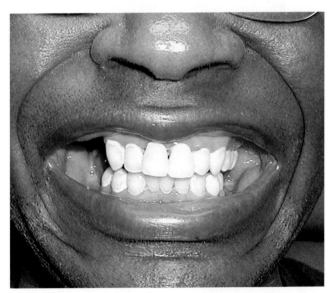

Figure 20-19. Trismus after total parotidectomy and postoperative radiation therapy for an adenoid cystic carcinoma.

and fibrosis or other scarring. Radiation therapy may contribute significantly to this problem. Trismus usually improves with mouth-opening exercises. Some patients may benefit from physical therapy or the use of a commercially available mouth-opening device (e.g., Therabite [Atos Medical, Hörby, Sweden]).

Hypertrophic Scar and Keloid

For the majority of patients, the parotidectomy incision heals well and is cosmetically acceptable as a result of concealment in the natural skin creases. Care must be taken during wound closure to carefully realign the wound to avoid the malpositioning of the earlobe. Hypertrophic scarring or keloid will rarely complicate healing (Figure 20-20). Scar revision, steroid injections, and other therapies are treatment options for the management of hypertrophic scars.

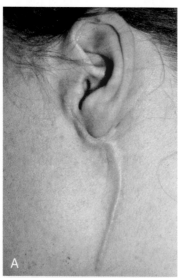

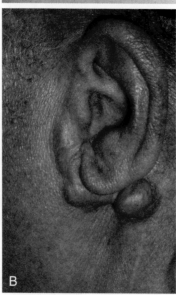

Figure 20-20. A, Hypertrophic scar after parotidectomy. **B,** Keloid after parotidectomy.

Amputation Neuroma of the Greater Auricular Nerve

An amputation neuroma (Figure 20-21) will occasionally form at the severed end of the greater auricular nerve after parotidectomy.[68,69] The diagnosis of an amputation neuroma is usually clinical. Patients may complain of localized or radiating pain related to the mass. A tender nodule usually less than 1 cm in diameter is palpable over the upper border of the sternocleidomastoid muscle. Palpation of the mass usually elicits tenderness and paresthesias.[68] Eddey[51] reported a 3.8% incidence of neuroma formation after parotidectomy. Hobsley[68] reported seven amputation neuromas that were diagnosed an average of 4 years after surgery. The incidence of this problem may be reduced with recent trends to preserve the greater auricular nerve during parotidectomy. Simple excision of the neuroma is usually curative.

Expected Sequelae

The expected sequelae of parotidectomy are as follows:
- Some degree of sensory loss in the distribution of the greater auricular nerve
- Soft-tissue deficit in the area of resection
- Scar

Sensory Loss in the Distribution of the Greater Auricular Nerve

All patients should be informed that sensory loss in the distribution of the greater auricular nerve to some degree is an expected sequela of parotidectomy. The posterior branch of this nerve can be preserved.[70,71]

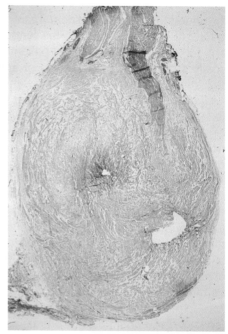

Figure 20-21. Excised amputation neuroma of the greater auricular nerve.

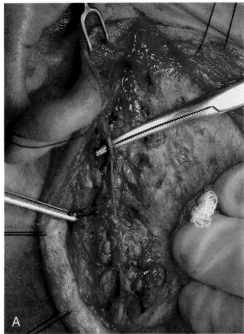

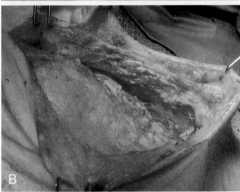

Figure 20-22. Preservation of the posterior branch of the greater auricular nerve. **A,** Nerve dissected circumferentially. **B,** Nerve undermined with a cuff of parotid tissue. This method avoids nerve stretch injury and contributes to improved facial contour.

In the authors' experience, this is possible in more than 50% of cases (Figure 20-22). The area of sensory loss decreases, and, with time, the sensory deficit becomes less noticeable to the patient.[72] Only approximately 25% of patients complained of this symptom when they were questioned postoperatively in the series reported by Eddey.[51] Patients with a sensory deficit should be cautioned about the possibility of unnoticed injury to the ear by thermal or other trauma (Figure 20-23).[73]

Soft-Tissue Deficit

A soft-tissue deficit in the area of resection is another expected sequela of parotidectomy. Most patients are not disturbed by this, and few request consideration for reconstructive surgery for its correction. This deformity is more severe after total or radical parotidectomy (Figure 20-24), and primary reconstruction may be beneficial to restore facial contour. Multiple reconstructive

procedures have been proposed for correction when the defect is significant, including fat graft,[74,75] microvascular muscular free flaps,[76] sternocleidomastoid muscle rotational flaps,[77,78] and fillers (e.g., AlloDerm [LifeCell, Branchburg, NJ]).

Scar

After parotidectomy, the wound generally heals with an inconspicuous scar. Careful placement of the incision parallel to relaxed skin tension lines contributes to optimal scar concealment. For young patients and women without a prominent preauricular crease, an incision behind the tragus may offer better camouflage for the scar line (Figure 20-25).

Tumor Recurrence

Recurrent tumor is a dreaded late complication of parotidectomy. Some malignant parotid tumors are known to have a relatively high rate of recurrence. Recurrences are more likely with higher tumor stage and higher histopathologic grade and among those patients with preoperative facial nerve paralysis.[79-81] Long-term follow up is necessary, particularly for adenoid cystic carcinoma and acinic cell carcinoma, because late recurrence can occur with these parotid malignancies.[79] Postoperative radiation therapy has been shown to reduce the risk of local recurrence of select malignant parotid neoplasms as compared with surgery alone.[81-83]

The recurrence of pleomorphic adenoma occurs less than 1% of the time after formal parotidectomy.[84,85] Alternatively, the enucleation of pleomorphic adenomas results in recurrence rates of 30% to 50%.[84,86,87] Recurrences after partial parotidectomy tend to occur later than those that occur after enucleation.[88] Recurrent pleomorphic adenoma may also occur as a result of tumor rupture and spillage during surgery with wound seeding.[89] The majority of recurrent pleomorphic adenomas are multifocal.[84,88,89] The average interval between the initial surgery and the identification of tumor recurrence is 10 years or more.[90,91] Both physical examination and imaging studies tend to underestimate the extent of disease (Figure 20-26).

Total parotidectomy with facial nerve preservation is recommended for the management of the first recurrence of pleomorphic adenoma.[24,84,88] Niparko and colleagues[92] reported a 53% incidence of control of initial recurrences with long-term follow up. Fee and colleagues[24] showed diminished control rates with subsequent recurrences after the initial recurrence. Increased risks of both temporary and permanent facial nerve paralysis occur with surgery for recurrent pleomorphic adenoma.[24,88] The excision of the old scar tract or of areas of skin adhering to the tumor may be necessary to ensure complete tumor resection (Figure 20-27). En bloc

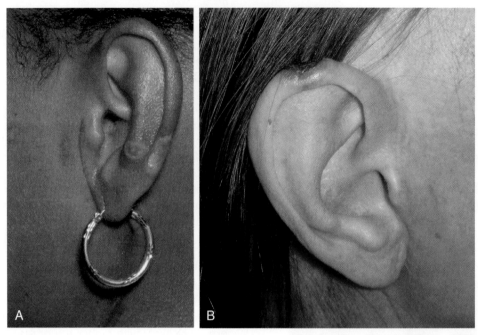

Figure 20-23. A, Burn to the pinna after parotidectomy. **B,** Dog bite of pinna. The patient was unaware of this injury, which was sustained while playing with a frisky puppy.

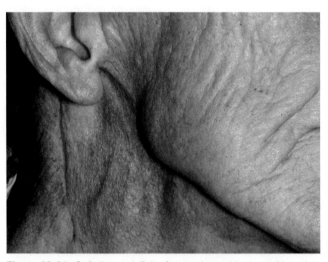

Figure 20-24. Soft-tissue deficit after total parotidectomy. Note the infra-auricular and facial depression.

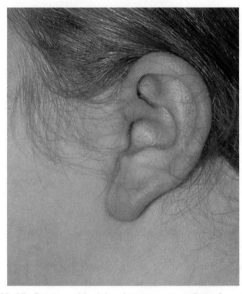

Figure 20-25. Posttragal incision for scar camouflage for a 15-year-old girl requiring a parotidectomy for a benign salivary neoplasm.

tumor resection with facial nerve sacrifice and immediate facial nerve grafting may be necessary for confluent recurrences that encase the facial nerve.[84,92,93]

Postoperative radiation therapy appears to be beneficial after the resection of recurrent pleomorphic adenoma.[94–96] Radiation therapy has been shown to be effective for those patients with microscopic residual pleomorphic adenoma after the surgical resection of recurrence but not for patients with residual gross disease after excision.[95] Patients must be informed that

radiation therapy carries with it a low risk of subsequent radiation-induced malignancy.[97]

COMPLICATIONS OF SUBMANDIBULAR GLAND EXCISION

Hemorrhage from the facial artery and the anterior facial vein can occur intraoperatively, and it can be vigorous. When hemorrhage occurs intraoperatively, care must be exercised to avoid injury to nerves in proximity to the bleeding vessel. The careful identification, division, and

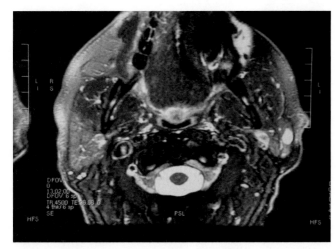

Figure 20-26. Coronal magnetic resonance image demonstrating the multifocal recurrence of pleomorphic adenoma of the left parotid.

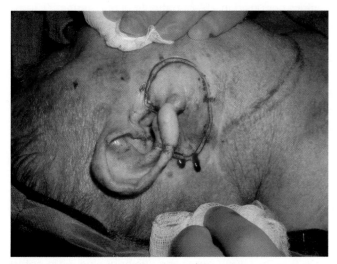

Figure 20-27. Excision of skin with a frozen-section margin for a patient with a recurrent malignant parotid cancer.

ligature of blood vessels are important to prevent this complication. Wound hematoma formation can occur postoperatively, and it can result in significant swelling of the floor of the mouth and tongue displacement, which may cause upper-airway obstruction.[98] The incidence of hematoma varies between 2% and 10%.[99–101] The treatment of hematoma consists of wound exploration, hematoma evacuation, and the control of bleeding vessels.

Infection can occur after submandibular gland excision, and the incidence of this complication varies from 2% to 9%.[33,99–101] This condition occurs more often than it does after parotidectomy, probably because infected tissues are more commonly involved.[102] Like parotidectomy, submandibular gland excision is considered to be a clean surgical procedure. Perioperative antibiotics are not used routinely if no infection exists before surgery.[33] The management of infection includes

the drainage of abscess, if present, and the administration of antibiotics.

The most common complication of submandibular gland excision is injury to the marginal mandibular branch of the facial nerve.[98,99] The impairment of lower-lip depressor function results from injury to this nerve. Bilateral injury of this nerve can result in oral incompetence. The marginal mandibular branch of the facial nerve is located deep to the platysma muscle and to the superficial layer of the deep cervical fascia. The best way to avoid injury to this nerve is with knowledge of the anatomy of the region and the nerve and with the careful elevation of the nerve out of the field of surgery. Care must be taken to carefully plan and perform the incision to avoid injury to the nerve. Incision of the superficial layer of the deep cervical fascia is performed inferior to the nerve. The facial vein is divided, and, because the marginal mandibular nerve is superficial to the vein, the superior segment of the vein can be used as a sling to elevate the fascia and nerve superiorly with protection of the nerve. Anatomic variability of the nerve must be considered.[103–104] Temporary paralysis of the marginal mandibular nerve is usually related to nerve stretch injury from retraction or operative manipulation. The incidence of temporary marginal mandibular nerve paresis varies between 10% and 30%.[98–101,105] Permanent nerve paralysis is rare,[98,100,101,105,106] but it may occur after inadvertent nerve transection, injury from electrocautery, or ligature entrapment of the nerve.

Injury to the lingual nerve, which results in sensory loss of the anterior two thirds of the ipsilateral tongue, is an uncommon complication. Injury to this nerve has been reported to occur in 3% to 6% of cases.[99,105,106] The careful identification and protection of the lingual nerve is important to avoid nerve injury. Chronic inflammation of the gland may result in difficulty separating the lingual nerve from the gland. Particular care must be taken to avoid nerve injury during the division of the submandibular ganglion. Lingual neuralgia can result if a ligature is placed too close to the main trunk of the nerve.[107]

Hypoglossal nerve injury, which causes ipsilateral tongue paralysis, is a rare complication of submandibular gland excision.[95,106] This nerve should also be carefully identified and preserved during dissection. The nerve is in close proximity to the lingual veins, and, if it is obscured, it may be injured during the control of hemorrhage from these vessels.[105] If it is divided, the nerve should be repaired to minimize denervation atrophy of the ipsilateral tongue.

Unusual complications of submandibular gland excision include xerostomia,[108,109] gustatory sweating,[110,111] toxic shock syndrome,[112] and mylohyoid nerve injury.[113,114] Complications of the residual submandibular duct after gland excision include retained calculi[99] and chronic inflammation.[115]

A noticeable scar can occur after submandibular gland excision, but this can be avoided with proper incision placement, the avoidance of wound-edge injury during retraction, and meticulous wound closure. Hypertrophic scarring and keloid formation are unusual complications of wound healing.

COMPLICATIONS OF SIALENDOSCOPY

Diagnostic and therapeutic sialendoscopy has recently become more popular as a minimally invasive approach to the evaluation and management of parotid and submandibular duct disorders. Complications are reported to occur in less than 10% of cases and are usually minor.[116–120] Stricture of the salivary duct orifice is an unusual complication of sialendoscopy, but it can occur if dilation and manipulation of the orifice are traumatic.

Salivary duct perforation can occur, but it can be avoided by the careful advancement of the endoscope within the duct, with adherence to endoscopic principles that include advancement under the direct visualization of the lumen and no forceful advancement. Salivary duct perforation can result in infection or duct stenosis. If a perforation is suspected during sialendoscopy, the procedure should be aborted, and the patient should be carefully observed for the development of infection. Infection is unusual after sialendoscopy with the routine administration of perioperative antibiotics.

All patients develop transient salivary gland swelling related to duct irrigation with saline during the procedure (Figure 20-28). This swelling is accompanied by mild pain and usually resolves within 1 to 2 days. Gentle gland massage and warm heat application are beneficial.

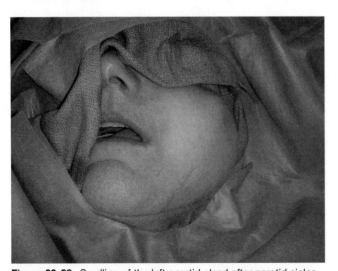

Figure 20-28. Swelling of the left parotid gland after parotid sialendoscopy for iodine[131] sialadenitis.

Unusual complications of sialendoscopy include temporary lingual nerve paresthesia, ranula formation, and the impaction of instruments in the duct.[116–118]

COMPLICATIONS OF SUBMANDIBULAR SIALODOCHOTOMY

Select sialoliths of the submandibular duct near the gland hilum that are not amenable to sialendoscopic management by retrieval or laser lithotripsy can be managed by sialodochotomy and transoral removal.[121,122] Stone palpability appears to be an important factor that influences the success of this approach.[123]

Complications of this procedure include temporary swelling of the floor of the mouth, the submandibular gland, and the tongue. This swelling usually resolves after several days. Stenosis of the newly created duct ostium occurred in 2% of patients in one series.[121] Temporary lingual nerve dysfunction is common as a result of the manipulation of this nerve, which is in proximity to the submandibular duct; however, permanent injury of the lingual nerve is unusual.[121–123] Ranula formation or salivary duct stenosis can also occur, but these are unusual complications.[122]

QUALITY OF LIFE

In general, modern surgery of the salivary glands is safe and well tolerated. However, formal studies that examine quality of life after salivary gland surgery are limited. Nitzan and colleagues[124] performed a quality-of-life study involving patients who underwent parotidectomy for benign and malignant neoplasms. Their results indicate that, although postoperative sequelae were noted in the majority of patients, parotidectomy did not seem to severely affect quality of life. Only 10% of their patients had some degree of permanent facial nerve impairment, yet facial function had the highest importance of all sequelae to the patients. The dominant sequelae were a change in appearance, altered sensation, pain, and gustatory sweating. These sequelae were considered, in general, to be somewhat important. There was no difference in quality-of-life scores between patients with benign as compared with malignant neoplasms.

Beutner and colleagues[125] assessed quality of life in 34 patients who underwent lateral parotidectomy. Surgery-affected changes in quality of life were assessed with two questionnaires. The results indicated that patients had no significant alterations in quality of life at 1 year after lateral parotidectomy.

As discussed previously in this chapter, the preservation of the posterior branch of the greater auricular nerve is advocated to reduce postoperative sensory loss after parotidectomy. Yokoshima and colleagues[126] demonstrated improved quality of life among patients who had this nerve preserved as compared with patients who had to sacrifice this nerve. Patients with greater auricular nerve preservation show quicker and more complete sensory recovery as compared with patients who have undergone nerve division.[127]

A number of studies have shown that facial contour and patient satisfaction can be improved with sternocleidomastoid muscle transposition.[77,78,128,129] In addition, the superficial musculoaponeurotic system flap has been successfully used to maintain facial contour with parotidectomy.[130]

Most patients are satisfied with the cosmetic appearance of the parotidectomy incision. For most patients, proper surgical planning allows for scar concealment in natural skin creases or along lines of relaxed skin tension. Further scar concealment can be accomplished with a modified face-lift incision.[131] Other modifications include a minimal incision for select patients with small, superficial neoplasms of the parotid gland.[132] These modifications are good options for optimizing patient satisfaction, provided that surgical access to the parotid gland is not compromised.

REFERENCES

1. Uchida Y, Minoshima S, Kawata T, et al: Diagnostic value of FDG-PET and salivary scintigraphy for parotid tumors. *Clin Nucl Med* 2005;30:170–176.
2. Otsuka H, Graham MM, Kogame M, et al: The impact of FDG-PET in the management of patients with salivary gland malignancy. *Ann Nucl Med* 2005;19:691–694.
3. Frable MAS, Frable WJ: Fine-needle aspiration biopsy of salivary glands. *Laryngoscope* 1991;101:245–249.
4. Shaha AR, Webber C, DiMaio T, et al: Needle aspiration biopsy in salivary gland lesions. *Am J Surg* 1990;160:373–376.
5. Alphs HH, Eisele DW, Westra WH: The role of fine needle aspiration in the evaluation of parotid masses. *Curr Opin Otolaryngol Head Neck Surg* 2006;14:62–66.
6. Yamaguchi KT, Strong MS, Shapshay SM, et al: Seeding of parotid carcinoma along Vim-Silverman needle tract. *J Otolaryngol* 1979;8:49–52.
7. Nettle WJS, Orell SR: Fine needle aspiration in the diagnosis of salivary gland lesions. *Aust N Z J Surg* 1989;59:47–51.
8. Mavec P, Eneroth CM, Franzen S, et al: Aspiration biopsy of salivary gland tumors. *Acta Otolaryngol* 1964;58:472–484.
9. Bahar G, Dudkiewicz M, Feinmesser R, et al: Acute parotitis as a complication of fine-needle aspiration in Warthin's tumor: A unique finding of a 3-year experience with parotid tumor aspiration. *Otolaryngol Head Neck Surg* 2006;134:646–649.
10. Feldman PS, Kaplan MJ, Johns ME, et al: Fine-needle aspiration in squamous cell carcinoma of the head and neck. *Arch Otolaryngol* 1983;109:735–742.
11. Lam KH, Wei WI, Ho HC, et al: Whole organ sectioning of mixed parotid tumors. *Am J Surg* 1990;160:377–381.
12. Zbaren P, Stauffer E: Pleomorphic adenoma of the parotid gland: Histopathologic analysis of the capsular characteristics of 218 tumors. *Head Neck* 2007;29:751–757.
13. Love JT, Marchbanks JR: Injury to the facial nerve associated with the use of a disposable nerve stimulator. *Otolaryngology* 1978;86:61–64.
14. Chase SG. Hughes GB, Dudley AW: Neuropathologic changes following direct current stimulation of the rat sciatic nerve. *Otolaryngol Head Neck Surg* 1984;92:615–617.
15. Terrell JE, Kileny PR, Yian C, et al: Clinical outcome of continuous facial nerve monitoring during primary parotidectomy. *Arch Otolaryngol Head Neck Surg* 1997;123:1081–1087.
16. Witt RL: Facial nerve monitoring in parotid surgery: The standard of care? *Otolaryngol Head Neck Surg* 1998;119:468–470.
17. Lowry TR, Gal TJ, Brennan JA: Patterns of use of facial nerve monitoring during parotid gland surgery. *Otolaryngol Head Neck Surg* 2005;133:313–318.
18. Langdon JD: Complications of parotid gland surgery. *J Maxillofac Surg* 1984;12:225–229.
19. Laccourreye H, Laccourreye O, Lauchois R, et al: Total conservative parotidectomy for primary benign pleomorphic adenoma of the parotid gland: A 25-year experience with 229 patients. *Laryngoscope* 1994;104:1487–1494.
20. Bron LP, O'Brien CJ: Facial nerve function after parotidectomy. *Arch Otolaryngol Head Neck Surg* 1997;123:1091–1096.
21. Guntinas-Lichius O, Kick C, Klussmann JP, et al: Parotidectomy for benign parotid disease at a university teaching hospital: Outcome of 963 operations. *Laryngoscope* 2006;116:534–540.
22. Bova R, Saylor A, Coman WB: Parotidectomy: Review of treatment and outcomes. *Aust N Z J Surg* 2004;74:563–568.
23. Gaillard C, Perie S, Susini B, et al: Facial nerve dysfunction after parotidectomy: The role of local factors. *Laryngoscope* 2005;115:287–291.
24. Fee WE, Goffinet DR, Calcaterra TC: Recurrent mixed tumors of the parotid gland—Results of surgical therapy. *Laryngoscope* 1978;88:265–273.
25. Ward CM: Injury of the facial nerve during surgery of the parotid gland. *Br J Surg* 1975;62:401–403.
26. Perzik SL: Parotidectomy in inflammatory lesions. *Am J Surg* 1961;102:769–776.
27. Beahrs OH, Devine KD, Woolner LB: Parotidectomy in the treatment of chronic sialoadenitis. *Am J Surg* 1961;102:760–768.
28. Arriaga MA, Myers EN: The surgical management of chronic parotitis. *Laryngoscope* 1990;100:1270–1275.
29. Sobol SM, May M, Mester S: Early facial reanimation following radical parotid and temporal bone tumor resections. *Am J Surg* 1990;160:382–386.
30. Jackson LL, Gourin CG, Thomas DS, et al: Use of the harmonic scalpel in superficial and total parotidectomy for benign and malignant disease. *Laryngoscope* 2005;115:1070–1073.
31. Fee WE, Jr, Handen C: Parotid gland surgery using the Shaw hemostatic scalpel. *Arch Otolaryngol* 1984;110:739–741.
32. Ramadan HH, Wax MA, Itani M: The Shaw scalpel and development of facial nerve paresis after superficial parotidectomy. *Arch Otolaryngol Head Neck Surg* 1998;124:296–298.
33. Johnson JT, Wagner RT: Infection following uncontaminated head and neck surgery. *Arch Otolaryngol Head Neck Surg* 1987;113:368–369.
34. Kaufman T, Eichenlaub EH, Levin M, et al: Tobacco smoking: Impairment of experimental flap survival. *Ann Plast Surg* 1984;13:468–472.
35. Rees TD, Liverett DM, Guy CL: The effect of cigarette smoking on skin-flap survival in the face lift patient. *Plast Reconstr Surg* 1984;73:911–915.
36. Maharaj M, Diamond C, Williams D, et al: Tisseel to reduce postparotidectomy wound drainage: Randomized, prospective, controlled trial. *J Otolaryngol* 2006;35:36–39.
37. Mandour MA, El-Sheikh MM, El-Garem F: Tympanic neurectomy for parotid fistula. *Arch Otolaryngol Head Neck Surg* 1976;102:327–329.
38. Ananthakrishnan N, Parkash S: Parotid fistulas: A review. *Br J Surg* 1982;69:641–643.
39. Burch RJ: Spontaneous closure of a parotid gland fistula with the aid of banthine: Report of a case. *Oral Surg* 1953;6:1191–1194.
40. Cecil AB, Martin GW: Banthine as an adjunct in the treatment of salivary fistulae. *Am J Surg* 1956;91:421–422.

41. Talmi YP, Finkelstein Y, Zohar Y: Reduction of salivary flow with transdermal scopolamine: A four-year experience. *Otolaryngol Head Neck Surg* 1990;103:615–618.

42. Chadwick SJ, Davis WE, Templer JW: Parotid fistula: Current management. *South Med J* 1979;72:922–926.

43. Ellies M, Gottstein U, Rohrbach-Volland S, et al: Reduction of salivary flow with botulinum toxin: Extended report on 33 patients with drooling, salivary fistulas, and sialadenitis. *Laryngoscope* 2004;114:1856–1860.

44. Marchese-Ragona R, Marioni G, Restivo DA, et al: The role of botulinum toxin in post parotidectomy fistula treatment. *Am J Otolaryngol* 2006;27:221–224.

45. Minor V: Eines neues verfahren zu der klinischen untersuchung der schweissabsonderung. *Dtsch Z Nervenheilkd* 1928;101:302–308.

46. Laage-Hellman JE: Gustatory sweating and flushing after conservative parotidectomy. *Acta Otolaryngol* 1957;48:234–252.

47. Glaister DH, Hearnshaw JR, Heffron PF, et al: The mechanism of post-parotidectomy gustatory sweating (the auriculotemporal syndrome). *Br Med J* 1958;2:942–946.

48. Spiro RH, Martin H: Gustatory sweating following parotid surgery and radical neck dissection. *Ann Surg* 1967;165:118–127.

49. Hays LL, Novack AJ, Worsham JC: The Frey syndrome: A simple, effective treatment. *Otolaryngol Head Neck Surg* 1982;90:419–425.

50. Kidd HA: Diseases of the parotid and the Frey syndrome. *Br J Hosp Med* 1969;2:1513–1522.

51. Eddey HH: Parotid tumors: A review of 138 cases. *Aust N Z J Surg* 1970:40:1–14.

52. Singleton CT, Cassisi NJ: Frey's syndrome: Incidence related to skin flap thickness in parotidectomy. *Laryngoscope* 1980;90:1636–1639.

53. Kornblut AD, Westphal P, Miehlke A: A reevaluation of the Frey syndrome following parotid surgery. *Arch Otolaryngol* 1977;103:258–261.

54. Guntinas-Lichius O, Gabriel B, Klussmann JP: Risk and facial palsy and severe Frey's syndrome after conservative parotidectomy for benign disease: Analysis of 610 operations. *Acta Otolaryngol* 2006;126:1104–1109.

55. Dulguerov P, Quinodoz D, Cosendai G, et al: Prevention of Frey syndrome during parotidectomy. *Arch Otolaryngol Head Neck Surg* 1999;125:833–839.

56. Sinha UK, Saadat D, Doherty CM, et al: Use of AlloDerm implant to prevent Frey syndrome after parotidectomy. *Arch Facial Past Surg* 2003;5:109–112.

57. Govindaraj S, Cohen M, Genden EM, et al: The use of acellular dermis in the prevention of Frey's syndrome. *Laryngoscope* 2001;111:1993–1998.

58. Boles R: Parotid neoplasms: Surgical treatment and complications. *Otolaryngol Clin North Am* 1977;10:413–420.

59. May JS, McGuirt WF: Frey's syndrome: Treatment with topical glycopyrrolate. *Head Neck* 1989;11:85–89.

60. Beerens AJ, Snow GB: Botulinum toxin A in the treatment of patients with Frey syndrome. *Br J Surg* 2002;89:116–119.

61. Laccourreye O, Akl E, Gutierrez-Fonseca R, et al: Recurrent gustatory sweating (Frey syndrome) after intracutaneous injection of botulinum toxin type A: Incidence, management, and outcome. *Arch Otolaryngol Head Neck Surg* 1999;125:283–286.

62. Laskawi R, Drobik C, Schonebeck C: Up-to-date report of botulinum toxin type A treatment in patients with gustatory sweating (Frey's syndrome). *Laryngoscope* 1998;108:381–384.

63. Sessions RB, Roark DT, Alford BR: Frey's syndrome—a technical remedy. *Ann Otol Rhinol Laryngol* 1976;85:734–739.

64. Wallis KA, Gibson T: Gustatory sweating following parotidectomy: Correction by a fascia lata graft. *Br J Plast Surg* 1978;31:68–71.

65. Boddie AW, Guillamondegui OM, Byers RM: Gustatory rhinorrhea developing after radical parotidectomy—A new syndrome. *Arch Otolaryngol* 1976;102:248–250.

66. Stevens HE, Doyle PJ: Bilateral gustatory rhinorrhea following bilateral parotidectomy: A case report. *J Otolaryngol* 1988;17:191–193.

67. Hamilton RB, Nettle WJS: Gustatory rhinorrhea after radical parotidectomy. *Scand J Plast Reconstr Hand Surg* 1990;24:163–166.

68. Hobsley M: Amputation neuroma of the great auricular nerve after parotidectomy. *Br J Surg* 1972;59:735–736.

69. Moss CE, Johnston CJ, Whear NM: Amputation neuroma of the great auricular nerve after operations on the parotid gland. *Br J Oral Maxillofac Surg* 2000;38:537–538.

70. Hui Y, Wong DS, Wong LY et al: A prospective controlled double-blind trial of great auricular nerve preservation at parotidectomy. *Am J Surg* 2003;185:574–579.

71. Vieira MBM, Maia AF, Ribeiro JC: Randomized prospective study of the validity of the great auricular nerve preservation in parotidectomy. *Arch Otolaryngol Head Neck Surg* 2002;128:1191–1195.

72. Ryan WR, Fee WE: Great auricular nerve morbidity after nerve sacrifice during parotidectomy. *Arch Otolaryngol Head Neck Surg* 2006;132:642–649.

73. Brown AMS, Wake JC: Accidental full thickness burn and the ear lobe following division of the great auricular nerve at parotidectomy. *Br J Oral Maxilliofac Surg* 1990;28:178–179.

74. Walter C: The free dermis fat transplantation as adjunct in the surgery of the parotid gland. *Laryngol Rhinol* 1975;54:435–440.

75. Nosan DK, Ochi JW, Davidson TM: Reservation of facial contour during parotidectomy. *Otolaryngol Head Neck Surg* 1991;104:293–298.

76. Baker DC, Shaw WW, Conley J: Reconstruction of radical parotidectomy defects. *Am J Surg* 1979;138:550–554.

77. Bugis SP, Young JEM, Archibald SD: Sternocleidomastoid flap following parotidectomy. *Head Neck* 1990;12:430–435.

78. Chow TL, Lam CY, Chiu PW, et al: Sternomastoid-muscle transposition improves cosmetic outcome of superficial parotidectomy. *Br J Plast Surg* 2001;54:409–411.

79. Spiro RH, Huvos AG, Strong EW: Cancer of the parotid gland: A clinicopathological study of 288 primary cases. *Am J Surg* 1975;130:452–459.

80. Woods JE: The facial nerve in parotid malignancy. *Am J Surg* 1983;146:493–496.

81. Matsuba HM, Thawley SE, Devineni VR, et al: High-grade malignancies of the parotid gland: Effective use of planned combined surgery and irradiation. *Laryngoscope* 1985;95:1059–1063.

82. Sullivan MJ, Breslin K. McClatchey KD, et al: Malignant parotid gland tumors: A retrospective study. *Otolaryngol Head Neck Surg* 1987;97:529–533.

83. North CA, Lee DJ, Piantadosi S, et al: Carcinoma of the major salivary glands treated by surgery or surgery plus postoperative radiotherapy. *Int J Radiat Oncol Biol Phys* 1990;18:1319–1326.

84. Conley J, Clairmont AA: Facial nerve in recurrent benign pleomorphic adenoma. *Arch Otolaryngol* 1979;105:247–251.

85. Maynard JD: Management of pleomorphic adenoma of the parotid. *Br J Surg* 1988;75:305–308.

86. Kirklin JW, McDonald JR, Harrington SW, et al: Parotid tumors: Histopathology, clinical behavior and end results. *Surg Gynecol Obstet* 1951;92:721–733.

87. Krolls SO, Boyers RC: Mixed tumors of salivary glands. *Cancer* 1972;30:276–281.

88. Maran AGD, Mackenzie IJ, Stanley RE: Recurrent pleomorphic adenomas of the parotid gland. *Arch Otolaryngol* 1984;110:167–171.

89. Myssiorek D, Ruah CB, Hybels RL: Recurrent pleomorphic adenomas of the parotid gland. *Head Neck* 1990;12:332–336.

90. Olsen KD, Daube JR: Intraoperative monitoring of the facial nerve: An aid in the management of parotid recurrent pleomorphic adenomas. *Laryngoscope* 1994;104:229–232.

91. Zbaren P, Tschumi I, Nuyens M, et al: Recurrent pleomorphic adenoma of the parotid gland. *Am J Surg* 2005;189:203–207.

92. Niparko JK, Beauchamp ML, Krause CJ, et al: Surgical treatment of recurrent pleomorphic adenoma of the parotid gland. *Arch Otolaryngol Head Neck Surg* 1986;112:1180–1184.

93. Work WP, Batsakis JG, Bailey DG: Recurrent benign mixed tumor and the facial nerve. *Arch Otolaryngol* 1976;102:15–19.

94. Dawson AK: Radiation therapy in recurrent pleomorphic adenoma of the parotid. *Int J Radiot Oncol Biol Phys* 1989;16:819–821.

95. Samson MJ, Metson R, Wang CC, et al: Preservation of the facial nerve in the management of recurrent pleomorphic adenoma. *Laryngoscope* 1991;101:1060–1062.

96. Chen AM, Garcia J, Bucci MK, et al: Recurrent pleomorphic adenoma of the parotid gland: Long-term outcome of patients treated with radiation therapy. *Int J Radiat Oncol Biol Phys* 2006;66:1031–1035.

97. Dawson AK, Orr JA: Long-term results of local excision and radiotherapy in pleomorphic adenomas of the parotid. *Int J Radiat Oncol Biol Phys* 1985;11:451–455.

98. Kennedy PJ, Poole AG: Excision of the submandibular gland: Minimizing the risk of nerve damage. *Aust N Z J Surg* 1989;59:411–414.

99. Milton CM, Thomas BM, Bickerton RC: Morbidity study of submandibular gland excision. *Ann R Coll Surg Engl* 1986;68:148–150.

100. Smith WP, Markus AF, Peters WJN: Submandibular gland surgery: An audit of clinical findings, pathology and postoperative morbidity. *Ann R Coll Surg Engl* 1986;75:164–167.

101. Bates D, O'Brien CJ, Tikaram K, Painter DM: Parotid and submandibular sialadenitis treated by salivary gland excision. *Aust N Z J Surg* 1998;68:120–124.

102. King GD: Complications in the management of surgical disease of the major salivary glands. *Surg Clin North Am* 1968;48:477–482.

103. Ziarah HA, Aktinson ME: The surgical anatomy of the mandibular distribution of the facial nerve. *Br J Oral Surg* 1978;19:159–170.

104. Nelson D, Gingross R: Anatomy of the mandibular branch of the facial nerve. *Plast Reconstr Surg* 1979;64:479–482.

105. Ichimura K, Nibu K, Tanaka T: Nerve paralysis after surgery in the submandibular triangle: Review of University of Tokyo experience. *Head Neck* 1997;19:48–53.

106. Ellies M, Laskawi R, Arglebe C: Surgical management of non neoplastic diseases of the submandibular gland. *Int J Oral Maxillofac Surg* 1996;25:285–289.

107. Blake P: Excision of the submandibular gland: Minimizing the risk of nerve damage (comment). *Aust N Z J Surg* 1989;59:894.

108. Cunning DM, Lipke N, Wax MK: Significance of unilateral submandibular gland excision on salivary flow in noncancer patients. *Laryngoscope* 1998;108:812–815.

109. Jacob RF, Weber RS, King GE: Whole salivary flow rates following submandibular gland resection. *Head Neck* 1996;18:242–247.

110. Young AG: Unilateral sweating of the submental region after eating. *Br Med J* 1956;2:976–979.

111. Bailey BM, Pearce DE: Gustatory sweating following submandibular salivary gland removal. *Br Dent J* 1985;158:17–18.

112. Fornadley JA, Gomez PJ, Crane RT, et al: Toxic shock syndrome following submandibular gland excision. *Head Neck* 1990;12:66–68.

113. Adjei SS, Hammersley N: Mylohyoid nerve damage due to excision of the submandibular salivary gland. *Br J Oral Maxillofac Surg* 1989;27:209–211.

114. Marinho ROM, Tenant CJ: Paresthesia of the cutaneous branch of the mylohyoid nerve after removal of a submandibular salivary gland. *J Oral Maxillofac Surg* 1997;55:170–171.

115. Hiatt WR, Castner DV: Chronic inflammation of residual submaxillary gland duct: Report of case. *J Oral Surg* 1967;25:550–551.

116. Marchal F, Dulguerov P, Becker M, et al: Submandibular diagnostic and interventional sialendoscopy: New procedure for ductal disorders. *Ann Otol Rhinol Laryngol* 2002;111:27–35.

117. Marchal F, Dulguerov P, Becker M, et al: Specificity of parotid sialendoscopy. *Laryngoscope* 2001;111:264–271.

118. Nahlieli O, Baruchin AM: Long-term experience with endoscopic diagnosis and treatment of salivary gland inflammatory diseases. *Laryngoscope* 2000;110:988–993.

119. Ziegler CM, Steveling H, Seubert M, et al: Endoscopy: A minimally invasive procedure for diagnosis and treatment of diseases of the salivary glands. *Br J Oral Maxillofac Surg* 2004;41:1–7.

120. Koch M, Zenk J, Bozzato A, et al: Sialoscopy in cases of unclear swelling of the major salivary glands. *Otolaryngol Head Neck Surg* 2005;133:863–868.

121. Zenk J, Constantindis J, Al-Kadah B, et al: Transoral removal of submandibular stones. *Arch Otolaryngol Head Neck Surg* 2001;127:432–436.

122. McGurk M, Makdissi J, Brown JE: Intra-oral removal of stones from the hilum of the submandibular gland: Report of technique and morbidity. *Int J Oral Maxillofac Surg* 2004;33:683–686.

123. Park JS, Sohn JH, Kim JK: Factors influencing intraoral removal of submandibular calculi. *Otolaryngol Head Neck Surg* 2006;135:704–709.

124. Nitzan D, Kronenberg J, Horowitz Z, et al: Quality of life following parotidectomy for malignant and benign disease. *Plast Reconstr Surg* 2004;114:1060–1067.

125. Beutner D, Wittekindt C, Dinh S, et al: Impact of lateral parotidectomy for benign tumors on quality of life. *Acta Otolaryngol* 2006;126:1091–1095.

126. Yokoshima K, Nakamizo M, Ozu C, et al: Significance of preserving the posterior branch of the great auricular nerve in parotidectomy. *J Nippon Med Sch* 2004;71:323–327.

127. Hui Y, Wong DSY, Wong LY, et al: A prospective controlled double-blind trial of great auricular nerve preservation at parotidectomy. *Am J Surg* 2003;185:574–579.

128. Kim SY, Mathog RH: Platysma muscle-cervical fascia-sternocleidomastoid muscle (PCS) flap for parotidectomy. *Head Neck* 1999;21:428–433.

129. Osborne RF, Tan JW, Hamilton JS, et al: Bipedicled sternocleidomastoid muscle flap for reconstruction of tail of parotid defects. *Laryngoscope* 2004;114:2045–2047.

130. Meninquad JP, Bertolus C, Bertrand JC: Parotidectomy: Assessment of surgical technique including facelift incision and SMAS advancement. *J Craniomaxillofac Surg* 2006;34:34–37.

131. Terris DJ, Tuffo KM, Fee WE: Modified facelift incision for parotidectomy. *J Laryngol Otol* 1994;108:574–578.

132. Marti-Pages C, Garcia-Diez L, Garcia-Arana D, et al: Minimal incision in parotidectomy. *Int J Oral Maxillofac Surg* 2007;36:72–76.

CHAPTER 21

Complications of Surgery of the Parapharyngeal Space

Eric J. Moore and Kerry D. Olsen

The minimization of complications of surgery of the parapharyngeal space entails accurate preoperative evaluation and the selection of an appropriate surgical procedure. Parapharyngeal neoplasms include both benign and malignant processes. Because most parapharyngeal neoplasms are benign and because patients rarely die of them, low morbidity and mortality rates are expected.[1] The goals of minimally morbid surgery in the parapharyngeal space are the excellent visualization of tumor, the preservation of surrounding nerves and vessels, the control of bleeding, and the complete removal of the tumor. The operation should be planned so that it can be easily extended to adjacent regions, if necessary. Some morbidity, such as that resulting from planned cranial nerve resection, is expected.[2] True complications should be exceedingly rare. Unfortunately, there are potential disastrous complications that can occur when operating in the parapharyngeal space. Complications usually result from unfamiliarity with the anatomy, improper preoperative assessment, poor patient selection, improper surgical approach, or a combination of these. This chapter will help prepare the surgeon by discussing both the common and the rare complications of surgery of the parapharyngeal space. Management will be discussed, but emphasis will be placed on preventive measures to decrease operative morbidity.

ANATOMY

The anatomy of the parapharyngeal space is complicated. Failure to appreciate the anatomic relationships can lead to the selection of an incorrect surgical approach. The result may be inadequate access, which may result in difficult tumor removal, damage to vital structures, or tumor spillage and thus recurrent neoplasms.

The parapharyngeal space is actually a potential space that is often described as an inverted pyramid with its base at the skull. The superior limit of the parapharyngeal space is a portion of the temporal bone and not the floor of the middle cranial fossa, which is the superior boundary of the infratemporal fossa. These areas are often confused with one another in the literature. The posterior wall is formed by the fascia over the spinal column and the paraspinal muscles. Another firm border is the lateral wall, which is defined by the fascia overlying the medial pterygoid muscle, the ramus of the mandible, and the deep lobe of the parotid gland. The inferior border is composed of the posterior belly of the digastric muscle and the greater cornu of the hyoid bone. The medial border consists of the fascia over the superior constrictor muscle and the tensor and levator palatini muscles. The inferior and medial borders constitute the less-rigid surfaces of the parapharyngeal space (Figure 21-1).

Fascia that extends from the styloid process to the tensor veli palatini muscles divides the parapharyngeal space into an anterolateral or prestyloid compartment and a posterolateral or retrostyloid compartment. The contents of these compartments are shown in Table 21-1. An excellent review of the pertinent anatomy of the parapharyngeal space is found in the article by van Huijzen.[3]

TUMORS

Tumors involve the parapharyngeal space as primary neoplasms, by direct extension from adjacent regions, or by metastatic disease to involved lymph nodes. Tumors of the parapharyngeal space usually present as asymptomatic masses noted by the patient or the physician at the angle of the mandible or as an asymmetry of the tonsil or the soft palate. Tumors may become quite large before they cause any symptoms. Patients may present with symptoms of dysphagia, hoarseness, pain, globus pharyngeus, or ear fullness.

The most common primary tumors are salivary gland neoplasms that originate from the deep lobe of the parotid gland or from minor salivary glands. In addition, neurogenic tumors (primarily neurilemomas and paragangliomas) often occur in this area. A list of reported benign and malignant parapharyngeal neoplasms is given in Table 21-2.

The histologic findings and the extent of the tumor should dictate treatment. Complications are far more likely with malignant lesions that extend into or that metastasize to the parapharyngeal space and with vascular lesions. Tumors may extend into the nasopharynx, the mandible, the oropharynx, the maxilla, and the oral cavity. Tumors from the parapharyngeal space can also extend intracranially through the jugular foramen or into the retropharyngeal space. Adequate preoperative imaging is essential for the delineation of the tumor and for the anticipation of potential complications. Fine-needle aspiration may offer additional information that

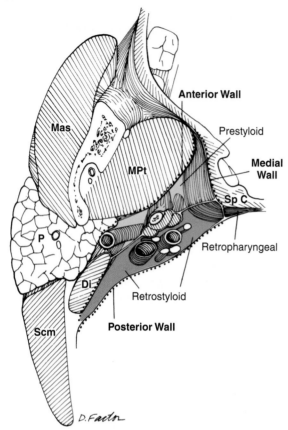

Figure 21-1. Anatomic borders of the parapharyngeal space *(area outlined by dots). Di,* Digastric muscle; *Mas,* masseter muscle; *Mpt,* medial pterygoid muscle; *P,* parotid gland; *Scm,* sternocleidomastoid muscle; *Spc,* superior constrictor muscle. (Courtesy of the Mayo Foundation, Rochester, Minn.)

TABLE 21-1   Contents of the Prestyloid and Poststyloid Compartments of the Parapharyngeal Space

Structure	Prestyloid Compartment	Poststyloid Compartment
Arteries	Internal maxillary artery Ascending pharyngeal artery	Internal carotid artery
Veins	—	Internal jugular vein
Nerves	Auriculotemporal nerve	Cranial nerves IX, X, XI, and XII
Lymph nodes	None	Cervical sympathetic chain
Glomus bodies	None	Present
Parotid gland	Deep lobe	Present

can guide the surgeon with regard to the selection of appropriate therapy.[4]

SURGICAL APPROACHES

Although many surgical approaches have been described for the treatment of parapharyngeal lesions, the vast majority of tumors in this area can be treated with the cervical–parotid approach, with or without minor variations.[5] The four most commonly applied operations are as follows:

1. Cervical
2. Cervical–parotid (Figure 21-2)
3. Cervical–parotid with a lateral or midline mandibulotomy (Figure 21-3)
4. Transoral

The mandibulotomy approach can be used with or without splitting the lip.[6] The transoral approach has been reported to be effective for removing select benign, minor salivary tumors that originate high in the parapharyngeal space.[7] However, this approach provides poor exposure, a lack of wide access to regional vessels and nerves, and a high risk of tumor spillage with possible recurrence. An incorrect approach can result in significant morbidity and mortality.

The authors' most commonly used surgical approaches for parapharyngeal lesions are the cervical–parotid approach and the cervical–parotid approach with midline mandibulotomy. The cervical–parotid approach is used for deep-lobe parotid neoplasms, extraparotid salivary tumors, and most neurogenic tumors. This approach can be combined with a craniotomy for tumors that extend intracranially; intracranial extension is then treated during the same operation. The cervical approach with midline mandibulotomy is used for highly vascular tumors that extend into the superior parapharyngeal space and for tumors confined to the superior parapharyngeal region (i.e., the Eustachian tube and the skull base). This procedure is indicated for tumors that have invaded the skull base or the vertebral bodies. In these cases and in those with obvious intracranial extension, the operation is performed in conjunction with a neurosurgeon.

REPORTED COMPLICATIONS

Complications of surgical approaches in the parapharyngeal space have been reported in a few large series in the literature.[1,2,6,7] Surgical complications can result in expected sequelae from the resection of cranial nerves as a planned part of tumor resection. This can occur frequently in operations of parapharyngeal space

TABLE 21-2   Neoplasms of the Parapharyngeal Space

Source	Benign	Malignant
Salivary gland	Pleomorphic adenoma Warthin tumor Oncocytoma Benign lymphoepithelial lesion	Adenoid cystic carcinoma Acinic cell carcinoma Adenocarcinoma Mucoepidermoid carcinoma Carcinoma ex pleomorphic adenoma
Neurogenic	Neurilemoma Neurofibroma Vagal paraganglioma Carotid body tumor	Neurofibrosarcoma
Other	Lymphatic malformation Hemangioma Rhabdomyoma Meningioma Teratoma Branchial cleft cyst Lipoma Venous malformation Leiomyoma Hemangioepithelioma	Lymphoma Rhabdomyosarcoma Plasmacytoma Fibrosarcoma Fibrous histiocytoma Hemangiopericytoma Liposarcoma

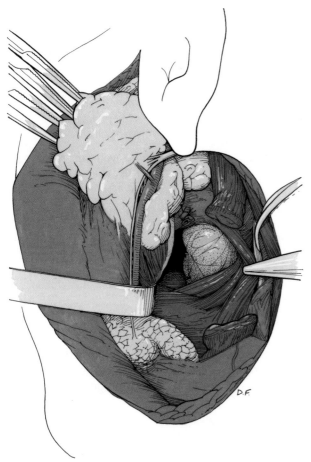

Figure 21-2. Portion of the cervical–parotid approach to the parapharyngeal space. (Courtesy of the Mayo Foundation, Rochester, Minn.)

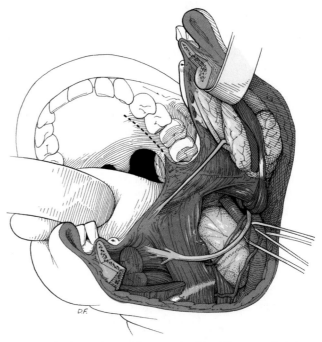

Figure 21-3. Cervical–parotid approach with midline mandibulotomy. (Courtesy of the Mayo Foundation, Rochester, Minn.)

masses, and it can result in both temporary and permanent morbidity.[2] The most frequently reported unexpected complications of surgery in the parapharyngeal space include tumor spillage (20%), first-bite pain (12%), trismus and law pain (4%), temporary facial paresis (4%), palatal weakness (2.7%), and cerebrospinal fluid (CSF) leak (2%).[1,2,4,7] Wound infection, orocutaneous fistula, hemorrhage, compromised airway, surgical-incision morbidity, and complications of catecholamine-secreting tumors are rare.

Fortunately, most operations in the parapharyngeal space are for primary benign neoplasms and have low expected morbidity. By contrast, cancers that extend into the parapharyngeal space or into the infratemporal fossa are associated with significantly higher morbidity after attempts at removal.[8] Reported complications have included major vessel injury, stroke, and death. Table 21-3 lists the reported complications and sequelae of surgery in the parapharyngeal space. Specific complications and steps to avoid them are addressed in the sections that follow.

RECURRENT TUMOR

The most common tumor encountered in the parapharyngeal space is a pleomorphic adenoma that arises from the deep lobe of the parotid gland or from a minor salivary gland (Figures 21-4 and 21-5). It is often necessary to operate on the capsule of a pleomorphic adenoma in the parapharyngeal space. Recurrent pleomorphic adenoma results from tumor spillage and inadequate excision. Tumor recurrence in the parapharyngeal space may not be recognized until 10 or even 20 years after the first operation. Operation for recurrent parapharyngeal pleomorphic adenoma poses a greater risk of injury to the facial nerve, and it should always be performed by an experienced surgeon with the aid of facial nerve monitoring. The surgical goal should be to remove the lesion intact without rupture, but this is sometimes not possible. In one reported series of parapharyngeal space tumors, tumor rupture or spillage was the most common complication, occurring in 37 of 172 patients. Of these 37 patients, 12 were noted to have tumor recurrence.[4] Tumor spillage can be lessened when the surgical exposure is improved. The surgeon can divide the stylomandibular ligament; remove or mobilize the submandibular gland; excise the superficial lobe of the parotid gland and the upper neck lymphatics; and remove the styloid process, the posterior belly of the digastric muscle, and the styloid musculature when necessary to lessen the chance of tumor compression and rupture (Figure 21-6). In addition, the mastoid tip can be removed, and mandibulotomy and the removal of the pterygoid plates can also be performed if tumor access is inadequate. Transoral open biopsy of parapharyngeal space tumors for diagnosis should not be performed because of the high rate of tumor spillage and recurrence.

Malignant tumors, paragangliomas, and neuromas also can recur after surgical removal (Figure 21-7). Difficulty

TABLE 21-3   Complications of Surgery in the Parapharyngeal Space

Complication	Sequelae
Recurrent tumor	Additional treatment Death
Nerve injury: cranial nerves VII, IX, X, and XII Greater auricular nerve Inferior alveolar nerve Cervical sympathetic chain	Aspiration Dysphonia Dysarthria Velopharyngeal insufficiency Horner syndrome Facial paralysis Facial numbness Shoulder dysfunction
Vessel injury: carotid artery, jugular vein	Hemorrhage Stroke Death
Airway compromise	Emergency tracheotomy Death
Mandibular osteotomy	Tooth loss Malunion Nonunion
Catecholamine-secreting tumor	Hypertensive crisis
Parotid gland complications	Frey syndrome Soft-tissue depression Salivary fistula First-bite pain
Cerebrospinal fluid leakage	Rhinorrhea Wound drainage Meningitis
Infection	Delayed wound healing Abscess Fistula
Other	Seroma Scar Thrombophlebitis Pneumonia Pulmonary embolism Myocardial infarction

with bleeding or extension of the tumor into the jugular foramen may prevent total removal. The recurrence of malignant tumor portends a poor prognosis.

NERVE INJURY

Operation on tumors of the parapharyngeal space and the skull base can cause injury to cranial nerves. In addition, the histologic features and the extent of the

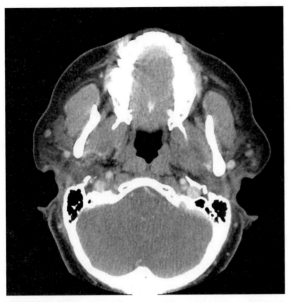

Figure 21-4. Axial computed tomography scan with contrast of a left parapharyngeal pleomorphic adenoma.

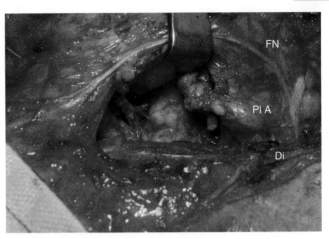

Figure 21-6. Cervical–parotid approach to the left parapharyngeal pleomorphic adenoma demonstrating tumor above the digastric muscle. Note the displaced superficial and deep parotid gland and the inferior division of the facial nerve. *Di,* Digastric muscle; *FN,* facial nerve, *Pl A,* pleomorphic adenoma.

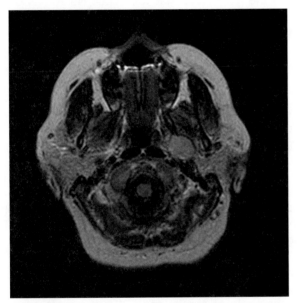

Figure 21-5. Magnetic resonance image of the same patient as shown in Figure 21-4 demonstrating a left parapharyngeal pleomorphic adenoma.

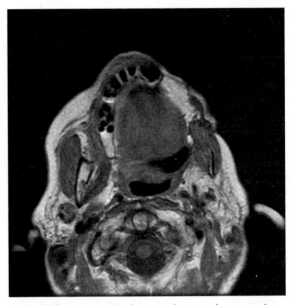

Figure 21-7. Recurrent extensive parapharyngeal sarcoma in a patient who has undergone previous pharyngeal/buccal resection, free-tissue reconstruction, and radiation therapy.

tumor may necessitate the resection of cranial nerves and result in expected morbidity. If possible, attempts should be made to preserve cranial nerves unless doing so would necessitate leaving gross tumor behind. For cases in which the resection of cranial nerves is planned, the early institution of speech and swallowing therapy and other forms of physical therapy can greatly improve the rehabilitation of the patient.[2] In addition, preoperative discussion of expected postoperative sequelae will greatly enhance the understanding and recovery of the patient.

Cranial Nerve VII

Mild paresis of the facial nerve (cranial nerve VII) is common after parapharyngeal space operations. With the use of regional landmarks, the identification of this cranial nerve is straightforward, and the use of a nerve monitor is usually not necessary. For recurrent tumors and to avoid excessive postoperative scarring, facial nerve monitoring, magnification, and the use of a nerve stimulator may be beneficial. With the cervical–parotid approach, the lower division of the facial nerve is isolated, and mild temporary paresis of the mandibular branch of the facial nerve is common. Deep-lobe parotid tumors often require an initial superficial parotidectomy for the exposure and mobilization of the facial nerve, and temporary paresis can occur. This paresis may be prolonged or more debilitating in the elderly patient, and temporary or permanent facial reanimation procedures may be required. The surgeon must be assured that the nerve is intact at the end of the procedure.

If the facial nerve is divided, a primary anastomosis without tension should be performed. If a segment of nerve is missing, then an interposition graft should be immediately placed with the use of the greater auricular nerve or the sural nerve. Some recovery of function is expected to return to the grafted nerve within 1 year. When the facial nerve must be transposed because of intracranial tumor extension, meticulous technique and the preservation of the large cuff of normal tissue around the nerve in the stylomastoid foramen region are helpful to minimize postoperative facial weakness. If continuity of the facial nerve is lost, eye protection can be aided by performing a lateral tarsorrhaphy or by inserting a gold weight in the upper lid. If the nerve is intact but the patient has upper-division weakness, the usual measures to ensure eye protection are adequate. Permanent injury to cranial nerve VII during parapharyngeal surgery is extremely rare, except for cases of malignant neoplasms that involve the parotid gland.

Cranial Nerve IX

During the cervical–parotid approach and always with the cervical approach with midline mandibulotomy, cranial nerve IX is visualized. Division of the nerve generally causes minimal sequelae, but its sensory innervation should be preserved, if possible. Cranial nerve IX injury could lead to a delay in identifying subsequent lesions located in the sensory distribution of this nerve. In addition, the division of this nerve may contribute to some of the pain symptoms that are common after surgery for neoplasms of the parapharyngeal space. Physicians should be aware of lesions in the parapharyngeal space that preoperatively may cause glossopharyngeal neuralgia with associated asystole, bradycardia, and convulsions.[8] These symptoms can be relieved with the removal of the parapharyngeal lesion.

Cranial Nerve XI

Accessory nerve (cranial nerve XI) injury can cause significant shoulder pain and disability. If the accessory nerve is divided during tumor removal, primary reanastomosis can be performed. If the nerve is resected and grafting is not possible, then an early physical therapy program should be initiated to prevent adhesive capsulitis of the glenohumeral joint.

This therapy is especially essential if postoperative radiation therapy is planned.

Cranial Nerve XII

If cranial nerve XII alone is divided during a surgical procedure in the parapharyngeal space, problems associated with its loss are usually minimal. If swallowing and talking are impaired, therapy usually aids recovery. The loss of cranial nerve XII and X together can cause significant problems with speech and swallowing that may require long-term therapy and the use of a gastrostomy tube for enteral nutrition supplementation.

Sympathetic Plexus

The sympathetic plexus can be injured during operations in the parapharyngeal space and result in Horner syndrome (ipsilateral ptosis, meiosis, and anhidrosis). The greater auricular nerve is often divided during the cervical–parotid approach, and patients should be told about the numbness that will occur. Neuromas of the greater auricular nerve are rarely a problem, and they may be excised, if indicated.

Cranial Nerve X

Injury to the vagus nerve (cranial nerve X) in the parapharyngeal space can cause significant morbidity. Dysphagia, aspiration, and dysphonia may result. These problems are less pronounced if the patient had vagal neuropathy that developed slowly before the surgery. Transection of the normally functioning nerve above the inferior (nodose) ganglion during surgery is especially debilitating because of the additional loss of the parapharyngeal branches and the superior laryngeal nerve. The vagus nerve should be preserved whenever possible.

Division of the vagus nerve generally occurs during the resection of vagal paragangliomas and neurilemomas. Neurilemoma of cranial nerve X is the most common parapharyngeal neurogenic tumor.[9] Because it is generally large when detected, its size usually makes nerve preservation impossible. If the tumor originates below the level of the superior laryngeal nerve, this branch should be preserved. If the tumor grows off of the nerve in a polypoid manner, the nerve may be preserved. With neurofibromas and paragangliomas, vagus nerve preservation is rare.[10]

If the vagus nerve is paralyzed preoperatively as a result of tumor involvement, most patients will have compensated, and the morbidity of resection will be low. If the nerve is functioning preoperatively, then patients usually suffer from dysphagia, velopharyngeal insufficiency, and aspiration postoperatively. Dysphonia may be mild or severe. Younger patients will compensate for the unilateral loss of the nerve better than older patients will. Patients may benefit from adjunctive measures of vocal-cord medialization with injectable material or laryngeal framework surgery. Palatal adhesion or pharyngeal flap surgery may benefit patients with significant velopharyngeal insufficiency. In general, the vigorous and early institution of speech and swallowing therapy should be instituted as the first intervention, with more aggressive measures employed after a period of observation and spontaneous recovery. This is particularly true if cranial nerve X is divided but cranial nerves XII and IX remain intact. Young patients may have dysphonia but very little dysphagia or aspiration. If the vagus nerve is intact postoperatively but paralysis is noted later, the surgeon should wait at least a year before permanently augmenting or medializing the vocal cord, because spontaneous recovery may occur.

When cranial nerve X division is performed and cranial nerve XII is also sacrificed, most patients will have significant difficulty with swallowing. These patients should have a feeding tube placed and oral feeding withheld. A tracheostomy tube may be necessary to facilitate pulmonary toilet in selected patients with significant aspiration. They may benefit from vocal-cord augmentation at the time of surgery. The tracheostomy tube should be changed slowly to an uncuffed metal tube, then plugged during the day, and then plugged during both the day and the night. It should be removed only when the patient can tolerate secretions without aspiration. Oral feeding should be withheld until the patient is able to swallow saliva without difficulty. The use of dynamic video swallow study and the assistance of a skilled speech therapist is essential to maximal rehabilitation. Feeding tubes are often necessary for several weeks or months after hospital discharge for elderly patients with multiple cranial neuropathies. Swallowing techniques such as those applied for patients with partial laryngeal procedures are useful. Compensation for the unilateral loss of the vagus and hypoglossal nerves occurs with time and therapy.

VESSEL INJURY

Carotid artery injury is the greatest potential risk of operation in the parapharyngeal space. Uncontrolled bleeding can cause death from hemorrhage or stroke. Parapharyngeal tumors can involve the jugular vein, the internal and external carotid arteries, and the vertebral artery. Vessel injury is uncommon, occurring in 0% to 2% of patients as reported in large series.[1,2] Vessel injury is more likely with paragangliomas, recurrent tumors, malignant tumors, after previous surgery and radiation therapy, and among elderly patients with tortuous carotid arteries.

An accurate radiographic assessment preoperatively is essential to minimize vascular morbidity during surgery.

Whenever radiographic studies show bone erosion of the cervical vertebrae or the skull base, the involvement of the vertebral arteries should be considered. Formal angiography should be performed preoperatively in all of these cases and in all cases of vascular parapharyngeal lesions (Figure 21-8). Conventional angiography and a balloon-occlusion study with xenon flow and the clinical observation of the patient's neurologic status should be performed. The results of these studies help determine whether the carotid artery can be resected with minimal morbidity. The embolization of lesions preoperatively is done for vascular lesions that extend intracranially. It is most important that the surgeon have a plan in place preoperatively to deal with vascular injury. The management of carotid injury is discussed more in depth elsewhere in this text. Attempts are always made to maintain or restore flow in the carotid artery. It is possible to isolate the internal carotid artery

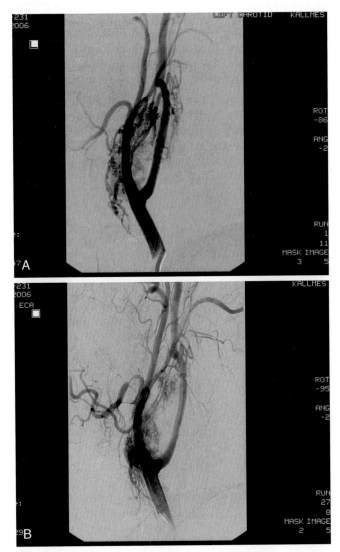

Figure 21-8. Angiogram of a patient with a left carotid body tumor. Note the characteristic splaying of the internal and external carotid arteries. **A,** The tumor before embolization. **B,** The same tumor after embolization and before removal.

proximally and distally to the level of the skull base through the cervical approaches; if artery control above the skull base is necessary, a partial petrous bone resection and a middle fossa craniotomy must be performed.

COMPROMISED AIRWAY

A large parapharyngeal tumor may impinge on the oral airway by displacing the pharyngeal wall medially (Figure 21-9). In this case, an initial tracheotomy may be required. After the cervical–parotid approach, unrecognized bleeding with subsequent hematoma can compromise the airway. An emergency tracheotomy may be necessary. Meticulous attention to hemostasis before closure with adequate wound irrigation and inspection is essential. Suction drainage is recommended for all cases of parapharyngeal tumor removal to prevent complications of airway compromise. Portable suction can be used to maintain constant negative pressure on the drains even when the patient is ambulant.

With the midline mandibulotomy approach, an initial tracheotomy is performed as a result of anticipated postoperative airway swelling. A cuffed tracheostomy tube is inserted initially, and, after several days, it is changed to a smaller cuffless tube, which remains in place for 3 to 5 days or until the edema subsides sufficiently to allow the tube to be safely plugged. When the cuffless tube can be plugged continuously for 24 hours, it is removed if the patient shows no signs of aspiration or wound complications and if he or she is swallowing well.

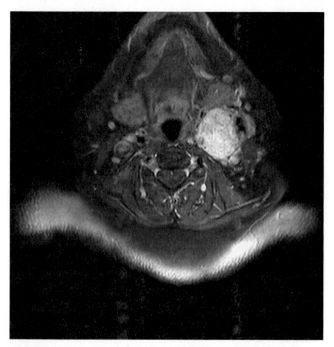

Figure 21-9. Magnetic resonance image of a patient with a left glomus vagale tumor. Note the displacement of the adjacent vascular structures laterally.

MANDIBULAR OSTEOTOMY COMPLICATIONS

The mandible can be divided in many areas for exposure of the parapharyngeal space. Midline mandibular osteotomy allows for excellent access to the superior parapharyngeal space and for the preservation of the inferior alveolar nerve. If, during a cervical approach, mandibular osteotomy is necessary, the mandible can be divided in a favorable direction and then plated after tumor removal. However, this approach is rarely necessary.

With the midline mandibular osteotomy approach, it is possible to preserve the lower incisors (provided that the patient is not edentulous). If the teeth are not too close together, the osteotomy site can be placed between the incisor teeth, and the teeth can be preserved. The osteotomy site is outlined after exposure of the underlying bone, and the mandible is divided with a saw in a stairstep manner. The final superior cut is made between the teeth with an osteotomy. If the incisor teeth are too close together, one tooth is removed, and the extraction site is used for the osteotomy. With the mandibular swing approach, the submandibular duct must be preserved with the mandible to prevent chronic obstructive symptoms of the submandibular gland. The lingual and hypoglossal nerves should also be identified and preserved.

Many osteotomy complications can occur, including the loss of incisor teeth, malunion, and nonunion. A panoramic radiograph should be taken preoperatively if there is concern about periapical disease.[11] There are several ways to reconstruct the mandible to avoid nonunion and malunion. Two reconstruction plates or a single compression plate can be placed along the lower border. A lingual splint can be fashioned and fixated to the mandible to improve stabilization. Before mandible fixation, a drill is used to remove irregular bone edges so that reapproximation can be tight and secure. Intermaxillary fixation is not necessary if fixation is stable. The mucosa is meticulously approximated around the osteotomy site to avoid exposed bone, and patients are tube fed for 2 weeks.

CATECHOLAMINE-SECRETING TUMORS

All patients with parapharyngeal space paragangliomas should be screened for possible catecholamine production. Glomus jugulare tumors, carotid body tumors, and vagal paragangliomas all can secrete catecholamines.

Historic points that may indicate catecholamine production include labile hypertension, headaches, tremulousness, or diaphoresis. Routine preoperative quantitative 24-hour urine studies should be done to determine levels of vanillylmandelic acid, metanephrine, dopamine, epinephrine, and norepinephrine. Serum catecholamine levels can also be analyzed. Although vagal paraganglioma catecholamine-secreting tumors are rare, they have been reported.

If a secreting tumor is found, preoperative blockade with propranolol and phenoxybenzamine can prevent intraoperative arrhythmias and hypertensive crisis. Failure to discover a secreting tumor preoperatively can have dire consequences during the surgical removal of the tumor.

PAROTID GLAND PROBLEMS

With the removal of parapharyngeal tumors, the lower portion of the parotid gland is often mobilized. For deep-lobe parotid tumors, a total parotidectomy may be done. Therefore many parapharyngeal surgical complications are similar to those of parotid gland operations. Soft-tissue depression at the angle of the mandible as a result of the removal of the gland, numbness from the division of the greater auricular nerve, and gustatory sweating (Frey syndrome) are common. A salivary fistula is rare; it is usually controlled with pressure and drainage.

Mobilization of the lower portion of the parotid gland commonly causes "first-bite pain." Patients describe sudden, severe pain in the parotid region after the ingestion of certain foods, but the pain subsides after the initial episode. This type of pain also occurs after neck dissection when the inferior portion of the parotid gland is removed. Patients are instructed to continue to chew through the pain and to chew gum for physiotherapy. The pain usually subsides within several weeks of the operation.

CEREBROSPINAL FLUID LEAK

CSF leakage through the wound or via the Eustachian tube are possible after the removal of parapharyngeal tumors that extend to the jugular foramen, that extend intracranially, or that cause the destruction of the cervical vertebrae. CSF leakage is most likely to occur after the removal of tumors that extend intracranially, and patients may also develop meningitis. In a report of neuromas removed from the jugular foramen region, there was a 40% incidence of CSF leakage postoperatively.[12] One group reported decreasing this rate to 4% for similar tumors by employing a three-layer closure with watertight dural closure, fibrin glue, and reinforcement with vascularized temporalis muscle.[13] For tumors that extend intracranially, after tumor removal, the watertight closure of the dura is performed with magnification. If a dural defect exists, a fascia lata graft is harvested and sewn to the dural edges. Fibrin glue, muscle, or fat can be used to reinforce a tenuous closure. For severe defects, a vascularized rotation or a microvascular graft can be employed. Lumbar drainage is used for several days if there is a high risk of leakage of CSF.

If a parapharyngeal tumor causes cervical bone destruction, tumor involvement of the spinal cord dura mater is possible. Collaboration with a neurosurgeon should be undertaken in all of these cases.

INFECTION

The removal of large parapharyngeal tumors by the cervical–parotid approach leaves a significant dead space that is prone to seroma formation and infection. A broad-spectrum antibiotic regimen is employed for several days postoperatively until the drains are removed. It is essential to maintain constant suction drainage to collapse the cavity that is left by the tumor to prevent the formation of a seroma or hematoma.

With the mandibular swing approach, the addition of metronidazole to a cephalosporin is used for prophylaxis. Antibiotics are continued for 7 days postoperatively.

QUALITY OF LIFE WITH PARAPHARYNGEAL TUMORS

The complexity and diversity of the surgical procedures performed in the parapharyngeal space can also cause complications that are common to all operations. These include thrombophlebitis, pulmonary embolism, stroke, myocardial infarction, and death. Postoperative fever as a result of atelectasis or aspiration is common, especially with the mandibular midline osteotomy approach. This approach also causes prolonged facial edema, which, if not discussed preoperatively, can be alarming to patients. Difficulty with deglutition also occurs until swelling resolves.

It is extremely rare for a patient to die as a result of an untreated benign parapharyngeal tumor.[14] The vast majority of these tumors are benign. Parapharyngeal tumors may be discovered during a routine physical examination or after an imaging study without the patient's knowledge of a problem. Neurogenic parapharyngeal tumors can be present for years without causing any deficits. Gradual paralysis is often less debilitating than a sudden loss of nerve function at the time of the operation. It is important during patient selection to weigh the potential risks of the operation against the risks of inaction. For elderly patients, observation with serial examination, imaging, or both may be preferable to tumor removal. This is particularly relevant if the tumor is likely neurogenic and demonstrates minimal growth over time.

For young patients, nerve tumors are normally removed to prevent the loss of multiple nerves in the future. Parapharyngeal vagal paragangliomas can extend intracranially and cause significant morbidity. For these patients, careful removal preceded by appropriate preoperative evaluation and imaging to determine the extent of the tumor is preferable to observation. However, surgery may not be without some expected morbidity. Patients should be appropriately counseled about the potential neurologic deficits that may result as well as the postoperative rehabilitation plan. Patients who are well informed about expected sequelae from nerve deficits will be better prepared to deal with them after the operation and less inclined to harbor resentment toward the surgeon about problems that they did not expect.

The timely institution of speech and swallowing rehabilitation can facilitate recovery among patients after the resection of neurogenic tumors. Laryngoplasty with injectable material or laryngeal framework medialization can improve dysphonia and aspiration in selected patients with vocal cord paralysis.[15] Unilateral palatal adhesion has been shown to improve velopharyngeal incompetence and speech in patients with glossopharyngeal nerve sacrifice.[16]

AVOIDANCE OF COMPLICATIONS

In general, patients with parapharyngeal tumors recover and achieve an excellent quality of life when they have outstanding preoperative, operative, and postoperative care. Accurate preoperative assessment is essential to avoid complications. Both computed tomography scanning and magnetic resonance imaging help determine the extent of the lesion and the possibility of intracranial extension, and they delineate vascular and nonvascular masses. The displacement of the carotid vessels (anteriorly by neurogenic tumors, posteriorly by salivary tumors) can give clues regarding the origin of the tumor. Angiography can define vascular tumors and provide information about carotid blood flow. Fine-needle aspiration can provide helpful information about

parapharyngeal tumors, and it can be performed safely. Cranial nerve monitoring can decrease the incidence of nerve injury in tumors that extend intracranially.

A well-prepared and experienced surgeon can expect to operate in the parapharyngeal space with minimal morbidity and excellent outcomes as long as complications are anticipated and appropriate steps for prevention are taken.

REFERENCES

1. Olsen KD: Tumors and surgery of the parapharyngeal space. *Laryngoscope* 1994;104:1–28.
2. Cohen SM, et al: Surgical management of parapharyngeal space masses. *Head Neck* 2005;27(8):669–675.
3. van Huijzen C: Anatomy of the skull base and the infratemporal fossa. *Adv Otorhinolaryngol* 1984;34:242–253.
4. Hughes KV, et al: Parapharyngeal space neoplasms. *Head Neck* 1995;17(2):124–130.
5. Malone JP, et al: Safety and efficacy of transcervical resection of parapharyngeal space neoplasms. *Ann Otol Rhinol Laryngol* 2001;110(12):1093–1098.
6. Baek CH, et al: New modification of the mandibulotomy approach without lip splitting. *Head Neck* 2006;28(7):580–586.
7. Carrau RL, et al: Management of tumors arising in the parapharyngeal space. *Laryngoscope* 1990;100:583–589.
8. Sobol SM, et al: Glossopharyngeal neuralgia-asystole syndrome secondary to parapharyngeal space lesions. *Otolaryngol Head Neck Surg* 1982;90:16–19.
9. Mikaelian DO, et al: Parapharyngeal schwannomas. *Otolaryngol Head Neck Surg* 1981;89:77–81.
10. Green JDJ, et al: Neoplasms of the vagus nerve. *Laryngoscope* 1988;98:648–654.
11. Cohen JI, et al: The mandibular swing stabilization of the midline mandibular osteotomy. *Laryngoscope* 1988;98:1139–1142.
12. Roland P, et al: Neuromas of the skull base. *Otolaryngol Head Neck Surg* 1986;94:539–547.
13. Ramina R, et al: Reconstruction of the cranial base in surgery for jugular foramen tumors. *Neurosurgery* 2005;56(2 Suppl):337–343.
14. Shahab R, et al: How we do it: A series of 114 primary pharyngeal space neoplasms. *Clin Otolaryngol* 2005;30:364–367.
15. Netterville J, et al: Rehabilitation of cranial nerve deficits after skull base surgery. *Laryngoscope* 1993;102:45–54.
16. Netterville JL, Vrabec JT: Palatal adhesions. *Arch Otolaryngol Head Neck Surg* 1994;120:218–221.

CHAPTER 22

Complications of Lip Surgery

Mark G. Shrime, David P. Goldstein, Jonathan C. Irish, and Patrick J. Gullane

Cancer of the lip accounts for approximately 30% of all oral cancers and affects approximately 1.8 per 100,000 people in the United States.[1] More than 90% of lip cancers are squamous cell carcinomas, with the vast majority occurring on the lower lip. Major causes include solar radiation exposure and tobacco abuse. Fortunately, the majority of patients present during the early stages of their disease, thereby allowing for less-complicated forms of surgical reconstruction.

Critical to successful lip surgery is the maintenance of near-normal anatomic and physiologic function. Complications arise when the maintenance of normal lip functional anatomy is compromised. Many factors play a role; these can be divided into patient-related factors (e.g., poor nutritional status, comorbidities, prior radiation therapy) and surgeon-related factors (e.g., in the planning or execution of the reconstruction). As a result, a thorough understanding of the anatomy, physiology, and function of the lips is essential.

ANATOMY AND PHYSIOLOGY

The embryologic development of the upper lip begins at about 6 to 7 weeks of gestation, when the medial nasal prominences merge with each other and with a contribution from the frontonasal prominence. These structures merge to form an intermaxillary segment that ultimately gives rise to the philtrum of the upper lip, the middle portion of the upper jaw and its associated gingiva, and the primary palate. The lateral parts of the upper lip, the upper jaw, and the secondary palate develop at the same time from the maxillary prominences. The lower lip is formed by the end of the fifth week of gestation as the mandibular prominences of the first branchial arch merge, giving rise to the lower jaw, the lower lip, and the lower part of the face. In contrast with the embryologic development of the upper lip, there is no intervening mesenchymal segment during lower-lip formation. The presence of a midline soft-tissue structure (the philtrum) in the upper lip creates an esthetic symmetry that must be recreated during any planned lip reconstructive procedures. It may also form an embryologic barrier to contralateral lymphatic drainage and consequent regional metastases.

Anatomically the lips are formed from muscular folds of the orbicularis oris muscle that surround the mouth, and they are covered externally by skin and internally by mucous membrane. The primary function of the orbicularis oris is to produce direct lip closure. The muscle has three main fiber types: the superficial fibers produce protrusion, approximation, and pursing of the lips, whereas the deep and oblique fibers join the risorius and buccinator muscles and are responsible for closely applying the lips against the maxillary and mandibular alveolar ridges. This lip–alveolus approximation is imperative for the clearance of food and saliva from the gingivobuccal sulcus.

As mentioned, the orbicularis oris muscle interdigitates with the muscles of facial expression on its deep surface. The levator labii superioris is the major elevator of the upper lip, whereas the zygomaticus major draws the angle of the mouth upward and backward. Retraction of the lip is performed by the risorius; the major lip depressors include the depressor labii inferioris, the depressor anguli oris, and the platysma muscle. Karapandzic flap and Gillies fan flap reconstruction of the lip require myotomy of the interdigitations of these facial muscles; this myotomy may adversely affect postoperative lip function. In addition, motor function of the lip is supplied by the buccal and mandibular branches of the facial nerve; sensory innervation is distributed through the maxillary and mandibular divisions of the trigeminal nerve. Denervation of the lip after attempted reconstruction is another important etiologic factor in postoperative lip dysfunction.

Knowledge of the vascular anatomy of the lip is imperative for the surgeon when planning Karapandzic flap, Gillies fan flap, or Abbé–Estlander flap reconstructions of the lip. The lips are supplied by the paired facial arteries, which are branches of the external carotid artery system. The superior and inferior labial artery branches course within the substance of the orbicularis oris muscle approximately 6 mm from the vermilion surface. The labial arteries are the major contributors to the vascular arcade around the oral cavity stoma, with minor contributions from the terminal branches of the mental artery, the infraorbital artery, the sphenopalatine artery, and the septal branches of the ethmoidal artery. It should be noted that previous flap reconstruction may temporarily reduce the continuity of the perioral vascular arcade and that a hiatus of at least 3 months is therefore recommended before any surgical revision should be considered.

Normal lip function and oral sphincter competence are essential for deglutition. Lip pliability and normal muscle function are required for the entry of food and liquid into the upper digestive system and for the production of normal speech. The lip also plays a clear role in the portrayal of emotion through facial animation.

COMPLICATIONS OF LIP SURGERY

Since the first mention of lip reconstruction by Celsius in 60 AD, myriad lip reconstruction techniques have been described. Complications resulting from the surgical reconstruction of the lip are the result of a failure to adhere to several important principles during preoperative planning, of a failure of technique during the operative procedure itself, or of a failure to follow several critical aspects of postoperative care. Complications of lip surgery that arise during the operative procedure itself are of two different broad types: those that are specific to the type of flap chosen for reconstruction and those that are not.

Although the reported incidence of local postoperative complications after lip reconstruction is low, oral dysfunction and poor esthetic appearance are difficult to quantify, and they are rarely included in most series that analyze the results of lip reconstruction. More important than the surgeon's ability to recognize and treat complications of the lip is the ability to prevent them in the first place.

Preoperative Considerations

The primary goal of surgery for cancer of the lip is disease eradication. Reconstruction is obviously a secondary consideration, but this in no way diminishes its import. The maintenance of oral-sphincter competence and the restoration of a cosmetically acceptable lip appearance must be addressed by the reconstructive surgeon. The ideal procedure will leave a patient cancer-free while producing normal-looking lip architecture with adequate stoma size, a good sulcus, a natural-appearing vermilion border, some sensory function, good muscle tone, an acceptable color match with the surrounding tissues, and maintained lip functions (i.e., the admission of food, mastication without drooling, the performance labial consonant articulation).

Meticulous preoperative planning is an essential step in the prevention of postoperative surgical complications. The planned use of the simplest reconstructive flap after adequate oncologic resection will optimize the final esthetic and functional results. The preferred tissues for lip reconstruction are as follows, in order of preference: the remaining portions of the resected lip, the opposite lip, the adjacent cheek, and, as a last resort, distant flaps.[2] The surgeon should favor single-stage reconstruction rather than multistage procedures. The motor and anatomic rehabilitation of the resected lip where flap reconstruction is necessary is best if full-thickness flaps of skin, muscle, and mucosa are used. If oncologically feasible, the surgeon should avoid extending the resection to the lateral commissure, because reconstruction of this lip site is difficult, and postoperative function is unsatisfactory.

As previously mentioned, complications in lip surgery may be the result of both surgeon-related and patient-related factors. The latter are extremely important, and the final outcome of lip reconstruction is often determined by the following:

- The size of the lip defect to be reconstructed
- The age, sex, and nutritional status of the patient
- The previous exposure of the site to radiation therapy
- Other comorbidities that can interfere with wound healing

Of these factors, the complication rate of lip surgery is most heavily dependent on the extent of surgical resection required and, therefore, on the size of the lesion to be resected. As a result, complications of lip surgery are generally low after surgery for T1 and T2 neoplasms. Care must be taken in all cases to adhere to careful reconstructive principles.

Nutritional deficiency in head and neck cancer may predispose patients to an increased incidence of postoperative complications. Nutritional deficiency in this population group may occur as a direct result of the presence of tumor, as a side effect of treatment, or as a consequence of associated systemic disease. The incidence of malnourishment is higher among patients with larger tumors. These patients may require more radical operative procedures, and, therefore, they may be more prone to postoperative complications.[3] The preoperative optimization of nitrogen balance and nutritional status will inevitably reduce postoperative complication rates related to infection and poor wound healing.[4]

Myriad causes of immunodeficiency can adversely influence healing after lip reconstructions. Both major causes of immunodeficiency (e.g., human immunodeficiency virus infection,[5,6] certain immunosuppressive drugs[7]) and less well-defined causes (e.g., diabetes mellitus[8]) have been associated with poor wound healing. The minimization of these immunosuppressive triggers with strict postoperative glycemic control, the reduction of immunosuppression (as much as possible), and the treatment of human immunodeficiency virus infection can improve wound healing. In addition, the issue of tobacco in wound healing merits discussion. Although the majority of lip cancers are thought to be related to exposure to sunlight, there is some correlation between carcinomas of the lip and tobacco use. Perioperative smoking significantly increases the patient's risk of cardiopulmonary complications, infections, and impaired wound healing.[9] The cessation of smoking for 4 weeks preoperatively may obviate these complications, but even former smokers may still suffer increased reconstructive complications.[10]

Intraoperative Considerations

Flap-Related Considerations

Surgical resections of the lip can cover a range from the precancerous or in situ carcinoma requiring a vermilionectomy to medium lip defects (less than one third of the lower lip or one fourth of the upper lip) to large lip defects (up to two thirds of upper or lower lip) to total lip defects requiring a free flap reconstruction. Each type of defect requires different reconstructive strategies and carries its own set of postoperative morbidities and complications. Although this chapter focuses on reconstruction after the resection of primary tumors of the lip, the principles outlined here apply to all surgery of the lip, including the incisions used for access to the oral cavity and the oropharynx.

Vermilionectomy or "lip shave" is indicated for the treatment of premalignant lesions of the lip and for carcinoma in situ. Some authors advocate the procedure as an adjunct during any resection of the lip for carcinoma as a result of the fact that about 7% of patients will develop a subsequent lip cancer and because approximately 5% of patients have multicentric disease at the time of their first procedure.[11] With this procedure, the red margin of the lip is resected with a variable amount of underlying muscle, depending on the depth of the extension of the lesion. The red lip margin is then reconstituted with the advancement of oral mucosa. The major postoperative shortfalls after this procedure are related to cosmetic appearance and include entropion and an overly red appearance of the lip that differs from the opposite lip. Entropion may result as the reconstructed lip is pulled inward, thereby causing a loss of natural lip fullness. In addition, if a substantial amount of underlying muscle is also resected, there can be a significant loss of lip convexity. The end result can be an unnaturally thin lip. Occasionally, depending on the advancement techniques used, hairs on the margin of the newly reconstructed lip can be a source of irritation. Designing a posteriorly based advancement flap of buccal and labial mucosa can prevent these cosmetic defects; further advancement may be obtained with the use of intraoral lateral-releasing incisions. Functional defects of the lip are rare after vermilionectomies.

Lesions that result in medium-sized defects of the lip (up to one third of the lower lip and up to one fourth of the upper lip) can usually be managed with a wedge or shield type of excision with primary closure. With larger lesions (especially along the lower lip), a W-plasty approach may be beneficial, because a shield or V-excision can lead to the loss of lower-lip projection. As previously implied, the incidence and severity of postoperative dysfunction as well as poor esthetic results increase with the extent of the primary resection required. The narrowing of the oral stoma can become clinically apparent (Figure 22-1).

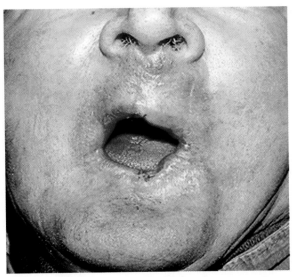

Figure 22-1. Microstomia after lower-lip reconstruction for a defect involving more than two thirds of the lower lip.

Microstomia is more than simply a cosmetic issue; it can also result in significant functional disturbance, interfering with oral competence, articulation, and even the ability of the patient to insert dental appliances. Microstomia as a result of properly chosen wedge resections of the lip, however, rarely results in a functional deficit, especially if close attention is paid intraoperatively to the reapposition of the orbicularis oris myotomy.

The upper lip is less amenable to V-excision and primary repair. Esthetically, the loss of the normal overhang of the upper lip on the lower lip becomes apparent, and even small excisions near the midline of the upper lip can cause especially obvious deformities because of the presence of the philtrum. In addition, compensatory movement of the remaining lip is limited as a result of the anchoring of soft tissue around the maxilla. Multiple procedures have been proposed for the reconstruction of the upper lip, including V-Y advancement flaps,[12] island pedicled flaps,[13] and other local flaps.[14-16] Because the number of upper lip cancers is small, these techniques are often reported in very small series.

Large defects of the lip involve less than two thirds of the upper or lower lip. Reconstruction of large lip defects are, in general, limited to the following three broad categories:

1. Those that involve lip-switch flaps (e.g., Abbé flaps, Estlander flaps)

2. Those that involve the rotation of tissue around the lip (e.g., Gillies fan flaps, Karapandzic flaps)

3. Those that involve sliding horizontal cheek flaps (e.g., Burrows flaps, Bernard flaps, Johanson flaps).

Barring the Karapandzic technique, all reconstructive modalities for large lip defects require the denervation of a segment of the lip, which may impair ultimate lip function. It is apparent (and well demonstrated by electromyogram studies) that muscle function and innervation of the rotated lip segment do recover. The reinnervation process may take several months, and full dynamic function of the reconstituted lip may not be realized for up to 1 year. Reconstructive modalities that involve the use of nonmuscularized adynamic tissue to replace resected muscularized dynamic lip, however, always carry a risk that the patient is never afforded true dynamic mobility of that segment of the lip. Patients who fail to develop reinnervation of the lip-switch or rotation flaps are particularly prone to oral incompetence, drooling, poor speech articulation, and oral dysphagia.

For larger lesions, lip-switch reconstructions are often employed. However, significant microstomia may result. The reconstructive surgeon must be cognizant of the fact that the incision on the pedicled side of a lip-switch flap can only be brought to within 6 mm of the vermilion border to preserve the labial artery. Lip-switch flaps from the lower to the upper lip are often functionally and esthetically less successful because of the requirement to maintain the symmetry of the Cupid's bow and its midline relationship to the nose. As a result, midline defects of the upper lip are significantly more prone to postoperative cosmetic deformity (Figure 22-2).

The major rotation flaps (e.g., Karapandzic flap, Gillies fan flap) involve the rotation of tissue around the lip and require the repositioning of the lip commissure into the upper or lower lip. The resultant rounded appearance is esthetically displeasing (Figure 22-3). In addition, the lip's role in the maintenance of oral competence and articulation is often lost. The effacement of the normal lip commissure often necessitates secondary procedures for its

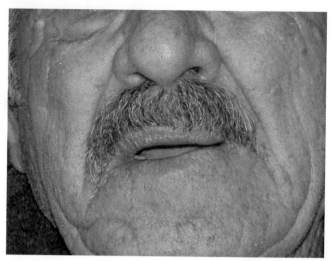

Figure 22-3. Blunting of the right oral commissure after reconstruction of a lower-lip defect with an Estlander flap.

recreation. As with all lip reconstructions, the preservation of the vascular arcade and the pedicle during the flap elevation is critical. If the preservation of the neurovascular bundle is accomplished, the Karapandzic flap offers the advantage over other rotational flaps of an innervated, vascularized, and competent oral sphincter. When the Karapandzic flap is used for defects of more than 75% of the length of the lip, however, the resultant oral microstomia causes serious functional limitations.

The sliding horizontal cheek flaps of Bernard and Burrow tend to defunctionalize the lower lip, because they replace dynamic tissue with adynamic adjacent tissue. The Meyers modification of the Bernard flap, in which the orbicularis oris is not sectioned, can result in improved postoperative function. The Johanson flap, which is another sliding flap, has the distinct advantage of preserving the oral commissure and the attachments of the buccinator, the zygomaticus, the risorius, and the depressor attachments to the orbicularis oris. The disadvantage of this flap is the loss of sensation and the slight microstomia that can result. Despite these limitations, however, the functional and aesthetic quality of reconstructions obtained from these sliding flaps is often superior to that obtained with the use of distant flaps. In addition, because the upper lip is not as functionally dynamic as the lower lip, the use of nonmuscular sliding flaps (e.g., the cheek-based nasolabial flap) in its reconstruction poses less of a problem.

Total lip defects, including maxillary involvement in upper-lip carcinoma and mandibular involvement in lower-lip tumors, may require the use of regional or free flap reconstruction. Total lower-lip defects may either be restored with bilateral inferiorly based nasolabial flaps or with free-tissue transfer. Limitations include the lack of a red lip margin, a central lip depression, and the lack of dynamic tone (Figure 22-4). Free flap reconstruction

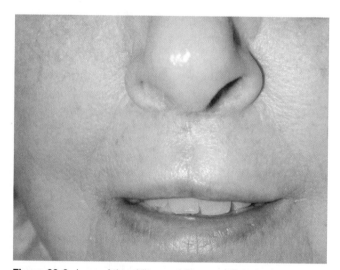

Figure 22-2. Loss of the philtrum of the upper lip after resection of the middle third of the lip.

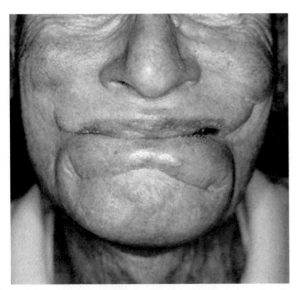

Figure 22-4. Absence of the vermilion border after reconstruction of a total lower-lip defect with bilateral nasolabial flaps.

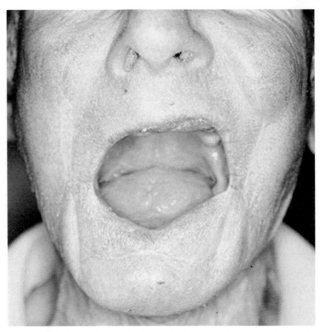

Figure 22-5. Notching and a loss of volume of the central lower lip after wedge resection.

offers the ability to use thin, pliable tissue for reconstruction; this benefit is not afforded by the regional flaps. Serious esthetic and functional complications from the use of free tissue, however, include poor color match, scarring, and the lack of kinetic activity, which results in speech impairment, oral incompetence, and trismus. The reconstruction of the underlying hard tissues is of utmost cosmetic importance. For example, inadequate tissue volume and a failure to reconstruct the anterior mandibular arch in lower-lip resections will result in an "Andy Gump" cosmetic deformity. The failure of the vascular pedicle in free flap reconstruction, although rare (<2%), can result in significant postoperative morbidity.

Non–Flap-Related Considerations

Attention to specific intraoperative details, regardless of the type of flap used, will significantly decrease postoperative patient morbidity. As previously mentioned, the surgeon's primary consideration is the complete surgical resection of the tumor. From a reconstructive standpoint, the surgeon must always consider the presence of residual or recurrent tumor as a cause of postoperative wound breakdown. During the reconstruction, the vermilion surface and its border with the skin and the internal surface of the lip must, whenever possible, be reconstituted or preserved. The three-layer closure of the mucosa, the orbicularis oris muscle, and the skin, with key suture placement in the vermilion border, is critical for good postoperative cosmesis. The failure to reappose the orbicularis oris muscle completely will result in a notch or "whistle" deformity (Figure 22-5) and possibly result in sphincter incompetence, with resulting drooling and lip malposition. The muscle and deep wound layers must absorb most of the wound tension. Reliance on the epidermal

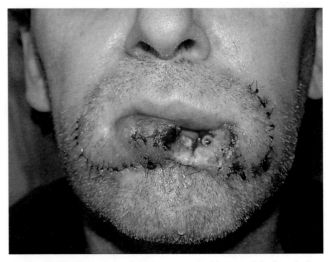

Figure 22-6. Necrosis and dehiscence of a Karapandzic flap during the early postoperative period.

suture for strength often gives rise to scar widening or wound breakdown, with the possibility of the development of wound infection (Figure 22-6). Postoperative wound dehiscence is best managed with local wound care and secondary closure at the earliest opportunity. For major reconstructions, wound breakdown can lead to bone exposure with resulting osteomyelitis, especially in the patient who has undergone radiation. Although myocutaneous flaps and free flaps have a high rate of survival, wound breakdown can occur as a result of poor recipient tissue viability, vascular insufficiency, or an inadequate watertight intraoral closure leading to salivary contamination.

Postoperative Considerations

Attentive postoperative care and early intervention at the first sign of complications are important aspects of the treatment of the patient with lip cancer. Perioperative antibiotics and good local wound care are essential to prevent local wound breakdown and infection.[17,18] Nutritional intake, smoking cessation, and the management of immunosuppression during the perioperative phase are important for good wound healing. For large lip defects, supplemental nasogastric tube feeding is often beneficial. A soft diet during the postoperative phase reduces wound tension and can prevent wound dehiscence. Because as many as 14% of patients with primary resections of lip carcinomas experience a recurrence within the remaining lip, careful follow up is essential, and readiness for a salvage surgical procedure for recurrent or residual disease is vital.[19]

REFERENCES

1. Baker SR: Risk factors in multiple carcinomas of the lip. *Otolaryngol Head Neck Surg* 1980;88:248–251.
2. Gullane PJ, Martin GF: Minor and major lip reconstructions. *J Otolaryngol* 1983;12:75–82.
3. Flynn MB, Leightty FF: Preoperative outpatient nutritional support of patients with squamous cancer of the upper aerodigestive tract. *Am J Surg* 1987;154:359–362.
4. Arnold M, Barbul A: Nutrition and wound healing. *Plast Reconstr Surg* 2006;117:42S–58S.
5. Eriguchi M, Takeda Y, Yoshizaki I, et al: Surgery in patients with HIV infection: Indications and outcome. *Biomed Pharmacother* 1997;51:474–479.
6. Morandi E, Merlini D, Salvaggio A, et al: Prospective study of healing time after hemorrhoidectomy: Influence of HIV infection, acquired immunodeficiency syndrome, and anal wound infection. *Dis Colon Rectum* 1999;42:1140–1144.
7. Dean PG, Lund WJ, Larson TS, et al: Wound-healing complications after kidney transplantation: A prospective, randomized comparison of sirolimus and tacrolimus. *Transplantation* 2004;77:1555–1561.
8. Hoogwerf BJ: Postoperative management of the diabetic patient. *Med Clin North Am* 2001;85:1213–1228.
9. Moller A, Tonneson H: Risk reduction: Perioperative smoking intervention. *Best Pract Res Clin Anaesthesiol* 2006;20:237–248.
10. Spear SL, Ducic I, Cuoco F, et al: The effect of smoking on flap and donor-site complications in pedicled TRAM breast reconstruction. *Plast Reconstr Surg* 2005;116:1873–1880.
11. Baker SR, Krause CJ: Carcinoma of the lip. *Laryngoscope* 1980;90:19–27.
12. Carvalho LM, Ramos RR, Santos ID, et al: V-Y advancement flap for the reconstruction of partial and full thickness defects of the upper lip. *Scand J Plast Reconstr Surg Hand Surg* 2002;36:28–33.
13. Kaufman AJ, Grekin RC: Repair of central upper lip (philtral) surgical defects with island pedicle flaps. *Dermatol Surg* 1996;22:1003–1007.
14. Włodarkiewicz A, Wojszwiłło-Geppert E, Placek W, Roszkiewicz J: Upper lip reconstruction with local island flap after neoplasm excision. *Dermatol Surg* 1997;23:1075–1079.
15. Ergun SS: Reconstruction of the labiomental region with local flaps. *Dermatol Surg* 2002;28:863–865.
16. Sarifakioglu N, Aslan G, Terzloglu A, et al: New technique of one-stage reconstruction of a large full-thickness defect in the upper lip: Bilateral reverse composite nasolabial flap. *Ann Plast Surg* 2002;49:207–210.
17. Johnson JT, Myers EN, Thearle PB, et al: Antimicrobial prophylaxis for contaminated head and neck surgery. *Laryngoscope* 1984;94:46–51.
18. Johnson JT, Yu VL: Antibiotic use during major head and neck surgery. *Ann Surg* 1988;207:108–111.
19. Palleta FX, Coldwater K, Booth F: Treatment of leukoplakia and carcinoma in situ of the lower lip. *Ann Surg* 1957;145:74–80.

CHAPTER 23

Complications of Surgery of the Oral Cavity

Jay O. Boyle and Vincent Reid

Squamous cell carcinoma of the oral cavity is caused by exposure to tobacco and alcohol and, in some patients, infection with human papilloma virus.[1] The disease occurs most commonly during the sixth, seventh, and eighth decades of life. The age and the lifestyle habits of patients with oral cancer contribute to significant comorbidities that predispose these patients to surgical complications.[2] Although oral cancer accounts for only 3% of new cancer cases in the United States, one third of all head and neck cancers occur in the oral cavity, where surgically based therapy is favored.[3] This is in contrast with cancers of the pharynx and larynx, where radiation-based therapies are frequently used because of a favorable balance of oncologic control and treatment morbidity. Consequently, most patients with oral cancer will require surgery to minimize the incidence and manage the occurrence of complications.

The oral cavity is a critically important organ for speech, mastication, deglutition, facial expression, and aesthetics. Complications of oral cavity surgery cause significant morbidity and decrease the patient's quality of life (QOL). This chapter focuses on complications of surgery for oral cancer. The discussion includes complications related to the mandible, the maxilla, and the soft tissues of the oral cavity.

When considering the adverse effects of surgery, a distinction between sequelae and complications must be made. However, the boundary is indistinct for many postsurgical events. In general, complications are unexpected outcomes after oral surgery that are distinct from the expected, planned sequelae of the surgical manipulation of the oral tissues. It is critical to understand that the prevention of complications through careful operative technique and excellent planning is much preferred to managing complications. This chapter includes strategies for preventing common complications as well as diagnostic and management strategies.

Some of the most important complications of oral cancer surgery involve complications of surgery on the mandible. Three common mandibular surgeries are the mandibulotomy for access to the posterior oral cavity, the pharynx, or the infratemporal fossa; the marginal mandibulectomy for tumors that abut the alveolar ridge; and the segmental resection for gross bone involvement of the mandible.

COMPLICATIONS OF MANDIBULOTOMY

When to Perform a Mandibulotomy

Mandibulotomy is an excellent approach to the posterior oral cavity, the pharynx, and the infratemporal fossa. This approach should be selected whenever tumors in this region cannot be adequately viewed and when tumors can be safely removed en bloc through the open mouth. Examples include T2 through T4 tumors of the far posterior lateral tongue and of floor of the mouth, especially those with tonsillar pillar involvement. In the oropharynx, cancer and even early tumors can rarely be completely removed en bloc with a cuff of normal tissue through the open mouth. Mandibulotomy is rarely necessary for large benign tumors of the deep lobe of the parotid, but it is often necessary for malignant tumors. To avoid healing complications and fractures, avoid performing mandibulotomy when marginal mandibulectomy is also needed.[4] The healing of the mandibulotomy site will be compromised in the irradiated mandible. Fortunately most mandibulotomies are median or paramedian, and often the dose of radiation to the oral cavity or the oropharynx is the least in the anterior mandibular arch.[5]

Precautions and Prevention of Possible Complications

Mandibulotomy sites may be irradiated postoperatively without undue risk of wound complications. Never perform a blind resection of cancer perorally when the tumor could be well visualized with mandibulotomy. For most cancer patients, the aesthetic and functional results are satisfactory; the adequate resection of the cancer is of paramount importance.

The rate of nonhealing of the osteotomy site and fibrous union is 7%.[6] It is caused principally by the instability of the repaired osteotomy, which is attributable to poor fixation and sometimes to infection.

Poor fixation can be a result of the geometry of the mandibulotomy or inappropriate fixation. Fixation can be performed equally well with wires or miniplates, but most surgeons prefer the precision of plating osteotomies.[7]

Instability can result from too few plates or screws or their inappropriate placement. In general, miniplates work well to provide three-dimensional fixation. At least two screws are required on each side of the osteotomy in each plate, and at least two miniplates are necessary to secure the osteotomy site in three dimensions. One miniplate is placed on the buccal surface of the mandible, and one is placed on the inferior surface. Technical aspects of placing the plates and screws are critical to the stability of the repair. Plates must be carefully bent to match the contour of the bone. Guide holes for the screws must be drilled to the proper depth and with the appropriate diameter drill bit. Screws must be tight, but they must not be stripped. If the screw hole is stripped during insertion then a "safety screw," which is slightly larger in diameter, is necessary. Compression plates are reported to improve stability and healing, but they are bulkier, they may be palpable, and they are slightly more difficult to apply accurately.[8] As a result of a small amount of bone loss from the osteotomy, the author prefers to place the screw holes after the osteotomy to maximize the stability of the repair; however, some surgeons prefer the precise realignment of the occlusion that may be augmented by placing the screw holes before osteotomy. Irradiation may increase the risk of nonunion, but this is debated in the literature.[9]

Proper Orientation and Geometry of the Osteotomy Site

Proper orientation and geometry of the osteotomy site will help to prevent nonunion complications by ensuring both the alignment and the stability of the osteotomy. Usually access to the pharynx and the posterior oral cavity is best achieved just lateral to the midline, so it is convenient to perform the osteotomy between the canine and the lateral incisor[10] (Figure 23-1).

This osteotomy site (see Figure 23-1) provides an advantage in that the tooth roots are moving away from each other as they travel caudally, thus reducing the chance of root injury and tooth loss.[11] Midline access may be best achieved through midline osteotomy between the central incisors, but the loss of one or both of the incisors may occur as a result of root injury or the loss of supporting bone at the osteotomy site. Using a thin saw blade and a straight cut reduces the chances of this complication. The bone cut should be performed carefully with copious irrigation to prevent heat from saw friction from destroying the nearby osteocytes that are necessary for bone formation and healing.

Stepped Osteotomy

Performing a stepped osteotomy in which the forces of mastication drive the osteotomy together (favorable orientation) can improve the alignment and stability of the repair. The author prefers a single-angle step anteriorly at a 45-degree angle (see Figure 23-1). This provides a favorable orientation, and, as compared with a square-notched osteotomy, it is less likely to damage the tooth roots, it is easier to perform, and it is less likely to fracture.

Osteomyelitis or Irradiation

Nonhealing fibrous union is more common after osteomyelitis or irradiation. Good soft-tissue coverage is necessary to provide a watertight mucosal repair and to cover the hardware adequately, especially if postoperative irradiation is a possibility.[12,13]

Exposed Hardware

If there is exposed hardware intraorally or externally, the wound will not heal, and osteomyelitis, screw loosening, plate extrusion, and nonunion are likely (Figure 23-2). If there is inadequate soft-tissue coverage for the hardware, then a local, regional, or free flap should be considered to ensure healing. If the hardware becomes exposed intraorally or externally, all hardware from the osteotomy should be removed. If the bone is not healed, then external fixation, splints, or intermaxillary fixation (IMF) may be necessary. Exposed intraoral hardware will often lead eventually to orocutaneous fistula.

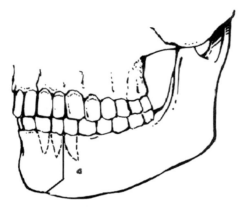

Figure 23-1. Bony cuts for paramedian mandibulotomy between the lateral incisor and the canine with a 45-degree step in the favorable orientation for forces of mastication.

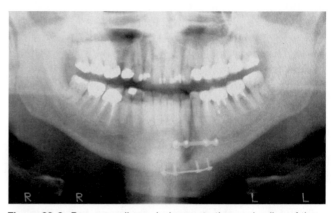

Figure 23-2. Panorex radiograph demonstrating nonhealing of the mandibulotomy site with loose screws and plates.

Intermaxillary Fixation

IMF with arch bars or Ivey loops and bands or wires will improve the chances of the osteotomy healing and the normalization of occlusion, especially if there are concomitant fractures, previous radiation, suboptimal soft-tissue healing, or other risks of poor healing. Dental splints may be useful to restore occlusion and orientation in complex cases; they are prepared preoperatively. If all conditions are favorable, IMF is not mandatory after mandibulotomy reconstruction.

Care After Osteotomy

Mandibulotomy patients require a pureed diet for 4 to 6 weeks after osteotomy to prevent the forces of mastication from disrupting the rigid fixation. For about 3 weeks, saline irrigation or antiseptic mouthwash should be prescribed four to five times daily until the mucosal wound is healed. A panorex radiograph at 8 weeks can help identify plate, screw, healing, or alignment problems. Pain, infection, exposed hardware, malocclusion, changes in occlusion, and instability of the osteotomy site suggest nonunion.

Lingual Nerve Injury

Lingual nerve injury can occur with mandibulotomy as a result of its anatomic location spanning the space between the lingual aspect of the ascending ramus of the mandible and the tongue musculature posteriorly. Because many patients who require mandibulotomy for cancer also require neck dissection, it can be useful to perform the neck dissection first and to tag the lingual nerve with a vessel loop for its careful preservation during dissection of the floor of the mouth later. A few patients may develop burning paresthesia of the tongue after the repair of the floor of the mouth as a result of lingual nerve injury. The nerve is wrapped around the Warthin duct of the submandibular gland in the floor of the mouth, and it can be injured with sutures when the defect is being closed. This paresthesia is permanent and should be avoided.

Mental Nerve Injury

The partial lower cheek flap and the midline lip-splitting incision are generally necessary for mandibulotomy, but the mental nerve can be preserved. Mental nerve injury causes permanent numbness of the lower lip and chin and contributes to drooling problems that are disturbing to patients. If the nerve is transected accidentally, it should be repaired primarily. The lip-splitting incision should be directly in the midline and straight down through the chin pad to best preserve symmetry. Complex incisions or incising around the chin pad do not improve the cosmetic or functional

results. Great care is necessary to reapproximate the vermilion border in younger patients, because even minimal offset is noticeable. It is advisable to create thin hash marks on the skin before incision to ensure good landmarks for accurate reconstruction at the closure. It is critical to close the orbicularis oris muscle layer as a separate layer. If there is dehiscence of this layer, the complication appears as a subcutaneous space where the muscle is absent in the midline, and oral competence may be compromised in some patients. It is sometimes possible to perform mandibulotomy without the lip-splitting incision through a visor-type approach. Only in some patients with a favorable orientation of tumor and a large mouth can adequate access to the tumor be accomplished without lip splitting.[14]

Marginal Mandibular Nerve Injury

Marginal mandibular nerve injury can occur during the lower cheek-flap development. The author prefers to identify and preserve the nerve to facilitate its protection. Incising the submandibular fascia, ligating the facial vein, and retracting the nerve superiorly may also protect the nerve. The complication of marginal nerve injury causes the elevation of the ipsilateral lower lip with mouth opening or smiling. This is not only a cosmetic problem but also a functional problem as a result of lip biting. As with most nerve injuries, there is no effective therapy, and avoidance is critical.

COMPLICATIONS OF MARGINAL MANDIBULECTOMY

When to Perform a Marginal Mandibulectomy

Marginal mandibulectomy is necessary when the tumor abuts the mandible. If there is cortical invasion, then a segmental mandibulectomy is indicated. Marginal mandibulectomy is commonly performed for cancer of the floor of the mouth or buccal mucosa cancer that involves the gingiva.[15]

The procedure involves the en bloc resection of the tumor and of the alveolar ridge of the mandible with the soft-tissue tumor. The inferior border is preserved for adequate bone strength to allow for the forces of mastication. Several complications may occur.

Fracture

The most severe complication that can occur is subsequent fracture as a result of an inadequate amount of bone stock remaining on the inferior border. To avoid this complication, care and judgment must be exercised at the time of operation.

The long edentulous mandible will lose the entire alveolar ridge to resorption, and the remaining bone is likely to be too thin for safe marginal mandibulectomy. Similarly, previously irradiated bone offers much less resistance to penetration by cancer, heals poorly, and may not withstand the forces of mastication after marginal mandibulectomy as well as nonirradiated bone.[16] Therefore, one should avoid marginal mandibulectomy in the mandible that is both weakened by previous radiation and very thin as a result of the resorption of the alveolar ridge.

Reverse marginal mandibulectomy involves the partial-thickness resection of the inferior border of the mandible for advanced neck disease that abuts the lower border of the mandible. Because most of the bone strength comes from the lower border, its resection significantly weakens the bone. Segmental resection should be considered rather than extensive lower-border marginal mandibulectomy, especially in the edentulous bone.

Some surgeons advocate supporting the residual mandible after marginal mandibulectomy with a reconstruction plate. These heavy plates can be fashioned to fit the bony contour and fixed with screws. The advantage of added strength should be balanced with the potential problems of drilling screw holes in the mandible and the need for good soft-tissue coverage. If the reconstruction plate becomes exposed as a result of poor tissue coverage it will need to be removed, and this may cause added trauma to the already compromised mandible. Reconstruction plates are usually palpable and sometimes visible under the thin skin of older patients.

Injury of Inferior Alveolar Nerve and Artery in the Canal

During marginal mandibulectomy, the inferior alveolar nerve and artery can be injured in the canal. Especially posteriorly and medially, the canal is high in the bone and easy to enter during marginal mandibulectomy. Closer to the mental foramen, the canal is more inferiorly and anteriorly oriented within the mandible. To preserve sensation to the lip and the endosteal blood supply, it is useful to observe caution to preserve the canal and its nerve and artery. In general, sacrifice of the artery will not condemn the bone as long as the periosteal blood supply is largely intact.

Iatrogenic Fracture

Iatrogenic fracture during marginal mandibulectomy is common. A lack of care with the osteotome, poor bone quality, and overaggressive resection are the main causes. To prevent iatrogenic intraoperative fracture, the surgeon must ensure complete cortical excision with the

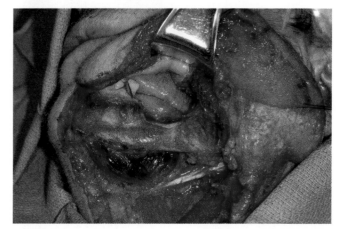

Figure 23-3. Marginal mandibulectomy demonstrating the smooth contours of the osteotomy.

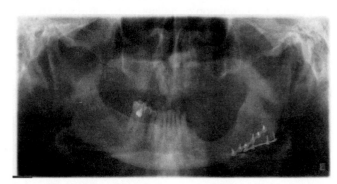

Figure 23-4. Marginal mandibulectomy with a fracture of the angle of the mandible plated and healed 8 weeks postoperatively.

sagittal saw or a small cutting burr, and he or she must rely on the osteotome only for completing the minimal residual bone adherences. If the osteotome is used in a prying fashion or with too much force (especially at the angle of the mandible), then fractures can occur. Making a smooth, curved resection rather than one with right angles will also reduce the risk of fracture (Figure 23-3). If intraoperative fracture occurs, it should be plated with miniplates (Figure 23-4). Excellent soft-tissue coverage should be ensured, and IMF should be considered. A liquid diet for 3 weeks and then a pureed diet for 3 weeks are prudent to ensure healing. Iatrogenic fractures are commonly in an unfavorable orientation with regard to the direction of the forces of mastication.

Loss of Adjacent Teeth

The loss of adjacent teeth months after marginal mandibulectomy may occur. This is typically the result of injury to the tooth root, not leaving enough bone around adjacent teeth, or prying on the teeth with osteotomies during surgery. To protect adjacent teeth, the osteotomy should be planned for the center of a tooth socket rather than between the sockets of intact teeth. A marginal resection that passes between sockets is likely to eventually cause a loss of the adjacent tooth, either from bone resorption or root damage.

COMPLICATIONS OF SEGMENTAL MANDIBULECTOMY

When to Perform a Segmental Mandibulectomy

Segmental mandibulectomy is indicated for the resection of tumors with gross bone invasion. The cancellous bone of the mandible offers no barrier to the progression of squamous cancer through the bone. Discontinuity of the mandible presents significant problems with occlusion, mastication, the position of the chin, oral competency, and pain. For these reasons, reconstruction of the jaw after segmental mandibulectomy is preferred. The most common and effective mandibular reconstruction is with free-tissue transfer, such as a fibular or scapular free flap. Reconstruction plates without bone grafts will invariably extrude if they span the anterior arch, but they may work well for small, lateral defects if they are covered by regional or free flaps. Free bone grafts of rib or iliac crest may suffice for some small, lateral defects when there is excellent soft tissue and no radiation, but they are much less reliable than free-tissue transfer. Trays filled with cancellous bone and distraction osteogenesis may be options for young patients with benign problems, but they work poorly for the cancer population. The choice of mandibular reconstruction is complex and beyond the scope of this chapter, but the following factors need to be considered:

- The portion of the mandible that is affected
- Previous or postoperative radiation
- The availability of reconstructive expertise
- Functional and aesthetic considerations

Obviously, many complications of segmental mandibulectomy revolve around reconstruction.

Soft-Tissue–Only Reconstructions

Older patients with lateral bony defects may be left with soft-tissue–only reconstructions if they are poor candidates for lengthy, free flap surgery; if they have poor vessels or are edentulous; or if they have extensive, soft-tissue reconstructive requirements. It is optimal in this situation to resect the entire ascending ramus of the mandible and to disarticulate the temporomandibular joint to prevent the pain associated with the subsequent medialization of the remnant mandible by the unopposed action of the lateral pterygoid muscle, which inserts near the condyle. If left unreconstructed, the chin position will drift toward the defect over time as a result of the unopposed action of the contralateral pterygoid muscles. Few patients will be able to chew solid food in this case. Sometimes a dental prosthesis, called a *guide plane,* can direct

the teeth back onto occlusion for mastication; however, most patients with unreconstructed lateral defects will achieve only a very soft diet. However, this may be preferable to the long and difficult management of a failed bone reconstruction in a poor candidate. It is almost never acceptable to not reconstruct the anterior arch of the mandible. The resulting "Andy Gump" deformity causes drooling, an inability to articulate speech, and severe aesthetic compromise. This defect is to be avoided if at all possible.

OSTEORADIONECROSIS

Osteoradionecrosis (ORN) after mandibular surgery of any kind, especially dental extraction, may occur after radiation.[17] The cause is the necrosis and infection of irradiated bone as a result of poor blood supply and healing. The risk is related to the dose of radiation, which is usually highest posteriorly, near the molars in patients with oropharynx cancer.[5] It may be prevented by careful extraction techniques, including perioperative antibiotics, the careful debridement of any bone spicules or fragments at the time of extraction, the careful reapproximation of soft-tissue coverage, postoperative antibiotic irrigations, and, possibly, perioperative hyperbaric oxygen treatments. Hyperbaric oxygen should be avoided if there is known cancer in the body, because it can accelerate tumor growth. Preradiation dental evaluation should identify and remove obviously septic teeth before radiation. Routine complete exodontia is rarely necessary and should not be automatically performed for all patients. Experience with selecting teeth for extraction in irradiated bone and knowledge of the radiation dose to the bone is important. In some cases, it may be preferable to allow a tooth to extrude rather than to extract it. In experienced hands, the rate of ORN can be extremely low.[5]

The diagnosis of ORN is made clinically. The hallmarks are a nonhealing surgical site, pain, exposed bone, odor, trismus, and evidence of necrotic bone on panorex radiograph (Figure 23-5). After significant necrosis

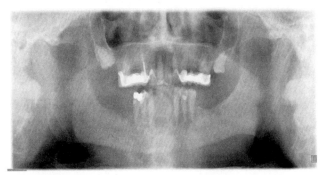

Figure 23-5. Panorex radiograph demonstrating osteoradionecrosis of the mandible from mid body to mid body. This condition requires mandibulectomy.

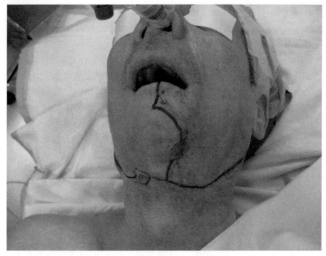

Figure 23-6. Preoperative photograph of a patient with osteoradionecrosis with multiple orocutaneous fistulae, a poor condition of the recipient tissues before mandibulectomy, and fibula free flap reconstruction.

occurs, it is irreversible. If the nonhealing site can be identified early, a few patients can improve with the aggressive debridement of bone spicules, oral and topical antibiotics, and aggressive cleansing. Unfortunately, most cases will progress to frank ORN with the development of mental nerve deficits, pain, cutaneous fistulae, and, if untreated, eventual fracture.

The controversy regarding the efficacy of hyperbaric oxygen for ORN continues despite the early closure of a randomized, prospective clinical trial demonstrating worse outcomes for ORN patients who received it.[18–20] The only effective treatment is mandibulectomy of the affected bone, typically with fibula or scapula free flap reconstruction.[21–23] This procedure is fraught with complication risk as a result of the condition of the recipient bed. The tissues are typically inflamed from infection and fistula (Figure 23-6), and the recipient tissues are already badly damaged from irradiation. There may already be a history of surgery in the neck and absent or poor recipient vessels. The patient may be in a poor nutritional state. Optimizing the operative condition of the patient with antibiotics and nutritional supplementation is wise before mandibulectomy. Intraoperatively, it is critical to excise the bone back to good, healthy, bleeding, viable bone, otherwise the ORN will persist at the margins, and poor healing of the bone will ensue. Excellent soft-tissue coverage is necessary. One cannot overemphasize the value of the prevention of ORN of the mandible.

COMPLICATIONS OF MAXILLECTOMY

When to Perform a Maxillectomy

Maxillectomy is a common operation for tumors of the palate, the upper gingiva, the nasal cavity, and the sinuses. Oronasal fistula is expected in all but the smallest

resections of the upper alveolar ridge. This defect is best handled by a dental prosthesis or an obturator. A few patients with no teeth or extensive resections have trouble retaining the prosthesis, but most function well both aesthetically and functionally. Osseointegrated implants can be placed to assist with holding the prosthesis in difficult cases.

Ectropion

After maxillectomy, ectropion can occur if there is a subciliary extension of the Webber–Ferguson incision. Scar tissue pulls down on the rim of the lower lid, thereby causing increased scleral show. Exposure keratopathy can occur in severe cases. A transconjunctival approach may reduce ectropion. If the incision is extended superiorly to the brow (i.e., the Lynch extension), then a W-plasty near the medial canthus will help prevent webbing in this area (Figure 23-7). The lateral rhinotomy portion is performed on the side wall of the nose rather than in the nasolabial crease to preserve the cosmetic unit of the lateral nose.

Epiphora

Epiphora is common but avoidable after maxillectomy. The lacrimal duct is usually divided in maxillectomy, and it should be identified, filleted open, and secured with absorbable suture (Figure 23-8). Alternatively, the lacrimal punctum can be cannulated with a lacrimal tube and the ends tied together in the nose. After several weeks, the knot can be cut intranasally and the tube removed; this ensures the patency of the lacrimal system. Laser-assisted dacrocystorhinostomy can be performed if delayed obstruction occurs. A few patients may develop recurrent abscess in the lacrimal duct related to poor flow and bacterial contamination.

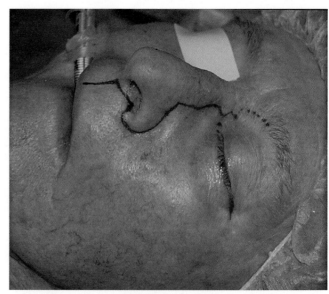

Figure 23-7. Incision planning for maxillectomy demonstrating a W-plasty at the medial canthus to prevent webbing deformity.

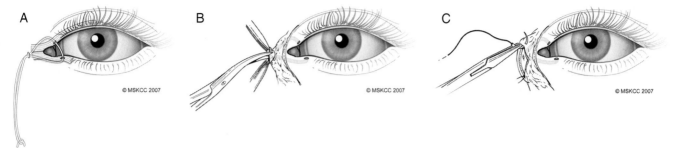

Figure 23-8. Illustration of **A,** a lacrimal tube. **B,** The opening of the lacrimal duct. **C,** Suturing the duct open to prevent stenosis and epiphora. (Reprinted with permission from Memorial Sloan-Kettering Cancer Center.)

Ipsilateral Eustachian Tube Dysfunction

Maxillectomy usually results in ipsilateral Eustachian tube dysfunction, and subsequent irradiation can amplify this problem. Patients with borderline hearing, with ipsilateral hearing loss in their best ear, or with recurrent acute otitis media require a tympanostomy tube in the ipsilateral tympanic membrane. The incidence of a chronic draining ear after tympanostomy tube placement is at least 25%. Patients should be warned of this possible complication.

Trismus

Trismus may occur after any oral surgery that involves the pterygoid muscles or after which there is disuse of the temporomandibular joint. Trismus causes many functional problems for eating, hygiene, examination, dental work, and airway management. Maxillectomy is the classic example of an oral operation that leads to trismus. All patients will experience scar tissue and inflammation of the pterygoids, which is reversible with stretching exercises; however, those patients who require postoperative radiation are at the highest risk for developing clinically significant trismus.[24] The early mobilization of the temporomandibular joint is critically important for trismus prevention.[25] Within several weeks of surgery or radiation, a dedicated regimen of stretching needs to be instituted. Several techniques are useful, including the use of tongue depressors of serially increasing size inserted between the incisors or the molars.[26] Patients need to know that trismus that occurs 1 year after treatment will be permanent and that there is no good surgical or medical therapy. Aggressive encouragement will lead to good compliance with trismus exercises and a low incidence of severe trismus, even after surgery and radiation. Some patients with severe trismus may have a component of muscle spasm that can be improved with the injection of botulinum toxin.

OROCUTANEOUS FISTULA

Orocutaneous fistula occurs most frequently after the composite resection of the tongue, floor of mouth, and mandible with neck dissection. Causative factors include the stage of the tumor and the amount of tissue

resected; the completeness of the reconstruction; and patient factors such as age, comorbidities, previous treatment, nutritional status, thyroid function, steroid use, and oral hygiene. Typically this complication is heralded by fever, pain, erythema, and an elevated white blood cell count. Clinical vigilance and early recognition can lead to rapid management and the minimization of adverse sequelae. Sometimes the use of perioperative antibiotics can blunt the usual signs and symptoms; the presence of systemic antibiotic treatment should be considered when making the clinical diagnosis.

Fluid Collection From and Care of an Orocutaneous Fistula

When the diagnosis of fluid collection is suspected, a computed tomography scan may demonstrate its presence, but more often there is just tissue edema on the computed tomography scan. The neck wound can be aspirated with a needle if there is fluctuance, but often there may be no frank collection in the fistula. Examination of the oral wound is likely to demonstrate dehiscence and an opening into the neck below. The neck wound needs to opened to allow the egress of pus and saliva, or a frank abscess, cellulitis, and sepsis will ensue. The wound should be opened as anteriorly as possible, with adequate drainage of the area of inflammation to help prevent the involvement of the carotid artery in the fistula tract and subsequent carotid rupture, which is often fatal.[27] By diverting the fistula flow anteriorly, the carotid artery can be spared from exposure to saliva. The opening of the wound needs to be large enough to allow for excellent drainage of the wound; it should be at least 2 cm to 4 cm, and, frequently, a much larger opening is necessary. The goal is that the skin opening be larger than the oral opening so that the shape of the fistula cavity is that of a cone with the tip facing upward. If the oral wound is larger than the skin wound, then additional subcutaneous undermining will occur as a result of the accumulation of secretions and pus unless the skin is opened wider. In addition to wound opening, the patient must receive nothing by mouth, the wound should be cultured and irrigated (if necessary), and wound packing should occur two to three times daily. The packing should help reduce oral contamination into the fistula superiorly and facilitate egress inferiorly. Strip packing is available in various sizes, and it is ideal for this purpose. If there is necrotic tissue, it should be debrided. If there is foul odor, a Dakin solution of sodium hypochlorite on the packing can temporarily help sterilize the wound, but it may inhibit healing if it is used very long.[28] Systemic antibiotics should be administered for 7 to 10 days or until there is no evidence of cellulitis or purulence on the wound. Ancef and Flagyl may suffice, or they may be altered according to bacterial culture speciation and sensitivity reports as they become available.

Closing the skin surgically is never helpful because of continued contamination from the mouth. Closing the oral opening with sutures is rarely helpful. Flap reconstruction is not indicated unless there is major tissue loss and a very clean recipient bed.[29] Surgery to divert the fistula anteriorly or to cover the carotid artery without necessarily closing the orocutaneous fistula is sometimes useful to minimize saliva contact with the carotid artery and to avoid carotid artery rupture.[30,31] In general, careful wound care will allow the fistula to heal over several weeks. The wound will slowly granulate in from the deeper aspect and, finally, the skin will close last. The packing is gradually reduced over time to allow for closure. In the nonirradiated patient, a small, well-cared-for fistula may heal in 7 days. More commonly, however, large, irradiated wounds may take weeks to months to slowly granulate over time.

Reasons for a Nonhealing Fistula

Clinicians should remain aware of several well-described reasons for a nonhealing fistula. Most important is the presence of tumor. Tumor at the edges of a wound will never heal; biopsies of nonhealing fistulae are indicated to rule out cancer. A patient in negative nitrogen balance will heal very slowly. Adequate, enteral nutrition by percutaneous endoscopic gastrostomy tube is necessary. Distal obstruction of the pharynx will divert more material into the fistula and prevent closure. The presence of a foreign body (e.g., nonabsorbable suture material, exposed hardware) will inhibit wound closure. An often overlooked wound-healing problem is a low thyroid hormone level, which is common among patients with head and neck cancer, often as a result of neck irradiation. Always check the serum thyroid-stimulating hormone level, and prescribe Synthroid, if appropriate.

AIRWAY COMPLICATIONS

Airway complications after oral surgery are rare, but they can be fatal. Most are caused by the unexpected compromise of the airway as a result of a foreign body, hemorrhage, hematoma, swelling, or mucus obstruction.

During the immediate postoperative period, oral surgery patients may be difficult to intubate because of swelling, flaps, or trismus. Mask ventilation may be impossible as a result of any of the aforementioned factors plus the discontinuity of the mandible, which inhibits the mask seal and promotes the collapse of the airway in the anteroposterior dimension. Bilateral vocal cord paralysis is a rare cause of airway compromise among these patients, but it may be precipitated by bilateral neck dissection and carotid sheath dissection, previously unrecognized unilateral vocal cord paralysis of unknown cause, previous head and neck surgery, or endotracheal tube trauma.

Prevention of Airway Emergencies

The prevention of airway emergencies is best accomplished with the appropriate aggressive use of tracheostomy at the time of surgery. The indications for tracheostomy should be individualized for each patient (Figure 23-9). Absolute indications for tracheostomy include free flap reconstruction of the oral cavity or the oropharynx and surgery for patients who cannot be nonintubated, such as those with permanent, severe trismus and nasopharynx stenosis. Tracheostomy should be considered for the presence of a foreign body (e.g., bolster, keel, stent) left in the mouth or pharynx and for in any patient in whom the surgeon suspects that airway compromise may occur. Relative indications for tracheostomy are factors that contribute to airway compromise in the oral surgery patient. The use of IMF after oral cancer surgery can contribute to difficulty with rapid oral intubation. Rubberbands can be removed faster than dental wires in an emergency. Any patient with IMF should have appropriate instrumentation at the bedside to open the IMF urgently if there are vomiting or airway problems. Trismus is a common problem among patients with head and neck cancer, and this factor should be considered as part of the airway management of these patients. Any time that

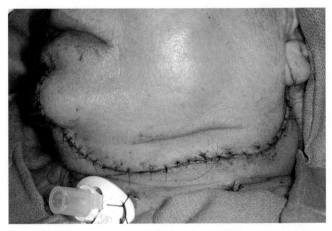

Figure 23-9. Tracheostomy after the resection of a posterior oral cavity tumor that may lead to airway compromise.

surgery extends into the pharynx, there is a risk of hemorrhage, hematoma, or swelling that could impair respiration. Previous radiation may have already compromised the pharyngeal lumen and predisposed the tissues to swelling from surgery. In the heavily treated patient, even neck surgery or minor oral surgery can induce unexpected swelling and airway distress.

A bolster for an oral skin graft should always be sewn to the oral tissue to prevent migration to the pharynx and aspiration. Meticulous care is necessary to prevent the leaving of surgical gauze in the pharynx. Never pack the pharynx unless pharyngeal hemorrhage is being controlled, in which case a tracheostomy is indicated. Any sizable resection of the posterior oral tongue could result in hematoma from the lingual artery branches and airway distress. Segmental mandibulectomy leaves the patient with an incomplete mandibular arch and the risk of pharyngeal airway collapse. Patients with short, heavy necks or the severe restriction of extension as a result of arthritis or hardware may benefit from prophylactic temporary tracheostomy if they are cannot be intubated. Obstruction of the pharyngeal or glottic airway can be caused by plugging with thick mucus or dried crusts after oral surgery. This is more likely to occur among irradiated patients who are receiving nothing by mouth in whom thick oral secretions can form heavy crusts. These patients require humidified air and saline rinses and gargles to ensure a patent airway and clean, healthy mucosa. Patient-controlled suction is useful for those who are unable to manage their own secretions well.

Use of Medications

Medications to dry the secretions may worsen the problem by making them thicker, drier, and harder to mobilize; thus these medications should be avoided. Appropriate perioperative antibiotics include 24 hours of intravenous Cephazolin and metronidazole to minimize cellulitis and abscess formation. Occasionally steroids may be useful to decrease edema of the oral tissues, the uvula, or the pharynx; however, their actions may be short lived or incomplete, and they should not be used instead of tracheostomy to manage a borderline airway.

Postoperative Diet

Great care is required with the management of the postoperative diet of patients with oral cancer. The temporary aspiration of thin liquids or the frank aspiration of foodstuffs may be absent, mild, or severe, depending on the patient's age, his or her previous treatments, and the amount of resection. A previously heavily treated patient with baseline tenuous swallowing may be severely affected by even minor oral surgery. Therefore oral surgery patients should be started on conservative diets such as thick liquids, full liquids, or purees and

monitored for signs of aspiration, which could lead to airway compromise or pneumonia. If there is baseline swallowing impairment or early difficulties with swallowing, then patients should receive nothing by mouth until they have been assessed by a speech–language pathologist or with a flexible endoscopic evaluation of swallowing with sensory testing examination. Severe swallowing compromise should be treated with aggressive swallowing therapy, percutaneous gastrostomy feeding to maintain nutritional status, and hydration during the healing process.

All precautions for the patient's airway should be rigorously maintained. Unexpected patient death from airway compromise is a devastating complication that is usually avoidable.

WOUND INFECTION

Wound infections occur in approximately 6% of contaminated operations on patients with head and neck cancer. This relatively low rate is attributable to the gentle handling of tissues, a good blood supply in head and neck tissues, prophylactic antibiotics, and advanced reconstructive practices that minimize fistula formation. Head and neck wound infections are polymicrobial, with aerobes, anaerobes, and gram-positive and gram-negative bacteria reflecting the pharyngeal flora. Several regimens of prophylactic antibiotics have proven to be effective for reducing postoperative wound infections. One widely used and cost-effective combination is Cephazolin and metronidazole. Prophylactic antibiotics must be started 1 hour preoperatively; no advantage has been shown for treatments beyond 24 hours. Antifungal and gram-negative coverage are unnecessary.[32]

Cellulitis presents as wound erythema, edema, and tenderness. There may be fever and an elevated white blood cell count. Cultures reveal gram-positive organisms such as *Streptococcus* and *Staphylococcus* species. Cellulitis typically responds within 24 hours to first-generation cephalosporins given intravenously or orally. Deep wound infections and abscesses tend to harbor β-lactamase–producing anaerobic bacteria. Fluid collections should be aspirated (at a minimum) or surgically drained and left open to heal by second intention with packing. Antibiotic choice should be dictated by the results of the culture and sensitivity testing of wound cultures.

QUALITY OF LIFE

Treatment for patients with cancer of the head and neck can have a significant impact on their physical, psychological, and social functioning.[33] As survival rates after the treatment of squamous cell carcinoma of the oral cavity (SCCOC) have improved during recent years, the focus of outcomes research has shifted to issues related to the QOL. Alterations of functions such as mastication, speech, taste, swallowing, oral sensation, and continence can have a devastating impact on the QOL.[34] Because of this, treatment—even when it successfully eliminates the neoplastic process—often has significant associated morbidity. The disabilities associated with the treatment of advanced oropharyngeal cancer can often seem worse to the patient than the untreated malignancy.[35] Traditional outcome measures such as overall survival, disease-free survival, and tumor recurrence are often meaningless to patients. Most patients are concerned with their ability to return to pre-illness levels of functioning and psychological well-being.[35] As a result of the association of SCCOC with smoking and drinking, most patients are also forced to live with the stigma of knowing that their prior behavior most likely contributed to their current status. The impact of SCCOC and its therapies on the overall QOL of these unfortunate patients is currently under investigation. It is clear that avoiding the complications of oral cancer surgery is paramount to maintaining the QOL.

REFERENCES

1. Blot WJ, McLaughlin JK, Winn DM, et al: Smoking and drinking in relation to oral and pharyngeal cancer. *Cancer Res* 1988;48(11):3282–3287.
2. Piccirillo JF: Importance of comorbidity in head and neck cancer. *Laryngoscope* 2000;110(4):593–602.
3. Jemal A, Siegel R, Ward E, et al: Cancer statistics—2007. *CA Cancer J Clin* 2007;57(1):43–66.
4. Wang CC, Cheng MH, Hao SP, et al: Osteoradionecrosis with combined mandibulotomy and marginal mandibulectomy. *Laryngoscope* 2005;115(11):1963–1967.
5. Sulaiman F, Huryn JM, Zlotolow IM: Dental extractions in the irradiated head and neck patient: A retrospective analysis of Memorial Sloan-Kettering Cancer Center protocols, criteria, and end results. *J Oral Maxillofac Surg* 2003;61(10):1123–1131.
6. Nam W, Kim HJ, Choi EC, et al: Contributing factors to mandibulotomy complications: A retrospective study. *Oral Surg Oral Med Oral Pathol Oral Radiol Endod* 2006;101(3):e65–e70.
7. Shah JP, Kumaraswamy SV, Kulkarni V: Comparative evaluation of fixation methods after mandibulotomy for oropharyngeal tumors. *Am J Surg* 1993;166(4):431–434.
8. McCann KJ, Irish JC, Gullane PJ, et al: Complications associated with rigid fixation of mandibulotomies. *J Otolaryngol* 1994;23(3):210–215.
9. Altman K, Bailey BM: Non-union of mandibulotomy sites following irradiation for squamous cell carcinoma of the oral cavity. *Br J Oral Maxillofac Surg* 1996;34(1):62–65.
10. Dai TS, Hao SP, Chang KP, et al: Complications of mandibulotomy: Midline versus paramidline. *Otolaryngol Head Neck Surg* 2003;128(1):137–141.
11. Pan WL, Hao SP, Lin YS, et al: The anatomical basis for mandibulotomy: Midline versus paramidline. *Laryngoscope* 2003;113(2):377–380.
12. Store G, Boysen M: Mandibular access osteotomies in oral cancer. *ORL J Otorhinolaryngol Relat Spec* 2005;67(6):326–330.
13. Eisen MD, Weinstein GS, Chalian A, et al: Morbidity after midline mandibulotomy and radiation therapy. *Am J Otolaryngol* 2000;21(5):312–317.
14. Baek CH, Lee SW, Jeong HS: New modification of the mandibulotomy approach without lip splitting. *Head Neck* 2006;28(7):580–586.
15. Shaha AR: Marginal mandibulectomy for carcinoma of the floor of the mouth. *J Surg Oncol* 1992;49(2):116–119.
16. Song CS, Har-El G: Marginal mandibulectomy: Oncologic and nononcologic outcome. *Am J Otolaryngol* 2003;24(1):61–63.
17. Celik N, Wei FC, Chen HC, et al: Osteoradionecrosis of the mandible after oromandibular cancer surgery. *Plast Reconstr Surg* 2002;109(6):1875–1881.
18. Annane D, Depondt J, Aubert P, et al: Hyperbaric oxygen therapy for radionecrosis of the jaw: A randomized, placebo-controlled, double-blind trial from the ORN96 study group. *J Clin Oncol* 2004;22(24):4893–4900.
19. David LA, Sandor GK, Evans AW, et al: Hyperbaric oxygen therapy and mandibular osteoradionecrosis: A retrospective study and analysis of treatment outcomes. *J Can Dent Assoc* 2001;67(7):384.
20. Rogers SN: Does the Annane paper (2004) signal the end of HBO for ORN? *Br J Oral Maxillofac Surg* 2005;43(6):538–539.
21. Ang E, Black C, Irish J, et al: Reconstructive options in the treatment of osteoradionecrosis of the craniomaxillofacial skeleton. *Br J Plast Surg* 2003;56(2):92–99.
22. Shaha AR, Cordeiro PG, Hidalgo DA, et al: Resection and immediate microvascular reconstruction in the management of osteoradionecrosis of the mandible. *Head Neck* 1997;19(5):406–411.
23. Curi MM, Oliveira dos Santos M, Feher O, et al: Management of extensive osteoradionecrosis of the mandible with radical resection and immediate microvascular reconstruction. *J Oral Maxillofac Surg* 2007;65(3):434–438.
24. Sakai S, Kubo T, Mori N, et al: A study of the late effects of radiotherapy and operation on patients with maxillary cancer: A survey more than 10 years after initial treatment. *Cancer Res* 1988;62(10):2114–2117.
25. Cohen EG, Deschler DG, Walsh K, et al: Early use of a mechanical stretching device to improve mandibular mobility after composite resection: A pilot study. *Arch Phys Med Rehabil* 2005;86(7):1416–1419.
26. Buchbinder D, Currivan RB, Kaplan AJ, et al: Mobilization regimens for the prevention of jaw hypomobility in the radiated patient: A comparison of three techniques. *J Oral Maxillofac Surg* 1993;51(8):863–867.
27. Upile T, Triaridis S, Kirkland P, et al: The management of carotid artery rupture. *Eur Arch Otorhinolaryngol* 2005;262(7):555–560.
28. Wilson JR, Mills JG, Prather ID, et al: A toxicity index of skin and wound cleansers used on in vitro fibroblasts and keratinocytes. *Adv Skin Wound Care* 2005;18(7):373–378.
29. Chun JK, Senderoff DM: Microsurgical reconstruction of difficult orocutaneous fistulas. *Ann Plast Surg* 1996;36(4):417–424.
30. Hillerman BL, Kennedy TL: Carotid rupture and tissue coverage. *Laryngoscope* 1982;92(9 Pt 1):985–988.
31. Coleman JJ, III: Treatment of the ruptured or exposed carotid artery: A rational approach. *South Med J* 1985;78(3):262–267.
32. Johnson JT, Yu VL: Antibiotic use during major head and neck surgery. *Ann Surg* 1988;207(1):108–111.
33. Alsarraf R, Coltrera MD, Deleyiannis FW, et al: Quality of life in head and neck cancer. *Laryngoscope* 2000;110(3 Pt 3):4–7.
34. Argerakis GP: Psychosocial considerations of the post-treatment of head and neck cancer patients. *Dent Clin North Am* 1990;34(2):285–305.
35. Deleyiannis FW, Coltrera MD, Weymuller EA Jr: Quality of life of disease-free survivors of advanced (stage III or IV) oropharyngeal cancer. *Head Neck* 1997;19(6):466–473.

CHAPTER 24

Dental Complications

Brian L. Schmidt

Dental complications of head and neck surgery are common, and they can have a profoundly negative impact on the quality of life of head and neck surgery patients. Complications can develop directly from treatment for an unrelated problem (e.g., tooth displacement during direct laryngoscopy) or inappropriate treatment for an injury that involves the dentition (e.g., an infected mandible fracture as a result of a retained carious tooth).

Not all dental complications can be avoided. However, the incidence of dental complications can be significantly reduced with the careful evaluation of the dentition before treatment is provided. Of particular note for the patient with head and neck cancer is that the maintenance of the dental status is critical for maintaining the quality of life.[1]

A proper evaluation requires the provider to have a clear understanding of the dentition and its supporting structure as well as the ability to perform a clinical examination and to interpret dental radiographs. The complications that will be discussed in this chapter include osteonecrosis after bisphosphonate therapy, dental complications as a result of radiation therapy, osteoradionecrosis, malocclusion after mandibular osteotomy or resection, and dental complications after trauma.

OSTEONECROSIS AFTER BISPHOSPHONATE THERAPY

Head and neck surgeons are often consulted to manage complications that result from treatment for cancer. Osteonecrosis of the jaws has recently been recognized as a complication among patients receiving bisphosphonate therapy for metastatic bone lesions and for the prevention of osteoporosis.

In 2003, Marx[2] reported in a letter to the *Journal of Oral and Maxillofacial Surgery* the association between bisphosphonates and jaw osteonecrosis. Ruggiero and colleagues[3] confirmed the role of bisphosphonate therapy in the development of jaw osteonecrosis in their report of 63 cases.

Bisphosphonates are commonly used to treat patients with malignancies. The American Society of Clinical Oncology has recommended the use of bisphosphonates for moderate to severe hypercalcemia associated with malignancies as well as for breast carcinoma,[4] multiple myeloma,[5] and metastatic osteolytic lesions.

Bisphosphonates inhibit osteoclasts. The drugs are not metabolized; rather, they are excreted by the kidneys, and their half-life is thought to be years. The intravenous preparations are pamidronate (Aredia) and zoledronic acid (Zometa). The oral preparations are alendronate (Fosamax), risedronate (Actonel), and ibandronate (Boniva).

Ruggiero and colleagues[3] found that less than 10% of patients who developed jaw osteonecrosis as a result of bisphosphonate therapy were diagnosed with osteoporosis and were receiving an oral preparation (alendronate). Marx and colleagues[6] found that 2.5% of patients with jaw osteonecrosis were receiving alendronate alone. They also found that the mean duration of time from the commencement of bisphosphonate therapy to the recognition of exposed bone was 14.3 months for patients taking pamidronate alone, 12.1 months for patients changed from pamidronate to zoledronate, and 9.4 months for patients receiving zoledronate alone.[6] Ruggiero and colleagues[3] found that the duration of bisphosphonate therapy ranged from 6 to 48 months.

Clinical Findings

Jaw osteonecrosis is not associated with infection; therefore antibiotics should not be considered a first-line treatment. On pathologic evaluation, Ruggiero and colleagues[3] found that the osteonecrotic specimens consisted of necrotic bone associated with bacterial debris and granulation tissue and that the culture results showed only normal oral flora.[3] Presenting symptoms typically include pain and exposed bone at the site of a previous tooth extraction. Spontaneous bone exposure, particularly in the posterior lingual aspect of the mandible, can also occur (Figure 24-1).

Fourteen percent of patients have no history of a recent dentoalveolar procedure yet developed spontaneous exposure and necrosis of the alveolar bone.[3] About 70% of patients with jaw osteonecrosis present with exposed bone and pain, whereas 30% of patients present with asymptomatic exposed bone.[6] Approximately 70% of cases involve the mandible exclusively, slightly less than 30% involve the maxilla, and less than 5% involve both the maxilla and the mandible.[6] The posterior mandible and maxilla are the most commonly involved sites.

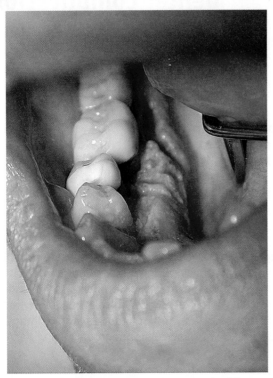

Figure 24-1. Bisphosphonate-induced osteonecrosis of the mandible. The most common site for exposed necrotic bone is the lingual aspect of the mandible. In this case, the exposure developed spontaneously. (Courtesy of Dr. Robert Ord, Baltimore, Md.)

Prevention

The prevention of osteonecrosis as a result of bisphosphonate treatment requires close communication among the oncologist, the surgeon, and the dentist. Before the initiation of bisphosphonate therapy, the patient should be evaluated by a dentist as well as an oral and maxillofacial surgeon. The examination should include a physical examination in combination with a panoramic radiograph and appropriate periapical radiographs.

Because the recognition of jaw osteonecrosis is a recent finding, an appropriately designed study has not been completed to definitively dictate methods of prevention. The following recommendations are based on clinical experience and available relevant publications. All dental and oral surgical treatment should be completed before starting the bisphosphonate therapy. The goal of dental treatment is the elimination of dental infection as well as the prevention of the need for tooth extraction after the commencement of bisphosphonate therapy. Because dental surgery clearly leads to jaw osteonecrosis, all dental surgery should be completed before beginning the bisphosphonate therapy. Third molars that are completely covered with soft tissue and bone can be left in place. If a third molar is exposed to the oral cavity, however, extraction before the commencement of bisphosphonate therapy is indicated.

Bisphosphonate therapy can typically be started approximately 1 month after invasive surgical procedures such as tooth extraction, periodontal surgery, and root canal therapy. Noninvasive dental care such as restoration, cleaning, and fitting for dentures can be performed after the administration of bisphosphonate therapy.

Antibiotics are not necessary for noninvasive dental procedures. For invasive dental procedures, prophylactic antibiotics should be used. Penicillin is the first choice. For the penicillin-allergic patient, quinolones and metronidazole are appropriate choices.[6] Routine dental surveillance should be performed approximately every 6 months after bisphosphonate therapy has been started.

Treatment

There is no effective treatment for bisphosphonate-induced jaw osteonecrosis. After bone exposure is recognized, the patient should be referred to an oral and maxillofacial surgeon.

It is critical to differentiate the underlying mechanisms and treatment regimens for osteoradionecrosis from bisphosphonate-induced osteonecrosis. Osteoradionecrosis affects localized regions of the mandible, and it is the consequence of radiation-induced hypocellularity and poor tissue oxygenation. Bisphosphonate-induced osteonecrosis (in contrast with localized radiation damage), affects the entire maxilla and mandible. In cases of bisphosphonate-induced osteonecrosis, attempts to reduce or cover the exposed bone with local flaps have been ineffective and can produce a considerable worsening of symptoms.

Because the entire mandible and maxilla are affected by the bisphosphonate therapy, debridement to viable, bleeding bone is not possible. Rather, debridement often results in further bone exposure.

Hyperbaric oxygen (HBO) therapy does not have a role in the management of bisphosphonate-induced jaw osteonecrosis. The practitioner is often faced with the decision of whether to cease treatment with the bisphosphonate.

The benefit of bisphosphonate therapy for controlling metastatic malignancies is clear. The half-life of bisphosphonates is years; therefore there is no clear reason to cease therapy if there is concern regarding bone metastasis. Treatment should be focused on the elimination of pain and the prevention of the progression of bone exposure. Pathologic fractures have not been typically encountered among these patients. In the report by Marx and colleagues of 97 patients with osteonecrosis treated with the authors' recommended regimen, there was no case of mandible fracture.[6] Fistula formation can occur, but the natural history of the fistulae in bisphosphonate-induced osteonecrosis is not clear. Sharp bony projections can produce significant pain and can be rounded off. However, the debridement of exposed bone should be avoided.

If secondary infection is suspected, penicillin can be prescribed in addition to rinses with 0.12% chlorhexidine (Peridex). If symptoms persist, then surgical resection can be considered. However, the outcomes of surgical resection and reconstruction in cases of bisphosphonate-induced osteonecrosis are unclear.

DENTAL AND JAW COMPLICATIONS AS A RESULT OF RADIATION THERAPY

Prevention of Dental Complications Associated With Radiation Therapy

The head and neck surgeon can significantly reduce the incidence of osteoradionecrosis by instituting strict preventative measures before starting radiation therapy. As soon as the patient is diagnosed with cancer, the dental status of the patient must be considered, and the patient should be evaluated by a dentist who is familiar with the management of head and neck cancer. Patients must be evaluated by a dentist before surgery or radiation therapy. Patients referred for dental evaluation after surgery are extremely difficult to examine and treat.

The dental evaluation should involve a clinical dental examination, a panoramic radiograph, and, possibly, a series of bitewing and periapical radiographs. Attention must be directed to dental caries, odontogenic infections, periodontal disease, and impacted or partially exposed teeth. If the restoration of teeth with caries cannot be completed, then the teeth should be extracted. Teeth with evidence of pulpal infection or teeth that are periodontally involved should be extracted. Any tooth that cannot be maintained for the life of the patient should be removed. Mandibular teeth that will receive 60 Gy or more of radiation should be removed.[7] Necessary dental surgical treatment must be completed as soon as possible before radiation therapy to allow for adequate healing. It is best if the extractions can be performed at the time of surgical resection.

The patient should also have a prophylactic dental cleaning. Fluoride trays should be fabricated, and daily fluoride treatment will be required for the life of the patient. During radiation treatment, topical 1% sodium fluoride gel should be applied daily using trays for both the upper and the lower teeth. The trays are left in place for 5 minutes, and the patient should avoid eating or drinking for 30 minutes after treatment.

Radiation Caries

Radiation caries are a result of xerostomia and direct damage to the tooth structures, the dentin, and the enamel (Figure 24-2). The vascularity of the tooth is significantly reduced. The enamel can be lost, and the dentin becomes black. Patients who have had radiation therapy can be treated with general dental care. Radiation caries should be treated early with caries excavation and the replacement of lost tooth structures.

Xerostomia

Xerostomia is a very common complication among patients receiving radiotherapy for head and neck cancer. Patients report changes in both the quantity and quality of their saliva during and after radiation therapy. Xerostomia has a dramatic effect on the quality of life and affects taste, speech, swallowing, and overall discomfort, because these oral functions depend on normal salivary flow.

The normal salivary flow is approximately 0.3 to 0.5 ml/minute, whereas xerostomic patients typically have a flow of less than 0.1 ml/minute. Patients with xerostomia will often complain of dryness, fissures at the lip commissures, atrophy of the tongue surface, burning of the tongue, and difficulty wearing dentures.

Salivary changes also contribute to dental caries after radiation therapy. The degree of xerostomia correlates with both the amount of glandular tissue radiated and the total dose, primarily to the major salivary glands.[8]

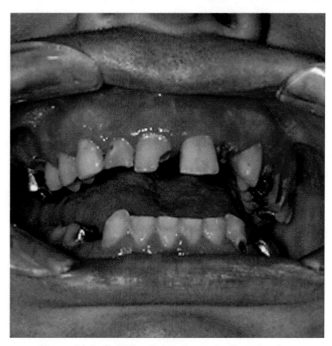

Figure 24-2. Radiation-induced xerostomia and caries.

The acinar portion of the salivary glands is radiosensitive, with the serous acini being more sensitive than the mucinous acini. The ductal portion of the glands is relatively radioresistant.

Intensity-modulated radiation therapy with the sparing of the submandibular gland appears to reduce the incidence and intensity of xerostomia.[9,10] Pilocarpine has been approved for postradiation xerostomia; it can be administered at a dose of 5 mg orally three times a day to improve salivary flow. Pilocarpine administration during radiation therapy does not ameliorate xerostomia or mucositis.[11] The administration of amifostine during radiotherapy appears to reduce xerostomia.[12–14]

Trismus

Limited jaw opening is a significant complication after radiation therapy. Radiation-induced fibrosis of the pterygomasseteric sling (including the masseter and medial pterygoid muscles) and fibrosis of the mucosa limit mouth opening. Trismus can be especially difficult for patients who require a maxillary obturator, because they may experience difficulty inserting the obturator. Trismus can also prevent adequate oral hygiene, including the application of daily fluoride; this may lead to radiation caries. In some cases, trismus is associated with osteoradionecrosis, and the treatment of the osteoradionecrosis may improve the limited mouth opening.

There are few treatment options for patients who have trismus as a result of muscle and mucosal fibrosis alone. The resection of the mucosa and muscle and their replacement with vascularized tissue offers little improvement. Temporomandibular joint surgery is not indicated for the treatment of radiation-induced trismus.

The prevention of trismus during radiation therapy is critical. Before starting radiation therapy, the patient must be taught aggressive jaw-opening exercises using either tongue blades or a TheraBite (Atos Medical, Horby, Sweden). Before the commencement of radiation therapy, the patient must be told of his or her maximum jaw opening. This measurement can either be in terms of millimeters (if using the TheraBite appliance) or in terms of the number of tongue blades. Throughout treatment, the patient must use this measurement as a goal to reach each day. Jaw-opening exercises should be performed three times per day. Patients will often be discouraged by the fact that their jaw opening is significantly restricted in the morning. However, they will find that, as the day progresses and they perform the jaw-opening exercises, they are able to attain a significantly wider opening. The patient should be seen by the head and neck surgeon during radiation therapy to confirm that mouth opening is being addressed.

Osteoradionecrosis

Osteoradionecrosis is one of the most difficult complications that the head and neck surgeon will encounter after radiation therapy. Osteoradionecrosis is not a bone infection; rather, it is hypovascular, hypoxic, and hypocellular bone as a consequence of radiation therapy.[7] These pathologic processes are progressive with time. Vascularity to the bone and soft tissues does not improve as the time after radiation therapy increases. The patient's risk for developing osteoradionecrosis increases with time after radiation therapy.

Osteoradionecrosis can develop spontaneously; however, it is most commonly precipitated by tooth extraction. The surgical trauma after the extraction of a tooth leads to progressive necrosis in the region of the extraction (Figure 24-3).

HBO has been used to prevent and treat osteoradionecrosis. It can be administered in a monoplace or multiplace chamber. Standard treatment involves the patient breathing 100% oxygen at 2.4 atmospheres for 90 minutes. Although there continues to be controversy regarding the efficacy of HBO for preventing osteoradionecrosis, data from a randomized prospective clinical trial supports the use of HBO before dental extraction.[15]

If dental extractions are required after the completion of radiation therapy, the 20/10 HBO protocol as described by Marx and colleagues[15] should be used. The protocol consists of 20 HBO sessions before surgery followed by 10 sessions after surgery. At the time of the extractions, periosteal stripping of the alveolar bone should be minimized. Although the primary closure of the mucosa is ideal, it should not be achieved at the expense of the periosteal coverage of the alveolar bone.

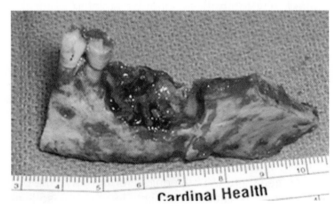

Cardinal Health

Figure 24-3. Osteoradionecrosis of the mandible after the removal of a mandibular molar. This patient required mandibular resection for osteoradionecrosis. The necrotic bone developed at the site of extraction. Resection was performed to remove all of the necrotic bone to the point of bleeding bone margins.

The management of osteoradionecrosis depends on the stage of presentation. The head and neck surgeon must always consider the possibility of recurrent tumor when faced with osteoradionecrosis. Ten percent of patients with osteoradionecrosis have a recurrence of the cancer or a new primary cancer.[16] The molar region of the mandible is the most common site affected.[16,17]

A number of staging systems are available for osteoradionecrosis.[18–20] The most commonly used is the classification system proposed by Marx.[19] In this classic manuscript, Marx describes an osteoradionecrosis treatment protocol using HBO therapy based on three stages. HBO therapy as described by Marx[15,21] has been shown to be an integral part of the effective management of osteoradionecrosis, depending on the stage.[22–24]

For stage I, the patient is treated with 30 HBO dives. The treatment objective is a decrease in the amount of exposed bone, the resorption of nonviable bone, and the absence of inflammation. Local debridement can then be performed, and this should be followed by 10 more HBO dives. If the patient does not respond to this regimen, then he or she is classified as stage II and undergoes surgical debridement followed by 10 additional dives. Stage III osteoradionecrosis is defined as exhibiting one of the following: (1) pathologic fracture; (2) orocutaneous fistula; or (3) osteolysis to the inferior border of the mandible. Also, stage II patients who do not respond to surgical debridement and HBO are classified as stage III. Stage III patients will require mandibular resection and microvascular reconstruction using both bone and soft tissue.

The principles of the surgical management of osteoradionecrosis involve the complete resection of the necrotic segment and the reconstruction of the hard and soft tissues. In many cases, both oral and facial soft-tissue coverage will be required. Careful surgical planning is necessary for the treatment of osteoradionecrosis. The native tissues have lost their regenerative capacity as a result of the radiation. Complications that result from the management of osteoradionecrosis are significant and can include the progression of the osteonecrosis, orocutaneous fistula, and nonhealing wounds. The viability of the mucosa and the mandibular bone need to be carefully assessed during presurgical planning and at the time of surgery to determine the appropriate margins of resection. The extent of bone necrosis can best be assessed with the use of plain radiographs such as a panoramic radiograph. Attention should be directed to establishing the correct occlusion after resection. All necrotic bone and mucosa should be replaced with vascularized tissue. Any extractions performed at the time of reconstruction

carry a risk for additional osteoradionecrosis at a separate site and should only be performed after careful consideration.

One particularly challenging situation is the development of bilateral osteoradionecrosis in the region of the angles (Figure 24-4). The management of the intervening viable mandible must be carefully considered.

MALOCCLUSION AFTER MANDIBULAR OSTEOTOMY OR RESECTION

Strict attention to the dentition is required when planning the surgical disruption of mandibular continuity. Quality-of-life studies have demonstrated that one of patients' primary complaints after head and neck surgery is difficulty chewing.[25]

The occlusion should be carefully evaluated before surgery, and it should be considered when planning the osteotomies. Consultation with the patients' dentist should be obtained to determine the status of the entire dentition. A panoramic radiograph and, in many cases, preoperative dental casts should be obtained to assess dental health, tooth position, and the occlusion. The placement of maxillary and mandibular arch bars at the time of the operation is required.

In the case of a mandibular resection, any form of intermaxillary fixation that does not involve the use of arch bars is inadequate as a result of the rotation of the remaining mandibular segment. The patient should be placed in intermaxillary fixation when adapting the reconstruction plate. A preoperative model can be generated from a computed tomography scan, and then the plate can be appropriately contoured before the operation (Figure 24-5). At the time of the operation, after the completion of the mandibular osteotomy, the patient should be placed into intermaxillary fixation. The contour of the plate should be carefully evaluated on the proximal and distal segments of bone before the plate is rigidly secured. After the placement of rigid fixation, the patient should be removed from fixation and the occlusion checked. If the occlusion is not acceptable, then the plate must be removed, recontoured, and replaced.

A mandibulotomy consisting of either a single or double osteotomy can be used to provide access to parapharyngeal lesions. Again, preoperative dental assessment is critical, and it has been shown to improve the postoperative occlusion of patients undergoing mandibulotomy.[26]

The planned osteotomy should be at a site where there will be adequate interdental bone after the completion of the osteotomy; otherwise tooth devitalization can occur. The proximal osteotomy should be placed anterior to the mental foramen, whereas the proximal osteotomy is placed superior to the lingula. Rigid fixation plates can then be placed across the osteotomy sites. An acrylic lingual splint is often recommended to prevent lingual torquing and the rotation of the lesser mandibular segment.

A review of 313 mandibulotomies demonstrated osteotomy-related complications in 20% of cases.[26]

Postoperative temporomandibular joint edema can result in postoperative occlusal discrepancies similar to the process that can occur after orthognathic surgery.[27] Mild interocclusal elastics for 2 to 3 weeks can be used to guide the mandible to the correct occlusion as the edema resolves.

Patients should be followed closely during the first 4 to 6 weeks after surgery to confirm that the occlusion is correct or improving. Minor corrections of the occlusion

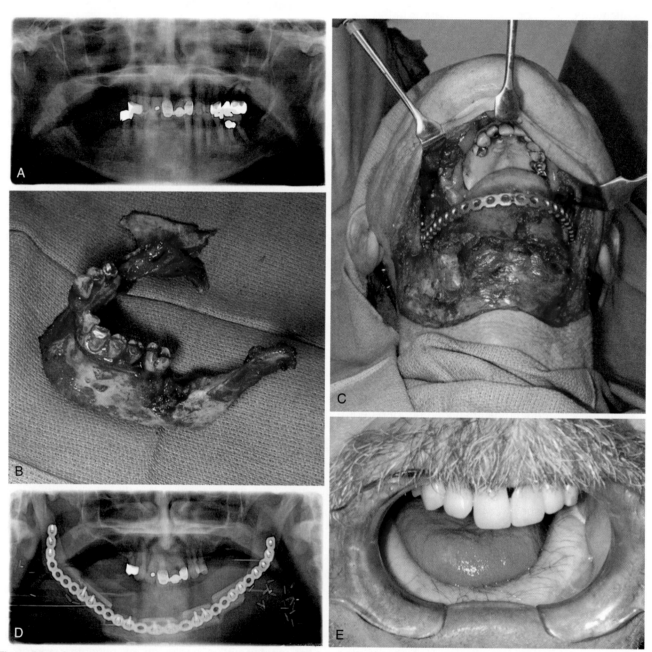

Figure 24-4. Surgical management of a patient with bilateral mandibular osteoradionecrosis. The patient had received radiation therapy for tonsillar squamous cell carcinoma. Subsequently, the patient had bilateral mandibular molars extracted and then developed osteoradionecrosis at both sites. **A,** Panoramic radiograph demonstrating osteolysis bilaterally in the molar regions involving the entire vertical height of the mandible. The patient had significant pain. The surgical plan involved the resection of the necrotic and intervening portions of the mandible. **B,** Resected mandible with obvious pathologic fracture and osteoradionecrosis. **C,** Mandibular reconstruction with a reconstruction plate. A free fibula flap was then used to reconstruct bone and soft tissue. **D,** Panoramic radiograph at 3 months after reconstruction demonstrating the healing fibula free flap. **E,** Intraoral view at 3 months after reconstruction demonstrating the adequate healing of the oral mucosa.

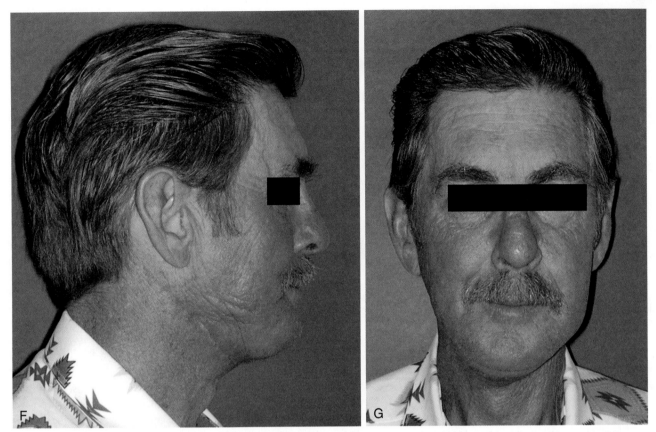

Figure 24-4. cont'd **F,** Lateral facial view at 3 months showing adequate mandibular projection. **G,** Frontal facial view at 3 months after reconstruction demonstrating appropriate aesthetics.

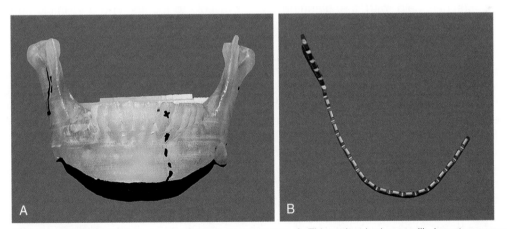

Figure 24-5. Mandibular model generated from a computed tomography scan. **A,** This patient had a mandibular osteosarcoma that required a resection of approximately 60% of the mandible. A mandibular model was generated from the computed tomography scan. **B,** The reconstruction plate was then accurately contoured using the mandibular model, and it could be used at the time of resection and reconstruction.

can be obtained with the use of arch bars and elastics. The significant medial muscle pull on the osteotomized segment can result with medial displacement and a resultant open-bite deformity (Figure 24-6). Such a complication requires a corrective mandibular osteotomy procedure.

DENTAL COMPLICATIONS ASSOCIATED WITH HEAD AND NECK TRAUMA

Dental complications associated with head and neck trauma are common and can result from the inadequate or inappropriate management of the dentition after trauma. A complete dental assessment should be

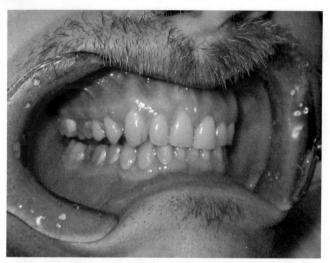

Figure 24-6. Development of a malocclusion after a mandibulotomy for access to a parapharyngeal tumor. Three months after surgery, the patient had a malocclusion with an open bite on the right-hand side. Rigid fixation was used in this case. The malocclusion was progressive and ultimately required reoperation to correct it.

performed as part of the head and neck examination. An account of all fractured or missing teeth must be made.

The dentition is critical to establishing proper jaw relationships. The viability and long-term prognosis of the dentition should be determined before commencing treatment. The dentition needs to be assessed on the basis of periodontal health, supporting alveolar bone, caries, and potential fracture. An evaluation of preoperative dental casts can help with the planning of surgery.

The status of the teeth should be assessed on the basis of a clinical examination and with a panoramic radiograph as well as a series of periapical radiographs. The teeth should be assessed for fractures of the enamel and dentin. If the crown is mobile, a root fracture is likely. The status of the tooth pulp relative to the fracture should be assessed. Each tooth should be checked for intrusion or displacement. Anterior teeth can be intruded superiorly along the long axis of the tooth. Significant information can be gained through the auditory and tactile response when tapping on the crown of involved teeth. Mechanical, thermal, and electric testing can be performed to determine pulpal vitality.

Dentoalveolar Trauma

Crown fractures represent more than half of dental injuries.[28] Root fractures can involve any portion of the root. When making a decision about treatment, it is essential to determine the location of the fracture. Both a luxation injury and an alveolar process fracture can present like a root fracture.[29]

Patients with root fractures will typically present with the displacement of the tooth and pain on biting. An undiagnosed root fracture will result in continued pain.

If a root fracture is suspected, then a radiograph can be taken at an appropriate angle to demonstrate the fracture line. A radiograph will most predictably disclose the fracture if the central beam is directed within a maximum of a 15- to 20-degree deviation from the fracture plane. A fracture in the apical one third will most likely be seen with an occlusal radiograph, whereas bisecting-angle radiographs are best for disclosing more coronally located fractures.

The location of the root fracture determines the treatment and the possible prognosis. The healing of the fracture line with calcified tissue is the optimal outcome. The prognosis is best for teeth with only slight fragment dislocation or immature root formation.[30,31]

If the fracture is at the gingival margin, the tooth is best managed by removing the crown. The tooth can possibly be restored by placing a post and orthodontically extruding the root, and this should be followed by coronal restoration. Fractures that are between 5 mm below the alveolar bone and the apex may be considered for conservative management. An apically positioned fracture with minimal displacement and little mobility may not require splinting. Displacement should be immediately reduced with apical pressure, and an acid-etch or resin splint may then be applied. Clinical studies are not available to recommend a splinting time that will allow for healing. However, the splint should be maintained for 2 to 3 months.

Regardless of the approach taken with a root fracture, the patient must be educated with regard to the importance of dental hygiene. The patient should keep the splint and the remaining teeth clean. Without proper dental hygiene, gingival inflammation may lead to the destruction of the periodontal apparatus and the apical migration of the periodontal attachment, a complication that could result in tooth loss.

Root resorption is a possible complication after root fracture. Root resorption can be classified as either root surface resorption or root canal resorption. Root surface resorption is also known as *external root resorption,* and it occurs most commonly after intrusive injuries. Root canal resorption, which occurs less commonly, is also known as *internal root resorption.* After dentoalveolar injuries, patients should be followed closely by their dentist to identify and potentially treat these complications of root fractures. Avulsion (the complete displacement of the tooth) is very common among pediatric patients sustaining dentoalveolar trauma. Typically these injuries involve maxillary central incisors.

The viability of the tooth will depend on the periodontal cells that remain on the root surface. These cells can be maintained by placing the tooth in either Hanks balanced salt solution (Biosure, Grass Valley, CA) or ViaSpan (DuPont Pharmaceuticals, Wilmington, DE). Other solutions that can serve as storage material are milk, saline, and saliva.

Early replantation and stabilization for 7 to 10 days are critical for tooth viability (Figure 24-7). The critical time for tooth replantation is not entirely clear, but it is likely in the range of 1 to 2 hours. Replantation failures can occur early or late. Late failures are typically manifested as root resorption. Fractures involving the alveolar process should be digitally reduced and rigidly stabilized for approximately 4 weeks to allow for bone healing. If the fracture is apical to the tooth roots, then the pulpal blood supply will likely be maintained. For cases in which the fracture runs through the tooth roots and the alveolar process, the risk for internal or external resorption is high.

Mandible Fracture

The management of the teeth in the line of fracture can be a source of complication in the management of a mandibular fracture. Mandibular fractures associated with teeth are associated with a higher rate of infection as compared with fractures in edentulous areas.[32]

Contamination of the fracture occurs through an infected pulp chamber as a result of caries or the migration of saliva and oral bacteria through a disrupted periodontal ligament. Caries is responsible for 83% of mandibular fracture infections associated with the teeth in the line of fracture.[33] If the teeth are to be retained, the rate of infection can be reduced with the administration of antibiotics. The retention of teeth

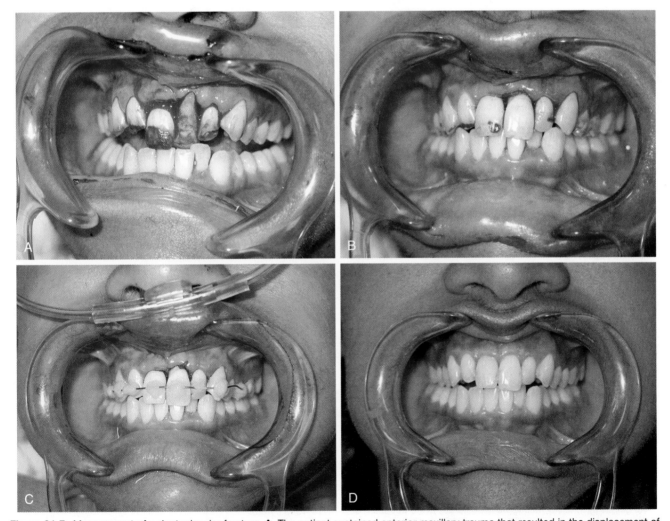

Figure 24-7. Management of a dentoalveolar fracture. **A,** The patient sustained anterior maxillary trauma that resulted in the displacement of the central incisors and the left lateral incisor. **B,** Digital pressure was used to reduce the maxillary teeth. Care was taken to reestablish the preinjury occlusion. **C,** A rigid wire was used with acrylic to splint the teeth together for 10 days. **D,** Three months after the removal of the splint, all teeth remained vital, and the final occlusion was appropriate. (Courtesy of Dr. Brian Bast, San Francisco, Calif.)

can aid in the stabilization of the fracture. Furthermore, the removal of impacted molars can produce significant distraction of the fracture and lead to an open fracture by tearing the mucosa. If there is no clear evidence of caries, periapical radiolucency, significant periodontal disease, or root fracture, then a tooth in the line of a mandible fracture should most likely be retained.[34,35]

One of the primary complications of the management of a mandible fracture is malocclusion. Maxillary and mandibular arch bars are required to establish the occlusion before addressing the fractured segments. When tightening the intermaxillary fixation, care must taken to not overtighten the wires. Because the arch bars are on the buccal aspect of the occlusion, such overtightening causes the buccal displacement of the inferior border and the decreased lingual contact of bone.[36] Accurate contouring of the plate is required to prevent malocclusion. The rigidity of rigid fixation plates leads to a higher rate of malocclusion when using rigid internal fixation.[37,38] Minor occlusal discrepancies can be corrected during the postoperative period with elastics when semiflexible systems are used.[39] With rigid fixation systems, however, the use of elastics will result in tooth movement. Therefore a significant malocclusion after the repair of a mandible fracture with rigid fixation will require reoperation.

REFERENCES

1. Duke RL, Campbell BH, Indresano AT, et al: Dental status and quality of life in long-term head and neck cancer survivors. *Laryngoscope* 2005;115:678.
2. Marx RE: Pamidronate (Aredia) and zoledronate (Zometa) induced avascular necrosis of the jaws: A growing epidemic. *J Oral Maxillofac Surg* 2003;61:1115.
3. Ruggiero SL, Mehrotra B, Rosenberg TJ, et al: Osteonecrosis of the jaws associated with the use of bisphosphonates: A review of 63 cases. *J Oral Maxillofac Surg* 2004;62:527.
4. Hillner BE, Ingle JN, Berenson JR, et al: American Society of Clinical Oncology guideline on the role of bisphosphonates in breast cancer: American Society of Clinical Oncology Bisphosphonates expert panel. *J Clin Oncol* 2000;18:1378.
5. Berenson JR, Hillner BE, Kyle RA, et al: American Society of Clinical Oncology clinical practice guidelines: The role of bisphosphonates in multiple myeloma. *J Clin Oncol* 2002;20:3719.
6. Marx RE, Sawatari Y, Fortin M, et al: Bisphosphonate-induced exposed bone (osteonecrosis/osteopetrosis) of the jaws: Risk factors, recognition, prevention, and treatment. *J Oral Maxillofac Surg* 2005;63:1567.
7. Marx RE, Stern D: *Oral and maxillofacial pathology: A rationale for diagnosis and treatment,* Chicago, 2003, Quintessence Pub Co, p vi.
8. Eisbruch A, Kim HM, Terrell JE, et al: Xerostomia and its predictors following parotid-sparing irradiation of head-and-neck cancer. *Int J Radiat Biol Phys* 2001;50:695.
9. Saarilahti K, Kouri M, Collan J, et al: Sparing of the submandibular glands by intensity modulated radiotherapy in the treatment of head and neck cancer. *Radiother Oncol* 2006;78:270.
10. Pacholke HD, Amdur RJ, Morris CG, et al: Late xerostomia after intensity-modulated radiation therapy versus conventional radiotherapy. *Am J Clin Oncol* 2005;28:351.
11. Scarantino C, LeVeque F, Swann RS, et al: Effect of pilocarpine during radiation therapy: Results of RTOG 97-09, a phase III randomized study in head and neck cancer patients. *J Support Oncol* 2006;4:252.
12. Brizel DM, Wasserman TH, Henke M, et al: Phase III randomized trial of amifostine as a radioprotector in head and neck cancer. *J Clin Oncol* 2000;18:3339.
13. Wasserman T, Mackowiak JI, Brizel DM, et al: Effect of amifostine on patient assessed clinical benefit in irradiated head and neck cancer. *Int J Radiat Oncol Biol Phys* 2000;48:1035.
14. Jellema AP, Slotman BJ, Muller MJ, et al: Radiotherapy alone, versus radiotherapy with amifostine 3 times weekly, versus radiotherapy with amifostine 5 times weekly: A prospective randomized study in squamous cell head and neck cancer. *Cancer* 2006;107:544.
15. Marx RE, Johnson RP, Kline SN: Prevention of osteoradionecrosis: A randomized prospective clinical trial of hyperbaric oxygen versus penicillin. *J Am Dent Assoc* 1985;111:49.
16. Thorn JJ, Hansen HS, Specht L, et al: Osteoradionecrosis of the jaws: Clinical characteristics and relation to the field of irradiation. *J Oral Maxillofac Surg* 2000;58:1088.
17. Beumer J, Harrison R, Sanders B, et al: Osteoradionecrosis: Predisposing factors and outcomes of therapy. *Head Neck Surg* 1984;6:819.
18. Schwartz HC, Kagan AR: Osteoradionecrosis of the mandible: Scientific basis for clinical staging. *Am J Clin Oncol* 2002;25:168.
19. Marx RE: A new concept in the treatment of osteoradionecrosis. *J Oral Maxillofac Surg* 1983;41:351.
20. Epstein JB, Wong FL, Stevenson-Moore P: Osteoradionecrosis: Clinical experience and a proposal for classification. *J Oral Maxillofac Surg* 1987;45:104.
21. Myers RA, Marx RE: Use of hyperbaric oxygen in postradiation head and neck surgery. *NCI Monogr* 1990;(9):151.
22. McKenzie MR, Wong FL, Epstein JB, et al: Hyperbaric oxygen and postradiation osteonecrosis of the mandible. *Eur J Cancer B Oral Oncol* 1993;29B:201.
23. Epstein J, van der Meij E, McKenzie M, et al: Postradiation osteonecrosis of the mandible: A long-term follow-up study. *Oral Surg Oral Med Oral Pathol Oral Radiol Endod* 1997;83:657.
24. van Merkesteyn JP, Bakker DJ, Borgmeijer-Hoelen AM: Hyperbaric oxygen treatment of osteoradionecrosis of the mandible: Experience in 29 patients. *Oral Surg Oral Med Oral Pathol Oral Radiol Endod* 1995;80:12.
25. Rogers SN, O'Donnell J P, Williams-Hewitt S, et al: Health-related quality of life measured by the UW-QoL—Reference values from a general dental practice. *Oral Oncol* 2006;42:281.
26. Dubner S, Spiro RH: Median mandibulotomy: A critical assessment. *Head Neck* 1991;13:389.
27. Fernandez Sanroman J, Gomez Gonzalez JM, Alonso Del Hoyo J, et al: Morphometric and morphological changes in the temporomandibular joint after orthognathic surgery: A magnetic resonance imaging and computed tomography prospective study. *J Craniomaxillofac Surg* 1997;25:139.
28. Andreasen JO, Andreasen FM: *Essentials of traumatic injuries to the teeth: A step-by-step treatment guide,* ed 2, Copenhagen, 2000, Munksgaard, p 188.
29. Andreasen FM, Andreasen JO: Diagnosis of luxation injuries: The importance of standardized clinical, radiographic and photographic techniques in clinical investigations. *Endod Dent Traumatol* 1985;1:160.
30. Jacobsen I: Root fractures in permanent anterior teeth with incomplete root formation. *Scand J Dent Res* 1976;84:210.
31. Zachrisson BU, Jacobsen I: Long-term prognosis of 66 permanent anterior teeth with root fracture. *Scand J Dent Res* 1975;83:345.
32. Passeri LA, Ellis E 3rd, Sinn DP: Complications of nonrigid fixation of mandibular angle fractures. *J Oral Maxillofac Surg* 1993;51:382.
33. Melmed EP, Koonin AJ: Fractures of the mandible: A review of 909 cases. *Plast Reconstr Surg* 1975;56:323.
34. Neal DC, Wagner WF, Alpert B: Morbidity associated with teeth in the line of mandibular fractures. *J Oral Surg* 1978;36:859.

35. Marker P, Eckerdal A, Smith-Sivertsen C: Incompletely erupted third molars in the line of mandibular fractures: A retrospective analysis of 57 cases. *Oral Surg Oral Med Oral Pathol* 1994;78:426.

36. Ellis E 3rd, Tharanon W: Facial width problems associated with rigid fixation of mandibular fractures: Case reports. *J Oral Maxillofac Surg* 1992;50:87.

37. Theriot BA, Van Sickels JE, Triplett RG, et al: Intraosseous wire fixation versus rigid osseous fixation of mandibular fractures: A preliminary report. *J Oral Maxillofac Surg* 1987;45:577.

38. Zachariades N, Papademetriou I, Rallis G: Complications associated with rigid internal fixation of facial bone fractures. *J Oral Maxillofac Surg* 1993;51:275.

39. Schilli W: Compression osteosynthesis. *J Oral Surg* 1977;35:802.

CHAPTER 25

Complications in Cleft Lip and Palate Surgery

Jennifer L. Rhodes and David Alan Staffenberg

The successful repair of a cleft lip and palate requires a thorough understanding of the deformity and craniofacial growth as well as the implementation of sound plastic surgery principles and judgment (Figure 25-1). When the repair falls short of expectation, a secondary deformity results, and revision may be indicated. Even for cases in which the deformity may be well understood and strict adherence to plastic surgery principles is assured, the growth of the repair may not match that of the child, and a secondary deformity will result. In any case, the primary repair is the cleft surgeon's best chance of achieving the desired goals. The goals of cleft lip and palate surgery include the following:

1. A symmetric lip with a natural-appearing cupid's bow and continuity of the orbicularis oris muscle

2. A fully intact palate reconstruction

3. The repair of the levator veli palatini with the competence of the velopharyngeal closure for speech

4. A united alveolar arch that allows for the retention of permanent dentition

5. Normal dental occlusion

6. A normal relationship of the maxilla and mandible with each other as well as with the lips and nose

7. A straight nose with an open airway

Virtually all cleft lip and palate deformities undergo primary repair during infancy to minimize early functional problems and to assist with social acceptance and maternal bonding. Complications of cleft lip and palate surgery include the following:

1. Direct complications of the surgery, including complications of wound healing

2. Deformities that result from primary repair, including suboptimal functioning

Patient expectations are high, and secondary corrections are often more challenging than the initial repair as a result of the presence of scar and further distortion of the abnormal anatomy. A cleft lip repair should ultimately be unrecognizable by a peer at conversational distance. The goal of a palate repair is the separation of the oral and nasal cavities to eliminate the nasal regurgitation of fluids while also allowing for the production of normal speech.

Before formulating a plan for treatment, a detailed and systematic evaluation of the child must be performed. Although many cleft lip and palate patients have an isolated defect, associated anomalies do occur, and a thorough examination of the entire body is mandatory. When treating these children, their feeding ability, dentition, hearing, speech, and psychosocial development require frequent monitoring by professionals from several disciplines. It is crucial that a multidisciplinary cleft lip and palate team collaborate in this comprehensive evaluation and that they also provide the ongoing treatment to maximize the continuity of care.

As a point of reference, the general timeline for the management of the typical cleft lip and palate should be as follows: cleft lips are repaired in a single stage at 2 to 3 months of age, and cleft palates are repaired in a single stage at 8 to 9 months of age.

EARLY COMPLICATIONS OF CLEFT REPAIR

Early complications of cleft lip and palate repair include bleeding, respiratory obstruction, wound infection, and dehiscence. Noteworthy bleeding is extremely unusual, but it may lead to respiratory compromise, so immediate attention is required and may necessitate an immediate return to the operating room. Respiratory obstruction is also quite rare, but a careful postoperative assessment must be made before transferring children from the recovery room. Children with other anomalies like Robin sequence are predisposed to airway obstruction and must be carefully evaluated. Wound healing problems are also uncommonly seen.

Robin Sequence

Careful evaluation and planning are crucial to securing optimal form and function while also minimizing morbidity and mortality. Managing the cleft palate in an infant with Robin sequence is a special challenge in terms of surgical timing, the possible need for additional surgery, and technical issues of the repair itself. Nasopharyngoscopy while the patient is awake is essential to evaluate the patency of the airway. In cases of Robin sequence with severe micrognathia, glossoptosis, and upper airway obstruction, a variety of procedures are available to address the airway. Typically tracheostomies are performed. In the authors' practice, other procedures are attempted that are meant to

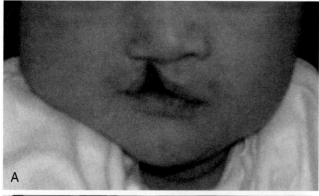

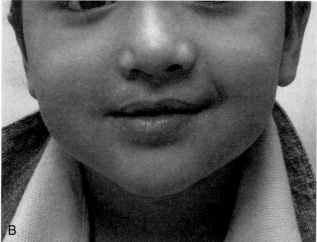

Figure 25-1. A, Incomplete right unilateral cleft lip and palate. **B,** The same patient 4 years after the primary repair of the right unilateral cleft lip by rotation advancement, cleft palate, and primary rhinoplasty.

obviate the need for tracheostomies and gastrostomies and their attendant risks as well as the resulting speech and swallowing delays. These additional procedures may include glossopexies and lip–tongue adhesions. Neonatal distraction osteogenesis for mandibular advancement is gaining in popularity, and the authors prefer to use internalized devices. The details of this technique are beyond the scope of this chapter, but they can be reviewed elsewhere. In less severe cases of Robin sequence with mild to moderate micrognathia, positioning the child in the decubitus or prone position or placing a soft nasopharyngeal tube may be adequate for short-term airway management. Because repair of the cleft palate itself may contribute to the airway obstruction in such cases, the palatoplasty is occasionally delayed until the child is 18 months old.

Wound Infection

Wound infection among these patients is quite rare, but it may require a course of antibiotics. Dehiscence is also quite unusual, but it can be expected when inadequate dissection and mobilization are performed and excessive tension is placed on the repair. The key to

successful cleft surgery is the amount of mobilization of soft tissue that is possible while preserving vascularity. In the rare case of a dehiscence that is recognized during the immediate postoperative period, a return to the operating room should be considered so that further mobilization can minimize the excessive tension. Beyond the immediate postoperative period, the dehiscence should be allowed to heal by secondary intention. When the induration is resolved (typically 6 weeks later), the resulting deformity can be repaired.

SECONDARY DEFORMITIES

Secondary deformities may be seen immediately after the primary repair or after a period of growth. It is evident that the deformity must be recognized and properly diagnosed to allow for its correction. The evaluation of a secondary deformity of a cleft lip must be done carefully, because the successful correction of secondary deformities is frequently more challenging than the primary repair. The correction of secondary deformities is considered for all age groups. A delay in presentation is frequently seen, because many cleft patients have been incorrectly told that any improvement after the initial repair is not possible. Needless to say, this misinformation is quite distressing.

Evaluation

The physical examination of the child's face in both repose and animation is central to the accurate diagnosis of any secondary deformity. The status of the soft tissue, muscle, and bone must be assessed. The lips are scrutinized for an unnatural appearance, any vertical or horizontal asymmetries, the misalignment of the white roll (or the vermilion–cutaneous junction), any distortion of the Cupid's bow, deficiency of the tubercle or the philtral column, a notch or whistle deformity, an insufficient vestibule, or cosmetically unacceptable scarring. The alignment and repair of the orbicularis oris musculature can be evaluated by asking the patient to purse the lips or whistle; the muscle will bulge on either side of the repair site when it is not in continuity. The nasal evaluation should assess the adequacy of the airway, the symmetry of the nostrils and their bases, the nasal tip, any deviation of the septum, the presence of a vestibular web, the length of the columella, and the adequacy of the lining. The palate should be inspected for the presence of fistula. The findings must be correlated with any underlying skeletal deformity, because maxillary hypoplasia or malposition contributes significantly to the secondary problems that are commonly seen.[1]

When the deformity has been defined, the cause of the deformity must be diagnosed. It may result from inherently dysmorphic tissues or uncorrected or undercorrected components of the original deformity, or it may be iatrogenic in nature.

An integrated treatment plan can now be developed with input from the entire cleft lip and palate team. The following basic guidelines, which are also applied to the primary repair, will help ensure optimal results[2]:

- Know the normal anatomy.
- Return the normal landmarks to their normal positions.
- Do not remove any tissue until it is absolutely certain that it will not be useful.
- Rearrange excess tissue to supplement deficient areas.
- Replace lost tissue with similar tissue whenever possible.
- Treat each case individually.

Secondary Lip Deformities

Timing

The timing of the surgery is an important variable in a growing child as opposed to a mature patient. The expected pattern of growth and the development of each facial component must be considered, and any interference with growth must be minimized. Functional problems such as difficulties with speech or eating should be addressed expediently. In addition, the severity of the deformity will affect the psychosocial development of the child and must be considered. Although the initial repair is generally performed during the first year of life, secondary repairs are commonly performed just before the child starts school to minimize any psychosocial concerns. Children are especially vulnerable at school age, because peer interactions begin to develop. The final surgery usually takes place during adolescence, when craniofacial growth is complete, because teens become even more self-aware and more vocal with regard to their appearance.[3]

Most secondary corrections in young children are performed under general anesthesia to allow for careful planning and marking. As with the initial repair, landmarks are identified, marked in ink, and tattooed with methylene blue and a 25-gauge needle before local infiltration. A combination of 0.5% lidocaine and 1:200,000 epinephrine provides a "dry" field as a result of hemostasis and postoperative analgesia.

Horizontal Excess

Horizontal excess can be seen after a bilateral cleft lip repair and occurs when the dimensions of the new philtrum were designed to be too wide during the primary repair. If the orbicularis oris muscle fibers are not reunited during the initial surgical repair, a gradual widening of the philtrum will occur. Correction involves the alignment of the muscular fibers and the resection of

sufficient lip tissue so that the resulting scars simulate the philtral columns. The new philtrum should be designed to be slightly narrower than ultimately desired in anticipation of continued stretching.

Tight Lip and/or Horizontal Deficiency

The appearance of a tight lip after cleft lip repair is often accentuated by underlying maxillary hypoplasia. Care must be taken to distinguish between maxillary retrusion (requiring a maxillary osteotomy and advancement) and a horizontal soft-tissue deficiency of the lip. A tight upper lip is more common after repair of a bilateral cleft lip, which can be caused by a congenital deficiency of tissue or overresection during the primary repair (Figure 25-2).

For a significant deformity, an Abbe flap is an excellent solution, and it will simulate the philtrum and tubercle when it is placed in the midline.[4-6] The use of the lower lip flap helps to minimize the disproportion of the lips by reducing the relative excess of the lower lip while augmenting the upper lip. The skin flap should be designed to fit the dimensions of a normal philtrum. Up to one third of the lower lip's length can be harvested, using the labial vessels for the blood supply. Ivy loops can be used to protect the flap from disruption; they can be tied loosely enough to allow the child to insert a spoon or straw while preventing the overstretching of the pedicle. The pedicle is usually divided 7 to 10 days later at the time of the septorhinoplasty.

Long Lip/Vertical Excess

The term *lip length* refers to the distance from the Cupid's bow to the base of the columella. A disproportionately long upper lip in the vertical dimension is frequently

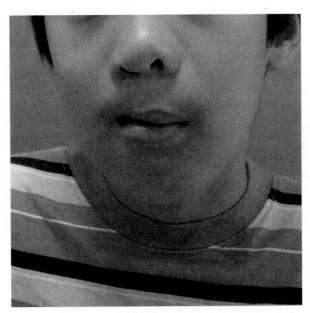

Figure 25-2. Severe deficiency of the right lateral lip element after rotation–advancement repair referred for correction.

seen after a bilateral cleft lip repair. When anatomic landmarks are minimally distorted, correction may be achieved by a full-thickness horizontal excision of tissue from the perialar region.[7]

It is very unusual for a rotation–advancement repair to produce a lip with vertical excess. However, when this is seen, it is usually the result of overrotation during the initial repair, and it may be corrected by the takedown of the repair with partial derotation of the medial segment. It may be necessary to shorten the vertical height of the lateral element to match the new rotation edge. This is accomplished by a horizontal excision under the alar base.[2]

Short Lip and/or Vertical Deficiency

When the distance of the Cupid's bow to the base of the columella or ala is deficient as compared with the noncleft side, it is said to be "short." If the disparity is very minor, a diamond-shaped excision, reopening the scar with a back cut, or a Z-plasty may be sufficient.[3] With unilateral repairs, a severe discrepancy is usually the result of a failure to adequately lengthen the lip at the primary repair. It is most frequently seen after a straight-line repair, such as those described by Rose-Thompson.[8] The excision of the scarred tissue and re-repair with the rotation–advancement technique usually corrects the problem (Figure 25-3).

A common myth is that a short cleft lip repair will improve with time; however, if inadequate lip length is achieved in the operating room, it will *not* improve with time. Alternatively, if proper symmetry was achieved during the repair, a temporary vertical deficiency may be seen, and it is usually maximal at 6 to 8 weeks after surgery. This is the result of scar contracture during the inflammatory phase of wound healing, and it will resolve with the maturation of the wound as long as the

muscular elements of the initial repair were performed correctly.[9] If this relaxation does not occur and the discrepancy is severe, the cause is likely to be the inadequate rotation of the medial lip element or an incomplete muscular repair at the initial operation. The repair must be reopened and any abnormal muscular attachments taken down. The upper fibers of the orbicularis should be anchored to the periosteum of the nasal spine, the horizontal fibers should be united across the cleft, and the lower fibers should be directed into the tubercle. After the muscular repair is completed, rerotation of the medial lip element is recommended.[2] A short lip can also be seen after rotation–advancement repairs of extremely wide clefts (Figure 25-4). Orthopedic treatment or lip adhesion in anticipation of the primary repair may be used to reduce the likelihood of this condition.[10,11]

A short lip after a bilateral cleft lip repair is uncommon and may be the result of an inadequate muscle repair, partial muscle dehiscence, or a greater deficiency of tissue. Although Z-plasties and V-Y advancements may provide length, an Abbe flap may provide the best correction.[4]

Tight Lip and/or Horizontal Deficiency

In the noncleft individual, the upper lip is more prominent than the lower lip. When the horizontal length of the upper lip is deficient as compared with the lower lip, it is considered tight. It must be stressed again that all of the tissues must be evaluated properly. The upper lip will appear to be less prominent than the lower when there is maxillary retrusion. This condition may be seen when the tension of the cleft lip repair restricts the subsequent sagittal growth of the maxilla, thereby leading to malocclusion. The malocclusion is usually corrected at skeletal maturity with a maxillary osteotomy. A tight upper lip is usually the result of a bilateral cleft lip. The

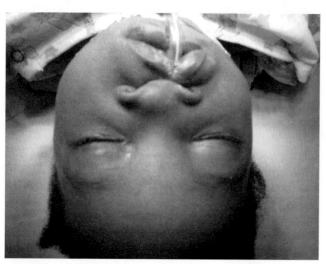

Figure 25-3. Extremely short lip resulting from a right unilateral cleft lip repair.

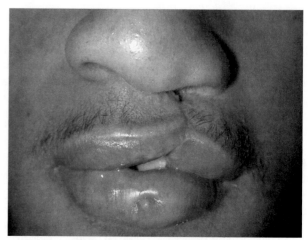

Figure 25-4. Short lip with a misalignment of the Cupid's bow and a notch at the free border of the vermilion after the rotation–advancement repair of a left unilateral cleft lip.

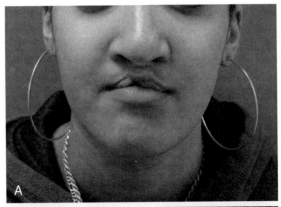

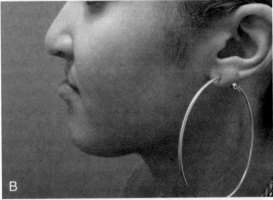

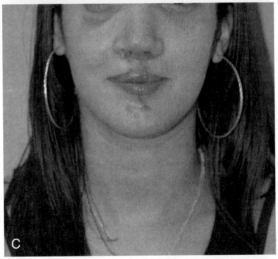

Figure 25-5. A and **B,** Horizontally tight upper lip after the repair of a bilateral cleft lip and primary rhinoplasty by another surgeon. **C,** The same patient 20 days after secondary rhinoplasty and division and the inset of an Abbe flap.

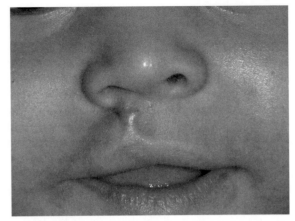

Figure 25-6. Red, raised, thick scar approximately 5 weeks after a right unilateral cleft lip repair.

the lateral advancement flap is used to fill the entire defect produced by the rotation of the medial segment, an oblique scar is produced that crosses the natural location of the philtral column. However, the C-flap is brought under the columella to fill this defect, and the resulting scar is oriented in a more vertical position, precisely where one would expect to find the contralateral philtral column.[12]

Keloid scars are rare in cleft repair, although hypopigmented, hypertrophic, or widened scars are the cause of some disappointment. It is not uncommon for scars to become red, raised, and firm during the weeks after surgery, and the authors encourage the use of paper tape for 3 months postoperatively (Figure 25-6). Sunscreen on the maturing scar is also employed. Wide scars may be seen after any repair technique, and they may require revision for satisfactory improvement. It is important to understand that a widened scar may be the result of an inadequate muscle repair across the cleft and that a full-thickness revision may be required. For hypertrophic scars, dermabrasion has been used with varying results. The erbium-doped yttrium aluminum garnet laser or the pulsed dye (i.e., 585-nm) laser may helpful for hypertrophic or erythematous scars.[13,14]

MISPLACED OR ABSENT LIP LANDMARKS

Deformities of the Vermilion Border and the White Roll

It is critical that the peaks of the Cupid's bow be at the same height as the contralateral side, because the misalignment of the vermilion border or the white roll by as little as 1 mm is noticeable at conversational distance.[3] The surgical recreation of the peaks of the Cupid's bow can be accomplished with a Gillies procedure, which consists of a triangular excision above the white line that is then closed horizontally.[15]

lower lip appears to be relatively prominent, but proper correction is directed to the upper lip rather than just performing a lower lip reduction. The Abbe flap is most useful for these cases (Figure 25-5).

Unfavorable Scars

The position and orientation of a scar dictates its esthetic impact, and careful planning at the time of primary repair is critical to optimize cosmesis. During rotation–advancement procedures, for example, when

Vermilion Deformities

Vermilion deformities may be caused by the inadequate approximation of the marginal portion of the deep orbicularis at the primary repair, but they may also result from the excessive resection of the vermilion border. The most common secondary deformity seen is a notch or whistle deformity at the free vermilion border of the repair site. Other deformities include deficiencies of the central tubercle or the lateral vermilion border (Figure 25-7). Vermilion deficiencies are more commonly seen after bilateral cleft repairs as a result of inherent tissue deficiency.

In the case of a very mild notching, when the lateral lip element appears to have a relative excess of vermilion, a horizontal elliptical excision at the wet–dry border may be all that is required. A V-Y or a double V-Y advancement is often a useful technique. When a paucity of vermilion is present, options for reconstruction include a free tongue graft from the lateral aspect of the tongue (harvested below the papillary line) or a pedicled tongue flap from the tip.[6,16] Major deficiencies will require a vermilion flap from the lower lip or a cross-lip flap.[3,17,18] A Kapetansky flap (i.e., a musculomucosal pendulum flap) using local transposition flaps may also be appropriate.[2,19]

Misalignment of the vermilion border, which is known as "red flare," is usually corrected with a Z-plasty.[2] If further augmentation is required, a tunnel can be created along the horizontal length of the tubercle at the junction of the dry and wet mucosa in the plane that is superficial to the orbicularis oris muscle. Temporoparietal fascia, dermal fat grafts, acellular allogeneic dermis, and fat injections have all been used reliably and can provide a natural appearance.[3,20–22]

BONE GRAFTING OF THE ALVEOLUS

Postoperative complications can occur, and the bone graft may become exposed as a result of poorly designed or executed flaps with poor blood supply, excessive tension, mobility of the maxillary segments, or trauma. Avoidance of these complications is the best approach and includes meticulous attention to oral hygiene preoperatively and immobilization of the premaxilla with orthodontic bands or arch bars. Intentionally collapsing or avoiding expansion at the level of the alveolar cleft increases the success of the soft-tissue coverage of the bone grafts. When the exposure of the bone graft is apparent, conservative therapy consisting of antibiotics and soft diet may minimize graft loss.[23] Even with uneventful healing, some graft resorption may occur, which results in a notching of the alveolus or a recurrence of the nasolabial fistula, and further surgery is required for correction (Figure 25-8). Secondary surgery, when needed, is recommended no earlier than 6 weeks after the primary surgery.

RESIDUAL SKELETAL DEFORMITIES

The correction of a skeletal deformity in the maxilla of cleft lip and palate patients requires close cooperation between the surgeon and the orthodontist. Although the

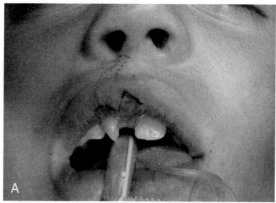
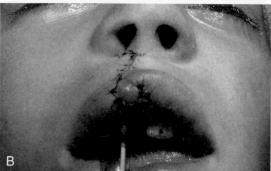

Figure 25-7. A, Secondary deformity of a right unilateral cleft after rotation–advancement repair. Note the irregularity of the wet–dry vermilion. The plan for an asymmetric Z-plasty correction is shown in ink. **B,** The same patient seen at the completion of the revision. Note the corrected alignment of the vermilion. Some distortion as a result of local infiltration is seen.

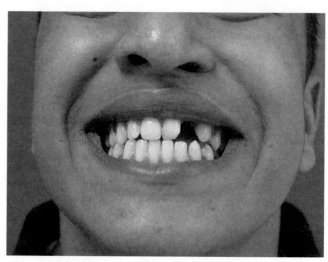

Figure 25-8. A patient referred for alveolar bone grafting after the primary attempt failed.

clinical presentation is variable, the maxilla of these children is frequently deficient in both the vertical and the anteroposterior dimensions. Concomitant nasal, mandibular, or chin abnormalities frequently exist as well, and a complete evaluation is crucial. Cephalometric examination allows for a comparison with age- and sex-matched controls, and it is essential for planning. Complications of orthognathic surgery include hemorrhage, infection, segmental necrosis, relapse, injury to dentition, persistent malocclusion, and hypernasal speech. This topic is beyond the scope of this chapter.

ORONASAL FISTULAS

Oronasal fistulas of as small as 5 mm may result in regurgitation, halitosis, poor oral hygiene, gingival and mucosal irritation, and problems with the development of normal speech.[24] Surprisingly, the reported incidence is as high as 20%. The most common locations are the incisive foramen and the junction of the hard and soft palate. A basic principle of fistula repair is that the flaps be designed to be relatively large in size to maximize their blood supply and to allow for closure with minimal tension. A two-layered closure is preferred. Lining flaps are usually obtained from the nasal cavity or the vomer, although turnover flaps are often the most useful. The palatal mucoperiosteum on one side is turned over to provide closure of the nasal lining, and a mucoperiosteal flap is transposed from the contralateral side to close the oral lining. If the surgeon is unable to maximize the vascularity of the flap and minimize tension, recurrence of the fistula is likely. The greater the number of attempts at closure, the higher the likelihood of failure with regional palatal tissue.[25]

The closure of larger oronasal fistulae remains a frustrating problem as a result of the paucity of local tissue (Figure 25-9). The use of regional tissues (e.g., tongue flaps, facial artery musculomucosal flaps) has been successful.[26,27] Temporalis flaps have also been applied to large palatal fistulae.[28] For extreme cases, free-tissue transfer may be necessary. Finally, an obturator can be constructed by a prosthodontist as a less-satisfying solution.

VELOPHARYNGEAL INCOMPETENCE

Although cleft palate repair restores anatomic continuity, some patients will develop hypernasal speech and compensatory misarticulations. Hypernasal speech may result from unrepaired cleft palates, significant oronasal fistulae, or velopharyngeal incompetence (VPI). VPI results from poor function of the levator veli palatini, from the inadequate repair or tethering of the palate, or from a deep posterior pharyngeal wall with a relatively short palate. Velopharyngeal closure may also be limited by tonsillar hypertrophy. VPI manifests with hypernasality, nasal emission, imprecise consonant production, decreased vocal intensity, and short phrases. It may also result from physiologic dysfunction (e.g., neurogenic paresis). Diagnosis is made by a speech pathologist only after a complete evaluation that includes nasoendoscopy with or without videofluoroscopy. Dynamic studies provide information about the functional anatomy of the soft palate as well as the degree of the medial and lateral excursion of the pharyngeal walls during speech.

The goal of surgical intervention among patients with VPI is to provide a mechanism for functional speech. Depending on the patient's anatomy, the surgical management of VPI usually consists of posterior pharyngeal wall augmentation, pharyngeal flap, sphincter pharyngoplasty, or palatal revision (Figure 25-10). When there

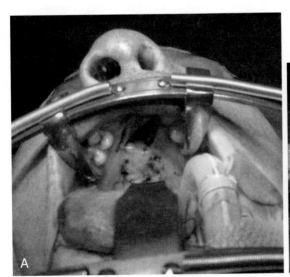
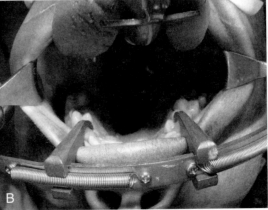

Figure 25-9. A, Anterior oronasal fistula in combination with an ungrafted alveolar cleft and a nasolabial fistula. **B,** Large oronasal fistula referred years after necrosis of the hard palate.

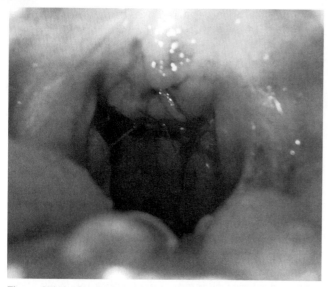

Figure 25-10. Completed sphincter pharyngoplasty (a tongue retractor is seen at the bottom of the photo).

is good mobility of the palate and the discrepancy between the palate and the posterior wall of the pharynx is small, palatal lengthening with a Furlow double-opposing Z-plasty may provide adequate palatal length to eliminate the VPI. [29–31]

When the soft palate is short as a result of intrinsic tissue deficiency or scarring and when it has poor mobility, a superiorly based musculomucosal flap is commonly employed. The flap is developed from the posterior pharyngeal wall incorporating the superior constrictor muscle, turned anteriorly at the tubercle of the atlas, and inset into the dorsum of the soft palate.[32] The nasopharynx is now obturated centrally, and velopharyngeal competence depends on the adequate medial excursion of the lateral pharyngeal wall. Because the amount of excursion is established from preoperative dynamic studies, the width of the flap can be individually tailored. If the flap is too narrow, the correction of VPI will not be achieved. If the flap is too wide, the patient can become a mouth breather, exhibiting hyponasality and possibly developing obstructive sleep apnea. Immediate postoperative complications include bleeding and airway obstruction; therefore the authors observe patients overnight after surgery in an intensive care unit setting. Patients with velocardiofacial syndrome may have anomalies of the carotid arteries that may cause these arteries to be damaged during pharyngeal flap elevation. Preoperative magnetic resonance angiography and careful palpation of the posterior pharyngeal wall before incision are recommended.[33]

For patients with either poor medial excursion or paradoxic movement of the lateral pharyngeal wall and good mobility of the palate on the basis of nasopharyngoscopy, a sphincter pharyngoplasty may be used. The

technique that is most commonly used today elevates superiorly based flaps bilaterally from the posterior tonsillar pillars, including the palatopharyngeus muscle. The flaps are brought across the posterior pharyngeal wall in a transverse incision at the caudal edge of the adenoid and sutured together to augment the Passavant ridge and to produce a central sphincter that is no more than 5 mm in diameter. Although the circumferential area of the nasopharynx is decreased by the operation, the newly created sphincter provides dynamic function for most patients.[34]

DISCUSSION

The optimal care of cleft lip and palate patients requires careful planning during the initial repair to minimize secondary deformities and functional limitations. The surgeon must be able to identify potential complications before they occur, to recognize complications when they do occur, and to institute a plan to correct them. In cleft surgery, both form and function are paramount; growth adds a unique dimension to the care of these patients. Because of the changes that may occur with growth, these patients must be followed until craniofacial maturity. The importance of caring for these patients throughout in an organized multidisciplinary cleft lip and palate team cannot be overemphasized. The regular surveillance of each patient's progress by this team of professionals will promptly identify secondary deformities and allow for an individualized plan for their correction.

REFERENCES

1. Bardach J, Salyer KE: Correction of secondary unilateral cleft lip deformities. In Bardach J, Salyer KE, editors: *Surgical techniques in cleft lip and palate,* Chicago, 1987, Yearbook Medical Publishers.
2. Millard DR Jr: *Cleft craft—The evolution of its surgery. I: The unilateral deformity,* Boston, 1976, Little, Brown.
3. Staffenberg DA, Wood RJ: Secondary deformities of cleft lip repair. In Aston S, Beasley R, Thorne C, editors: *Grabb and Smith's plastic surgery,* ed 5, Philadelphia, 1997, Lippincott-Raven Publishers.
4. Abbé R: A new plastic operation for the relief of deformity due to double harelip. *Med Rec* 1898;53:477.
5. Schuh FD, Crikelair GF, Cosman B: A critical appraisal of the Abbé flap in secondary cleft lip deformity. *Br J Plast Surg* 1970;23:142.
6. Millard DR Jr: *Cleft craft—The evolution of its surgery. II: Bilateral and rare deformities,* Boston, 1977, Little, Brown.
7. Webster JP: Crescentic peri-alar cheek excision for upper lip flap advancement with a short history of upper lip repair. *Plast Reconstr Surg* 1955;16:434.
8. Thompson JE: An artistic and mathematically accurate method of repairing the defect in cases of harelip. *Surg Gynecol Obstet* 1912;14:498.
9. Millard DR Jr: Unilateral cleft lip deformity. In McCarthy JF, editor: *Plastic surgery,* vol 4, Philadelphia, 1990, WB Saunders.
10. Millard DR Jr, Latham RA: Improved primary surgical and dental treatment of clefts. *Plast Reconstr Surg* 1990;86:856.
11. Grayson BH, Cutting CB: Presurgical nasoalveolar orthopedic molding in primary correction of the nose, lip, and alveolus of infants born with unilateral and bilateral clefts. *Cleft Palate Craniofac J* 2001;38(3):193–198.

12. Bardach J, Salyer KE: *Surgical techniques in cleft lip and palate,* ed 2, St Louis, 1991, Mosby Yearbook.

13. Nocini PF, D'Agostino A, Trevisiol L: Treatment of scars with Er: YAG laser in patients with cleft lip: A preliminary report. *Cleft Palate Craniofac J* 2003;40(5):518–522.

14. Sawcer D, Lee HR, Lowe NJ: Lasers and adjunctive treatments for facial scars: A review. *J Cutan Laser Ther* 1999;1(2):77–85.

15. Gillies H, Kilner TP: Harelip operations for the correction of secondary deformities. *Lancet* 1932;2:1369.

16. Cohen SR, Kawamoto HK Jr: The free tongue graft for correction of secondary deformities of the vermilion in patients with cleft lip. *Plast Reconstr Surg* 1991;88:613.

17. Kawamoto HK Jr: Correction of major defects of the vermilion with a cross-lip vermilion flap. *Plast Reconstr Surg* 1979;64(3): 315–318.

18. Wagner JD, Newman MH: Bipedicled axial cross-lip flap for correction of major vermilion deficiency after cleft lip repair. *Cleft Palate Craniofac J* 1994;31(2):148–151.

19. Hirano A: Tulip flap for reconstruction of the central tubercle in cleft lip patients. *Plast Reconstr Surg* 1998;102(7):2511–2512.

20. Chen PK, Noordhoff MS, Chen YR, et al: Augmentation of the free border of the lip in cleft lip patients using temporoparietal fascia. *Plast Reconstr Surg* 1995;95(5):781–789.

21. Patel IA, Hall PN: Free dermis-fat graft to correct the whistle deformity in patients with cleft lip. *Br J Plast Surg* 2004;57(2):160–164.

22. Rohrich RJ, Reagan BJ, Adams WP Jr, et al: Early results of vermilion lip augmentation using acellular allogeneic dermis: An adjunct in facial rejuvenation. *Plast Reconstr Surg* 2000;105(1): 409–416.

23. Wolfe SA, Price GW, Stuzin JM, et al: Alveolar and anterior palatal clefts. In McCarthy J, editor: *Plastic surgery,* Philadelphia, 1990, WB Saunders.

24. Bajaj AK, Wongworawat AA, Punjabi A: Management of alveolar clefts. *J Craniofac Surg* 2003;14(6):840–846.

25. Schultz RC: Cleft palate fistula repair: Improved results by the addition of bone. *Arch Otolaryngol Head Neck Surg* 1989;115(1):65–67.

26. Pribaz J, Stephens W, Crespo L, et al: A new intraoral flap: Facial artery musculomucosal (FAMM) flap. *Plast Reconstr Surg* 1992;90(3):421–429.

27. Cleft palate. In Georgiade GS, Riefkohl R, Levin LS, editors: *Plastic, maxillofacial, and reconstructive surgery,* Baltimore, 1997, Williams & Wilkins.

28. Furnas D: Temporal osteocutaneous island flaps for complete reconstruction of cleft palate defects. *Scand J Plast Reconstr Surg Hand Surg* 1987;21(1):119–128.

29. Furlow LT Jr: Furlow palatoplasty for management of velopharyngeal insufficiency: A prospective study of 148 consecutive patients (discussion). *Plast Reconstr Surg* 2005;116(1):81–84.

30. Sommerlad BC, Mehendale FV, Birch MJ, et al: Palate re-repair revisited. *Cleft Palate Craniofac J* 2002;39(3):295–307.

31. Lindsey WH, Davis PT: Correction of velopharyngeal insufficiency with Furlow palatoplasty. *Arch Otolaryngol Head Neck Surg* 1996;122(8):881–884.

32. Shprintzen RJ, Lewin ML, Croft CB, et al: A comprehensive study of pharyngeal flap surgery: Tailor made flaps. *Cleft Palate J* 1979;16(1):46–55.

33. Sloan GM: Posterior pharyngeal flap and sphincter pharyngoplasty: The state of the art. *Cleft Palate J* 2000;37(2):112–122.

34. Witt PD, Marsh JL, Arlis H, et al: Quantification of dynamic velopharyngeal port excursion following sphincter pharyngoplasty. *Plastic Reconstr Surg* 1998;101:1205–1211.

CHAPTER 26

Temporomandibular Joint Surgery

M. Anthony Pogrel

BACKGROUND

The temporomandibular joint (TMJ) is the most complex joint in the human body. It is a small joint that both hinges (in the initial mouth opening) and translates or slides forward (in the wider opening), and it is one of the only three joints in the body (the others being the knee and sternoclavicular joints) to have a meniscus or fibrocartilage to divide the joint into an upper and lower compartment. To coordinate these intricate movements, the lateral pterygoid muscle divides so that part is inserted into the anterior pole of the mandibular condyle, and a small slip of the muscle is inserted into the anterior attachment of the meniscus so that the condyle and the meniscus move in unison. As if this was not complex enough, it is also the only joint in the body where, if one side moves, the other side has no option but to move as well.

Therefore in many ways it is not surprising that it is a joint that is prone to many different types of problems. It is also, interestingly enough, the only joint in the body that is not treated primarily by orthopedic surgeons but rather by dentists or maxillofacial or head and neck surgeons.

The types of problems suffered by the TMJ include the following:
- Ankylosis
- Trauma
- Acute arthritides
- Degenerative joint disease
- Internal derangement

Ankylosis

The term *ankylosis* denotes restricted movement in the joint, and it can be bony or fibrous. Bony ankylosis often results from childhood trauma, particularly when the meniscus is damaged (e.g., intracapsular fracture) and the bone of the condyle contacts the bone of the glenoid fossa; the resultant hemarthrosis organizes and ossifies. Fibrous ankylosis is also often as a result of trauma.

Trauma

Fractures of the neck of the mandibular condyle are among the most common single type of mandibular fracture encountered today, composing approximately 20% of mandibular fractures.[1] Open reduction and internal fixation are complicated by the fact that the mandible is at its thinnest at this point, and access is made difficult by the presence of the facial nerve. Most cases are still treated with a closed reduction, and resultant malocclusion, restricted motion, or both are not uncommon. Intracapsular fractures are less common but more problematic to treat, and they may lead to ankylosis if the disc is damaged and the condyle head comes into contact with the roof of the glenoid fossa.

Acute Arthritides

Rheumatoid arthritis can affect the TMJ. It is essentially the same disease with the same symptoms as are found in other joints. The TMJ is rarely affected in isolation. Condylar resorption often results, leaving a resultant retrognathism and an anterior open bite.

Degenerative Joint Disease

Also referred to as *osteoarthritis,* degenerative joint disease is essentially a wear-and-tear phenomenon caused by excessive loading of the joints. Because the TMJ is not normally a weight-bearing joint (the weight is actually taken on the teeth), the pattern of disease is somewhat different from that seen in other joints. Pain, limited mobility, and crepitation within the joints are the common symptoms. It can affect the TMJ alone, and it often is at its peak when patients are between the ages of 40 and 55 years. It often "burns itself out" after this time as the condyle remodels, becomes smaller, and no longer suffers excessive forces.[2]

Internal Derangement

Internal derangement is a catchall phrase to describe incoordination between the condyle head, the meniscus, and the roof of the glenoid fossa. The most common single internal derangement is a partial or complete anteromedial dislocation of the meniscus that causes pain and limited movement of the jaw, often with joint noises such as clicking and popping. The pain is probably caused primarily by the richly innervated (from the auricular temporal nerve) retrodiscal tissues being pulled anteriorly by the disc and compressed between the condyle head and the glenoid fossa.

NONSURGICAL MANAGEMENT

Most cases of TMJ dysfunction can be managed non-surgically. Surgery should only be contemplated when a reasonable trial of nonsurgical treatment has failed. Most nonsurgical treatment is generally provided by a specialized dentist and consists of treatment that can include the following:

- Physical therapy
- Occlusal treatment
- Muscle relaxation
- Pain medication
- Psychotherapy and counseling

For reasons that are unclear, women present for the management of TMJ conditions more frequently than men do, although some studies have shown that the incidence of the problem within the population does not have much of a gender bias.[4] It is possible that, although the incidence is the same, women either have more severe problems or are perceived in that way such that women present for treatment more often. It is felt that about 70% of patients with TMJ problems can be helped by nonsurgical treatment to the extent that further treatment is not required. For those who are not helped by nonsurgical treatment, a variety of surgical options have been explored over the years.

Physical Therapy

Physical therapy includes joint exercises to coordinate joint movements between one side and the other and also within the joint itself. Heat in the form of moist heat or ultrasound can also be used to cause the relaxation of the muscles (particularly the lateral pterygoid muscle) to allow for some discal repositioning to occur.

Occlusal Treatment

Many patients are given a splint or bite-raising appliance to wear in the mouth, and, although their mode of action is still unknown, these appliances are successful in many cases.[3] There are many different designs of splints, including those placed in the upper jaw, those placed in the lower jaw, those reproducing cuspal patterns, those that are flat on their occlusal surface, those that attempt to only occlude on the front teeth, those that only occlude on the back teeth, those that try to reposition the mandible, and those that do not. It is likely that the main actions of these splints are to disocclude the teeth, to break up any abnormal proprioceptive input, and, by physically separating the teeth, to decrease the loading of the TMJ.

Muscle Relaxation

Muscle relaxation can be provided in many ways, including muscle-relaxing medications, trigger joint injections, yoga, and other contemplative exercises. Many patients do suffer from muscle spasms and muscle tension, which probably exacerbate any discal mobility or displacement.

Pain Medication

Pain medications include narcotic analgesics and anti-inflammatory agents. Tricyclic antidepressant medications given in doses below those required for their anti-depressant action have been shown to be effective for TMJ conditions.

Psychotherapy and Counseling

Many patients show signs of depression, tension, anger, and other psychological issues, and it is sometimes difficult to know which came first, the psychological problems or the TMJ problems. Nevertheless, psychological counseling can be very helpful for many patients.

TEMPOROMANDIBULAR JOINT SURGERY

If nonsurgical treatments have failed, surgical treatment can be performed. The history of TMJ surgery is not a very happy one. There are inherent difficulties with operating on the TMJ, including difficult access: one can really only approach the joint from the lateral side because of vital structures being present on all other sides. In addition, the margin for error is small, because the auditory apparatus is posterior to the joint, vital blood vessels and nerves run on the medial surface,[5] and, anteriorly, the lateral pterygoid muscle and the trigeminal nerve can be located. The joint is also small and complex, and branches of the facial nerve run in close proximity to it and limit access. Until recently, it was also difficult to image the joint to know exactly what was wrong, so much of the surgery being performed was exploratory in nature. Since the 1980s, however, computed tomography scans have been able to show the bony structure of the joint in details, and magnetic resonance images can accurately show the position of the meniscus, although they cannot always demonstrate perforation.[6] Diagnostic arthroscopy has also been attempted to gain further information about the pathology present in the joint.[7] Nevertheless, despite all of these aids, the results are still unpredictable, which is why surgery is only attempted when nonsurgical treatments have failed. It is often stated that, with TMJ surgery, approximately 70% of patients receive up to a 70% improvement. Essentially what this means is that nobody is completely cured (i.e., they always have joints that must be treated with care) and that, in 30% of patients, the surgery fails to produce any relief and may actually make matters worse.

Over the years, the following surgical protocols have been attempted:
- Arthroscopic surgery
- Extra-articular procedures
- Operations on the joint itself

Arthroscopic Surgery

With the advent of arthroscopic surgery for the treatment of other joints, it has also been attempted for use with the TMJ. However, its use has been limited by the small size of the instrument that has to be used; the difficulty of access (one can only really approach the joint from the lateral aspect, although attempts have been made to approach it through the external auditory meatus); and the fact that miniaturized surgical instruments are only now becoming available and may still not be satisfactory. Nevertheless, attempts have been made through an arthroscope to irrigate the joint to wash out various cytokines, to lyse adhesions, to surgically reposition the meniscus, and to surgically smooth irregularities of the condyle head.[8,9] In general, the results have been unpredictable.

Extra-Articular Procedures

Because of the difficulty of operating on the joint itself, some surgeons perform surgery outside of the joint. These approaches can help some TMJ problems in the following ways:
- The condylotomy (open or closed variety) can be performed.[10] This involves sectioning through the condyle neck or the ascending ramus of the mandible and allowing the condyle to take up a more physiologic position. It can be used in some cases of meniscal displacement to allow the condyle to reposition itself on the meniscus.
- Sectioning the pterygoid plates from the base of the skull and through a Le Fort I level maxillary osteotomy approach and then fracturing them posteriorly to shorten the lateral pterygoid muscles has been performed, thereby alleviating meniscal displacement.
- For cases of severe ankylosis of the joint, surgical treatment can consist of a gap arthroplasty carried out in the ascending ramus of the mandible and away from the joint to create an artificial joint inferior to the original one.[11] This can be quite successful, but it will result in an asymmetric pattern of opening. Because recurrent ankylosis is quite frequent, however, a gap arthroplasty may avoid this problem. Autogenous material is generally placed within the gap to prevent any bony fusion. This can be either temporalis muscle brought in from above or masseter muscle brought in from above or below.

- Eminectomy is another extra-articular procedure that can be used for chronic dislocation of the jaw, and it has also been claimed to have been successful for some cases of internal derangement.[12]

Operations on the Joint Itself

Surgical procedures on the TMJ are normally carried out via a preauricular incision, which is often combined with a temporal extension to allow for superior access and for the use of a temporalis muscle or fascial flap for reconstruction, if required.[13] Other approaches have been described that involve entering through the external auditory canal (the endaural approach)[14] and via a postauricular incision, where the external ear is retracted forward and the condyle is approached from a posterolateral position.[15] The condyle is approached in layers, with care taken to avoid trauma to the tragal cartilage as well as to the facial nerve. The most posterior branch of the facial nerve is the zygomaticotemporal branch, and, unfortunately, its position is variable and can be anywhere from 0.8 cm to 3.5 cm anterior to the anterior concavity of the external auditory canal as measured along the arch of the zygoma.[13] As a result of the position of the facial nerve, dissection along the arch of the zygoma must be subperiosteal, because the nerve lies just supraperiosteally. If present, the capsule of the joint is conventionally approached through a T-shaped incision, with the horizontal arm of the T along the arch of the zygoma and the vertical arm of the T over the center of the joint and down the condyle neck.[16] When the joint cavity has been entered, the surgical procedure performed depends on the underlying pathology.

For cases of ankylosis, the ankylotic mass is usually excised using a combination of drills and chisels. Sometimes the joint can be reconstructed with the use of autogenous tissue with the remnants of the condyle stump and a reconstructed meniscus.[17] If it is not possible to reconstruct the joint using local autogenous tissues, then a new joint can be constructed with either a costochondral graft or a prosthetic joint. Currently there are two prosthetic joints approved by the U.S. Food and Drug Administration that have been approved for long-term use: the TMJ Concept (TMJ Concepts, Inc., Camarillo, CA) and the Christiansen joint (TMJ Implants, Inc., Golden, CO).[18,19] However, there are few long-term follow-up studies regarding the use of these prostheses.

Surgical treatment for a joint affected by rheumatoid arthritis may involve synovectomy, arthroplasty, or condylectomy and possible reconstruction with a costochondral graft or a prosthetic joint. Treatment for degenerative joint disease will normally involve an arthroplasty to recontour the condyle head, the repair or removal of any meniscal remnants, and the replacement of the meniscus as appropriate.[20]

Treatment for the recurrent dislocation of the condyle can take a number of forms, depending on the surgeon's philosophy.[21] Some surgeons like to augment the eminence to prevent dislocation either with a bone graft, a cartilage graft, or a prosthesis. Others like to reduce bony interferences so that the condyle can slide forward and backward without dislocating; this could include either an arthroplasty or a condylectomy to reduce the height of the joint or an eminectomy to reduce the height of the eminence. Additionally, condylar motion can be restricted by the injection of autogenous blood into the joint or by a capsular plication procedure. The injection of sclerosing solution to restrict joint movement has also been described.

The surgical management of the internal derangement of the joint remains problematic. If the problem is acute and a dislocated meniscus is diagnosed, this can sometimes be repositioned surgically and stabilized in its correct position either with sutures or screws of various kinds.[22] More commonly, when the meniscus is chronically displaced, it cannot be repositioned; it must be removed and is generally replaced. This is often combined with an arthroplasty if there is felt to be decreased joint space, which many feel exacerbates the problems with internal derangement.[20]

The exact function of the meniscus in the joint is still unknown, although it does divide the joint into a lower compartment where rotation takes place and an upper compartment where forward movement of the whole joint occurs. Additionally, it probably has some type of shock-absorbing properties. It is known that, when the meniscus is removed and not replaced, patients actually do well for several years, but they do seem to have a higher incidence of degenerative joint disease in later life,[23] and most authorities recommend replacement of the meniscus. Replacement with alloplastic materials has been unsuccessful and has actually caused many complications[24,25]; now only autogenous materials are recommended for the replacement of the joint. Among the materials that have been described are a locally obtained temporalis fascia, a muscular flap, or both, which can be either pedicled or free and can be passed either over or under the arch of the zygoma; a cartilage graft, which can be obtained from the nasal septum or the concha of the ear; or a dermis graft.[20] Success has been claimed with the use of all of these materials.

COMPLICATIONS OF TEMPOROMANDIBULAR JOINT SURGERY

Complications of TMJ surgery can be essentially subdivided into the following five categories:

1. Patient selection and the selection of the appropriate surgical procedure
2. Complications specific to arthroscopy
3. Perioperative complications of open joint surgery
4. Postoperative complications
5. Long-term complications

Patient Selection and the Selection of the Appropriate Surgical Procedure

Patient selection may be more critical for TMJ surgery than for other forms of maxillofacial or head and neck surgery. The reasons for this are somewhat unclear, but they may revolve around the fact that patients often have pain that does not correspond with a preoperative pathologic or imaging diagnosis, the fact that the pain is often poorly localized, and the fact that, with the complex structure of the TMJ, it may be difficult to accurately identify the exact cause of a problem. It is particularly important to differentiate articular pathology from within the joint itself from neuromuscular and fibromyalgia-type symptoms. Additionally, patients may suffer from headache-like symptoms, migraine-type symptoms, and variants of atypical facial pain. For the majority of these conditions, TMJ surgery has no role and could aggravate the symptoms. In general terms, the more that the pain and symptoms are directly localized to the TMJ, the greater the possibility of a successful surgical result. The more that the symptoms are diffuse and radiating and not specifically confined to the TMJ, the greater the possibility of failure.

If possible, surgery should be tailored to the pathology identified. Ankylosis surgery should be designed to release the ankylosis and reconstruct the joint in a way as to minimize the chances of reankylosis. Surgery for degenerative joint disease should be primarily aimed at an arthroplasty to smooth the joint and then to repair or replace the meniscus as appropriate. Internal derangement surgery is probably the most difficult to standardize, because it may consist of elements of surgery to release the slip of lateral pterygoid muscle inserted into the disc, the surgical repositioning or replacement of the disc, and a possible increase in joint space to prevent further compression of the new or reconstructed disc. In the absence of discernible pathology, surgery for pain alone has a relatively low success rate, and it can lead to a dependent patient whose management can become an issue that can lead to repeated surgeries and the concept of the "TMJ cripple" (Figure 26-1).

Complications Specific to Arthroscopy

TMJ arthroscopy was introduced in the United States in the mid 1980s[26] and rose to prominence during the late 1980s and the early 1990s; it is still carried out today,

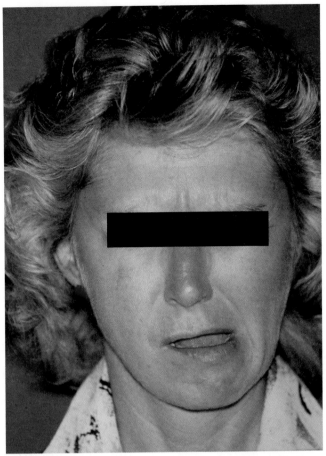

Figure 26-1. Photographs of a patient who has had a total of 23 temporomandibular joint operations: 13 on one side and 10 on the other. She has permanent facial nerve weakness and a malocclusion with facial symmetry. She shows many of the problems of a temporomandibular joint patient who has undergone multiple operations.

Infection is a possibility with any surgical procedure. After arthroscopy, treatment would consist of antibiotics and appropriate drainage, if necessary.

The breakage of instruments during arthroscopic procedures has been described, because the instruments that have been developed are extremely fragile and slender. The breakage of an instrument in the joint could lead to the need for open joint surgery to recover the instrument from either the upper or lower joint compartment, as appropriate[27,28] (Figure 26-2).

Entry into the middle cranial fossa with arthroscopic instruments has been described during arthroscopic surgery, because, in some patients, the roof of the glenoid fossa or the floor of the middle cranial fossa is extremely thin, particularly if there was preexisting joint pathology present.[29] This will necessitate open surgery and a possible bone-grafting procedure to be carried out on the defect, with possible meningeal repair if the meninges have been violated.

Penetration of the auditory apparatus has also been described with arthroscopic surgery. This can involve the external auditory meatus, which may be lacerated, or the middle ear, where the displacement of the ossicles has been documented; this may require the removal and alloplastic replacement of the ossicles and of the conducting mechanism of the middle ear.[30–32] In one case, the problem was noted when middle-ear structures were viewed through the arthroscope.[33] Lacerations of the external auditory meatus are normally treated conservatively, and they rarely require suturing. However, they may require the application of Gelfoam (Johnson & Johnson, New Brunswick, NJ) or a similar

although on a more selective group of patients than was previously considered. This is because a magnetic resonance image gives almost as much diagnostic information as arthroscopy, and the results of arthroscopic surgery have been mixed. Nevertheless, there are a number of complications that are specifically related to the arthroscopic surgery of the TMJ.

Bleeding is a possibility with any surgical procedure, and it can be particularly worrisome with arthroscopic surgery. Because it is essentially closed surgery, it is difficult to access the bleeding vessels quickly. Bleeding can result from the penetration of the temporal vessels that are superficial to the joint. This is usually not of serious clinical significance, because these vessels are fairly superficial, and they can be accessed without too much difficulty. Bleeding from the medial aspect of the joint, however, can be very serious, because it can involve the middle meningeal artery, which may run within 2 mm of the medial joint surface; surgical access to this area is time consuming and difficult.[5]

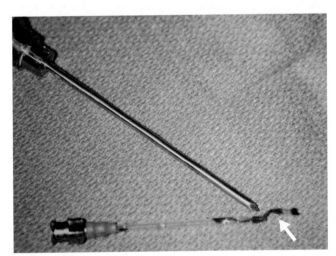

Figure 26-2. An Angiocath-type cannula that was used as an outflow port for temporomandibular joint arthroscopies. Note that the cannula has been almost totally transected *(arrow)* by contact with the arthroscope trochar. If total transection had occurred, open joint surgery would have been necessary to recover the broken fragments. (Arthroscope produced by Karl Storz Endoscopy, Culver City, CA.)

hemostatic and bandage-type agent in addition to antibiotic eardrops.

Among the surgical procedures performed with the use of an arthroscope are laser procedures, particularly those involving the holmium:yttrium-aluminum-garnet laser.[9,34,35] This laser will penetrate water, but it is absorbed by color (particularly red), and it will vaporize tissues while passing through the irrigating solution in the joint. If the laser beam is allowed to pass extraarticularly, however, serious complications have been reported, including damage to the external auditory meatus, the middle ear, the middle cranial fossa, and the brain itself, leading to serious consequences that require consultation with an otologist or a neurosurgeon.

Perioperative Complications of Open Joint Surgery

Bleeding during open TMJ surgery is often troublesome, because it can obscure the operative field, which is usually small and deeply placed. When approaching the joint, bleeding can arise from the superficial temporal artery and its branches. As one approaches the capsule, there is a particularly troublesome small transverse facial branch that, if it is not recognized and ligated before the capsule is approached, can retract when incised and cause troublesome hemorrhage. For obvious reasons, hemorrhage must be identified and treated. Otherwise, the joint is obscured, and the surgery becomes very difficult. For surgery in which the medial confines of the joints are approached (i.e., ankylosis release and the removal of a medially displaced meniscus), the middle meningeal artery can be near[5] (Figure 26-3). Bleeding from this vessel can be a major problem, because hemorrhage in this area is very difficult to control. Treatment may require the dislocation of the mandible or even a condylotomy to expose the area adequately. The old solution of placing a sharpened matchstick into the foramen spinosum by which the middle meningeal artery leaves the skull is not practiced today (even using an updated equivalent of a sharpened matchstick),[36] but if the middle meningeal artery is detached from the base of the skull, neurovascular intervention may be necessary. Damage to both an artery and a vein that are close to each other can result in healing with the formation of an arteriovenous fistula. This is rarely of medical significance in that it does not place any significant load on the cardiovascular system, but it normally comes to light in the form of a very disturbing pulsatile tinnitus. This symptom normally warrants reexploration with clipping of the fistula or embolization via interventional radiology.[37,38]

Facial nerve involvement is a constant risk in any open TMJ surgery. The zygomaticotemporal branches are at particular risk, but even other branches may be affected

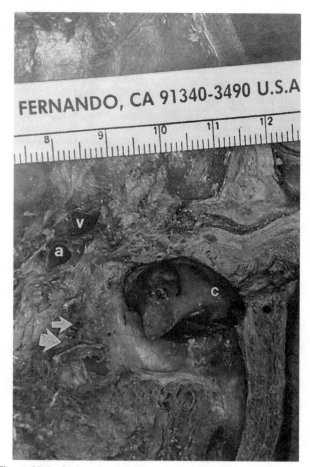

Figure 26-3. Cadaveric photograph of the structures medial to the temporomandibular joint. *a,* Carotid artery; *c,* condyle; *v,* jugular vein; *small arrow,* middle meningeal artery; *large arrow,* trigeminal nerve.

on occasion, usually secondarily as a result of pressure or hemorrhage. The position of the zygomaticotemporal branch as it crosses the arch of the zygoma has been studied, but unfortunately it lies in a variable position, and it can be anything from 8 mm to 35 mm in front of the anterior concavity of the external auditory canal[13] (Figure 26-4). The branches can rarely be identified during the surgery. Fortunately most cases of facial nerve involvement are only temporary, but estimates have shown a rate of approximately 10% involvement after TMJ surgery; of those, about 10% of cases are permanent, for a 1% rate of some type of permanent facial nerve involvement (Figure 26-5). The rate of nerve involvement increases with repeat surgery as a result of the restriction of the nerve branches by scar tissue from previous surgery. Surgical intervention to identify and repair these smaller branches of the facial nerve is virtually never successful and can make matters worse, so it is therefore not generally advised.

Damage to the auriculotemporal nerve is frequent with open joint surgery, resulting in some paresthesia over the lower part of the earlobe and the skin anterior to the ear. In some cases, this is even deliberate during the

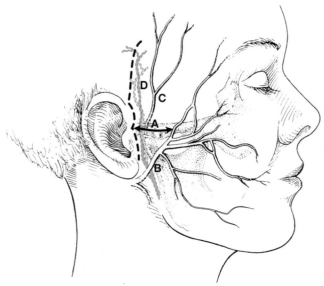

Figure 26-4. Facial nerve branches *(B),* the auricular–temporal nerve *(C),* and the superficial temporal vessels *(D)* in the region of the temporomandibular joints. The most posterior of the facial nerve branches is the zygomaticotemporal. As it crosses the arch of the zygoma, it can be anywhere between 8-mm and 35-mm anterior to the tympanic plate *(A).*[13]

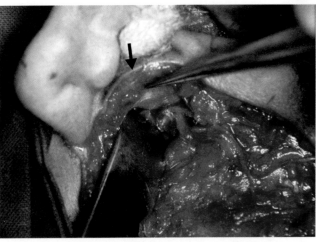

Figure 26-6. Clinical photograph to show the position of the auriculotemporal nerve *(arrowed)* as it passes behind the temporomandibular joint and gives branches to the joint itself and to the retrodiscal tissues.

surgery, because most of the innervation of the joint itself is carried by the auriculotemporal nerve. Destroying this nerve also denervates, to a certain extent, the TMJ, and this may enhance pain control[39] (Figure 26-6).

Damage to the inferior alveolar nerve has been reported after TMJ surgery, with resulting paresthesia over the lower jaw and the lower lip on the affected side. Two possible mechanisms have been invoked. The first involves the hemorrhage and compression of the inferior alveolar nerve as it passes medial to the joint, and the second involves the use of a clamp on the angle of the mandible to distract the condyle head to allow the joint surgery to be performed. If the clamp is inadvertently applied with the medial point over the lingula, direct damage to the inferior alveolar nerve can occur[40] (Figure 26-7).

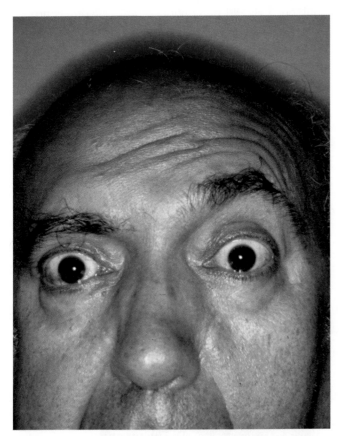

Figure 26-5. Permanent forehead weakness after temporomandibular joint surgery. Note the lack of forehead wrinkling on the paralyzed right side. Weakness of the zygomaticotemporal and orbital branches of the facial nerve are the most frequently seen.

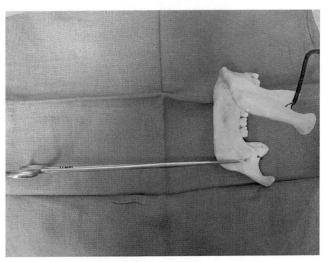

Figure 26-7. In vitro illustration of how a clamp can inadvertently damage the inferior alveolar nerve if it is used to distract the mandibular condyle.

Perforation into the middle cranial fossa is not unknown during TMJ surgery. It normally results from complex procedures such as ankylosis release or from cases involving considerable degenerative joint disease or other arthritic disease affecting the glenoid fossa as well as the condyle head.[41] In these cases, the glenoid fossa is normally reconstructed with a bone graft that would often be taken from an adjacent outer layer of the cranium. If the meninges are perforated, a neurosurgical consultation is necessary for meningeal repair or patching.

Perforation of the external auditory meatus is normally treated by suturing and the application of a Gelfoam dressing and antibiotic eardrops. An aural–temporomandibular fistula can occasionally develop and require secondary closure.[42] Perforation of the tympanic membrane of the middle ear is a major complication of TMJ surgery. It is probably most frequent when the approach to the joint goes through the parotid gland, because it is possible to become disoriented during the approach. If the approach is made posteriorly down the tragal cartilage with the forward retraction of the parotid gland and all surgery is carried out in an anterior direction, the likelihood of this occurring should be much less. If perforation of the middle ear does occur, a consultation with an otologist is necessary. Occasionally this complication results in a conductive hearing loss that is severe enough to require repair and the possible replacement of the ossicles of the middle ear with alloplastic replacements.[43]

After the reconstruction of the meniscus by means of a temporalis muscle or fascia flap, there is frequently a depression over the temporal region above the zygoma, which can occasionally be troublesome to patients (Figure 26-8). This normally occurs when a full-thickness temporalis flap is used, and it can usually be avoided with the use of a partial-thickness flap. Normally this is something that patients can tolerate or hide with hair styling. However, if treatment is required, techniques have been described to recontour the depression previously occupied by the temporal muscle either with a dermal fat graft from the abdomen or with an alloplastic implant of some type, which can be placed against the skull and under the soft tissues of that region. Acrylic resin has been the most frequently advocated alloplast.[44]

Infection after open TMJ surgery is remarkably rare, because this is a normally clean, uncontaminated surgery without involvement of the oral cavity. Prophylactic antibiotics effective against staphylococci are normally employed, and a suitable regimen would be one dose of antibiotics given intravenously at the start of the surgery and one additional dose given 4 to 6 hours later. Antibiotics should be continued until any drains are removed, if they have been used. If no drains are used,

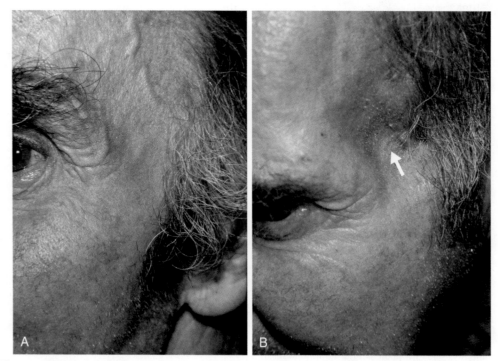

Figure 26-8. A, The appearance of the patient's temporal region before the reconstruction of the temporomandibular joint with a temporalis muscle and fascia flap. **B,** The postoperative appearance, with a marked depression visible *(arrow)* when a full-thickness temporalis flap was used. This can be masked with a soft-tissue or alloplastic graft.

then the initial two doses of antibiotics should be adequate.

Postoperative Complications

On occasion, some perioperative complications may not become apparent until the postoperative period. This includes facial nerve involvement and middle ear involvement. Facial nerve involvement may not be apparent for several hours, and it may be masked by any swelling that is present. Similarly, any hearing loss may be masked by the dressings the patient wears, and patients may be somewhat sedated during the immediate postoperative period. If either of these complications are recognized, they should be managed appropriately during the postoperative period. Other postoperative complications include malocclusions, which are not infrequent after TMJ surgery (Figure 26-9). With any other joint surgery in the body, if the postoperative position of the bone is a millimeter or two away from the preoperative position, this is not usually of any consequence. However, when this occurs in the TMJ, a difference in the occlusion of even 0.1 mm can be very apparent to the patient. For this reason, most patients with teeth will be placed in arch bars prophylactically, and guiding elastics can be used quite aggressively during the postoperative period if there is any sign of a malocclusion developing. In this way, most malocclusions can be prevented or treated, particularly with some physical therapy to train the neuromuscular apparatus to close into the previous occlusion. If a malocclusion becomes established after TMJ surgery, it may be necessary to accept it and to treat the patient secondarily with either orthodontic treatment to reposition the teeth or occlusal rehabilitation or orthognathic surgery to reposition the jaws to accommodate the change in occlusion.

A further postoperative complication is the occasional development of Frey syndrome (gustatory sweating) as a result of the perforation of the capsule of the parotid gland and the involvement of the parotid in the approach to the TMJ (Figure 26-10). The sympathetic nerve fibers supplying the sweat glands of the skin of the face (via the external carotid artery, the middle meningeal artery, and the auricular temporal nerve) become damaged and receive cross innervation to the parasympathetic fibers from the otic ganglion via the auriculotemporal nerve to become the secretor motor fibers to the parotid gland. In this case, the stimulation of the parasympathetic fibers can cause skin sweating, also known as *Frey syndrome.* After TMJ surgery, the area affected by Frey syndrome is usually relatively small (as compared with parotid surgery), but the treatment principles remain the same.[45] The frequency of the condition really depends on how well patients are questioned or tested (e.g., with the starch–iodine test using tincture of iodine with glycerin and wheat starch), but it may be present in up to 20% of TMJ surgery patients postoperatively (see Figure 26-10). Treatment can be medical, with the use of topical sialagogues or parasympathetic-blocking medications applied to the skin (e.g., scopolamine, glycopyrrolate cream)[46]; it can be surgical, with a tympanic neurectomy; or it can be local, with the insertion of a subdermal free dermis graft to block the nerve impulses.[46–50] Botulinum toxin[50] given by subdermal injection and oral glycopyrrolate[51] have also been used effectively.

Postoperative parotid complications can occur after TMJ surgery, particularly when the approach is made through the parotid gland. Parotid fistulae and sialoceles have been reported after TMJ surgery.[52] Fistulae normally close spontaneously, particularly if an antisialagogue is

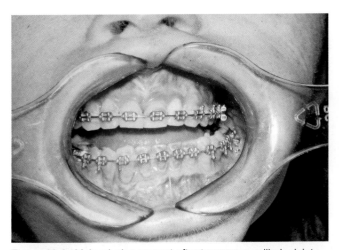

Figure 26-9. Malocclusion present after temporomandibular joint surgery. The most common malocclusion is a lateral open bite on the side opposite from the surgery as a result of the shortening of the ramus and the condyle on the operated side.

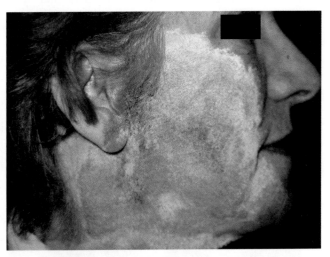

Figure 26-10. Frey syndrome (gustatory sweating) visualized by means of a starch–iodine test for a patient who is chewing after temporomandibular joint surgery. This starch–iodine test shows brown in the area demonstrating the gustatory sweating.

used to decrease secretions. Atropine or scopolamine can be used in the short term for this purpose. Similarly, sialoceles often improve spontaneously; however, if they persist, injection with a sclerosing agent (e.g., sodium tetradecyl) or surgical removal can be employed. Needle drainage and a pressure dressing coupled with an antisialagogue can also be used.

Long-Term Complications

Ankylosis or reankylosis is a problem after TMJ surgery. It normally occurs when there is a possibility of bone-on-bone contact; therefore the use of a suitable barrier within the joint to replace the disc should theoretically prevent this occurrence, but it is still reported. It is a known risk of any surgery that is performed to release ankylosis that the joints have a propensity to reankylose (Figure 26-11). After the joint has reankylosed, repeated surgery is the only possible solution. In this case, one would take prophylactic measures to prevent a secondary ankylosis, either by employing bisphosphonates intravenously or orally[53–56] during the postoperative period or by using radiation therapy to inhibit heterotropic bone formation. The protocol is similar to that used for the prevention of heterotropic bone formation in the hip in that a single dose of 500 cGy to 700 cGy of radiation is given to the joints 24 to 72 hours postoperatively.[57,58] For obvious reasons, the eye must be protected during the radiation therapy. Both of these protocols have been shown to decrease the incidence of reankylosis.

Alloplastic implants used in various types of TMJ reconstruction have been shown to be a cause of long-term complications. In particular, the Proplast Teflon TMJ disc replacement (Vitek, Inc., Houston, TX) (Figure 26-12) that was used during the 1980s caused a prolific giant-cell reaction with subsequent fibrosis, ankylosis, and bone

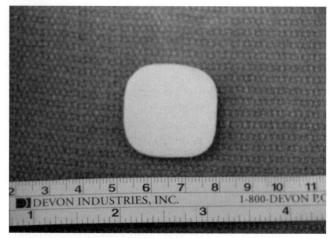

Figure 26-12. A Proplast Teflon implant used as a meniscal replacement during the 1980s (Vitek II implant).

loss in both the condyle and glenoid fossa (Figures 26-13 and 26-14). The implant itself was removed from the market in 1990, and most patients who received this implant have now had it removed and have been subsequently treated.[24] Every year, however, one or two patients appear who still have this implant in place. In those cases, it is mandatory to image the joint with both a panoramic x-ray and a computed tomography scan, and it is almost certainly advisable to remove the alloplastic meniscus and replace it with an autogenous product, even if it appears to be asymptomatic.[25] Silastic disc replacements (Dow-Corning, Midland, MI) (temporary and permanent) were also used (Figures 26-15 and 26-16), but they have now been withdrawn from the market. The Silastic could fragment (Figure 26-17) and potentially cause problems.

The two alloplastic joint replacements that are currently approved by the U.S. Food and Drug Administration do not have long-term studies associated with

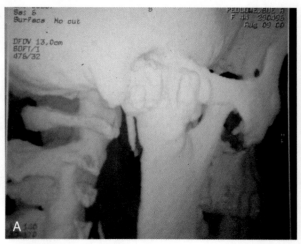
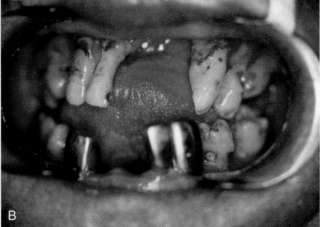

Figure 26-11. A, A three-dimensional computed tomography reconstruction of an ankylosed left temporomandibular joint with extensive heterotrophic bone formation. **B,** In the same patient, this shows the amount of mandibular opening.

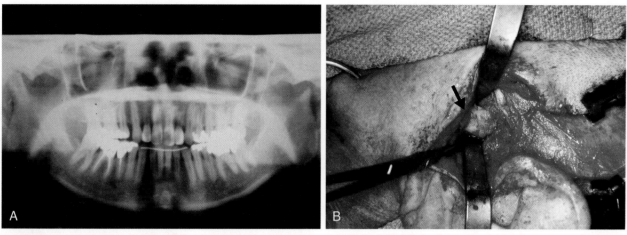

Figure 26-13. A patient with a Proplast Teflon implant in the left temporomandibular joint **(A)** that has caused total destruction and reabsorption of the joint *(arrow)* **(B)**.

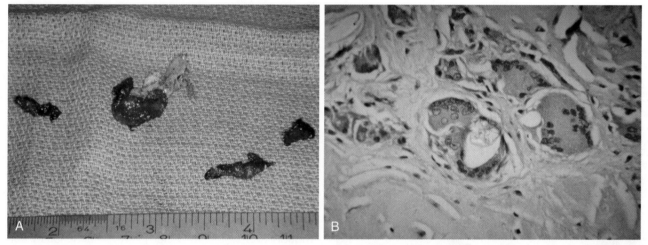

Figure 26-14. A, The appearance of the Proplast Teflon implant shown in Figure 26-13 on removal. Note the exuberant granulation tissue adherent to the fragmented implant. **B,** The histologic appearance of the specimen from part **A,** showing an exuberant giant-cell reaction.

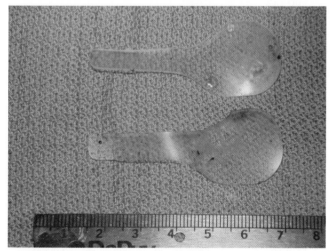

Figure 26-15. Temporary Silastic disc replacements that were fitted during the late 1980s and the early 1990s. The larger portion of the Silastic was placed in the disc compartment. The extension protruded through the skin and was used to remove the implant after about 6 weeks, when it was hoped that a fibrous capsule would have formed around it to become a new disc.

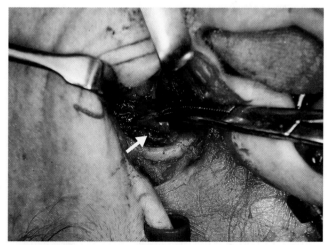

Figure 26-16. A Silastic interpositional implant *(arrow)* being removed from the temporomandibular joint space.

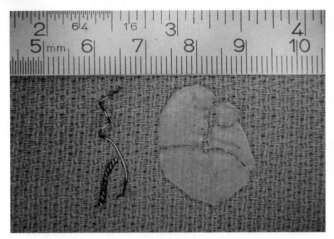

Figure 26-17. Appearance of a fragmented Silastic disc replacement that had to be removed surgically.

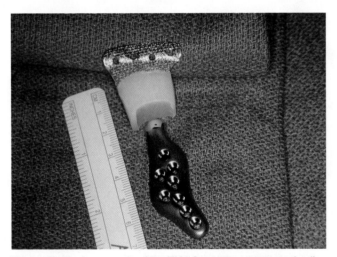

Figure 26-18. An example of the TMJ Concepts custom-made alloplastic mandibular condyle and glenoid fossa replacement. The custom joint is made from a lithographic model generated from a three-dimensional computed tomography scan.

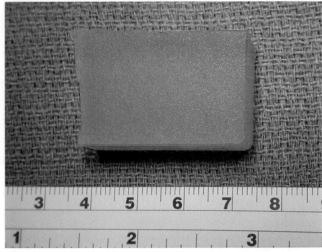

Figure 26-19. A 15-mm Silastic block that makes a suitable spacer when an alloplastic joint has to be removed and before a new replacement (either another alloplastic joint or a costochondral graft) is used.

Unfortunately, one of the most challenging long-term complications of TMJ surgery is persistent pain. All patients with this problem should be fully evaluated postoperatively by a multidisciplinary TMJ team that includes a nonsurgical TMJ specialist with suitable pharmacologic, psychological, and physical therapy support. One should be wary of rushing in to repeat any surgical procedures, because there is a danger of creating the long-term "TMJ cripple" who has had multiple TMJ procedures carried out, who still has persistent pain, and who now has malocclusion-restricted joint motion and possible facial nerve weakness. In some cases, the exact reason for the persistent pain cannot be determined and does not appear to have an anatomic or pathologic basis. In these cases, surgery should not be performed.

them, and their life expectancy is probably 15 to 20 years[18,19] (Figure 26-18). Failures are being reported with these devices that can necessitate their removal. In general, if removal is indicated, this is carried out surgically. A decision must later be made regarding the placement of some kind of spacer into the resulting cavity or to let it heal and then reassess the situation for further joint replacement. Providing the surgical field is clean without any perforations or infection, it is probably advantageous to use some kind of spacer to hold the joint space open so that reoperation can be carried out in a physiologically normal field without scarring and malocclusion. A suitable spacer can be a block of Silastic as long as it is for short-to medium-term use only. A 15-mm block of Silastic makes a very suitable spacer, as does a reshaped Silastic testicular implant (Figure 26-19).

REFERENCES

1. Vetter JD, Topazian RG, Goldberg MH, et al: Facial fractures occurring in a medium-sized metropolitan area: Recent trends. *Int J Oral Maxillofac Surg* 1991;20(4):214–216.
2. Toller PA: Osteoarthrosis of the mandibular condyle. *Br Dent J* 1973;134(6):223–231.
3. Al-Ani MZ, Davies SJ, Gray RJ, et al: Stabilisation splint therapy for temporomandibular pain dysfunction syndrome. *Cochrane Database Syst Rev* 2004;(1):CD002778.
4. Rieder CE, Martinoff JT, Wilcox SA: The prevalence of mandibular dysfunction. Part I: Sex and age distribution of related signs and symptoms. *J Prosthet Dent* 1983;50(1):81–88.
5. Talebzadeh N, Rosenstein TP, Pogrel MA: Anatomy of the structures medial to the temporomandibular joint. *Oral Surg Oral Med Oral Pathol Oral Radiol Endod* 1999;88(6):674–678.
6. Dolan EA, Kim HG, Nokes SR, et al: Correlation of magnetic resonance imaging and surgical findings in patients with meniscal perforation. *J Craniomandib Disord* 1989;3(3):174–178.
7. Smolka W, Iizuka T: Arthroscopic lysis and lavage in different stages of internal derangement of the temporomandibular joint: Correlation of preoperative staging to arthroscopic findings and treatment outcome. *J Oral Maxillofac Surg* 2005;63(4):471–478.

8. McCain JP, Podrasky AE, Zabiegalski NA: Arthroscopic disc repositioning and suturing: A preliminary report. *J Oral Maxillofac Surg* 1992;50(6):568–580.

9. McCain JP, Sanders B, Koslin MG, et al: Temporomandibular joint arthroscopy: A 6-year multicenter retrospective study of 4,831 joints. *J Oral Maxillofac Surg* 1992;50(9):926–930.

10. Werther JR, Hall HD, Gibbs SJ: Disk position before and after modified condylotomy in 80 symptomatic temporomandibular joints. *Oral Surg Oral Med Oral Pathol Oral Radiol Endod* 1995;79(6):668–679.

11. Roychoudhury A, Parkash H, Trikha A: Functional restoration by gap arthroplasty in temporomandibular joint ankylosis: A report of 50 cases. *Oral Surg Oral Med Oral Pathol Oral Radiol Endod* 1999;87(2):166–169.

12. Williamson RA, McNamara D, McAuliffe W: True eminectomy for internal derangement of the temporomandibular joint. *Br J Oral Maxillofac Surg* 2000;38(5):554–560.

13. Al-Kayat A, Bramley P: A modified pre-auricular approach to the temporomandibular joint and malar arch. *Br J Oral Surg* 1979;17(2):91–103.

14. Dias AD: A truly endaural approach to the temporo-mandibular joint. *Br J Plast Surg* 1984;37(1):65–68.

15. Walters PJ, Geist ET: Correction of temporomandibular joint internal derangements via the posterior auricular approach. *J Oral Maxillofac Surg* 1983;41(9):616–618.

16. MacFarlane WI: Recurrent dislocation of the mandible: Treatment of seven cases by a simple surgical method. *Br J Oral Surg* 1977;14(3):227–229.

17. Kaban LB, Perrott DH, Fisher K: A protocol for management of temporomandibular joint ankylosis. *J Oral Maxillofac Surg* 1990;48(11):1145–1152.

18. Christensen RW, Alexander R, Curry JT, et al: Hemi and total TMJ reconstruction using the Christensen prostheses: A retrospective and prospective evaluation. *Surg Technol Int* 2004;12:292–303.

19. Mercuri LG, Wolford LM, Sanders B, et al: Long-term follow-up of the CAD/CAM patient fitted total temporomandibular joint reconstruction system. *J Oral Maxillofac Surg* 2002;60(12):1440–1448.

20. Pogrel MA, Kaban LB: The role of a temporalis fascia and muscle flap in temporomandibular joint surgery. *J Oral Maxillofac Surg* 1990;48(1):14–19.

21. Pogrel MA: Articular eminectomy for recurrent dislocation. *Br J Oral Maxillofac Surg* 1987;25(3):237–243.

22. Mehra P, Wolford LM: The Mitek mini anchor for TMJ disc repositioning: Surgical technique and results. *Int J Oral Maxillofac Surg* 2001;30(6):497–503.

23. Eriksson L, Westesson PL: Long-term evaluation of meniscectomy of the temporomandibular joint. *J Oral Maxillofac Surg* 1985;43(4):263–269.

24. U.S. Food and Drug Administration: www.fda.gov/cdrh/consumer/tmjupdate/TMJupdate.html#questionVitek.

25. Kearns GJ, Perrott DH, Kaban LB: A protocol for the management of failed alloplastic temporomandibular joint disc implants. *J Oral Maxillofac Surg* 1995;53(11):1240–1249.

26. Murakami K, Ono T: Temporomandibular joint arthroscopy by inferolateral approach. *Int J Oral Maxillofac Surg* 1986;15(4):410–417.

27. McCain JP, de la Rua H: Foreign body retrieval: A complication of TMJ arthroscopy: Report of a case. *J Oral Maxillofac Surg* 1989;47(11):1221–1225, 1228–1229.

28. Tarro AW: Instrument breakage associated with arthroscopy of the temporomandibular joint: Report of a case. *J Oral Maxillofac Surg* 1989;47(11):1226–1229.

29. McCain JP: Arthroscopy of the human temporomandibular joint. *J Oral Maxillofac Surg* 1988;46(8):648–655.

30. Schickinger B, Gstoettner W, Cerny C, et al: Variant petrotympanic fissure as possible cause of an otologic complication during TMJ arthroscopy: A case report. *Int J Oral Maxillofac Surg* 1998;27(1):17–19.

31. Sugisaki M, Ikai A, Tanabe H: Dangerous angles and depths for middle ear and middle cranial fossa injury during arthros-

copy of the temporomandibular joint. *J Oral Maxillofac Surg* 1995;53(7):803–810.

32. Tsuyama M, Kondoh T, Seto K, et al: Complications of temporomandibular joint arthroscopy: A retrospective analysis of 301 lysis and lavage procedures performed using the triangulation technique. *J Oral Maxillofac Surg* 2000;58(5):500–506.

33. Van Sickels JE, Nishioka GJ, Hegewald MD, et al: Middle ear injury resulting from temporomandibular joint arthroscopy. *J Oral Maxillofac Surg* 1987;45(11):962–965.

34. Koslin MG: Proper use of the holmium:YAG laser. *J Oral Maxillofac Surg* 1993;51(3):339.

35. Koslin MG, Martin JC: The use of the holmium laser for temporomandibular joint arthroscopic surgery. *J Oral Maxillofac Surg* 1993;51(2):122–124.

36. Cillo JE Jr, Sinn D, Truelson JM: Management of middle meningeal and superficial temporal artery hemorrhage from total temporomandibular joint replacement surgery with a gelatin-based hemostatic agent. *J Craniofac Surg* 2005;16(2):309–312.

37. Kornbrot A, Shaw AS, Toohey MR: Pseudoaneurysm as a complication of arthroscopy: A case report. *J Oral Maxillofac Surg* 1991;49(11):1226–1228.

38. Martin-Granizo R, Caniego JL, de Pedro M, et al: Arteriovenous fistula after temporomandibular joint arthroscopy successfully treated with embolization. *Int J Oral Maxillofac Surg* 2004;33(3):301–303.

39. Bradley PF: Conservative treatment for temporomandibular joint pain dysfunction. *Br J Oral Maxillofac Surg* 1987;25(2):125–137.

40. Heffez L, Blaustein D: Diagnostic arthroscopy of the temporomandibular joint. Part I: Normal arthroscopic findings. *Oral Surg Oral Med Oral Pathol* 1987;64(6):653–670.

41. Cillo JE, Sinn DP, Ellis E 3rd: Traumatic dislocation of the mandibular condyle into the middle cranial fossa treated with immediate reconstruction: A case report. *J Oral Maxillofac Surg* 2005;63(6):859–865.

42. Sinn DP, Tharanon W, Culbertson MC Jr, et al: Surgical correction of an aural-temporomandibular joint fistula with a temporalis flap. *J Oral Maxillofac Surg* 1994;52(2):197–200.

43. Loughner BA, Larkin LH, Mahan PE: Discomalleolar and anterior malleolar ligaments: Possible causes of middle ear damage during temporomandibular joint surgery. *Oral Surg Oral Med Oral Pathol* 1989;68(1):14–22.

44. Cheung LK, Samman N, Tideman H: The use of mouldable acrylic for restoration of the temporalis flap donor site. *J Craniomaxillofac Surg* 1994;22(6):335–341.

45. Swanson KS, Laskin DM, Campbell RL: Auriculotemporal syndrome following the preauricular approach to temporomandibular joint surgery. *J Oral Maxillofac Surg* 1991;49(7):680–682.

46. Hays LL: The Frey syndrome: A review and double blind evaluation of the topical use of a new anticholinergic agent. *Laryngoscope* 1978;88(11):1796–1824.

47. Parisier SC, Binder WJ, Blitzer A, et al: Evaluation of tympanic neurectomy and chorda tympanectomy for gustatory sweating and benign salivary gland disease. *Ear Nose Throat J* 1978;57(5):213–223.

48. Parisier SC, Blitzer A, Binder WJ, et al: Evaluation of tympanic neurectomy and chorda tympanectomy surgery. *Otolaryngology* 1978;86(2):ORL308–ORL321.

49. Bonanno PC: Re: Dermis-fat graft after parotidectomy to prevent 'Frey's syndrome and the concave deformity.' *Ann Plast Surg* 1994;33(2):235.

50. Ferraro G, Altieri A, Grella E, et al: Botulinum toxin: 28 patients affected by Frey's syndrome treated with intradermal injections. *Plast Reconstr Surg* 2005;115(1):344–345.

51. Edick CM: Oral glycopyrrolate for the treatment of diabetic gustatory sweating. *Ann Pharmacother* 2005;39(10):1760.

52. Hutchison IL, Ryan D: A parotid fistula and sialocele complicating temporomandibular joint surgery. *Br J Oral Maxillofac Surg* 1989;27(3):203–208.

53. Haran M, Bhuta T, Lee B: Pharmacological interventions for treating acute heterotopic ossification. *Cochrane Database Syst Rev* 2004;(4):CD003321.

54. Licata AA: Discovery, clinical development, and therapeutic uses of bisphosphonates. *Ann Pharmacother* 2005;39(4):668–677.

55. Schuetz P, Mueller B, Christ-Crain M, et al: Amino-bisphosphonates in heterotopic ossification: First experience in five consecutive cases. *Spinal Cord* 2005;43(10):604–610.

56. Wilkinson JM, Stockley I, Hamer AJ, et al: Biochemical markers of bone turnover and development of heterotopic ossification after total hip arthroplasty. *J Orthop Res* 2003;21(3):529–534.

57. Padgett DE, Holley KG, Cummings M, et al: The efficacy of 500 CentiGray radiation in the prevention of heterotopic ossification after total hip arthroplasty: A prospective, randomized, pilot study. *J Arthroplasty* 2003;18(6):677–686.

58. Stein DA, Patel R, Egol KA, et al: Prevention of heterotopic ossification at the elbow following trauma using radiation therapy. *Bull Hosp Jt Dis* 2003;61(3–4):151–154.

CHAPTER 27

Complications of Surgery of the Oropharynx

Karen T. Pitman

The spectrum of surgery for tumors of the oropharynx ranges from transoral resections with primary closures to complex resections and reconstructive procedures. To understand and appreciate the sequelae and complications that can occur as a result of these procedures, a fundamental knowledge of the anatomy and function of the oropharynx is essential.

This chapter is limited to a discussion of the procedures that are designed specifically for neoplasms of the oropharynx and transoropharyngeal approaches to the parapharyngeal region (Box 27-1). Other operations for the oropharynx are considered elsewhere in this book.

SURGICAL ANATOMY

The oropharynx extends from the plane of the hard palate superiorly to the plane of the hyoid bone inferiorly. It communicates with the nasopharynx above, the hypopharynx inferiorly, and the oral cavity anteriorly. Subsites of the oropharynx are the tonsils, the tonsillar pillars, the soft palate, the base of the tongue, and the posterior pharyngeal wall.

The roof of the oropharynx is formed anteriorly by the pharyngeal portion of the soft palate, but it is incomplete posteriorly, communicating with the nasopharynx via the nasopharyngeal isthmus. The lateral and posterior margins of the isthmus are formed by fibers of the palatopharyngeus muscle, which encircle the pharynx inside the superior constrictor and form Passavant ridge, against which the soft palate impinges when elevated by the levator palati muscle. Other fibers of the palatopharyngeus muscle form the posterior tonsillar pillar. Any surgery that disrupts the musculature of the soft palate in any way will inevitably lead to some degree of velopharyngeal incompetence and Eustachian tube dysfunction.

Anteriorly the oropharynx communicates with the oral cavity via the oropharyngeal isthmus, which is bordered by the soft palate above, the anterior tonsillar pillars laterally, and the dorsum of the tongue at the circumvallate papillae. The lateral walls of the oropharynx are delineated by the anterior and posterior tonsillar pillars, which are mucosal folds overlying the palatoglossus and the palatopharyngeus muscles, respectively, with the tonsillar fossa occupying the space between these two pillars. Deep to the mucosa, the lateral wall consists of the superior constrictor, the upper fibers of the middle constrictor, and the palatoglossus, palatopharyngeus, salpingopharyngeus, and stylopharyngeus muscles. The posterior wall of the oropharynx is related to the second and third cervical vertebrae and consists of mucosa, constrictor muscle, and the buccopharyngeal and prevertebral fascia.

FUNCTION

Normal oropharyngeal anatomy and function are vital for speech and swallowing. Any distortion of the anatomy can profoundly affect these complex and vital processes. During the oral phase of swallowing, food is forced by the tongue through the oropharyngeal isthmus into the oropharynx, thereby initiating the involuntary phase. The palatoglossus muscles contract and prevent the reflux of food into the oral cavity. The larynx rises against the epiglottis, which is pushed backward and downward by the movement of the tongue base. The nature of the bolus determines its subsequent progress. If the bolus is liquid or semiliquid, the thrust of the tongue is sufficient to propel it into the esophagus. If it is solid, the pharyngeal muscles need to contract to push the food into the esophagus. The distortion of normal oropharyngeal anatomy can cause dysphagia, dysarthria, aspiration, or reflux through an incompetent nasopharyngeal or oropharyngeal isthmus.

TREATMENT STRATEGIES FOR OROPHARYNGEAL CANCER

Before the clinical experience with organ-preservation protocols during the late twentieth century, surgery with adjuvant radiation was the standard of care for oropharyngeal carcinoma. Clinical trials that have examined combinations of radiation therapy with or without concurrent chemotherapy as primary therapy have demonstrated favorable oncologic and functional outcomes. Accordingly, organ preservation strategies have gained popularity, and, today, several treatment algorithms are available, depending on the TNM stage. These include primary radiation or surgery for early-stage lesions and combinations of chemotherapy and radiation with or without brachytherapy for advanced disease. Clinical studies suggest that oncologic outcomes are similar for surgery with adjuvant radiation and combinations of chemoradiation. Treatment decisions are increasingly made on the basis of the functional outcome of patients

---

BOX 27-1 Surgical Approaches to the Oropharynx

1. Transoral resection
2. Mandible-sparing procedures
   - Lateral pharyngotomy
   - Transhyoid pharyngotomy
3. Mandible-splitting procedures
   - Lateral mandibulotomy
   - Anterior mandibulotomy
4. Mandible resection
   - Segmental mandibulectomy
5. Transpharyngeal approaches
   - Transpharyngeal styloid process resection
   - Transpharyngeal approach to the parapharyngeal space
   - Transpalatal approach to the nasopharynx

---

treated with primary surgery as compared with chemoradiation. The patient's pretreatment comorbidity and functional status[1] as well as the capabilities of the treatment team also factor into treatment decisions.

OROPHARYNGEAL CANCER AND QUALITY OF LIFE

Regardless of the cause, derangements of normal oropharyngeal function negatively affect perceptions of the quality of life. Studies that have specifically examined the pretreatment functioning of patients with oropharyngeal cancer show that oropharyngeal lesions do affect function and that differences in the level of dysfunction are variable, depending on the site and stage of the tumor.[1,2] Many studies that have examined oropharyngeal function relative to treatment for oropharyngeal tumors have compared posttreatment function with that of normal subjects or have not controlled for tumor stage. If pretreatment function was not assessed, the true impact of treatment cannot be assessed. Studies that have compared pretreatment and posttreatment oropharyngeal function provide clinicians with meaningful comparisons between treatment modalities. In studies that have controlled for these variables, outcomes for early-stage tumors have similar functional and global quality of life outcomes with either primary surgery or primary radiation. By contrast, patients with advanced-stage tumors show highly significant differences that favor nonoperative primary treatment.[3] Regardless of the primary treatment modality, head and neck surgeons must be familiar with the complications and sequelae of surgery for oropharyngeal neoplasms, because surgery will continue to have a significant role in their treatment.

SEQUELAE VERSUS COMPLICATIONS

A *sequela* is a logical consequence of a procedure, whereas a *complication* is an unexpected, untoward event. As technology and surgical technique improve, many of the postoperative outcomes that were formerly considered sequelae are now regarded as complications.

TRANSORAL RESECTION

Indications and General Principles

Transoral resection is usually reserved for very small, benign, or low-grade malignant tumors. Some cancers of the oropharynx are amenable to transoral resection, particularly small superficial exophytic cancers that arise on the posterior pharyngeal wall and soft palate. The key to successful transoral resection consists of the adequate exposure and illumination of the lesion. A variety of mouth gags, cheek retractors, and tongue depressors are used to obtain exposure. Excision is accomplished using a scalpel, electrocautery, or laser. After resection, the defect typically heals by secondary intention, although primary closure or a skin graft can be employed.

Complications

Complications of all of the procedures discussed can be divided into those that result from either achieving exposure, the resection, or the repair of the defect.

Exposure

The Davis–Crowe instrument opens the mouth, depresses the tongue, and maintains the position of the endotracheal tube. The most common complication associated with this instrument is contusion or laceration of the posterior pharyngeal wall caused by the blind insertion of the instrument without adequate visualization of the tip of the tongue blade. This can be remedied by carefully selecting a blade of appropriate length and inserting it under direct visualization with adequate illumination from a headlight. Temporomandibular joint dislocation is also possible and should be checked for after the instrument is removed from the mouth.

Another complication attributed to the Davis–Crowe retractor is paresthesia of the lingual or hypoglossal nerve resulting from prolonged pressure on the tongue during a long procedure. This may cause aberrations in mobility, taste, and tongue sensation that can persist for weeks after the procedure. Knowledge of this potential complication should remind the surgeon to periodically release the pressure during procedures that last for more than a few minutes.

Resection

Hemorrhage can present at the time of surgery or during the immediate postoperative period, or it may be delayed (secondary hemorrhage). Surgery of the base of the tongue is particularly vulnerable because of its rich blood supply. Although the use of electrocautery and the laser tend to minimize this complication, the size of the vessels in the tongue base precludes truly bloodless surgery.

If significant bleeding is encountered intraoperatively, cautery or ligation of the affected vessel is usually possible. However, if the bleeding site cannot be identified because of the retraction of the vessel, blind clamping or cautery should be avoided, and a deep, judiciously placed suture ligature should be used to control the retracted vessel. A similar approach should be adopted for postoperative or secondary hemorrhage. If perioperative hemorrhage cannot be controlled with these techniques, angiography with embolization or the open exploration of the neck and the ligation of the relevant external carotid artery branches may be necessary.

A problem unique to the surgery of the base of the tongue is the development of an interstitial hematoma, which can lead to significant swelling and airway obstruction. Hematoma occurs because bleeding from retracted blood vessels spreads between the muscle fibers. It is usually self-limiting as a result of the tamponade effect from the hematoma. Vessels characteristically cannot be identified for ligation, and the hematoma cannot be evacuated in the conventional sense. Therefore the best treatment is to protect the airway with a nasal trumpet or a tracheotomy and await spontaneous resolution, which normally occurs in 2 to 3 days.

The aspiration of blood or secretions during the perioperative period can result in pulmonary complications, and a throat pack is recommended for oropharyngeal procedures. The excision of small superficial lesions does not usually cause any alteration in oropharyngeal function, but through-and-through defects of the soft palate result in velopharyngeal incompetence with hypernasal speech and the reflux of food and liquids through the nose. Secondary Eustachian tube dysfunction is another sequela of the resection of the soft-palate musculature. The first-line treatment of velopharyngeal incompetence consists of the placement of an obturator or a prosthesis. Surgical reconstruction with local or regional flaps is considered if the patient cannot tolerate the obturator or if it is not effectively functioning. If sequelae of Eustachian tube dysfunction occur, myringotomy and the placement of a ventilation tube are recommended.

Some clinicians employ a carbon dioxide laser for transoral resection. Nonhealing ulcers, fistula formation, and osteonecrosis of the mandible have been described after laser excision.[4] Complications are more likely to occur as the indications for this technique are extended for more advanced lesions.[5]

Repair

Most defects after transoral resection can heal by secondary intention with no sequelae. If the musculature is damaged, however, the resultant scarring and contracture can cause distortion of the anatomy and may affect function. Velopharyngeal dysfunction, secondary Eustachian tube dysfunction, and dysphagia are possible. Circumferential dissection may result in nasopharyngeal stenosis; the avoidance of such defects is recommended.[6]

Scarring and wound contracture that occur with healing by secondary intention can be minimized using a skin graft to cover the postresection defect. A bolster is recommended to immobilize the graft for 5 days and can necessitate a tracheotomy. An alternative that may obviate the need for tracheotomy is to quilt the graft into place, but the survival of the skin graft is better when a bolster is used.

MANDIBLE-SPARING PROCEDURES

Lateral Pharyngotomy

Indications and General Principles

The lateral pharyngotomy approach (Figure 27-1, *A*) provides adequate exposure for the resection of small- to moderate-sized lesions of the base of the tongue,

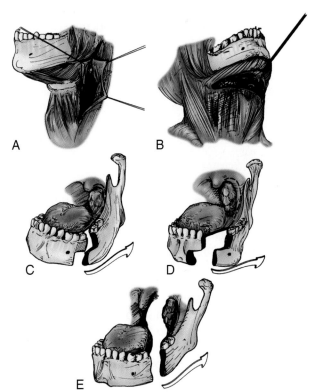

Figure 27-1. Surgical approaches to the oropharynx. **A,** Lateral pharyngotomy. **B,** Transhyoid pharyngotomy. **C,** Lateral mandibulotomy. **D,** Anterior mandibulotomy. **E,** Jaw–neck procedure.

the epiglottis, and the posterior and lateral pharyngeal walls. This approach can be combined with a neck dissection or extended superiorly by performing a mandibular osteotomy.

Complications

Exposure

Damage to the superior laryngeal or hypoglossal nerve by stretching or disruption can also result from exposure and result in temporary or permanent aspiration or dysarthria. Complications related to the carotid artery are rare but well documented, and they can be devastating to the patient. The carotid artery should be handled cautiously to minimize the likelihood of a dislodged atherosclerotic plaque, carotid artery spasm, or thrombosis.[7] The onset of symptoms can occur at the time of injury or a few hours to days after the procedure. The best treatment is prevention, with the surgeon being cognizant of the potential complication and ensuring that the retraction is gentle and that it is relaxed at regular intervals. The hyperextension of the neck and direct trauma by excessive retraction or manipulation should be avoided. Localizing neurologic symptoms or signs during the postoperative period should be evaluated with head computed tomography scanning, angiography, and appropriate consultation with vascular or neurosurgical colleagues.

Resection

Complications related to the resection are directly dependent on the site of resection and the size of the defect. Accordingly, large pharyngeal defects have a higher incidence of complications. Because lateral pharyngotomy is most commonly used for posterior and lateral pharyngeal wall cancers, hemorrhage and the aspiration of blood and secretions are the major concerns. Meticulous hemostatic dissection will minimize the chance of these problems.

Repair

The defect can be closed by primary repair, skin graft, or regional or free flap reconstruction. The most serious complication common to all three types of repair is a pharyngocutaneous fistula. Although many local and systemic factors may contribute to the formation of a fistula, the choice of the reconstructive procedure and the surgical technique are things that the surgeon can control. A poorly planned or executed reconstruction, impaired wound healing, and flap failure can lead to the formation of a fistula. The consequences of a fistula range from inconvenience to disaster, so every attempt should be made to prevent this complication. After it has occurred, a fistula should be treated aggressively with meticulous attention to detail and according to standard guidelines.

The treatment of a fistula consists of early identification. Early symptoms include cervical tenderness, erythema, fever, tachycardia, and malaise. An indirect fistula should be converted to a direct fistula by incising directly over the tract, diverting the saliva away from the great vessels, and ensuring that the neck flaps are not compromised. The majority will heal spontaneously with time and appropriate wound care. Surgical intervention is considered only if the fistula fails to close over a prolonged period of time.

Prevention is maximized with careful planning of the reconstruction and meticulous attention to the mucosal closure. If primary closure is not an option, a skin graft is the next consideration. The mucosal edges of the defect are sutured to the skin graft and to the tissues of the deep margin. For posterior pharyngeal wall defects, the graft is sutured to the prevertebral musculature so that the closure is stable and watertight. If the defect is larger, a regional flap can be used. A pectoralis major flap may be too bulky. Better options include a deltopectoral flap with a deepithelialized pedicle; a temporalis muscle flap; or a thin, pliable, free flap.

Carotid artery protection is advisable if a lateral pharyngotomy and a neck dissection are performed simultaneously. Some clinicians use a dermal skin graft, the pedicle of a myocutaneous flap, or the soft tissue of a free flap. Perioperative antibiotics may aid in diminishing the incidence of fistula formation,[8,9] with a 24-hour regimen probably being as effective as a 5-day course.[10] Rinsing the oral cavity with antimicrobial mouthwash 30 minutes before surgery and for the first few days postoperatively may also be effective.

Most techniques of pharyngeal reconstruction produce an adynamic, insensate region of the pharynx that contributes to the fixation of the larynx as well as an area that has lost its capacity for coordinated peristalsis. Significant dysphagia and aspiration can occur in these patients, and it is compounded if there is associated injury to the lower cranial nerves. There is no ready remedy for this problem except to use as thin and pliable a flap as possible and to begin comprehensive rehabilitation during the postoperative period. The removal of the tracheostomy before initiating swallowing is important, because the tracheostomy can compound the laryngeal fixation. The routine use of prophylactic cricopharyngeal myotomy has not been conclusively shown to improve the swallowing outcome in these cases.

Transhyoid Pharyngotomy

Indications and General Principles

The transhyoid pharyngotomy (Figure 27-1, B) has been advocated for cancer of the epiglottis, of the base of the tongue, and of the posterior pharyngeal wall.[11,12] Caution should be used for epiglottic and base of tongue lesions, because blind entry into the vallecula may violate the tumor.[13] The hyoid bone can be left intact, with the entire dissection being performed in the suprahyoid area, or the hyoid can be excised, thereby yielding improved exposure but a more challenging closure.

Complications

Exposure

Inadvertent stretching or severing of the hypoglossal or superior laryngeal nerves is possible. If the greater horns of the hyoid are left undissected, the likelihood of nerve damage is significantly less. The resultant dysarthria, dysphagia, and aspiration from this injury can be severe.

Resection

Complications are similar to those encountered with lateral pharyngotomy. For those patients in whom small tongue-base tumors are excised with the use of this approach, complications are not commonly encountered.[11]

Repair

The site of resection is repaired using the same principles as described for lateral pharyngotomy. Fistula formation, aspiration, and dysphagia are potential complications, and their management has already been described. The advantage of this technique is that the approach itself is relatively atraumatic, and primary closure results in no functional or anatomic impairment. Wound dehiscence and fistula formation at the site of incision are rare. A prophylactic tracheostomy should be strongly considered in the presence of perioperative edema or hemorrhage.

MANDIBLE-SPLITTING PROCEDURES

Mandibulotomy

Indications and General Principles

Anterior osteotomy is the procedure of choice when mandibulotomy is indicated to gain access to the oropharynx (Figure 27-1, D). Its major advantage over a lateral osteotomy is the preservation of the inferior alveolar nerve and the vascular bundle. It is typically outside of the radiation field, which is an important consideration if adjuvant radiation is part of the treatment. The osteotomy is placed anterior to the mental foramen in the symphyseal[14] or parasymphyseal[15] site. After the osteotomy has been performed, the mandible is displaced laterally by making an incision along the floor of the mouth (mandibular swing) or along the midline of the tongue (median labiomandibular glossotomy).[13,16,17]

The lateral mandibulotomy (Figure 27-1, C) was originally described by Trotter.[18] As a result of a lateral osteotomy,

the inferior alveolar nerve and the vascular bundle will be transected, thus causing numbness of the ipsilateral teeth, the alveolar ridge, and the mental skin. Although it has been suggested that the anesthesia can recover,[19] this is not routinely reported in the literature. This sequela is a significant disadvantage to this technique. The procedure may continue to have a role for larger lesions of the oropharynx when superior extension of the lateral pharyngotomy is required for access (e.g., tumors involving the posterior and lateral walls). The actual site of the osteotomy is dictated by the site of the tumor and whether the patient is dentulous or edentulous.

Complications

Exposure

Exposure of the osteotomy site is usually accomplished via a lip-splitting incision or a visor flap.[15] Osteotomy design is intended to maximize stability and minimize any dental trauma. The reconstruction plate can be bent, secured, and then removed before the osteotomy, which preserves normal dental occlusion. Removing a tooth at the osteotomy site will minimize the chance of damage to the adjacent tooth roots and teeth. Copious irrigation minimizes thermal damage from the saw and drill. A stairstep osteotomy is another technique to maximize postoperative stability. Some authors advocate a straight osteotomy between the teeth without extraction and report no increased dental trauma.[15] Because the mandible is swung laterally to obtain exposure, temporomandibular joint disruption and damage to the lingual nerve may result if care is not taken to avoid vigorous retraction.

Resection

Oropharyngeal tumors that require this approach are at an advanced stage and require more complicated resection and reconstruction. The incidence of wound dehiscence, hemorrhage, infection, and fistula formation tend to be higher than what is seen with early-stage tumors.[14]

Closure

Complications related to the closure of the osteotomy include those related to the closure of the mucosal defect and the repair of the osteotomy. Wound dehiscence, orocutaneous fistula, and infection are caused by the disruption of the closure of the floor of mouth. The key to prevention is to leave an adequate cuff of mucosa on the alveolar ridge when making the incision along the floor of the mouth (Figure 27-2). Meticulous closure of the mucosa is also important.

Unstable repair of the osteotomy can be associated with malunion, nonunion, osteomyelitis, and osteoradionecrosis. Several techniques have been suggested to prevent complications related to the healing of the osteotomy. The preservation of the mandibular

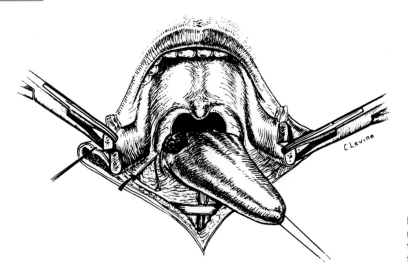

Figure 27-2. Technique for anterior osteotomy with mandibular swing. An adequate cuff of mucosa is left on the alveolar ridge *(arrow)* to enable a good anastomosis to be performed.

periosteum and the blood supply will improve chances of osteotomy healing. Accurate positioning of the plate and screw holes before the osteotomy is performed will ensure the exact reapproximation of the bone fragments. A stairstep design and the rigid fixation of the osteotomy improve the stability of the repair. Malunion and nonunion of the bone segments are more likely to occur if preoperative or adjuvant radiation therapy are planned.

Malunion or nonunion related to the instability of the reconstituted fragments, together with osteomyelitis or infection around the hardware that is used to stabilize the fragments, is a difficult problem (Figures 27-3 and 27-4).[17,20] Damage from the saw or inadequate soft-tissue coverage may also predispose a patient to osteomyelitis. After the diagnosis of infection has been confirmed, clinical treatment regimens vary, usually involving some combination of plate removal, the debridement of nonviable bone, antibiotics, and hyperbaric oxygen

according to individual practice patterns and the clinical scenario.

COMPOSITE RESECTION

Indications and General Principles

Composite resection and the *jaw–neck procedure* (Figure 27-1, *E*) are the names given to segmental mandibulectomy with incontinuity neck dissection and partial pharyngectomy. This procedure is the cornerstone of surgical treatment for advanced cancer of the oropharynx or for cases in which the mandible is directly involved with tumor.

The sequelae associated with this procedure in the past were primarily related to the large defects created and the limited reconstructive options available before the current reconstructive era. Primary closure, skin grafts, or regional flaps frequently resulted in the contracture and distortion of the oropharynx that led to significant

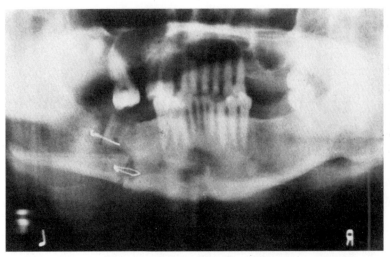

Figure 27-3. Malunion of a lateral mandibulotomy with early osteomyelitis.

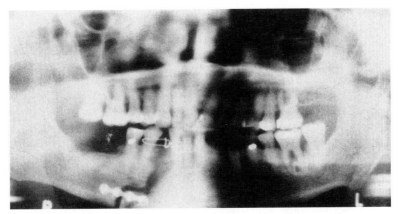

Figure 27-4. Nonunion and osteomyelitis with an anterior osteotomy.

problems with speech, mastication, deglutition, and cosmesis. In fact, the mandible was frequently sacrificed not for oncologic reasons but rather to facilitate exposure, resection, and closure. During the modern era, with excellent techniques for reconstructing both soft tissue and bone, these sequelae occur less frequently, and the rates of functional defects, cosmetic defects, and complications have declined significantly.

Complications

Exposure

The resection of a segment of the mandible concurrent with neck dissection facilitates exposure of the tumor and important structures. Oncologic resection and reconstruction are likewise facilitated. These resections are usually done for large oropharyngeal tumors that extend into the floor of the mouth and the submandibular triangle. Resection of the contents of the submandibular triangle together with the primary tumor (as opposed to the neck contents) will avoid any cutting into the primary tumor and thereby compromising the oncologic resection.

Resection

Intraoperative bleeding can arise from damage to the internal maxillary artery when performing the posterior osteotomy. It can be controlled by rotating the mandibular segment out of the way to gain access to the artery. Oozing from the pterygoid plexus of the veins usually responds to intraoperative packing and electrocautery.

During the early postoperative period, hemorrhage may manifest as increased drainage from the suction drains or as an accumulation under the skin flaps. Because flap necrosis and wound infection are consequences of hematoma formation,[21] the wound should be explored immediately, the hematoma evacuated, the bleeding points isolated and ligated, and fresh drains inserted. Inadequate evacuation of the hematoma or the premature removal of the drains can result in seroma formation,

which at the very least will require repeated needle aspiration and the application of a pressure dressing. Occasionally incision and drainage are indicated. Other complications that result from resection are related to the site and extent of the primary resection and neck dissection. Damage to associated cranial nerves contributes to dysphagia, dysarthria, and aspiration.

The extrusion of the free edge of the remaining mandibular segment through the skin (Figure 27-5) or into the oral cavity can be prevented by rounding off any sharp bone edges with a rongeur, a rasp, or a drill. If extrusion does occur postoperatively, open exploration and the amputation of any protruding segment should be performed. Osteomyelitis of the mandibular stump has been reported and is treated with debridement.[22]

The resection of the posterior segment of the mandible without bone reconstruction will result in varying degrees of mandibular migration and the collapse of the

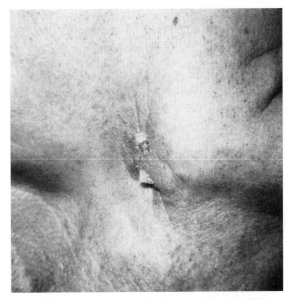

Figure 27-5. Protrusion of the posterior end of the mandible through the skin.

lateral wall of the oropharynx. If the angle and a small portion of the body are removed in an edentulous patient, the consequences are minimal. Larger resections can remove the support of the tongue, resulting in respiratory obstruction, sleep apnea, and possibly other functional problems.

Reconstruction

In the era preceding the development of the advanced reconstructive procedures that are available today, most composite defects were closed primarily. Primary closure can lead to the distortion of the pharynx, ipsilateral mandibular migration, and cosmetic deformity, which produces dysphagia, dysarthria, and difficulty with mastication. The solution to sequelae is the almost routine use of skin grafts, regional cutaneous flaps, and, more recently, myocutaneous and free flaps. These reconstructive procedures have reduced the distortion and functional deficits as well as the incidence of complications.

The incidence of pharyngocutaneous fistula, even in adequately reconstructed patients, is 10% to 30%. The vast majority heal with conservative therapy, whereas a small percentage will require surgical closure if conservative therapy fails. The consequences of a poorly managed fistula range from a prolonged hospital stay to flap necrosis, wound infection, and carotid rupture. Routine prophylactic coverage of the exposed great vessels should be strongly considered at the time of resection.[23]

Cosmetic outcome and dental occlusion in patients with teeth warrant the consideration of mandibular reconstruction in conjunction with the reconstruction of the mucosal defect. Various techniques including reconstruction plates,[4] autogenous free grafts, osteomyocutaneous flaps, regional flaps, and free flaps all have their advocates.[24] Decisions regarding whether the advantages of mandibular reconstruction outweigh the disadvantages are made by the treatment team.

The composite resection of oropharyngeal tumors invariably results in some degree of deglutition and speech impairment. The extent of functional disability depends on the amount of resected tissue and the type of reconstruction used to close the defect. Dysphagia after the composite resection of oropharyngeal tumors results in significant dysphagia that is multifactorial and that involves both the oral and pharyngeal phases of swallowing, which renders rehabilitation complicated and difficult. Articulation defects associated with the formation of speech fricatives require lingual–alveolar approximation. Functional parameters have been assessed after oropharyngeal resection, and they demonstrate that the degree of tongue mobility is the most significant variable for determining postoperative function.[25–27] Functional outcomes in dentate patients undergoing osseous free flap reconstruction and endosteal implants have been shown to achieve superior results in all parameters without prolonged hospitalization or a significant increase in complications as compared with other reconstructive procedures.[28,29]

TRANSPHARYNGEAL APPROACHES

Transpharyngeal Styloid Process Resection

Indications and General Principles

Originally described by Eagle in 1937,[30] the transpharyngeal approach for the resection of an elongated styloid process or a calcified stylohyoid ligament is a frequently performed procedure. After tonsillectomy, an incision is made through the tonsillar fossa directly over the elongated styloid process. The styloid process is dissected by means of sharp and blunt dissection, and the bone is fractured as superiorly as possible. Some authors believe that an external approach is safer.[31]

Complications

Inadvertent damage to the carotid artery system and the glossopharyngeal nerve are possible with blind dissection. The best treatment is prevention, ensuring that the dissection is kept subperiosteal. If significant hemorrhage is encountered, a cervical approach to identify and control the bleeding source is recommended. Damage to the glossopharyngeal nerve will become apparent postoperatively, and treatment is consultation for swallowing rehabilitation. Occasionally, after its division, the styloid process may be "lost" in the neck. This is of no consequence, and the fragment is best left alone rather than attempting a deep dissection to retrieve it with a concomitant risk of injury to the surrounding structures. Because transpharyngeal resection can result in the infection of the parapharyngeal space, prophylactic antibiotics should be used. The development of surgical emphysema has been cited as a rare complication of the transpharyngeal approach.[31] In a large series of more than 150 cases of transpharyngeal styloid excision, no complications of any consequence were recorded, thus supporting the claim that, if it is carefully performed, this is a reasonable approach to the styloid process.[32]

Transpharyngeal Approach to the Parapharyngeal Space

Indications and General Principles

Transoral, transpharyngeal resection of parapharyngeal space tumors should only be considered for very small tumors of the pharyngeal wall that can be adequately visualized. The limited and blind nature of the approach results in a significant risk for neural and vascular damage,[33,34] inadequate tumor resection,[35] and tumor spillage. The literature does contain reports of successful resections performed via this route.[35,36] In the hands of an experienced surgeon and with careful case selection, it may occasionally be feasible.

Transpalatal Approach to the Nasopharynx

Indications and General Principles

The transpalatal route provides a simple and direct approach to the anterior skull base that offers excellent exposure of the nasopharynx, the posterior pharyngeal wall, the sphenoid sinus, and the clivus. Therefore it can be used successfully for the excision of selected angiofibromas, clival chordomas, and nasopharyngeal malignancies as well as for the repair of choanal atresia and for access to the cervical spine. The principle of this approach is the elevation of palatal flaps to preserve the blood supply from the greater palatine arteries. This necessitates a midline palatal incision or a U-shaped incision to keep the flap pedicled on the greater palatine arteries bilaterally. The bony hard palate is then removed, depending on the access required.

Complications

Complications of the midline incision include palatal flap necrosis as a result of a severed greater palatine artery and the dehiscence of the soft-palate incision with the development of an oronasal fistula palatal shortening and velopharyngeal incompetence. Prevention consists of the meticulous three-layer closure of the palatal incision and the avoidance of undue nasopharyngeal packing, which may cause pressure necrosis and wound disruption. If a dehiscence develops, primary repair may be possible, but only under exceptional circumstances. Usually a prosthetic denture allows the defect to be obturated. Palatal shortening has been attributed to contracture after a simple midline incision, and it can be prevented by altering the incision to an S shape.[37]

REFERENCES

1. Borggreven PA, Verdonck-de Leeuw IM, Muller MJ, et al: Quality of life and functional status in patients with cancer of the oral cavity and oropharynx: Pretreatment values of a prospective study. *Eur Arch Otorhinolaryngol* 2007;264:651–657.
2. Mowry SE, Ho A, Lotempio MM, et al: Quality of life in advanced oropharyngeal carcinoma after chemoradiation versus surgery and radiation. *Laryngoscope* 2006;116:1589–1593.
3. Allal AS, Nicoucar K, Mach N, et al: Quality of life in patients with oropharynx carcinomas: Assessment after accelerated radiotherapy with or without chemotherapy versus radical surgery and postoperative radiotherapy. *Head Neck* 2003;25:833–840.
4. Guerry TL, Silverman S, Dedo HH: Carbon dioxide laser resection of superficial oral carcinoma. *Ann Otol Laryngol* 1986;95:547–555.
5. Fisher SE, Frame JW, Browne RM, et al: A comparative histological study of wound healing following CO_2 laser and conventional surgical excision of canine buccal mucosa. *Arch Oral Biol* 1983;28:287–291.
6. Nagorsky MJ, Sessions DG: Laser resection or early oral cavity cancer—Results and complications. *Ann Otol Rhinol Laryngol* 1987;96:556–560.
7. Miller DR, Bergstrom L: Vascular complications of head and neck surgery. *Arch Otolaryngol* 1974;100:136–140.
8. Robbins KT, Byers RM, Fainstein V, et al: Wound prophylaxis with metronidazole in head and neck surgical oncology. *Laryngoscope* 1988;98:803–806.
9. Becker GD, Parell GJ: Cefazolin prophylaxis in head and neck cancer surgery. *Ann Otol Rhinol Laryngol* 1979;88:183–186.
10. Johnson JT, Schuller DE, Silver F, et al: Antibiotic prophylaxis in high-risk head and neck surgery: One-day vs. five day therapy. *Otolaryngol Head Neck Surg* 1986;95:554–557.
11. Zeitels SM, Vaughn CW, Ruh S: Suprahyoid pharyngotomy for oropharyngeal cancer including the tongue base. *Arch Otolaryngol Head Neck Surg* 1991;117:757–760.
12. Zeitels SM, Vaughn CW, Toomey JM: A precision technique for suprahyoid pharyngotomy. *Laryngoscope* 1991;101:565–566.
13. Gluckman JL, Thompson R: Cancer of the oropharynx. In Suen JW, Meyers EM, editors: *Cancer of the head and neck*, New York, 1989, Churchill Livingstone.
14. Spiro GR, Gerold FP, Shah JP, et al: Mandibulotomy approach to oropharyngeal tumors. *Am J Surg* 1985;150:466–469.
15. McGregor IA, MacDonald DG: Mandibular osteotomy in the surgical approach to the oral cavity. *Head Neck Surg* 1983;5:457–462.
16. Martin H, Tollefsen HR, Gerold FP: Median labiomandibular glossotomy. *Am J Surg* 1971;102:753–759.
17. Tollefsen HR, Spiro RH: Median labiomandibular glossotomy. *Ann Surg* 1971;173:415–420.
18. Trotter W: Operations for malignant disease of the pharynx. *Br J Surg* 1929;16:485–495.
19. Pinsolle J, Siberchicot F, Emparanza A, et al: Approach to the pterygomaxillary space and posterior part of the tongue by lateral stair-step mandibulotomy. *Arch Otolaryngol Head Neck Surg* 1989;115:313–315.
20. Dawson DE, Gapany M, LaVelle WE: Titanium lag-screw osteosynthesis for the restoration of mandibular continuity in mandibular "swing" procedures. *Laryngoscope* 1990;100:1241–1244.
21. McGuirt WF, McCabe BF, Krause CJ: Complications of radical neck dissection: A survey of 788 patients. *Head Neck Surg* 1979;1:481–487.
22. LaFerriere KA, Sessions DG, Thawley SE, et al: Composite resection and reconstruction for oral cavity and oropharynx cancer. *Arch Otolaryngol* 1980;106:103–110.
23. Shumrick DA: Carotid artery rupture. *Laryngoscope* 1973;83:1051–1061.
24. Chow JM, Hill JH: Primary mandibular reconstruction using the AO reconstruction plate. *Laryngoscope* 1986;96:768–773.
25. Logemann JA, Bytell DE: Swallowing disorders in three types of head and neck surgical patients. *Cancer* 1979;44:1095–1105.
26. McConnel FMS, Teichenberg JF, Adler RK: A comparison of three methods of oral reconstruction. *Arch Otolaryngol Head Neck Surg* 1987;113:496–500.
27. Teichenberg J, Bowman J, Geopfert H: New test series for the functional evaluation of oral cavity cancer. *Head Neck Surg* 1985;8:9–20.
28. Komisar A: The functional results of mandibular reconstruction. *Laryngoscope* 1990;100:364–374.
29. Urken ML, Buchbinder D, Weinberg H, et al: Functional evaluation following microvascular oromandibular reconstruction of the oral cancer patient: A comparative study of Surgery of the oropharynx reconstructed and nonreconstructed patients. *Laryngoscope* 1991;101:935–950.
30. Eagle WW: Elongated styloid process: Report of two cases. *Arch Otolaryngol* 1937;25:584–587.
31. Strauss M, Zohar Y, Laurian N: Elongated styloid process syndrome: Intraoral vs. extraoral approach for styloid surgery. *Laryngoscope* 1985;95:976–979.
32. Eagle WW: Elongated styloid process: Symptoms and treatment. *Arch Otolaryngol* 1958;67:172–176.

33. Som PM, Biller HF, Lawson W: Tumors of the parapharyngeal space: Preoperative evaluation, diagnosis and surgical approaches. *Ann Otol Rhinol Laryngol* 1981;90(Suppl 80):3–15.

34. Carrau RL, Myers EN, Johnson JT: Management of tumors arising in the parapharyngeal space. *Laryngoscope* 1990;100:583–589.

35. Goodwin WJ, Chandler JR: Transoral excision of lateral pharyngeal space tumors presenting intraorally. *Laryngoscope* 1988;98:266–269.

36. McIlrath DC, Remine WH, Devine KD, et al: Tumors of the parapharyngeal region. *Surg Gynecol Obstet* 1963;116:88–94.

37. Kennedy DW, Panel ID, Holliday M: Transpalatal approach to the skull base. *Ear Nose Throat J* 1986;65:48–60.

CHAPTER 28

Complications of Tonsillectomy and Adenoidectomy

Thomas J. Ow and Sanjay R. Parikh

Tonsillectomy and adenoidectomy are among the most common procedures performed by the general and pediatric otorhinolaryngologist, numbering roughly 500,000 annually.[1] These surgeries are most often indicated to improve obstructive sleep apnea, recurrent pharyngitis, and recurrent otitis media with effusion. Failure to thrive, abnormal dentofacial growth, dysphagia, speech impairment, halitosis, persistent streptococcal colonization, recurrent peritonsillar abscess, and suspicion of malignancy are also relative indications for tonsillectomy, adenoidectomy, or both.[2]

The mortality rate of adenotonsillar surgery has been quoted between 1 in 16,000 and 1 in 35,000 cases, paralleling that of general anesthesia alone. Most deaths are the result of complications of general anesthesia or hemorrhage.[3]

Tonsillectomy and adenoidectomy have seen a tremendous evolution during the last two decades. Patient selection and preoperative evaluation have improved, the procedure has become largely ambulatory, and various new techniques have been developed.

This chapter addresses the intraoperative, short-term postoperative, and long-term postoperative complications associated with the surgical excision of the tonsils and the adenoids. High-risk groups and their specific considerations are described as well. Finally, the evolving attitudes and techniques for tonsillectomy and adenoidectomy are discussed as they relate to morbidity and mortality.

INTRAOPERATIVE COMPLICATIONS

Intraoperative Hemorrhage

The adenoid and tonsillar regions are richly vascularized, and bleeding during surgery is inevitable. Adequate control is usually achievable with routine surgical techniques, but severe bleeding can quickly create a life-threatening situation. Minimizing intraoperative hemorrhage and the accurate assessment of the volume lost is mandatory, especially when operating on a young child. Total blood volume is best estimated at 7.5 ml per 100 g of body weight. Estimated blood volume varies slightly by age, with the following calculations:

Newborns: 80 to 90 ml/Kg

Infants: 70 to 80 ml/Kg

Children: 70 ml/Kg

Calculating the maximal allowable blood loss preoperatively can help the surgeon to avoid complications from excessive bleeding. The following calculation is used:

$$\text{Maximal allowable blood loss} = ([\text{Estimated blood volume}] \times [\text{Hematocrit} - 25])/\text{Hematocrit}$$

This estimate provides the surgeon and anesthesiologist with guidelines for fluid management and indications for necessary blood transfusion.[3]

The adenoid bed receives its blood supply from the ascending pharyngeal, Vidian, and sphenopalatine arteries.[4] Injury to these large vessels is very rare during adenoidectomy, and bleeding usually occurs as a result of smaller venous or arterial branches. If the adenoid is resected in too deep of a plane, injury to the posterior pharyngeal wall musculature can cause bleeding. Hemostasis during adenoidectomy is usually obtained either with electrocautery under mirror visualization or with direct pressure with packing material. Most often gauze packing is used, and it may be dry or impregnated with topical vasoconstrictors. If bleeding persists, various hemostatic agents and packing materials are available.[3] If these methods fail to control hemorrhage, a posterior nasal pack may be necessary to maintain pressure in the nasopharynx for 24 to 48 hours. If the pack is not secured, if the patient is hemodynamically unstable, or if the patient is very young, then he or she should remain intubated. Observation in an intensive care setting while pressure is maintained at the bleeding site is recommended, and the patient should be stabilized with blood products and proper fluid management as necessary.

The tonsils are generally fed by larger-caliber arteries than those that feed the adenoid bed, and arterial bleeding is more common during tonsillectomy. The inferior tonsillar pole is fed by the tonsillar and ascending palatine branches of the facial artery and the tonsillar branches of the lingual artery. The middle tonsillar region is fed by the ascending pharyngeal artery, and the superior pole is supplied by the descending palatine artery.[4] Similar to the adenoid bed, careful dissection between the tonsil capsule and the pharyngeal muscle can minimize bleeding. Remnant tonsil can cause persistent bleeding, and injury to the deep musculature of the lateral pharyngeal wall can lead to large vessel disruption. When bleeding does occur, control is commonly achieved with brief periods of local pressure and packing, with or without vasoactive agents. Electrocautery is also often used to control bleeding. Alternatively, suture ligation of the offending vessels or of the region in the tonsillar fossa can be used to obtain hemostasis. Sutures in this region pose a risk of injuring the underlying facial, internal maxillary, or carotid arteries, which can lead to severe bleeding. If pseudoaneurysm develops, patients may present days after surgery with severe hemorrhage.[3]

Severe bleeding that is not controlled with local methods requires more extensive procedures. One option is neck exploration with the exposure of the carotid sheath and the ligation of the external carotid artery. During this procedure, the carotid bulb and the external and internal carotid artery should be explored to identify any injury to these structures.[5] When performing an external carotid artery ligation, at least two of the vessel's branches should be identified before artery ligation to adequately differentiate it from the internal carotid artery.[3] Another option for the diagnosis and possible management of persistent adenotonsillar bleeding is angiography. This procedure is absolutely necessary if external carotid ligation fails to control hemorrhage. Embolization is often therapeutic if a bleeding source can be identified.[5]

General Anesthesia

Adenotonsillar surgery poses many challenges to the anesthesiologist. The main issues involve the manner in which the airway is approached and protected, because the otorhinolaryngologist and anesthesiologist share the same working field. All patients undergoing adenoidectomy and tonsillectomy are typically intubated and under general anesthesia. Evaluation of the dentition before surgery by both the anesthesiologist and the otorhinolaryngologist is important. There is the potential for tooth dislodgement during intubation, during the placement and removal of the mouth gag, and during extubation. The patient can aspirate a tooth either before intubation or after extubation. If a tooth or a portion of a tooth is noted to be missing and cannot be accounted for, a chest radiograph should be obtained. To prevent this complication, loose teeth should be identified before

surgery, extremely loose teeth should be extracted at the commencement of surgery (permission should be obtained preoperatively in the informed consent), and the mouth gag should be carefully placed and positioned. Silk suture can be fastened to loose teeth to retrieve them if they are dislodged. The surgeon should carefully inspect the oral cavity and pharynx before extubation, especially if a tooth is missing. If a tooth is seen in the trachea or bronchus on the chest radiograph after extubation, bronchoscopy and retrieval are necessary.

During the operation, the endotracheal tube is at risk of kinking or dislodgement as the mouth gag is placed, positioned, or removed. If the oxygen saturation begins to decrease, if the patient's measured tidal volumes diminish, or if the airway pressures change without a known reason, obstruction or the accidental removal of the endotracheal tube should be suspected. If this complication is suspected, the mouth gag should be loosened, and laryngoscopy and the repositioning or replacement of the endotracheal tube may be urgently necessary.

Laryngospasm is also an important consideration for patients undergoing tonsillectomy and adenoidectomy. The topical application of 2% lidocaine or intravenous lidocaine before intubation can decrease the risk of this complication.[6] Should the patient develop laryngospasm, the obstruction can often be broken with positive pressure using mask ventilation. Sustained laryngospasm can be dangerous, causing hypoxemia and negative pressure pulmonary edema. If laryngospasm does not resolve quickly, succinylcholine can be given to relax the laryngeal musculature and release the obstruction. Before extubation, the surgeon should suction secretions and blood from the oral cavity and the oropharynx, and the patient should be fully awakened before the endotracheal tube is removed. The gastric contents do not need to be aspirated unless there is an excessive amount of blood loss. After extubation, the patient should be placed in the lateral decubitus position to best prevent aspiration and laryngospasm.

Technical Considerations

There are many technical pitfalls that the surgeon faces during the tonsillectomy procedure. When the patient is being prepared and draped, his or her eyes must be taped closed, and a head drape is placed. If a towel clip is used, care must be taken to protect the underlying skin and eyes. If cautery is used for dissection and coagulation, the soft tissues of the oral cavity and oropharynx must be protected from burns. Burns of the tongue, the buccal mucosa, the lips, and the palate are particularly painful. Insulated mouth gags are routinely used. If instruments such as clamps or a Hurd elevator are used during cautery coagulation, care must be taken to avoid conduction through the metallic instruments. This can result in burns to the tongue, the lips, or the oral commissure, which can be disfiguring and painful.

The use of electrocautery has become routine for adenotonsillectomy, which creates a risk of airway fire as a result of the proximity of the cautery tip to the endotracheal tube and airway. The hypopharynx should be packed with damp gauze, and air leakage around the endotracheal tube should be minimized. Ventilation should be maintained with a minimal concentration of inspired oxygen, preferably below 25%. Airway fire is a surprisingly rare complication of tonsillectomy.[7] If a fire occurs, a rapid response is necessary. Ventilation should be immediately halted, the endotracheal tube should be removed, and the fire should be extinguished by pouring water on the flames. Flammable drapes and materials should be removed. After the fire is extinguished, ventilation with 100% oxygen should be reestablished, and reintubation may be necessary. Laryngoscopy and bronchoscopy should then be performed for the assessment and clearance of debris from the trachea. A chest x-ray film should be ordered. Long-term intubation may be needed if significant pulmonary injury is present. Tracheostomy may be necessary if there is significant tracheal injury.[8]

To achieve hemostasis, some surgeons soak packing in vasoconstrictors to diminish intraoperative bleeding. Phenylephrine is one vasoconstrictor that is commonly used in otorhinolaryngology. The drug is an α-selective agonist, and, if available systemically, it may cause peripheral vasoconstriction, increased systemic vascular resistance, and decreased left ventricular performance with a resulting increase in pulmonary capillary pressure and edema. Phenylephrine has been contraindicated for adenotonsillectomy after reports of hypertension, pulmonary edema, and death associated with its use were reported. Strict guidelines for the use of this medication have been published to limit its application in otorhinolaryngologic surgery.[9] Although not well studied, oxymetazolone, which has been examined in endoscopic sinus surgery, may be a safe alternative.[10]

SHORT-TERM POSTOPERATIVE COMPLICATIONS

Postoperative Hemorrhage

Bleeding is the most common life-threatening complication after adenotonsillectomy. Recent literature suggests that the incidence is between 0.6% and 13%.[11,12] Reports vary widely on the basis of the criteria used to define post-tonsillectomy hemorrhage. Bleeding requiring major intervention (e.g., return to the operative suite, blood transfusion) appears to occur among 1% to 5% of patients.[11,13–19] The mortality from postoperative bleeding is estimated to be 0.002%.[20] Post-tonsillectomy hemorrhage is differentiated into primary bleeding (occurring within 24 hours of surgery) and secondary bleeding (occurring after 24 hours of surgery). Bleeding occurs most commonly between 5 and 9 days postoperatively.[11,13,16] The incidence of primary hemorrhage is much lower than that of secondary hemorrhage in the majority of large reports, but primary hemorrhage is often more severe.[20] Excessive postoperative bleeding from the adenoid bed is much less common than bleeding from the tonsillar fossae. Specific reports of isolated bleeding from adenoidectomy are scarce, but one study suggests a rate of 0.25% of cases.[19]

There are few risk factors for post-adenotonsillectomy bleeding that have been clearly identified. Most studies report that adult age poses a higher risk of bleeding,[14,16,18] although this has been contested.[13,15] Some studies have found bleeding to be more common among male patients.[13,19] One recent large retrospective study found no difference in bleeding among patients who received perioperative antibiotics, intraoperative injection of lidocaine with epinephrine, or bismuth placement in the operating room. Intraoperative blood loss, surgical technique, and surgery performed on an ambulatory basis did not appear to play a role in postoperative rates of hemorrhage, according to the study.[16] "Cold" instrument dissection has a higher rate of intraoperative blood loss as compared with "hot" electrocautery techniques, but most studies have failed to show a significant difference in postoperative hemorrhage between the two techniques.[16,21] Recently one prospective study and a large retrospective study have found an increase in secondary hemorrhage when bipolar diathermy was compared with cold steel dissection techniques.[14,22] When a patient presents with postoperative hemorrhage, swift and appropriate evaluation and management are crucial. In severe cases, airway management is an initial concern, and stabilization may be necessary with intubation or even tracheotomy. Large-bore intravenous access should be established, and appropriate resuscitative fluids should be administered. An initial hemodynamic assessment is of utmost importance and should include evaluation for signs and symptoms of hypovolemia during the taking of the history and the physical examination. It should be elicited whether the patient feels dizzy, lightheaded, or confused, and signs such as pallor and abnormalities in blood pressure and heart rate should be noted. It is important to attempt to quantify the blood loss while reviewing the history and to compare this with calculations of the patient's estimated blood volume. Initial laboratory evaluation includes a complete blood cell count, a prothrombin time, and a partial thromboplastin time as well as typing and cross matching for potential blood transfusion. Coagulopathies are a rare finding among patients with post-tonsillectomy hemorrhage.[15,23]

Management is dependent on the severity of bleeding. For patients who report a very small amount of bleeding on history and in whom no active bleeding or clot is seen on physical examination, a short period of observation with discharge home is appropriate if the patient is hemodynamically stable. If a clot is seen, some advocate complete suctioning of the clot for the proper assessment of active bleeding.[20] If active bleeding is seen, the severity is assessed. If bleeding is minimal, attempts can be made in cooperative patients to attain hemostasis using silver nitrate cautery or the application of pressure.[20] These patients should then be observed in the inpatient setting for 24 hours to ensure prolonged hemostasis.

Signs of significant bleeding necessitate a return to the operating room for examination under general anesthesia and control of the hemorrhage with either electrocautery or suture ligation of the bleeding vessels.[3,20] Rapid-sequence intubation is usually necessary due to the risk of aspiration from active bleeding or vomited blood. The endotracheal tube should be suctioned to remove all blood or a clot that may have been aspirated before intubation. The stomach should be adequately suctioned via gastric lavage to aid in quantifying the preoperative blood loss.[3] If bleeding cannot be controlled with standard measures, the throat should be packed, and external carotid artery ligation or angiography may be necessary, as previously described. Pseudoaneurysm of the external or internal carotid artery as a result of injury is a rare cause of late-onset severe bleeding,[24,25] and standard angiography, computed tomographic angiography, or magnetic resonance angiography may be necessary to make the diagnosis.

Respiratory Complications

Respiratory compromise after tonsillectomy can result from multiple causes. First, pulmonary edema may develop after the relief of chronic airway obstruction[26] — a condition termed *postobstructive pulmonary edema.* With chronic upper airway obstruction, there may be a compensated state of increased intrathoracic pressure. When the obstruction is relieved by intubation and/or adenotonsillectomy, the baseline intrathoracic pressure is suddenly decreased. This results in an increase in pulmonary venous return, pulmonary blood volume, pulmonary hydrostatic pressure, and the development of transudative pulmonary edema. This complication can be seen intraoperatively or hours after surgery.[3,27] A second cause of perioperative respiratory compromise is negative-pressure pulmonary edema. In this process, if a patient becomes acutely obstructed (e.g., during an episode of laryngospasm), the large negative inspiratory pressure created in the thoracic cavity as a result of the patient's respiratory efforts against an obstructed airway can draw transudate into the patient's pulmonary interstitium. This process will also lead to pulmonary edema.[26,27]

Postobstructive pulmonary edema and negative-pressure pulmonary edema have similar presentations, and swift recognition and treatment are important. These diagnoses should be considered if a patient exhibits respiratory distress during or after adenotonsillectomy, if frothy secretions are seen from the endotracheal tube or with coughing, or if chest radiography shows evidence of pulmonary infiltrates.[27] Patients with pulmonary edema may need to be treated with supplemental oxygen and diuretics. If respiratory compromise is severe, they may need to be observed in an intensive care setting and even require mechanical ventilatory support until the edema resolves.

Finally, patients undergoing adenotonsillectomy for obstructive sleep apnea have respiratory difficulty at baseline, and they may have significant respiratory compromise during the immediate period after their tonsils and adenoids are removed. Airway edema from surgery and recovery from general anesthesia can exacerbate the patient's premorbid conditions. Many of these patients have associated factors in addition to adenotonsillar hypertrophy that may contribute to their sleep apnea, including neuromuscular disease, craniofacial abnormalities, and morbid obesity. A patient's presurgical conditions must be examined to predict whether the patient will have respiratory difficulty in the postoperative setting. One study suggested that patients with asthma have an increased risk of respiratory complications after adenotonsillectomy.[28] Other studies have examined patients with severe apnea. Patients with very high respiratory distress indices on polysomnography (i.e., >30–40) have a significant decrease in their index after having their tonsils and adenoids removed. However, these patients may still have apnea indices that fall within the abnormal range,[29,30] and they may have significant obstructive sleep apnea after surgery. Patients with severe apnea, morbid obesity, craniofacial abnormalities, or neuromuscular disease are at particular risk of respiratory complications postoperatively.[31] Many of these high-risk groups are highlighted later in this chapter.

Dehydration, Emesis, and Pain

Dehydration

Fluid management plays an important role in any surgical setting, but hydration is particularly challenging among patients who undergo tonsillectomy and adenoidectomy. Postoperative dehydration is a common complication of adenotonsillectomy, causing extended hospital stays and readmissions.[32] The majority of patients undergoing this procedure are in the pediatric population, and adenotonsillectomy has become an ambulatory procedure at many centers. The surgery leaves large open wounds in the oropharynx, which create significant pain. Postoperative emesis is very common after this surgery. The management of patients after tonsillectomy and adenoidectomy is a balance between establishing and maintaining adequate oral fluid intake, avoiding excessive or persistent nausea and vomiting, and decreasing postoperative pain.

To properly replace surgical fluid losses both during and after surgery, one must calculate the patient's fluid deficit. Most patients begin surgery in a slightly dehydrated state as a result of maintaining an empty stomach preoperatively. The preoperative fluid deficit can be determined by multiplying the number of hours of fasting times the maintenance fluid requirement. Maintenance fluid requirements per hour are calculated on the basis of the patient's weight[33]:

4 cc/kg/h for the first 10 kg

+ 2 cc/kg/h for the next 10 kg

+ 1 cc/kg/h for each additional kilogram

When replacing these volume deficits, isotonic fluids should be used. The second consideration for fluid replacement is intraoperative blood loss. For each 1 cc lost, 3 cc of isotonic fluid should be used to replace the volume. In cases of severe bleeding, blood transfusion and volume expanders can be used to treat or avoid shock. When the total volume deficit has been calculated, half of the deficit should be infused over the first hour after surgery, and one quarter should be replaced over each of the next 2 hours. Replacement can be initiated intraoperatively to help reduce the postoperative fluid needs. When the patient begins to tolerate liquids adequately, the intravenous fluid can be stopped, and the patient can rely on his or her intrinsic thirst to maintain adequate hydration.

Adenotonsillectomy has become an ambulatory procedure at many institutions. For patients (particularly children) to be discharged after surgery, they must be able to maintain their fluid balance with adequate oral intake. Recent articles have examined the effect of oral fluid requirements postoperatively. Two recent studies showed that encouraging oral fluid and setting a goal amount postoperatively had no significant impact on the readmission rate. In fact, increased oral intake immediately after surgery may increase the rate of postoperative nausea and vomiting. Defining a mandatory volume of fluid consumed postoperatively delayed patient discharge with no improvement in patient outcome.[32,34]

Emesis

Protracted or recurrent nausea and vomiting are other common complications after tonsillectomy and adenoidectomy. The incidence of emesis after tonsillectomy ranges from 10% to 80% in the literature.[32,34–36] Nausea and vomiting after anesthesia is a well-recognized complication, but the incidence appears to be higher in the tonsillectomy population.[35] Management of these complications is therefore important for the fluid balance considerations previously detailed. Fluid losses from vomiting should be replaced at an equal ratio with isotonic fluid. Because the incidence is high, measures should be taken to prevent postoperative nausea. One recent meta-analysis supported the use of serotonergic agonists (e.g., ondansetron, dolasetron), metoclopramide, and steroids prophylactically. The use of steroids perioperatively in post-tonsillectomy patients has been analyzed carefully in recent literature. Perioperative steroid administration (i.e., usually one dose dexamethasone of 0.4–1 mg/kg to a maximum dose of between 10 mg and 25 mg before surgery) has been shown to be effective for decreasing both the incidence of postoperative emesis and the time to tolerating a soft or regular diet without any significant untoward effects.[37–39] Authors have also questioned routine gastric aspiration at the completion of tonsillectomy. Recent data shows that this practice does not have an effect on postoperative vomiting and nausea and that it does not decrease the use of antiemetics postoperatively.[36]

Pain

There is no question that tonsillectomy with adenoidectomy is associated with considerable pain. It is difficult to study postoperative pain, because there are few methods to measure it objectively, especially among the pediatric population. Adenoidectomy is less painful than tonsillectomy and often requires less aggressive management. Common medications used for analgesia include acetaminophen, narcotic medication, and nonsteroidal anti-inflammatory drugs (NSAIDs). Acetaminophen and acetaminophen with codeine are two of the most common medications used to control post-tonsillectomy pain. The addition of codeine has the possible benefit of increased analgesia, but, as a narcotic, it carries with it the potential side effects of constipation, nausea, vomiting, and respiratory depression. A recent study comparing acetaminophen plus codeine with acetaminophen alone showed no significant difference in postoperative pain control. The group taking acetaminophen alone displayed an increase in oral intake, and the acetaminophen with codeine group showed a trend toward (but not a significant difference in) increased nausea and vomiting.[40] NSAIDs offer another analgesic option, with ketorolac and ibuprofen being two of the most commonly used medications. These medications are attractive because they have anti-inflammatory and analgesic properties without the associated untoward effects of narcotics. Some authors have raised concern regarding the increased risk of bleeding with these medications as a result of their antiplatelet activity.[41–44] A recent systematic review in the Cochrane database reported that NSAIDs were not associated with an increased rate of bleeding in post-tonsillectomy patients and that they demonstrated a decreased rate of postoperative nausea and vomiting.[45]

There has been much debate regarding the role of perioperative antibiotics and their effect on postoperative pain. Early studies suggested that antibiotics decreased postoperative pain.[46] Recently large systematic reviews have shown that antibiotics have no effect on postoperative pain, but they may decrease the time it takes to return to normal diet.[47–49] The antibiotic regimen in these studies was often one intravenous dose of a penicillin class drug preoperatively with 5 to 7 days of oral penicillin, usually amoxicillin or amoxicillin/clavulanic acid.

One method otorhinolaryngologists have used to decrease perioperative pain is the injection of local anesthetic into the operative site or intraoperative packing with swabs soaked in local anesthetic. The medications described in the literature include lidocaine, bupivacaine, and ropivacaine, each with or without epinephrine. In general, reports of the response to these methods have varied.[50–54] One study reported no advantage to pain control with the application of local ropivacaine, yet measurable plasma levels of the drug were identified after injection of the local anesthetic intraoperatively, thus suggesting the potential for toxicity.[52] There is no consensus regarding whether these techniques significantly decrease postoperative pain, and there have been reports of complications as a result of their use. Epinephrine can potentiate preventricular ectopy and ventricular arrhythmias when it is used in conjunction with inhaled anesthetic agents.[55] There is one report of brainstem stroke after the injection of bupivacaine with epinephrine into the adenoid and tonsillar beds.[56]

Fever and Bacteremia

Fever after adenotonsillectomy is common, with a wide range in the incidence reported in the literature. Fever is one of the most common reasons for prolonged hospital stay,[57] and it exacerbates dehydration by increasing insensible fluid losses. Many studies report an incidence of more than 50%, but fever is usually low-grade and of little consequence.[58] The cause of fever in these patients is unclear. Although tonsillectomy appears to cause a transient bacteremia immediately after surgery, studies have shown a variable association between positive blood cultures and fever. Fever may be more related to an acute-phase reaction to surgical trauma than to bacterial infection.[58]

Transient bacteremia after tonsillectomy has been well documented and appears to occur during the immediate postoperative period in roughly 25% to 40% of patients.[59–61] The most common organisms isolated in these cases vary in the literature, and α-hemolytic streptococcus, *Haemophilus influenza, Staphylococcus aureus, Neisseria spp., Branhamella catarrhalis,* and diphtheroid species are among those listed.[58–61] Cultures of the tonsils from both the surface and the deep tissue have yielded similar bacteria.[57,58,60] Although bacteremia appears to be common, the presence of bacterial colonization of the tonsils and positive blood cultures after surgery do not seem to be more common among those patients who develop fever, which suggests that pyrexia in these patients is caused by other factors.[58]

The role of antibiotics in patients undergoing tonsillectomy is also unclear. The data regarding the use of perioperative antibiotics to reduce fever and bacteremia is limited, but some data does suggest that antibiotics decrease the incidence and severity of perioperative fever.[47,49] The regimen most often used is one dose of β-lactam or first-generation cephalosporin antibiotics intraoperatively with 5 to 7 days of amoxicillin during the postoperative period. Special consideration should be made for patients with endocardial disease.[60] The transient bacteremia common to this procedure can place patients with endocardial or cardiac valvular disease at risk for the development of bacterial endocarditis, and therefore prophylactic antibiotics are recommended. Patients should be evaluated preoperatively by their cardiologist to determine their risk of endocarditis and for antibiotic recommendations. The guidelines for prophylaxis against endocarditis during tonsillectomy and adenoidectomy for at-risk patients as suggested by the American College of Cardiology and the American Heart Association are listed as follows[62]:

Ampicillin: Adults, 2.0 g (children, 50 mg/kg) given intramuscularly or intravenously within 30 minutes before the procedure

If the patient is allergic to amoxicillin, ampicillin, and/or penicillin and is unable to take oral medications, use the following:

Clindamycin: Adults, 600 mg (children, 20 mg/kg) intravenously within 30 minutes before the procedure

-OR-

Cefazolin*: Adults, 1.0 g (children, 25 mg/kg) intramuscularly or intravenously within 30 minutes before the procedure

---

*Cephalosporins should not be used to treat patients with immediate-type hypersensitivity reactions to penicillins.

LONG-TERM POSTOPERATIVE COMPLICATIONS

Velopharyngeal Insufficiency

Velopharyngeal insufficiency (VPI) occurs when there is improper closure of the soft palate against the pharyngeal wall during speech and swallowing that results in regurgitation through the nasal cavity and hypernasal speech (rhinolalia aperta). VPI is mainly a complication of adenoidectomy. Tonsillectomy may cause VPI in the rare instance of significant palatal scarring. Transient VPI is common after adenotonsillectomy, and it usually resolves without intervention. Prolonged VPI that persists for months after surgery is less common. The true incidence varies in the literature greatly, with a range between 1 in 1200 and 1 in 10,000.[63,64] Reports vary on the basis of the duration of follow up as well as the method and timing of evaluation.

There are risk factors identified for the potential development of VPI after adenoidectomy. These include patients with neuromuscular disease or craniofacial disorders such as velocardiofacial syndrome, Treacher–Collins syndrome, or Pierre–Robin sequence.[27,63–65] Congenital palatal abnormalities can also put patients at risk of developing VPI. These conditions include overt cleft palate or submucous cleft palate, which can be identified by findings of a zona pellucida, a bifid uvula, an attenuated medium raphe, or a V-shaped notch of the hard palate.[27,66] Velopharyngeal disproportion, which has been described as the incompetence of velopharyngeal closure despite appropriate mobility and morphology of the palate, has also been found to contribute to VPI.[64] In some patients, VPI appears to be related to a behavioral disorder.[63] Some patients may also develop VPI if residual adenoid tissue is left in the nasopharynx and obstructs complete palatal closure.[67] This failure in technique should obviously be avoided, and it should be considered if apparently normal patients develop VPI. When considering adenoidectomy among patients with clinical risk factors for the development of VPI, special evaluation is necessary, and modifications of the adenoidectomy procedure may be indicated.

If patients have signs of VPI on examination or any of the clinical risk factors described above, appropriate preoperative assessment includes a formal evaluation by a speech therapist as well as videofluoroscopy and fiberoptic nasopharyngoscopy.[68] Videofluoroscopy may show the penetration of contrast into the nasal vault and provide a dynamic view of incomplete palatal closure. Nasopharyngoscopy may show a flattening of the superior surface of the soft palate or even a midline groove, and the soft palate may not contact the pharyngeal wall laterally or posteriorly with swallowing and phonation. With these evaluation techniques, the degree of adenoid hypertrophy as well as the degree of velopharyngeal incompetence can be assessed.[69,70] After the evaluation is complete, the risks and benefits of an adenoidectomy can be properly weighed. Among patients with a submucous cleft or mild insufficiency, a modified procedure (i.e., a superior adenoidectomy opening the nasal choanae but leaving a cuff of adenoid tissue inferiorly) can be considered.[65] The use of powered precision instruments as well as endoscopic transnasal techniques have been described recently for this procedure, with good results.[71–73]

In studies evaluating VPI after adenoidectomy, it appears that, in roughly 50% of patients, the symptoms will resolve with either observation alone or observation and speech therapy after 6 to 12 months.[63,64,74] Patients should be genetically evaluated for velocardiofacial (VCF) syndrome (chromosome 22q11). One study suggested that VCF syndrome is discovered in 25% of patients who develop VPI after adenoidectomy.[75] In persistent cases, speech therapy, prosthetic application, or surgical correction are treatment options. Palatal obturators and palatal lift devices can position the palate superiorly to allow for closure in patients with neurologic disease. This option is often employed in patients with contraindications to surgery.[69]

Corrective surgical technique is chosen on the basis of the endoscopic and videofluoroscopic findings.[69,76] Submucous clefts are treated with Furlow palatoplasty. Small defects in palatal closure can be treated with bulking injections, pharyngeal flap, or sphincter pharyngoplasty. In large gaps with good lateral pharyngeal wall motion, pharyngeal flaps are effective. For cases in which lateral pharyngeal wall motion is insufficient, sphincter pharyngoplasty is indicated.[69]

Nasopharyngeal and Oropharyngeal Stenosis

Stenosis of the nasopharynx or the oropharynx after adenotonsillectomy occurs when injury to the mucosal lining leads to extensive scar formation. In cases of nasopharyngeal stenosis, the overaggressive removal of lateral and inferior adenoid can lead to denuding of the soft palate, posterior tonsillar pillars, and posterior nasopharynx. As these injuries heal, circumferential scar or adhesion creates obstruction of the nasal airway. Similarly, oropharyngeal stenosis occurs when the anterior tonsillar pillars and the inferior tonsillar fossae adhere to the base of the tongue after extensive dissection of these regions.[77]

The injury leading to these serious complications after adenotonsillectomy can be the result of aggressive dissection of pharyngeal tissue or of extensive cautery or packing to control bleeding. Surgery in the presence of active infection or severe laryngopharyngeal reflux may also lead to nasopharyngeal or oropharyngeal stenosis. These complications are also more likely in revision surgery or surgery among patients who are prone to keloid formation.[27] Potassium–titanyl–phosphate laser adenotonsillectomy has been linked to a high incidence of choanal and nasopharyngeal stenosis, as well.[77,78]

Nasopharyngeal and oropharyngeal stenosis are very rare complications. Symptoms include difficulty handling nasal or pharyngeal secretions, nasal obstruction, mouth breathing, hyponasal speech, dysphagia, and obstructive sleep apnea. The presence of these symptoms after adenotonsillectomy warrants videofluoroscopy and nasopharyngoscopy.[27] The severity of these symptoms varies with the severity of stenosis.

Treatment for these patients is often difficult. Thin adhesions can be lysed, and stents can be used to prevent restenosis. For severe stenosis, thick scar can be removed with either transpalatal or endoscopic transnasal techniques. Denuded areas then need to be covered to prevent recurrent scar formation. This has been accomplished with skin grafts, Z-plasty local flaps, and local musculomucosal rotation flaps. Two described procedures that have achieved success are a bilobed palatal transposition flap[79] and a laterally based pharyngeal flap.[80] A recent report described good results with the use of the laser release of scarred tissue and prolonged obturator dilation in combination with the injection of mitomycin C for severe stenosis.[77]

Atlantoaxial Subluxation

The displacement of the first cervical vertebrae (C1) over the second cervical vertebrae (C2), which is also known as *atlantoaxial subluxation,* can have many potential causes, including traumatic dislocation, infectious osteomyelitis, or inflammatory arthritis.[81] In 1830, atlantoaxial subluxation was described by Bell as a consequence of the syphilitic ulceration of the pharynx, and 100 years later Grisel described a similar condition as a consequence of nasopharyngitis.[82] Thus the eponym "Grisel syndrome" is used to describe atlantoaxial subluxation without a history of trauma. Atlantoaxial subluxation has occurred among patients after adenotonsillectomy, but the cause of the complication is not known. Hypotheses suggest that infectious or inflammatory mediators create conditions that lead to laxity of the transverse ligament that supports the odontoid process against the anterior arch of C1. One theory is that an infectious process causes spasm of the paravertebral muscles, with resulting bony displacement. Other proposed mechanisms suggest that inflammation creates a hyperemic state in the paravertebral tissue, resulting in the decalcification of C1 and the weakening of the insertions of

the transverse ligament. Alternatively, inflammation may create laxity in the ligaments themselves.[82]

Atlantoaxial subluxation after tonsillectomy or adenoidectomy is rare, and it can occur either immediately after surgery or as a delayed complication. The condition occurs primarily among children. Patients with Down syndrome, Arnold–Chiari malformation, and achondroplasia are at increased risk.[81] Patients typically complain of a painful stiff neck, and examination shows significant cervical muscle spasm and torticollis, with the head tilted and turned to the opposite side. The atlantoaxial joint can be tender, and the spinous process of C2 may be deviated to the affected side.[82] The diagnosis can be confirmed with plain radiographs, but computed tomography scanning with contrast can give detailed views of the position of the bony structures, and a deep space neck abscess can be ruled out. The computed tomography scan will show a rotary subluxation with widening of the atlas–dens interval.[81,82] The subluxation has been classified into four types on the basis of severity[83] (Box 28-1), and this can be used to guide management.

Although neck pain is common after tonsillectomy and adenoidectomy, suspicion of Grisel syndrome should be high among patients with severe or persistent pain. Special attention should be paid to patients with significant torticollis, because atlantoaxial subluxation can have permanent restrictive or neurologic effects if treatment is delayed. For patients with rotational displacement but minimal anterior displacement of C1, treatment with bed rest, muscle relaxants, and soft cervical immobilization or cervical traction is advocated. For those cases involving significant anterior or posterior displacement of the atlas, if there are signs of osteopenia, osteomyelitis, or neurologic deficits or in cases of chronic subluxation, more aggressive treatment is recommended, including

---

BOX 28-1 Classification of Rotary Subluxation of C1 and C2

TYPE I
- Rotary fixation with no anterior displacement and with the odontoid acting as the pivot point

TYPE II
- Rotary fixation with anterior displacement of 3 mm to 5 mm and one lateral articular process acting as the pivot

TYPE III
- Rotary fixation with anterior displacement of more than 5 mm

TYPE IV
- Rotary fixation with posterior displacement

Adapted from Fielding JW: Atlantoaxial rotary deformities. *Orthop Clin North Am* 1978;9:955–967.

halo immobilization, C1–C2 fusion, and arthrodesis. In all cases, systemic antibiotics covering oropharyngeal aerobic and anaerobic pathogens should be administered, and neurosurgical consultation is necessary to aid in the diagnosis and management.[82]

HIGH-RISK GROUPS

Young Patients

Children who are less than 3 years old have been identified as a high-risk group for postoperative complications after adenotonsillectomy.[84,85] They have been shown to have a higher rate of postoperative respiratory complications. In one recent large study, nearly 10% of patients less than 3 years old had respiratory compromise after tonsillectomy and adenoidectomy, which was two times the rate found among patients between the ages of 3 and 5 years.[84] Respiratory complications included oxygen desaturation, the need for supplemental oxygen or diuretic therapy, apnea or increased work of breathing, and the need for intervention, including reintubation, the placement of a nasopharyngeal airway, or the use of continuous positive airway pressure. Chest radiograph changes, including atelectasis, effusion, pulmonary edema, pulmonary infiltrate, pneumothorax, and pneumomediastinum, were also recorded. Patients in this age group also appear to have a higher incidence of laryngospasm and poor oral intake postoperatively.[85] These complications lead to increased hospital stays. Young patients have a lower blood volume than older patients and therefore they are at higher risk for dehydration during the postoperative period. Intraoperative and postoperative bleeding can have more grave consequences. It is recommended that children who are less than 3 years old be routinely admitted for observation after tonsillectomy and adenoidectomy in light of the increased risk of a complicated course after surgery.[84]

Morbid Obesity

The prevalence of childhood and adult obesity has greatly increased over the last three decades. Morbid obesity is defined as an age- and gender-specific body mass index that is higher than the 95th percentile.[86] Obstructive sleep apnea in these patients is common, and the otorhinolaryngologist is often faced with the decision to perform adenotonsillectomy in the morbidly obese patient when tonsillar and adenoid hypertrophy is concurrently present. In addition to enlarged tonsils and adenoids, morbidly obese patients can have respiratory difficulty as a result of fat deposition in the pharyngeal musculature and the surrounding tissues, decreased chest-wall compliance, displacement of the diaphragm toward the chest cavity from increased abdominal adipose, decreased functional residual capacity, and increased lung atelectasis leading to a larger ventilation–perfusion mismatch.[87]

Because adenotonsillar hypertrophy is not the only contributor to obstructive symptoms, tonsillectomy and adenoidectomy should not be the only interventions considered for these patients. A multidisciplinary approach to the obese patient involving a pulmonologist, a nutritionist, and an internist or pediatrician is necessary. Before surgery, supportive measures should be undertaken, including weight loss, diet control, and continuous positive airway pressure ventilatory support during sleep. Surgical intervention beyond adenotonsillectomy may be necessary, including uvulopalatopharyngoplasty, tongue-base reduction, and various orthognathic procedures. Tracheostomy is an ultimate cure for severe cases that are unresponsive to other measures.[87]

Preoperative and postoperative polysomnography should be obtained for morbidly obese patients to assess the level of improvement after surgery. Adenotonsillectomy has been found to improve sleep apnea in morbidly obese children,[86] but residual obstruction may complicate the postoperative period and continue to affect the patient.[87] Postoperative complications in morbidly obese patients after adenotonsillectomy have not been well studied. Obese patients are at increased risk for cardiopulmonary complications after tonsillectomy. Further study is necessary to determine the best approach for the management of morbidly obese patients with obstructive sleep apnea and adenotonsillar hypertrophy.

Down Syndrome

Children with Down syndrome commonly present to the otorhinolaryngology office for the evaluation of sleep apnea. Adenotonsillar hypertrophy is common among this population, but other craniofacial abnormalities such as midface hypoplasia, micrognathia, narrow nasopharyngeal and oropharyngeal dimensions, and macroglossia exacerbate airway obstruction among patients with Down syndrome.[88,89] The disorder is also characterized by muscular hypotonia and obesity,[89] which contribute to sleep apnea. Patients with Down syndrome often require tonsillectomy and adenoidectomy to improve their condition. Preoperative polysomnography is important to characterize the patient's sleeping disorder and to assess severity.

General anesthesia for patients with Down syndrome can be challenging. In particular, airway management can be difficult as a result of the anatomic and physiologic abnormalities in this patient population. Patients with Down syndrome typically have a short neck, a large tongue, and a narrow laryngotracheal diameter.

They also have a higher incidence of atlantoaxial instability than the general population as well as a predisposition to upper respiratory tract infection and increased respiratory secretions.[88] All of these factors need to be considered when managing the airway for general anesthesia. Intubation may require endotracheal tubes one or two sizes smaller than those used for other patients matched for age. Air-leak tests should be performed to ensure that the appropriate-sized tube is being used.

Postoperative complications are increased among patients with Down syndrome. In particular, these patients require respiratory monitoring and support after surgery. Patients with Down syndrome have an increased incidence of structural cardiac defects, which can put them at risk for cor pulmonale.[89] A recent study found that patients with Down syndrome have an increased incidence of upper airway obstruction, oxygen desaturation, and postoperative stridor.[88] The study group also had a prolonged time to adequate oral intake after surgery as compared with control patients.[88] For these reasons, patients with Down syndrome often require continuous pulse-oximeter monitoring after surgery, and they commonly require supplemental oxygen and respiratory intervention. Intervention includes the placement of a nasopharyngeal airway and intermittent stimulation or repositioning to improve respiratory drive. Intravenous hydration is usually prolonged as a result of a longer period to oral intake. For these reasons, patients with Down syndrome often have a prolonged hospital course. Initial placement in an intensive care setting is recommended, especially if preoperative polysomnography demonstrates severe sleep apnea.

Neurologic and Neuromuscular Disease

Patients with neurologic and neuromuscular disease often have sleep-disordered breathing and sleep apnea. Depending on the neurologic disorder, patients may have significant hypotonia of the pharyngeal musculature, which exacerbates the effects of adenotonsillar hypertrophy. Polysomnography is necessary in these patients to differentiate central from obstructive sleep apnea.

Patients with neuromuscular disorders, cerebral palsy, and seizure disorders have been found to have a higher incidence of complications after tonsillectomy and adenoidectomy.[90,91] In this population, the patient's underlying disorder must be considered by the anesthesiologist when weighing the effects of induction agents, anesthetics, and paralytic medication. The management of the airway can be a challenge as a result of hypotonia, and postoperative respiratory support and prolonged intubation are often necessary. Extended observation, including intensive care monitoring, should be considered among patients with neurologic and neuromuscular disease, depending on the severity of the patient's condition.

Mucopolysaccharidoses

The mucopolysaccharidoses are a family of diseases that are caused by enzymatic defects that result in an accumulation of glycosaminoglycans in the cell lysosomes. The genetic defects specific to each of these disorders are inherited in an autosomal-recessive pattern, except for Hunter syndrome, which is X-linked. The metabolic disorder affects a variety of organ systems, and clinical manifestations vary, depending on the specific disease. Abnormalities of the upper airway are common and multifactorial in patients with these diseases. Patients can have abnormalities of the cervical vertebrae, including atlantoaxial instability, narrow tracheobronchial dimensions, a short neck, macroglossia, glottic and supraglottic abnormalities, a narrow nasopharynx, and a hypoplastic mandible. Glycosaminoglycans are progressively deposited in the tissues of the upper airway, and tonsillar and adenoid hypertrophy are common.[92]

Obstructive sleep apnea is common, and adenotonsillectomy is performed to help improve respiratory symptoms. Mask ventilation and intubation are usually difficult. Patients with lysosomal storage disorders often have significant cardiopulmonary disease, and postoperative care can be complicated by persistent airway obstruction, oxygen desaturation, and respiratory failure. Inpatient hospitalization is the usual course postoperatively, and there should be a low threshold for observation in an intensive care setting if obstructive sleep apnea or cardiopulmonary symptoms are significant.

Sickle Cell Disease

Sickle cell disease is an autosomal-recessive inherited disease that is caused by a gene mutation that creates a dysfunctional β-chain hemoglobin. Hypoxia, acidosis, hyperthermia, and hypovolemia can lead to the sickling of red blood cells and vaso-occlusive events. These events can create pain crises, acute chest syndrome, priapism, and stroke.[93] Obstructive sleep apnea is particularly dangerous in children with sickle cell disease, because oxygen desaturation and hypercarbia increase the likelihood of sickle cell crises. Polysomnography is therefore necessary in these patients if there is any suspicion that nighttime apnea could be exacerbating their disease.

Surgery in sickle cell patients is also challenging. Traditionally these patients are admitted 24 hours before surgery for aggressive hydration and blood transfusion, and postoperatively they are observed for an extended period with supplemental oxygen and further hydration in the hospital setting. The goal is to avoid sickle cell crises as a result of the potential hypoxia and hypoperfusion that can occur during general anesthesia and after adenotonsillectomy.[27,93] Recent studies have advocated less-aggressive measures, suggesting that preoperative admission and transfusion are only necessary for patients whose hemoglobin levels are less than 10 g/dl. In addition, extended hospital stay and supplemental oxygen do not seem to be necessary if oxygen saturation remains greater than 94%.[93] Less-aggressive preoperative and postoperative management does not appear to increase sickle-cell–related complications, and it may decrease blood-transfusion–related complications. Patients with severe obstructive sleep apnea, a hemoglobin S ratio of less than 40%, and an age of less than 4 years may benefit from the more traditional approach of transfusion, oxygen supplementation, and extended monitoring.[94]

Bleeding Disorders

von Willebrand Disease

von Willebrand factor (vWF) is a large adhesive glycoprotein found in plasma, platelets, and endothelial cells that plays a key role in platelet adhesion and acts as a carrier for coagulation factor VIII. von Willebrand disease (vWD) is the most common hereditary bleeding disorder, and it is a condition in which vWF is deficient or dysfunctional, thus resulting in platelet and coagulation dysfunction.[95] There are numerous genetic defects that result in this condition. The severity of bleeding among patients with vWD depends on the genetic defect that is present and whether the patient is a heterozygous or homozygous carrier of the deficient gene. The disorder can be classified into the following three main types, with further subclassification based on the genetic defect and the resulting deficiency or dysfunction of vWF[95,96]:

Type 1: The most common type of vWD (~75%), caused by a quantitative decrease in vWF.

Type 2: The second most common type of vWD (~20%), caused by a qualitative and quantitative decrease in vWF. It can be further subdivided as follows:
- *Type 2A:* A qualitative defect in which vWF–platelet interaction is dysfunctional
- *Type 2B:* A qualitative defect in which vWF has a higher affinity for its platelet-binding site, resulting in rapid clearance and often thrombocytopenia.
- *Type 2N:* A qualitative defect in which vWF does not bind to factor VIII and protect it from rapid degradation

Type 3: The least common type of vWD (~5%), caused by an absence of vWF.

The diagnosis of vWD involves assays for plasma vWF-mediated platelet function, vWF antigen level, and factor VIII level. Additional specialized tests may be indicated to assess the structure and distribution of vWF multimers or factor VIII binding activity.[95] Adenotonsillectomy carries an obvious risk of severe bleeding for patients with vWD. The raw surfaces left from the resection of the tonsils and the adenoids rely on proper thrombogenesis and coagulation to provide hemostasis after surgery. Patients undergoing surgery must be pretreated with either desmopressin or blood products containing vWF, factor VIII, or both.

Desmopressin acetate (1-desamino-8-D-arginine vasopressin) can be useful for patients with type 1 vWD. The exact mechanism of action of this drug is unclear, but the medication causes the release of preformed vWF from storage sites in endothelial cells and the release of factor VIII.[95,97] Desmopressin acetate is given at a dose of 0.3 mcg/kg in 50 ml of normal saline intravenously 30 to 60 minutes before surgery; another dose is given 12 to 24 hours after the procedure. Some authors advocate using desmopressin alone to maintain hemostasis during and after tonsillectomy.[98] The administration of desmopressin acetate after surgery is variable. Some authors suggest no further use of desmopressin acetate after the initial dose,[97] whereas others have advocated daily dosing until tonsillar eschars are healed.[98] Hyponatremia and tachyphylaxis are the main side effects of desmopressin acetate.[95] Hyponatremia is the result of the antidiuretic effects of vasopressin and the subsequent retention of free water. The electrolyte imbalance can be severe and may lead to seizures. Therefore the close monitoring of sodium levels and the administration of isotonic fluids postoperatively is crucial. Desmopressin acetate has a variable effect on patients with type 2A vWD, and it can cause a severe thrombocytopenia in patients with type 2B vWD. Therefore desmopressin acetate is not recommended in the management of these patients. For patients with type 3 vWD, desmopressin acetate is ineffective.[95]

Patients who fail to maintain hemostasis with desmopressin acetate or those with type 2 or 3 disease must rely on blood products such as factor VIII concentrate or cryoprecipitate, both of which are rich in vWF. These products are effective in decreasing bleeding complications when they are used perioperatively, but they carry the risk of transmitting blood-borne diseases (e.g., human immunodeficiency virus, hepatitis B, hepatitis C). Cryoprecipitate carries a higher risk of transmission than concentrated factor VIII.[95] Aminocaproic acid and tranexamic acid are antifibrinolytic medications that can be used intravenously as an adjunctive therapy to maintain hemostasis in patients with vWD after surgery. Aminocaproic acid is also available in an oral formulation, and tranexamic acid is available as a mouthwash. Both may be useful when patients return home postoperatively.[95]

Factor VIII and IX Deficiency

Deficiencies of coagulation factors VIII (hemophilia A) and IX (hemophilia B or Christmas disease) are sex-linked recessive bleeding diatheses. Autosomally inherited conditions resulting in deficiencies of factor V, VII, X, XI, and fibrinogen also exist, but they are much more rare than hemophilia A and B. These conditions are diagnosed by measuring coagulation factor assays. Factor VIII and IX deficiencies are present in 1 in 5000 and 1 in 30,000 male births, respectively.[99]

If adenotonsillectomy is found to be necessary for these patients, there is obviously a high risk for postoperative bleeding. For elective surgery, concentrates of factor VIII and factor IX are given to maintain hemostasis. A preoperative dose is infused to attain 80% to 100% of normal activity, and one half of this initial dose is given every 8 hours for hemophilia A and every 12 hours for hemophilia B on the basis of the different half-lives of factors VIII and IX, respectively.[99] Guidelines for maintaining hemostasis postoperatively have been largely empiric, and recent studies have examined low-dose intermittent factor replacement as well as the use of continuous infusion to avoid fluctuations in factor levels.[100,101] Patients with these diseases also develop antibodies that inhibit the transfused factors after they receive multiple infusions to treat their disorders. If significant inhibitors are present, porcine factor VIII and activated factor VII are available to maintain hemostasis. DDAVP and Amicar can be used adjunctively. Perioperative management of these patients can become very complex, and it must be individualized on the basis of the patient's factor deficiency, the severity of disease, the presence of inhibitors, and the history of previous treatment.[27,99] Close management with the patient's hematologist is mandatory.

Preoperative Testing

Bleeding dyscrasias are rare, but they have the potential to cause devastating complications among patients undergoing tonsillectomy and adenoidectomy. The usefulness of preoperative testing to identify patients with potential bleeding disorders has been debated. Most studies have concluded that finding abnormalities in prothrombin, partial thromboplastin, and bleeding times is nonspecific and not usually predictive of bleeding disorders and postoperative tonsillectomy bleeding.[102,103] The routine screening of patients for underlying bleeding disorders appears to create significant cost without an appreciable benefit. For these reasons, many authors support a careful history and physical examination with laboratory testing reserved for those patients at risk for or with findings suggestive of an underlying bleeding disorder.[103] Despite inconclusive evidence in support of the practice, routine testing is still common, perhaps as a result of medicolegal concerns.

RECENT ADVANCES IN TONSILLECTOMY AND ADENOIDECTOMY

Day-Case Tonsillectomy

Over the last two decades, adenotonsillectomy has become an ambulatory procedure at many centers, with the routine discharge of the patient shortly after surgery. The advantages of outpatient surgery include improved patient comfort and decreased hospital costs. Multiple studies have supported the safety of ambulatory tonsillectomy when patients are properly selected.[104–106] Patients should be considered for admission after surgery if they have significant comorbid conditions, such as significant asthma, developmental delay, neuromuscular disease, and severe upper airway obstruction. There are also social issues that may necessitate admission, such as residence a great distance from the hospital (e.g., >30 minutes to 1 hour away) or a family without a phone or automobile.[105] Very young patients should also be evaluated carefully, and there should be a low threshold for admission among this population.[107]

Recent studies suggest that patients originally scheduled for outpatient tonsillectomy are admitted after surgery at a rate of between 4% and 9%.[104–106] Patients stay in the hospital most commonly for respiratory complications (e.g., desaturation, stridor, or apnea requiring supplemental oxygen, nasopharyngeal airway, or reintubation), protracted nausea and vomiting, and inadequate oral intake. Primary hemorrhage occurs in roughly 1% to 6% of patients, but it appears that bleeding is recognized in 83% to 98% of patients in the recovery room before they are discharged.[104–106] Another 1% to 4% of patients are readmitted shortly after being discharged from the hospital, most commonly for decreased oral intake or fever and rarely for bleeding.[104–106] Recently, a systematic review of 17 articles suggested that day-case tonsillectomy was a safe procedure.[108] The complication rate noted in this study was 8.8% (95% confidence interval, 5.5%–12.1%), and the unplanned admission rate was 8.0% (95% confidence interval, 5.3%–10.7%). The review showed that patients who were less than 4 years old were at higher risk for complications and unplanned admission.

Controversy exists regarding the minimal time for observation after tonsillectomy and the minimum age for outpatient tonsillectomy. Early studies advocating outpatient tonsillectomy recommended a postoperative observation period of between 6 and 10 hours.[109–112] Recent studies have demonstrated safety with discharging patients after 3 to 5 hours[106] and even after less than 3 hours.[104] This decrease in observation time has a significant impact on hospital costs.[104] Studies have also examined the safety of performing day-case tonsillectomy for very young patients. Children 4 years old or younger have a significant increase in complications, particularly respiratory events.[104,107] It can be argued that even moderate bleeding in the very young patient can be devastating as a result of a decreased reserve, and it appears that respiratory complications play a large role in determining hospital admission in this patient population.[107] Currently it is generally accepted that hospital admission is strongly recommended for patients who are less than 3 or 4 years old. Complications are common, and the ability to predict a complicated postoperative course is difficult.[107] If day-case tonsillectomy is considered among patients who are less than 3 or 4 years old, the patients should be carefully selected and closely observed postoperatively before discharge.

New Techniques

The tonsillectomy procedure can be dated back to the Romans in the writings of Celsus during the first century AD. The removal of the tonsil with its capsule intact was first described near the turn of the nineteenth century.[113] During the last 10 to 20 years, there have been a large number of new techniques developed. The refinement of electrocautery dissection has led to the use of bipolar forceps, bipolar scissors, and microdissection with needle-tip cautery.[114,115] Various new modalities including the ultrasound harmonic scalpel, various laser devices, radiofrequency destruction, and microdebrider powered instrumentation have been employed to accomplish tonsillotomy and the tonsillectomy procedure.[116–120] Many of these techniques are not universally accepted and require further study to determine whether they have advantages that justify their use over traditional techniques. Two modalities—radiofrequency tonsillectomy or tonsillotomy (i.e., coblation) and microdebrider-assisted tonsillotomy—have gained rapid acceptance and received recent attention in the literature.

Coblation uses radiofrequency energy in a bipolar mode to energize ions in a conductive solution (i.e., saline) to form a small plasma field. The plasma has enough energy to break the tissue's molecular bonds. The temperature achieved with this process is approximately 45°C to 85°C, a temperature that is significantly lower than that produced by electrocautery techniques.[121] There are three ways in which radiofrequency energy has been employed to achieve tonsillar reduction surgery: (1) radiofrequency ablation; (2) subcapsular tonsillotomy; and (3) tonsillar dissection.[117] Radiofrequency ablation involves placing a probe into the tissue itself at several points within the tonsil. The tonsil is partially destroyed, and it undergoes further contraction during the postoperative period as the ablated tonsil heals. A subcapsular tonsillotomy technique (i.e., with coblation) has also been described in which the radiofrequency device is used to remove the tonsil, leaving only a thin layer of tonsillar tissue over the tonsillar capsule. Finally, the coblation device can also be used to dissect the tonsil free in an extracapsular plane as with standard cold and electrocautery techniques. Radiofrequency ablation of the adenoids has also been described.[122]

In recent studies, it appears that all three radiofrequency techniques (tonsillar radiofrequency ablation, coblator subcapsular tonsillotomy, and coblator tonsillectomy) lead to decreased pain and increased oral intake among patients as compared with those patients who have undergone standard electrocautery tonsillectomy.[123–126] When comparing these radiofrequency techniques with standard cold dissection tonsillectomy, some studies report improvements in pain and oral intake,[117] whereas others report no difference.[127,128] Intraoperative blood loss, primary and secondary hemorrhage rates, and the length of surgery with coblation techniques appear to be equal to those reported for electrodissection.[123–126] Finally, there are preliminary study results that address the efficacy of radiofrequency techniques. In one study, standard cold dissection tonsillectomy achieved a 100% reduction in tonsillar tissue at 12 weeks postoperatively, whereas subcapsular coblator tonsillotomy and radiofrequency ablation reduced tonsil bulk by 86% and 54%, respectively.[117] Another study suggests that roughly 4% of patients require tonsillectomy after subcapsular tonsillotomy with coblation.[129] The efficacy of radiofrequency techniques is just beginning to be established, but results are promising, and the reduction in postoperative pain appears to be significant.

A second technique that has been gaining popularity is the microdebrider-assisted tonsillotomy and adenoidectomy. The microdebrider is a device that makes use of a rapidly rotating blade that simultaneously cuts and suctions away the removed tissue. This optimizes precision and visualization while removing tonsil and adenoid tissue. Tonsillotomy involves removing tonsillar tissue without the violation of the tonsillar capsule, thereby avoiding the underlying pharyngeal musculature and larger proximal arteries. Multiple studies have reported improved postoperative pain, hydration, and return to normal activity with this technique as compared with electrocautery tonsillectomy.[120,130–133] Intraoperative bleeding appears to be slightly increased with this procedure,[130] but postoperative bleeding appears to be decreased substantially.[132] One study examined the usefulness of the procedure for patients who are less than 3 years old. Microdebrider tonsillotomy appeared to reduce the risk of postoperative bleeding and dehydration in this patient population, potentially lowering the threshold to use tonsil reduction surgery in young patients and increasing the percentage of young patients discharged on the day of surgery.[134]

The main disadvantages of the procedure are the cost of the microdebrider instruments and the increased risk of residual tonsillar tissue and tonsillar regrowth. One study suggested that patients undergoing microdebrider tonsillotomy were five times more likely to have residual tonsillar tissue at follow up than those undergoing traditional tonsillectomy.[133] Another recent study examining patients more than 1 year after the procedure found that only 0.46% of patients undergoing microdebrider tonsillotomy were found to have tonsillar regrowth.[132] The evidence that microdebrider tonsillotomy decreases post-tonsillectomy pain and dehydration is promising. However, additional studies are necessary to examine the significance of residual tonsil or tonsillar regrowth as well as the cost–benefit ratio when comparing the cost of powered instruments with the savings in decreased hospital stay and readmission rates.

CONCLUSION

Tonsillectomy and adenoidectomy are among the most common surgical procedures performed by the otorhinolaryngologist. Common complications, such as significant pain and dehydration, can increase hospital costs and decrease patient satisfaction. Rare complications, such as bleeding and respiratory failure after adenotonsillectomy, can be devastating. Careful preoperative evaluation and planning as well as swift recognition and action in the face of complications can significantly improve patient morbidity and mortality after tonsillectomy and adenoidectomy.

REFERENCES

1. Younis RT, Lazar RH: History and current practice of tonsillectomy. *Laryngoscope* 2002;112:3–5.
2. Darrow DH, Siemens C: Indications for tonsillectomy and adenoidectomy. *Laryngoscope* 2002;112(8 Pt 2 Suppl 100):6–10.
3. Randall DA, Hoffer ME: Complications of tonsillectomy and adenoidectomy. *Otolaryngol Head Neck Surg* 1998;118:61–68.
4. Janfaza P, Nadol JB Jr, Galla RJ, et al: Pharynx. In Janfaza P, Fabian RL, editors: *Surgical anatomy of the head and neck,* Philadelphia, 2001, Lippincott Williams & Wilkins.
5. Windfuhr JP: Indications for interventional arteriography in post-tonsillectomy hemorrhage. *J Otolaryngol* 2002;31(1):18–22.
6. Donlon JV, Doyle DJ, Feldman MA: Anesthesia for eye, ear, nose and throat surgery. In Miller RD, editor: *Miller's anesthesia,* ed 6, Philadelphia, 2005, Elsevier.
7. Mattucci KF, Militana CJ: The prevention of fire during oropharyngeal electrosurgery. *Ear Nose Throat J* 2003;82(2):107–109.
8. Rampill IJ: Anesthesia for laser surgery. In Miller RD, editor: *Miller's anesthesia,* ed 6, Philadelphia, 2005, Elsevier.
9. Jones J, Lyon G, Groudine S, et al: Phenylephrine advisory report. *Int J Pediatr Otorhinolaryngol* 1998;45:97–99.
10. Riegle EV, Gunter JB, Lusk RP, et al: Comparison of vasoconstrictors for functional endoscopic sinus surgery in children. *Laryngoscope* 1992;102(7):820–823.
11. Irani DB, Berkowitz RG: Management of secondary hemorrhage following pediatric adenotonsillectomy. *Int J Pediatr Otorhinolaryngol* 1997;40:115–124.
12. Tomkinson A, DeMartin S, Gilchrist CR, et al: Instrumentation and patient characteristics that influence postoperative hemorrhage rates following tonsil and adenoid surgery. *Clin Otolaryngol* 2005;30:338–346.
13. Collison PJ, Mettler B: Factors associated with post-tonsillectomy hemorrhage. *Ear Nose Throat J* 2000;79(8):640–649.
14. Lee MSW, Montague ML, Hussain SSM: Post-tonsillectomy hemorrhage: Cold vs. hot dissection. *Otolaryngol Head Neck Surg* 2004;131:833–836.
15. Liu JH, Anderson KE, Willging JP, et al: Posttonsillectomy hemorrhage. *Arch Otolaryngol Head Neck Surg* 2001;127:1271–1275.
16. Wei JL, Beatty CW, Gustafson RO: Evaluation of posttonsillectomy hemorrhage and risk factors. *Otolaryngol Head Neck Surg* 2000;123:229–235.
17. Windfuhr JP, Ulbrich T: Posttonsillectomy hemorrhage: Results of a three month follow-up. *Ear Nose Throat J* 2001;80(11):795–802.
18. Windfuhr JP, Chen YS: Incidence of post-tonsillectomy hemorrhage in children and adults: A study of 4,848 patients. *Ear Nose Throat J* 2002;81(9):626–634.
19. Windfuhr JP, Chen YS, Remmert S: Hemorrhage following tonsillectomy and adenoidectomy in 15,281 patients. *Otolaryngol Head Neck Surg* 2005;132:281–286.
20. Cressman WR, Meyer CM III: Management of tonsillectomy hemorrhage: Results of a survey of pediatric otolaryngology fellowship programs. *Am J Otolaryngol* 1995;16(1):29–32.
21. Haddow K, Montague ML, Hussain SS: Post-tonsillectomy hemorrhage: A prospective, randomized, controlled clinical trial of cold dissection versus bipolar diathermy dissection. *J Laryngol Otol* 2006;120(6):450–454.
22. Lowe D, van der Meulen J: Tonsillectomy technique as a risk factor for postoperative hemorrhage. *Lancet* 2004;364(9435):642–643.
23. Windfuhr JP, Yue-Shih C, Remmert S: Unidentified coagulation disorders in post-tonsillectomy hemorrhage. *Ear Nose Throat J* 2004;83(1):28–39.
24. Tovi F, Leiberman A, Hertzanu Y, et al: Pseudoaneurysm of the internal carotid artery secondary to tonsillectomy. *Int J Otorhinolaryngol* 1987;13(1):69–75.
25. Karas DE, Sawin RS, Sie KC: Pseudoaneurysm of the external carotid artery after tonsillectomy: A rare complication. *Arch Otolaryngol Head Neck Surg* 1997;123(3):345–347.
26. Mehta VM, Har-El G, Goldstein NA: Postobstructive pulmonary edema after laryngospasm in the otolaryngology patient. *Laryngoscope* 2006;116(9):1693–1696.
27. Cunningham MJ, Myers CM III: Tonsillectomy and adenoidectomy. In Josephson GD, Wohl DL, editors: *Complications in pediatric otolaryngology,* Boca Raton, Fl, 2005, Taylor and Francis Group.
28. Kalra M, Buncher R, Amin RS: Asthma as a risk factor for respiratory complications after adenotonsillectomy in children with obstructive breathing during sleep. *Ann Allergy Asthma Immunol* 2005;94(5):549–552.
29. Mitchell RB, Kelly J: Outcome of adenotonsillectomy for severe obstructive sleep apnea in children. *Int J Pediatr Otorhinolaryngol* 2004;68(11):1375–1379.
30. Tal A, Barr A, Leiberman A, et al: Sleep characteristics following adenotonsillectomy in children with obstructive sleep apnea syndrome. *Chest* Sept 2003;124(3):948–953.
31. Rosen GM, Muckle RP, Maholwald MW, et al: Postoperative respiratory compromise in children with obstructive sleep apnea syndrome: Can it be anticipated? *Pediatrics* 1994;93(5):784–788.
32. Messner AH, Barbita JA: Oral fluid intake following tonsillectomy. *Int J Pediatr Otorhinolaryngol* 1997;39(1):19–24.
33. Kaye AD, Kucera IJ: Intravascular fluid and electrolyte management. In Miller RD, editor: *Miller's anesthesia,* ed 6, Philadelphia, 2005, Elsevier.
34. Tabaee A, Lin JW, Dupiton V, et al: The role of oral fluid intake following adeno-tonsillectomy. *Int J Pediatr Otorhinolaryngol* 2006;70(7):1159–1164.
35. Kermode J, Walker S, Webb I: Postoperative vomiting in children. *Anaesth Intensive Care* 1995;23(2):196–199.
36. Jones JE, Tabaee A, Glasgold R, et al: Efficacy of gastric aspiration in reducing posttonsillectomy vomiting. *Arch Otolaryngol Head Neck Surg* 2001;127(8):980–984.

37. Bolton CM, Myles PS, Nolan T, et al: Prophylaxis of postoperative vomiting in children undergoing tonsillectomy: A systematic review and meta-analysis. *Br J Anaesth* 2006;97(5):593–604.

38. Heatley DG: Perioperative intravenous steroid treatment and tonsillectomy. *Arch Otolaryngol Head Neck Surg* 2001;127(8):1007–1008.

39. Goldman AC, Govindaraj S, Rosenfeld RM: A meta-analysis of dexamethasone use with tonsillectomy. *Otolayrngol Head Neck Surg* 2000;123(6):682–686.

40. Moir MS, Bair E, Shinnick P, et al: Acetaminophen versus acetaminophen with codeine after pediatric tonsillectomy. *Laryngoscope* 2000;110(11):1824–1827.

41. Splinter WM, Rhine EJ, Roberts DW, et al: Preoperative ketorolac increases bleeding after tonsillectomy in children. *Can J Anaesth* 1996;43(6):560–563.

42. Rusy LM, Houck CS, Sullivan LJ, et al: A double blind evaluation of ketorolac tromethmine versus acetaminophen in pediatric tonsillectomy: Analgesia and bleeding. *Anesth Analg* 1995;80(2):226–229.

43. Judkins JH, Dray TG, Hubbell RN: Intraoperative ketorolac and posttonsillectomy bleeding. *Arch Otolaryngol Head Neck Surg* 1996;122(9):937–940.

44. Gallagher JE, Blauth J, Fornadley JA: Perioperative ketorolac tromethamine and postoperative hemorrhage in cases of tonsillectomy and adenoidectomy. *Laryngoscope* 1995;105(6):606–609.

45. Cardwell M, Siviter G, Smith A: Non-steroidal anti-inflammatory drugs and perioperative bleeding in paediatric tonsillectomy. *Cochrane Database Syst Rev* 2005;18(2);CD003591.

46. Telian SA, Handler SD, Fleisher GR, et al: The effect of antibiotic therapy on recovery after tonsillectomy in children: A controlled study. *Arch Otolaryngol Head Neck Surg* 1986;112(6):610–615.

47. Iyer S, DeFoor W, Grocela J, et al: The use of perioperative antibiotics in tonsillectomy: Does it decrease morbidity? *Int J Pediatr Otorhinolaryngol* 2006;70(5):853–861.

48. Burkart CM, Steward DL: Antibiotics for reduction of posttonsillectomy morbidity: A meta-analysis. *Laryngoscope* 2005;115(6):997–1002.

49. Dhiwakar M, Eng CY, Selvaraj S, et al: Antibiotics to improve recovery following tonsillectomy: A systematic review. *Otolaryngol Head Neck Surg* 2006;134(3):357–364.

50. Egeli E, Harputluoglu U, Oghan F, et al: Does topical lidocaine with adrenalin have an effect on morbidity in pediatric tonsillectomy? *Int J Pediatr Otorhinolaryngol* 2005;69(6):811–815.

51. Kountakis SE: Effectiveness of perioperative bupivacaine infiltration in tonsillectomy patients. *Am J Otolaryngol* 2002;23(2):76–80.

52. Park AH, Pappas AL, Fluder E, et al: Effect of perioperative administration of ropivacaine with epinephrine on postoperative pediatric adenotonsillectomy recovery. *Arch Otolaryngol Head Neck Surg* 2004;30(4):459–464.

53. Hung T, Moore-Gillon V, Hern J, et al: Topical bupivacaine in paediatric day-case tonsillectomy: A prospective randomized controlled trial. *J Laryngol Otol* 2002;116(1):33–36.

54. Arikan OK, Ozcan S, Kazkayasi M, et al: Preincisional infiltration of tonsils with ropivacaine in post-tonsillectomy pain-relief: Double-blind, randomized, placebo-controlled intraindividual study. *J Otolaryngol* 2006;35(3):167–172.

55. Page PS, Kersten JR, Farber NE, et al: Cardiovascular pharmacology. In Miller RD, editor: *Miller's anesthesia,* ed 6, Philadelphia, 2005, Elsevier.

56. Alsaraff R, Sie KC: Brain stem stroke associated with bupivacaine injection for adenotonsillectomy. *Otolaryngol Head Neck Surg* 2000;122(4):572–573.

57. Zhao YC, Berkowitz RG: Prolonged hospitalization following tonsillectomy in healthy children. *Int J Pediatr Otorhinolaryngol* 2006;70(11):1885–1889.

58. Anand VT, Phillips JJ, Allen D, et al: A study of postoperative fever following paediatric tonsillectomy. *Clin Otolaryngol Allied Sci* 1999;24(4):360–364.

59. Soldado L, Esteban F, Delgado-Rodriguez M, et al: Bacteremia during tonsillectomy: A study of the factors involved and clinical implications. *Clin Otolaryngol Allied Sci* 1998;23(1):63–66.

60. Kaygusuz I, Gok U, Yalcin S, et al: Bacteremia during tonsillectomy. *Int J Pediatr Otorhinolaryngol* 2001;58(1):69–73.

61. Yildirim I, Okur E, Ciragil P, et al: Bacteremia during tonsillectomy. *J Laryngol Otol* 2003;117(8):619–623.

62. Dajani AS, Taubert KA, Wilson W, et al: Prevention of bacterial endocarditis: The recommendations of the American Heart Association. *Circulation* 1997;96(1):358–366.

63. Saunders NC, Hartley BE, Sell D, et al: Velopharyngeal insufficiency following adenoidectomy. *Clin Otolaryngol Allied Sci* 2004;29(6):686–688.

64. Stewart KJ, Ahmad T, Razzell RE, et al: Altered speech following adenoidectomy: A 20 year experience. *Br J Plast Surg* 2002;55(6):469–473.

65. Kakani RS, Callan ND, April MM: Superior adenoidectomy in children with palatal abnormalities. *Ear, Nose Throat J* 2000;79(4):300, 303–305.

66. Shprintzen RJ, Schwartz RH, Daniller A, et al: Morphologic significance of bifid uvula. *Pediatrics* 1985;75(3):553–561.

67. Ren YF, Isberg A, Henningsson G: Velopharyngeal incompetence and persistent hypernasality after adenoidectomy in children without palatal defect. *Cleft Palate Craniofac J* 1995;32(6):476–482.

68. Golding-Kushner KJ, Argamaso RV, Cotton RT, et al: Standardization for the reporting of nasopharyngoscopy and multiview videofluoroscopy: A report from an International Working Group. *Cleft Palate J* 1990;27:337–348.

69. Willging JP: Velopharyngeal insufficiency. *Int J Pediatr Otorhinolaryngol* 1999;49 Suppl 1:S307–S309.

70. Conley SF, Gosain AK, Marks SM, et al: Identification and assessment of velopharyngeal inadequacy. *Am J Otolaryngol* 1997;18(1):28–46.

71. Sorin A, Bent JP, April MM, et al: Complications of microdebrider-assisted powered intracapsular tonsillectomy and adenoidectomy. *Laryngoscope* 2004;114(2):297–300.

72. Stern Y, Segal K, Yaniv E: Endoscopic adenoidectomy in children with submucous cleft palate. *Int J Pediatr Otorhinolaryngol* 2006;70(11):1871–1874.

73. Shin JJ, Hartnick CJ: Pediatric endoscopic transnasal adenoid ablation. *Ann Otol Rhinol Laryngol* 2003;112(6):511–514.

74. Fernandes DB, Grobbelaar AO, Hudson DA, et al: Velopharyngeal incompetence after adenotonsillectomy in non-cleft patients. *Br J Oral Maxillofac Surg* 1996;34(5):364–367.

75. Perkins JA, Sie K, Gray S: Presence of 22q11 deletion in postadenoidectomy velopharyngeal insufficiency. *Arch Otolaryngol Head Neck Surg* 2000;126(5):645–648.

76. De Serres LM, Deleyiannis FW, Eblen LE, et al: Results with sphincter pharyngoplasty and pharyngeal flap. *Int J Pediatr Otorhinolaryngol* 1999;48(1):17–25.

77. Jones LM, Guillory VL, Mair EA: Total nasopharyngeal stenosis: Treatment with laser excision, nasopharyngeal obturators, and topical mitomycin-c. *Otolaryngol Head Neck Surg* 2005;133(5):795–798.

78. Giannoni C, Sulek M, Friedman EM, et al: Acquired nasopharyngeal stenosis: A warning and review. *Arch Otolaryngol Head Neck Surg* 1998;124:163–167.

79. Toh E, Pearl AW, Genden EM, et al: Bivalved palatal transposition flaps for the correction of acquired nasopharyngeal stenosis. *Am J Rhinol* 2000;14(3):199–204.

80. Cotton RT: Nasopharyngeal stenosis. *Arch Otolaryngol* 1985;111:146–148.

81. Onerci M, Ogretmenoglu O, Ozcan OE: Atlanto-axial subluxation after tonsillectomy and adenoidectomy. *Otolaryngol Head Neck Surg* 1997;116(2):271–273.

82. Battiata AP, Pazos G: Grisel's syndrome: The two-hit hypothesis—A case report and literature review. *Ear Nose Throat J* 2004;83(8):553–555.

83. Fielding JW: Atlantoaxial rotary deformities. *Orthop Clin North Am* 1978;9:955–967.

84. Statham MM, Elluru RG, Buncher R, et al: Adenotonsillectomy for obstructive sleep apnea syndrome in young children: Prevalence of pulmonary complications. *Arch Otolaryngol Head Neck Surg* 2006;132(5):476–480.

85. Mitchell RB, Kelly J: Outcome of adenotonsillectomy for obstructive sleep apnea in children under 3 years. *Otolaryngol Head Neck Surg* 2005;132(5):681–684.

86. Mitchell RB, Kelly J: Adenotonsillectomy for obstructive sleep apnea in obese children. *Otolaryngol Head Neck Surg* 2004;131(1):104–108.

87. Shine NP, Coates HL, Lannigan FJ: Obstructive sleep apnea, morbid obesity, and adenotonsillar surgery: A review of the literature. *Int J Pediatr Otorhinolaryngol* 2005;69(11):1475–1482.

88. Goldstein NA, Armfield DR, Kingsley LA, et al: Postoperative complications after tonsillectomy and adenoidectomy in children with Down syndrome. *Arch Otolaryngol Head Neck Surg* 1998;124(2):171–176.

89. Bower CM, Richmond D: Tonsillectomy and adenoidectomy in patients with Down syndrome. *Int J Pediatr Otorhinolaryngol* 1995;33(2):141–148.

90. Biavati MJ, Manning SC, Phillips DL: Predictive factors for respiratory complications after tonsillectomy and adenoidectomy in children. *Arch Otolaryngol Head Neck Surg* 1997;123(5):517–521.

91. Gerber ME, O'Connor DM, Adler E, et al: Selected risk factors in pediatric adenotonsillectomy. *Arch Otolaryngol Head Neck Surg* 1996;122(8):811–814.

92. Leighton SE, Papsin B, Vellodi A, et al: Disordered breathing during sleep in patients with mucopolysaccharidoses. *Int J Pediatr Otorhinolaryngol* 2001;58(2):127–138.

93. Duke RL, Scott JP, Panepinto JA, et al: Perioperative management of sickle cell disease children undergoing adenotonsillectomy. *Otolaryngol Head Neck Surg* 2006;134(3):370–373.

94. Halvorson DJ, McKie V, McKie K, et al: Sickle cell disease and tonsillectomy: Preoperative management and postoperative complications. *Arch Otolaryngol Head Neck Surg* 1997;123(7):689–692.

95. White GC Jr, Sadler JE: von Willebrand disease: Clinical aspects and therapy. In Hoffman R, Benz EJ Jr, Shattil SJ, et al, editors: *Hematology: Basic principles and practice,* ed 4, Philadelphia, 2005, Elsevier.

96. Shah SB, Lalwani AK, Koerper MA: Perioperative management of von Willebrand's disease in otolaryngologic surgery. *Laryngoscope* 1998;108(1):32–36.

97. Allen GC, Armfield DR, Bontempo FA, et al: Adenotonsillectomy in children with von Willebrand disease. *Arch Otolaryngol Head Neck Surg* 1999;125(5):547–551.

98. Derkay CS, Werner E, Plotnick E: Management of children with von Willebrand disease undergoing tonsillectomy. *Am J Otolaryngol* 1996;17(3):172–177.

99. Lozier JN, Kessler CM: Clinical aspects and therapy of hemophilia. In Hoffman R, Benz EJ, Shattil SJ, et al, editors: *Hematology: Basic principles and practice,* ed 4, Philadelphia, 2005, Elsevier.

100. Srivastava A, Chandy M, Sunderaj GD, et al: Low dose intermittent factor replacement for post-operative hemostasis in haemophilia. *Haemophilia* 1998;4:799–801.

101. Rochat C, McFadyen ML, Schwyzer R, et al: Continuous infusion of intermediate-purity factor VIII in haemophilia A patients undergoing elective surgery. *Haemophilia* 1999;5(3):181–186.

102. Zwack GC, Derkay CS: The utility of preoperative hemostatic assessment in adenotonsillectomy. *Int J Pediatr Otorhinolaryngol* 1997;39(1):67–76.

103. Derkay CS: A cost-effective approach for preoperative hemostatic assessment in children undergoing adenotonsillectomy. *Arch Otolaryngol Head Neck Surg* 2000;126(5):688.

104. Lalakea LM, Marquez-Biggs I, Messner AH: Safety of pediatric short-stay tonsillectomy. *Arch Otolaryngol Head Neck Surg* 1999;125:749–752.

105. Mills N, Anderson BJ, Barber C, et al: Day-stay pediatric tonsillectomy: A safe procedure. *Int J Pediatr Otorhinolaryngol* 2004;68:1367–1373.

106. Granell J, Gete P, Villafruela M, et al: Safety of outpatient tonsillectomy in children: A review of 6 years in a tertiary hospital experience. *Otolaryngol Head Neck Surg* 2004;131(4):383–387.

107. Ross AT, Kazahaya K, Tom LWC: Revisiting outpatient tonsillectomy in young children. *Otolaryngol Head Neck Surg* 2003;128(3):326–331.

108. Brigger MT, Brietzke SE: Outpatient tonsillectomy in children: A systematic review. *Otolaryngol Head Neck Surg* 2006;135(1):1–7.

109. Reiner SA, Sawyer WP, Clark KF, et al: Safety of outpatient tonsillectomy and adenoidectomy. *Otolaryngol Head Neck Surg* 1990;102:161–168.

110. Helmus C, Grin M, Westfall R: Same-day-stay adenotonsillectomy. *Laryngoscope* 1990;100:593–596.

111. Carithers JS, Gebhart DE, Williams JA: Postoperative risks of pediatric tonsiloadenoidectomy. *Laryngoscope* 1987;97:422–429.

112. Shott SR, Myer CM, Cotton RT: Efficacy of tonsillectomy and adenoidectomy as an outpatient procedure: A preliminary report. *Int J Pediatr Otorhinolaryngol* 1987;13:157–163.

113. Koempel JA: On the origin of tonsillectomy and the dissection method. *Laryngoscope* 2002;112(9):1583–1586.

114. Patel N, Kirkland P, Tandon P, et al: Comparison of bipolar scissors and bipolar forceps in tonsillectomy. *Ear Nose Throat J* 2002;81(10):714–717.

115. Perkins J, Dahiya R: Microdissection needle tonsillectomy and postoperative pain: A pilot study. *Arch Otolaryngol Head Neck Surg* 2003;129(12):1285–1288.

116. Unkel C, Lehnerdt G, Schmitz KJ, et al: Laser tonsillotomy for treatment of obstructive tonsillar hyperplasia in early childhood: A retrospective review. *Int J Pediatr Otorhinolaryngol* 2005;69(12):1615–1620.

117. Friedman M, LoSavio P, Ibrahim H, et al: Radiofrequency tonsillar reduction: Safety, morbidity, and efficacy. *Laryngoscope* 2003;113:882–887.

118. Kamal SA, Basu S, Kapoor L, et al: Harmonic scalpel tonsillectomy: A prospective study. *Eur Arch Otorhinolaryngol* 2006;263(5):449–454.

119. Leaper M, Mahadevan M, Vokes D, et al: A prospective randomised single blinded study comparing harmonic scalpel tonsillectomy with bipolar tonsillectomy. *Int J Pediatr Otorhinolaryngol* 2006;70(8):1389–1396.

120. Koltai PJ, Solares A, Koempel JA, et al: Intracapsular tonsillar reduction (partial tonsillectomy): Reviving a historical procedure for obstructive sleep disordered breathing in children. *Otolaryngol Head Neck Surg* 2003;129(5):532–538.

121. Woloszko J, Gilbride C: Coblation technology: Plasmamediated ablation for otolaryngology applications. In Anderson RR, Bartels KE, Bass LS, et al, editors: *Lasers in surgery: Advanced characterization, therapeutics, and systems.* Proc. SPIE May 2000;3907:306–316.

122. Timms MS, Ghosh S, Roper A: Adenoidectomy with the coblator: A logical extension of radiofrequency tonsillectomy. *J Laryngol Otol* 2005;119(5):398–399.

123. Glade RS, Pearson SE, Zalzal GH, et al: Coblation adenotonsillectomy: An improvement over electrocautery technique? *Otolaryngol Head Neck Surg* 2006;134(5):852–855.

124. Hall DJ, Littlefield PD, Birkmire-Peters DP, et al: Radiofrequency ablation versus electrocautery in tonsillectomy. *Otolaryngol Head Neck Surg* 2004;130(3):300–305.

125. Littlefield PD, Hall DJ, Holtel MR: Radiofrequency excision versus monopolar electrosurgical excision for tonsillectomy. *Otolaryngol Head Neck Surg* 2005;133(1):51–54.

126. Chang KW: Randomized controlled trial of coblation versus electrocautery tonsillectomy. *Otolaryngol Head Neck Surg* 2005;132(2):273–280.

127. Ragab SM: Bipolar radiofrequency dissection tonsillectomy: A prospective randomized trial. *Otolaryngol Head Neck Surg* 2005;133(6):961–965.

128. Philpott CM, Wild DC, Mehta D, et al: A double-blind randomized controlled trial of coblation versus conventional dissection tonsillectomy on post-operative symptoms. *Clin Otolaryngol* 2005;30:143–148.

129. Ericsson E, Graf J, Hultcrantz E: Pediatric tonsillotomy with radiofrequency technique: Long-term follow-up. *Laryngoscope* 2006;116:1851–1857.

130. Sobol SE, Wetmore RF, Marsh RR, et al: Postoperative recovery after microdebrider intracapsular or monopolar electrocautery tonsillectomy. *Arch Otolaryngol Head Neck Surg* 2006;132: 270–274.

131. Lister MT, Cunningham MJ, Benjamin B, et al: Microdebrider tonsillotomy vs electrosurgical tonsillectomy. *Arch Otolaryngol Head Neck Surg* 2006;132:599–604.

132. Solares CA, Koempel JA, Hirose K, et al: Safety and efficacy of powered intracapsular tonsillectomy in children: A multicenter retrospective case series. *Int J Pediatr Otorhinolaryngol* 2005;69:21–26.

133. Derkay CS, Darrow DH, Welch C, et al: Post-tonsillectomy morbidity and quality of life in pediatric patients with obstructive tonsils and adenoid: Microdebrider vs. electrocautery. *Otolaryngol Head Neck Surg* 2006;134(1):114–120.

134. Bent JP, April MM, Ward RF, et al: Ambulatory powered intracapsular tonsillectomy and adenoidectomy in children younger than 3 years. *Arch Otolaryngol Head Neck Surg* 2004;130: 1197–2000.

CHAPTER 29

Complications of Sleep Surgery

Eric J. Kezirian

Treatments for obstructive sleep apnea (OSA) include behavioral approaches, positive airway pressure, oral appliance therapy, and surgery. Positive airway pressure is recognized as the first-line treatment for most patients with OSA, but patients often do not tolerate this treatment modality, and they may consider other options, including surgery. The surgical treatment of sleep-disordered breathing can be directed at one or more of three potential regions of upper-airway narrowing and/or obstruction: the nose, the palate/tonsils, and the so-called hypopharynx (actually a portion of the oropharynx posterior to the tongue base and the hypopharynx). Box 29-1 presents the most common procedures that are available for the treatment of OSA.

This chapter describes the overall risk of perioperative complications after OSA surgery and then discusses specific potential complications of procedures directed at airway obstruction occurring at the levels of the palate and the hypopharynx. As described in Box 29-1, several procedures that are often performed for the treatment of OSA—including nasal procedures, tonsillectomy, tracheotomy, and maxillomandibular advancement—will not be explicitly discussed. The interested reader is directed to other chapters in this text for the discussion of specific complications of these procedures.

PERIOPERATIVE COMPLICATIONS

Incidence of Complications and Risk Factors

The anatomic and physiologic abnormalities associated with OSA pose independent risks of complications during the intraoperative and perioperative periods.[1–4] Anesthetics and narcotics increase upper-airway instability and suppress the respiratory drive. Postoperative edema after upper-airway surgery further raises the concern for complications. Although rare, airway obstruction leading to respiratory arrest and the need for reintubation or emergent tracheotomy most commonly occurs within hours of surgery.[1,3] Patients with OSA may be especially vulnerable to myocardial infarction or other cardiovascular events after surgery as a result of the association between OSA and cardiovascular disease.[2] Finally, all OSA surgical patients (particularly those undergoing concurrent tonsillectomy) are at risk for postoperative hemorrhage.

Nevertheless, serious perioperative complications related to sleep surgery appear to be uncommon. The risks of uvulopalatopharyngoplasty (UPPP) have been the most closely studied, because UPPP is the most common surgical procedure performed for the treatment of OSA. Early published data came from single-site case series[5–10]; these studies identified the perioperative risks but had limited generalizability and, because of their size, a limited ability to address potential risk factors for perioperative complications.

A larger, multisite, cohort study that included 3130 patients from all Veterans Affairs Medical Centers in the United States from 1991 to 2001 undergoing UPPP addressed these two weaknesses of the previous studies.[11] This study determined that the incidence of serious perioperative complication after UPPP (with or without other sleep-related surgeries performed concurrently) was 1.6%, including a 30-day mortality rate of 0.2%. Most of these complications were respiratory (1.1%), but patients also experienced cardiovascular complications (0.3%) and significant hemorrhage (0.3%). Subsequent analysis of this cohort revealed the following risk factors for complication: medical comorbidity, OSA severity (measured by the apnea–hypopnea index), and body mass index.[12] Concurrent hypopharyngeal procedures were associated with an increased risk of complications, but it was not possible to determine whether the risk of performing these procedures concurrently was higher than the cumulative risk when they were performed separately.

Perioperative Management

The recognition of perioperative risks and the adoption of management strategies can reduce the incidence of complications. Practice guidelines developed on the basis of expert opinion (as a result of the absence of systematic investigations) have been developed by the American Society of Anesthesiologists to address the unique challenges of patients with OSA.[13] Interested readers should consult this publication or the anticipated updates developed by its authors and other organizations. These guidelines address several issues that are not possible within the scope of this chapter, including preoperative screening and intraoperative and postoperative management.

BOX 29-1 Obstructive Sleep Apnea Surgical Procedures

PALATE
- Uvulopalatopharyngoplasty
- Uvulopalatal flap
- Transpalatal advancement pharyngoplasty
- Z-Palatoplasty
- Lateral pharyngoplasty
- Palate radiofrequency
- Laser-assisted uvulopalatoplasty

HYPOPHARYNX
- Genioglossus advancement
- Mortised genioplasty
- Tongue radiofrequency
- Midline glossectomy
- Lingual tonsillectomy
- Hyoid suspension
- Tongue suspension

SURGICAL PROCEDURES PERFORMED FOR THE TREATMENT OF OBSTRUCTIVE SLEEP APNEA BUT NOT DISCUSSED IN THE CHAPTER TEXT
- Nasal procedures
- Tonsillectomy
- Tracheotomy
- Maxillomandibular advancement

Although these are not discussed here in detail, certain points deserve mention. Airway management in patients with OSA requires close cooperation between the otolaryngology–head and neck surgery and anesthesia teams. A surgeon has typically performed in-office flexible fiber-optic examination of the patient's airway; a discussion of patient-specific anatomy may allow for the detection of patients who may present special challenges during intubation. The development of a plan and backup plans for successful intubation may require that the anesthesia team perform intubation and/or extubation with several precautions. Although none of these have been evaluated specifically for patients with OSA, these precautions may include the use of fiber-optic guidance for intubation and the performance of extubation in the operating room rather than in the recovery room and only after the patient is fully awake. This so-called "deep" extubation can minimize coughing, but it may leave a patient less able to protect his or her airway.

The ideal setting for postoperative monitoring is a subject of debate. The traditional view that any upper-airway surgery in patients with OSA mandates, at a minimum, overnight inpatient observation has been challenged, and the evidence neither confirms nor refutes this.[13] A case series has demonstrated the safety of outpatient palate surgery (including tonsillectomy) and nasal surgery among patients with OSA[14]; nevertheless, the evidence supporting an inpatient stay after one of the hypopharyngeal procedures is stronger.[13]

Continuous monitoring is essential for patients who are at significant risk of respiratory compromise or other perioperative complications. The best choice among various monitored settings has not been determined and likely varies according to patient, personnel, and institutional factors.

Although perioperative management is ultimately based on the nature of the surgical intervention, there are some common strategies. Airway management typically includes a combination of monitoring, corticosteroids administered for 24 hours to minimize edema, and the judicious use of narcotics to control pain aggressively while also avoiding excessive sedation and upper-airway muscle relaxation. The strict control of blood pressure, including the use of intravenous agents, can decrease the risk of bleeding and the resulting airway compromise. The benefits of close blood pressure control may be particularly important after hypopharyngeal procedures, because bleeding in this region can present more challenging airway compromise. The use of positive airway pressure during the perioperative period can effectively maintain upper-airway patency as a pneumatic splint and, perhaps, by decreasing edema. Although patients undergoing surgery are largely unable to tolerate positive airway pressure therapy, those patients with moderate to severe OSA should strongly consider perioperative use, if possible. Perioperative antibiotics can decrease the risk of infection and postoperative inflammation. Finally, histamine-receptor blockers or proton-pump inhibitors provide prophylaxis against stress gastritis or treatment for the extraesophageal acid reflux that commonly coexists.

COMPLICATIONS RELATED TO SPECIFIC PROCEDURES

The true incidence of procedure-specific complications—both major and minor—after specific procedures has often not been established. The figures presented here reflect the reported rates of complications, when available. In the absence of reported rates, the potential risks, avoidance strategies, and treatments for these complications are described.

Palate Surgery Including Uvulopalatopharyngoplasty, Uvulopalatal Flap, Lateral Pharyngoplasty, and Z-Palatoplasty

Hemorrhage and Wound Dehiscence

Palate surgery carries an unspecified risk of bleeding, and the risk is higher if tonsillectomy is also performed in the same setting. After UPPP with or without tonsillectomy, the incidence of substantial hemorrhage (i.e., >4 units of packed red blood cells) was 0.3% in the previously described cohort study,[11] but the incidence of hemorrhage of a lesser degree was unknown. It is important to note that it was not possible to determine the rates after procedures with and without tonsillectomy. Large case series have demonstrated that approximately 1% to 4% of patients who undergo tonsillectomy alone experience bleeding after surgery and that the risk may be higher among adults than children.[15]

Wound closure during palate surgery occurs along the soft palate, and, in cases with concurrent tonsillectomy, the closure of the tonsillar pillars (suture pharyngoplasty) can be performed. Wound closure involves coverage of exposed muscle tissue with mucosa, and wound dehiscence may be a contributing factor to bleeding after palate surgery, because it produces exposure of the vascular muscle layer. In addition to the bleeding risk, wound dehiscence also may compromise surgical results by reversing the repositioning of tissues that is sometimes performed during these palate procedures.

Wound tension along the palate is related to soft-palate thickness and the length of mucosa that can be closed over the residual soft-palate muscle. Tension can be minimized by preserving the mucosa, particularly the posterior mucosa along the nasal surface of the soft palate, during dissection; judicious thinning of the residual soft-palate bulk (when possible); and a two-layer suture closure. Although it has not been evaluated systematically, in the author's experience, wound dehiscence may be reduced with the use of two layers of absorbable sutures: one deep layer for the approximation of muscle tissue to decrease wound tension, in areas of significant tension (when possible), and a second layer that incorporates mucosa, submucosal tissue, and possibly muscle. Although the dehiscence of the superficial exposed layer of sutures may be unavoidable, the deep suture layer reduces the degree of wound dehiscence.

Wound closure along the tonsillar fossa is accomplished with suture pharyngoplasty, although there is greater tension promoting dehiscence as a result of the vector forces of the palatoglossus and palatopharyngeus muscles. Although the preservation of both mucosa and muscle tissue reduces the tension on the closure, a two-layer closure (particularly in the superior aspect of the tonsillar fossa) may prove useful.

Infection

Reactive edema, whether a result of the surgery or a tissue reaction to the suture material, is common. True infection, however, is rare but not impossible after palate surgery with or without tonsillectomy. Perioperative antibiotics are often used to decrease reactive edema after all palate procedures, and this may reduce the risk of infection as well. Mouthwashes or oral rinses containing ethanol or other mucosal irritants should be avoided until complete healing has occurred, because these will increase the degree of reactive edema. Some surgeons advocate antiseptic rinses such as chlorhexidine, but these have not been studied systematically.

Nasal Regurgitation and Velopharyngeal Insufficiency

Normal speech and swallowing depend in part on the function of the velopharyngeal sphincter. Sphincter closure is a complex motor process that requires the coordination of multiple muscles, and the required movements for speech and swallowing are distinct. Palate surgery involves the surgical removal and repositioning of palatal tissue, and it therefore can disrupt normal sphincter physiology. Velopharyngeal dysfunction can produce the nasal regurgitation of food or liquids with or without velopharyngeal insufficiency and the associated hypernasal speech. Symptoms of velopharyngeal dysfunction, especially the nasal regurgitation of liquids, are common during the first 2 weeks after surgery,[16] although most patients do not experience these problems. The resolution of edema and the recovery of muscle function during healing allows for recovery such that few patients have noticeable long-term dysfunction.

No large studies have considered the incidence of these potential complications, but, fortunately, permanent velopharyngeal insufficiency appears to be rare.[17,18] In one study, intermittent nasal regurgitation of liquids beyond three months postoperatively was reported by 10% (5 of 50) of patients after UPPP.[18a] These complications are likely related to the extent of palatal resection, the thickness and relative length of the residual soft-palate tissue, and the degree of postoperative fibrosis. There have been no direct comparisons of different methods for determining the extent of palatal resection in UPPP, and multiple palate surgery techniques have been developed.[19–22]

The uvulopalatal flap procedure was developed as an alternative to UPPP specifically for patients with relatively thin soft palates.[22] By performing less resection of tissue and using electrocautery sparingly, the incidence of nasal regurgitation and velopharyngeal insufficiency should be lower in this group of patients who otherwise may be at especially high risk for these complications. In the series of 80 patients described in the original article, no instances of these complications were reported.[22]

By contrast, the Z-palatoplasty creates a greater disruption of the velopharyngeal sphincter by dividing a portion of the soft palate in the midline and repositioning this tissue. Nasal regurgitation and possibly velopharyngeal insufficiency are expected to last for 1 to 3 months, although the long-term incidence of these sequelae has not been reported.[21]

For the treatment of velopharyngeal insufficiency and nasal regurgitation, the use of sphincter pharyngoplasty or pharyngeal flap surgeries,[23] palate pushback procedures, obturators, and Teflon paste injections[24,25] have been described. The author prefers sphincter pharyngoplasty using the technique described by Jackson and Silverton,[26] although the palatal fibrosis that occurs after palate surgery and the related limited ability to retract the soft palate superiorly can make the placement of the pharyngeal flaps at the level of the velopharynx challenging. The treatment of velopharyngeal dysfunction carries the risk of worsening underlying sleep-disordered breathing, and the balance between adequate volitional velopharyngeal closure and airway obstruction can be a delicate one.

Nasopharyngeal Stenosis

Nasopharyngeal stenosis after palate surgery is thought to result from cicatricial scarring after palate surgery; fortunately it is uncommon.[18] Several factors are felt to increase the risk of nasopharyngeal stenosis, including concurrent adenoidectomy, excessive thermal injury (either as a result of electrocautery or laser energy in laser-assisted uvulopalatoplasty), the aggressive excision of posterior tonsillar pillar tissue or the undermining of posterior pharyngeal wall tissue, wound dehiscence, infection, and tissue necrosis.[18,27,28] This complication is particularly problematic, because patients can experience the symptoms of velopharyngeal dysfunction with the resulting effects on speech and swallowing as well as airway obstruction. Strategies for prevention include the avoidance of the listed factors as well as techniques to minimize wound tension and dehiscence.

The treatment of nasopharyngeal stenosis is challenging. A grading system for this problem has been developed,[27] and results overall are better in less severe forms of stenosis. Treatment has been described using dilation, steroid injection, carbon-dioxide lasers to release fibrous scar tissue with or without the use of nasopharyngeal obturators[27,28] with or without the application of mitomycin C,[29] local flaps, pedicled flaps, and free-tissue transfer.[28,30–33] Multiple treatments are often required to obtain satisfactory results.

Changes in Speech

Palate surgery can produce changes in phonation, resonance, and articulation. Risks for these changes have been examined most closely for UPPP, and several studies have separately considered these potential changes with objective and subjective evaluation.[34] Overall the results have shown conflicting results without substantial changes across groups of patients.

Because UPPP does not involve the larynx, one may expect that there would be no changes in the voice, particularly with regard to the fundamental frequency. However, the fundamental frequency and other phonatory characteristics (e.g., the first and second formants) can be affected by upper-airway structure and muscle activity. Although one study showed a small increase in fundamental frequency and a diminution of the second formant in the sustained vowels /e/ and /u/,[35] others have not demonstrated any changes.[34]

Changes in the upper-airway dimensions can also affect resonance and produce hypernasality. Although hypernasality (including velopharyngeal insufficiency) may result in individual patients, in large series, this has not been shown objectively to occur.[34] Similarly, studies have shown little or no change in articulation.[34]

Taste Disturbance

Hypogeusia, or a diminished sense of taste, has been described after UPPP,[36] and it is thought to arise from two possible mechanisms. The placement of a mouth gag with pressure on the tongue during the procedure can create pressure-induced damage of the lingual nerve, and palate surgery can include the resection or injury of the taste receptors on the oral surface of the soft palate.[37]

One series reported five patients who complained of taste disturbance 3 months postoperatively from a series of 108 patients undergoing palate surgery.[38] Evaluation with an objective test of taste function demonstrated a loss of the sense of sweet taste in 4 of 5 patients and the loss of bitter sensation in 1 of 5 patients. The use of electrocautery (but not operative time or other operative variables) was associated with taste disturbance, which suggests that taste disturbance may be associated with surgical trauma to the palate taste receptors rather than lingual nerve injury. Spontaneous resolution was seen in 4 of 5 patients by 9 months after surgery.

Foreign-Body Sensation and Excessive Phlegm

Although they are considered minor, foreign-body sensation and excessive phlegm may be very bothersome. They are common during the perioperative period, but they can persist (although somewhat improved) over time. Their causes are likely multifactorial and complex. Some have suggested that these conditions are related to the disruption of normal mucus and saliva flow into the pharynx, and others have argued that they relate to the presence of scarring along the oral surface or the free edge of the soft palate (both of which are preferred to a suture line on the nasal surface of the soft palate to minimize the risk of the more serious complications listed previously).[39] No treatment has yet been curative.

Complications Related to Specific Palate Procedures: Palatal Advancement Pharyngoplasty

Oronasal Fistula

Oronasal fistula may occur after palatal advancement pharyngoplasty as a result of the dehiscence of the palatal suture line and/or partial flap necrosis; both of these events create a temporary fistula that can become permanent. The original technique[40] was modified specifically to decrease the rate of dehiscence by incorporating a small segment of palatal bone attached to the tensor veli palatini aponeurosis.[41] The largest case series, which combined patients from two centers who were treated with both the original and modified techniques, revealed an incidence of oronasal fistula of 13% (i.e., 6 of 47), with a higher rate seen among smokers. The authors report a lower rate with the modified technique, but data are not presented. Their treatment of oronasal fistula included the use of occlusive oral prostheses and minor wound revision. Healing occurred within 1 to 3 weeks in all 6 cases.[40]

Nasal Regurgitation and Velopharyngeal Insufficiency

Any increase in retropalatal airway space requires a corresponding increase in velopharyngeal sphincter function during speech and swallowing. After palatal advancement pharyngoplasty, nasal regurgitation occurred with some frequency (i.e., 3 of 30 [10%] in the previously cited series), but it did not persist over extended periods of time. Nasal regurgitation occurred more commonly with concurrent soft-palate resection (modified UPPP). Velopharyngeal insufficiency was not reported.[40]

Radiofrequency Palatoplasty

Radiofrequency energy has been used to treat the soft palate in selected patients suffering from less severe forms of sleep-disordered breathing, such as primary snoring, upper airway resistance syndrome, and mild obstructive sleep apnea. There are multiple available technologies that make use of radiofrequency energy for treatment, and they share certain characteristics. As compared with other palate procedures (e.g., UPPP), radiofrequency treatment creates less tissue injury and subsequent improvements in airway dimensions, and it also has a lower morbidity rate.

However, complications can occur with radiofrequency palatoplasty. Temperature-controlled and bipolar radiofrequency are designed to treat submucosal palate tissue while sparing the mucosa. Mucosal disruption and ulceration may result if the tissue injury involves the mucosa itself, and a fistula can develop if there is full-thickness injury. Infection and a thin soft palate may contribute to mucosal disruption and fistula. Regardless of the cause, mucosal disruption is typically associated with increased pain as a result of the exposure of underlying soft tissues. Uvular sloughing can occur if there is sufficient soft-palate tissue disruption that involves the base of the uvula, and dysphagia can result with excessive soft-palate or uvular edema.

A literature review categorized complications according to severity: minor (mucosal ulceration or uvular sloughing), moderate (hemorrhage, palatal fistula, nerve paresis or paralysis, or significant dysphagia), or major (serious infection requiring drainage or other significant airway compromise).[42] This review indicated that the overall rate of moderate or severe complications was 1.2% (8 of 669 patients), primarily involving fistulas that healed spontaneously; it was difficult to determine the incidence of minor complications, because these were not reported as thoroughly.

Laser-Assisted Uvulopalatoplasty

Many lasers, primarily the carbon-dioxide laser, have been used to treat the soft palates and uvulas of selected patients with sleep-disordered breathing, including OSA. Because this procedure requires the removal of at least a portion of the uvula and the soft palate, it has many of the same potential risks as UPPP. No large studies have determined their incidence after laser-assisted UPPP, but one study showed a 13% (9 of 69) incidence of nasal regurgitation and a 7% (5 of 69) incidence of speech disturbances.[42a] Complications, however, are likely to be related not only to the amount of tissue removed during the procedure but also to the thermal injury and associated fibrosis that occurs. Because no sutures are placed during the procedure, the results are based to some extent on healing patterns that can be unpredictable. There has been a general trend toward performing laser-assisted uvulopalatoplasty in a staged fashion, with multiple, less aggressive laser procedures. This may reduce the incidence of permanent complications.

HYPOPHARYNGEAL PROCEDURES

Several procedures to treat the so-called hypopharyngeal airway have been developed, and most have a unique set of potential complications. However, all of these procedures carry the risk of airway compromise during the perioperative period as a result of edema. Hypopharyngeal airway compromise should be considered more serious than that which occurs after palatal surgery, because there is less ability to bypass the airway obstruction with maneuvers such as placing a nasopharyngeal airway or opening the mouth to transition from nasal to oral breathing. For this reason, patients are routinely hospitalized for overnight observation after these procedures when perioperative corticosteroids are administered, except in the case of isolated tongue radiofrequency, which can be performed on an outpatient basis.

Genioglossus Advancement and Mortised Genioplasty

Three techniques have been described for the advancement of the genioglossus muscle attachment to the mandible lingual cortex: the genioglossus advancement procedure incorporating a rectangular[43] or circular[44] osteotomy and the mortised genioplasty.[45] These will be discussed together, although differences will be highlighted when appropriate.

Hematoma

These procedures require mandibular osteotomies and the resulting exposed bony edges, including the vascular marrow space. The potential hematoma of the floor of the mouth is noteworthy because it creates an associated posterior displacement of the tongue with airway compromise. The key to avoiding this airway compromise is prevention, because the treatment of the hematoma after it develops is difficult. Typically there is no discrete hematoma that can be evacuated with a drainage procedure; instead, the floor of the mouth typically has diffuse ecchymosis (Figure 29-1).

Prevention begins with aggressive intraoperative and perioperative blood pressure control. Intraoperative hemostasis is also valuable and can include the discrete cauterization of the genioglossus (genioglossus advancement) or the geniohyoid and/or the mylohyoid (mortised genioplasty) muscles if they are cut during the performance of the osteotomies. The mandibular marrow space may contain enlarged sinusoids. Hemostatic agents may be packed into these sinusoids or placed into the floor of mouth adjacent to the rotated bone fragment (genioglossus advancement) for purposes of tamponade and the promotion of hemostasis.

Dental Numbness or Paresthesias

The mandible and the lower dentition are supplied by the inferior alveolar neurovascular bundles traveling within the mandibular canal. Within the mandibular canal, the neurovascular bundles supply the molars and the premolars as well as the adjacent gingiva. The two terminal branches of the inferior alveolar nerve are the mental nerve, which emerges from the mental foramen to innervate the soft tissues of the chin and the lower lip, and the smaller incisive branch, which supplies the canine and incisor teeth with arterial and venous branches by traveling though the mandible in a superior, vertical direction. Both terminal branches are at risk for injury, with corresponding temporary or permanent sequelae.

The genioglossus advancement and mortised genioplasty procedures require osteotomies that unavoidably transect the incisive neurovascular bundles and that therefore produce numbness of the lower incisors. After these nerve injuries, the processes of nerve degeneration and recovery through reinnervation occur over time. The recovery of dental sensation generally occurs over 6 to 12 months, and, during this period, paresthesias or dental sensitivity to hot and cold temperatures may occur. A substantial minority of patients will experience some degree of permanent numbness of the affected teeth, although persistent paresthesias and sensitivities are even less common.

Mental Nerve Injury

The mental foramen is located lateral to the canine roots, and the mental nerve is therefore at risk for transection or traction injury during this procedure. Fortunately, careful dissection ensures that nerve transection is uncommon, but traction injury can produce similar temporary or permanent sequelae. Because osteotomies are performed medial to the canine roots during the genioglossus advancement procedure, mental nerve injury is typically related to the retraction of soft tissues and the associated stretch injury. However, the mortised genioplasty includes an osteotomy that is in closer proximity to the mental foramen and that likely places the nerve at higher risk for both transection and traction injury. Mental nerve injury produces chin and lower lip numbness, but the sensation of numbness is common in the perioperative period and is likely related to soft tissue edema. Typically numbness in this region resolves within weeks to months after the procedure.

Dental Injury

Both procedures require mandibular osteotomies that are performed in relative proximity to the dentition. The panoramic radiograph, or Panorex, is used most commonly for the radiographic evaluation of the maxilla and the mandible with the dentition. Key features of the panorex related to these procedures are the mandibular height, the length and orientation of the incisor and canine roots, and the evaluation for other dental or mandibular pathology. Certain patients will not be candidates for genioglossus advancement or mortised genioplasty as a result of a mandible without sufficient height, incisor roots that are excessively long, canine

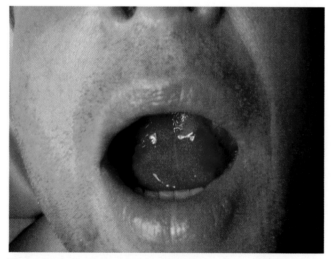

Figure 29-1. Ecchymosis of the floor of the mouth after genioglossus advancement. This moderate amount of ecchymosis produced no airway compromise. The picture was taken with the patient elevating the tongue to touch the hard palate and to thus allow visualization of the floor.

roots that are directed markedly inferomedially, or other abnormalities.

Despite all precautions taken during the performance of mandibular osteotomies and the presence of a panorex without the above-named findings, it is possible for the canines and/or incisors to be injured during this procedure. One advantage of the genioglossus advancement procedure performed using a rectangular osteotomy as compared to a circular osteotomy is that it is easier to adjust the dimensions of the osteotomy on the basis of the findings from the panorex image. Dental injury typically occurs as a result of direct or regional trauma to the teeth or the neurovascular supply, and some authors have advocated maintaining at least 5 mm of intact bone between the incisor root tips and the osteotomies.[46] There appears to be no universal relationship between direct dental trauma (or the lack thereof) and dental injury. In some cases, the root tips may be transected without adverse sequelae, and the opposite pattern can also be seen.[47] The latter situation may be related to events that affect the pulp chamber or other components of the dentition unrelated to direct trauma, but its basis is undetermined.

In cases of suspected dental injury, evaluation by a dental professional is valuable. A dental evaluation may include radiographs as well as a formal examination of dental health with pulp vitality testing. There are several techniques of pulp vitality testing that assess the health of the dental pulp using thermal, electric, or mechanical stimuli or the assessment of pulp blood flow.[48–50] The former group of stimuli-based tests depends on intact dental innervation and therefore is inaccurate after these procedures. Because the primary direct vascular supply to these teeth is also disrupted during the procedure, vitality testing based on pulp blood flow will also be affected. It is critical that a dental professional understands the nature of the mandibular osteotomies and the implications for vitality testing techniques. The comprehensive evaluation of dental health should also include direct inspection and radiographic examination for the early detection of the signs of permanent dental injury. The treatment of dental injury may require interventions such as endodontic therapy or dental extraction.

Incisional Dehiscence and Infection

Dehiscence of the gingivolabial incision can be associated with infection of the soft tissues, the hardware, or the mandible or the development of the "witch's chin" deformity. No studies have systematically evaluated techniques to reduce incisional dehiscence, but prevention can include a combination of careful incision closure and adjunctive measures such as dressings. The closure of the incision is similar to that performed after the use of a similar incision for the treatment of mandible fractures. Two techniques have been used widely, a one-layer closure incorporating mucosa and muscle and a two-layer closure with separate closure of the mentalis muscle with one or two interrupted sutures separate from the mucosal layer. Both techniques typically involve the use of absorbable sutures. Adjunctive measures include the use of a dressing to support the weight of the chin soft tissues by securing this dressing to the skin overlying the regions of the mandible.

The treatment of incisional dehiscence includes wound care and the use of antibiotics that are protective against oral flora. In cases of dehiscence, the wound should be probed gently. Wound care includes gentle rinsing after oral intake to prevent the collection of particles within the wound. For cases in which the mucosal dehiscence is noticeably smaller than the underlying cavity, thus creating a pocket, a portion of the mucosa should be opened to simplify wound care and to allow for healing by secondary intention. Healing generally occurs within 2 to 3 weeks, and, in some cases, the gentle debridement of the wound edges can facilitate this process. In cases involving the apparent infection of the hardware or a bony fragment, it may be possible to remove either or both of these at 6 weeks after surgery; at this time, fibrosis may prevent relapse of the soft tissues, although this has not been demonstrated conclusively. Because the hardware placed after mortised genioplasty contributes more substantially to mandibular stability, it should be removed after this procedure only after careful consideration.

Changes in the Appearance of the Lower Face and the Chin

These procedures effectively produce augmentation of the lower face. This augmentation is related to the size of the advanced mandibular segment and to the degree of advancement. The genioglossus advancement involves the augmentation of the facial profile in the symphyseal region of the mandible alone, whereas the mortised genioplasty requires the advancement of a larger segment of bone. The overall distance of advancement is greater in the former procedure, but the effective augmentation is lessened by the removal of the buccal cortex and the marrow space of the fragment. In addition, the lingual cortex fragment can be thinned to minimize the cosmetic impact. For both procedures, the mandible contour is largely maintained by the thick soft tissues that drape over the surgically altered mandible. All patients should understand that they will experience some degree of augmentation of the lower face after these procedures, although many patients consider this as cosmetically beneficial, particularly in those patients with some degree of mandibular insufficiency.

Mandible Fracture

Osteotomies unavoidably reduce the mandible's bony integrity. The genioglossus advancement is designed to leave intact the inferior border of the mandible, which comprises its thickest and strongest portion. Ideally at least 8 mm to 10 mm of the inferior border is left intact,[43] but mandible anatomy, including the lower incisor roots and the relative location of the genial tubercle, may dictate that a slightly smaller width of intact mandible be left along the inferior border (Figure 29-2). Intraoperative mandible fracture is rare but not impossible.[43] Instead, all patients are at increased risk for fracture after trauma postoperatively, and they should be counseled appropriately. The treatment of mandible fractures typically requires open reduction and internal fixation rather than the use of maxillomandibular fixation alone. Maxillomandibular fixation alone may be limited, because the extent of bony contact along fracture lines is reduced after these procedures.

Mortised genioplasty involves osteotomies through the inferior border of the mandible and therefore carries a greater potential risk of associated mandible fracture. Prefabricated plates have been developed for use in this procedure to maintain mandible strength, and no fractures were reported with their use in a series of more than 75 patients.[51]

Tongue Radiofrequency

Temperature-controlled and bipolar radiofrequency have also been used to treat the tongue in patients with OSA.[52–54] Treatment techniques vary, but, in general, submucosal tissue injury and subsequent fibrosis with less morbidity than electrocautery. However, complications are possible.

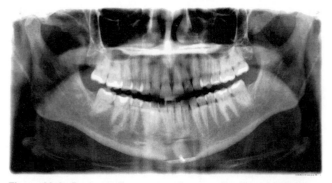

Figure 29-2. Postoperative panoramic x-ray showing mandibular osteotomy in close proximity to the inferior border of the mandible. This osteotomy location was, to some extent, dictated by the location of the genial tubercle and the genioglossus muscle attachments. No adverse sequelae resulted.

The literature review cited above also determined the rate of complications of moderate (hemorrhage, nerve paresis or paralysis, or significant dysphagia) or major (serious infection requiring drainage or other significant airway compromise) severity.[42] The overall rate of moderate or severe complications was 2.6% (38 of 1486 treatment sessions). Although two studies reported complication rates that were notably higher,[55,56] one of these described a novel and more aggressive treatment technique. This literature review also suggested that the routine use of perioperative steroids for isolated tongue radiofrequency treatment may be associated with a higher incidence of complications.[42]

Tongue Abscess and Mucosal Ulceration

All technologies generate submucosal thermal injury to the tongue, and infection is possible. Infection can arise as an abscess that either remains contained within the tongue or undergoes spontaneous drainage. The latter may be an underlying source for mucosal ulceration, but fortunately cases with spontaneous drainage are less likely to present with life-threatening airway compromise.

Preventive measures include the use of an antiseptic oral rinse before the procedure to decrease the bacterial load introduced to the tongue during the placement of the treatment probe. In addition, perioperative antibiotics directed against oral and pharyngeal flora may reduce the incidence of infection. As previously described, the avoidance of perioperative corticosteroids (unless other procedures such as uvulopalatopharyngoplasty are performed concurrently) may also reduce the risk of infection.

A tongue abscess, particularly ones that do not undergo spontaneous drainage, requires prompt recognition and treatment. Signs and symptoms of tongue abscess include airway compromise, pain, dysphagia, dysarthria, and neurologic sequelae such as tongue weakness, numbness, or tingling. Treatment can require incision and drainage, and airway intervention may be required.

Hypoglossal or Lingual Neurovascular Injury

Both the hypoglossal nerve and the lingual neurovascular bundles travel in the inferolateral portions of the tongue base.[57] The dorsal lingual arteries are branches of the lingual artery that travel from the lateral portion of the tongue toward the midline near the junction of the oral tongue and the tongue base. Both the hypoglossal and lingual nerves have branches that are directed toward the midline. Although neurovascular injury may be unavoidable in certain cases, the risk can be reduced by ensuring that radiofrequency energy is administered to the tongue base or vental tongue tissue, near the midline.

Neurovascular injury can produce airway compromise (as a result of hemorrhage and associated tissue edema), tongue weakness or numbness, and taste disturbance. Airway compromise requires close monitoring and, in some cases, emergent intervention, including tracheotomy. Neurologic injury is usually temporary, with recovery occurring over the course of days to weeks. However, this process can extend over months, or the damage may be permanent.

Acute Sialadenitis

Radiofrequency energy can be delivered to the ventral tongue with a transoral[54] or transcervical approach. This technique possesses the same set of potential complications as the treatment of the tongue base, but there is also the possibility of submandibular duct obstruction and an associated sialadenitis. Submandibular duct obstruction may occur as a result of soft-tissue swelling and the external compression of the duct lumen, or it may result from direct duct injury. The former is more common and typically resolves with conservative measures such as aggressive hydration, sialagogues, and warm compresses. Antibiotics may be necessary in selected cases.

Midline Glossectomy and Lingual Tonsillectomy

Several techniques have been described for midline glossectomy and lingual tonsillectomy.[58–62] The potential risks associated with midline glossectomy and lingual tonsillectomy are similar to the ones associated with tongue radiofrequency. Although these procedures have not been studied in as much detail, midline glossectomy and lingual tonsillectomy can be considered to have greater morbidity and more potential for airway compromise. Dysphagia is expected, and it typically improves within the first 2 weeks postoperatively. Because the tissue injury by necessity involves the mucosa, there may be a higher risk of bleeding but a lower risk of tongue abscess that remains confined with the substance of the tongue.

Hyoid Suspension

Two approaches for hyoid suspension have been described: the advancement and suspension to the inferior border of the mandible (with fascia lata the original technique,[63]) and the modified technique suspending to the superior border of the thyroid cartilage (with sutures[64] or wire fixation.[65]) The modified technique was developed on the basis of animal studies that demonstrated the benefits of the anterior advancement of the hyoid bone.[66] Although the original technique of the suspension to the mandible inferior border was abandoned by the original authors, multiple other suspension materials have been used for this approach.[67]

Seroma or Hematoma

Although bleeding is minimal, a passive or active suction drain can reduce the incidence of seroma or hematoma. Infection is rare, but it may occur in the setting of seroma or hematoma. Perioperative antibiotics directed against skin flora may be preventive, and treatment is best accomplished by aspiration or incision and drainage with culture-directed antibiotics.

Dysphagia

Dysphagia is not uncommon, and it can be related to the swelling of the pharyngeal soft tissues, the expansion in the pharyngeal dimensions that increases the forces required for airway protection during swallowing, and/or injury to the superior laryngeal or hypoglossal nerves. Hyoid suspension is beneficial for the treatment of OSA explicitly because the hyoid bone has multiple soft-tissue attachments, particularly the epiglottis (via the hyoepiglottic ligament) and the suprahyoid musculature (the hyoglossus, digastric, and geniohyoid muscles). The procedure advances and stabilizes the hyoid bone, thereby increasing the hypopharyngeal airway dimensions and reducing the tendency of these soft tissues to contribute to airway collapse. This increase in pharyngeal dimensions, however, necessitates greater forces and the mobilization of soft tissues to prevent aspiration during swallowing. A straightforward increase in pharyngeal dimensions would not be associated with a substantial risk of dysphagia; however, the mechanism by which this is accomplished in hyoid suspension (anterior advancement and the stabilization of soft tissues such as the epiglottis) makes airway protection during swallowing more difficult, because the parapharyngeal soft tissues become less mobile.

The superior laryngeal nerves are branches of the vagus nerve that travel lateral to the lesser cornua of the hyoid bone to provide motor (cricothyroid) and sensory innervation (glottic and supraglottic mucosa) to the larynx. The hypoglossal nerves have a variable location, but they are typically found superior to the hyoid bone. Nerve injury is therefore minimized by careful dissection directly over the hyoid bone without extending the dissection lateral to the lesser cornua of the hyoid bone. Although thermal nerve injury can occur, the complete transection of these nerves is rare.

Dysphagia usually resolves over the course of 2 to 14 days after surgery. Evaluation of the patient with dysphagia involves a complete examination, including fiberoptic endoscopy, to determine the extent of edema and the possible presence of neurologic injury. The formal evaluation of the swallowing function with either a functional endoscopic evaluation of swallowing or a barium swallow can be performed but is usually unnecessary. Although dysphagia carries an increased risk of aspiration pneumonia, empiric dietary restrictions (e.g., a thick liquid diet) until swallowing function returns are generally satisfactory precautions. In rare cases, the degree of hyoid advancement may be the major cause of dysphagia, and the release of the suspension sutures may be required to restore swallowing function.

Hyoid Fracture

Because this procedure requires dissection along the hyoid bone with anterior traction on the bone itself, hyoid fracture is possible. This complication may not be entirely preventable in certain cases of diminished preoperative bony integrity, but certain technical considerations may reduce the risk. The use of the pharmacologic paralysis of the patient, the dissection of the infrahyoid, and, in some cases, a portion of the suprahyoid musculature off the hyoid bone can minimize the force necessary to advance the hyoid. Fracture can be treated with the application of a titanium craniofacial plate to reestablish bony structure. For cases in which this is not possible or does not appear to be necessary, it is possible to suspend each segment of the hyoid bone superiorly, rather than using miniplate fixation.

Suspension Material Breakage

Depending on the technique, hyoid suspension has been described with the use of fascia lata (mandible), sutures (mandible or thyroid cartilage), or wire (thyroid cartilage). In all cases, the material used to suspend the hyoid bone may break. The authors of the original technique chose fascia lata for the suspension to the inferior border of the mandible, because other materials, including sutures, had an undesirable incidence of breakage in their experience.[64] In the revised technique of suspension to the thyroid cartilage, a total of four interrupted sutures or a single wire are placed to approximate the hyoid bone against the thyroid cartilage. Because the hyoid bone and the thyroid cartilage are directly approximated, fibrosis can support the hyoid advancement and suspension. The placement of multiple sutures on each side of the hyoid bone also limits the consequences of a single suture breakage as compared with the single piece of suspension material on either side of the hyoid bone during suspension to the mandible. Symptoms of suspension material breakage include a worsening of sleep-disordered breathing, pain, and dysphagia, but this event can also be asymptomatic. Treatment options include the removal of the suspension material or revision surgery to resuspend the hyoid bone.

Pharyngocutaneous Fistula

Fistula may occur if there is a violation of the pharyngeal mucosa during dissection or with the passage of sutures around the hyoid bone. Although the mucosal disruption is typically limited and heals spontaneously, the presence of the suture material can function as a foreign body to serve as a nidus for persistent infection and fistula. A fistula is characterized by mucoid or mucopurulent drainage from the neck incision that does not resolve with antibiotic therapy. Treatment typically requires wound exploration with the removal of the involved suture, which is most commonly a single suture.[68]

Tongue Stabilization

Dental Injury

Tongue stabilization involves the placement of a screw in the lingual cortex of the mandible, and cases of dental injury have been reported as a result of the direct placement of the screw into the dentition or because of neurovascular compromise. Treatment may require screw removal as well as evaluation and treatment by a dental professional, with possible endodontic therapy or dental extraction.

Suture Migration or Breakage

This procedure requires that a suture be passed through the tongue to support the tongue and to resist the prolapse that occurs during sleep with muscle relaxation. As a result of the tension forces produced during voluntary and involuntary tongue movements, suture migration and breakage have been reported.[69-71] The adverse effects of these changes are unclear, although presumably they would lessen the effectiveness of the procedure. Although there has been the suggestion that fibrosis can maintain tongue stabilization in the event of suture breakage, no studies have examined the development of fibrosis or the effects of suture migration and breakage.

Dysphagia and Dysarthria

Suture stabilization of the tongue can improve sleep-disordered breathing by limiting tongue mobility to maintain upper airway patency. However, the changes in tongue function can produce an associated dysphagia and dysarthria that improve over 3 to 4 weeks.[69-71] Although these can be permanent, the most common long-term noticeable change is a slight decrease in tongue protrusion.[72] Both of these potential effects may be related to the degree of suture tightening and stabilization. In severe cases, the suture can be cut to release the stabilization and to improve tongue mobility.

Infection

The transoral approach introduces some degree of contamination with oral flora. Early experience with this procedure demonstrated that oral antiseptic rinses and perioperative antibiotics can reduce the risk of infection.[69]

Hypoglossal or Lingual Neurovascular Injury

With the passage of a suture within the substance of the tongue, injury to the hypoglossal nerve or the lingual neurovascular bundles is possible. To capture and stabilize the tongue base, this procedure requires the placement of the suture toward the lateral portion of the tongue base, thus creating the potential complication risk. However, the incidence of this complication has not been determined.

Acute Sialadenitis

Sialadenitis can occur as a result of associated soft-tissue edema or direct injury of the submandibular gland or duct. The incidence of this complication has been reported to be between 9% and 11%.[69,71] This complication is usually temporary, although it can be permanent. Treatment is the same as was previously described for tongue radiofrequency.

REFERENCES

1. Connolly LA: Anesthetic management of obstructive sleep apnea patients. *J Clin Anesth* 1991;3:461–469.
2. Dart RA, Gregoire JR, Gutterman DD, et al: The association of hypertension and secondary cardiovascular disease with sleep-disordered breathing. *Chest* 2003;123:244–260.
3. Johnson JT, Braun TW: Preoperative, intraoperative, and post-operative management of patients with obstructive sleep apnea syndrome. *Otolaryngol Clin North Am* 1998;31:1025–1030.
4. Marrone O, Bonsignore MR: Pulmonary hemodynamics in obstructive sleep apnoea. *Sleep Med Rev* 2002;6:175–193.
5. Esclamado RM, Glenn MG, McCulloch TM, et al: Perioperative complications and risk factors in the surgical treatment of obstructive sleep apnea syndrome. *Laryngoscope* 1989;99: 1125–1129.
6. Haavisto L, Suonpaa J: Complications of uvulopalatopharyngoplasty. *Clin Otolaryngol* 1994;19:243–247.
7. Harmon JD, Morgan W, Chaudhary B: Sleep apnea: Morbidity and mortality of surgical treatment. *South Med J* 1989;82: 161–164.
8. Mickelson SA, Hakim I: Is postoperative intensive care monitoring necessary after uvulopalatopharyngoplasty? *Otolaryngol Head Neck Surg* 1998;119:352–356.
9. Riley RW, Powell NB, Guilleminault C, et al: Obstructive sleep apnea surgery: Risk management and complications. *Otolaryngol Head Neck Surg* 1997;117:648–652.
10. Terris DJ, Fincher EF, Hanasono MM, et al: Conservation of resources: Indications for intensive care monitoring after upper airway surgery on patients with obstructive sleep apnea. *Laryngoscope* 1998;108:784–788.
11. Kezirian EJ, Weaver EM, Yueh B, et al: Incidence of serious complications after uvulopalatopharyngoplasty. *Laryngoscope* 2004;114:450–453.
12. Kezirian EJ, Weaver EM, Yueh B, et al: Risk factors for serious complications after uvulopalatopharyngoplasty. *Arch Otolaryngol Head Neck Surg* 2006;132(10):1091–1098.
13. Gross JB, Bachenberg KL, Benumof JL, et al: Practice guidelines for the perioperative management of patients with obstructive sleep apnea: A report by the American Society of Anesthesiologists Task Force on Perioperative Management of patients with obstructive sleep apnea. *Anesthesiology* 2006;104:1081–1093, 1117–1118.
14. Hathaway B, Johnson JT: Safety of uvulopalatopharyngoplasty as outpatient surgery. *Otolaryngol Head Neck Surg* 2006;134: 542–544.
15. Windfuhr JP, Chen YS: Incidence of post-tonsillectomy hemorrhage in children and adults: A study of 4,848 patients. *Ear Nose Throat J* 2002;81:626–628, 630, 632.
16. Katsantonis GP, Walsh JK, Schweitzer PK, et al: Further evaluation of uvulopalatopharyngoplasty in the treatment of obstructive sleep apnea syndrome. *Otolaryngol Head Neck Surg* 1985;93:244–250.
17. Katsantonis GP, Friedman WH, Krebs FJ 3rd, et al: Nasopharyngeal complications following uvulopalatopharyngoplasty. *Laryngoscope* 1987;97:309–314.
18. Fairbanks DN: Uvulopalatopharyngoplasty complications and avoidance strategies. *Otolaryngol Head Neck Surg* 1990;102:239–245.
18a. Croft CB, Golding-Wood DG: Uses and complications of uvulo-palatophary. *J Laryngol Otol* 1990;104:871–875.
19. Fujita S, Conway W, Zorick F, et al: Surgical correction of anatomic abnormalities in obstructive sleep apnea syndrome: Uvulopalatopharyngoplasty. *Otolaryngol Head Neck Surg* 1981;89:923–934.
20. Cahali MB: Lateral pharyngoplasty: A new treatment for obstructive sleep apnea hypopnea syndrome. *Laryngoscope* 2003;113:1961–1968.
21. Friedman M, Ibrahim HZ, Vidyasagar R, et al: Z-palatoplasty (ZPP): A technique for patients without tonsils. *Otolaryngol Head Neck Surg* 2004;131:89–100.
22. Powell N, Riley R, Guilleminault C, et al: A reversible uvulopalatal flap for snoring and sleep apnea syndrome. *Sleep* 1996;19: 593–599.
23. Jackson IT, Kenedy D: Surgical management of velopharyngeal insufficiency following uvulopalatopharyngoplasty: Report of three cases. *Plast Reconstr Surg* 1997;99:1151–1153.
24. Altermatt HJ, Gebbers JO, Sommerhalder A, et al: Histopathologic findings in the posterior pharyngeal wall 8 years after treatment of velar insufficiency with Teflon injection. *Laryngol Rhinol Otol (Stuttg)* 1985;64:582–585.
25. Furlow LT Jr, Williams WN, Eisenbach CR Jr, et al: A long term study on treating velopharyngeal insufficiency by teflon injection. *Cleft Palate J* 1982;19:47–56.
26. Jackson IT, Silverton JS. The sphincter pharyngoplasty as a secondary procedure in cleft palates. *Plast Reconstr Surg* 1977;59:518–524.
27. Krespi YP, Kacker A: Management of nasopharyngeal stenosis after uvulopalatoplasty. *Otolaryngol Head Neck Surg* 2000;123: 692–695.
28. Van Duyne J, Coleman JA Jr: Treatment of nasopharyngeal inlet stenosis following uvulopalatopharyngoplasty with the CO2 laser. *Laryngoscope* 1995;105:914–918.
29. Jones LM, Guillory VL, Mair EA: Total nasopharyngeal stenosis: Treatment with laser excision, nasopharyngeal obturators, and topical mitomycin-c. *Otolaryngol Head Neck Surg* 2005;133:795–798.
30. Cotton RT: Nasopharyngeal stenosis. *Arch Otolaryngol* 1985;111: 146–148.
31. Ingrams DR, Spraggs PD, Pringle MB, et al: CO2 laser palatoplasty: Early results. *J Laryngol Otol* 1996;110:754–756.
32. Kazanjian VH, Holmes EM: Stenosis of the nasopharynx and its correction. *Arch Otolaryngol* 1946;44:376–386.
33. Stepnick DW: Management of total nasopharyngeal stenosis following UPPP. *Ear Nose Throat J* 1993;72:86–90.
34. Van Lierde KM, Van Borsel J, Moerman M, et al: Nasalance, nasality, voice, and articulation after uvulopalatopharyngoplasty. *Laryngoscope* 2002;112:873–878.
35. Brosch S, Matthes C, Pirsig W, et al: Uvulopalatopharyngoplasty changes fundamental frequency of the voice: A prospective study. *J Laryngol Otol* 2000;114:113–118.
36. Croft CB, Golding-Wood DG: Uses and complications of uvulo-palatopharyngoplasty. *J Laryngol Otol* 1990;104:871–875.
37. Nilsson B: The occurrence of taste buds in the palate of human adults as evidenced by light microscopy. *Acta Odontol Scand* 1979;37:253–258.

38. Li HY, Lee LA, Wang PC, et al: Taste disturbance after uvulopalatopharyngoplasty for obstructive sleep apnea. *Otolaryngol Head Neck Surg* 2006;134:985–990.

39. Powell N: Personal communication. Palo Alto, Calif, 2003.

40. Woodson BT, Robinson S, Lim HJ: Transpalatal advancement pharyngoplasty outcomes compared with uvulopalatopharyngoplasty. *Otolaryngol Head Neck Surg* 2005;133:211–217.

41. Woodson BT, Toohill RJ: Transpalatal advancement pharyngoplasty for obstructive sleep apnea. *Laryngoscope* 1993;103:269–276.

42. Kezirian EJ, Powell NB, Riley RW, et al: Incidence of complications in radiofrequency treatment of the upper airway. *Laryngoscope* 2005;115:1298–1304.

42a. Grontved AM, Karup P: Complaints and satisfaction after uvulopalatopharyngoplasty. *Acta Otolaryngol Suppl* 2000;543:190–192.

43. Li KK, Riley RW, Powell NB, et al: Obstructive sleep apnea surgery: Genioglossus advancement revisited. *J Oral Maxillofac Surg* 2001;59:1181–1185.

44. Lewis MR, Ducic Y: Genioglossus muscle advancement with the genioglossus bone advancement technique for base of tongue obstruction. *J Otolaryngol* 2003;32:168–173.

45. Hendler BH, Costello BJ, Silverstein K, et al: A protocol for uvulopalatopharyngoplasty, mortised genioplasty, and maxillomandibular advancement in patients with obstructive sleep apnea: An analysis of 40 cases. *J Oral Maxillofac Surg* 2001;59:892–899.

46. Bell WH, Proffitt WR, White RP: *Surgical correction of dentofacial deformities,* Philadelphia, 1980, WB Saunders, 1980.

47. Riley R: Personal communication. Burlingame, CA, 2003.

48. Petersson K, Soderstrom C, Kiani-Anaraki M, et al: Evaluation of the ability of thermal and electrical tests to register pulp vitality. *Endod Dent Traumatol* 1999;15:127–131.

49. Radhakrishnan S, Munshi AK, Hegde AM: Pulse oximetry: A diagnostic instrument in pulpal vitality testing. *J Clin Pediatr Dent* 2002;26:141–145.

50. Evans D, Reid J, Strang R, et al: A comparison of laser Doppler flowmetry with other methods of assessing the vitality of traumatised anterior teeth. *Endod Dent Traumatol* 1999;15:284–290.

51. Hendler B, Silverstein K, Giannakopoulos H, et al: Mortised genioplasty in the treatment of obstructive sleep apnea: An historical perspective and modification of design. *Sleep Breath* 2001;5:173–180.

52. den Herder C, Kox D, van Tinteren H, de Vries N: Bipolar radiofrequency induced thermotherapy of the tongue base: Its complications, acceptance and effectiveness under local anesthesia. *Eur Arch Otorhinolaryngol* 2006;263:1031–1040.

53. Powell NB, Riley RW, Guilleminault C: Radiofrequency tongue base reduction in sleep-disordered breathing: A pilot study. *Otolaryngol Head Neck Surg* 1999;120:656–664.

54. Riley RW, Powell NB, Li KK, et al: An adjunctive method of radiofrequency volumetric tissue reduction of the tongue for OSAS. *Otolaryngol Head Neck Surg* 2003;129:37–42.

55. Pazos G, Mair EA: Complications of radiofrequency ablation in the treatment of sleep-disordered breathing. *Otolaryngol Head Neck Surg* 2001;125:462–467.

56. Robinson S, Lewis R, Norton A, et al: Ultrasound-guided radiofrequency submucosal tongue-base excision for sleep apnoea: A preliminary report. *Clin Otolaryngol Allied Sci* 2003;28:341–345.

57. Lauretano AM, Li KK, Caradonna DS, et al: Anatomic location of the tongue base neurovascular bundle. *Laryngoscope* 1997;107:1057–1059.

58. Robinson S, Ettema SL, Brusky L, et al: Lingual tonsillectomy using bipolar radiofrequency plasma excision. *Otolaryngol Head Neck Surg* 2006;134:328–330.

59. Yonekura A, Kawakatsu K, Suzuki K, Nishimura T: Laser midline glossectomy and lingual tonsillectomy as treatments for sleep apnea syndrome. *Acta Otolaryngol Suppl* 2003:56–58.

60. Suzuki K, Kawakatsu K, Hattori C, et al: Application of lingual tonsillectomy to sleep apnea syndrome involving lingual tonsils. *Acta Otolaryngol Suppl* 2003:65–71.

61. Andsberg U, Jessen M: Eight years of follow-up—Uvulopalatopharyngoplasty combined with midline glossectomy as a treatment for obstructive sleep apnoea syndrome. *Acta Otolaryngol Suppl* 2000;543:175–178.

62. Fujita S, Woodson BT, Clark JL, et al: Laser midline glossectomy as a treatment for obstructive sleep apnea. *Laryngoscope* 1991;101:805–809.

63. Riley RW, Powell NB, Guilleminault C: Inferior sagittal osteotomy of the mandible with hyoid myotomy-suspension: A new procedure for obstructive sleep apnea. *Otolaryngol Head Neck Surg* 1986;94:589–593.

64. Riley RW, Powell NB, Guilleminault C: Obstructive sleep apnea and the hyoid: A revised surgical procedure. *Otolaryngol Head Neck Surg* 1994;111:717–721.

65. Hormann K, Baisch A: The hyoid suspension. *Laryngoscope* 2004;114:1677–1679.

66. Van de Graaff WB, Gottfried SB, Mitra J, et al: Respiratory function of hyoid muscles and hyoid arch. *J Appl Physiol* 1984;57:197–204.

67. Dattilo DJ, Kolodychak MT: The use of the Mitek Mini Anchor system in the hyoid suspension technique for the treatment of obstructive sleep apnea syndrome. *J Oral Maxillofac Surg* 2000;58:919–920.

68. De Vries N: Personal communication. Chicago, Ill, 2006.

69. Woodson BT: A tongue suspension suture for obstructive sleep apnea and snorers. *Otolaryngol Head Neck Surg* 2001;124:297–303.

70. Omur M, Ozturan D, Elez F, et al: Tongue base suspension combined with UPPP in severe OSA patients. *Otolaryngol Head Neck Surg* 2005;133:218–223.

71. Miller FR, Watson D, Malis D: Role of the tongue base suspension suture with The Repose System bone screw in the multilevel surgical management of obstructive sleep apnea. *Otolaryngol Head Neck Surg* 2002;126:392–398.

72. Woodson BT: Personal communication. Chicago, Ill, 2006.

PART 3
Larynx, Trachea, and Hypopharynx

CHAPTER 30

Complications of Endoscopy: Rigid and Flexible

Mark S. Courey

OVERVIEW AND PERSPECTIVE

Endoscopy of the upper aerodigestive tract involves indications, techniques, and procedures shared by the disciplines of otolaryngology–head and neck surgery, anesthesiology, gastroenterology, general surgery, pediatric surgery, thoracic surgery, pulmonary medicine, and speech–language pathology. Within otolaryngology–head and neck surgery, the indications, techniques, and procedures are divided among many surgeons from the various subspecialties including laryngology, bronchoesophagology, and head and neck surgery. With such a varied group of health-care providers performing overlapping procedures, it is no wonder that techniques and indications vary widely. As such, so do the potential complications.

This chapter is written from the perspective of an otolaryngologist–head and neck surgeon with subspecialization in laryngology/bronchoesophagology. While attempting to be inclusive of all endoscopy techniques, the chapter will concentrate on those complications encountered by the otolaryngologist–head and neck surgeon. In addition, the complications discussed will be limited to those that result from the endoscopy itself and will not include those that result from the disease process for which the endoscopy was performed. A discussion of complications of the individual disease processes for which endoscopy is performed is beyond the scope of this chapter.

A new appreciation for the function of the larynx and airway during the last 20 years together with developments in technology have revolutionized the practice of endoscopy. For example, it is now widely appreciated that voice quality is determined by the quality and characteristics of the vibrations of the vocal-fold mucosa.[1] It is understood that this mucosa includes both the epithelium and the superficial portion of the lamina propria, and it is further believed that the human adult lamina propria does not regenerate well. Therefore the inadvertent loss of the lamina propria from injudicious surgical techniques leads to a poor quality of vibrations and poor voice. Consequently it is no longer acceptable to remove benign laryngeal lesions without high magnification and modern surgical techniques involving precise dissection. These techniques have been made possible through the development of specialized instrumentation (e.g., the binocular laryngoscope, the miniaturization of laryngeal instrumentation) that is now widely available through many instrument companies.[2] These techniques have become standard training procedures in residency programs, and it is expected that otolaryngologists–head and neck surgeons treating benign laryngeal lesions or even early glottic cancers will employ these principles as the standard of care. These principles often lead to an increased frequency of suspension laryngoscopy as compared with direct laryngoscopy for diagnostic purposes. As such, it is pertinent to examine whether suspension laryngoscopy is associated with a different or a higher complication rate than diagnostic rigid laryngoscopy.

In addition to improvements in instrumentation for rigid endoscopy, improvements in instrumentation for flexible endoscopy have also changed practice standards, techniques, and potential complications.[3] Flexible endoscopes that employ fiber-optic technology to carry light into the upper aerodigestive tract and another set of fiber-optic rods to carry the image out to the human eye have been available for decades. As a result of limitations in light- and image-carrying capabilities with fiber-optic technology, the image produced was relatively dimly lit with reduced resolution. The revolution in the camera-chip industry has allowed for the production of miniature camera chips. These small chips can be placed at the distal end of a flexible telescope. Fiber-optic technology is still used to carry the light into the field, but the image is now captured distally and transmitted through electric circuitry out to a video monitor that may be recorded.

The "distal-chip" technology provides significantly improved resolution that can be highly magnified without significant image degradation. These improvements in resolution and magnification potentially allow for the more accurate identification of changes within the upper aerodigestive tract and for the performance of precise surgical treatment under conditions that permit flexible endoscopy. The chips have also been miniaturized so that they can fit comfortably through the nasal cavity. This allows for the performance of flexible endoscopic procedures with scopes of reduced diameter through the nasal cavity. Stimulation of the gag reflex is markedly reduced with these smaller endoscopes. This reduces the need for general sedation during flexible endoscopy of the upper aerodigestive tract. Studies have shown that sedation is the primary cause of complications during flexible endoscopy.[4–6] Studies have also shown that, at least for the upper gastrointestinal tract, the accuracy of endoscopy performed transnasally by experienced endoscopists is comparable to that performed with larger-caliper scopes that need to be placed transorally.[7,8] In addition, studies have shown that patients prefer the transnasal route without sedation to the transoral route.[7,8] For these reasons, it is likely that, as chip technology improves, transnasal endoscopy with minimal or no sedation will become the standard of care for endoscopy of the upper aerodigestive tract.

In addition to smaller endoscopes, instruments that are used through the side channels of these scopes are also evolving. Evaluation for Barrett esophagitis formerly required a four-quadrant mega-cup biopsy. This 2-mm biopsy cup required a large side port on the endoscope. The developing Oral CDx Brush Biopsy (CDx Laboratories, Suffern, NY) technology, which captures epithelial cells, now obviates the need for four-quadrant biopsy.[9] The endoscope side channels can be made smaller. These smaller endoscopes will lessen patient discomfort during the procedure but may result in different complications.

COMPLICATIONS OF LARYNGOSCOPY

Indirect Flexible Laryngoscopy

Indirect laryngoscopy is an office procedure that is commonly used by otolaryngologist–head and neck surgeons and speech pathologists to evaluate the structure and function of the larynx and the pharynx. Although it was originally developed and named for the purpose of laryngeal evaluation, it should now be recognized that the complete indirect flexible laryngoscopy procedure should include the evaluation of palatal, tongue-base, and lateral pharyngeal wall structure and function as well as that of the larynx. It makes sense to evaluate these regions simultaneously, because cranial nerve X (the vagus nerve) controls the muscular function of the palatal and pharyngeal wall musculature as well as the larynx. Therefore the evaluation of vocal-fold paralysis is not complete unless the function of other areas controlled by the nerve is also evaluated. Likewise, cranial nerve XII (the hypoglossal nerve) for tongue function exits the skull base only a few millimeters away from cranial nerve X, and it crosses the internal carotid artery near the vagus nerve, so its function should be evaluated as well. The function of both cranial nerves X and XII is critical for intact swallowing. Fiberoptic endoscopic examination of swallowing with or without sensory testing is accomplished with flexible transnasal laryngopharyngoscopy, and it has become a valuable tool in the hands of otolaryngologist–head and neck surgeons and speech–language pathologists for the diagnosis and management of patients with swallowing disorders.[10]

Regardless, flexible laryngoscopy (or laryngopharyngoscopy, as it is more aptly termed) is a relatively safe procedure that is associated with few complications, including epistaxis during passage through the nasal cavity, pain, and gagging.[11–13] If the endoscope is brought too near the larynx, it is possible to stimulate laryngospasm, but serious injury from this has not been reported.

The examination may be accomplished with or without local topical anesthesia. Lidocaine and Pontocaine are the most common agents used. If topical anesthesia with or without vasoconstriction is used, then complications from the anesthetic can occur. These include anaphylaxis or toxicity to the substance in sensitive patients and methemoglobinemia if Benzocaine or other topical anesthetics containing an aniline ring are used. The initial signs of lidocaine toxicity include nervousness, weakness, dizziness, nausea, and visual disturbances.[14] If they are unrecognized, these can progress on to seizures, cardiac toxicity, and death. Methemoglobinemia results from the binding of the aniline ring to hemoglobin molecules, thereby preventing oxygen binding and transfer. Patients can become cyanotic, and treatment involves replacing bound hemoglobin molecules with unbound molecules via a packed red blood cell transfusion or waiting for the natural process of hemoglobin replacement.[15] In general, however, topical agents for local anesthesia are safe and well tolerated. Toxicity does not usually occur unless the recommended dose of 7 mg/kg is exceeded; most patients require far less than this dose for nasal analgesia. Toxicity is influenced by factors that affect mucosal absorption. The simultaneous administration of vasoconstricting agents (e.g., epinephrine), which decrease absorption, lowers the risk of toxicity. Alternatively, conditions such as infection or open breaks in the mucosa, which increase vascularity and absorption, increase the risk of toxicity at lower-than-standard doses.[16]

Indirect Rigid Laryngoscopy

Rigid Hopkins rod telescopes for the performance of indirect laryngoscopy predate the use of flexible fiber-optic and "distal camera chip" technology. For indirect rigid laryngoscopy, high-quality glass rods are used to carry the light into the aerodigestive tract and carry the image out. These high-quality rod lenses provide excellent image resolution. A glass prism positioned at the distal end of the telescope allows for the deflection of the image through a series of angles without distortion. By changing the angle of deflection at the distal end of the scope, examiners can choose the scope that provides them with the most comfort during the patient examination. Typically, for laryngeal and pharyngeal examination, 70- and 90-degree prisms are most commonly used.[17] In addition, as a result of the excellent light and image resolution, a camera can be attached to the proximal eyepiece of the telescope to allow for the video recording of the examination.

Criticism of the indirect rigid examination technique stems from the fact that patients must extend their tongue for the examination. The tongue must be held in a semirigid position by either the patient or the examiner. This permits the patient to phonate only on vowels, without consonants. However, the careful examiner is still able to evaluate lateral pharyngeal wall function as well as tongue-base function. Although the main complication is gagging, most patients find the examination significantly less invasive than flexible endoscopy in the hands of an experienced endoscopist. The examination does not require local anesthesia, so it eliminates those attendant complications.

Direct Rigid Laryngoscopy

Direct rigid and microdirect rigid laryngoscopy are the procedures of choice for the diagnosis and surgical treatment of most laryngeal diseases. Direct rigid laryngoscopy can be undertaken with sedation and topical anesthesia or under general anesthesia with complete relaxation. Patients under local anesthesia are at risk for those complications discussed previously as well as the risks associated with sedation, whereas patients under general anesthesia are at risk for those complications associated with general anesthesia. Further, rigid direct laryngoscopy procedures can be divided into diagnostic procedures, which are often completed through small monocular laryngoscopes and are of short duration, and therapeutic procedures, during which larger laryngoscopes and suspension are employed to allow for improved operative field stabilization, binocular visualization, and bimanual manipulation and which are usually of longer duration. It is therefore valuable to evaluate complication types and incidences separately for these various procedures.

Generally direct rigid laryngoscopy is considered to be a safe procedure.[18] Complications can be divided into major and minor categories. Major complications include those that are life threatening, those that require hospitalization, those that involve cardiac complications, those that involve major bleeding, and those that require reintubation or tracheotomy for airway protection. Alternatively, minor complications such as mucosal ulcerations and/or lacerations, tongue or lip injury (e.g., hematoma, swelling), dental injury, and minor bleeding are usually self-limiting in nature. Regardless, each of these potential complications should

be discussed with the patient and specifically documented. A preoperative risk–benefit form is useful for this documentation (Figure 30-1).

Major complications have been identified primarily through retrospective reviews or case reports. No prospective study has identified any major complications after rigid laryngoscopy when a significant risk for airway obstruction was not present preoperatively.[19] One retrospective review did identify a 1.2% to 3% risk of reintubation among patients undergoing laryngoscopy and panendoscopy. This was greater than the risk of reintubation among patients undergoing other procedures under general anesthesia during the same time period (0.17%). However, the analysis did not indicate how many of these patients were suspected to be at high risk for airway obstruction as the primary indication for the endoscopy.[20] Another retrospective review of 589 patients treated at an outpatient facility revealed that nine patients required extended observation or admission. Five of these nine patients required reintubation in the operating room. The overall major complication rate is less than 1%; thus the procedure is relatively safe when it is undertaken with the appropriate precautions.[21]

It was originally held that patients undergoing microsurgery of the larynx through suspension laryngoscopy were at increased risk for cardiac complications. This was theorized to be as a result of vagal nerve stimulation during laryngeal instrumentation and suspension. Rigid guidelines for perioperative management with the routine use of electrocardiography were recommended.[22] This increased risk of cardiac complications, however, was not borne out by a later retrospective review.[23] Major complications of bleeding and airway obstruction have also been reported in retrospective case reviews and case reports by other authors. Recently two prospective studies were undertaken to review the incidence of complications from suspension laryngoscopy, and a combined analysis of 392 patients did not reveal any major complications from endoscopy. Therefore, when appropriate precautions are followed, the procedure is safe.[24,25]

With regard to minor complications, in one prospective study,[24] mucosal lesions of the oral cavity, the oropharynx, and the hypopharynx occurred in 75% of patients. Mucosal lesions were identified as bleeding, fissure formation, erosion, hematoma, and swelling. Within this group, erosions of the oral-cavity mucosa were identified as the most common minor complication of rigid endoscopy (33%). This was true for both therapeutic and diagnostic laryngoscopy. Erosion was most commonly found on the mucosa of the maxilla, and it was less commonly identified on the lateral surface of the tongue or along the inner surface of the mandible. In

**The University of California, San Francisco
Voice and Swallowing Center**

Date: _____

Impression:

_____
_____
_____

Goal: _____

_____
_____

Plan:

_____
_____
_____

Site:

_____
_____
_____

Alternatives:

_____
_____
_____

Risks and Possible Complications, including but not limited to:

☐ Death   ☐ Infection
☐ Chipped and/or avulsed tooth/teeth   ☐ Airway obstruction
☐ Altered taste   ☐ Need for tracheotomy
☐ Tongue numbness   ☐ Permanent hoarseness/whisper voice
☐ Voice may remain same or get worse   ☐ Oral tears/lacerations
☐ Reoccurrence of problem   ☐ May never be able to sing again
☐ Scarring   ☐ Other: _____
☐ Bleeding   ☐ Other: _____

Postoperative Plan:

____ Weeks voice rest   ____ Weeks gradual incremental increase in voice use

____ Months speaking and/or singing intervention

☐ The Patient or legal representative was given the opportunity to ask questions. Questions were answered and additional information was provided as needed.

The above risks (in addition to those discussed with me), benefits, alternatives, and consequences of no (or other) treatment have been explained to me. I understand there may be other unforeseen complications.

M.D. _____ Patient _____ Witness _____

Figure 30-1. Risk–benefit form for discussion with patients before endoscopy. (Developed in conjunction with Marge Middleton, RN, and Donna Offschanka, LPN, Vanderbilt University Voice Center, Vanderbilt University Medical Center, Nashville, Tenn.)

addition, hematoma occurred within the oral cavity in 8% of patients. Hematoma occurred most commonly in the tongue, followed by the maxillary mucosa, and it often took several weeks to resolve.

After the oral cavity, the oropharynx was the second most common site of mucosal injury (30%). In patients with oropharyngeal injury, hematoma accounted for the most common type of mucosal injury. Hematomas were most commonly identified within the soft palate. The lips were the third most common site of mucosal injury, accounting for 18% of all mucosal injuries, with the lower lip being injured more than twice as frequently as the upper lip (Figure 30-2).

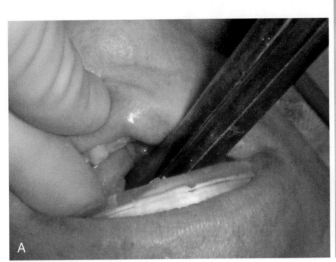
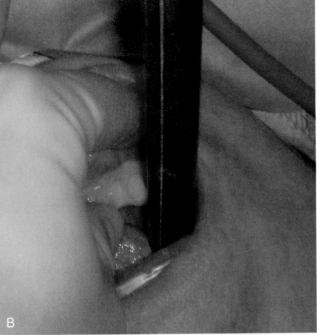

Figure 30-2. A, As the laryngoscope is inserted, the lower lip can be inadvertently trapped between the scope and the lower dentition, causing a laceration or hematoma. **B,** Using the appropriate hand position with the surgeon's nondominant hand allows for the protection of the lower lip. The thumb is used to open the mouth with pressure on the maxilla, and the index finger is used to distract the lower lip. This prevents the lip from becoming trapped against the lower dentition.

Only 1% of patients suffered a mucosal injury of the hypopharynx.

Minor bleeding was identified in only 7% of all patients undergoing suspension laryngoscopy. Dental injury was identified in 6.5% of patients. Nearly all patients suffering dental injury (92%) had preexisting dental disease. Loosening of a tooth was the most common type of dental injury, with tooth avulsion found in only a few patients. Injury to fillings or dental prostheses also accounted for one fourth of all dental injuries. The teeth that were the most commonly injured were located in the anterior portion of the mouth, with nearly half of the injuries identified in mandibular teeth. Most surgeons performing rigid endoscopy employ dental protection on the maxillary teeth. Routinely, little attention is paid to the lower jaw, and no protection is provided. In suspension laryngoscopy with binocular laryngoscopes, limitations for exposure are often encountered from a narrow mandibular arch. The wide binocular scope often hits either the inner surface of the mandible or the lateral incisors or molars, if present (Figure 30-3). This narrow area within the airway prevents the insertion of the scope, so the larynx cannot be well visualized. If the mandible is narrow, as the scope is inserted, the jaw is opened widely; however, the tip of the laryngoscope will not advance to the larynx. This problem can be overcome with the use of a narrow-angled binocular laryngoscope, but the working space within the scope is reduced as compared with more standard scopes[26]

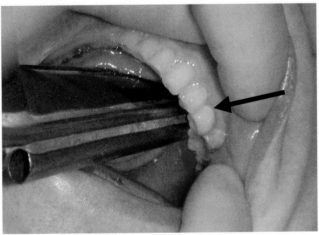

Figure 30-3. This photograph documents the mandibular arch or the mandibular dentition as the site of limitation during the insertion of a binocular laryngoscope. The binocular laryngoscope is abutting the first molar *(arrow)*. This is often the limiting site for the insertion of the laryngoscope, and, under force, it can result in injury to the tooth. If the tooth is not present, then the scope can rub against the mandible and cause erosion of the mucosa. This can be particularly problematic for patients who have undergone previous radiation therapy.

(Figure 30-4). In another prospective study of 53 patients, no dental injuries were identified.[25]

Temporary injury to either the lingual nerve or the hypoglossal nerve is a well-recognized complication of rigid endoscopy. Several reports discuss potential causes of injury to the lingual nerve. The most commonly accepted

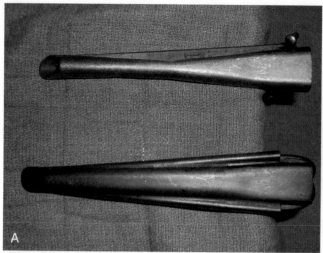

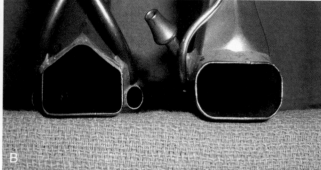

Figure 30-4. Comparison of binocular laryngoscopes. **A,** The scopes are viewed from the inferior aspect. The Ossoff–Pilling endoscope (Pilling–Weck, Canada; *top*) is narrower in the mid portion than the Modified Dedo (Pilling Surgical, Fort Washington, PA) laryngoscope *(bottom).* The narrow midportion allows for the passage of the laryngoscope in patients with a narrow mandibular arch. **B,** This view demonstrates the proximal openings of the endoscopes. Both scopes allow for binocular vision. The working space in the Ossoff–Pilling (Pilling Surgical, Fort Washington, PA) scope *(right)* is reduced as compared with the Modified Dedo endoscope *(left).*

mechanism of injury is the stretching of the lingual nerve caused by pressure of the suspended laryngoscope on the tongue or the retrolingual region.[27] One other retrospective review of 100 patients undergoing suspension laryngoscopy found that 18% of patients had paresthesia of the lingual nerve. The incidence in this series was significantly greater among women, and it was also related to the length of suspension time, with those who were suspended for more than 1 hour having a four-times greater risk of injury.[28] Two prospective studies also identified lingual nerve injury as a complication. The incidence varied widely from 2.6%[24] to 12.5%.[26] Rosen postulated that the variable incidence was the result of the more common use of larger binocular laryngoscopes in one study group as compared with the other. Regardless, in all studies, lingual nerve injuries appear to be transient and to resolve sometime between 11 days and 3 months postoperatively. Because the incidence is relatively high, transient injury should be discussed with the patient preoperatively.

BRONCHOSCOPY

Bronchoscopy is frequently performed by otolaryngologist–head and neck surgeons, pulmonologists, and thoracic surgeons. Each specialty has its own indications for the procedure and their own preferred techniques. The main indication for bronchoscopy within otolaryngology–head and neck surgery is surveillance for second primary upper aerodigestive tract malignancies. A subgroup of otolaryngologist–head and neck surgeons also elects to treat tracheal disease endoscopically. Commonly treated diseases include tracheal stenosis, recurrent respiratory papillomatosis within the trachea, vascular malformations,

and obstructing tumors. Bronchoscopy can be performed with flexible endoscopes or rigid techniques. The choice of endoscopes is related primarily to surgeon preference and the indications for the procedure.

For both flexible and rigid bronchoscopy, instrumentation of the airway increases the risk of airway obstruction. This can occur as a result of foreign body dislocation, edema in an already partially obstructed airway, or laryngospasm or bronchospasm in a patient with reactive airway disease. In addition, laryngeal and tracheal manipulation may lead to cardiac arrhythmias, or cardiac arrhythmias may be the result of periods of desaturation from either manipulation of the airway, hypoventilation, or sedation.

Flexible Bronchoscopy

The incidence of major complications from flexible bronchoscopy has been reported to be 0.08%, with a death rate of 0.01%.[29] Most complications can be prevented or successfully treated with careful patient selection and appropriate surgical and perioperative observation. Major complications include hemorrhage, pneumothorax, and cardiac arrhythmias.

Again, the majority of cardiac arrhythmias are associated with hypoventilation and oxygen desaturation. Rates have been reported to be as high as 40%.[30] During the procedure, the bronchoscope is usually passed through the endotracheal tube. This may result in significant obstruction of the tube leading to difficulty with ventilation. Alternatively, if the patient is not intubated, then sedation may lead to hypoventilation. In both circumstances, the careful monitoring of oxygen saturation and levels of carbon dioxide can decrease the likelihood of problems occurring.

Major hemorrhage from bronchoscopy is also rare, but it can occur from the biopsy of vascular lesions or inadvertent transtracheal or transbronchial injury to major blood vessels. In most cases, bleeding after biopsy is minor and resolves spontaneously with the application of topical vasoconstriction agents such as epinephrine, or it may require temporary pressure being applied with the bronchoscope. In any case, initial attempts at management should include the identification of the source. If the bleeding does not appear to be stopping spontaneously, then pressure should be applied with a bronchoscope while ventilation is maintained. If necessary, an external approach for the ligation of the involved blood vessels can be undertaken. Major hemorrhage from transbronchial injury to pulmonary arteries is rare but possible. Most surgeons consider the neodymium yttrium–aluminum–garnet laser the laser of choice for the management of endobronchial lesions.[31] Properties of this laser result in tissue penetration 4 mm beyond the tip of the laser fiber. The use of the laser fiber in a contact mode on the tracheal wall can result in thermal injury that extends beyond the bronchus. Therefore injury to major blood vessels, particularly the pulmonary arteries, is possible. If bleeding is not detected immediately, then delayed fatal hemorrhage may occur 1 to 2 weeks after treatment as a result of delayed vessel rupture.

Pneumothorax has been reported in a small group of patients after bronchoscopy. This rare complication may occur as a result of high-pressure ventilation or endobronchial biopsy. The use of ultrathin bronchoscopes that extend the surgical ability into the distal pulmonary tissue may be associated with an increased incidence of pneumothorax from injury to the visceral pleura.[32] Most patients with pneumothorax will be symptomatic, and the use of routine chest x-ray for the postoperative management of patients undergoing flexible bronchoscopy is of questionable benefit.[33,34]

Rigid Bronchoscopy

Since the introduction of flexible bronchoscopy, the frequency of rigid bronchoscopy has decreased. As a diagnostic procedure for the surveillance of second primary tumors in patients with head and neck carcinoma, rigid bronchoscopy can be replaced by telescopic bronchoscopy.[35] Telescopic bronchoscopy performed with a 50-cm 0- or 30-degree telescope through the laryngoscope allows for the excellent visualization of the airway as well as the opportunity for photographic documentation when combined with a still or video camera. This technique is not associated with complications.

Rigid bronchoscopy for the management of endobronchial lesions can be associated with the same complications as flexible bronchoscopy. As with flexible bronchoscopy, complications occur as a result of hypoventilation or vagal stimulation leading to cardiac arrhythmias and from the instrumentation of the airway during biopsy or the removal of tissue leading to injury of the tracheal bronchial tree. In all cases, prompt recognition significantly improves the chance of successful management.

ESOPHAGOSCOPY

Rigid Esophagoscopy

With the advent of flexible esophagoscopes, the use of rigid esophagoscopy is significantly less common. A review of the literature suggests that the most common indication for rigid esophagoscopy is foreign-body removal.[36] However, multiple studies have indicated that flexible esophagoscopy may be equally as effective for removing foreign bodies.[37,38] In general, the primary complication of rigid esophagoscopy is the perforation of the esophagus as a result of instrumentation. The reported incidence from retrospective reviews in diagnostic esophagoscopy ranges from 0% to 1.3%.[39] The risk of perforation is increased in the presence of tumors, strictures, and longstanding foreign bodies, and it is reported to occur between 0% and 6.8% of the time.[38–40] Airway obstruction from laryngospasm with postobstructive pulmonary edema in patients having foreign bodies removed has also been reported.[41]

The management of esophageal perforations remains controversial. It is universally acknowledged that the prompt recognition and initiation of treatment are associated with the most favorable outcomes. However, the mortality rate from esophageal perforation still remains between 13% and 20%.[42] Chest x-ray films demonstrating pneumomediastinum and/or contrast esophagrams demonstrating leakage are often helpful for confirming suspected esophageal perforation. During the procedure, the experienced endoscopist should recognize the shiny gray appearance of the prevertebral fascia. Small perforations of the esophagus from biopsy often heal spontaneously with conservative measures, including parenteral nutrition, antibiotics, and observation.[43] Perforations from instrumentation that cause larger disruptions involving the mucosal and muscular layers rarely heal adequately without direct layered repair.[44–46] For cases of larger perforations caused by the rigid endoscope being placed through the wall of the esophagus, attempted conservative management often results in prolonged hospitalizations, unnecessary delays in definitive management, and reductions in survival.[46]

Flexible Esophagoscopy

Flexible esophagoscopy is commonly carried out under local anesthesia with sedation. The majority of complications are therefore related to the effects of sedation or anxiety around the procedure. Sedation and anxiety have been linked to periprocedural shifts in blood pressure producing either hypotension or anxiety-induced hypertension.[47,48] In addition, asymptomatic cardiac arrhythmias are common, and they are also believed to be the result of sedation or anxiety related to the procedure.[49] Regardless, these complications are usually transient; they resolve after the procedure is terminated, and they do not result in clinically significant complications. The risk of myocardial infarction is estimated by the American Society for Gastrointestinal Endoscopy to be 0.002%, yet it is common practice to avoid instrumentation among patients who have unstable angina or recent myocardial infarction unless the information is critical to their current management.

Respiratory depression as a result of excessive sedation often leads to respiratory compromise and hypoventilation. This occurs in as many as 80% of patients who are undergoing gastroscopy. It may not only be the result of sedation; it may also be aggravated by protective laryngeal closure during instrumentation.[50] Recently, the development of esophagoscopes, which are smaller and may be passed transnasally, has been shown to be associated with a reduced need for sedation during the endoscopic procedure. This is critical, because the majority of complications resulting from flexible esophagoscopy are caused by the required sedation for the transoral route of scope passage. Prospective series have demonstrated that, in experienced hands, the visual and biopsy findings from esophagoscopy with reduced-diameter endoscopes are comparable with the findings obtained when the examination was performed with larger-diameter endoscopes. In addition, patients preferred the transnasal route without sedation to the transoral route. Thus it appears that, with the development of high-quality, small-diameter esophagoscopes, the transnasal route without sedation is gaining more acceptance than the standard transoral route as a result of patient tolerance, comfort, and a reduced risk of complications, at least for diagnostic esophagoscopy.

As with rigid esophagoscopy, esophageal perforation is the most worrisome direct complication of esophageal instrumentation. Again, perforation can occur at any level along the pharyngeal or esophageal lumen. Perforations within the hypopharynx are most commonly the result of difficulties passing the endoscope, whereas perforations of the esophagus are usually related to the underlying disease process for which the esophagoscopy was undertaken. The risk of perforation may be slightly less with flexible esophagoscopy than rigid esophagoscopy. Large retrospective series demonstrate a perforation rate for flexible esophagoscopy of between 0.01% and 0.03%[51,52] and of 0.04% for rigid esophagoscopy.[51] Analysis of the literature bears out these relatively similar rates of perforation, because perforation is most commonly associated with esophageal diseases rather than esophagoscopy in a normal esophagus. In addition, smaller retrospective series demonstrate a lower perforation rate of flexible esophagoscopy as compared with rigid esophagoscopy during foreign-body removal; however, these differences are not statistically significant.[36] Regardless of the cause of perforation, management strategies, which have previously been discussed, are unchanged, and their prompt recognition is the key to a successful outcome.

CONCLUSION

Endoscopic approaches for the evaluation and therapeutic treatment of the upper aerodigestive tract are relatively safe. Appropriate precautions need to be undertaken, particularly with regard to the choice of patients and the use of sedation. For endoscopy as a whole, complications caused by sedation or anesthesia are more common than complications directly related to the passage of the endoscope. Technologic advances in scope design and development as well as improved appreciation for the physiologic function of the upper aerodigestive tract have resulted in changes in endoscopic techniques. With large-diameter laryngoscopes, minor complication rates involving mucosal erosions or tongue paresthesias may be slightly higher. These complications are self-limiting in nature and have no adverse implications for long-term outcomes. Flexible endoscopic instruments with distal-chip cameras have greatly improved the visualization of the esophagus and trachea without significantly altering the frequency or types of complications. This is largely because complications from esophagoscopy and bronchoscopy are more commonly related to the disease process for which the endoscopy is undertaken rather than to the procedure itself.

REFERENCES

1. Johns MM, Garrett CG, Hwang J, et al: Quality-of-life outcomes following laryngeal endoscopic surgery for non-neoplastic vocal fold lesions. *Ann Otol Rhinol Laryngol* 2004;113(8):597–601.
2. Shapshay SM, Healy GB: New microlaryngeal instruments for phonatory surgery and pediatric applications. *Ann Otol Rhinol Laryngol* 1989;98(10):821–823.
3. Berci G, Paz-Partlow M: Electronic imaging in endoscopy. *Surg Endosc* 1988;2(4):227–233.
4. Chak A, Rothstein RI: Sedationless upper endoscopy. *Rev Gastroenterol Disord* 2006;6(Suppl 1):S3–S11.
5. Conigliaro R, Rossi A: Italian Society of Digestive Endoscopy (SIED) Sedation Commission: Implementation of sedation guidelines in clinical practice in Italy: Results of a prospective longitudinal multicenter study. *Endoscopy* 2006;38(11):1137–1143.
6. Yagi J, Adachi K, Arima N, Tanaka S, et al: A prospective randomized comparative study on the safety and tolerability of transnasal

esophagogastroduodenoscopy. *Endoscopy* 2005;37(12): 1226–1231.

7. Thota PN, Zuccaro G Jr, Vargo JJ Jr, et al: A randomized prospective trial comparing unsedated esophagoscopy via transnasal and transoral routes using a 4-mm video endoscope with conventional endoscopy with sedation. *Endoscopy* 2005;37(6):559–565.

8. Dean R, Dua K, Massey B, et al: A comparative study of unsedated transnasal esophagogastroduodenoscopy and conventional EGD. *Gastrointest Endosc* 1996;44(4):422–424.

9. Halum SL, Postma GN, Bates DD, et al: Incongruence between histologic and endoscopic diagnoses of Barrett's esophagus using transnasal esophagoscopy. *Laryngoscope* 2006;116(2):303–306.

10. Langmore SE: Evaluation of oropharyngeal dysphagia: Which diagnostic tool is superior? *Curr Opin Otolaryngol Head Neck Surg* 2003;11(6):485–489.

11. Aviv JE, Kaplan ST, Thomson JE, et al: The safety of flexible endoscopic evaluation of swallowing with sensory testing (FEESST): An analysis of 500 consecutive evaluations. *Dysphagia* 2000;15(1): 39–44.

12. Cohen MA, Setzen M, Perlman PW, et al: The safety of flexible endoscopic evaluation of swallowing with sensory testing in an outpatient otolaryngology setting. *Laryngoscope* 2003;113(1):21–24.

13. Aviv JE, Murry T, Zschommler A, et al: Flexible endoscopic evaluation of swallowing with sensory testing: Patient characteristics and analysis of safety in 1,340 consecutive examinations. *Ann Otol Rhinol Laryngol* 2005;114(3):173–176.

14. Labedzki L, Ochs HR, Abernethy DR, et al: Potentially toxic serum lidocaine concentrations following spray anesthesia for bronchoscopy. *Klin Wochenschr* 1983;61(7):379–380.

15. Hegedus F, Herb K: Benzocaine-induced methemoglobinemia. *Anesth Prog* 2005;52(4):136–139.

16. Ameer B, Burlingame MB, Harman EM: Rapid mucosal absorption of topical lidocaine during bronchoscopy in the presence of oral candidiasis. *Chest* 1989;96(6):1438–1439.

17. Berci G, Calcaterra T, Ward PH: Advances in endoscopic techniques for examination of the larynx and nasopharynx. *Can J Otolaryngol* 1975;4(5):786–792.

18. Leipzig B, Zellmer JE, Klug D: The role of endoscopy in evaluating patients with head and neck cancer: A multi-institutional prospective study. *Arch Otolaryngol* 1985;111(9):589–594.

19. Robinson PM: Prospective study of the complications of endoscopic laryngeal surgery. *J Laryngol Otol* 1991;105(5):356–358.

20. Hill RS, Koltai PJ, Parnes SM: Airway complications from laryngoscopy and panendoscopy. *Ann Otol Rhinol Laryngol* 1987;96(6):691–694.

21. Armstrong M, Mark LJ, Snyder DS, et al: Safety of direct laryngoscopy as an outpatient procedure. *Laryngoscope* 1997;107(8): 1060–1065.

22. Strong MS, Vaughan CW, Mahler DL, et al: Cardiac complications of microsurgery of the larynx: Etiology, incidence and prevention. *Laryngoscope* 1974;84(6):908–920.

23. Wenig BL, Raphael N, Stern JR, et al: Cardiac complications of suspension laryngoscopy: Fact or fiction? *Arch Otolaryngol Head Neck Surg* 1986;112(8):860–862.

24. Klussmann JP, Knoedgen R, Wittekindt C, et al: Complications of suspension laryngoscopy. *Ann Otol Rhinol Laryngol* 2002;111(11): 972–976.

25. Rosen CA, Andrade Filho PA, Scheffel L, et al: Oropharyngeal complications of suspension laryngoscopy: A prospective study. *Laryngoscope* 2005;115(9):1681–1684.

26. Weed DT, Courey MS, Ossoff RH: Microlaryngoscopy in the difficult surgical exposure: A new microlaryngoscope. *Otolaryngol Head Neck Surg* 1994;110(2):247–252.

27. Gaut A, Williams M: Lingual nerve injury during suspension microlaryngoscopy. *Arch Otolaryngol Head Neck Surg* 2000; 126(5):669–671.

28. Tessema B, Sulica L, Yu GP, et al: Tongue paresthesia and dysgeusia following operative microlaryngoscopy. *Ann Otol Rhinol Laryngol* 2006;115(1):18–22.

29. Credle WF Jr, Smiddy JF, Elliott RC: Complications of fiberoptic bronchoscopy. *Am Rev Respir Dis* 1974;109(1):67–72.

30. Katz AS, Michelson EL, Stawicki J, et al: Cardiac arrhythmias: Frequency during fiberoptic bronchoscopy and correlation with hypoxemia. *Arch Intern Med* 1981;141(5):603–606.

31. Shapshay SM, Dumon JF, Beamis JF Jr: Endoscopic treatment of tracheobronchial malignancy: Experience with Nd-YAG and CO_2 lasers in 506 operations. *Otolaryngol Head Neck Surg* 1985;93(2):205–210.

32. Oki M, Saka H, Kitagawa C, et al: Visceral pleural perforation in two cases of ultrathin bronchoscopy. *Chest* 2005;127(6):2271–2273.

33. Milam MG, Evins AE, Sahn SA: Immediate chest roentgenography following fiberoptic bronchoscopy. *Chest* 1989;96(3):477–479.

34. Izbicki G, Shitrit D, Yarmolovsky A, et al: Is routine chest radiography after transbronchial biopsy necessary? A prospective study of 350 cases. *Chest* 2006;129(6):1561–1564.

35. Ku PK, Tong MC, Kwan A, et al: Modified tubeless anesthesia during endoscopy for assessment of head and neck cancers. *Ear Nose Throat J* 2003;82(2):121–125.

36. Berggreen PJ, Harrison E, Sanowski RA, et al: Techniques and complications of esophageal foreign body extraction in children and adults. *Gastrointest Endosc* 1993;39(5):626–630.

37. Brady PG, Johnson WF: Removal of foreign bodies: The flexible fiberoptic endoscope. *South Med J* 1977;70(6):702–704.

38. Herranz-Gonzalez J, Martinez-Vidal J, Garcia-Sarandeses A, et al: Esophageal foreign bodies in adults. *Otolaryngol Head Neck Surg* 1991;105(5):649–654.

39. Wilson JA, Murray JA, von Haacke NP: Rigid endoscopy in ENT practice: Appraisal of the diagnostic yield in a district general hospital. *J Laryngol Otol* 1987;101(3):286–292.

40. Kubba H, Spinou E, Brown D: Is same-day discharge suitable following rigid esophagoscopy? Findings in a series of 655 cases. *Ear Nose Throat J* 2003;82(1):33–36.

41. Mehta VM, Har-El G, Goldstein NA: Postobstructive pulmonary edema after laryngospasm in the otolaryngology patient. *Laryngoscope* 2006;116(9):1693–1696.

42. Jones WG Jr, Ginsberg RJ: Esophageal perforation: A continuing challenge. *Ann Thorac Surg* 1992;53(3):534–543.

43. Huber-Lang M, Henne-Bruns D, Schmitz B, et al: Esophageal perforation: Principles of diagnosis and surgical management. *Surg Today* 2006;36(4):332–340.

44. Brinster CJ, Singhal S, Lee L, et al: Evolving options in the management of esophageal perforation. *Ann Thorac Surg* 2004;77(4):1475–1483.

45. Nesbitt JC, Sawyers JL: Surgical management of esophageal perforation. *Am Surg* 1987;53(4):183–191.

46. Eroglu A, Can Kurkcuogu I, Karaoganogu N, et al: Esophageal perforation: The importance of early diagnosis and primary repair. *Dis Esophagus* 2004;17(1):91–94.

47. Pristautz H, Biffl H, Leitner W, et al: Influence of an antiarrhythmic premedication on the development of premature ventricular contractions during fiberoptic gastroduodenoscopy. *Endoscopy* 1981;13(2):57–59.

48. Sturges HF, Krone CL: Cardiovascular stress of peroral gastrointestinal endoscopy. *Gastrointest Endosc* 1973;19(3):119–122.

49. Hart R, Classen M: Complications of diagnostic gastrointestinal endoscopy. *Endoscopy* 1990;22(5):229–233.

50. Bell GD, Reeve PA, Moshiri M, et al: Intravenous midazolam: A study of the degree of oxygen desaturation occurring during upper gastrointestinal endoscopy. *Br J Clin Pharmacol* 1987;23(6):703–708.

51. Silvis SE, Nebel O, Rogers G, et al: Endoscopic complications: Results of the 1974 American Society for Gastrointestinal Endoscopy Survey. *JAMA* 1976;235(9):928–930.

52. Schiller KF, Cotton PB, Salmon PR: The hazards of digestive fibre-endoscopy: A survey of British experience. *Gut* 1972;13(12):1027.

CHAPTER 31

Complications of Percutaneous Gastrostomy

Rohan R. Walvekar and Robert L. Ferris

OVERVIEW

Disorders of the upper aerodigestive tract may render swallowing function or airway protection inadequate or unsafe. In addition, many head and neck cancer patients suffer from poor nutrition, which is a problem both before and after therapy.[1] The surgical treatment of head and neck cancer alters the upper aerodigestive tract both anatomically and physiologically, affecting swallowing function and nutritional status. Nonsurgical treatment in the form of radiation therapy and chemotherapy may be used as the primary treatment modality.

Radiation therapy is often associated with mucositis, dysphagia, loss of taste, and anorexia. In fact, about 60% of patients have significant weight loss during radiation treatment. Chemoradiation and hyperfractionated radiation therapy are usually associated with even more treatment-related side effects and greater impairment of swallowing function.[2] Other conditions (e.g., vagus nerve injury, recurrent laryngeal nerve injury) may induce aspiration and necessitate a gastrostomy to facilitate enteral feeding.

Impact of Malnutrition on Patients

The impact of malnutrition on patient outcomes is significant. It has been reported that a progressive involuntary weight loss of more than 10% of the body weight over 6 months and a body mass index of 20 or less are prognostic markers for increased surgical complication rates and mortality.[3] Surgical therapy for the treatment of head and neck cancer affects nutrition and consequently affects treatment outcomes.

Providing Adequate Nutritional Support

Adequate nutritional support must be provided to preserve or improve function, to hasten recovery, and to reduce complications.[4] Piquet and colleagues[5] studied the role of early nutritional intervention via percutaneous endoscopic gastrostomy (PEG) among patients undergoing radiation therapy for oropharyngeal cancer and suggested that the early nutritional support prevents or corrects nutritional deficiencies and helps to maintain a desirable weight throughout the course of treatment. Nutritional support must be provided by the enteral route whenever possible, because it has fewer complications, it is easy to administer, and it has better intestinal use as compared with parenteral nutrition. Such nutritional support also prevents intestinal atrophy and promotes immune function, and it is more economical than total parenteral nutrition.[4]

Several routes of gastrointestinal access for enteral nutrition have been described.[6] Traditionally, surgical (open) gastrostomy and nasogastric tube placement were the preferred approaches for enteral alimentation.[6] Currently PEG has become the preferred method of providing long-term enteral nutrition, for several reasons. Open gastrostomy requires general anesthesia and has higher morbidity, mortality, and complication rates as compared with PEG.[7,8] Nasogastric tube placement can also be associated with multiple problems (e.g., laryngeal irritation, persistent gastroesophageal reflux, nasal alar necrosis, sinusitis, inadvertent removal, patient dissatisfaction, patient discomfort).[8] As a result, PEG has become the preferred approach for providing enteral nutrition among patients with head and neck cancer.[5]

PERCUTANEOUS ENDOSCOPIC GASTROSTOMY

PEG was introduced in 1980 by Gauderer and Ponsky.[9] In 1986, Ruppin and Lux[10] confirmed the safety and usefulness of the PEG procedure for patients with head and neck cancer.

Percutaneous Endoscopic Gastrostomy Techniques

There are many techniques and approaches to the PEG procedure. The most widely used method is called the *pull method* or the *standard Ponsky technique*.[10] Russell[11] introduced a modification of this technique called the *push method,* which is used less frequently but has the advantage of avoiding the transoral passage of the PEG tube. In 1983, Ho[12] described another technique called *percutaneous radiologic gastrostomy (PRG)* or *percutaneous fluoroscopic gastrostomy,* which is used by interventional radiologists and allows for the percutaneous placement of the feeding tube under fluoroscopic guidance.

The basic principle common to all techniques of PEG tube placement is gastric insufflation, which brings the stomach into contact with the abdominal wall. Then percutaneous placement of a cannula, a guide suture, or a wire is performed to enable the gastrostomy tube to be introduced into the stomach.[7] The procedure is as follows:

- Pass the flexible endoscope transorally into the stomach.
- Insufflate the stomach with air.
- Identify the proposed percutaneous endoscopic gastrostomy site by manual palpation and endoscopic confirmation of the desired site through the visualization of a finger depression of the anterior gastric wall (Figure 31-1).

Pull Method

With the pull method, a guide wire is passed transabdominally under endoscopic visualization. This guide wire is then grasped with a snare through a port on the endoscope and subsequently advanced retrograde through the patient's mouth. This leaves the remaining end to exit the patient through the abdominal wall (Figure 31-2, A).

Next, a no. 18 or no. 20 Fr gastrostomy tube is secured to the oral end of the guide wire, and the PEG tube is advanced through the mouth, the esophagus, the stomach, and the anterior abdominal wall. The PEG tube is advanced by pulling the extra-abdominal end of the guide wire to advance the tube out through the gastrostomy (Figure 31-2, B).

Push Method

In principle, the PRG is similar to the push technique, but additional guidance is obtained with either ultrasound or fluoroscopy.[13,14] With the push method, four T-fasteners are placed before the gastrostomy tube is inserted. This secures the stomach to the anterior abdominal wall; otherwise the stomach would be displaced internally while pushing the gastrostomy tube into it. Next a short guide wire is passed transabdominally into the stomach under endoscopic view (Figure 31-3, A). Serial dilatation then helps with the creation

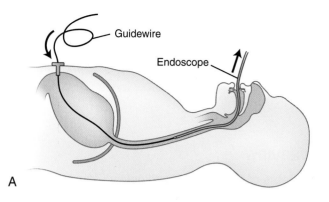
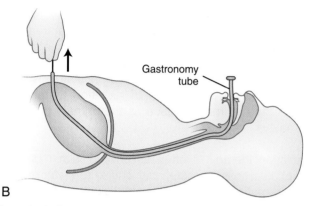

Figure 31-2. Pull technique. **A,** Retrograde advancement of guidewire with endoscope. **B,** Traction on guidewire to facilitate advancement of gastronomy tube.

of a stomal tract. A no. 18 Fr gastrostomy tube is inserted (or "pushed") over the guide wire using gentle force and a twisting motion (Figure 31-3, B).

Comparison of the Pull and Push Techniques

Prospective, randomized, controlled studies have generally shown that the techniques are equivalent in terms of safety and the success of placement.[7] The Ponsky and Gauderer technique (i.e., the pull method), however, is technically easier to perform and more widely practiced. The Russell technique (i.e., the push method) is associated with a lower incidence of certain complications.[7,15] For example, with the push technique, the rate of wound infection and the risk of tumor seeding of the gastrostomy site are decreased, because the contaminated oropharyngeal area is bypassed.[7] In fact, all reported cases of tumor formation at the PEG site in patients with head and neck cancer have been associated with the use of the pull technique, which suggests that this technique is associated with the direct implantation of tumor cells carried from the primary tumor to the gastrostomy site.[7,16]

Both techniques for PEG placement are contraindicated in several situations (Box 31-1). Percutaneous radiologic gastrostomy can be useful when PEG placement is contraindicated, and it is particularly helpful

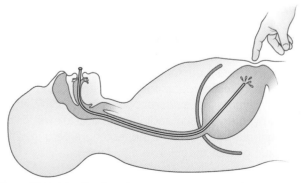

Figure 31-1. Identification of the percutaneous endoscopic gastrostomy placement site. Fiberoptic esophagoscope allows direct visualization of finger from gastric lumen.

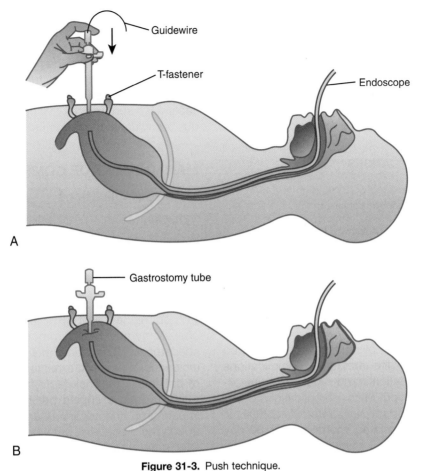

Figure 31-3. Push technique.

BOX 31-1 **Contraindications for Percutaneous Endoscopic Gastrostomy Placement**

ABSOLUTE CONTRAINDICATIONS

- The presence of a large, obstructing pharyngeal or esophageal lesion
- The inability to transilluminate the abdominal wall as a result of morbid obesity, ascites, or interposition of the colon
- Intra-abdominal infection
- A history of subtotal gastrectomy
- Gastric "pull-up" (i.e., after total pharyngectomy for hypopharyngeal cancer)

RELATIVE CONTRAINDICATIONS

- Severe emphysema
- Trismus
- High transverse stomach
- Coagulopathy
- Esophageal stricture
- Megacolon
- Cirrhosis
- Hepatomegaly
- Previous upper abdominal surgery

when bypassing an obstructing tumor or a stenosis of the upper digestive tract. During PRG, the stomach can be insufflated via a small-bore (i.e., no. 5 Fr or no. 6 Fr) nasogastric tube so that obstructing lesions can be navigated successfully.[14] Like the push technique, PRG avoids oropharyngeal contamination with

a resulting lower site infection rate and a reduced chance of the tumor seeding of the gastrostomy site.[14] The visualization of relevant abdominal anatomy facilitates accurate tube placement.[14] Percutaneous radiologic gastrostomy allows for greater flexibility with scheduling, because it can be performed as an outpatient procedure without deep sedation, thereby reducing the risk of airway compromise among patients with bulky head and neck tumors.[14,17]

Disadvantages of the PRG include the fact that a smaller-bore gastrostomy tube is usually inserted. This may limit feedings and medication administration, and it may also lead to more frequent occlusion.[2] Another risk associated with PRG that is not shared by PEG is the low dose of fluoroscopic radiation exposure, except for cases in which ultrasound guidance is used. This dose is minimal as compared with the diagnostic radiation doses received by most patients with head and neck cancer.[17]

COMPLICATIONS OF PERCUTANEOUS ENDOSCOPIC GASTRONOMY

Schapiro and Edmundowicz[18] classified PEG-related complications as either major or minor. Box 31-2 summarizes the common complications encountered with

BOX 31-2 Complications of Percutaneous Endoscopic Gastrostomy Placement

MINOR COMPLICATIONS

- Peristomal wound infection and/or granulations
- Tube obstruction
- Tube fragmentation and/or fungal colonization
- Tube migration into the small bowel
- Leakage around the percutaneous endoscopy gastrostomy
- Prolonged ileus

RELATIVE CONTRAINDICATIONS

- Peritonitis
- Premature removal
- Perforation of related abdominal organs
- Aspiration
- Tube migration through the gastric wall
- Gastrocolic-cutaneous fistula
- Hemorrhage
- Necrotizing fasciitis
- Tumor implantation in the stoma site

PEG placement. Overall complication rates have ranged from 4% to 23.8%. Major, life-threatening complications occur in 1% to 5% of patients and require hospitalization or surgical intervention. Minor complications occur more frequently and reportedly vary from 5% to 20%.[7,19] The rates of procedure-related mortality and 30-day mortality attributable to PEG placement are very low

(0%–2% and 1.5%–2.1%, respectively).[19] Reports show that mortality after PEG tube placement is less than 1%, and complications after PEG tube placement occur between 5% and 15% of the time.[7] Complication rates for percutaneous gastrostomy tubes placed endoscopically are similar to those of tubes placed radiographically.[7,20] Table 31-1 summarizes the complication rates for various techniques of gastrostomy tube placement.

MANAGEMENT OF COMPLICATIONS

Major Complications

Aspiration

Foutch[20] reported aspiration to be the most commonly reported major complication. The incidence of PEG-related aspiration is reported to be between 0.3% and 1.0%.[19,21] Tracheopulmonary aspiration is a common occurrence in the patient with head and neck cancer, with an incidence of 58% among patients with a tracheostomy and of 23% among patients without a tracheostomy.[22] It would be reasonable to expect a higher incidence of procedure-related aspiration in this subset of patients. Other risk factors for intraprocedural aspiration include a supine position, sedation, neurologic impairment, and advanced age.[19] Aspiration can occur during the procedure, but it has also been reported at a later date as a result of oropharyngeal aspiration, the

TABLE 31-1 Comparative Data for Gastrostomy Placement[a]

Author	Year of Publication	Approach	Number of Patients	Success Rate (%)	Major Complications (%)	Minor Complications (%)	Tube-Related Complications (%)
Gibson[b]	1992	PEG-HNC	114	93	0.9	4.4	
Gibson[b]	1992	PEG-Control	220	97	1.9	13.1	
Riley[c]	1992	PEG-HNC	46	77	20.6	36	
Deutsch[d]	1992	PRG	68	100	4.7	7.8	
Grant[e]	1993	PEG	598	99.4	1.3	3.7	
Wollman[f]	1995	Surgical	4	100	25	0	
Wollman, meta-analysis[f]	1995	Surgical	721	100	19.9	9	
Wollman[f]	1995	PEG	35	94	14	9	3
Wollman, meta-analysis[f]	1995	PEG	4194	95.7	9.4	5.9	16
Wollman[f]	1995	PRG	33	100	12	18	3
Wollman, meta-analysis[f]	1995	PRG	837	99.2	5.9	7.8	12.1

TABLE 31-1 Comparative Data for Gastrostomy Placement[a]—cont'd

Author	Year of Publication	Approach	Number of Patients	Success Rate (%)	Major Complications (%)	Minor Complications (%)	Tube-Related Complications (%)
Bell[g]	1995	PRG	519	95.1	1.3	2.9	8
Beaver[h]	1998	PRG	92	98	1	13	13
Righi[i]	1998	PRG	56	98.2	1.8	10.9	
Cosentini[j]	1998	PEG	24	100	17	33	12
Cosentini[j]	1998	Surgical	14	100	14	43	7
Cosentini[j]	1998	PRG	44	100	11	36	20
Dewald[k]	1999	PRG	701	95.6	0.5	5.3	13.5
de Baere[l]	1999	PRG	500	99	1.4	5.4	17.6
Deurloo[m]	2001	PRG	118	97	6	15	1
Neeff[n]	2003	PEG	56	89	3.6	7	
Neeff[n]	2003	PRG	18	100	5.6	39	

PEG, Percutaneous endoscopic gastrostomy; *PEG-Control,* percutaneous endoscopic gastrostomy, control; *PEG-HNC,* percutaneous endoscopic gastrostomy, head and neck cancer; *PRG,* percutaneous radiologic gastrostomy.

[a]This table compares percutaneous endoscopic gastrostomy, surgical gastrostomy, and percutaneous radiologic gastrostomy.

[b]Gibson SE, Wenig BL, Watkins JL: Complications of percutaneous endoscopic gastrostomy in head and neck cancer patients. *Ann Otol Rhinol Laryngol* 1992;101:46–50.

[c]Riley DA, Strauss M: Airway and other complications of percutaneous endoscopic gastrostomy in head and neck cancer patients. *Ann Otol Rhinol Laryngol* 1992;101:310–313.

[d]Deutsch LS, Kannegieter L, Vanson DT: Simplified percutaneous gastrostomy. *Radiology* 1992;184:181–183.

[e]Grant JP: Percutaneous endoscopic gastrostomy: Initial placement by single endoscopic technique and long-term follow up. *Ann Surg* 1993;217(2):168–174.

[f]Wollman B, D'Agostino HB, Walus-Wigle JR, et al: Radiologic, endoscopic, and surgical gastrostomy: An institutional evaluation and meta-analysis of the literature. *Radiology* 1995;197:699–704.

[g]Bell SD, Carmody EA, Yeung EY, et al: Percutaneous gastrostomy and gastrojejunostomy: Additional experience in 519 procedures. *Radiology* 1995;194:817–820.

[h]Beaver ME, Myers JN, Griffenberg L: Percutaneous fluoroscopic gastrostomy tube placement in patients with head and neck cancer. *Arch Otolaryngol Head Neck Surg* 1998;124:1141–1144.

[i]Righi PD, Reddy DK, Weisberger EC, et al: Radiologic percutaneous gastrostomy: Results in 56 patients with head and neck cancer. *Laryngoscope* 1998;108:1020–1024.

[j]Cosentini EP, Sautner T, Gnant M, et al: Outcomes of surgical, percutaneous endoscopic, and percutaneous radiological gastrostomies. *Arch Surg* 1998;133:1076–1083.

[k]Dewald CL, Hiette PO, Sewall LE, et al: Percutaneous gastrostomy and gastrojejunostomy with gastropexy: Experience in 701 procedures. *Radiology* 1999;211:651–656.

[l]de Baere T, Chapot R, Kuoch V, et al: Percutaneous gastrostomy with fluoroscopic guidance: Single-center experience in 500 consecutive cancer patients. *Radiology* 1999;210:651–654.

[m]Deurloo EE, Schultze Kool LJ, Kroger R, et al: Percutaneous radiological gastrostomy in patients with head and neck cancer. *Eur J Surg Oncol* 2001;24(1):94–97.

[n]Neeff M, Crowder VL, McIvor NP, et al: Comparison of the use of endoscopic and radiologic gastrostomy in a single head and neck cancer unit. *ANZ J Surg* 2003;73:590–593

reflux of feedings, and delayed gastric emptying.[18] Aspiration can be reduced by avoiding oversedation during the procedure, minimizing air insufflation in the stomach, and thoroughly aspirating gastric contents beforehand.[19] A newer technique of unsedated transnasal PEG placement is associated with a lower risk of aspiration.[23]

Aspiration can also be reduced by placing the gastrostomy tube for gravity drainage or suction for 12 hours after placement. In addition, careful attention should be paid to tube-feeding instructions, including the routine measurement of gastric residuals, the elevation of the head during feeding and for 2 hours after bolus feeding, the avoidance of oversedation, and the aggressive medical management of documented gastroesophageal reflux.[18]

Peritonitis

Peritonitis is a serious and potentially fatal complication of PEG placement with an incidence of between 0.55% and 1.3%.[19] Ehrsson and colleagues[24] retrospectively studied 156 patients with head and neck cancer who had a PEG. Procedure-related fatal complications in all cases were related to gastric leakage and peritonitis. Post-PEG peritonitis manifests itself as diffuse abdominal pain, fever, leukocytosis, and ileus. It can be caused by the premature removal or displacement of the tube, the unrecognized perforation of the gastrointestinal tract lumen, or the leakage of gastric contents around the gastrostomy tube site.[18] Peritoneal leakage seems to be lower after the pull technique. For comparison, the introducer or push technique has a mechanically suboptimal internal anchoring device, and the no. 16 Fr peel-away sheath leaves a larger hole for the gastrostomy tube. Consequently, a greater risk may exist for peritoneal leakage and peritonitis.[25] The delayed onset of peritonitis may occur during the tube change, perhaps as a result of a preexisting disruption of the gastrointestinal tract[26] or of small-bowel injury during tube removal without endoscopic assistance.[27]

The incidence of transient subclinical pneumoperitoneum during PEG placement is as high as 56%,[20] and it is usually not of any clinical significance. However, it does limit the usefulness of plain radiographs for evaluating suspected peritonitis.[19] Fluoroscopic imaging of the PEG tube with the infusion of water-soluble contrast is useful for detecting a leak as well as for confirming proper tube placement. In the case of an active leak, a computed tomography scan is helpful for delineating the course of the gastrostomy tube and its relationship with the small bowel and the colon.[18] When patients present with signs of peritonitis with an active leak, proper management includes the administration of broad-spectrum antibiotics, surgical exploration, and conversion to an open gastrostomy using a purse-string suture.[7,18,19]

Premature Removal of the Gastrostomy Tube

The premature or inadvertent removal of the PEG tube within the first 7 days after insertion and before the adherence of the gastric serosa to the parietal peritoneum is a very serious complication[28] that is reported to occur in up to 7.8% of cases.[29] Consequences include intraperitoneal spillage and the subsequent development of intra-abdominal sepsis and its associated complications. Percutaneous endoscopic gastrostomy tube maturation tends to occur within 7 to 10 days after insertion, and it may be delayed for up to 4 weeks in the presence of malnutrition, ascites, or corticosteroid treatment.[19] In most cases, the premature removal of the PEG tube can be managed nonoperatively. In the absence of signs and symptoms of peritoneal involvement, the PEG tube can be replaced within 1 week of dislodgement.[29] Galat and colleages,[28] reporting about the placement of 271 PEG tubes, listed an incidence of 1.8% of premature dislodgement within 7 days; immediate replacement was performed using the retrograde string technique under endoscopic control and avoiding laparotomy. Marshall and colleagues[30] found

evidence of intraperitoneal contamination in one patient 2 to 4 days after the removal of the gastrostomy at laparotomy. If the recognition of the accidental dislodgement is delayed, management should consist of nasogastric suction for 48 hours and intravenous antibiotics followed by repeat PEG placement 7 to 10 days later.[30] If the patient shows evidence of peritoneal contamination, surgical exploration is recommended. Recently the laparoscopic replacement of the PEG tube has been described.[31] Laparoscopic exploration is less morbid than laparotomy while still allowing for a wide visualization of the peritoneal cavity, the closure of the gastrostomy, the irrigation of the peritoneal cavity, and the placement of new enteral access.[29]

Various preventive measures have been suggested to reduce the incidence of premature removal, especially for patients who may be prone to pulling out their own tubes. Such patients should undergo PEG only if T-fasteners are used.[29] A randomized comparison study of patients undergoing PRG showed that PRG without T-fasteners was associated with a 10% incidence of serious technical complications. Thus the authors recommended the routine use of T-fastener gastropexy.[32] Additional sutures that anchor the tube to the abdominal wall, cutting the tube down to 6 to 8 inches (thus avoiding excess length that provides a "handle"), the use of abdominal binders, and low-profile PEG buttons that lay flush with the skin can reduce the risk of future inadvertent removal.[18,19,29]

Migration of the Gastrostomy Tube and Buried Bumper Syndrome

The term *buried bumper syndrome* refers to the partial or complete growth of gastric mucosa over the internal bolster, or bumper, and it has been reported to occur in 0.3% to 6.1% of cases.[19,33] It usually occurs after 4 months of use, but it can be seen as a delayed complication as well.[23,34] Frascio and colleagues[35] reported this complication 7 years after PEG placement. The mechanism for this syndrome is excessive traction on the internal retaining bumper of certain types of gastrostomy tubes.[18] This complication can be prevented by using balloon-tipped replacement tubes inserted 3 to 6 months after PEG placement in patients requiring long-term feeding as opposed to using tubes with a mushroom-like round tip or a four-wing tip.[34] Vargo and Ponsky[36] recommended that an additional 1.5 cm be allowed between the external bumper of the PEG tube and the skin to prevent the migration of the tube.

Buried bumper syndrome is diagnosed on physical examination.[34] Symptoms can range from abdominal pain or feeding difficulties to frank peritonitis.[18] A case of significant bleeding as a result of tube migration has been reported.[37] There are various internal and external techniques that have been used to manage this condition.

The basic principle that is common to all is the replacement of the tube while minimizing trauma to the PEG tract.[19] Surgical removal was reasonable for the management of this complication. Ma and colleagues[38] introduced the "needle-knife" technique with which the gastric mucosa over the embedded internal bumper is endoscopically incised, thus allowing the internal bumper to be removed endoscopically and the residual portion of the tube to be removed via the external route. Recently neodymium-doped yttrium–aluminum–garnet lasers have been used to incise the gastric mucosa instead of the needle sphincterotome.[39] Other techniques of removing the internal bumper include grasping with a snare or forceps, dilatation using a balloon dilator either externally or endoscopically, push and pull "T" techniques with a tube fragment grasped in a snare, extraction using the tapered tip of a new PEG tube, external incision on the abdominal wall, and the extraperitoneal removal of the internal bumper.[33] With the advent of the softer, collapsible internal bumpers, nonsurgical removal with external traction has become possible for buried bumpers, thereby reserving surgical or endoscopic removal for cases in which the internal bumper breaks off or is retained in the abdominal or gastric wall during external traction.[40]

Perforation

Esophageal and posterior pharyngeal perforation can occur during upper endoscopy or gastrostomy tube insertion, especially among patients with malignancies of these areas.[18] Esophageal perforation can be complicated by life-threatening mediastinitis that may present in a delayed fashion.[41] The removal of the PEG tube is also associated with complications, and it must be performed with endoscopic assistance. Intestinal obstruction by retained internal bumper separated from the PEG tube during the removal of an old pull-through gastrostomy tube has been reported.[42] Small-bowel perforation is also seen as a consequence of tube migration caused by peristalsis. The contact of the balloon-tip catheter with the small bowel for long periods may cause pressure necrosis and perforation. Complications of long-term PEG tubes (e.g., gastrointestinal erosion, small-bowel perforation) can be avoided by the proper maintenance of the gastrostomy tube with routine evaluations to identify cracks, to confirm proper fit, and to look for signs of wear and tear.[42]

Gastrocolocutaneous Fistula

Evans and Serpell[43] reported the first case of gastroenterocutaneous fistula, which can present acutely with symptoms of colonic perforation or obstruction or chronically with symptoms of a partial intestinal obstruction. Yoshihiro and colleagues[44] reported a cologastric fistula complicated by a colonic perforation 2 years after PEG placement that was diagnosed during tube replacement. Gastrocolocutaneous fistula can

occur when the colon is inadvertently punctured partially or completely during placement or as a result of the erosion of the PEG tube into a juxtaposed colon.[19] This complication can be diagnosed with a gastrograffin study via the PEG tube or with a barium enema. The latter can also be used to evaluate the persistence of a fistula after treatment. The clinician must suspect a fistulous communication with the colon if patients present with excessive diarrhea, fecal vomiting, or fecal aspiration from a PEG tube.[44] Management is nonsurgical and involves the removal of the tube, which usually results in the spontaneous closure of the gastrocolic and colocutaneous fistulas within several hours.[18,19,26] Surgical treatment may be required if patients have signs of peritonitis, difficulty with diarrhea, or an immature tract.[18] This complication can be prevented by avoiding an excessive insufflation of air that causes gastric rotation that exposes the posterior gastric wall and tents up the transverse colon. A well-defined transillumination site and the direction of the needle perpendicular to the abdominal wall further decrease the likelihood of this complication.[44] Foutch[20] recommends the elevation of the head of the bed during placement to displace the colon inferiorly. In addition, he indicates that the use of an aspirating syringe filled with saline can identify intervening bowel between the skin and the stomach if air bubbles appear in the syringe before endoscopic visualization of the needle in the gastric lumen; this is called the *safe-track technique*.[20]

Hemorrhage

Significant bleeding during PEG insertion is uncommon, occurring in 1% of cases.[19] Risk factors include anticoagulation and the previous anatomic alteration of abdominal structures.[19,45] A fatal retroperitoneal hemorrhage believed to be related to altered surgical anatomy[46] as well as a case of fatal aortic perforation from a retained and impacted PEG flange have been reported.[47] In most situations, hemorrhage occurs as a result of trauma to gastric mural vessels, from ulceration of the gastric wall at the G-tube site, or from the contralateral wall by the retaining bumper or by concomitant peptic ulcer disease (15%). The avoidance of excessive traction on the G-tube can reduce the risk of ulceration.[18] Kanie and colleagues[48] also observed that histamine blockers did not reduce gastric ulcers among these patients; rather the occurrence of gastric ulcers appeared to be related to the shape of the tube within the internal gastric cavity. A protrusion of the internal gastric bumper of more than 5 mm was found to be a relevant factor for the development of gastric ulcers.[48] Ulla and colleagues[49] reported upper gastrointestinal bleeding related to the extrusion of an internal gastric bumper of more than 5 mm. Esophagitis associated with reflux disease is a common occurrence, and it has been associated with upper gastrointestinal bleeding in patients with PEG. Histamine blockers are not effective in this situation.[50] Traumatic passage of the string, the guide wire, or the feeding tube can also cause lower esophageal ulcerations and bleeding.[51] Fortunately the endoscopic evaluation of acute gastrointestinal bleeding after PEG seems to be very well tolerated. The endoscopist should inspect the upper gastrointestinal tract and the gastrostomy site with the external manipulation of the G-tube to visualize the mucosa under the retaining bumper, which is often the site of bleeding.[20]

Necrotizing Fasciitis

Necrotizing fasciitis is a relatively uncommon, severe, and frequently fatal soft-tissue infection.[52] There have been a few reports that have described it as a complication of PEG placement. The characteristic clinical manifestations include a rapidly spreading infection with high fever, localized pain, cellulites, and edematous soft tissue with subcutaneous emphysema.[18,53] The skin near the PEG site is usually abnormal, demonstrating induration, ecchymosis, crepitance, or bulla.[18] Necrotizing fasciitis presenting within 72 hours of tube placement occurs as a result of an inadequate abdominal skin incision that does not allow for adequate wound drainage and as a consequence of ischemic necrosis of the gastric mucosa as a result of excessive traction on the gastrostomy tube.[54] In their series, McLean and colleagues[55] reported this complication to be seen in a delayed fashion, and the proposed mechanism was tube dislodgement with the subsequent leakage of nonsterile feedings. Yusoff and Ormonde[53] reported a variation of this clinical presentation in which a subcutaneous leak into the anterior abdominal wall tissues presented as a less severe form of necrotizing fasciitis. The causative organisms in these infections are most commonly *Streptococcus pyogenes* and group A β-hemolytic *Streptococcus*[52]; however, a wide range of organisms can be responsible.[53] Antibiotic therapy should be directed at the most common organisms and should cover a broad spectrum of anaerobes. A meta-analysis of randomized controlled trials showed that antibiotic prophylaxis in the form of a single dose of broad-spectrum antibiotic 30 minutes before PEG reduces the incidence of peristomal wound infections.[56] The diagnosis of necrotizing fasciitis is a clinical one that can be confirmed by subcutaneous emphysema on a plain abdominal x-ray scan. A computed tomography scan may be useful to identify a leaking gastrostomy tube and to rule out intra-abdominal abcesses.[55] Treatment includes a combination of early and aggressive surgical debridement, broad-spectrum antibiotics, and intensive supportive care including modalities such as hyperbaric oxygen.[18,57] Some authors recommend a second surgical exploration with repeated debridement followed by appropriate coverage of the large abdominal wall defects after the infection has been controlled. This may include local flaps, free-tissue transfers, split-thickness skin grafts, and vacuum dressings.[55]

Tumor Implantation at the Percutaneous Endoscopic Gastrostomy Site

The spread of cancer from the upper aerodigestive tract to a gastrostomy stoma was first reported in 1977 by Algaratham[58]; in 1996, Schneider and Loggie[59] reported the first successful surgical resection of a PEG site metastasis. The true incidence of PEG site metastasis is difficult to gauge, because many patients succumb to widespread disease before the clinical detection of these cases. A large autopsy study of 832 cases reported a prevalence of 1.3%.[7] To date, 25 cases of cancer metastasis to the gastrostomy site have been reported.[60] Almost all of these cases involved advanced (stage III and IV) squamous cell carcinomas of the head and neck region. PEG site metastases tend to become evident 8 months (range, 2–24 months) after gastrostomy tube placement.[61] They are not always associated with signs and symptoms of involvement of the gastrointestinal tract. The most common symptoms include epigastric pain, ulceration, erythematous lesions, and peristomal drainage. There may be associated nausea, vomiting, postprandial bloating, obstruction, perforation, and bleeding.[60] These metastatic lesions may present in a similar fashion to granulation tissue (Figure 31-4). It is important to consider the biopsy of lesions that occur at the PEG site to rule out metastatic tumor.[59]

PEG site metastasis is associated with a poor prognosis. In most cases, the identification of this condition is accompanied by evidence of synchronous distant metastasis, especially in the lung.[61] A study by Adelson and colleagues[62] found that, when a PEG site metastasis was identified more than 10 months after tube placement, 100% of patients had synchronous distant metastasis (as compared with 24% when the PEG site metastasis was identified before 10 months). The median survival of a patient with gastric metastasis from a head and neck cancer, however, is approximately 6 months.[60] An exception to this rule is the patient who

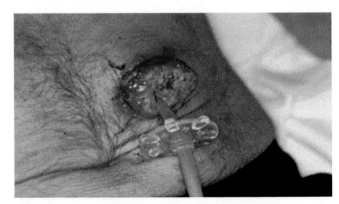

Figure 31-4. Cutaneous abdominal wall metastasis. (From Cruz I, Mamel JJ, Brady PG, Cass-Garcia M: Incidence of abdominal wall metastasis complicating PEG tube placement in untreated head and neck cancer. *Gastrointest Endosc* 2005;62(5):708–711. With permission from the American Society for Gastrointestinal Endoscopy.)

underwent surgical resection successfully and had a prolonged disease-free survival.[59]

The postulated mechanisms for PEG site metastasis include the implantation of tumor cells along the path where the instruments for insertion have injured the tissues.[60] This theory is favored by the fact that all PEG site metastases to date have occurred with the pull technique, which is associated with oropharyngeal contamination and contact with tumor cells if the PEG placement is done before tumor extirpation. Adelson and colleagues[62] recommend the push technique to prevent this complication. However, there is considerable evidence that PEG site metastasis is primarily related to the hematogenous or lymphatic spread of circulating tumor cells. This implies that the method of tube placement does not alter or affect the risk of PEG site metastasis.[61]

A recommendation for minimizing the risk of PEG site metastasis is to place the PEG tube after the resection of the primary cancer. This is also advocated because it is associated with fewer complications, and it reduces the risk of airway complications that can occur if tube placement is attempted under sedation, especially among patients who have advanced oral cancer.[63] If PEG placement is indicated before surgical resection or chemoradiation, several authors recommend using the push technique or performing laparoscopic or open gastrostomy tube placement, with meticulous care taken to keep the surgical sites and the equipment separate.[62] Although PEG site metastasis is associated with a poor prognosis, surgical resection and the establishment of an alternative enteral access are recommended whenever feasible.

Minor Complications

There is no uniform list of minor complications nor is there a standardized format for reporting minor complications. However, some commonly occurring minor complications are listed here to facilitate early treatment and to reduce the morbidity associated with them.

Peristomal Wound Infections and Granulations

Peristomal wound infections are one of the most common complications of PEG.[56] The incidence of this complication is reported to be between 4.3% and 16%.[56] Other studies suggest that as many as 30% of patients with PEGs will develop wound infections,[19] and about 3% to 8% will develop local cellulitis or abscess formation.[56] It must be borne in mind that some of these infections can progress to give rise to a more serious complication (i.e., necrotizing fasciitis). There are several factors that contribute to PEG site infections, including preexisting infections and nosocomial colonization.[18] Patients with compromised immune function from various conditions (e.g., diabetes, obesity, poor nutritional status, malignancy, chronic corticosteroid therapy) are also at increased risk for infection.[18,19] Excessive pressure between external and internal bolsters is associated with a higher infection rate, so avoiding excessive traction on the gastrostomy tube can reduce PEG site infections. An adequate skin incision at the PEG site (i.e., 1–2 mm larger than the dimension of the tube) also helps to reduce traction on the PEG tube and maceration of the skin.[18,19] Various regimens of oral decontamination have been tried without an effect on the incidence of PEG site infections.[18] However, antibiotic prophylaxis given 30 minutes before the procedure is effective for reducing the relative and absolute risks of infection by 73% and 17.5%, respectively.[56] The introducer technique is also associated with a lower incidence of infection, because it avoids oral contamination as compared with the pull technique.[19]

Chronic infection and irritation lead to granulation tissue, which is also commonly seen at the PEG insertion site. This granulation tissue tends to be a source of great discomfort to long-term patients. A long-term survey of patients showed that up to 67% of patients developed granulation tissue.[64] Persistent granulations that do not respond to conservative treatment or that recur should be biopsied, because they may harbor metastatic tumor. Granulation tissue can be treated with various techniques such as cauterization with silver nitrate, electrocautery, laser ablation, or surgical excision.

Deterioration of the Gastrostomy Tube

With the growing number of PEG placements, it is important to define clinical indicators for tube replacement. Tube deterioration leads to decreased structural integrity and luminal patency, thereby increasing the number of tube-clearing interventions.[65] Deterioration can ultimately result in the fragmentation of the tube with the passage of internal retaining devices into the stomach, and small-bowel obstruction and even fatal peritonitis can result. In these situations, observation is recommended, but a failure to pass the bumper in 2 to 3 weeks must be evaluated radiologically. If the bumper gets impacted at the ileocecal valve, then colonoscopic removal or laparotomy is indicated.[18] Tube deterioration is multifactorial. Dwell time, tube material, and fungal colonization are all important determinants of tube deterioration. Iber and colleagues[66] found dwell time to be an important determinant of tube failure. They reported a 37% rate of fungal tube failure with the tube in situ at 250 days, and this increased to 70% at 251 to 450 days.[66] Fungal colonization of the tube is one of the most important factors for tube deterioration. A prospective randomized controlled comparison showed that silicone PEG tubes are associated with more short-term complications and fail sooner than polyurethane tubes.[65] However, polyurethane tubes are not resistant to fungal colonization.[67] Histologic studies have demonstrated actual fungal growth into the tube wall that leads to brittleness, dilatation, cracking, and eventual puncture of the tube. No treatment has been shown to be useful.[19] The reason for such aggressive colonization is that the PEG tube serves as the ideal incubator for the *Candida* biofilm, with a high humidity level, a temperature of close to 36°C to 37°C, and the regular provision of fresh culture medium; in addition, the organisms that colonize the PEG tubes are inaccessible to the host's defense mechanisms.[65]

Until better tube materials are developed that are more resistant to fungal colonization, it seems reasonable to perform regular tube checks to assess the need for replacement. Exit-site complications and tube-related complications are indications for gastrostomy tube replacement. Other indications for tube replacement include evidence of fungal colonization (commonly seen as inconsistently sized brown or creamy patches within the tube walls that are resistant to flushing) and changes in the integrity of the tube wall (evidenced by bubbles, dilatation, or blockage to the flow of feeds). The use of polyurethane tubes will also reduce the need for frequent tube changes.[67] In some cases, the repair of the external portion of the tube or the placement of a new tube within the existing one corrects leakage-related issues until a formal tube replacement can be performed.[18]

Leakage Around the Gastrostomy Tube

The reported incidence of leakage around PEG site is 1% to 2%. A recent study shows that 56% of patients receiving long-term home enteral nutrition have problems related to leakage or tube breakdown.[61] Risk factors include PEG site infections, increased gastric acid secretions, excessive cleansing with hydrogen peroxide, buried bumper syndrome, side torsion of the tube, and the absence of an external bolster to stabilize the tube.[64] Peristomal leakage tends to occur more frequently with the pull technique as compared with the push technique.[2] The leaking PEG site must be evaluated for infection, ulceration, or a buried bumper. Remedial measures include proton pump inhibitor therapy to reduce gastric acid secretion. Side torsion can be minimized by clamping the device, thereby reducing the resultant enlargement of the tract and ulceration. A low-profile button can accomplish the same result.[19] Gentle traction of the PEG tube often resolves the leak; however, significant traction may lead to necrosis and worsening of the leak.[18] Usually the replacement of the PEG tube with a larger one is unrewarding.[18,19] The removal of the tube for several days may allow the stoma to shrink, but, in some cases, a new anatomic site may need to be selected for repeat PEG.[18] After the primary cause of stomal leakage is addressed, local skin irritation should be treated with either stoma adhesive powder, zinc oxide, or cleansing with hydrogen peroxide.

Allowing the site to remain open to air will often resolve the dermatitis.[18,19]

Tube Migration Into the Small Bowel

PEG tube migration is an unusual complication of PEG.[18] An external bumper is necessary to prevent the migration of the tube with peristalsis. If the external bumper anchoring the tube is not secure, it may allow the tip of the tube to migrate with gastric motility as far as the fourth part of the duodenum at the duodenojejunal flexure, where it can lodge.[42] Consequences of tube migration include emesis if a distended balloon-tip PEG tube is impacted at the pylorus, irritation of the small bowel leading to gastrointestinal erosion and perforation, and retrograde jejunoduodenal intussusception with bowel ischemia.[18,42] Tube migration can be prevented with certain precautions. During tube replacement, a Foley catheter can lead to tube migration. This can be resolved by applying an external bolster to the catheter, using a replacement gastrostomy tube with an external retaining device, or replacing it with a gastrostomy button.[18] Alternatively, the Foley catheter must be used temporarily until a proper replacement is available. Placing the PEG tube properly to allow for a snug fit of the internal and external retaining devices to the gastric wall and the anterior abdominal wall and keeping the tube held in position with a 0 silk tie will reduce the chance of tube migration. Another suture anchoring the external bumper to the skin provides further protection against tube migration.[42]

Prolonged Ileus and Other Miscellaneous Complications

A prolonged ileus can be observed in 1% to 2% of patients undergoing PEG placement. Tube feeding can be established 3 hours after placement. However, when prolonged ileus is present, it must be managed conservatively. Acute gastric distention after PEG placement can be decompressed by simply uncapping the PEG tube.[19] There are some miscellaneous complications that are worth reviewing. An unusual complication of aortogastric fistula was described by Ware and colleagues,[18] and it led to a fatal hemorrhage in a 4-year-old child. Subcutaneous emphysema has also been described after PEG. It is important to differentiate benign subcutaneous emphysema from that associated with the onset of the more serious necrotizing fasciitis.[18,52] Gastric volvulus after PEG placement results from excessive air inflation at the time of the gastrostomy and the entrance of the PEG site at the posterior wall of the stomach, which, together with minimal adhesion around the stomach, facilitates torsion and volvulus.[68] This can be prevented by avoiding excessive air insufflation and carefully identifying the anterior wall of the stomach during PEG. In the event that this does occur, treatment is surgical, with a mini laparotomy and the revision of the gastrostomy site.[68,69]

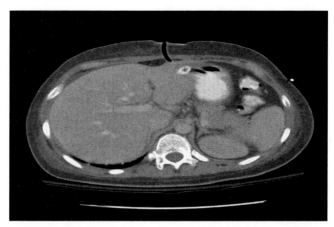

Figure 31-5. Liver injury during percutaneous endoscopic gastrostomy placement.

The liver may also be injured during the insertion of the PEG (Figure 31-5).[70]

QUALITY OF LIFE AND PERCUTANEOUS ENDOSCOPIC GASTRONOMY PLACEMENT

There is very little information regarding health-related quality of life (HRQOL) among patients with PEG placements. The assessment of HRQOL in this group offers special challenges as a result of the heterogeneity of diseases and the substantial cognitive and intellectual impairments seen in this patient population.[71] Quality of life (QOL) has become essential in all situations in which the disease or its treatment is likely to induce physical, emotional, cognitive, social, family, or professional impairment. It is important to validate PEG placement by evaluating treatment-related side effects and potential complications with regard to their impact on HRQOL. Large retrospective studies have shown that the overall mortality rates for patients who have PEG placement are between 59% and 63% at 1 year after the procedure.[72] This is not surprising, because most often PEG placement is for palliation or adjuvant to cancer treatment. However, this does raise questions regarding the benefit that PEG provides to this subgroup of patients. The American Gastroenterology Association has recommended that PEGs be placed only in patients who have a life expectancy of more than 30 days. The indications for PEG placement need to be reviewed closely, and a part of the decision-making process regarding PEG placement should involve the potential effects on the patient's QOL.

Klose and colleages[72] prospectively studied the effects of PEG placement on QOL and nutritional status. PEG compensated for gross nutritional deficiencies, and the Gastrointestinal Quality of Life Index was used to assess QOL. Subjective assessments related to PEG were assessed with an additional four questions (i.e.,

the PEG QOL Index). An unrestricted QOL could be maintained in 61% of the patients. Bannerman and colleagues[68] also showed that PEG placement had a positive influence on HRQOL. Although the QOL was found to be poorer among this group as compared with the general population (as can be expected), a positive effect was seen among 55% of patients and 80% of caregivers. Most patients reported that they could cope with the care of the gastrostomy and the administration of feeds adequately.[71]

Among patients with head and neck cancer, an emerging problem is the increasing incidence of treatment-related pharyngoesophageal stenosis associated with organ-sparing chemoradiotherapy regimens. Dysphagia occurs in up to 50% of patients receiving chemoradiotherapy. PEG placements are often indicated for these patients in anticipation of feeding difficulties. Severe treatment-related side effects such as mucositis, xerostomia, and poor oral intake compounded by dependence on the PEG can result in irreversible changes in the oropharyngeal mucosa leading to stenosis and fibrosis. An imperative part of "up front" PEG placement should be the ongoing encouragement of oral intake to avoid this complication and early PEG-tube dependence. Patients must be constantly coached by the health-care team to continue oral intake for as long as possible throughout treatment.[73]

REFERENCES

1. Hujala K, Sipila J, Pulkkinin J, et al: Early percutaneous endoscopic gastrostomy nutrition in head and neck cancer patients. *Acta Otolaryngol* 2004;124(7):847–850.
2. Tucker AT, Gourin CG, Ghegan MD, et al: "Push" versus "pull" percutaneous endoscopic gastrostomy tube placement in patients with advanced head and neck cancer. *Laryngoscope* 2003;113: 1898–1902.
3. Allison SP: Malnutrition, disease, and outcome. *Nutrition* 2000; 16(7–8):590–593.
4. Beer KT, Krause KB, Zuercher T, et al: Early percutaneous endoscopic gastrostomy insertion maintains nutritional state in patients with aerodigestive tract cancer. *Nutr Cancer* 2005;52(1): 29–43.
5. Piquet MA, Ozsahin M, Larpin I, et al: Early nutritional intervention in oropharyngeal cancer patients undergoing radiotherapy. *Support Care Cancer* 2002;10(6):502–504.
6. de Baere T, Chapot R, Kuoch V, et al: Percutaneous gastrostomy with fluoroscopic guidance: Single-center experience in 500 consecutive cancer patients. *Radiology* 1999;210:651–654.
7. Lin HS, Ibrahim HZ, Kheng JW, et al: Percutaneous endoscopic gastrostomy: Strategies for prevention and management of complications. *Laryngoscope* 2001;111:1847–1852.
8. Bhama JK, Haas MK, Fisher WE: Spread of a pharyngeal cancer to the abdominal wall after percutaneous endoscopic gastrostomy. *Surg Laparosc Endosc Percutan Tech* 2001;11:375–378.
9. Ruppin H, Lux G: Percutaneous endoscopic gastrostomy in patients with head and neck cancer. *Endoscopy* 1986;18(4): 149–152.
10. Gauderer MW, Ponsky JL, Izant RJ Jr: Gastrostomy without laparotomy: A percutaneous endoscopic technique. *J Pediatr Surg* 1980;15(6):872–875.
11. Russell TR, Brotman M, Norris F: Percutaneous gastrostomy: A new simplified and cost-effective technique. *Am J Surg* 1984; 148(1):132–137.

12. Ho CS: Percutaneous gastrostomy for jejunal feeding. *Radiology* 1983;149:595–596.

13. Deurloo EE, Schultze Kool LJ, Kroger R, et al: Percutaneous radiological gastrostomy in patients with head and neck cancer. *Eur J Surg Oncol* 2001;24(1): 94–97.

14. Beaver ME, Myers JN, Griffenberg L: Percutaneous fluoroscopic gastrostomy tube placement in patients with head and neck cancer. *Arch Otolaryngol Head Neck Surg* 1998;124:1141–1144.

15. Kozarek RA, Ball TJ, Ryan JA: When push comes to shove: a comparison between two methods of percutaneous endoscopic gastrostomy. *Am J Gastroenterol* 1986;81:642–645.

16. Lee DS, Mohit-Tabatabai MA, Rush BF, et al: Stomal seeding of head and neck cancer by percutaneous endoscopic gastrostomy tube placement. *Ann Surg Oncol* 1995;2:170–173.

17. Righi PD, Reddy DK, Weisberger EC, et al: Radiologic percutaneous gastrostomy: Results in 56 patients with head and neck cancer. *Laryngoscope* 1998;108:1020–1024.

18. Schapiro GD, Edmundowicz SA: Complications of percutaneous endoscopic gastrostomy. *Gastrointest Endosc Clin N Am* 1996;6(2):409–422.

19. Lynch CR, Fang JC: Prevention and management of complications of percutaneous endoscopic gastrostomy (PEG) tubes. *Practical Gastroenterology* 2004;66–76. (http://www.healthsystem.virginia.edu/internet/digestive-health/nutritionarticles/lyncharticle.pdf)

20. Foutch PG: Complications of percutaneous endoscopic gastrostomy and jejunostomy: Recognition, prevention, and treatment. *Gastrointest Endosc Clin N Am* 1992;2:231–248.

21. Grant JP: Percutaneous endoscopic gastrostomy: Initial placement by single endoscopic technique and long-term follow up. *Ann Surg* 1993;217(2):168–174.

22. Muz J, Mathog RH, Nelson R, et al: Aspiration in patients with head and neck cancer and tracheostomy. *Am J Otolaryngol* 1989;10(4): 282–286.

23. Dumortier J, Lapalus MG, Pereira A, et al: Unsedated transnasal PEG placement. *Gastrointest Endosc* 2004;59(1):54–57.

24. Ehrsson YT, Langiuseklof A, Bark T, et al: Percutaneous endoscopic gastrostomy (PEG): A long-term follow-up study in head and neck cancer patients. *Clin Otolaryngol* 2004;29:740–746.

25. Peterson TI, Kruse A: Complications of percutaneous endoscopic gastrostomy. *Eur J Surg* 1997;163:351–356.

26. Gauderer MW, Stellato TA, Wade DC: Complications related to gastrostomy button placement. *Gastrointest Endosc* 1993;39:467

27. Lattuneddu A, Morgagni P, Benati G, et al: Small bowel perforation after incomplete removal of percutaneous endoscopic gastrostomy catheter. *Surg Endosc* 2003;17:2028–2031.

28. Galat SA, Gerig KD, Porter JA, Slezak FA: Management of premature removal of the percutaneous gastrostomy. *Am Surg* 1990;56(11):733–736.

29. Pofahl WE, Ringlod F: Management of early dislodgement of percutaneous gastrostomy tubes. *Surg Laparosc Endosc Percutan Tech* 1999;9(4):253–256.

30. Marshall JB, Bodnarchuk G, Barthel JS: Early accidental dislodgement of PEG tubes. *J Clin Gastroenterol* 1994;18:210–212.

31. Blocksom JM, Sugawa C, Tokioka S, et al: Endoscopic repair of gastrostomy after inadvertent removal of percutaneous endoscopic gastrostomy tube. *Surg Endosc* 2004;18:868–870.

32. Thornton FJ, Fotheringham T, Haslam PJ, et al: Percutaneous radiological gastrostomy with and without T-fastener gastropexy: A randomized comparison study. *Cardiovasc Intervent Radiol* 2002;25:467–471.

33. Strock P, Weber J: Buried bumper syndrome. *Endoscopy* 2005; 37:279.

34. Gencosmanoglu R, Koc D, Tozun N: The buried bumper syndrome: migration of internal bumper of percutaneous endoscopic gastrostomy tube into the abdominal wall. *J Gastroenterol* 2003; 38:1077–1080.

35. Frascio F, Giacosa A, Piero P, et al: Another approach to the buried bumper syndrome. *Gastrointest Endosc* 1995;41:505–508.

36. Vargo JJ, Ponsky JL: Percutaneous endoscopic gastrostomy: Clinical applications. *Medscape Gastroenterology eJournal* 2000;2(4). Available at http://www.Medscape.com/viewarticle/407957.

37. Anagnostopoulos GK, Kostopoulos P, Arvanitidis DM: Buried bumper syndrome with a fatal outcome, presenting as a gastrointestinal bleeding after percutaneous endoscopic gastrostomy placement. *J Postgrad Med* 2003;49(4):325–327.

38. Ma MM, Semlacher EA, Fedorak RN, et al: The buried gastrostomy bumper syndrome: Prevention and endoscopic approaches to removal. *Gastrointest Endosc* 1995;41:508–511.

39. Obed A, Hornung M, Schlottmann K, et al: Unnecessary delay of diagnosis of buried bumper syndrome resulting in surgery. *Eur J Gastroenterol Hepatol* 2006;18:789–792.

40. Vu CF: Buried bumper syndrome: Old problems, new tricks. *J Gastroenterol Hepatol* 2002;17:1125–1128.

41. Papakonstantinou K, Karagiannis A, Tsirantonaki M, et al: Mediastinitis complicating a percutaneous endoscopic gastrostomy: A case report. *BMC Gastroenterol* 2003;6:3–11.

42. Bumpers HL, Collure WD, Best IM, et al: Unusual complications of long-term percutaneous gastrostomy tubes. *J Gastrointest Surg* 2003;7(7):917–920.

43. Evans PM, Serpell JW: Small bowel fistula: a complication of percutaneous endoscopic gastrostomy. *Aust N Z J Surg* 1994;64(7): 518–520.

44. Yoshihiro K, Harushi U, Yoshiaki K, et al: Cologastric fistula and colonic perforation as a complication of percutaneous gastrostomy. *Surg Laparosc Endosc* 1999;9(3):220–222.

45. Younossi ZM, Strum WB, Schatz RA, et al: Effect of combined anticoagulation and low dose aspirin in upper gastrointestinal bleeding. *Dig Dis Sci* 1997;42(1):79–82.

46. Lau G, Lai SH: Fatal retroperitoneal hemorrhage: an unusual complication of percutaneous endoscopic gastrostomy. *Forensic Sci Int* 2001;116:69–75.

47. Robinson SR, Johnston P, Wyeth JW: Aortic perforation due to an impacted percutaneous endoscopic gastrostomy gastric flange: Case report. *ANZ J Surg* 2001;71:71–72.

48. Kanie J, Akatsu H, Suzuki Y, et al: Mechanism of development of gastric ulcer after percutaneous endoscopic gastrostomy. *Endoscopy* 2002;34:480–482.

49. Ulla JL, Alvarez V, Carpio D, et al: Upper gastrointestinal bleeding in a patient with balloon bumper PEG feeding tube. *Surg Laparosc Endosc Percutan Tech* 2005;115(2):94.

50. Dharmarajan TS, Yadav D, Adiga GU, et al: Gastrostomy, esophagitis, and gastrointestinal bleeding in older adults. *J Am Med Dir Assoc* 2004;5(4):228–232.

51. Cappell MS: Esophageal bleeding after percutaneous endoscopic gastrostomy. *J Clin Gastroenterol* 1998;10(4):383–385.

52. Balbierz JM, Ellis K: Streptococcal infection and necrotizing fasciitis—Implications for rehabilitation: A report of 5 cases and review of literature. *Arch Phys Med Rehabil* 2005;85:1205–1209.

53. Yusoff IF, Ormonde DG: Subcutaneous leak with subcutaneous emphysema. *Gastrointest Endosc* 2000;51(1):88–90.

54. Chung RS, Schetzer M: Pathogenesis of complications of percutaneous endoscopic gastrostomy: A lesson in surgical principles. *Am Surg* 1990;56:134–137.

55. McLean AA, Miller G, Bamboat ZM, et al: Abdominal wall necrotizing fasciitis from dislodged percutaneous endoscopic gastrostomy tubes: A case series. *Am Surg* 2004;70(9):827–831.

56. Sharma VK, Howden CW: Meta-analysis of randomized controlled trials of antibiotic prophylaxis before percutaneous endoscopic gastrostomy. *Am J Gastroenterol* 2000;95(11):3133–3136.

57. Lalwani AK, Kaplan MJ: Mediastinal and thoracic complications of necrotizing fasciitis of the head and neck. *Head Neck* 1991;13(6):531–539.

58. Alagaratnam TT, Ong GB: Wound implantation—a surgical hazard. *Br J Surg* 1977; 64(12):872–875.

59. Schneider AM, Loggie BW: Metastatic head and neck cancer to the percutaneous endoscopic gastrostomy exit site: A case report and review of literature. *Am Surg* 1997;63(3):481–486.

60. Thakore JN, Mustafa M, Suryaprasad S, et al: Percutaneous endoscopic gastrostomy associated gastric metastasis. *J Clin Gastroenterol* 2003;37(4):307–311.

61. Brown MC: Cancer metastasis at percutaneous endoscopic gastrostomy stomata is related to the hematogenous or

lymphatic spread of circulating tumor cells. *Am J Gastroenterol* 2000;95(11):3288–3291.

62. Adelson RT, Ducic Y: Metastatic head and neck carcinoma to a percutaneous endoscopic gastrostomy site. *Head Neck* 2005;27(4):339–343.

63. Chandu A, Smith ACH, Douglas M: Percutaneous endoscopic gastrostomy in patients undergoing resection for oral tumors: A retrospective review of complications and outcomes. J *Oral Maxillofac Surg* 2003;61:1279–1284.

64. Crosby J, Duerksen D: A retrospective survey of tube-related complications in patients receiving long-term home enteral nutrition. *Dig Dis Sci* 2005;50:1712–1717.

65. Blacka J, Donoghue J, Sutherland M, et al: Dwell time and functional failure in percutaneous endoscopic gastrostomy tubes: A prospective randomized-controlled comparison between silicon polymer and polyurethane percutaneous endoscopic gastrostomy tubes. *Aliment Pharmacol Ther* 2004;20:875–882.

66. Iber F, Livak A, Patel M: Importance of fungus colonization in failure of silicone rubber percutaneous gastrostomy tubes PEGS. *Dig Dis Sci* 1996;411:226–231.

67. Trevisani L, Sartori S, Rossi MR, et al: Degradation of polyurethane gastrostomy devices: What is the role of fungal colonization? *Dig Dis Sci* 2005;50:463–469.

68. Sookpotarom P, Vejchapipat P, Chongsrisawat V, et al: Gastric volvulus caused by percutaneous endoscopic gastrostomy: A case report. *J Pediatr Surg* 2005;40:E21–E23.

69. Deutsch LS, Kannegieter L, Vanson DT: Simplified percutaneous gastrostomy. *Radiology* 1992;184:181–183.

70. Gubler C, Wildi SM, Bauerfeind P: Liver injury during PEG placement: a report of two cases. *Gastrointest Endosc* 2005;61(2):346–348.

71. Bannerman E, Pendlebury J, Phillips F, et al: A cross-sectional and longitudinal study of health-related quality of life after percutaneous gastrostomy. *Eur J Gastroenterol Hepatol* 2000;12(10):1101–1109.

72. Klose J, Heldwein W, Rafferzeder M, et al: Nutritional status and quality of life in patients with percutaneous endoscopic gastrostomy (PEG) in practice: Prospective one-year follow-up. *Dig Dis Sci* 2003;48(10):2057–2063.

73. Gougen LA, Posner MR, Norris CM, et al: Dysphagia after sequential chemoradiation therapy for advanced head and neck cancer. *Otolaryngol Head Neck Surg* 2006;134:916–922.

Complications of Intubation and Emergency Airway Management

M. Boyd Gillespie, Brian Craig, and Stephen F. Dierdorf

The likelihood of a serious airway complication in normal patients undergoing routine, elective procedures is quite low. The increasing prevalence of obesity, the more aggressive surgical management of head and neck cancer and reconstructive facial surgery, and the aging of the population, however, have created new challenges for airway management. Early intervention by the otolaryngologist after an emergency airway has been established can reduce the likelihood of long-term airway complications. It is not unusual for a critically ill patient to recover from a serious medical or surgical illness but to be left with a severely limiting airway complication (e.g., tracheal stenosis).

The incidence of difficult airway management among patients presenting for elective surgery has been defined by several studies. These studies suggest an incidence of difficult tracheal intubation of 1% to 2% and the incidence of ventilation difficulty to be less than 1%.[1,2] Others report the incidence of difficult tracheal intubation to be as high as 13%.[3] Difficult tracheal intubation is also associated with a greater incidence of airway injury.[4]

The incidence of difficult tracheal intubation outside of the operating room is not well known, but it may be 3% to 5% in the emergency department.[5] The intubation of patients in the intensive care unit (ICU) may be difficult in 12% of patients, with significant complications occurring in 28%.[6] Airway emergencies often prevent many of the airway examination and evaluation procedures that are possible for elective airway management, and therefore the prediction of airway difficulty is less certain. Healthcare providers with airway-management expertise are not always readily available in emergent situations, and the inexperience of the provider may increase the risk of airway injury. The emergency management of the airway may be required before the patient arrives at the hospital (prehospital), in the emergency department, in the hospital ward, in the ICU, or in the operating room. The development of effective supraglottic airway devices during the past 10 years has lessened the need for emergent tracheal intubation by inexperienced providers. Out-of-hospital tracheal intubation is a highly controversial issue, and the complication rate may be high.[7] A modern approach to emergency airway management may entail the insertion of a supraglottic device (e.g., laryngeal mask airway [LMA (LMA North America, San Diego, CA)], Combitube [Tyco-Kendall Mansfield, MA]) and effective ventilation being established until a provider with expertise in tracheal intubation can be present. Cooperative efforts among paramedics, emergency physicians, anesthesiologists, and otolaryngologists can improve training and reduce the risk of serious airway complications.[8] The formation of a "difficult airway team" composed of anesthesiologists with special expertise in airway techniques is effective for managing unanticipated airway problems in the operating room.[9] The presence of an otolaryngologist with airway expertise is invaluable when invasive techniques may be required.

AIRWAY EVALUATION

There is no single examination or evaluation technique that reliably predicts difficulty with airway management and tracheal intubation. Consequently, there are many airway evaluation techniques. Patients with a history of difficult airway management are often aware of previous problems. It is important during the airway evaluation to differentiate potential difficult ventilation from difficult intubation. However, a normal airway examination should not provide a false sense of security; preparations for alternative management techniques should always be made.[10]

The most commonly used method for airway evaluation is the Mallampati classification in which the patient is asked to open the mouth and protrude the tongue.[11] A more accurate assessment may be the modified Mallampati, also known as the *Friedman tongue position score,* which is used in sleep apnea assessment and in which the patient opens the mouth without protruding the tongue (Figure 32-1). These scoring systems estimate the size of the tongue relative to the oral cavity and may indicate whether the displacement of the tongue by the laryngoscope blade may be difficult. Other factors that influence the airway examination include the state and occlusion of the dentition, the mouth opening, the thyromental and sternomental distance, the cervical range of motion, the neck length and thickness, the presence of a beard, and the body mass index. The thyromental distance assesses the mandibular space and indicates the relative ease of tongue displacement. If the distance from the mentum to the thyroid cartilage is less

Tongue Sizes

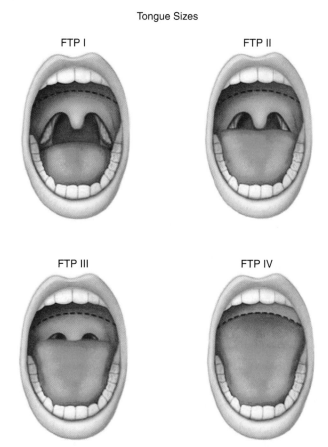

Figure 32-1. The Friedman tongue position evaluates the size of the tongue in relation to the overall airway volume.

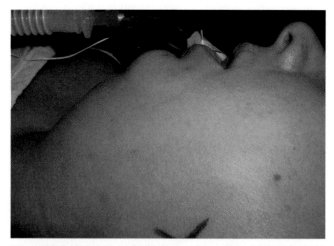

Figure 32-2. A physical feature suggestive of difficult laryngoscopy includes a convex thyromental angle.

than 6 cm, rigid laryngoscopy may be difficult (Figure 32-2). Sternomental distance reflects head and neck mobility. If the distance from the mentum to the manubrium is less than 13.5 cm, laryngoscopy may be difficult. Identifying the cricothyroid membrane in every patient is useful in the event that an emergent invasive airway procedure becomes necessary (Figure 32-3).

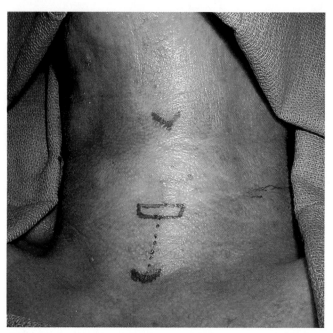

Figure 32-3. Palpable landmarks of the upper airway for emergency tracheotomy planning include the thyroid notch, the cricothyroid space, and the sternal notch.

Despite a multifactorial evaluation technique, many cases of difficult mask ventilation and difficult tracheal intubation cannot be predicted.[12]

PREVENTION OF COMPLICATIONS

The consequences of the lost airway with the inability to ventilate are dire, and they all too frequently cause death or permanent neurologic disability. Alternative techniques for ventilation and tracheal intubation have been developed to provide the practitioner with additional methods should primary airway techniques fail. The successful outcome of an airway emergency depends on timely and effective intervention.

Difficult Airway Guidelines

Several professional societies representing medical specialties involved with airway management have developed guidelines for emergency airway management. These guidelines are directed at aiding physicians with making sound clinical decisions in a timely manner to avoid the devastating consequences of inadequate ventilation and hypoxemia that can lead to death or permanent neurologic injury. Guideline development is based on a thorough analysis of published scientific material and comprehensive expert opinion. As new information accrues, guidelines must be methodically reviewed and periodically updated. The American Society of Anesthesiologists published the first societal difficult airway guidelines in 1993, and they were subsequently updated in 2003.[13,14] Societies in France, Canada, and Italy have also developed guidelines for the management of the difficult airway.[15] Proof of the efficacy of the guidelines is difficult to obtain, but there is evidence that the incidence of significant airway events during the induction phase of anesthesia has decreased significantly since the introduction of the guidelines.[16]

Tracheal Intubation Technique

Tracheal intubation is most commonly performed with rigid direct laryngoscopy. Although there are a variety of laryngoscope blades available, most can be classified as either straight blade (e.g., Miller and Wisconsin blades) or curved (e.g., Macintosh blade). These blades are designed to provide a line-of-sight axis for the visualization of the glottis by pushing the anterior tongue to the left side of the mouth and displacing the base of the tongue into the retromandibular space. An enlarged tongue (as may occur with lingual tonsillar hypertrophy or obesity), abnormal dentition, poor mouth opening, or decreased cervical range of motion may complicate this technique and render tracheal intubation difficult or impossible (Figure 32-4). As the degree of difficulty for rigid direct laryngoscopy increases, the risk of injury to the upper airway also increases.

Alternative Ventilation and Intubation Techniques

Laryngeal Mask Airway

The invention of the LMA introduced a new class of airways: the supraglottic airways. When correctly positioned, the LMA rests directly above the glottic inlet, thereby bypassing structures of the mouth and pharynx and providing a patent airway. Insertion of the LMA is done by propelling the device along the surface of the hard and soft palate and into the hypopharynx with the

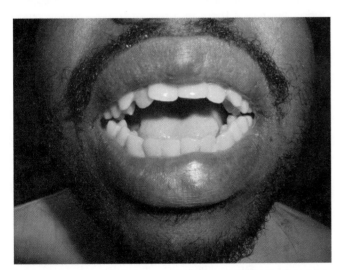

Figure 32-4. Trismus presents a possible contraindication to orotracheal intubation.

index finger. After the LMA is positioned, the cuff is inflated, and a seal is established around the glottis that permits spontaneous or positive-pressure ventilation. When the LMA is inserted with the cuff deflated, only minimal mouth opening is required, and the device conforms to the patient's airway anatomy.

Since the introduction of the LMA into clinical practice in the United States in 1992, the device has proven to be reliable and extremely effective, with only a minimal risk of complications for emergency intubation. The success of the original or classic LMA gave rise to different models, most notably the intubating LMA. Most practitioners find the intubating LMA easier to insert than the classic LMA. The intubating LMA has a wide-bore airway shaft that permits the passage of tracheal tubes with an internal diameter as large as 9 mm. The intubating LMA is a dual-purpose airway in that it provides an avenue for ventilation as well as a guide for tracheal intubation. The C-trach is an intubating LMA with a fiber-optic imaging bundle. A small screen can be attached to the C-trach for the direct imaging of the glottic inlet. Many other supraglottic airways have been introduced into clinical practice. Some are for ventilation only, and others provide a route for intubation. Currently the intubating LMA is the most mature, with a large body of published experience discussing its use.

Flexible Fiberscopes

A flexible fiberscope was first used for tracheal intubation during the late 1960s. Since that time, the technologic development of flexible fiberscopy has been substantial. The most recent advance was the introduction of the video fiberscopes. These fiberscopes provide a wide-angle, high-resolution image of the airway, and they are invaluable for the tracheal intubation of patients with pharyngeal or laryngeal cancer and patients who have sustained upper airway trauma. The primary advantages of the flexible fiberscope are that the device conforms to the patient's anatomy and that it can be navigated through the most anatomically abnormal airways. The flexible fiberscope can also be used as a diagnostic tool for the examination of the airway when the origin of the abnormality is not known. The disadvantage of the flexible fiberscope is that it cannot provide ventilation. Many anesthesiologists are now highly skilled in the use of the flexible fiberscope, and the instrument has become a mainstay for airway management in the operating room.

Rigid Fiber-optic Laryngoscopes

Fiber-optic and digital imaging systems have been applied to rigid direct laryngoscopes to improve image quality and reduce the need for a line-of-sight axis to visualize the glottic inlet. The risk of trauma to the teeth and pharynx is reduced by indirect imaging techniques. These systems have proven especially useful for the tracheal intubation of morbidly obese patients. Some manufacturers produce interchangeable systems that permit for a rapid transition from rigid laryngoscopy to flexible fiberscopy.

Airway Device Cuffs

Most airway devices—whether tracheal tubes or supraglottic airways—have a cuff that, when inflated, provides an airtight seal in the airway and permits positive-pressure ventilation. Ideally the cuff pressure should not exceed 25 cm of water. Inflation of the cuff above the pressure required to "just seal" the device incurs the risk of excessive pressure against the wall of the airway. Minor side effects include tracheal tube cuff herniation and sore throat. More severe complications include airway wall necrosis and damage to nerves within the airway wall. Necrosis leads to scarring and a decrease in the diameter of the airway lumen. The cuff of any airway device must be carefully inflated to a pressure that minimizes the risk of excessive intracuff pressures. Although the routine pressure monitoring of airway devices is not standard practice, it may be indicated for patients with airway devices that will be in place for prolonged periods of time.

Nitrous oxide diffuses into air-filled spaces 30 times faster than nitrogen can diffuse out of the space. Any air-filled space exposed to nitrous oxide will consequently either expand or undergo a significant pressure increase, depending on the compliance of the space. If inhaled nitrous oxide is used during the administration of anesthesia, the pressure can increase in tracheal tube and supraglottic airway devices to very high levels. This problem can be avoided by eliminating nitrous oxide from the anesthetic or filling the tracheal tube cuff with saline or a mixture of nitrous oxide and oxygen.[17]

Extubation Techniques

Current studies indicate that the risk of a lost airway may be greater at the time of extubation than at the time of intubation. There are no completely reliable indicators for safe extubation. Physiologic indicators include satisfactory arterial blood gas values, a low alveolar–arterial oxygen gradient, adequate neuromuscular function to provide a normal tidal volume and vital capacity, the clearance of hypnotic drugs, and an unobstructed upper airway. Temporary deflation of the tracheal tube cuff and an audible leak around the deflated cuff generally indicate that any laryngeal swelling has diminished enough to permit extubation. Before extubation, any equipment or devices required for reintubation should be at the bedside, and their proper function should be ensured. Direct inspection of the airway with a flexible fiberscope or a rigid laryngoscope may be indicated if obstructive lesions are suspected. If the previously mentioned requirements have been met and there is still any doubt about the patient's ability to tolerate extubation, an airway exchange catheter can be inserted into the trachea via the tracheal tube before extubation. Should reintubation be necessary, a new tracheal tube can be passed over the airway exchange catheter.

Indications for Reintubation

Failure to tolerate tracheal extubation can be caused by poor respiratory control, poor gas exchange at the alveolar–capillary interface, inadequate neuromuscular function to generate an adequate minute ventilation, and airway obstruction. Airway obstruction is the most uncertain, because the other functions can be quantified before extubation. An obstructive lesion that is bypassed by an airway device can certainly obstruct the airway after the device is removed.

COMPLICATIONS OF INTUBATION

Head and Face

Ocular Injury

Significant ocular injury during airway management is rare, but, when it occurs, it can be painful and uncomfortable. Injury can occur during the intubation process from direct trauma to the eye from the laryngoscope or the laryngoscopist's fingers. The most common manifestation of eye injury is corneal abrasion. The incidence of clinically significant corneal abrasion is 0.06% to 0.17%,[18] although diagnosis by fluorescein staining has a much higher incidence. Care must be taken to avoid eye contact during laryngoscopy and intubation. The eyes should be protected after intubation if the patient is heavily sedated or anesthetized. A bland lubricant can be applied to the eyes before the lids are taped shut. Hard-shelled eye protectors are indicated during surgery if there is a risk of trauma to the eyes. Postoperative patients with corneal abrasions usually complain of severe eye pain and photophobia. Treatment consists of antibiotic ointment and patching of the eye if pain is severe. Topical local anesthesia provides short-term relief of pain.

Epistaxis

Epistaxis is a frequent complication of a traumatic nasotracheal intubation. To reduce the risks of this complication, efforts should be made to have patients stop taking anticoagulants before surgery, to correct thrombocytopenia with a platelet transfusion (>60 K/cm^3), and to reduce systemic hypertension. The resultant bleed is usually self-limited, but it may increase the risk of aspiration and the loss of airway during an awake fiber-optic intubation on a patient with a difficult airway.

The following steps should be taken during nasotracheal intubation to reduce the risk of this complication:

1. The anterior nasal cavity should be visually inspected with an adequate light source to assess for significant septal deviations or inferior turbinate hypertrophy that may impede the placement of the nasotracheal tube.

2. Both nasal cavities should be thoroughly decongested with four to five squirts of oxymetazoline spray directed at the lateral wall of the nasal cavity or with oxymetazoline-soaked pledgets 5 minutes before intubation.

3. The nasal cavity is then anesthetized and serially dilated with silicone nasal airway trumpets of increasing diameter that are coated with lidocaine jelly.

4. The nasal trumpets and the endotracheal tube should be advanced along the floor of the nose parallel to the hard palate and not directed superiorly, where trauma to the middle turbinate and the skull base can result.

5. If there is significant resistance to the nasal trumpets of the nasotracheal tube, the dilation steps should be repeated on the opposite side to assess for easier passage.

6. The smallest-diameter nasotracheal tube that will allow for adequate ventilation should be selected.

7. The nasotracheal tube should be well lubricated with lidocaine jelly or surgical lubricant and passed smoothly and rapidly with gentle pressure into the nasopharynx before attempting to guide the tube with the fiber-optic scope.

If epistaxis does occur during nasotracheal intubation, oropharyngeal suctioning should be immediately performed to prevent aspiration and to improve the visualization of the airway with a fiber-optic scope. The airway should be secured as rapidly as possible. The nasal cavity should be flooded with oxymetazoline spray, and gentle pressure should be applied to the soft nasal dorsum. After the airway is secure and the patient is under general anesthesia, an absorbable packing material can be placed around the nasotracheal tube to promote hemostasis.

Nasal Alar Necrosis

Ulceration and necrosis of the nasal ala are frequently overlooked complications of nasotracheal intubation. Although these injuries have little functional consequence, necrosis and ulceration of the soft triangle of the nasal ala may cause significant cosmetic deformity as a result of the notching and retraction of the nasal rim. Repair of the defect is difficult to achieve; therefore emphasis is placed on the prevention of this complication.

Nasal alar ulceration and necrosis can occur within the first 24 hours of intubation. The nasotracheal tube should be secured with either tape or a columellar suture in a fashion that secures the tube caudally and medially away from the nasal rim. If contact between the nasotracheal tube and the nasal rim is noted, an effort should be made to provide a buffer with a petroleum gel gauze wrap around the tube. The nasal rim should be assessed at least twice a day for the erythema and indentation that precede ulceration. If these early signs of pressure necrosis are noted, the nasotracheal tube should be repositioned or replaced with a smaller tube or an orotracheal tube. If ulceration is noted, the tube should be removed and the nasal rim managed with antibiotic ointment until healing has occurred. Patients with a persistent deformity should be referred to an experienced rhinoplastic surgeon for further management.

Rhinosinusitis

Rhinosinusitis is a recognized complication of prolonged nasotracheal intubation as a result of the mechanical obstruction of the sinus ostia by the nasotracheal tube. Rhinosinusitis may also occur among orotracheally intubated patients as a result of the obstruction of the sinus ostia from positional edema of the nasal cavity, a lack of nasal airflow, and the accumulation of nasal secretions caused by reduced mucociliary clearance as a result of pharyngeal obstruction from the orotracheal tube. The incidence of sinusitis may approach 20% among patients in the ICU who are intubated for more than 5 days.[19] In a study of 351 patients in the ICU with fever of unknown origin (FUO) examined by sinus plain films and follow-up sinus aspiration, van Zanten and colleagues[20] found sinusitis to be the sole cause of fever in 16% of patients and a contributing cause in 14%. Up to one third of intubated ICU patients with FUO may therefore have clinically significant sinusitis. Immunocompromised patients or those with head injury with blood in the sinuses may be at particular risk for clinically significant sinusitis.[21]

The early recognition and management of nosocomial sinusitis in the ICU population may have a profound impact on patient outcome. Nasotracheally intubated patients in the ICU with FUO who are screened and treated for sinusitis have been shown to have significantly lower rates of ventilator-associated pneumonia and higher 2-month survival rates as compared with control patients not evaluated for sinusitis.[22] Intubated patients with FUO should be evaluated by nasal endoscopy, if feasible, and imaging of the maxillary sinus with plain films, computed tomography (CT) scanning, or ultrasound imaging. The visualization of purulence in the middle meatus on nasal endoscopy is the greatest positive predictor for positive culture on maxillary sinus aspiration.[23] Patients with evidence of sinus opacification, purulent sinus discharge, or both should be managed with the removal of the mechanical obstruction (e.g., nasotracheal tube, nasogastric tube); aggressive nasal irrigation with saline spray three times a day; nasal decongestion acutely (i.e., oxymetazoline twice daily for 3 days) and chronically (i.e., nasal steroid spray daily for 2 to 3 weeks); and a broad-spectrum antimicrobial. Strong consideration should be given to performing a maxillary sinus aspiration and lavage on the most opacified side to obtain material for culture given the diversity and resistance profile of nosocomial infections. *Pseudomonas* and *Klebsiella,* however, are the dominant causative species among this population.[20] Maxillary sinus puncture can be performed with a large-bore needle (i.e., 18 gauge) sublabially through the canine fossa or transnasally through the inferior meatus 1 cm to 2 cm behind the nasal vestibule.

Patients who do not respond to initial interventions may require a sinus CT scan to assess the response to therapy as well as the opacification of additional sinuses (e.g., frontal, sphenoid). Intraoperative endoscopy and sinusotomy are recommended if there is a concern of sepsis, abscess, meningitis, or an unusual organism (e.g., fungal).

Cervical Spine Injury

Cervical spine injury during tracheal intubation in patients without cervical pathology is exceedingly rare. The risk of spinal cord injury from airway management in patients with known neck injury is also unlikely when a practitioner experienced with airway management is available.[24] The intubation of patients with cervical spine injury is complicated by the need to maintain the head in a neutral position and by the limitations of mouth opening and cervical mobility that a hard cervical collar produces.[25] Rigid direct laryngoscopy can be performed if the head is maintained in a neutral position. Alternative intubation techniques include the intubating LMA, the C-trach LMA, flexible fiber-optic assisted laryngoscopy, or rigid laryngoscopy with modified laryngoscope blades.[26]

Oral Complications

Oral and Pharyngeal Edema and Laceration

Direct trauma to the soft tissues of the oral cavity and oropharynx during intubation may result in laceration, ulceration, and edema. Typically these injuries are the result of trauma from the leading edge of the laryngoscope, but they may also result from an intubating stylet or a poorly positioned endotracheal tube. The application of a thin layer of lubricating jelly to the lips

and the laryngoscope may reduce the tendency of tissue to catch on the edge of the scope. Soft-tissue trauma is rare if the patient is fully relaxed, if the appropriate-sized laryngoscope with a strong light source is used, and if an assistant is available to retract the lips or to provide cricoid pressure, as indicated. Oral and pharyngeal lacerations rarely need repair, and they can be managed with saline gargles and lubricating or anesthetic gels.

Uvular edema and necrosis are frequent causes of sore throat and odynophagia after intubation. These effects most likely result from pressure on the uvula by the endotracheal tube during the operative procedure. Examination is notable for an edematous uvula that is either erythematous or pale, with necrotic debris. Treatment with saline gargles, oral antibiotics and analgesics, and a steroid taper pack provide comfort and promote healing. In rare cases, greatly enlarged uvulas that cause significant gagging or supine orthopnea require surgical amputation.

Dental Injury

Injury to the teeth, gums, and lips is relatively common during laryngoscopy. Although rarely life-threatening unless teeth are aspirated, these injuries produce discomfort for patients. Claims for dental injury may be the most numerous of liability claims against anesthesiologists. The largest reported series detected an incidence of dental injury requiring treatment of 1 in every 4500 anesthetic treatments. If the cases not requiring treatment were included, there can be little doubt that the incidence would be much higher. Risk factors for perianesthetics injuries include tracheal intubation, coexisting poor dentition, and difficult laryngoscopy.[27] The reported incidence of dental trauma from tracheal intubation during emergency conditions ranges from 0.5% to 3.7%.[28] The most commonly injured teeth are the upper incisors and crowns. The lower incisors are more frequently injured during emergent endointubation; this may be the result of other attempted airway maneuvers before intubation.[29] Dental injury can also occur during patient awakening as the patient bites on the endotracheal tube. The practice of using hard oral airways as bite blocks should be discouraged, because teeth can be dislodged when the patient bites. Bite blocks should be made of soft, compressible material and positioned between the occlusal surfaces of the molars.

Combitube Injuries

The esophageal–tracheal Combitube is primarily used for difficult intubations or in "cannot ventilate, cannot intubate" situations.[30] The Combitube is a double-lumen tube that is an improved variant of the esophageal obturator. One tube is patent and can serve as a tracheal tube if the Combitube is inadvertently inserted into the trachea. The Combitube is designed to be passed blindly into the esophagus, at which point a distal balloon is inflated with 15 ml of air and a proximal pharyngeal balloon is inflated with 100 ml of air. The primary tube is sealed at the end, and there are a series of openings that are more proximal. After the two balloons seal the esophagus and the pharynx, ventilation occurs through the fenestrations in the tube that are situated adjacent to the glottic inlet. The Combitube is simple to insert and requires only minimal training for the user to become proficient. After the Combitube is placed and secured, the device is very stable. The device is quite popular with paramedics and combat medics as a result of its reliability and stability under adverse conditions.[31,32] Although it is meant for short-term use, prolonged ventilation via the Combitube has been reported. A tracheostomy can be performed with the Combitube in place if a more definitive airway is required.

Reported complications from the use of the Combitube include pharyngeal and esophageal trauma that may include laceration.[33] Although not a common practice, the Combitube has been used for airway management among patients undergoing elective surgery. Because the pharyngeal cuff is a high-volume, high-pressure cuff, a postoperative sore throat is to be expected.

Supraglottic Airways

The versatility and reliability of the LMA led to a proliferation in the development of many types of supraglottic airways. Some of these devices have undergone rigorous scientific investigation, whereas others have had only cursory examination. These devices have an airway shaft and some type of mechanism, usually an inflatable balloon, to provide an airtight seal in the hypopharynx. Most complications are the result of forceful insertion with subsequent trauma to the pharynx or the larynx or the overinflation of the cuff causing excessive pressure against the pharyngeal mucosa and its underlying structures. Injuries to the lingual nerve, the hypoglossal nerve, the recurrent laryngeal nerve, and the glossopharyngeal nerve have been reported with the use of supraglottic airways. Nerves may be injured by pressure from the airway shaft on the tongue or pressure from the cuff of the device against the pharyngeal wall. Some neuropraxias resolve spontaneously, whereas others may require surgical palliation.[34,35] Proper sizing and minimal cuff inflation of the supraglottic airway may minimize the risk of pressure-related complications.

Glottic Complications

Glottic Soft-Tissue Trauma

Direct injury to the soft tissues of the larynx may occur as a result of a traumatic intubation resulting in laryngeal edema, hematoma, or laceration. Soft-tissue injuries of the larynx are most commonly the result of the forceful advancement of the endotracheal tube or of an exposed stylet. If trauma is suspected at the time of anesthesia, direct laryngoscopy should be performed to directly assess the extent of injury. Tissue flaps should be reapproximated with endolaryngeal instruments, and they may require trimming if they are obstructing the airway. Vocal-fold hematomas should be drained by laryngeal needle or microscissors followed by gentle pressure with an oxymetazoline-soaked pledget to avoid airway obstruction at extubation or chronic hoarseness from the formation of a hemorrhagic polyp or vocal-fold fibrosis (Figure 32-5).

If not recognized at the time of surgery, patients with glottic soft-tissue trauma may present with stridor, dysphonia, sore throat, odynophagia, or dysphagia after extubation. Patients with stridor and air hunger should be immediately evaluated with fiber-optic laryngoscopy to rule out the need for reintubation. Unfortunately there is no rule regarding when to reintubate a patient with airway obstruction. Typically, if there is significant edema with a glottic airway of less than 4 mm (e.g., the diameter of a standard flexible endoscope) and the work of breathing is increased, reintubation should be performed in a controlled fashion, with a surgical airway set available. Less severe cases can be managed with intensive care monitoring, intravenous steroids (i.e., 10 mg of dexamethasone every 8 hours for 24 hours), cool mist humidity, saline gargles, and helium and/or oxygen (heliox) inhalation. Hematomas or lacerations large enough to result in dyspnea or dysphonia are best managed with timely surgical drainage, the reapproximation of tissue flaps, or both. Small lacerations and

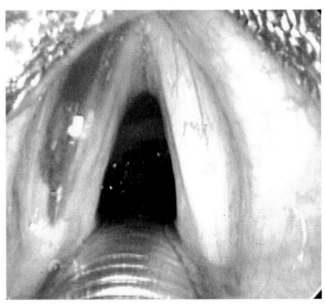

Figure 32-5. Hematoma of the left vocal cord after traumatic intubation.

hematomas that cause only sore throat or mild dysphagia can typically be observed, with improvement expected over 24 to 48 hours.

Vocal-Process Granulomas

Vocal-process granulomas are nonneoplastic inflammatory lesions that are often referred to as *intubation granulomas.* Vocal-process granulomas are reparative processes that consist of hyperplastic squamous epithelium overlying an infiltrate of acute and chronic inflammatory cells and fibroblasts without the typical mononuclear or multinucleated histiocytes that are seen in true granulomatous processes.[36] The most common cause of the lesion is the ulceration of the posterior vocal cord adjacent to the vocal process from endotracheal tube trauma, laryngopharyngeal reflux, or voice abuse.[37] Intubation trauma is generally assumed to be the underlying cause if the patient was intubated within 3 months of presentation. Patients typically present with raspy or breathy dysphonia, cough, foreign-body sensation, and, more rarely, dysphagia or dyspnea. Flexible laryngoscopy typically reveals a fleshy, pale to pink exophytic growth in the posterior third of the vocal fold adjacent to the vocal process. Computed tomography is not required for diagnosis, but it may reveal perichondritis of the arytenoid cartilage and rule out the possibility of tumor invasion of the thyroarytenoid or the paraglottic space.

The treatment of vocal-process granulomas is predominantly medical; therefore empiric therapy aimed at addressing the underlying cause can be instituted without biopsy in low-risk individuals when the history is consistent with the diagnosis. Treatment consists of a steroid taper pack, inhaled topical steroids, an aggressive antireflux regimen (i.e., a proton-pump inhibitor taken twice daily with a type 2 histamine blocker taken at bedtime), and voice therapy in patients with abusive or hyperfunctional vocal characteristics. Direct laryngoscopy with the removal of the lesion is recommended for patients who present with stridor or dyspnea or with atypical symptoms such as otalgia and odynophagia; for individuals at high risk for head and neck cancer (e.g., tobacco and alcohol users); and for patients who do not respond to medical treatment or who demonstrate a progression of the lesion after 4 to 6 weeks of medical therapy. Surgery should focus on obtaining sufficient material for pathologic diagnosis as well as the conservative debridement of the base of the lesion with sharp dissection. Treating the base of the lesion with a 1-cc injection of triamcinolone solution (i.e., 40 mg/ml) or topical mitomycin C (i.e., 1 cc of 0.4 mg/ml solution) on a pledget for 5 minutes may reduce the recurrence of the lesion. Overly aggressive resection results in additional tissue trauma and ongoing inflammation that can cause recurrence.

Vocal-Fold Motion Impairment

Breathy dysphonia after extubation may indicate vocal-fold motion impairment. The diagnosis is confirmed by flexible endoscopy, which most commonly demonstrates an immobile vocal fold in the paramedian or lateral position with a persistent glottic gap during adduction (sustained vowel articulation). Vocal-fold motion impairment from endotracheal tube trauma is most commonly the result of vocal-cord paralysis/paresis and rarely the result of arytenoid dislocation.

Vocal-Fold Paralysis and Paresis

Intubation-related vocal-fold paresis and paralysis are most commonly attributed to a high-riding endotracheal tube with an inflated cuff at the level of the subglottis that results in a pressure neuropraxia of the recurrent laryngeal nerve as it enters the posterior endolarynx adjacent to the cricothyroid joint.[21] The injury is best prevented by ensuring that the cuff of the tube is inserted beyond the subglottis and that the minimal cuff inflation volumes needed to eliminate air leak are maintained at pressures of less than 25 mm Hg (i.e., tracheal capillary perfusion pressure). The risk of paralysis also increases with chronic pressure from the endotracheal tube in the posterior glottis; therefore tracheotomy should be considered for patients requiring a prolonged intubation of more than 10 days.

Patients with unilateral vocal-fold paralysis and paresis after intubation typically present with a low-volume, breathy voice that fatigues with repeated use. Dysphagia (especially with liquids) and cough during swallow are less common and may indicate an associated injury of the internal branch of the superior laryngeal nerve. Flexible laryngoscopy typically reveals a vocal fold in the paramedian or lateral position that may be slightly flaccid or bowed with incomplete glottic closure on full adduction (e.g., sustained vowel articulation). The integrity of the internal branch of the superior laryngeal nerve can be tested by tapping the ipsilateral supraglottis with the scope to elicit the glottic closure reflex and cough. In the majority of cases, it is advisable to rule out silent aspiration with the assessment of the patient's swallow by a speech pathologist with either a modified barium swallow or a flexible endoscopic evaluation of swallow. Rigid videostroboscopy is helpful for differentiating between vocal-fold paralysis and arytenoid dislocation as well as for documenting subtle changes in mobility during a period of observation.

The early treatment of vocal-fold paralysis and paresis is indicated among patients who have evidence of aspiration, who have difficulty communicating as a result of the loss of the voice, or who require a strong cough for adequate pulmonary toilet (e.g., thoracic and cardiac surgical patients). Observation alone is indicated in less

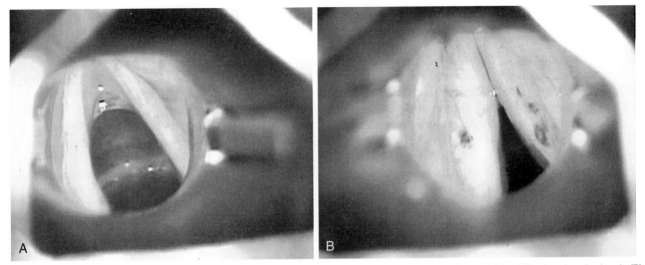

Figure 32-6. A paralyzed left vocal cord with vocalis atrophy and bowing **(A)** is rehabilitated with the injection of lyophilized cadaveric dermis **(B)**.

severe cases, because the majority of intubation-related paralyses will demonstrate gradual improvement over time. The initial treatment of vocal-fold paralysis and paresis consists of the injection of a resorbable implant (e.g., autologous fat, gelatin sponge, lyophilized cadaveric dermis, hyaluronic acid gel) either transorally or percutaneously in the office or operating room setting (Figure 32-6). The temporary implants provide vocal rehabilitation while allowing time for neural recovery or full denervation atrophy to occur. Patients with preoperative evidence of aspiration will require repeat swallowing assessment and therapy to ensure the safety of their diets. Patients may additionally benefit from voice therapy to prevent the onset of maladaptive vocal strain. If no improvement in vocal-fold mobility is documented after 6 to 12 months of observation, patients may benefit from medialization laryngoplasty with a permanent implant if sufficient denervation atrophy has occurred. Laryngeal electromyography may be performed if more prognostic information is desired.

Bilateral vocal-fold paralysis is rarely caused by intubation alone unless the patient has a preexisting vocal-cord paralysis from another cause. Therefore patients with a history of unilateral vocal-fold paralysis require careful intubation technique and management. Bilateral vocal-fold paralysis may present acutely with airway distress and stridor at extubation or in a delayed fashion with a chief complaint of dyspnea and air hunger. Voice and swallow are typically asymptomatic. Patients with acute presentation may require reintubation followed by intravenous steroids (10 mg of dexamethasone every 8 hours), with a repeated attempt at extubation in 24 hours. Patients who fail a second extubation attempt or who have severe obstruction should proceed to tracheotomy. The decision of when and how to intervene is more challenging with chronic bilateral vocal-fold paralysis. In general, the reestablishment of a patent

airway is indicated if the maximal glottic aperture is less than 4 mm (e.g., the diameter of the standard flexible endoscope) or the maximal mid-inspiratory effort on a flow-volume loop is less than 1.5 L/s (Figure 32-7). The patient will have to decide between a tracheostomy tube, which preserves the voice and provides an excellent airway, or a glottic-enlargement technique (e.g., partial cordectomy, arytenoidectomy, arytenoid lateralization), which avoids a tracheostomy tube albeit with a loss of voice and a less optimal airway. Patients with less severe symptoms may be closely observed over time, but they will have to limit their activity levels. In addition, these patients should always have an active prescription of oral steroids on hand and an emergency

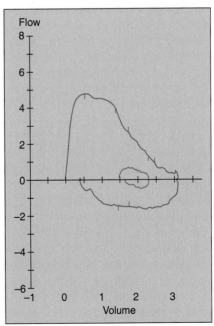

Figure 32-7. The flow-volume loop of a patient with bilateral vocal cord immobility demonstrates a critical reduction and flattening in inspiratory airflow (area below zero).

number to call in the event of sudden airway distress from an upper respiratory infection or laryngitis.

Arytenoid Dislocation

Arytenoid dislocation is a rare disorder that may result from intubation trauma. In the largest reported series of arytenoid dislocations in 63 patients, 80% were the result of a traumatic intubation, whereas the remaining 20% were the result of external trauma.[38] The disorder is more frequently observed among females (60%), perhaps as a result of the placement of endotracheal tubes that are too large for the glottic aperture.[38] Although rare, the possibility of arytenoid dislocation should be considered whenever vocal-fold immobility is observed after extubation. Early diagnosis and intervention allow for the optimal repositioning of the arytenoid and increase the likelihood of sustaining joint mobility by preventing the onset of ankylosis.

Rigid videostroboscopy is superior to flexible endoscopy for the diagnosis of arytenoid dislocation. Unlike flexible endoscopy, rigid videostroboscopy improves the ability to visualize subtle differences between vocal-fold levels, which occur more frequently with dislocation as compared with paralysis. In addition, videostroboscopy may provide information about the mechanism of injury and the direction in which force should be applied during closed reduction. An anteromedial inferiorly displaced vocal process with a shortened vocal fold likely indicates an anterior dislocation that occurred during intubation, whereas a posterolateral superiorly rotated vocal process is most commonly the result of a posterior dislocation from an extubation injury. A fine-cut laryngeal CT scan without contrast may confirm the diagnosis; however, a normal CT is not adequate to rule out the disorder. Laryngeal electromyography may be valuable for differentiating arytenoid dislocation from nerve injury, but up to 40% of patients with dislocation have a coexisting laryngeal nerve paresis or paralysis as determined by laryngeal electromyography.[38]

Diagnostic laryngoscopy with the palpation of the arytenoid may also be helpful for differentiating between vocal-fold paralysis and arytenoid dislocation. The arytenoid of a paralyzed vocal fold is supple and allows for the gentle displacement of the vocal process when nudged by a suction tip, whereas the dislocated arytenoid demonstrates reduced mobility. The closed reduction of posterior dislocations can be managed by placing a Miller no. 3 laryngoscope in the ipsilateral pyriform sinus and applying gentle anterosuperior pressure. Anterior dislocations are reduced with gentle posterolateral pressure from a Hollinger laryngoscope.[39] The goal of closed reduction is the reestablishment of the medially rotated vocal process at a level equal to the opposing fold. If there is a concern that the joint is hypermobile and that it may redislocate, then the injection of an absorbable material (e.g., autologous fat, gelatin sponge, lyophilized cadaveric dermis, hyaluronic gel) lateral to the joint and the vocal process may improve the orientation and stability of the arytenoid. Approximately 70% of patients will have voice improvement after closed reduction, but most patients will continue to have some degree of vocal impairment, which may improve with voice therapy.[38] Patients who have no improvement may benefit from open surgical repair (e.g., type I laryngoplasty, arytenoid adduction, arytenoidopexy) to improve the height of the vocal process.

Glottic Stenosis

Indwelling endotracheal tubes frequently induce the ulceration of the thin mucosa overlying the laryngotracheal cartilages as a result of pressure necrosis. These ulcerations can be demonstrated within the first 24 hours after intubation, and they increase in frequency and severity with time.[40] The ulcerations may be exacerbated by repeated trauma from excessive tube mobility or from ongoing chemical injury from laryngopharyngeal reflux. In an autopsy study of 41 intubated patients, mucosal ulcers were found at the level of the epiglottis in 12%, at the level of the posterior glottis in 51%, and in the trachea at the level of the endotracheal tube cuff in 15%.[41] If extubated within a timely fashion, most of these injuries are asymptomatic and will spontaneously reepithelialize. When the depth of injury extends to the submucosa and the perichondrium, healing will occur by fibrosis and scar contracture, thereby leading to laryngotracheal stenosis.

The risk of laryngotracheal stenosis is best managed by prevention. A 2% incidence of laryngotracheal stenosis has been observed among patients who are intubated for less than 6 days, whereas the incidence increases to 12% among patients who are intubated for more than 10 days.[42] A study of 280 patients examined by endoscopy fewer than 6 months after an ICU admission found evidence of laryngotracheal stenosis in 7% of patients.[43] The major risk factor for stenosis identified with multiple logistic regression analysis was an intubation time of more than 11 days. In an effort to reduce the incidence of long-term laryngotracheal stenosis, current evidence largely supports tracheotomy for patients who will likely require mechanical ventilation for more than 10 days.[44]

Intubation-related glottic stenosis typically presents weeks to months after intubation as the scar tissue forms and slowly occludes the glottis.[45] Symptoms most commonly include exertional dyspnea, stridor, and dry cough, with lesser degrees of vocal impairment. Glottic stenosis from intubation is almost always located posteriorly as a result of pressure on this region from the endotracheal tube.[46] Direct laryngoscopy or videostroboscopy may demonstrate reduced vocal-fold mobility, thickened interarytenoid tissue, and/or adhesions between the vocal processes. The degree of functional impairment should be assessed with flow-volume loops. Patients with maximum inspiratory flows of less than 1.5 L/s are highly impaired and may require airway enlargement.

The condition may be confused with vocal-fold paralysis if the scar tissue is not obvious; therefore a confirmation of the diagnosis generally requires intraoperative laryngoscopy. When glottic stenosis is suspected, the surgeon and the anesthesiologist must work as a team to determine the optimal method of airway management. If the patient has favorable anatomy for direct laryngoscopy, the airway can be safely managed with the induction of anesthesia followed by direct laryngoscopy with ventilation via a small cuffed or cuffless endotracheal tube or jet ventilation. Patients with challenging anatomy for laryngoscopy (e.g., obesity, large tongue, small mandible, anterior larynx) are best managed by awake fiber-optic intubation if the glottic aperture permits or awake tracheotomy. After the airway is established, glottic stenosis is diagnosed with the gentle lateral palpation of the vocal process with a suction tip. If the vocal fold is not supple or if the entire larynx shifts with palpation, stenosis is likely present. Inspection of the entire airway with a rigid fiber-optic telescope will magnify offending scar tissue and often reveal coexisting distal subglottic or tracheal stenoses.[47]

The treatment of glottic stenosis depends on the severity of disease. The classification scheme of Bogdasarian and Olsen[48] classifies posterior glottic stenosis into the following four categories:

1. Interarytenoid synechia with posterior sinus tract

2. Posterior commissure scar without a posterior tract

3. Posterior commissure scar with a unilaterally fixed arytenoids

4. Posterior commissure scar with bilaterally fixed arytenoids

Thin webs and scar bands between the vocal processes respond well to endoscopic division with either laser or cold techniques (Figure 32-8). The application of a topical mitomycin-C–soaked pledget (0.4 mg/cc) for 5 minutes followed by a saline rinse has been reported to reduce restenosis.[49] Posterior commissure scar bands without tracts may require the elevation of a mucosal flap with the division of scar followed by laryngeal dilation. Posterior bands with arytenoid fixation can be treated endoscopically with posterior cordectomy or arytenoidectomy. If scar tissue extends into the subglottis, open surgery with laryngofissure, scar excision, and posterior cricoid split with cartilage graft may be necessary. Open surgery is usually preceded by tracheotomy, because most patients will require a laryngeal keel (e.g., preformed keel, latex finger cot) for 2 to 3 weeks postoperatively. Alternatively, tracheotomy provides an excellent airway and good voice for patients with bilateral fixation or complicated glottic

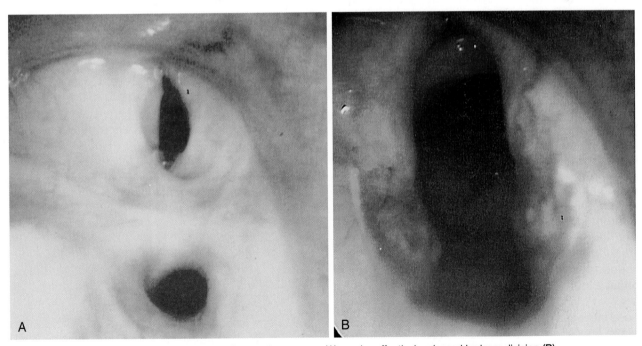

Figure 32-8. A scar between the vocal processes **(A)** can be effectively released by laser division **(B)**.

or subglottic stenoses. All patients should be treated with aggressive reflux management before and after surgical management given the high rates of reflux disorders in this patient population.

Tracheal Complications

Tracheal Stenosis

Endotracheal intubation is the most common cause of stenosis of the subglottis and trachea.[50] The pathophysiology involves ischemia of the tracheal wall from pressure necrosis as a result of contact with the endotracheal tube and cuff. Pressures exceeding the capillary perfusion pressure of 25 mm Hg can result in ulceration and chondritis, with subsequent granulation tissue and fibrosis leading to progressive cicatricle obliteration of the tracheal lumen.[46] Risk factors for the development of tracheal stenosis include prolonged intubation, high cuff pressures, oversized endotracheal tubes, and associated medical comorbidities such as diabetes, sepsis, and hypotension.[46] The likelihood of stenosis is reduced by systematic checks of endotracheal tube cuff pressure, with the ideal pressure remaining below 25 mm Hg. The movement of the tube should be minimized with adequate taping, and tracheotomy should be performed if an intubation of more than 10 days is anticipated.

Some degree of tracheal stenosis has been noted in up to 10% of patients with prolonged intubation.[51] The vast majority of these lesions are clinically insignificant; however, a small percentage of patients will experience progression of the stenosis that usually becomes clinically evident when the airway is narrowed by 50% or more.[21] Symptomatic patients typically experience progressive dyspnea on exertion with or without biphasic stridor that can be mistaken for a wheeze. Many patients will present after unsuccessful treatment with bronchodilator therapy. Laryngotracheal stenosis should be highly suspected in any patient with a history of intubation and progressive dyspnea that is not explained by other medical conditions. Longer lesions can be visualized with plain-film x-ray scans (Figure 32-9), but the length of the lesion and the degree of stenosis are better assessed with a fine-cut CT scan. The classic flow-volume loop demonstrates a fixed, extrathoracic obstruction with flattening of the inspiratory and expiratory loops. The diagnosis is confirmed by flexible or rigid bronchoscopy, which can characterize the maturation of the scar as well as the presence of synchronous lesion from the glottis to the segmental bronchi (Figure 32-10).

Limited stenoses of less than 1 cm in length may be amenable to endoscopic techniques such as the creation of four-quadrant radial incisions with a carbon dioxide laser

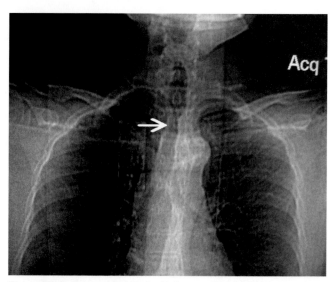

Figure 32-9. Dyspneic patient with low cervical tracheal stenosis noted on a chest x-ray film. Arrow denotes tracheal narrowing.

followed by dilation with rigid bronchoscopy, Jackson dilators, or balloon dilation (Figure 32-10). The application of topical mitomycin C potentially reduces the rate of restenosis.[49] Tracheal resection and anastomosis are currently the preferred methods for the management of longer lesions.[52] The accessibility of the lesion to transcervical repair must be assessed preoperatively by bronchoscopy and imaging. Lesions that are less than 3 cm in length can usually be excised without release, whereas lesions that are longer than 3 cm typically require the transection of the suprahyoid muscles and hyoid osteotomy at the lesser cornu for sufficient tension-free closure. When subglottic stenosis is present, the cricoid ring anterior to the cricothyroid joint is resected with subsequent thyrotracheal anastomosis. The tracheostomy stoma should be included in the resection, if present. Anastomosis is performed with circumferential, interrupted, submucosal 3.0 polyglactin 910 sutures with two 2.0 silk-stay sutures placed laterally between tracheal rings above and below the anastomosis. Preferably no tracheotomy will be performed, and the patient is extubated immediately after surgery. The patient's head is kept flexed with a reminder stitch between the chin

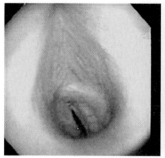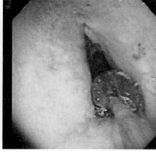

Figure 32-10. High tracheal stenosis with attempted treatment with balloon dilation.

and chest for 5 to 7 days postoperatively. Airway stenting via a tracheotomy tube or a T-tube is often required for patients with long stenotic segments (i.e., >6 cm), associated laryngeal stenosis or tracheomalacia, poor surgical risk, or ongoing tracheal inflammatory disease. Indwelling tracheal stents are not recommended for benign tracheal stenosis as a result of the high rates of occlusion from granulation tissue, retained secretions, and stent fracture.[53]

Tracheomalacia

Prolonged intubation by both endotracheal and tracheostomy tubes is a recognized cause of tracheomalacia, a condition that is characterized by the weakness and collapse of a segment of the trachea caused by the weakening of the cartilage, of the longitudinal elastic fibers of the membranous tracheal wall, or of both.[54] Tracheomalacia more commonly occurs in the setting of prolonged intubation, high-dose steroid exposure, smoking history, chronic obstructive pulmonary disease, and obstructive sleep apnea.[54] Symptoms include dyspnea, cough, increased sputum production, wheezing, and stridor. The current gold standard for diagnosis is flexible bronchoscopy in the spontaneously ventilating patient with the demonstration of a luminal collapse of more than 50%. The collapse is more pronounced on expiration, with inward bulging of the membranous wall and flattening of the tracheal rings. Recent studies have suggested that a collapse of more than 50% on expiratory dynamic spiral CT scanning demonstrates excellent correlation with bronchoscopic findings for the diagnosis of tracheomalacia.[55,56] Flow-volume loops demonstrate decreased forced expiratory volume in 1 second, with rapid decreases in flow and relatively normal inspiratory loops.[54]

Intubated patients with underlying lung disease who require high pressures for ventilation are at the greatest risk for tracheomalacia. As airway pressures increase, the cuff pressure must also increase to maintain a seal. This can lead to a destructive cycle of progressive increases in cuff pressures and tube sizes, with resulting enlargement and weakening of the trachea. If a patient in this situation requires ongoing intubation, there are two options for management[21]:

1. Perform a tracheotomy and insert a flexible armored endotracheal tube with an adjustable flange (e.g., Bivona) so that the cuff position can be moved up or down by 2 cm on a daily basis, thereby limiting the trauma to any one tracheal site.

2. Convert to high-frequency ventilation, which obviates the need for a tube cuff in many patients.

Many adults with tracheomalacia are incidentally diagnosed at the time of bronchoscopy for other pulmonary disease, and they require no specific therapy. Symptomatic patients with short-segment malacia (<6 cm) who are good surgical candidates may be amendable to resection and anastomosis. Unfortunately, most patients with symptomatic tracheomalacia are poor surgical candidates as a result of extensive collapse involving the bronchi, associated stenotic lesions, severe underlying pulmonary disease, and other medical conditions (e.g., obesity, diabetes, obstructive sleep apnea). Poor surgical candidates may improve with continuous positive airway pressure devices alone, or they may require stenting of the weak segment with a tracheotomy tube or a T-tube.

EMERGENCY SURGICAL AIRWAY MANAGEMENT

Indications and Techniques for Emergency Surgical Airway Management

The creation of an emergency surgical airway is indicated for patients with upper airway obstruction who cannot be ventilated and intubated by other means. Common reasons for failure to intubate include difficult anatomy, upper airway edema, obstructing mass lesion, severe oropharyngeal hemorrhage, and maxillofacial or neck trauma.[57] A surgical airway should be attempted after one or two attempts at intubation by an experienced endoscopist if the patient cannot be ventilated or if the patient is rapidly decompensating from the lack of an airway.

The three principal techniques for establishing a surgical airway include cricothyroidotomy, tracheotomy, and needle cricothyroidotomy. Emergency cricothyroidotomy is a highly effective means of establishing a surgical airway, with success rates ranging from 88% to 100%.[57] Cricothyroidotomy has been advocated as the emergency surgical airway procedure of choice because it is fast and less bloody, it has better palpable landmarks, and it is easier to teach to nonsurgical personnel.[58] Less is known about the role of tracheotomy in the emergency situation; however, 100% of patients were successfully cannulated by tracheotomy in one case series of emergency airway procedures.[57] Although percutaneous dilation tracheotomy has gained acceptance in the elective setting, the use of this technique is discouraged in the emergency situation as a result of the lack of bronchoscopic visualization.[44] Needle cricothyroidotomy with jet ventilation has been proposed as an alternative method to establish an emergency airway; this may be especially useful as an initial intervention until a surgical airway can be established.[21,57]

Complications of Emergency Surgical Airways

Emergency surgical airways frequently result in complications as a result of the factors that surround the emergency scenario itself, including the need for haste, operator stress, poor patient anatomy (e.g., obesity, short neck), poor visualization, and the lack of appropriate equipment. Complications occur in 13% to 40% of cases of emergency cricothyroidotomy.[59–63] The complication rate of emergency tracheotomy is estimated to be three times greater than the 15% complication rate observed for elective tracheotomy.[64] In addition, higher complication rates are observed for emergency surgical airways performed in the inpatient setting as compared with the emergency room, perhaps as a result of the younger, predominantly male trauma population that requires surgical airway establishment in the emergency room suite.[57]

Failure to Establish an Airway

The most devastating potential complication of emergency surgical airway procedures is the failure to establish an airway. Experiences with the techniques in the nonemergent setting will likely improve surgical success; however, all physicians and emergency personnel should be familiar enough with airway anatomy to at least attempt to place a surgical airway if the situation dictates. Although not every surgical airway will be successful, failure to try will lead to certain anoxic brain injury or death in most instances.

Surgical airways can fail despite the successful opening of the airway if the surgical opening cannot be cannulated. False passage and an inability to intubate can occur if the intubating tube is too large to fit through the surgical opening or if excessive force is used for tube insertion (Figure 32-11). The average height of the adult cricothyroid membrane is 9 mm; therefore the use of a small cuffless tracheotomy tube (i.e., No. 4 Shiley [Nellcor Puritan Bennett, Boulder, CO], 5.0-mm internal diameter Portex [Smiths Medical, Watford, UK]) or a No. 6 cuffless endotracheal tube (i.e., 8.2-mm outer diameter) will increase the likelihood of a successful cannulation.

The recommended technique involves grasping the laryngotracheal complex with the nondominant hand and making a long vertical incision through the skin and the subcutaneous fat. Finger or blunt dissection is performed to the level of the cricothyroid space or the tracheal rings. A generous incision is made until an air gurgle is heard. The hole is maintained with a finger until it can be cannulated with a small uncuffed endotracheal or tracheotomy tube.

Hemorrhage

Brisk hemorrhage is frequently encountered during the placement of an emergency surgical airway, and it is of secondary importance to the establishment of a patent airway. Bleeding should be anticipated, and it is best ignored or rapidly managed with a combination of surgical hemostats and strong suction. Common sources of bleeding include the skin, the anterior jugular veins, the thyroid gland, and the tracheal mucosa. The risk of

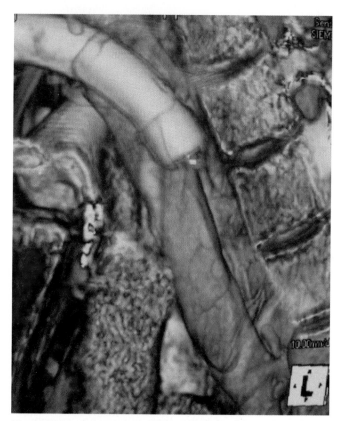

Figure 32-11. Traumatic tracheostomy tube insertion through the posterior tracheal wall into the upper esophagus.

bleeding is reduced with the use of a vertical incision over the laryngotracheal complex, thereby avoiding the lateral great vessels. Subcutaneous tissue is thinnest over the cricothyroid space, and entering the airway through this space avoids the thyroid isthmus. When the airway is secure and the patient is successfully ventilating, bleeding vessels can be individually ligated or cauterized. If the tube makes access to the bleeding sites difficult, the wound should be packed with an absorbable surgical dressing or iodoform gauze. If bleeding persists, manual pressure can be applied to the wound and the patient transported to the operating room for wound exploration. Therapeutic bronchoscopy with airway lavage and suctioning may be needed to remove blood and clot from the airway (Figure 32-12).

A high innominate artery is usually below the level of the cricothyroid space, and it can be easily palpated and avoided. However, the innominate artery may be at risk for delayed hemorrhage if a tracheotomy is placed low in the neck. An anteriorly rotated tracheotomy tube or an excessively inflated tracheotomy cuff may cause pressure erosion of the anterior tracheal wall with the subsequent formation of a tracheoinnominate fistula. Often patients will present after a brief, brisk, sentinel bleed through their tube or stoma. These patients should be hemodynamically stabilized and the airway inspected with flexible endoscopy with the tracheostomy tube in

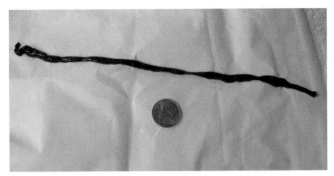

Figure 32-12. Occlusive bronchial clot removed with therapeutic bronchoscopy.

situ. If an anterior erosion, a large clot, or an active bleed is visualized, a cardiovascular surgery consult should be obtained. Angiography can alternatively be used to establish the diagnosis if the patient is stable and the diagnosis is highly suspected. If the patient presents with a massive active bleed consistent with the diagnosis, an endotracheal tube should be passed through the stoma distal to the bleeding site and the cuff fully inflated. Finger dissection should then be attempted between the trachea and the sternum in an effort to manually compress the innominate against the posterior sternum. Emergent sternotomy with the ligation of the innominate is indicated.

Subcutaneous Emphysema and Pneumothorax

Patients with upper airway obstruction often generate greatly negative intrathoracic pressures in the attempt to ventilate across the obstruction. When a surgical wound is created in the neck and dissection performed to the level of the airway, negative mediastinal pressures may pull air into the neck and mediastinum, resulting in a rupture of a mediastinal bleb into the pleural space and causing a pneumothorax. Alternatively, ventilating a tube placed in a false passage forces air into the neck and the mediastinum. The aggressive advancement of an endotracheal tube into the airway may result in a tracheobronchial tear and a pneumothorax.

Subcutaneous emphysema is usually benign if the airway is established; however, the expansion of air within the neck before airway cannulation can rapidly transform an urgent airway into an emergent airway as a result of the obliteration of landmarks, the deviation of the airway, and pneumothorax. The risk of this complication is especially high with a poorly placed needle cricothyroidotomy as a result of the ability to deliver large volumes of air rapidly with jet ventilation. The demonstration of air bubbles in a saline-filled syringe on the end of the catheter can help to confirm successful placement in the airway before jet ventilation. After an airway is established, subcutaneous emphysema can be managed with antibiotic prophylaxis and a cervical pressure dressing. If the subcutaneous emphysema worsens or fails to resolve within 24 to 48 hours, bronchoscopy or wound exploration should be performed as a result of the likelihood of a tracheal injury requiring a muscle patch.

The presence of breath sounds should be confirmed over both lung fields after a surgical airway is established. If the patient is stable but breath sounds cannot be heard, the patient should be suctioned, the endotracheal tube repositioned, and the patient reauscultated. If sounds still cannot be heard, an anteroposterior chest film should be obtained. If breath sounds cannot be heard and the patient is requiring high ventilatory pressures or is experiencing a loss of blood pressure, a tension pneumothorax should be suspected and presumptively treated. A large-bore angiocatheter should be placed through the second intercostal space. A loud hiss with the reestablishment of a normal airway and blood pressure is noted if the diagnosis was correct. A chest tube should then be placed in the ipsilateral pleural space in a timely fashion.

Infection

Emergency surgical airways are usually performed in a nonsterile field, thereby increasing the risk of local wound infection. The surgical wound should be thoroughly irrigated with saline after the procedure, followed by gram-positive antibiotic therapy until the first tracheotomy change in 5 to 7 days. Local would infections are generally minor and rarely result in abscess or cellulitis. They can be successfully treated with broad-spectrum antibiotics and local wound care.

Subglottic and Tracheal Stenosis

Subglottic and tracheal stenosis are the most common chronic complications of emergency surgical airways. Jackson[65] discouraged the use of cricothyroidotomy, because the subglottis is the narrowest portion of the laryngotracheal airway, the subglottic tissues are intolerant of contact with a tracheotomy tube, and damage to the cricoid cartilage and the cricothyroid membrane disrupt the only complete ringlike support of the airway. However, Jackson observed high rates of subglottic stenosis in his series as a result of the use of metal tracheotomy tubes in a predominantly pediatric population with underlying inflammatory diseases of the laryngotracheal complex (e.g., diphtheria, tuberculosis). Large retrospective studies of elective cricothyroidotomy demonstrate rates of subglottic stenosis of less than 1% when it is performed in adults without laryngotracheal inflammation.[66,67] Consideration should be given to converting a cricothyroidotomy to a tracheotomy if the patient requires the tube for more than 1 week.[57] Subglottic stenosis after emergency cricothyroidotomy was observed in 5% (1 of 21) to 13% (2 of 15) of survivors in two case series that assessed for this complication[57,60]; therefore the overall risk of this complication is thought to be acceptable given the clinical indications.

Bronchoscopic evaluation after the placement of an emergency surgical airway may identify fractured or displaced cartilaginous fragments that should be surgically reduced or debrided to prevent long-term tracheal stenosis and tracheomalacia. Patients with emergency surgical airways who require prolonged tracheotomies encounter similar rates of tracheal stenosis and tracheomalacia as compared with patients with prolonged intubation. When encountered, these conditions are managed in a similar fashion to that previously described.

CONCLUSION

Intubation and emergency airway management are areas of critical concern to the otolaryngologist–head and neck surgeon. An understanding of the potential complications of these techniques and of the factors that cause them can help them to be avoided or managed appropriately.

REFERENCES

1. Rose DK, Cohen MM: The airway problems and predictions in 18,500 patients. *Can J Anaesth* 1994;41:372–383.
2. El-Ganzouri AR, McCarthy RJ, Tuman KJ, et al: Preoperative airway assessment: Predictive value of a multivariate risk index. *Anesth Analg* 1996;82:1197–1204.
3. Heidegger T, Gerig HJ, Ulrich B, et al: Validation of a simple algorithm for tracheal intubation: Daily practice is the key to success in emergencies—An analysis of 13,248 intubations. *Anesth Analg* 2001;92:517–522.
4. Domino KB, Posner KL, Caplan RA, et al: Airway injury during anesthesia. *Anesthesiology* 1999;91:1703–1711.
5. Levitan RM: Myths and realities: The "difficult airway" and alternative devices in the emergency setting. *Acad Emerg Med* 2001;8:829–832.
6. Jaber S, Amraoui J, Lefrant J-Y, et al: Clinical practice and risk factors for immediate complications of endotracheal intubation in the intensive care unit: A prospective, multiple center study. *Crit Care Med* 2006;34:2355–2361.
7. Wang HE, Yealy DM: Out-of-hospital endotracheal intubation: Where are we? *Ann Emerg Med* 2006;47:532–541.
8. Kovacs G, Law JA, Ross J, et al: Acute airway management in the emergency department by non-anesthesiologists. *Can J Anaesth* 2004;51:174–180.
9. Parmet JL, Colonna-Romano P, Horrow J, et al: The laryngeal mask airway reliably provides rescue ventilation in cases of unanticipated difficult tracheal intubation along with difficult mask ventilation. *Anesth Analg* 1998;87:661–665.
10. Yentis SM: Predicting difficult intubation—Worthwhile exercise or pointless ritual? *Anaesthesia* 2002;57:105–109.
11. Mallampati SR, Gatt SP, Gugino LD, et al: A clinical sign to predict difficult tracheal intubation: A prospective study. *Can Anaesth Soc J* 1985;32:429–434.
12. Langeron O, Masso E, Hurauz C, et al: Prediction of difficult mask ventilation. *Anesthesiology* 2000;92:1229–1236.
13. American Society of Anesthesiologists Task Force on Management of the Difficult Airway: Practice guidelines for management of the difficult airway. *Anesthesiology* 1993;78:597–602.
14. American Society of Anesthesiologists Task Force on Management of the Difficult Airway: Practice guidelines for management of the difficult airway. *Anesthesiology* 2003;98:1269–1277.
15. Henderson JJ, Popat MT, Latto P, et al: Difficult Airway Society guidelines for management of the unanticipated difficult intubation. *Anaesthesia* 2004;59:675–694.

16. Peterson GN, Domino KB, Caplan RA, et al: Management of the difficult airway. *Anesthesiology* 2005;103:33–39.
17. Combes X, Schauvilege F, Peyrouset O, et al: Intracuff pressure and tracheal morbidity. *Anesthesiology* 2001;95:1120–1124.
18. Roth S, Thisted RA, Erickson JP, et al: Eye injuries after nonocular surgery: A study of 60,965 anesthetics from 1988 to 1992. *Anesthesiology* 1996;85:1020–1027.
19. Deutschman CS, Wilton P, Sinow J, et al: Paranasal sinusitis associated with nasotracheal intubation: A frequently unrecognized and treatable source of sepsis. *Crit Care Med* 1986;14:111–114.
20. van Zanten AR, Dixon JM, Nipshagen MD, et al: Hospital-acquired sinusitis is a common cause of fever of unknown origin in orotracheally intubated critically ill patients. *Crit Care* 2005;9: R583–R590.
21. Weymuller EA Jr: Complications of intubation and emergency airway management. In Eisele DW, editor: *Complications in head and neck surgery,* St Louis, 1993, Mosby-Year Book.
22. Holzapfel L, Chastang C, Demingeon G, et al: A randomized study assessing the systematic search for maxillary sinusitis in nasotracheally mechanically ventilated patients: Influence of nosocomial maxillary sinusitis on the occurrence of ventilator-associated pneumonia. *Am J Respir Crit Care Med* 1999;159: 695–701.
23. Skoulas IG, Helidonis E, Kountakis SE: Evaluation of sinusitis in the intensive care unit patient. *Otolaryngol Head Neck Surg* 2003;128:503–509.
24. Crosby E: Airway management after upper cervical spine injury: What have we learned? *Can J Anaesth* 2002;49:733–744.
25. Goutcher CM, Lochhead V: Reduction in mouth opening with semi-rigid cervical collars. *Br J Anaesth* 2005;95:344–348.
26. Bilgin H, Bozkurt M: Tracheal intubation using the ILMA, C-trach, or McCoy laryngoscope in patients with simulated cervical spine injury. *Anaesthesia* 2006;61:685–691.
27. Warner ME, Benenfeld SM, Warner MA, et al: Perianesthetic injuries: Frequency, outcomes, and risk factors. *Anesthesiology* 1999;90:1302–1305.
28. Tam AYB, Lau FL: A prospective study of tracheal intubation in an emergency department in Hong Kong. *Eur J Emerg Med* 2001;8: 305–310.
29. Givol N, Gershtansky Y, Halamish-Shani T, et al: Perianesthetic dental injuries: Analysis of incident reports. *J Clin Anesth* 2004;16:173–176.
30. Mort TC: Laryngeal mask airway and bougie intubation failures: The Combitube as a secondary rescue device for in-hospital emergency airway management. *Anesth Analg* 2006;103: 1264–1266.
31. Rabitsch W, Moser D, Inzunza MR, et al: Airway management with endotracheal tube versus Combitube during parabolic flight. *Anesthesiology* 2006;105:696–702.
32. Gabrielli A, Layon AJ, Wenzel V, et al: Alternative ventilation strategies in cardiopulmonary resuscitation. *Curr Opin Crit Care* 2002;8:199–211.
33. Stoppacher R, Teggatz JR, Jentzen JM: Esophageal and pharyngeal injuries associated with the use of the esophageal-tracheal Combitube. *J Forensic Sci* 2004;49:586–591.
34. Brimacombe J, Clarke G, Keller C: Lingual nerve injury associated with the ProSeal laryngeal mask airway: A case report and review of the literature. *Br J Anaesth* 2005;95:420–423.
35. Chan TV, Grillone G: Vocal cord paralysis after laryngeal mask airway ventilation. *Laryngoscope* 2005;115:1436–1439.
36. Devaney KO, Rinaldo A, Ferlito A: Vocal process granuloma of the larynx—Recognition, differential diagnosis and treatment. *Oral Oncol* 2005;41:666–669.
37. Havas TE, Priestley J, Lowinger D: A management strategy for vocal process granulomas. *Laryngoscope* 1999;109:301–306.
38. Rubin AD, Hawkshaw MJ, Moyer CA, et al: Arytenoid cartilage dislocation: A 20-year experience. *J Voice* 2005;19:687–701.
39. Sataloff RT: Arytenoid dislocation: Techniques of surgical reduction. *Operative Tech Otolaryngol Head Neck Surg* 1998;9:196–202.
40. Donnelly WH: Histopathology of endotracheal intubation: An autopsy study of 99 cases. *Arch Pathol* 1969;88:511–520.

41. Stauffer JL, Olson DE, Petty TL: Complications and consequences of endotracheal intubation and tracheotomy: A prospective study of 150 critically ill adult patients. *Am J Med* 1981;70:65–76.
42. Whited RE: A prospective study of laryngotracheal sequelae in long-term intubation. *Laryngoscope* 1984;94:367–377.
43. Esteller-More E, Ibanez J, Matino E, et al: Prognostic factors in laryngotracheal injury following intubation and/or tracheotomy in ICU patients. *Eur Arch Otorhinolaryngol* 2005;262:880–883.
44. McWhorter AJ: Tracheotomy: Timing and techniques. *Curr Opin Otolaryngol Head Neck Surg* 2003;11:473–479.
45. Gardner GM: Posterior glottic stenosis and bilateral vocal fold immobility. *Otolaryngol Clin North Am* 2000;33:855–878.
46. Sue RD, Susanto I: Long-term complications of artificial airways. *Clin Chest Med* 2003;24:457–471.
47. Lorenz RR: Adult laryngotracheal stenosis: Etiology and surgical management. *Curr Opin Otolaryngol Head Neck Surg* 2003;11:467–472.
48. Bogdasarian RS, Olson NR: Posterior glottic stenosis. *Otolaryngol Head Neck Surg* 1980;88:765–772.
49. Rahbar R, Shapshay SM, Healy GB: Mitomycin: Effects on laryngeal and tracheal stenosis, benefits and complications. *Ann Otol Rhinol Laryngol* 2001;110:1–6.
50. George M, Lang F, Philippe P, et al: Surgical management of laryngotracheal stenosis in adults. *Eur Arch Otorhinolaryngol* 2005;262:609–615.
51. Herrington HC, Weber SM, Andersen PE: Modern management of laryngotracheal stenosis. *Laryngoscope* 2006;116:1553–1557.
52. Gavilan J, Toledano A, Cerdeira MA, et al: Tracheal resection and anastomosis. *Operative Tech Otolaryngol Head Neck Surg* 1997;8:122–129.
53. Rampey AM, Silvestri GA, Gillespie MB: Combined endoscopic and open approach to the removal of expandable metallic tracheal stents. *Arch Otolaryngol Head Neck Surg* 2007;133:37–41.
54. Carden KA, Boiselle PM, Waltz DA, et al: Tracheomalacia and tracheobronchomalacia in children and adults. *Chest* 2005;127:984–1005.
55. Hein E, Rogalla P, Hentschel C, et al: Dynamic and quantitative assessment of tracheomalacia by electron beam tomography: Correlation with clinical symptoms and bronchoscopy. *J Comput Assist Tomogr* 2000;24:247–252.
56. Heussel CP, Hafner B, Lill J, et al: Paired inspiratory/expiratory spiral CT and continuous respiration cine CT in the diagnosis of tracheal instability. *Eur Radiol* 2001;11:982–989.
57. Gillespie MB, Eisele DW: Outcomes of emergency surgical airway procedures in a hospital-wide setting. *Laryngoscope* 1999;109:1766–1769.
58. Milner SM, Bennett JDC: Emergency cricothyrotomy. *J Laryngol Otol* 1991;105:883–885.
59. Erlandson MJ, Clinton JE, Ruiz E, et al: Cricothyroidotomy in the emergency department revisited. *J Emerg Med* 1989;7:115–118.
60. Salvino CK, Dries D, Garnelli R, et al: Emergency cricothyroidotomy in trauma victims. *J Trauma* 1993;34:503–505.
61. DeLaurier G, Hawkins ML, Treat RC, et al: Acute airway management: Role of cricothyroidotomy. *Am Surg* 1990;56:12–15.
62. McGill J, Clinton JE, Ruiz E: Cricothyroidotomy in the emergency department. *Ann Emerg Med* 1982;11:361–364.
63. Fortune JB, Judkins DG, Scanzaroli D, et al: Efficacy of prehospital surgical cricothyrotomy in trauma patients. *J Trauma* 1997;42:832–836.
64. Yarrington CT: Complications of tracheostomy. *Arch Surg* 1965;91:652–655.
65. Jackson C: High tracheostomy and other errors, the chief cause of laryngeal stenosis. *Surg Gynecol Obstet* 1921;32:392–398.
66. Brantigan CO, Grow JB: Cricothyroidotomy: Elective use in respiratory problems requiring tracheotomy. *J Thorac Cardiovasc Surg* 1976;71:72–81.
67. Boyd AD, Romita MC, Conlan AA, et al: A clinical evaluation of cricothyroidotomy. *Surg Gynecol Obstet* 1979;149:365–368.

CHAPTER 33

Complications of Laryngeal Surgery

Richard V. Smith

The larynx is a complex organ that serves many functions in humans. For many species, the larynx is primarily used to separate the respiratory tract from the digestive tract, thus performing the critical function of aspiration prevention. The human species has highly developed the speech functions of the larynx, and many think of speech as the primary function of the larynx. Human voices and the ways that people speak often help to define their individuality. In addition to speech generation, the larynx has essential relationships to breathing and swallowing. Therefore, when one performs surgery on the larynx for benign or malignant conditions, he or she must be acutely aware of the potential effects on all of these functions. A perturbation of any one of these important tasks may have a marked impact on a patient.

Surgical procedures have an expected set of sequelae as well as an unexpected set of complications related to the intervention. This chapter will focus predominantly upon the latter, mentioning expected changes only as they relate to complications. Surgery on the larynx may be generally divided into those procedures that address malignant conditions and those that address benign disease processes, although there is certainly some overlap. Extensive resections may be required for certain benign conditions, and, conversely, limited resections are indicated for certain malignancies. For the purpose of this chapter, in accordance with that delineation, the complications will be separated into those related to laryngeal cancer surgery and those that occur after phonosurgery, particularly as they relate to vocal-fold immobility. Because the reasons for these surgeries are very different, the expectations of the patient and the physician are also quite different.

COMPLICATIONS OF LARYNGEAL CANCER SURGERY

There are many surgical procedures that are performed to address cancer of the larynx. These surgeries range from partial cordectomies to total laryngectomies. Many procedures have been described to provide adequate oncologic results and to maximize function, and there has been an expanding focus on endoscopic techniques to manage laryngeal cancer. It is generally thought that endoscopic partial laryngectomies will reduce the complication rates of partial laryngeal procedures. This section will discuss the complications of total laryngectomy and partial laryngectomy, including those of open and endoscopic procedures.

Despite the focus on surgical complications, the paradigm shift in the United States has been away from primary surgery to manage laryngeal cancer. Many head and neck surgeons advocate the appropriate use of primary surgery (both conservation and total laryngectomy procedures) for carefully selected patients. However, most patients will currently be treated with nonsurgical, "organ-sparing" therapy that consists of primary radiotherapy or combined chemotherapy and radiotherapy rather than primary surgery, particularly for advanced-stage disease.[1] However, these treatment strategies are not without impact to the patient, and they can produce both systemic toxicities and local toxicities in the head and neck. The addition of concurrent chemotherapy to radiotherapy doubles the most commonly measured acute toxicities, including grade 3 and 4 mucositis (43%) and pharyngoesophageal problems (35%), and it also adds grade 3 and 4 hematologic (47%) and nausea and/or vomiting (20%) toxicities as compared with radiotherapy alone.[2] The most common long-term sequelae of this therapy include dysphagia, hypopharyngeal and/or esophageal stenosis, the need for long-term gastrostomy, voice changes, xerostomia, and aspiration.[3-6] In addition to the complications of the therapy itself, salvage surgery in the postchemoradiotherapy patient is fraught with additional risk, such as a doubling of the rate of fistula formation.[7] Even nonmajor head and neck surgery after chemotherapy is affected, with a significant elevation in risk for postoperative wound infection.[8] It is important for the head and neck surgeon to be aware of these consequences to adequately assess the risks and benefits of surgical and nonsurgical therapy for laryngeal cancer. It is also imperative to be aware of the risks of this nonsurgical approach so that one may adequately counsel the patient regarding which treatment paradigm is right for him or her.

Pharyngocutaneous Fistula

Pharyngocutaneous fistula is the most troubling complication after total and open partial laryngectomy. Although this has been a clinically important problem since the advent of total laryngectomy, its incidence has increased after the adoption of chemotherapy and radiotherapy and the abandonment of primary total laryngectomy to manage advanced laryngeal cancer (Figure 33-1). Fistula rates vary greatly across reported series, occurring in as few as 5% to more than 50% of cases. Potential predisposing factors to fistula development are listed in Table 33-1. Matikie and colleagues[9] have provided a nice summary of the topic in their review of pharyngocutaneous fistula.

The presence of a fistula should be suspected if there is a fever spike during the early postoperative period,[10] although this may not be clearly identified until a week or more after surgery. This will often be heralded by a tense, warm, erythematous region in the suprastomal region or the lateral neck, or it may simply present as an innocuous wound separation with subsequent salivary drainage. Krouse and Metson[11] have advocated the routine use of a barium swallow to identify those who are at risk for fistula formation, documenting a sinus tract in 20% of their patients. However, a more detailed analysis showed that 100% (4 of 4) of patients with sinus tracts longer than 2 cm developed a fistula as compared with 17% (1 of 6) of patients with sinus tracts shorter than 2 cm. Although more problematic after total laryngectomy, pharyngocutaneous fistula remains a problem after partial procedures as well, as demonstrated by the 50% fistula rate after near-total laryngectomy reported by Gavilán and colleagues.[12] This complication has also been reported after endoscopic laser resection.[13]

Although many factors have been thought to contribute to the development of pharyngocutaneous fistula, only a subset—ranging from early feeding to concomitant neck surgery and pharyngeal closure techniques—are controllable at the time of surgery or during the early postoperative period. More recent series have debunked some of the previous reports for causative factors of fistula formation. Soylu and colleagues[14] retrospectively analyzed 295 patients and reported a fistula rate of 12.5% (37 patients). They failed to demonstrate a statistically significant association between early feeding, prior radiotherapy (as a result of limited number of patients), prior tracheotomy, accompanying neck dissection, or surgical technique and fistula development. The only statistically significant causative factors were suture type, with Vicryl (Ethicon, Somerville, UT) having a lower fistula rate than catgut, and T stage, with T3 and T4 tumors having 2.5 times the fistula rate of T2 tumors. There was a trend toward decreased fistula formation using a T pharyngeal closure (8.5%) as compared with a vertical closure (12.8%), but this difference was not statistically significant. In their series, only

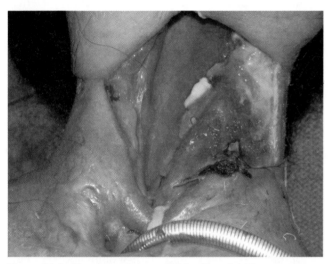

Figure 33-1. Pharyngocutaneous fistula after a total laryngectomy. This patient had an earlier large fistula repaired with a pectoralis myocutaneous flap closure with the subsequent loss of the skin paddle and the distal muscle, leaving the defect shown.

TABLE 33-1 Proposed Factors Related to Pharyngocutaneous Fistula Development After Total Laryngectomy

Systemic	Local	Technical	Tumor Factors
Liver disease	Neck dissection	Suture material	T stage
Anemia	Preoperative tracheotomy	Closure (T vs. linear)	Residual disease
Malnutrition (low albumin)	Preoperative radiotherapy	Devascularization	
Hypothyroidism	Postoperative radiotherapy	Early feeding	
Chronic obstructive pulmonary disease		Postoperative vomiting	
Immunosuppression		Tight mucosal closure	
Peripheral vascular disease		Prolonged operative time	
Diabetes			

21 patients had received preoperative radiotherapy, thus limiting any conclusions in that group. The recommendations were to use careful surgical technique and to begin early postoperative feeding at 3 days. Saydam and colleagues[15] studied a series of 48 patients who began oral clear liquid feedings on postoperative day 1, and they reported a fistula rate of 12.5%. They also found no association between early oral feeding and fistula development, but they did find an association between pharyngeal resection at the time of total laryngectomy (4 of 13) and fistula formation ($P = .04$) as compared with no pharyngeal resection (2 of 35).

Comorbidity has been demonstrated to be an independent factor for survival in cancer, and surgeons have also been assessing the general medical health of the patient as a risk factor for fistula formation. Cavalot and colleagues[16] evaluated medical comorbidities in 293 patients undergoing total laryngectomy. They evaluated the association between fistula formation and diabetes, liver disease, chronic anemia, and other local factors, such as closure technique, radiotherapy, tracheotomy, and neck dissection. They reported a correlation between diabetes, liver disease, chronic anemia, and preoperative radiotherapy and fistula development ($P \leq .001$ in all cases). In this series, there was no association with Vicryl sutures, intraoperative blood transfusion, or preoperative tracheotomy. As can be appreciated, despite large series, there are conflicting results regarding which factors are associated with fistula formation.

More recent series have used large databases or meta-analysis to evaluate risk factors for fistula formation. In their study of 2063 laryngectomy patients in the Department of Veterans Affairs database, Schwartz and colleagues[17] identified preoperative radiotherapy, prolonged operative time, low albumin level, and diabetes as independent factors associated with postoperative complications. Wound complications in this study included superficial and deep wound infections, wound dehiscence, and frank fistula. In this study, fistula was not separated during the analysis. Factors that were not associated with wound complications were concomitant neck dissection, myofascial flap use, patient age, alcohol use, and smoking status. The odds ratios for the associated factors varied from 1.48 (i.e., thrombocytosis) to 2.10 (i.e., operative time >10 hours). Combinations of risks factors also increased the rate of wound complications as demonstrated by the change from 6.3% for patients with no factors to 13.7% for patients with low albumin and/or preoperative radiotherapy *or* diabetes to 21.7% for patients with low albumin and/or preoperative radiotherapy *and* diabetes.

A meta-analysis of fistulas was performed by Paydarfar and Birkmeyer[18] by examining studies from 1970 through 2003. Only 26 of the 65 studies evaluated met their strict inclusion criteria. This analysis showed a low postoperative hemoglobin level (<12.5 g/dl; relative risk [RR], 2.10), preoperative radiotherapy (RR, 2.28), radiotherapy and neck dissection (RR, 2.96), and prior tracheotomy (RR, 1.60) to all have a statistically significant elevation with regard to the relative risk of fistula formation. Although comorbid illness had an RR of 2.26, there was a great degree of heterogeneity among studies, thus limiting its statistical significance. The dose of radiotherapy and time from completion to surgery did not affect the relative risk. This is somewhat counterintuitive, and its relevance may have fallen as a result of other uncontrollable variables.

Other factors may also be contributory. A study of 472 patients from five Danish head and neck oncology centers noted an increase in the fistula rate from 12% in 1987 to 30% in 1997, with a corresponding decrease in the annual rate of laryngectomy by 40%. The authors postulated that this increase in fistula rate may be related to a decrease in surgical volume and experience.[19] In addition, positive surgical resection margins seem to contribute to fistula formation, more than tripling the fistula rate from 11% in patients with negative surgical margins to 38% in those with positive surgical margins.[20]

The management of pharyngocutaneous fistula can be quite prolonged and daunting. The optimal management, of course, is to avoid a fistula. Because many laryngeal cancer patients will have undergone preoperative chemotherapy and radiotherapy, meticulous tissue handling is essential during the surgery. Care must be taken to avoid significant crush injury to the tissues, to excise questionably viable mucosa, and to avoid unnecessary tension on the pharyngeal closure. The closure type, as demonstrated in the previously cited studies, has little to do with fistula formation, but tenuous sutures (i.e., those that are too close to the margin of the tissue) and widely spaced sutures are likely to contribute.

The prevention of fistula formation in salvage total laryngectomy may include the routine use of a myogenous pectoralis major flap for the enhancement of the closure.[21] In a study of 223 total laryngectomy patients, Smith and colleagues[21] noted a reduction in fistula formation from 23% to less than 1% with the routine use of pectoralis myogenous flaps to cover the pharyngeal closure. A recent study has even advocated the routine use of free flaps to reinforce the suture line, noting that, although the fistula rate of 30% was unchanged with salvage laryngectomy, the severity of the fistulas was markedly decreased in the free flap group.[22]

When a fistula occurs, conservative management is appropriate. Routine wound care with wet-to-dry dressings is the mainstay of therapy. In general, in the absence of major vessel exposure, dressing changes and meticulous wound care will result in spontaneous closure through

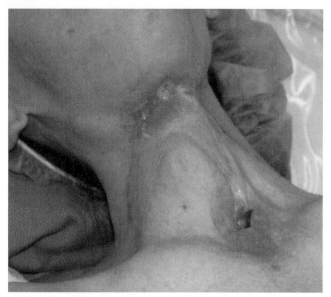

Figure 33-2. Same patient as seen in Figure 33-1 after allowing the wound to heal with secondary intention after wet-to-dry dressings, gastrostomy alimentation, and topical platelet-derived growth factor application.

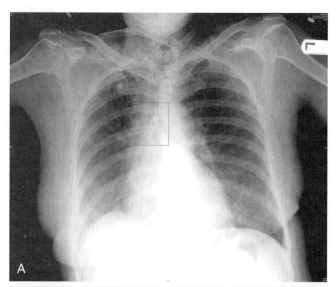

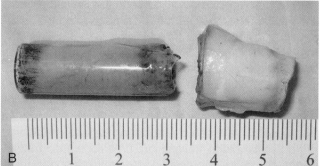

Figure 33-3. A, Aspiration of crack pipe following total laryngectomy (box surrounds pipe in right mainstem bronchus). **B,** Crack pipe after removal with rigid bronchoscopy.

healing from secondary intention (Figure 33-2). Such a closure may take several months. For patients in whom little wound closure is accomplished with wound care or in whom the carotid artery or the jugular vein is exposed, surgical closure with a flap is indicated. Galli and colleagues[23] noted that, in two thirds of their patients, fistulas closed spontaneously with wound care, and they advocated a "wait-and-see" policy for a month before proceeding to flap closure. Flap closure may employ a pectoralis myocutaneous flap or a free flap, such as a radial forearm flap, a lateral arm flap, or a gastroomental flap.

It is important to rule out any metabolic contributions to the fistula formation (e.g., hypothyroidism, severe malnourishment) as well as persistent tumor. Additional techniques to assist with the closure and to minimize wound contamination include the use of a salivary bypass tube, the placement of a suction sump drain into the pharynx through the neck, the use of stomal bags, the use of biologic response modifiers to improve granulation tissue formation,[24] or the injection of fibrin sealant into the fistula site.[25] The important management skills for this complication include patience, communication of the problem and its solutions to the patient and his or her family, careful wound care, and the judicious use of additional surgery when there is a significant delay in healing or concern about carotid artery or jugular vein integrity.

Dysphagia and Aspiration

Although dysphagia can occur after total laryngectomy, this problem is most often discussed after open or endoscopic partial laryngectomy. Aspiration in these cases is intimately involved with the dysphagia, and it can be a major morbidity of partial laryngectomy. Aspiration in patients who have received a total laryngectomy is either related to leakage around a tracheoesophageal voice prosthesis, a pharyngocutaneous fistula, or foreign-body aspiration (Figure 33-3). Dysphagia after total laryngectomy is most often related to stenosis of the neopharynx as either a consequence of a tight surgical closure, cicatricial scar formation at the pharyngeal suture line, or stenotic healing of a pharyngocutaneous fistula. Pharyngeal stenosis is best prevented by avoiding the primary closure of a narrow pharynx. A pharyngeal width of at least 3 cm to 4 cm should be maintained, if oncologically feasible, for closure. Flap augmentation should be employed as needed to create an adequate pharyngeal lumen. When a stenosis does occur, serial bougie dilations are required to break the stenosis and to provide a patent pharyngoesophageal conduit. Particularly after chemoradiotherapy, however, the pharyngeal musculature may be scarred, fibrosed, or otherwise rendered nonfunctional, and dysphagia may persist despite an adequate pharyngeal lumen. In severe cases of stenosis, if repeated dilations provide only temporary relief, pharyngostomy or pharyngectomy with flap reconstruction is warranted.

After partial laryngectomy, some degree of dysphagia and aspiration are expected after most procedures, with the incidence and severity often increasing with the amount of tissue removed from the larynx. For instance, aspiration after supracricoid laryngectomy with cricohyoidopexy is frequently more severe than cricohyoidoepiglottopexy, which in turn is more severe than endoscopic resections. The advent of endoscopic partial laryngectomy has decreased the risk of long-term aspiration, particularly for supraglottic laryngectomy. Open vertical laryngectomy posed a lower threat of long-term aspiration than supraglottic laryngectomy, and endoscopic resection has further lowered the risk, with reports of aspiration in open procedures ranging from 1.3% to 21% (median, 13%) and those in endoscopic procedures ranging from 1.7% to 10% (median, 5%).[26] The addition of radiation therapy after partial laryngectomy increases the risk of aspiration and swallowing problems. This appears to be dose dependent, with severe complications related to a postoperative dose of 60 Gy to the larynx as compared with 50 Gy.[27]

Many of the contraindications to open supraglottic laryngectomy (e.g., advanced age, limited pulmonary reserve or function) are less critical when employing endoscopic surgical techniques. This is in large part because of the more limited resection volume, which involves resecting only those tissues required for an adequate margin, as compared with the open techniques, which require the resection of the entire supraglottic unit to minimize the chance of prolonged arytenoid edema (Figure 33-4). These factors allow for a sensate recovery of the remaining supraglottic tissues, thereby minimizing the risk of aspiration. In their report of transoral carbon-dioxide laser supraglottic laryngectomy, Rudert and colleagues[28] noted aspiration in 12.5% of their patients. Bernal-Sprekelsen and colleagues[26] studied factors that were predictive of aspiration in 210 patients undergoing carbon-dioxide laser resection of laryngeal and hypopharyngeal tumors. The need for gastrostomy was present in 6% of patients and correlated significantly with the supraglottis and the hypopharynx (as compared with the glottis, $P = .002$), advanced tumor stage ($P = 0.002$), patient age (>65 years old, $P = .02$), and postoperative radiotherapy ($P = .04$). In addition, the need for tracheotomy for aspiration-related pulmonary toilet similarly correlated with tumor location and locally advanced disease. Occasional cough after oral intake was noted among 19% of patients with endoscopic glottic resections as compared with 27% of patients undergoing supraglottic resection, with pneumonia rates of 1.7% and 5.8%, respectively. No patients undergoing glottic resections required a gastrostomy, and 1 patient required a definitive tracheotomy. Of the patients undergoing supraglottic resection, 6 required gastrostomy (4 were temporary), and 4 required tracheotomy (2 were temporary).

Another study of complications after the transoral resection of 275 laryngeal and hypopharyngeal tumors reported pneumonia in 6% of patients, with the larynx and the hypopharyngeal primary sites not being separated.[13] In that study, complications were significantly

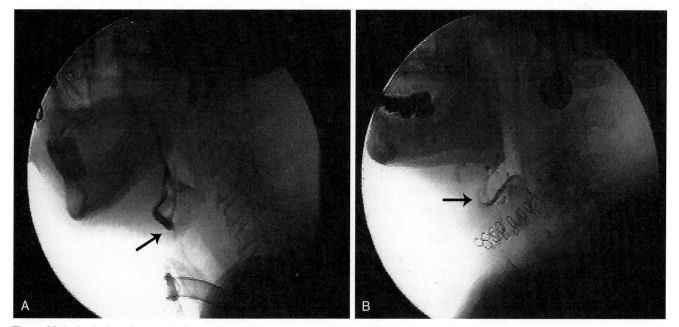

Figure 33-4. Aspiration of contrast after supraglottic laryngectomy. **A,** A modified barium swallow demonstrating the contrast lining the total supraglottic defect with the penetration of the glottis *(arrow)* and a tracheotomy tube in place. **B,** A modified barium swallow after endoscopic supraglottic laryngectomy. Note less tissue loss as outlined by the barium, no penetration *(arrow),* and the presence of a staple on the skin (swallowing study preformed on postoperative day 3).

associated with tumor extension ($P < .0001$), diabetes mellitus ($P = .01$), and less surgical experience ($P < .0001$). The total complication rate in that series was 18.9 %, with 9.8% considered major and 9.1% considered minor. Additional complications encountered included postoperative bleeding (8%), dyspnea (1.8%), emphysema (1%), local infection (0.3%), cutaneous fistula (0.3%), and airway fire (0.3%).

Dysphonia

Alteration in voice is commonly encountered after partial laryngectomy and is expected, although the severity can be of varying degrees. Total laryngectomy carries the obvious result of severe dysphonia and total aphonia in the absence of tracheoesophageal puncture (TEP) or esophageal speech development. Interestingly, however, speech results after radical radiotherapy and successful TEP reconstruction after total laryngectomy are not significantly different. This was studied in a cohort of 34 men, 12 of whom received radical radiotherapy, 12 who received total laryngectomy with TEP, and 10 normal controls.[29] There were no significant differences in acoustic or temporal measures between the radiotherapy and surgical groups, although there was a significant perceptual difference between the two, particularly as compared with the normal controls. The lack of acoustic differences is not what one would expect, but it does point to the complexity of voice production and highlights the fact that the presence of the organ does not guarantee its function. Speech after near-total laryngectomy remains limited as compared with partial laryngectomy, although it can be produced in 90% of patients by 6 months, with the development of hands-free conversation among half of these patients.[12]

The voice results after endoscopic partial laryngectomy have been found to be quite good in several studies. In a study of quality of life and functional outcomes after the treatment of early glottic cancer, Smith and colleagues[30] noted no difference between endoscopic resection and radiotherapy with respect to speech and quality of life, among other factors. When comparing transoral laser microsurgery and open frontolateral partial laryngectomy, Reker[31] demonstrated improved phonatory ability after laser resection, with only 18% of laser-resection patients having a poor-quality voice as compared with 62% of patients who were treated with the open approach. Clearly the benefit of laser resection is in a decreased removal of uninvolved tissue, thus limiting the block-type resection used in open techniques that were originally employed to minimize prolonged tracheotomy or aspiration. Several authors have compared the voice results after laser resection with those that occur after radiation therapy.[32,33] The voice changes after laser resection are similar to those found

after radiotherapy, with no significant difference between the two. Voice changes are expected after endoscopic resection or open resection with adequate reconstruction, but marked dysphonia and aphonia are relatively uncommon.

Medical Complications

Endocrine

Endocrine complications associated with laryngeal cancer surgery are related to the local effects of the resection and the inclusion of the paratracheal and paraesophageal tissues with the nodal dissection. One must always keep a high level of suspicion for hypothyroidism, particularly in cases of pharyngocutaneous fistula formation. In addition, radiation therapy has been shown to predispose patients to hypothyroidism as well. If surgical salvage for radiation failure is performed, the risk of hypothyroidism is greater, with undiagnosed hypothyroidism in 28% of patients (18.6% with subclinical hypothyroidism and 9.6% with clinical manifestations of the disorder).[34] Gal and colleagues[35] studied risk factors for hypothyroidism after laryngectomy in 136 patients (with 37.5% developing hypothyroidism) and found that female sex ($P = .005$), preoperative radiotherapy ($P = .002$), thyroid gland invasion ($P = .0003$), nodal metastases ($P = .002$), and postoperative fistula ($P = .01$) were all significantly associated with hypothyroidism. Interestingly, the greatest risk of hypothyroidism extends from the immediate postoperative period up to 14 months after the surgery. Aimoni and colleagues[36] found that none of the 30 patients in their study of hypothyroid patients after salvage laryngectomy had perioperative hypothyroidism, but 13% were hypothyroid 1 year after the surgery. Physicians from the Cleveland Clinic have identified a cumulative risk of hypothyroidism that lasts for several years after cancer treatment.[37]

Hypoparathyroidism develops immediately after surgery. To monitor for its development, calcium levels should be checked during the early postoperative period, and the patient should be monitored for signs of hypocalcemia, such as circumoral tingling, digital paresthesias, and Chvostek or Trousseau signs. Immediate repletion with calcium should be initiated, with vitamin D analogues administered as well. This complication occurs primarily after paratracheal neck dissection, when the parathyroid glands are either devascularized or included in the resected tissue. It is incumbent on the surgeon to minimize the chance of hypoparathyroidism by carefully dissecting these tissues and preserving the blood supply to the parathyroid glands. If parathyroid resection is noted and the gland is not involved with the tumor, then autologous reimplantation should be performed using the sternocleidomastoid muscle as the recipient site. Because the early postoperative patient may not be able to talk, and therefore may be unable to report symptoms of hypocalcemia, the surgeon must be vigilant regarding the diagnosis of this complication.

Cardiovascular and Respiratory

Cardiovascular and pulmonary complications—either as exacerbations of preexisting conditions or as new events—are not uncommon after laryngeal cancer surgery. Buitelaar and colleagues[38] studied cardiovascular and respiratory complications in 469 patients undergoing primary surgery for head and neck cancer, 31% of whom had laryngeal cancer surgery. Cardiovascular complications occurred in 12% of patients (most commonly heart failure), and respiratory complications occurred in 11% of patients (most commonly pneumonia). Risk factors for cardiovascular complications included advanced age, pulmonary disease, alcohol abuse, and tumor location (i.e., oral cavity, oropharynx, hypopharynx, or supraglottis). The majority (81%) of these complications occurred within the first 4 postoperative days. Alternatively, pulmonary complications were associated with preexisting pulmonary disease, prior myocardial infarction, or advancing American Society of Anesthesiologists grade. The majority (60%) of pulmonary complications occurred within the first 4 postoperative days, with an additional 18% occurring within 5 to 7 days. Another study of pulmonary complications after major head and neck surgery identified postoperative pulmonary complications in 47% of patients, with the majority developing pneumonia.[39] A 5-day course of postoperative intravenous amoxicillin and clavulanic acid had no effect on the infection rate, which was significantly related to poor preoperative pulmonary function and postoperative atelectasis, thus leading the authors to their recommendation to routinely use incentive spirometry postoperatively. Studies of endoscopic resections, including that of Laccourreye and colleages,[27] show a lower rate of pneumonia of roughly one quarter of that found in the previously cited studies. These complications are best prevented by avoiding overly aggressive hydration intraoperatively and postoperatively, by avoiding the intraoperative aspiration of blood during the transection of the trachea and the creation of the stoma, and by employing early mobilization and incentive spirometry.

Stenosis

Laryngeal Stenosis

Laryngeal stenosis may occur after open or endoscopic partial laryngectomy. This may take the form of cicatricial fibrotic stenosis or severe postoperative laryngeal remnant edema. Horizontal supraglottic partial laryngectomy (Figure 33-5) and vertical laryngectomy (Figure 33-6) can both have this complication. Persistent laryngeal edema was more commonly observed after open partial laryngectomy, potentially related to the disruption of the local lymphatic pathways after significant dissection external to the defect and

tumor as well as the greater degree of tissue removal routinely performed using the open techniques.

Varying rates of these complications have been reported. Vilaseca-González and colleagues[13] noted airway edema or stenosis in 1.8% of patients undergoing the carbon-dioxide laser resection of laryngeal and hypopharyngeal tumors, whereas Laccourreye and colleagues[27] reported a 4.4% incidence of laryngeal stenosis after partial laryngectomy with postoperative radiotherapy. The management of this complication involves the division of the stenosis and subsequent dilation. This is commonly performed endoscopically, with a carbon-dioxide laser and microsurgical techniques. Endoscopic therapy may need to be performed more than once to achieve the adequate opening of the airway and the excision of the stenosis. For more severe cases of glottic stenosis, however, an open approach with interposition grafts or stent placement may be required. For cases of impending airway obstruction or failed endoscopic management, tracheotomy is the definitive treatment.

Tracheostomal Stenosis

Tracheostomal stenosis after total laryngectomy may occur at any point after surgery. Generally this is a slowly progressive process that can be managed in the office with a stomal tube that has been specially designed for laryngectomees to account for the anatomic and geometric changes that occur after total laryngectomy and tracheostoma creation (Figure 33-7). Predisposing factors can be the presence of a tube postoperatively causing local inflammation and fibrosis at the stoma, postoperative radiotherapy to the stoma and skin for close surgical margins or other tumor characteristics, or tracheoesophageal prosthesis placement. The basic tissue event is necrosis of the tracheal mucosa or the adjacent skin edge with the development of a localized perichondritis that can then result in fibrosis of the involved area. Kou and colleagues[40] retrospectively studied 207 laryngectomy patients, reporting an overall incidence of stomal stenosis in 13% of patients. Although stenosis occurred more frequently among patients undergoing primary tracheoesophageal punctures or pectoralis flap pharyngeal reconstruction, those patients who had had a stomal infection, and women, only stomal infection and female gender were significant factors on multivariate analysis.

Stomal narrowing can be quite severe and requires urgent management with a surgical incision and dilation of the stoma. Long-term management may take the form of a lifelong silastic stomal tube, but this has the distinct disadvantage of limiting or eliminating prosthetic speech rehabilitation; therefore surgical correction is often recommended. This will require some form of a stomaplasty with local tissue advancement, either in the form of Z-plasty closure or advancement flaps after the removal of the stenotic tracheal segment.

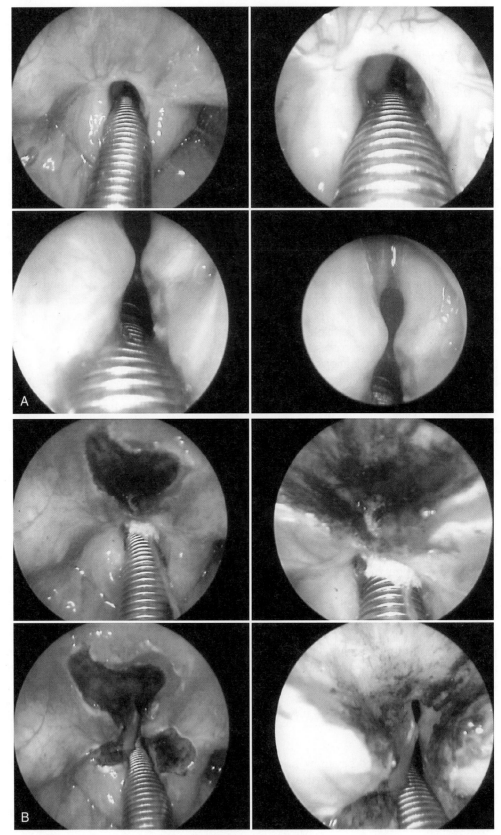

Figure 33-5. A, Symptomatic supraglottic stenosis after endoscopic supraglottic laryngectomy. **B,** Airway opened after the radial division of the stenosis with a carbon-dioxide laser, thus providing lasting symptomatic relief.

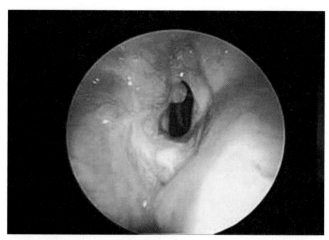

Figure 33-6. Asymptomatic anterior glottic webbing after carbon-dioxide laser resection of true vocal-fold carcinoma with mid vocal-fold laryngeal granulation tissue that was removed endoscopically.

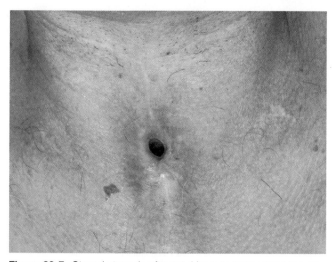

Figure 33-7. Stomal stenosis after total laryngectomy requiring stomaplasty.

Many surgeons use a Z-plasty, placing the central limb along the axis of the tracheocutaneous junction. This has the added advantage of breaking the fibrotic ring and redirecting the scarring forces more favorably. Severe recurrent stenosis may also require more extensive surgery, potentially including free flap reconstruction.[41]

Vascular and Lymphatic Complications

Vascular and lymphatic consequences of laryngeal cancer surgery are rare, and they are related primarily to associated central compartment neck dissections. In the absence of such dissections, the carotid sheath structures are relatively isolated from the resection plane, and the thoracic duct is similarly outside of the surgical field. When a central compartment neck dissection (either upper mediastinal or paratracheal) is included, major vascular injury is a potential complication. Most often this would be a consequence of direct vascular injury during the surgery or delayed injury and bleeding as a result of

a pharyngocutaneous fistula. Direct vascular injury must be repaired immediately, or the vessel must be ligated, if appropriate. The superior thyroid and the superior laryngeal vessels are the most likely vessels involved in direct injury, and these vessels should be suture ligated at their proximal stump rather than controlled with electrocautery. Delayed bleeding may be the result of arterial or, less commonly, venous vessel wall injury after fistula formation or from the innominate artery in the case of a tracheoinnominate fistula, an exceedingly rare result of long-term tracheotomy. Bleeding may also occur as a consequence of the endoscopic laser resection of laryngeal tumors caused by the incomplete control of the arterial vessels during resection. Vilaseca-González and colleagues reported an 8% incidence of postoperative hemorrhage. Only a minority of these patients had self-limiting bleeds (25%), and the remainder (75%) had life-threatening bleeding that required a return to the operating room. The hemorrhage was controlled by electrocautery in the majority (15 of 16) of patients, and 1 patient required vessel embolization. Careful control of intraoperative bleeding during endoscopic resection is essential, and the use of vascular clips should be routine for the superior laryngeal vessels or the lingual artery.

Lymphatic injury is possible after associated central compartment neck dissection. Its management is discussed in detail in the chapter on neck surgery (Chapter 36), and it is related to thoracic duct injury on the left or the major lymphatic ducts present in the lower neck on the right. Briefly, however, care must be taken when dissecting the medial aspect of level IV on either the right or left side, because the lymphatic structures may be visualized before their interruption. Should lymph be present after dissection, the optimal management is at the time of primary surgery, and time should be taken to suture ligate the area to prevent leakage. Unnecessary dissection and sutures in the area may exacerbate the injury, thereby complicating management. Some surgeons recommend using surgical clips rather than sutures to avoid additional injury. Other forms of management may be employed if the leak is discovered during the postoperative period; these may include compressive dressings, dietary modifications, or sclerosing agents.

Tracheoesophageal Puncture Complications

Speech rehabilitation after total laryngectomy has evolved from esophageal speech to an electrolarynx to tracheoesophageal speech and potentially to other devices, such as palatal prostheses. The mainstay of speech rehabilitation at this time is tracheoesophageal speech through a low-pressure, one-way valve voice prosthesis (i.e., TEP). The correct identification of appropriate candidates is required to avoid unnecessary failure of the rehabilitation. Patient factors such as poor eyesight and poor dexterity from diseases such as rheumatoid arthritis can be contraindications for placement, because the patient cannot adequately care for the prosthesis. Other factors, such as age, prelaryngectomy communication status,[42] and cognitive factors[43] have been associated with successful speech rehabilitation as well.

Complications related to TEP can occur early or late after the procedure (Box 33-1), and they can involve either primary (i.e., at the time of total laryngectomy) or secondary (i.e., delayed) punctures. There has been debate during the past regarding whether primary TEP had higher complication rates than secondary TEP, but most studies have failed to demonstrate a significant difference, and many surgeons perform primary TEP. In fact, Cheng and colleagues[44] have demonstrated excellent voice results in 80% of patients with primary TEP as compared with 50% after secondary TEP. Complications have also changed somewhat as surgeons have moved toward the placement of indwelling speech devices.[45] As a complication, leakage is only appropriate defined during the early postoperative period, because late leakage signals the incompetence of the TEP valve, and it is the primary sign for prosthesis replacement among patients with indwelling devices.

Total complications are reported in many cases of TEP, up to 40% or more in some series. Albirmawy and colleages[46] reported a 19% incidence of dysphonia/aphonia, a 19% incidence of peristomal cellulitis, and a 25% incidence of inflammation during the early postoperative period after primary TEP. They also noted a 19% incidence of granulation tissue formation during the late postoperative period. In that study, late complications after secondary TEP were granulation tissue in 23% and stenosis in 26%. Calder and colleages[47] reviewed their experience in 100 TEP patients, documenting an overall complication rate of 45%, with 35% of patients requiring at least one admission related to TEP complications and only 67% vocalizing with the valve. As in other series, granulation tissue was the most common complication, occurring in 20% of patients, with fistula enlargement and valve loss each occurring in 16% of patients.

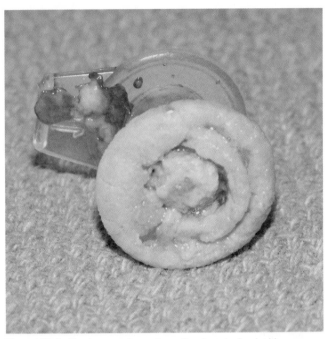

Figure 33-8. Tracheoesophageal prosthesis colonized with *Candida*, demonstrating the total involvement of the esophageal flange and hood.

When complications do occur after TEP, the primary treatment is the removal of the prosthesis. Complications such as leakage and *Candida* overgrowth (Figure 33-8) can be managed with removal and the immediate replacement of a new prosthesis. Others, such as granulation tissue, are often managed with the prosthesis in place and the cauterization of the surrounding tissue. Dysphonia or aphonia after TEP may be related to the hypertonicity of the pharyngeal segment, thus requiring pharyngeal plexus neurectomy,[48] botulinum toxin A injection,[49,50] cricopharyngeal myotomy, or systemic muscle relaxants. The in situ management of an enlarged and incompetent fistula may be accomplished with the injection of materials such as a polysaccharide gel[51] or autologous fat[52] into the surrounding tissue to reduce the diameter and patency of the fistula. The remainder of the complications will often require the removal of the TEP, secondary healing of the fistula site, and a secondary puncture. Patients in whom the fistula is allowed to close must be cautioned against aspiration during the healing phase. The sequential downsizing of red-rubber catheters placed through the fistula can minimize aspiration risks, but most patients can be managed without a tube, with care taken during eating and the avoidance of water and very thin liquids during the healing process. The fistula in some patients will not close in this fashion, and a surgical procedure will be required to close the patent fistula site (Figure 33-9). Because many patients have undergone radiotherapy to the area, this procedure can be quite challenging and may require flap closure.

BOX 33-1 Complications of Tracheoesophageal Puncture and/or Prosthesis

EARLY	LATE
• Leakage	• Leakage
• Dysphonia/aphonia	• Dysphonia/aphonia
• Local inflammation	• Granulation tissue
• Crusting	• Candidal colonization
• Peristomal cellulitis	• Stomal stenosis
• Esophageal perforation	• Migration/extrusion
• Dental complications from insertion	• Persistent fistula
	• Dysphagia
	• Esophageal stenosis

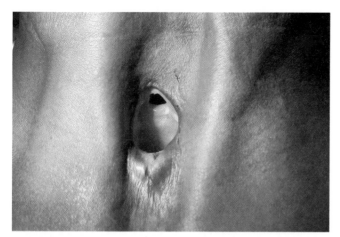

Figure 33-9. Persistent dilated tracheoesophageal puncture fistula requiring surgical closure.

Closure with local tissue is usually the first step to avoid the potential sequelae of oversized reconstruction tissue in the stomal region, and this may include the placement of a dermal graft[53] (either autologous or acellular processed dermis) as an intermediate third layer between the esophageal and tracheal mucosa. More complicated defects or failed initial closures may require a regional flap or a free flap to successfully close a persistent fistula.

COMPLICATIONS OF PHONOSURGERY

Phonosurgery represents the vast majority of procedures meant to address phoniatric functional aspects of the larynx. These procedures, although meant to improve the voice, all have the capability to worsen it and to produce significant dysphonia or hypophonia. These procedures include transoral microsurgery for lesion or polyp removal, laryngeal framework surgery (e.g., thyroplasty, arytenoid adduction), and injection vocal-fold augmentation. Because the main complication of microsurgery for polyp and nodule removal is dysphonia, most of the complications discussed pertain to procedures for managing vocal-fold immobility. Complications that can occur after phonosurgery are presented in Box 33-2.

Surgical techniques have improved with the advent of surgical microscopes and magnification with telescopes. In addition, the routine use of angled telescopes (i.e., 0, 30, 70, and 120 degrees) permits intralaryngeal manipulation and surgery to occur with greater precision. It is generally felt that significant declines in vocal function after phonosurgery for lesion excision are related to the violation of the deep layer of the Reinke's space, allowing for the formation of scar tissue between the vocal ligament and the overlying mucosa. This in turn inhibits the mucosal wave that is required for normal voice production. The obvious goal of this

---

BOX 33-2 Complications of Phonosurgery

EXTERNAL APPROACH: MEDIALIZATION LARYNGOPLASTY AND/OR ARYTENOID ADDUCTION

Early
- Airway edema
- Overmedialization
- Vocal fold hemorrhage
- Supraglottic edema
- Aspiration
- Hematoma
- Soft-tissue cellulitis
- Seroma
- Implant infection

Late
- Poor voice quality
- Glottic stenosis
- Implant extrusion
- Implant migration
- Soft-tissue scarring

ENDOSCOPIC APPROACH: INJECTION LARYNGOPLASTY AND MICROLARYNGOSCOPY

Early
- Aspiration
- Donor-site hematoma
- Vocal-fold hematoma
- Glottic edema

Late
- Implant migration
- Injection granuloma (Teflon)
- Vocal-fold deposits
- Injection absorption
- Poor voice quality
- Anterior web/glottic stenosis

---

type of surgery is to avoid the involvement of the deep layers of the Reinke's space when mucosal incisions are required. The hydrodissection of the Reinke's space in the area of the surgery will facilitate the accomplishment of that goal.

Dysphonia

Because phonosurgery is performed predominantly to address voice problems with the expectation of an improved voice, the complications of a worsened voice and dysphonia are particularly distressing. Additionally, because vocal improvement is the expectation of this surgery, a stable voice is also often considered a failure. Therefore, it is extremely important to educate the patient to ensure realistic surgical expectations. In addition, the surgeon must carefully explain the postoperative voice changes that occur and that often involve a fluctuating voice for the first few weeks or months.

Dysphonia can be implied by the need for the revision of a thyroplasty implant. According to a survey of 1039 otolaryngologists who performed medialization laryngoplasty or arytenoid adduction, only 5.4% of patients required revision phonosurgery.[54] Complications of this study were associated with experience, with a higher complication rate seen among surgeons performing the procedure fewer than 10 times. Failure of medialization and its causes were evaluated by Woo and colleages,[55] who noted three major types of failure. In their series of 20 patients undergoing revision surgery, 55% (11 of 20) were caused by a persistent posterior glottic gap, 30% (6 of 20) were related to implant mal-position or inadequate size, and 10% (2 of 20) were the result of an increased glottal gap as caused by muscle atrophy. Methods to correct these problems were revision medialization (11 of 20), arytenoid adduction (12 of 20), lipoinjection (2 of 20), and implant removal (4 of 20), ultimately leading to an improved voice in 75% (15 of 20) of patients. More uncommon causes of dysphonia after implant medialization include thyroid cartilage window migration[56] and implant displacement after endotracheal intubation for an abdominal procedure.[57] Whatever the cause, medialization laryngoplasty does have an incidence of postoperative dysphonia and the potential need for revision. This must be kept in mind when counseling the patient preoperatively.

Injection into the vocal fold for the management of vocal-fold immobility is also a common treatment, often being performed in the office under local anesthesia. Many compounds have been used for this purpose, including Teflon, autologous fat, Gelfoam, dermis, and collagen. The techniques are somewhat different for the different materials, and they are beyond the scope of this chapter. The voice results, although generally excellent, can be suboptimal in certain cases, and they may be related to surgeon technique or underlying anatomic changes. Ford and colleagues[58] reported excellent voice results using injectable collagen, but 29% of patients undergoing injection to manage a scarred vocal fold had only transient (7%) or no improvement (22%) in their voice. Two cases of a firm submucosal deposit forming after collagen injection were reported by Anderson and Sataloff.[59] Both patients had interruption of the mucosal wave by the deposit, and they were treated with the microscopic removal of the deposit with the subsequent return of a normal voice. Hypersensitivity to dermal collagen has long been a concern as well, with initial reports advocating hypersensitivity skin testing before injection laryngoplasty. A recent report by Luu and colleagues[60] demonstrated that this skin testing is not required, with no episodes of hypersensitivity noted among 895 patients undergoing 1290 injections. In a report of 80 patients, fat injection met with variable success, with initial and overall success rates of 96% and 77%, respectively, suggesting that resorption over time compromises the speech results of the technique.[61] Overall many surgeons prefer medialization techniques for the definitive management of vocal-fold immobility as a result of their more predictable success.

Airway Compromise

Airway compromise is a potentially life-threatening complication of phonosurgery. Airway edema causes this compromise during the immediate postoperative period. When open techniques are used, airway compromise is more common after arytenoid adduction than medialization laryngoplasty. Management may require steroid therapy, tracheotomy, implant removal, arytenoid adduction suture release, or endotracheal intubation. Tucker and colleagues[62] reported an incidence of airway obstruction among 10% of their patients, all of which were related to hematoma and all of whom required tracheotomy to secure the airway. Weinman and Maragos[63] reviewed 332 patients who underwent a total of 630 thyroplasty procedures. Twenty of these patients required tracheotomy, and 7 required an unplanned tracheotomy for perioperative airway compromise after appropriate medical management, with a median time of 9 hours after surgery until the development of stridor. All patients requiring tracheotomy received arytenoid adduction as part of their procedure, with none developing airway compromise after medialization alone. Abraham and colleagues[64] also noted an increased risk of airway complications among patients with accompanying arytenoid adduction, reporting a 2% tracheotomy incidence in this group. Rosen's survey[54] of otolaryngologists performing phonosurgery revealed that 14% of respondents had experienced a patient with postoperative airway compromise. In that study, 2.8% of patients after medialization laryngoplasty and 6.2% of patients after arytenoid adduction had airway compromise postoperatively. More than half of the patients in each group were observed and managed medically. Airway compromise is a rare complication of injection procedures, but it is not unheard of. Laccourreye and colleagues[61] reported one case of airway compromise requiring tracheotomy out of 80 patients receiving autogenous fat injection laryngoplasty.

Infection

Infection after phonosurgery is quite rare. It occurs predominantly after medialization procedures using implants, because the implants act as a nidus of infection. This complication is more likely in the event of the transgression of the laryngeal mucosa, exposing the implant to laryngopharyngeal secretions, or as a consequence of an operative site hematoma, which provides an optimal medium for bacterial growth. In either case, systemic antibiotics should be given, and the implant likely needs to be removed. Cases of soft-tissue infection and abscess formation also necessitate incision and drainage. If the implant is unaffected, antibiotics and observation are appropriate, with the removal of the implant being necessary only if it is obviously involved with the infection.

Aspiration

Aspiration as a result of vocal-fold immobility is not an uncommon finding, and, in some cases, it may represent the primary indication for medialization. There is debate regarding whether arytenoid adduction surgery is required to address this issue or whether medialization alone is sufficient. Many patients have experienced a resolution of swallowing difficulties and aspiration after medialization alone. Cummings and colleagues[65] report the subjective improvement of dysphagia and aspiration in 85% and 88% of their patients, respectively, after hydroxylapatite medialization thyroplasty. The radiographic analysis of aspiration and laryngeal penetration has been performed by Nayak and colleagues.[66] Videofluoroscopic swallowing studies were performed in 14 patients who received medialization thyroplasty and 53 patients who underwent injection augmentation for unilateral vocal-fold paralysis. Postoperative laryngeal penetration and aspiration was present in 45% and 24% of patients, respectively, with aspiration noted as being associated with other pharyngeal transport abnormalities, swallowing delay, or limited laryngeal elevation, all of which are problems associated with the process that led to the vocal-fold immobility. Therefore, one should clinically assess the preoperative swallowing status of these patients before counseling them about the likelihood of the resolution of their swallowing problems after surgery, because the successful elimination of aspiration is not guaranteed. The size of the glottal gap has been shown by Fang and colleagues[67] to predict aspiration, with patients having larger glottal gaps aspirating before surgical correction. In contrast with Nayak's report, the successful closure of the glottal gap with autologous fat both alleviated aspiration and improved breath control.

Implant Extrusion

Implant extrusion is a possible complication of either injection laryngoplasty or medialization laryngoplasty. Fortunately this is an uncommon event in both circumstances. Extrusion after medialization laryngoplasty is thought to occur less commonly if a window of the thyroid ala is medialized with the implant superficial to it or by maintaining the integrity of the inner thyroid perichondrium. The widespread use of the Montgomery implant system, however, has changed that practice, because the inner perichondrium is intentionally divided and the thyroid ala window is removed. Silastic is the most commonly used implant material at present, but other materials have been advocated as well, including hydroxylapatite, titanium, and Gore-Tex, with no significant difference in results.[68] These materials may have different extrusion rates, but data is limited. Tucker and colleagues[62] published their complication rate in 1993, reporting an extrusion rate of 6.7% using Silastic implants, and, in 1995, Cotter and colleagues[69] reported an extrusion rate of 8.6%. Tucker's group advocated maintaining the integrity of the thyroid perichondrium to assist with preventing the migration of their individually carved implants. Other reports show lower

rates of implant extrusion of approximately 3%.[64] Rosen[54] noted an extrusion rate of 0.8% after medialization laryngoplasty (implant type unknown), with 92% of these extruding into the airway. Extruded implants must be removed either through the standard transcervical approach or with an endoscopic technique.[70]

Although not typically considered extrusion, injectables may also extrude into the lumen (Figure 33-10). Hsiung and Pai[71] reported the extrusion of autogenous fat in 3 of the 101 patients in their series. This would likely be related to the more superficial injection of fat into the vocal fold as compared with the deeper injections used for Teflon and Gelfoam. Additional complications from autogenous fat can occur at the harvest site, including harvest-site hematoma. Laccourreye and colleagues[61] noted a 4% incidence of harvest-site hematoma, a 4% incidence of intracordal cyst development, and a 1% incidence of fat extrusion at the injection site.

Teflon-injection laryngoplasty is, by and large, something of historical concern. Teflon has been clearly associated with injection-site granulomas, which may cause airway obstruction and other local problems. These granulomas may extend into the supraglottis or the subglottis and act as an extruded implant.[72] Should this occur, the granuloma must be removed either through an external approach[73] or endoscopically using microsurgical techniques and laser removal. These granulomas may occur many years after the initial injection; therefore all clinicians must be aware of this complication and its management.

Stenosis

Glottic stenosis is predominantly a complication of microlaryngoscopy with the excision of lesions such as nodules or papillomas. It is quite unlikely after medialization techniques unless inadvertent entry into the

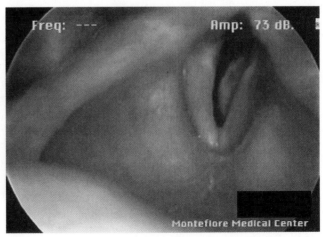

Figure 33-10. Subglottic extension of the Cymetra injection during medialization laryngoplasty of the left vocal fold.

laryngeal airway takes place. In this circumstance, mucosal healing and fibrosis can lead to some stenosis, although it is rare. Microsurgical techniques to remove cysts, nodules, or other mucosal processes, however, can predispose patients to glottic stenosis if bilateral surgery is performed in the anterior glottis, particularly when this involves the anterior commissure. Bilateral surgery in the anterior commissure promotes stenosis through the gradual healing of the vocal folds in an anterior-to-posterior direction, bringing the vocal folds into apposition as they heal (Figure 33-11). This complication should be carefully avoided, because it can be quite difficult to correct, potentially requiring multiple surgeries, tracheotomy, stent placement, or other treatments. Recent efforts to improve the endoscopic management of glottic stenosis have included the use of topical mitomycin C applied to the wound after the division of the stenosis. This antiproliferative agent, which was initially used for cancer treatments, inhibits fibroblast function, potentially setting up the wound for favorable healing without excessive deep fibrosis and scarring. Perepelitsyn and Shapshay[74] evaluated endoscopic stenosis management with a carbon-dioxide laser demonstrating a significant increase in successful endoscopic management with dilation and mitomycin C (75%) as compared with laser and dilation (15%) and laser, dilation, and steroid injection (18%). The use of mitomycin C has become relatively commonplace, and

it does seem to have a positive impact on the success of the endoscopic management of stenosis.

Airway Fire

A chapter about the complications of laryngeal surgery would not be complete without the mention of airway fires. The oxygen-rich environment of the airway during surgery creates the potential for laser fire whenever laser laryngoscopy is performed. Fortunately the development of and the adherence to laser safety principles throughout the past several decades have minimized this life-threatening complication. Fried,[75] in his 1984 survey of otolaryngologists performing laser laryngoscopy, found that 23% of the physicians experienced complications of this procedure. The most frequent complication was endotracheal tube ignition, with others including facial burns, pneumothorax, and subcutaneous emphysema. The incidence of this complication has been dramatically reduced as a result of the increased awareness of this potential problem and the development of laser tubes that will resist ignition. The operating surgeon must be aware of the variety of laser tubes available, because not all tubes are appropriate for all laser frequencies. Management requires the discontinuation of the respiratory circuit with the immediate removal of the fuel for the fire (i.e., the endotracheal tube), the extinguishment of the fire, and the reestablishment of an adequate airway. The

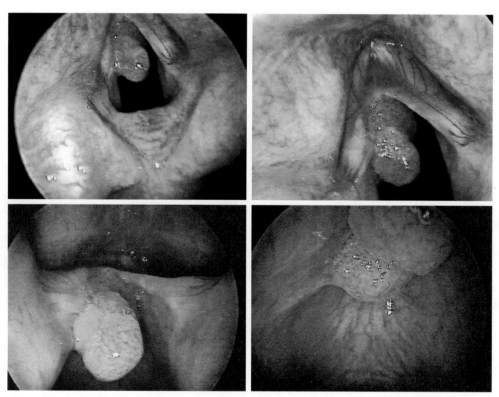

Figure 33-11. Anterior webbing after the removal of benign vocal nodules 8 years before the development of left vocal-fold T1 squamous cell carcinoma. Photo panels depict different telescope angles (0, 30, 70, and 120 degrees).

airway may deteriorate several hours after the burn as a result of tissue edema.

Quality of Life

It is common sense that the quality of life after laryngeal surgery will be negatively affected by complications. What is also common sense is that the quality of life will also be enhanced by less-aggressive surgery with similar outcomes.[76] Therefore the migration of laryngeal cancer surgery toward endoscopic techniques, when appropriate, would be expected to further improve quality of life, provided that similar disease control results. In fact, a direct comparison of voice quality and quality of life among patients treated with endoscopic surgery or radiation therapy for early glottic cancer shows no difference between the two groups.[77] McNeil's study[78] of unaffected volunteers reported a willingness of patients to accept lower cure rates for laryngeal preservation. However, Otto and colleagues[79] assessed patients who had already undergone laryngectomy and found that only 20% would trade their voices for a lower cure rate. Alternatively, health-care providers perceived that patients would be willing to make that trade in 46% of cases, highlighting the danger of inferring treatment without involving the patient. Additionally, when global quality-of-life scores are used, there is no overall difference in quality of life between total laryngectomy and chemoradiation therapy for advanced laryngeal cancer.[80] Vilaseca and colleagues[81] have also demonstrated that the long-term overall quality of life in the laryngectomy patient is not decreased as compared to patients without laryngectomy, although certain domains, such as physical function and voice handicap, are worse among the laryngectomy patients.

Quality-of-life assessments for benign laryngeal surgery have focused more on the development of reliable questionnaires and objective testing. Murry and colleagues[82] found that objective and subjective ratings of voice quality did not always correlate with quality-of-life measures. Johns and colleagues[83] documented a significant quality-of-life improvement with laryngeal microsurgery for vocal fold cysts and polyps, although it was less favorable for vocal-fold scarring. Interestingly, a recent report showed similar improvements in quality of life using three instruments when comparing voice therapy or surgery for benign voice disorders.[84] These results highlight the need for additional studies regarding how laryngeal surgery affects the quality of life of these patients.

CONCLUSION

Complications after laryngeal surgery for benign and malignant conditions can be severe and occasionally life-threatening. Most can be avoided if careful attention is paid to meticulous surgical technique. The early recognition and management of the complication will minimize its significance and impact. The laryngeal surgeon should possess a detailed knowledge of the surgical anatomy of the larynx, because many complications are related to anatomic factors. All surgeons, no matter how skilled, will experience a complication at some point. The recognition and proper management of that complication is the hallmark of an excellent surgeon.

REFERENCES

1. Pfister DG, Laurie SA, Weinstein GS, et al: American Society of Clinical Oncology clinical practice guideline for the use of larynx-preservation strategies in the treatment of laryngeal cancer. *J Clin Oncol* 2006;24:3693–3704.
2. Forastiere AA, Goepfert H, Maor M, et al: Concurrent chemotherapy and radiotherapy for organ preservation in advanced laryngeal cancer. *N Engl J Med* 2003;349:291–1098.
3. Smith RV, Kotz T, Beitler JJ, et al: Long-term swallowing problems after organ preservation therapy with concomitant radiation therapy and intravenous hydroxyurea: Initial results. *Arch Otolaryngol Head Neck Surg* 2000;126:384–389.
4. Franzmann EJ, Lundy DS, Abitbol AA, et al: Complete hypopharyngeal obstruction by mucosal adhesions: A complication of intensive chemoradiation for advanced head and neck cancer. *Head Neck* 2006;28:663–670.
5. Akst LM, Chan J, Elson P, et al: Functional outcomes following chemoradiotherapy for head and neck cancer. *Otolaryngol Head Neck Surg* 2004;131:950–957.
6. Woodson GE, Rosen CA, Murry T, et al: Assessing vocal function after chemoradiation for advanced laryngeal carcinoma. *Arch Otolaryngol Head Neck Surg* 1996;122:858–864.
7. Weber RS, Berkey BA, Forastiere A, et al: Outcome of salvage total laryngectomy following organ preservation therapy: The Radiation Therapy Oncology Group trial 91-11. *Arch Otolaryngol Head Neck Surg* 2003;129:44–49.
8. Penel N, Fournier C, Lefebvre D, et al: Previous chemotherapy as a predictor of wound infections in nonmajor head and neck surgery: Results of a prospective study. *Head Neck* 2004;26:513–517.
9. Matikie AA, Irish J, Gullane PJ: Pharyngocutaneous fistula. *Curr Opin Otolaryngol Head Neck Surg* 2003;11:78–84.
10. Friedman M, Venkatesan TK, Yakovlev A, et al: Early detection and treatment of postoperative pharyngocutaneous fistula. *Otolaryngol Head Neck Surg* 1999;121:378–380.
11. Krouse JH, Metson R: Barium swallow is a predictor of salivary fistula following laryngectomy. *Otolaryngol Head Neck Surg* 1992;106:254–257.
12. Gavilán J, Herranz J, Pim P, et al: Speech results and complications of near-total laryngectomy. *Ann Otol Rhinol Laryngol* 1996;105:729–733.
13. Vilaseca-González I, Bernal-Sprekelsen M, Blanch-Alejandro J-L, et al: Complications in transoral CO2 laser surgery for carcinoma of the larynx and hypopharynx. *Head Neck* 2003;25:382–388.
14. Soylu L, Kiroğlu M, Aydoğan B, et al: Pharyngocutaneous fistula following laryngectomy. *Head Neck* 1998;20:22–25.
15. Saydam L, Kalcioglu T, Kizilay A: Early oral feeding following total laryngectomy. *Am J Otolaryngol* 2002;23:277–281.
16. Cavalot AL, Gervasioa C-F, Nazionale G, et al: Pharyngocutaneous fistula as a complication of total laryngectomy: Review of the literature and analysis of case records. *Otolaryngol Head Neck Surg* 2000;123:587–592.
17. Schwartz SR, Yueh B, Maynard C, et al: Predictors of wound complications after laryngectomy: A study of over 2000 patients. *Otolaryngol Head Neck Surg* 2004;131:61–68.
18. Paydarfar JA, Birkmeyer NJ: Complications in head and neck surgery: A meta-analysis of postlaryngectomy pharyngocutaneous fistula. *Arch Otolaryngol Head Neck Surg* 2006;132:67–72.

19. Grau C, Johansen LV, Hansen HS, et al: Salvage laryngectomy and pharyngocutaneous fistulae after primary radiotherapy for head and neck cancer: A national survey from DAHANCA. *Head Neck* 2003;25:711–716.

20. Markou KD, Vlachtsis KC, Nikolaou AC, et al: Incidence and predisposing factors of pharyngocutaneous fistula formation after total laryngectomy: Is there a relationship with tumor recurrence? *Eur Arch Otorhinolaryngol* 2004;261:61–67.

21. Smith TJ, Burrage KJ, Ganguly P, et al: Prevention of postlaryngectomy pharyngocutaneous fistula: The Memorial University experience. *J Otolaryngol* 2003;32:222–225.

22. Fung K, Teknos TN, Vandenberg CD, et al: Prevention of wound complications following salvage laryngectomy using free vascularized tissue. *Head Neck* 2007;29:425–430.

23. Galli J, DeCorso E, Volante M, et al: Postlaryngectomy pharyngocutaneous fistula: Incidence, predisposing factors, and therapy. *Otolaryngol Head Neck Surg* 2005;133:689–694.

24. Jakubowicz D, Smith RV: The use of becaplermin the closure of pharyngocutaneous fistulae. *Head Neck* 2005;27:433–438.

25. Farrag TY, Boahene KD, Agrawal N, et al: Use of fibrin sealant in closing mucocutaneous fistulas following head and neck cancer surgery. *Otolaryngol Head Neck Surg* 2007;137:159–161.

26. Bernal-Sprekelsen M, Vilaseca-González I, Blanch-Alejandro J-L: Predictive values for aspiration after endoscopic laser resections of malignant tumors of the hypopharynx and larynx. *Head Neck* 2004;26:103–110.

27. Laccourreye O, Hans S, Borzog-Grayeli A, et al: Complications of postoperative radiation therapy after partial laryngectomy in supraglottic cancer: A long-term evaluation. *Otolaryngol Head Neck Surg* 2000;122:752–757.

28. Rudert HH, Werner JA, Höft S: Transoral carbon dioxide laser resection of supraglottic carcinoma. *Ann Otol Rhinol Laryngol* 1999;108:819–827.

29. Finizia C, Dotevall H, Lundström E, et al: Acoustic and perceptual evaluation of voice and speech quality: A study of patients with laryngeal cancer treated with laryngectomy vs irradiation. *Arch Otolaryngol Head Neck Surg* 1999;125:157–163.

30. Smith JC, Johnson JT, Cognetti DM, et al: Quality of life, functional outcome, and cost of early glottic cancer. *Laryngoscope* 2003;113:68–76.

31. Reker U: Phonatory ability after surgery of vocal cord carcinoma of limited extension: A comparison between transoral laser microsurgery and frontolateral partial laryngeal resection. *Adv Otorhinolaryngol* 1995;49:215–218.

32. Tamura E, Kitahara S, Ogura M, et al: Voice quality after laser surgery or radiotherapy for T1a glottic carcinoma. *Laryngoscope* 2003;113:910–914.

33. Delsupehe KG, Zink I, Lejaegere M, et al: Voice quality after narrow-margin laser cordectomy compared with laryngeal irradiation. *Otolaryngol Head Neck Surg* 1999;121:528–533.

34. Lo Galbo AM, de Bree R, Kuk DJ, et al: The prevalence of hypothyroidism after treatment for laryngeal and hypopharyngeal carcinomas: Are autoantibodies of influence? *Acta Otolaryngol* 2007;127:312–317.

35. Gal RL, Gal TJ, Klotch DW, et al: Risk factors associated with hypothyroidism after laryngectomy. *Otolaryngol Head Neck Surg* 2000;123:211–217.

36. Aimoni C, Scanelli G, D'Agostino L, et al: Thyroid function studies in patients with cancer of the larynx: Preliminary evaluation. *Otolaryngol Head Neck Surg* 2003;129:733–738.

37. Mercado G, Adelstein DJ, Saxton JP, et al: Hypothyroidism: A frequent event after radiotherapy and after radiotherapy with chemotherapy for patients with head and neck carcinoma. *Cancer* 2001;92:2892–2897.

38. Buitelaar DR, Balm AJM, Antonini N, et al: Cardiovascular and respiratory complications after major head and neck surgery. *Head Neck* 2006;28:595–602.

39. Ong S-K, Morton RP, Kolbe J, et al: Pulmonary complications following major head and neck surgery with tracheotomy: A prospective, randomized, controlled trial of prophylactic antibiotics. *Arch Otolaryngol Head Neck Surg* 2004;130:1084–1087.

40. Kuo M, Cho CM, Wei WI, et al: Tracheostomal stenosis after total laryngectomy: An analysis of predisposing clinical factors. *Laryngoscope* 1994;104:59–63.

41. Gal TJ, Jones LM: Reconstruction of recalcitrant stenosis of the laryngectomy stoma using the radial forearm free flap. *Am J Otolaryngol* 2007;28:52–54.

42. Jacobson MC, Franssen E, Birt BD, et al: Predicting postlaryngectomy voice outcome in an era of primary tracheoesophageal fistulization: A retrospective evaluation. *J Otolaryngol* 1997;26:171–179.

43. Ho TP, Gray J, Ratcliffe AA, et al: Does cognitive function influence alaryngeal speech rehabilitation? *Head Neck* 2006;28:413–419.

44. Cheng E, Ho M, Ganz C, et al: Outcomes of primary and secondary tracheoesophageal puncture: A 16-year retrospective review. *Ear Nose Throat J* 2006;85:262–267.

45. Stafford FW: Current indications and complications of tracheoesophageal puncture for voice restoration after laryngectomy. *Curr Opin Otolaryngol Head Neck Surg* 2003;11:89–95.

46. Albirmawy OA, Elsheikh MN, Saafan ME, et al: Managing problems with tracheoesophageal puncture for alaryngeal voice rehabilitation. *J Laryngol Otol* 2006;120:470–477.

47. Calder N, MacAndie C, MacGregor F: Tracheoesophageal voice prostheses complications in north Glasgow. *J Laryngol Otol* 2006;120:487–491.

48. Singer MI, Blom ED, Hamaker RC: Pharyngeal plexus neurectomy for alaryngeal speech rehabilitation. *Laryngoscope* 1986;96:50–53.

49. Crary MA, Glowasky AL: Using botulinum toxin A to improve speech and swallowing function following total laryngectomy. *Arch Otolaryngol Head Neck Surg* 1996;122:760–763.

50. Hamaker RC, Blom ED: Botulinum neurotoxin for pharyngeal constrictor muscle spasm in tracheoesophageal voice restoration. *Laryngoscope* 2003;113:1479–1482.

51. Luff DA, Izzat S, Farrington WT: Viscoaugmentation as a treatment for leakage around the Provox 2 voice rehabilitation system. *J Laryngol Otol* 1999;113:847–848.

52. Laccourreye O, Papon JF, Brasnu D, et al: Autogenous fat injection for the incompetent tracheoesophageal puncture site. *Laryngoscope* 2002;112:1512–1514.

53. Rosen A, Scher N, Panje WR: Surgical closure of persisting failed tracheoesophageal voice fistula. *Ann Otol Rhinol Laryngol* 1997;106:775–778.

54. Rosen CA: Complications of phonosurgery: Results of a national survey. *Laryngoscope* 1998;108:1697–1703.

55. Woo P, Pearl AW, Hsiung MW, et al: Failed medialization laryngoplasty: Management by revision surgery. *Otolaryngol Head Neck Surg* 2001;124:615–621.

56. Rosen CA, Murry T, DeMarino DP: Late complication of type I thyroplasty: A case report. *J Voice* 1999;13:417–423.

57. Ayala MA, Patterson MB, Bach KK: Late displacement of a Montgomery thyroplasty implant following endotracheal intubation. *Ann Otol Rhinol Laryngol* 2007;116:262–264.

58. Ford CN, Bless DM, Loftus JM: Role of injectable collagen in the treatment of glottic insufficiency: A study of 119 patients. *Ann Otol Rhinol Laryngol* 1992;101:237–247.

59. Anderson TD, Sataloff RT: Complications of collagen injection of the vocal fold: Report of several unusual cases and review of the literature. *J Voice* 2004;18:392–397.

60. Luu Q, Tsai V, Mangunta V, et al: Safety of percutaneous injection of bovine dermal crosslinked collagen for glottic insufficiency. *Otolaryngol Head Neck Surg* 2007;136:445–449.

61. Laccourreye O, Papon JF, Kania R, et al: Intracordal injection of autologous fat in patients with unilateral laryngeal nerve paralysis: Long-term results from the patient's perspective. *Laryngoscope* 2003;113:541–545.

62. Tucker HM, Wanamaker J, Trott M, et al: Complications of laryngeal framework surgery (phonosurgery). *Laryngoscope* 1993;103:525–528.

63. Weinman E, Maragos NE: Airway complications in thyroplasty surgery. *Laryngoscope* 2000;110:1082–1085.

64. Abraham MT, Gonen M, Kraus DH: Complications of type I thyroplasty and arytenoid adduction. *Laryngoscope* 2001;111: 1322–1329.

65. Cummings CW, Purell LL, Flint PW: Hydroxylapatite laryngeal implants for medialization: Preliminary report. *Ann Otol Rhinol Laryngol* 1993;102:843–851.

66. Nayak VK, Bhattacharyya N, Kotz T, et al: Patterns of swallowing failure following medialization in unilateral vocal fold immobility. *Laryngoscope* 2002;112:1840–1844.

67. Fang TJ, Li HY, Tsai FC, et al: The role of glottal gap in predicting aspiration in patients with unilateral vocal paralysis. *Clin Otolaryngol Allied Sci* 2004;29:709–712.

68. Nouwen J, Hans S, De Mones E, et al: Thyroplasty type I without arytenoid adduction in patients with unilateral laryngeal nerve paralysis: The Montgomery implant versus the Gore-Tex implant. *Acta Otolaryngol* 2004;124:732–738.

69. Cotter CS, Avidano MA, Crary MA, et al: Laryngeal complications after type I thyroplasty. *Otolaryngol Head Neck Surg* 1995;113:671–673.

70. Halum SL, Posta GN, Koufman JA: Endoscopic management of extruding medialization laryngoplasty implants. *Laryngoscope* 2005;115:1051–1054.

71. Hsiung MW, Pai L: Autogenous fat injection for glottic insufficiency: Analysis of 101 cases and correlation with patients' self-assessment. *Acta Otolaryngol* 2006;126:191–196.

72. Nakayama M, Ford CN, Bless DM: Teflon vocal fold augmentation: Failures and management in 28 cases. *Otolaryngol Head Neck Surg* 1993;109:493–498.

73. Netterville JL, Coleman JR Jr, Chang S, et al: Lateral laryngotomy for the removal of Teflon granuloma. *Ann Otol Rhinol Laryngol* 1998;107:735–744.

74. Perepelitsyn I, Shapshay SM: Endoscopic treatment of laryngeal and tracheal stenosis—Has mitomycin C improved the outcome? *Otolaryngol Head Neck Surg* 2004;131:16–20.

75. Fried MP: A survey of the complications of laser laryngoscopy. *Arch Otolaryngol* 1984;110:31–34.

76. DeSanto LW, Olsen KD, Perry WC, et al: Quality of life after surgical treatment of cancer of the larynx. *Ann Otol Rhinol Laryngol* 1995;104:763–769.

77. Loughran S, Calder N, MacGregor FB, et al: Quality of life and voice following endoscopic resection or radiotherapy for early glottic cancer. *Clin Otolaryngol* 2005;30:42–47.

78. McNeil BJ, Weichselbaum R, Pauker SG: Speech and survival: Tradeoffs between quality and quantity of life in laryngeal cancer. *N Engl J Med* 1981;305:982–987.

79. Otto RA, Dobie RA, Lawrence V, et al: Impact of laryngectomy on quality of life: Perspective of the patient versus that of the health care provider. *Ann Otol Rhinol Laryngol* 1997;106:693–699.

80. Hanna E, Sherman A, Cash D, et al: Quality of life for patients following total laryngectomy vs chemoradiation for laryngeal preservation. *Arch Otolaryngol Head Neck Surg* 2004;130:875–879.

81. Vilaseca I, Chen AY, Backscheider AG: Long-term quality of life after total laryngectomy. *Head Neck* 2006;28:313–320.

82. Murry T, Medrado R, Hogikyan ND, et al: The relationship between ratings of voice quality and quality of life measures. *J Voice* 2004;18:183–192.

83. Johns MM, Garrett CG, Hwang J, et al: Quality-of-life outcomes following laryngeal endoscopic surgery for non-neoplastic vocal fold lesions. *Ann Otol Rhinol Laryngol* 2004;113:597–601.

84. Steen IN, MacKenzie K, Carding PN, et al: Optimising outcome assessment of voice interventions, II: Sensitivity to change of self-reported and observer-rated measures. *J Laryngol Otol* 2008;122(1):46–51.

CHAPTER 34

Complications of Tracheostomy and Tracheal Surgery

Ivan H. El-Sayed, Amol M. Bhatki, and Nissim Khabie

The recorded history of tracheotomy traces back to two ancient Egyptian tablets (3600 BC.) and to the Rig Veda (circa 2000 BC), a sacred Hindu medical text.[1] The first procedure is attributed by Galen to Asclepiades of Bithynia during the first century BC, and Alexander the Great is thought to have performed a tracheotomy on one of his soldiers. The procedure failed to gain acceptance in the Western world, however, and it was regarded by physicians with disdain throughout the middle ages, because it was widely believed that incisions into cartilage could never heal. Interest in the tracheotomy was revived during the Renaissance, and the techniques and instrumentation associated with the procedure began to evolve.[1] Only 28 successful tracheotomies are recorded before 1825. The first reported successful tracheotomy was performed in 1546 by Antonio Muos Brasovolvo.[2] Sanctorious (1561–1636) introduced the use of a trocar, which he left in place for several days after the procedure. Marco Aurelio Serverino successfully treated patients with airway obstruction during the diphtheria epidemic of 1610. In 1718, Lorenz Heister championed the term *tracheotomy* and campaigned for its use. In 1730, George Martine introduced a double cannula for ease of cleaning.[1] The first successful pediatric tracheotomy was on a 7-year-old boy to remove a bean, and it was performed by St. Germain en Lay in Caron in 1766. During the early nineteenth century, again spurred by diphtheria, the tracheotomy came to the forefront as Bretonnear and Troussear demonstrated its efficacy to relieve airway obstruction.[2] However, issues regarding patient selection and the timing of tracheotomy were not defined, and it was a generally held belief that tracheotomy should be reserved until the last possible moment. Furthermore, physicians were unable to manage and recognize complications such as pneumothorax and obstructing granulomas. As a result of the poor timing, the lack of antibiotics, and the inability to manage complications, tracheotomy had a high mortality rate of 75% during the 1800s.[1]

Chevalier Jackson's methodic work standardized the technique while reducing the mortality rate to 0.5%.[1] Having become an accepted surgical procedure for emergent airway obstruction, indications for tracheotomy expanded with the introduction of positive-pressure respiratory ventilation.[3] The era of the elective tracheotomy was initiated to facilitate mechanical ventilation and to prevent complications of long-term oral intubation.[4,5] As the incidence of tracheotomies increased, a new set of complications became apparent that were related to high-pressure cuffs and rigid tubing, including postintubation stenosis, tracheomalacia, ulceration granuloma, tracheoesophageal fistula, and innominate artery fistula. Further technologic advancement helped alleviate these complications with the introduction of soft tracheotomy tubes and low-pressure cuffs.

With the advancement of surgical techniques and the knowledge gained from recent studies, percutaneous dilatational tracheotomy (PDT) has gained acceptance and is becoming an accepted method of elective tracheotomy. Percutaneous tracheotomy was first described by Shelden and colleagues[6] in 1957. Toy and Weinstein[7] modified the technique by applying the guide-wire principle of Seldinger in 1969. Technical difficulties and anatomic uncertainty, however, prevented the wide use of this technique. Ciaglia and colleagues[8] described successful PDT by serially dilating over the guide wire. Wang and colleagues[9] noted a high complication rate in a series of 7 patients, and they therefore condemned this procedure by "relegating [it] to the waste pile of many other previously failed techniques." However, several larger studies have since shown an excellent safety record, especially when PDT is performed with bronchoscopic guidance.[10–15] In addition, three meta-analyses show a lower overall complication rate when comparing PDT with standard surgical tracheotomy.[10,13,16] The skepticism is now fading, and PDT is becoming popular as a safe, cost-effective, and efficient way of providing elective tracheotomy to critically ill patients.

No discussion of tracheotomy is complete without the mention of terminology. *Tracheotomy* properly refers to an operation in which an incision is made in the trachea.[2] *Tracheostomy* refers to a procedure in which the epithelial lining of the skin of the neck is sutured or approximated with the epithelium of the trachea. This can be accomplished either by raising a flap of the anterior tracheal wall or skin and closing it to its counterpart or by bringing the distal end of the transected trachea (i.e., after laryngectomy) to anastomose with the skin. The opening is referred to as a *tracheal stoma* or a *tracheostoma*. Although clarification of the terminology may seem trivial, poor standardization of terminology surrounding surgical airways is a potential source of error in airway management. To improve communication among providers and during emergencies at the authors' institution, an airway form has been instituted, and it is posted at the bedside of every patient with a surgical airway to identify the type of airway and the means of patient ventilation in the event of an emergency (Figure 34-1).

Medical advances also introduced a better ability to deal with tracheal disease related to intubation, tracheostomy, and other diseases. Rigid and flexible

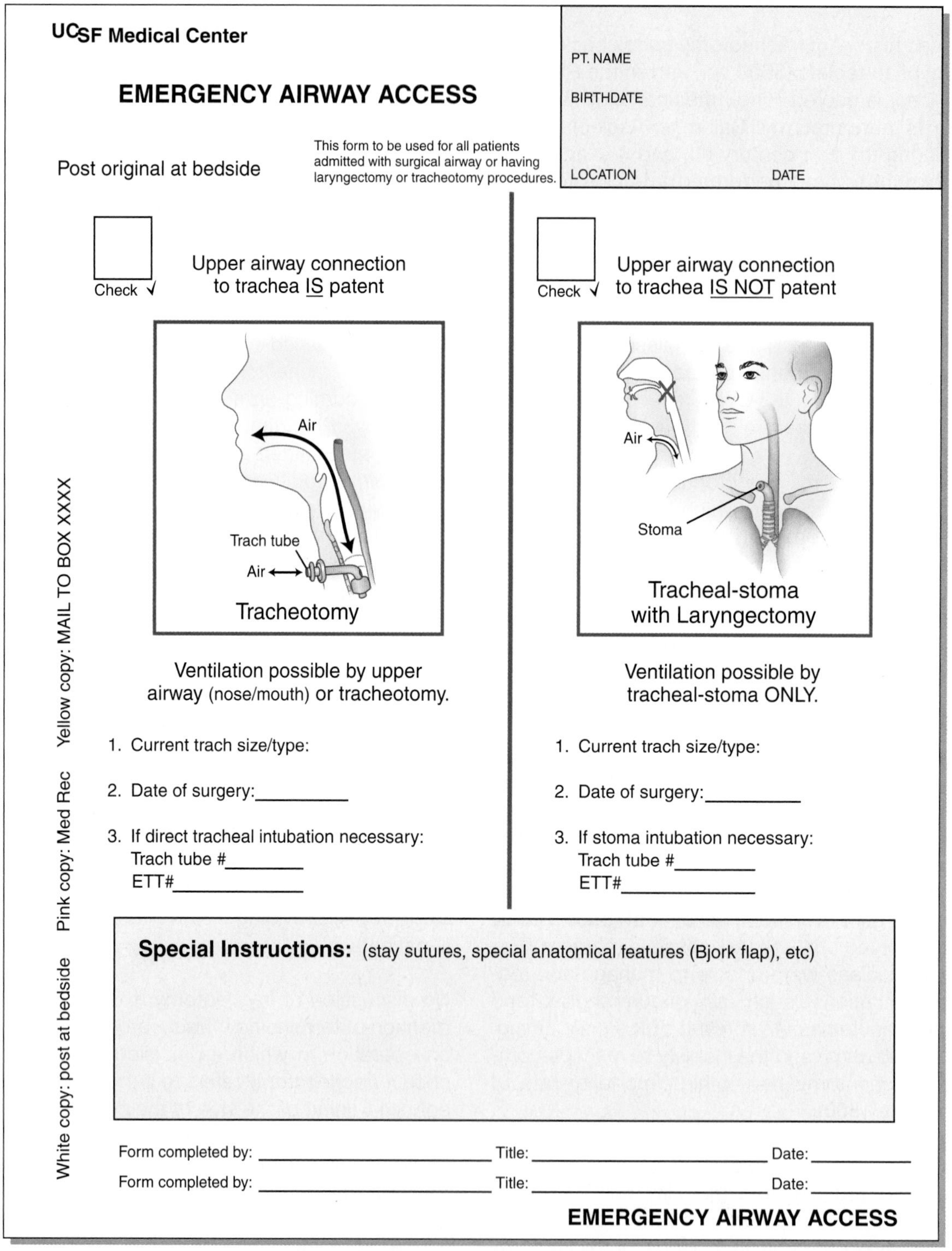

UCSF Medical Center

EMERGENCY AIRWAY ACCESS

Post original at bedside

This form to be used for all patients admitted with surgical airway or having laryngectomy or tracheotomy procedures.

PT. NAME
BIRTHDATE
LOCATION DATE

Check √ Upper airway connection to trachea IS patent

Tracheotomy

Ventilation possible by upper airway (nose/mouth) or tracheotomy.

1. Current trach size/type:
2. Date of surgery:__________
3. If direct tracheal intubation necessary:
   Trach tube #________
   ETT#_____________

Check √ Upper airway connection to trachea IS NOT patent

Tracheal-stoma with Laryngectomy

Ventilation possible by tracheal-stoma ONLY.

1. Current trach size/type:
2. Date of surgery:__________
3. If stoma intubation necessary:
   Trach tube #________
   ETT#_____________

Special Instructions: (stay sutures, special anatomical features (Bjork flap), etc)

Form completed by: ______________ Title: ______________ Date: ________
Form completed by: ______________ Title: ______________ Date: ________

EMERGENCY AIRWAY ACCESS

White copy: post at bedside Pink copy: Med Rec Yellow copy: MAIL TO BOX XXXX

Figure 34-1. The Emergency Airway Access form is designed to convey important information efficiently to first responders in the event of the loss of a surgical airway. The form is posted at the bedside of all patients with a tracheotomy or laryngectomy in the authors' institution to help clinicians to understand important airway alterations. The form serves to do the following: (1) to efficiently identify the airway in emergent situations; (2) to standardize terminology; and (3) to identify patients for whom oral intubation is impossible.

bronchoscopy, laser bronchoscopy, intraluminal stents, and open tracheal resections or stenting have recently evolved to aid in the management of a host of disorders across the age spectrum. This chapter provides an overview of the important complications of tracheotomy and tracheal surgery encountered by head and neck surgeons.

TRACHEOTOMY INDICATIONS

Indications for tracheotomy are upper-airway obstruction, the need for pulmonary toilet, and respiratory insufficiency. Although these three issues can often be initially addressed with short-term endotracheal intubation, long-term management requires assessment for a tracheotomy. Among intubated patients, the benefits of a tracheotomy as compared with a prolonged translaryngeal intubation include the following: improved patient comfort with a decreased need for sedatives; improved pulmonary toilet; decreased airway resistance; enhanced patient mobility; reduced ventilator-associated pneumonia; a secure airway; increased potential for oral intake and speech; accelerated ventilator weaning; and the potential ability to transfer ventilator-dependent patients from the intensive care unit.[17] Importantly, complications from the prolonged orotracheal intubation that include laryngeal or tracheal mucosal injury and that give rise to vocal-fold paralysis, ulcers, granulomas, or secondary stenosis can also be avoided.

The optimal timing for tracheotomy is controversial and evolving. Older studies found that injuries related to oral intubation were related to pressure necrosis in the glottis and at the site of the cuff.[18] With the introduction of low-pressure cuffs, tracheal injuries from the cuffs of oral endotracheal tubes and tracheotomy tubes are greatly reduced. Lindholm[19] discovered 1 death among 120 children that was a likely complication of prolonged oral intubation as a result of the small caliber of the tubes. Currently tracheotomies are generally performed after 7 to 14 days in critically ill patients to avoid complications associated with long-term intubation.[20] However, Rumbak and colleagues[21] recently reported that early tracheotomy in the intensive care unit (defined as an early percutaneous tracheotomy within 48 hours of intubation), in contrast with delayed tracheotomy at 14 to 16 days, greatly diminished the time in the intensive care unit, the time on mechanical ventilation, the cumulative frequency of pneumonia (5% vs. 25%), the mortality rate (31.7% vs. 61.7%), and accidental extubation (0 vs. 6). Overall, the early tracheotomy group spent less time in the intensive care unit (5 vs. 16 days) and less time on the ventilator (7.6 vs. 17.4 days).[21] Although further research is needed, a paradigm shift to early tracheotomy may be on the horizon.[22]

SURGICAL AIRWAY TECHNIQUES

Cricothyroidotomy

Cricothyroidotomy is generally performed as an emergent procedure for upper-airway obstruction when intubation is either contraindicated or has failed. This procedure may also be used when access to the tracheal rings is limited (e.g., rheumatoid arthritis, achondroplasia) or when the extension of the neck is contraindicated and tracheotomy cannot be adequately performed.

In an emergency, this direct approach is advantageous over a formal tracheotomy. With the patient supine and the neck extended, a horizontal skin incision is made over the cricothyroid membrane. The incision is then sharply continued through this membrane in a horizontal fashion, and the airway is cannulated with a small-diameter tracheotomy tube (e.g., No. 4) or a small endotracheal tube. A tracheal hook can be used to superiorly elevate the cricoid cartilage and to facilitate tube placement. Although this "slash" incision provides direct access to the airway, the anterior jugular veins, the cricothyroid muscle, and the superior laryngeal nerves are at risk. Some surgeons use a midline vertical skin incision to minimize inadvertent injury to these structures.[23] In such circumstances, the soft tissues of the neck are retracted laterally until the cricothyroid membrane is identified and horizontally incised.

Open Tracheotomy

So long as the requisite lighting, equipment, and ancillary staff are available, the procedure can be performed in either the operating room or the intensive care unit. The patient lies supine with the neck in mild extension. Landmarks including the laryngeal prominence, the cricoid cartilage, and the jugular notch are identified and marked. Local anesthetic containing epinephrine is infiltrated subcutaneously. The fraction of inspired oxygen is decreased to the lowest tolerated level to minimize the risk of airway fire if electrocautery is used. A vertical or horizontal incision is made between the cricoid cartilage and the jugular notch. Subcutaneous fat is incised in the midline. The strap muscles are then separated in the midline and retracted laterally. If the thyroid isthmus impedes access to the airway, it is next bluntly dissected away from the trachea and divided with electrocautery or suture ligated. When electrocautery is no longer necessary, the patient can then be preoxygenated on 100% oxygen. A tracheal hook may be placed to elevate and stabilize the cricoid, if necessary, and a transverse incision is made between the second and third tracheal rings. An inferiorly based U-shaped flap (i.e., a Björk flap) can be created and sutured to the skin to maintain patency in the event of accidental postoperative decannulation. Alternatively, retention sutures can be placed to accomplish the same objective. The tested tracheotomy tube is then inserted under direct visualization with minimal force. The tube is attached to the respiratory circuit, and the cuff is inflated. Bilateral chest rise, adequate tidal volumes, and positive tracing on capnometry all indicate proper tube placement. The tube is secured in place with sutures and firmly tied with twill ties (Figure 34-2).

Percutaneous Tracheotomy

There are several techniques by which to perform percutaneous tracheotomy. Examples include the rapid percutaneous tracheotomy, the Griggs guide-wire dilating forceps method, the Fantoni translaryngeal technique, and the Ciaglia percutaneous dilatational tracheotomy.[14] The authors' group prefers the Ciaglia method and uses the Blue Rhino Percutaneous Tracheostomy Introducer Set (Cook Critical Care, Bloomington, IN).

The procedure can be performed at the bedside in the intensive care unit or in the operating room. A history and physical examination are performed to identify concerning features such as a history of tracheotomy or neck surgery, the inability to palpate the trachea, a low-lying cricoid, or an anomalous innominate artery. The neck is placed in extension, and 100% oxygen is delivered. Additional intravenous sedation may be necessary. Neck landmarks are identified, local anesthesia with epinephrine is injected subcutaneously, and the site is prepared and draped. A transverse 1.5-cm skin incision is made one-finger's-width above the sternal notch just inferior to the palpable cricoid ring. Blunt dissection of the subcutaneous tissue identifies the investing fascia and will allow for the passage of the dilator. A bronchoscope connected to a video screen is inserted into the endotracheal tube, and the intensive care staff monitors the vital signs, including the pulse oximetry, continuously. The endotracheal tube is withdrawn under direct vision to the level of the subglottis, transilluminating the incision site. The trachea is palpated with a mosquito clamp, and the site of palpations is identified with the bronchoscope. The introducer needle is inserted into the trachea in the midline approximately 1.5 cm below the cricoid ring. Video bronchoscopy confirms the entrance of the needle into the airway without injury to the posterior tracheal wall. Before the needle is removed, a J-tipped wire is inserted through the needle into the distal airway over which a 14-Fr introducer dilator is gently inserted into the tracheal lumen. The 8-Fr guiding catheter and the Blue Rhino dilator further gently dilate the tracheal opening with firm pressure. The Blue Rhino dilator has a lubricating substance on it that is activated immediately before its use with sterile saline. The tracheotomy tube, preloaded with a tapered dilator, is then passed into the defect and inserted into the trachea. After proper tube

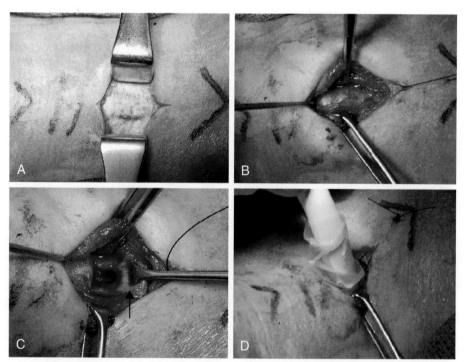

Figure 34-2. Tracheotomy. **A,** After a vertical incision, the subcutaneous tissue is dissected until the investing fascia of the strap muscles is identified. Care is taken to avoid traumatizing the anterior jugular veins. **B,** The midline raphe is identified, and the strap muscles are sequentially retracted laterally. If the thyroid isthmus is obstructing access, it is also divided and suture ligated. **C,** A horizontal incision is made between the second and third tracheal rings. Subsequently, an inferiorly-based, U-shaped Björk flap *(arrow)* is sutured to the inferior skin. **D,** The tracheotomy tube is then inserted into the trachea under direct visualization. The circuit is connected, and the balloon is inflated. Bilateral chest rise, the detection of carbon dioxide on capnometry, and the adequate delivery of tidal volumes confirm positioning.

placement is confirmed by the passage of the broncho-scope through the tracheotomy tube, the endotracheal tube is removed, and the tracheotomy tube is secured in place.

COMPLICATIONS OF TRACHEOTOMY

Intraoperative Complications of Tracheotomy

Several possible intraoperative complications may arise during the performance of a surgical airway. These include premature airway obstruction, paratracheal insertion, hemorrhage, and intraoperative airway fire. The overall incidence of tracheotomy complications is about 15%, with a two- to five-times higher rate for emergent procedures.[24,25]

Premature Airway Obstruction (Loss of Airway)

The best approach to the management of the difficult airway is to recognize the situation early and to anticipate the worst-case scenario, thereby minimizing the risk of complete airway obstruction precipitated by failed intubation, oversedation, neoplasm, or infection. The patient, when possible, should be psychologically prepared while instrumentation is procured and tested in advance. Intravenous steroids, racemic epinephrine, and helium and oxygen treatments are interventions that may be useful temporarily. Also, continuous positive airway pressure (CPAP) may allow for temporary mechanical stenting of the airway. It is important to minimize airway trauma with repetitive intubation attempts or blind nasal intubations that can create edema or bleeding and induce laryngeal airway obstruction.

In the event of airway obstruction with failed intubation, alternative methods of tracheal intubation should be considered. This may include an intubating laryngeal mask airway, rigid bronchoscopy with a ventilating bronchoscope, and transtracheal needle jet ventilation. Forethought along with cooperation and communication between the surgeon and the anesthesiologist is essential for success. If the patient is maintaining a satisfactory airway, it is important to allow him or her to continue to do so. Paralytic agents should generally be avoided in this situation. A surgical airway should be obtained after reasonable attempts to secure the airway transorally have failed or if the patient's cardiopulmonary status deteriorates.

Paratracheal Insertion

The creation of a false passage as a result of improper tube insertion not only compromises airway security, but it can also lead to the collateral damage of adjacent tissues. Failure to ventilate the lungs immediately after the insertion of the tracheotomy tube suggests tube misplacement. This may occur anterior to the trachea within the soft tissues of the neck. Alternatively, the tube may perforate through the posterior tracheal wall into the mediastinum or the esophagus. Paratracheal insertion can occur either during the initial operative placement of the tube or during replacement after accidental dislodgement or routine tracheotomy tube changes.

Several maneuvers allow for the confirmation of proper tube placement. First, after the tracheal incision is made, the tracheotomy tube should be inserted into the trachea under direct vision. Rotation of the wrist allows the tube to follow its curve into the airway. Second, after the anesthesia circuit is reconnected, adequate ventilation is indicated by the detection of carbon dioxide with capnometry as well as tidal volumes commensurate with preoperative levels. Simultaneously, the surgeon can inspect for a symmetric chest rise. Third, suction tubing should pass easily into the trachea without resistance. The development of subcutaneous emphysema or a pneumothorax can also be an indicator of paratracheal insertion.

Esophageal perforation is an uncommon complication. When suspected, management includes endoscopic evaluation to assess the location and extent of the perforation. The tube should be positioned distal to the site of injury. A nasogastric tube should be placed under endoscopic guidance, and systemic antibiotics should be administered. Conservative management should result in the closure of small defects. Larger defects or the presence of a persistent tracheoesophageal fistula require surgical exploration and repair.

Special consideration is given to PDT. The use of the video fiber-optic bronchoscope during PDT is especially important to prevent paratracheal insertion or esophageal perforation. In a prospective trial, Cole and colleagues[26] reported three misplaced tubes (one resulting in death) in 32 patients without bronchoscopic assistance as compared with only two minor complications in 23 procedures performed with bronchoscopic assistance. Kost[14] reported a low 6.5% complication rate in 309 patients with the Ciaglia method and the Blue Rhino single dilator using bronchoscopy. The use of the video endoscope appears to be essential to ensuring the proper placement of the tube during the procedure.

Intraoperative Hemorrhage

Bleeding during tracheotomy may be significant, and it may cause both intraoperative and postoperative difficulties. The causes of bleeding are related to surgical technique as well as to inherent predisposing patient factors. Anticoagulants and antiplatelet agents significantly increase the risk of hemorrhage. Elective cases should therefore be delayed until the effects of these agents have waned. Often patients requiring tracheotomy are critically ill and have multisystem pathology. Coagulopathies that result from liver, bone marrow, or consumptive problems should be corrected whenever possible. Management includes the administration of fresh frozen plasma, coagulation factors, platelet transfusion, or intramuscular vitamin K and the topical application of coagulants such as thrombin or absorbable hemostatic packing. In emergent situations, however, the surgeon must be prepared to deal with potential bleeding.

Anatomic discrepancies may also contribute to intraoperative hemorrhage. The paired anterior jugular veins, which run within the investing cervical fascia, are variable in their course, and they are a common site of bleeding.[27,28] In 30% of cases, a duplicate anterior jugular vein is present, and these veins sometimes cross the midline.[29] Before the dissection of this fascial layer, these veins should be identified and avoided or, alternatively, ligated. Deeper in the neck, 1% to 8% of individuals may have a thyroid ima artery that courses along the anterior trachea.[30] This vessel must be identified and controlled, because the proximal portion may retract into the lower neck or the mediastinum and continue to bleed. Furthermore, the thyroid isthmus, which is a vascular structure, is often divided to gain tracheal access. Hemostasis of the cut edges of the isthmus either by electrocautery[31] or suture ligation[32] minimizes bleeding. Alternatively, some surgeons simply retract the thyroid isthmus,[33] but this approach increases the risk of airway obstruction of the newly formed tracheotomy opening in the event of accidental decannulation.

The identification of a high-riding innominate artery is of utmost importance during tracheotomy (Figure 34-3). Although uncommon, the innominate artery, which is the first branch of the aortic arch and which travels anterior to the cervical trachea before dividing into the right common carotid and the right subclavian arteries, may cross the cervical trachea.[34] By palpation of the suprasternal soft tissues preoperatively and intraoperatively for a pulsatile mass, the identification of this vessel avoids catastrophic hemorrhage and possible death from its inadvertent injury. Among patients who are suspected of having a high-riding innominate artery, preoperative imaging with ultrasound or computed tomography scanning can identify the vessel. If the vessel is identified intraoperatively, a sternocleidomastoid muscle interposition flap can be used to separate the tracheostomy tube from the vessel to prevent vessel erosion.

Intraoperative Airway Fire

Airway fire is a rare but devastating complication of tracheotomy. The combination of an endotracheal tube, a high flow of oxygen, and electrocautery provide combustible material, an oxidizer, and an ignition source, respectively. Although the flammability of common inhaled anesthetics is insignificant,[35] the high frequency of laser and electrocautery in the airway

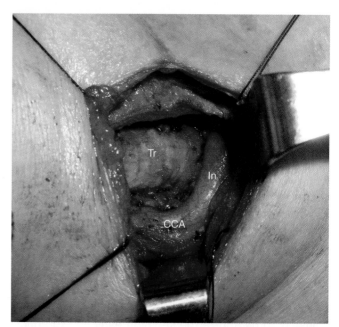

Figure 34-3. Intraoperative identification of a high-riding innominate artery. The central neck is shown here after thyroidectomy and central neck dissection. The innominate artery *(In)* is seen crossing the trachea *(Tr)* at the fifth tracheal ring, after which it divides into the common carotid artery *(CCA)* and the right subclavian artery (not shown).

necessitates an understanding of fires and prevention strategies.

Electrocautery, which is a ubiquitous tool in the operating room, is a frequent cause of operating room fires. The tip of this instrument can reach 1670°F (910°C); this, in combination with an alternating current, can lead to sparking.[36] Thus direct contact with an oxygen-rich environment or combustible materials is not necessary. From 1987 to 2006, at least 24 cases of airway fires specifically related to tracheotomy were reported, all of which involved electrocautery.[37] In many cases, cautery was used to incise the trachea or obtain hemostasis after tracheal opening. Cautery should be used with great caution after the trachea is exposed and not at all after the trachea is incised.

Endotracheal tubes, which are often made of polyvinyl chloride, are flammable and can ignite in oxygen environments of as low as 25%.[36] Their shape along with airflow from the ventilation circuit facilitates rapid ignition with the expulsion of heat, flames, and fumes both proximally and distally (i.e., the "blowtorch effect"), resulting in severe burns of the upper and lower airways.

Although some speculate that an inflated cuff distal to the operative site obviates the risk of fire, oxygen flowing at even low volumes within the tube can precipitate combustion. With a low ignition coefficient, oxygen is ignitable at 26% concentration.[37] As reported by the Emergency Care Research Institute, 74% of all surgical fires occurred in an oxygen-rich environment, with approximately one third occurring in the airway.[38] Often patients requiring tracheotomy have comorbid conditions that require a higher fraction of inhaled oxygen, thus increasing the risk of ignition. In addition to oxygen, inhaled anesthetic agents such as nitrous oxide carry the same risk of flammability and should be avoided.[39] Other combustible materials such as drapes, rubber, paper, and gauze are often present in the operative field. These materials also serve as potential fuels, and therefore electrocautery should be used cautiously in their presence. Of notable interest is that volatile skin preparation agents that contain isopropyl alcohol evaporate into flammable vapors that are combustible with electrosurgery and that have caused operating room fires.[39,40]

Several key measures are necessary to prevent fires in the operating room. Foremost is effective communication with the anesthesiologist. Flammable vapors can be dispersed through a hole in the tube or after the cuff is let down, or they may accumulate in the spaces below the drapes around the neck. Care should be taken to allow 3 minutes to elapse after the application of alcohol-based preparatory solutions before the use of electrocautery. The patient should be on the lowest concentration of oxygen that is safely tolerated (preferably less than 40%). In addition, nitrous oxide should be avoided. The operative field should be free of loose drapes, gauze, and other combustible material. Electrocautery should be avoided after the trachea is exposed. Hemostasis necessitating electrocautery should be obtained before the tracheal incision.

If an airway fire occurs, immediate and decisive action by both the anesthesiologist and the surgeon is necessary. The endotracheal tube should be immediately withdrawn and ventilation ceased. The airway circuit should be removed from the anesthesia machine. Any burning material should be extinguished, and oxygen should be delivered by mask ventilation until the trachea can be intubated.[37] Thereafter the entire upper aerodigestive tract should be carefully inspected for thermal injury. Antibiotics and steroids can be administered, depending on the extent of the injury.

Early Postoperative Complications of Tracheotomy

Hemorrhage

Hemorrhage is the most common complication during the early postoperative period, with a reported incidence ranging between 0.8% and 5.7%.[13,24,41] However, most bleeding is minor, and it results from inadequate intraoperative hemostasis. Elevated venous pressure from coughing can increase the risk. Management includes the packing of the wound with Nu-Gauze or hemostatic material (i.e., SurgiCel [Johnson and Johnson, Somerville, NJ],

Avitene [C. R. Bard, Inc., Murray Hill, NJ], Gelfoam [Pfizer, Inc., New York, NY]) and the correction of a coagulopathy, if present. The use of tissue sealant is not recommended. If bleeding is refractory to these techniques, the patient should be returned to the operating room for thorough evaluation of the wound and definitive control of the source of bleeding (Figure 34-4).

Tube Obstruction

Tube obstruction is the second most common complication during the early postoperative period. With an incidence that ranges from 0.3% to 2.7%,[24,42] this specific complication carries with it a high mortality rate. Among pediatric patients, tube obstruction comprises one third of all early complications.[43] Tube obstruction within the first 24 hours is likely the result of a blood clot or a mucous plug, partial tube dislodgement, or tube impingement on the posterior tracheal wall. Routine care should include intensive care unit observation and monitoring, humidification, regular cleaning or replacement of the inner cannula (in adults), and frequent suctioning. Nursing staff members should be instructed about the importance of diligent tracheotomy care and monitoring to prevent this complication.

Accidental Decannulation

Accidental decannulation or tube dislodgment is the third most common complication during the early postoperative period among patients undergoing tracheotomy, with an incidence of approximately 0.3% to 1.5%.[24,42] Several factors—including tube length, the thickness of the neck, the site of the tracheotomy, and the effectiveness of securing the tube—can contribute to dislodgment.

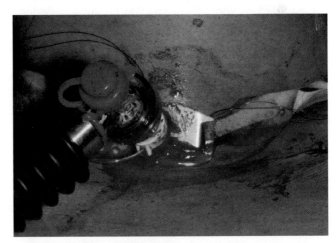

Figure 34-4. Postoperative hemorrhage. Hemorrhage can range from scant to gross bleeding. Bright red blood or copious dark blood clot formation around the stoma indicate a significant bleed. Initial inspection around the tracheotomy tube may identify the bleeding source while protecting the airway. The use of electrocautery should be avoided in ventilated patients requiring oxygen supplementation. If the bleeding cannot be controlled, then the patient must be taken back to the operating room, where adequate lighting, suction, and equipment are available for the inspection, clamping, and suture ligation of significant vessels.

The length and the curvature of the tracheotomy tube have historically been uncontrollable variables. Standard tracheotomy tubes stocked by hospitals and emergency rooms may not accommodate patients with large tumors or obese necks or burn patients with progressive soft-tissue edema. The Rusch tube (Willy Rusch, Stuttgart, Germany) was the first tube to provide an accommodating adjustable flange. However, several brands now offer adjustable tubes or a wide range of extended-length tubes such as Bivona and Portex (Smiths Medical, United Kingdom) and Shiley (Nellcore, Hayward, CA).

The surgeon may minimize the risk of accidental tube dislodgement by ensuring the proper placement of the tracheotomy, appropriately sizing the tracheotomy tube, and securing the tracheotomy to the patient's neck. The tracheotomy incision should be made between the second and fourth tracheal rings to allow for an adequate distance from the subglottic region; this ensures that the stoma will not descend into the thorax after the patient's neck is flexed. The distance from the tracheal wall to the skin increases more distally in the trachea. Further, variability exists between patients on the basis of the thickness of the skin and the subcutaneous tissue and the slope of the angle of the trachea away from the skin as it descends into the thorax (Figure 34-5). The selection of a tracheotomy tube of appropriate size, length, and angulation is important to ensure a proper fit for a given patient with minimal adjacent mucosal trauma. The tracheotomy tube must then be secured in place with nonabsorbable sutures through four points of the faceplate. Twill ties provide further security and should be placed snugly with the patient's neck in the neutral position. When concern for tube dislodgement exists, the creation of a permanent tracheostomy, as described by Eliachar and colleagues,[44] may be warranted. Alternatively, a Björk flap or lateral tracheal stay sutures are also useful for patients who are at risk for decannulation.

Pneumothorax

The incidence of pneumothorax after adult tracheotomy is between 0% and 5%.[41,45-47] Berg and colleagues[46] propose three pathophysiologic mechanisms. The first involves direct injury to the pleura, because the pleural cupula extends into the root of the neck. A second theory suggests that air may dissect through the deep layer of the middle cervical fascia, thus leading to pneumomediastinum. If air ruptures the mediastinal pleura, then a pneumothorax results. The third possibility is that a ruptured alveolar bleb can also result in a pneumothorax. Clinical signs of pneumothorax, such as tachycardia (pulse >120 bpm), oxygen desaturation, decreased breath sounds, dyspnea, subcutaneous emphysema, and chest pain, may be present during the postoperative period.[41]

Routine postoperative chest radiographs are traditionally advocated to evaluate for pneumothorax, pneumomediastinum, and tube position. However, several recent studies have argued against the benefits of this practice. Barlow and colleagues[47] retrospectively reviewed 100 adult tracheotomies and found 2 cases of pneumothorax. Both patients had risk factors or signs and symptoms of pneumothorax postoperatively. Two additional retrospective studies revealed pneumothorax rates of 1.2% and 1% in 250 and 100 patients, respectively.[41,45] In patients with clinically significant pneumothoraces, clinical signs were present, and chest radiograph confirmed the diagnosis and guided management. However, there was a higher rate of pneumothorax for urgent or emergent procedures.[41] In lieu of this evidence, routine chest radiography is not recommended, and it can be reserved for patients who exhibit signs or symptoms of pneumothorax, pediatric

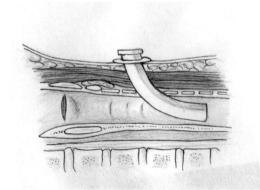
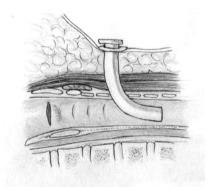

Figure 34-5. Anatomic variation of the relation of the trachea to the skin. The thickness of the skin and the subcutaneous tissues can vary from thin to thick necks. The angle of the trachea can vary, thereby increasing the distance from the skin to the trachea as it descends into the chest. In addition to the outer and inner diameters, tracheotomy tubes also vary in overall, proximal, and distal lengths as well as the angle of the proximal tracheotomy tube to the faceplate. The selection of appropriately sized tubes to match a patient's anatomy can reduce unplanned dislodgement and unnecessary mucosal trauma. (Artwork by Belinda Hahn.)

patients, urgent or emergent scenarios, or technically difficult cases.

Infection

Stomal cellulitis is the most common manifestation of tracheotomy wound infection, and it occurs in 2.4% to 6.6% of patients.[13,41] The source is likely the repeated contamination of the wound from secretions and saliva. Dressing changes, topical antimicrobial solutions, and broad-spectrum systemic antibiotics against staphylococci and gram-negative rods are the treatment. Abscess formation is relatively rare, and it is managed with adequate surgical drainage in addition to the previously described interventions.

Reports of rare but severe infectious complications of tracheotomy, such as osteomyelitis of the clavicle, mediastinitis, and necrotizing fasciitis, have been reported.[48–50] The early identification of these problems will minimize mortality. Prior radiation therapy, diabetes mellitus, an immunocompromised state, and malnutrition are all predisposing factors. For osteomyelitis, soft-tissue swelling or abscess and associated pain, especially in the clavicular head, may be early signs. Computed tomography and radionuclide bone scans are useful for diagnosis. Long-term parenteral antibiotics directed against the causative organism are the mainstay of treatment. For mediastinitis and necrotizing fasciitis, antibiotics alone may be insufficient, and surgical drainage and debridement are often necessary to remove loculated infections and devitalized tissue.[48,49] Infections of this magnitude may also require the removal of the tracheotomy tube and replacement with an endotracheal tube to improve wound drainage and minimize repeated contamination.

Postobstructive Pulmonary Edema

Negative-pressure pulmonary edema (NPPE) is defined as a noncardiogenic process in which a transudation of fluid into the pulmonary interstitium occurs in response to the generation of markedly negative intrathoracic pressures.[51] NPPE develops in two clinical scenarios. The more common type I occurs immediately after the onset of an acute upper airway obstructive process (e.g., laryngospasm, epiglottitis). Type II occurs after the relief of chronic upper airway obstruction, such as immediately after surgery for adenotonsillar hypertrophy or a laryngeal neoplasm.[51] Postobstructive pulmonary edema is estimated to occur among 11% of patients requiring active intervention for acute upper airway obstruction.[52]

The generation of highly negative intrathoracic pressures serves as the stimulus for the development of NPPE. Forceful inspiration against a closed glottis enhances venous return with a simultaneous increase in pulmonary microvascular hydrostatic pressure. This increased pressure favors a transudation of fluid into the

pulmonary interstitial space and results in pulmonary edema.[51] Laryngospasm is the most common cause of NPPE. However, it is unclear why only a minority of individuals with laryngospasm will progress to clinically significant pulmonary edema.[51]

Of supreme importance to the management of post-obstructive pulmonary edema is the maintenance of a high clinical index of suspicion, because the majority of negative outcomes are linked to a delay in diagnosis and appropriate intervention. The onset of pulmonary edema can be immediate or within hours of the obstructive event. In addition to the establishment of an airway and supplemental oxygen, the majority of cases will require mechanical ventilation with positive end-expiratory pressure from 5 cm H_2O to 10 cm H_2O. In less severe cases, continuous CPAP has been used successfully.[51] Resolution typically occurs within 24 hours, but the incidence of severe morbidity or death can range from 11% to 40%.[51,53,55]

Post-Tracheotomy Apnea

Apnea after tracheotomy has been reported, predominantly among patients suffering from obstructive sleep apnea who have become dependent on the hypoxic stimulation of the respiratory centers.[56] Sudden relief of the obstruction in conjunction with sedation may blunt the respiratory drive, resulting in periods of apnea despite systemic hypercapnia. Patients undergoing tracheotomy for obstructive sleep apnea should therefore be monitored postoperatively in the intensive care unit. If apnea is present, it should be managed with ventilation.

Late Postoperative Complications of Tracheotomy

Hemorrhage

Delayed bleeding after tracheotomy often results simply from stomal granulation tissue. Because of the possibility of massive hemorrhage from innominate artery erosion, however, the investigation of the source of any bleeding is mandatory. With the improved design of tracheotomy tubes and increased attention to surgical technique, the incidence of massive hemorrhage has decreased to less than 1%.[24,41]

Although venous injury may occur, the cause of massive hemorrhage during the late postoperative period is typically related to the erosion of the innominate artery. Tracheoinnominate fistula (TIF) is a rare but devastating complication of tracheotomy.[57] If a patient has immediate intervention when a TIF occurs, the rate of survival is reported as 14.3%.[58] Of patients who will develop a TIF, most (78%) do so within the first 3 weeks after tracheotomy[59]; therefore one must act with a high index of suspicion when investigating bleeding or hemoptysis in a tracheotomy patient to appropriately identify the source of any sentinel hemorrhage. Erosion of the anterior tracheal wall by the tube tip or cuff is the proposed mechanism for innominate artery rupture.[60] The tracheal wall and the intervening cartilage are devitalized by pressure from the tracheotomy tube, thus causing exposure of the innominate artery. Oshinsky and colleagues[60] found the innominate artery to vary in position from the sixth to thirteenth tracheal ring. Although it is recommended to never place the tracheotomy below the fifth tracheal ring, the variable location of the innominate artery can put any patient at risk for this complication.

In a patient with a tracheotomy, bleeding should be investigated by fiber-optic bronchoscopy with careful evaluation of the anterior tracheal wall. If erosion or necrosis is present, the patient must immediately be evaluated under general anesthesia in conjunction with a thoracic surgeon, with the patient prepared for mediastinal exploration and thoracotomy. After the tracheotomy tube is removed, an endotracheal tube is passed beyond the suspected site of injury. The artery is explored and, in the elective scenario, repaired or bypassed.[61] Surgical repair of the tracheal site should also include reinforcement with an interpositioned muscle flap.[62]

In the case of massive arterial hemorrhage, bleeding is minimized by direct digital pressure on the anterior wall of the trachea or the tracheostomal tract.[63] With the surgeon's finger in place, an endotracheal tube is then immediately passed beyond the bleeding site to secure the airway and to prevent blood from entering the lungs. If both a finger and a tube cannot be accommodated, the surgical site can be widened, or the cuff of the endotracheal tube can be inflated at the site of maximal injury, thus providing tamponade.[57] The patient is stabilized hemodynamically, and a satisfactory airway is assumed before the patient is transported to the operating room. The vertical extension of the stoma site inferiorly and partial sternotomy provide access for innominate artery division. Simple repair of the innominate artery results in high rebleeding rates (60%) and higher mortality (90%).[64] By contrast, the division of the innominate artery reduces rebleeding to 7%, with resulting improvement in long-term survival to 64%; ensuing neurologic or vascular compromise is rare.[64] As mentioned previously, tracheal repair with an interpositioned muscle flap is also required.

Infection

Clinically relevant tracheotomy site infections occur in 0.4% to 6.6% of cases.[13,24,41] The technique of tracheotomy may influence this incidence. A recent meta-analysis demonstrated a statistically significant reduction in the odds ratio for wound infection for PDT as compared with standard open surgical tracheotomy.[13] At any rate, infections are often easily treated with local wound care and systemic antibiotic therapy. Significant sequelae of infection such as granulation tissue and laryngeal and tracheal stenosis, however, are predisposed to occur.

A tracheostomy results in the bacterial contamination of the wound and the airway. Sasaki and colleagues[65] demonstrated the exponential growth of bacteria in tracheotomized dogs that were subjected to experimental subglottic injuries. By contrast, bacteria levels remained low among nontracheotomized controls. These findings suggest that the contaminated wound from tracheotomy can ascend and secondarily infect the larynx, especially if previous injuries from intubation exist.[65] This process then contributes to the formation of suprastomal granulation tissue and laryngeal stenosis.

Granulation tissue may cause bleeding, airway obstruction, and delayed wound healing after tracheotomy decannulation. In addition to occurring at the stoma, granulation tissue may develop on the anterior tracheal wall at the tip of the tracheotomy tube or on the posterior wall superior to a tube fenestram if a fenestrated tube is present. A higher incidence of granulation tissue formation and resultant mortality are seen among the pediatric population, as described later in this chapter.[43,66]

Small amounts of granulation tissue in the peristomal region may be sharply excised and followed by chemical cautery with silver nitrate. More involved areas are best managed by exposure with either a bronchoscope or a microscope-aided suspension subglottic scope and excision with a carbon-dioxide laser.[67] If direct access is not possible, a neodymium– or holmium–yttrium–aluminum–garnet laser may be delivered through a flexible fiber-optic scope.

Tracheocutaneous Fistula

Tracheocutaneous fistulas (Figure 34-6) can result from the incomplete healing of the tracheotomy wound as a result of patient metabolic factors or from the mechanical forces keeping the airway patent. Van Hueren[68] identified 2 fistulas in 150 patients (1.3%) having percutaneous tracheotomy. Among children, the condition has been associated with the method of tracheotomy, with a higher incidence seen when a "starplasty" procedure is used.[69] Patient factors include a longstanding stoma with a well-epithelized tract, a history of diabetes mellitus, obesity, hypothyroidism, or another metabolic condition. Among patients with chronic respiratory insufficiency (e.g., chronic obstructive pulmonary disease), the stoma may fail to heal as a result of the increased pulmonary demand. Among these patients, the persistent tracheal opening may benefit the patient by decreasing respiratory dead space, and the patients may ultimately benefit from a permanent tracheostomy. Management is on a case-by-case basis, depending on

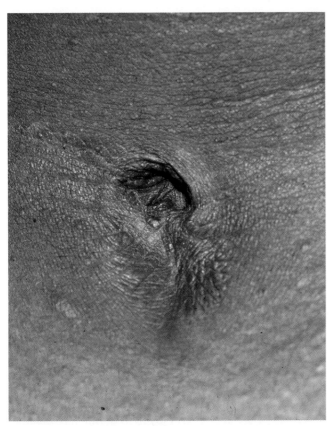

Figure 34-6. Tracheocutaneous fistula. A persistent fistula can develop with epithelialization of the tract. Poor wound healing or increased ventilatory needs may contribute to tract formation.

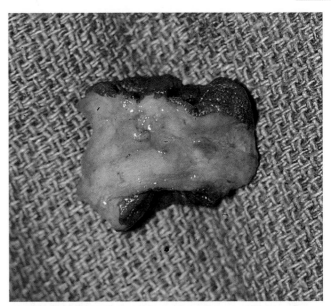

Figure 34-7. Excised fistula tract. The epithelialized tract is completely removed from the skin to the trachea, and the wound can be sutured closed in layers. A dressing with ointment-coated gauze can be placed, and the patient is instructed to hold pressure over the dressing during phonation and with coughing to help prevent air escape through the wound during the healing process.

the cause. Optimizing the patient's medical status is important. Cauterization[70] or the resection of an epithelized tract (Figure 34-7) and surgical closure may be necessary.[69,71,72]

Tracheoesophageal Fistula

Acquired tracheoesophageal fistula is a rare complication of tracheostomy, occurring in less than 0.5% of patients.[73,74] It is often associated with severe circumferential malacia of the trachea. Tracheoesophageal fistulas range from approximately 1.5 cm to 4 cm in length.[75] Pressure necrosis results from high cuff pressures or poorly positioned tracheotomy tubes, and repair requires addressing both problems at the same time. These lesions can be fixed in a single-stage or a two-stage procedure.[76] The lesion can be approached anteriorly or through a lateral approach. If a laryngotracheal reconstruction is needed, a multi-stage approach may be required.[77] Single-stage repairs have a complication rate of 25% to 50%.[76] Complications are related to excess tension at the tracheal anastomosis and inflammation of the tissue and the anastomotic site.[76] Complications of the repair include subcutaneous emphysema, tracheal stenosis, pneumonia, or a recurrent tracheoesophageal fistula.

Tracheal Stenosis

Tracheal stenosis is a well-known complication of tracheotomy and orotracheal intubation that occurs in approximately 1% of patients with a tracheotomy.[78] The cause is damage to the tracheal wall with resultant scarring. A 50% narrowing of the airway is necessary for a patient to become symptomatic.[79] Stenosis may occur as a result of the following three mechanisms:

1. Granuloma formation

2. A posteriorly depressed flap or anterior tracheal wall into the tracheal lumen

3. Anterolateral stenosis

The sites of obstruction include the glottis, the subglottis, the stoma, and the infrastomal trachea. Glottic injuries are related to the pressure from the endotracheal tube, whereas subglottic, stomal, and infrastomal lesions could result from the oral endotracheal tube or the tracheotomy tube. Subglottic stenosis occurs in the setting of a high tracheotomy or as a result of the superior erosion of the tracheotomy tube into the cricoid ring. This is more likely to occur in older kyphotic patients. The older literature elucidated the role of rigid tubing and high-pressure cuffs as major causes of stenosis. Rigid tubes do not conform to the patient's anatomy, and they can erode into the tracheal wall. Unfortunately the incidence of tracheal stenosis has not significantly diminished after the introduction of low-pressure, large-volume cuffs, perhaps as a result of the misuse of low-pressure cuffs and long periods of intubation.[80]

Granulation tissue can be identified while the tracheotomy tube is still in place, or it may be noted weeks to months after decannulation. It results from mucosal injury and ulceration. As the exuberant healing proceeds, it may obstruct the airway. The curve of the tube can depress the tracheal wall flap above the stoma into the airway. If this is prolonged, the flap may remain in place and even become calcified after the removal the tube, thereby causing obstruction at the stoma. The selection of a tracheotomy tube that properly fits the airway is important to ventilate adequately without side walling the tube and also to decrease unnecessary tracheal cartilage and mucosal injury (see Figure 34-5). The authors prefer to minimize the use of fenestrated tubes in favor of smaller-diameter, nonfenestrated tubes or the use of alternative types of tracheotomy tubes such as the Montgomery long-term cannula (Boston Medical, Boston, MA) or the Olympic button (Olympic Medical, Seattle, WA).

Anterolateral tracheal stenosis is the most common form of stenosis. The cause is thought to be an excessive opening of the tracheal wall caused either by the erosion of the tracheotomy tube toward the side, bacterial superinfection, or retropulsion of the tracheotomy as a result of the excessive weight of the connected tubing. Whatever the cause, the stoma is large as compared with the trachea. The anterior wall of the trachea then narrows as it scars, pulling the two lateral walls into a classic triangular "A" shape that is recognizable on bronchoscopy.[81]

Infrastomal stenosis is thought to result from high pressure or poorly fitting cuffs. Cooper and Grillo[82] found that a cuff pressure of 25 cm incited ulceration and tracheal injury, which were followed by cicatricial stenosis and airway obstruction. It is thought that injury results from pressure necrosis caused by the occlusion of the capillary blood blow. In addition, rigid tubes were designed without regard for the shape of the trachea, and the cuffs were formerly round and filled to a high volume. Grillo introduced a latex cuff that would continually conform to the shape of the trachea with a low pressure. Technical difficulties with the manufacturing, storage, and expense of latex cuffs made them impractical. The shapes of the cuff and the tracheotomy tube are also important. Because the inner trachea is elliptical (being wider at the sides), round cuffs exert more pressure at the anterior wall. Large-volume cuffs can create a seal over a large surface area and thus decrease the chance of focal necrosis. Current cuffs are made of nondistensible plastic that have a lower safety profile than latex and that can become high-pressure cuffs with overinflation. Therefore

it is important to understand that the cuff should be inflated only to the minimum amount necessary to create a seal.[79]

Tracheomalacia and trachiectasis also occur, and their exact causes are unknown.[79] This problem is associated with the need for an excessive cuff volume to create a seal. The site of the cuff should be changed by altering the tube length. The authors prefer to use large foam cuff tubes (i.e., Bivona [Smiths Medical, Inc., St. Paul, MN]) in these cases to prevent the progression of the malacia. Another alternative is placing a double cuff tube to broaden the area of the seal and to limit focally high pressure on the trachea. Care must be taken to attempt to prevent increasing the size of the defect with frequent monitoring to ensure low cuff volumes.

Percutaneous Tracheotomy

Patient Selection

When evaluating a patient for PDT, there are several contraindications that one must consider. The percutaneous procedure should not be performed on children.[14] Also, children have pliable laryngeal and tracheal cartilage that is predisposed to structural airway collapse.[14] PDT is best employed in controlled, elective situations. Patients with unprotected airways, hemodynamic instability, and impending airway obstruction are not good candidates. Anatomic factors also play a role. Severe thyromegaly, anatomic distortion of the midline neck, and the presence of vascular or pulsatile masses also prohibit safe PDT.[14–16]

Although not absolute contraindications, several other scenarios must be specially considered. A history of tracheostomy was initially considered to be a contraindication. However, Meyer and colleagues[83] recently reported a series of 14 patients safely undergoing PDT with a history of tracheotomy. The authors' experience suggests that these patients should be selected carefully, because the dense scar tissue that forms after a tracheotomy can impede the proper placement of the needle into the trachea. The surgeon should be prepared to convert the procedure to an open bedside tracheotomy, if necessary. Patients with a high oxygen requirement or a positive end-expiratory pressure of more than 20 cm of water may become hypoxic during the procedure as a result of airway obstruction by the dilator or of the loss of air through the tracheotomy. Uncorrected coagulopathy (i.e., international normalized ratio <2.0) or thrombocytopenia (i.e., <50,000) may lead to postoperative hemorrhage. Furthermore, obese patients with short necks (i.e., 2.5 cm from the cricoid to the sternal notch) and patients without palpable landmarks pose technical challenges.[14–16] Obese patients (i.e., body mass index >27.5 kg/m^2) undergoing PDT have a 2.7-fold increase in overall complications and a 4.9-fold increase in serious complications such as the loss of the airway, hemorrhage, pneumothorax, and death.[84] Although PDT can be performed in these circumstances, a detailed understanding of the potential complications along with the surgeon's personal experience and sound judgment dictate the best approach.[85]

Percutaneous Dilatational Tracheotomy Complications

Many of the previously mentioned intraoperative and postoperative complications associated with traditional open tracheotomy can also occur in PDT. The overall complication rates appear to be similar, and they range from 0% to 14%.[12,14–16,86] Furthermore, these rates are significantly reduced with the use of single-dilator systems and bronchoscopic assistance.[14] The most common complications of transient hypoxemia, cuff puncture, and resistance to insertion are probably related to the technique of PDT. Other complications of bleeding, infection, the loss of the airway/accidental decannulation, and tracheal stenosis are comparable.[13,14] In a meta-analysis of randomized controlled trials of PDT by Delaney and colleagues,[13] a statistically significant reduction in clinically relevant wound infections was seen among patients undergoing PDT as compared with surgical tracheotomy. Those authors also confirmed that the time of translaryngeal intubation before tracheotomy was also significantly less. Although bleeding, paratracheal insertion, and loss of airway are commonly raised concerns with PDT, the large study confirmed no statistically significant differences in these parameters as compared with standard surgical tracheotomy.[13] Other authors have concurred that the safety profile of PDT is equivalent and may even be superior to that of surgical tracheotomy.[10,13,16] In addition, PDT has the added benefits of lower overall cost and logistical constraints.

There are special complications that are particularly unique to PDT. The problem of paratracheal tube insertion has essentially ceased since the introduction of bronchoscopic assistance by Paul and colleagues.[87] Posterior tracheal wall perforation can occur during the needle puncture of the anterior wall. Subcutaneous emphysema can result after a tracheal wall injury from the dilation procedure or from a false passage. Pneumothorax or pneumomediastinum can subsequently result. The benefits of visual confirmation have made video bronchoscopy an essential part of the procedure. However, the presence of the fiber-optic scope in the tracheotomy tube obstructs ventilation and makes it difficult to perform the procedure on patients with high oxygen requirements or high positive end-expiratory pressures.

Several case reports describe tracheal stenosis as a result of tracheal ring fractures incurred during the performance of PDT.[88–90] A recent report also suggests that suprastomal tracheal stenosis is increased after PDT. Koitschev and colleagues[91] reported 23% (n = 105) of patients had grade II (i.e., >50% of the lumen) suprastomal stenosis after PDT as compared with 7.3% (i.e., n = 41) after standard tracheotomy. Interestingly, there was a difference between the grade of stenosis and the timing of the examination in the PDT group and not in the surgical tracheotomy group. The median time to examination for grade II stenosis was 92 days versus 46.5 days for grade I stenosis as compared with 60.5 (i.e., grade I) and 69 days (i.e., grade II) for the surgical tracheotomy group. Since long-term follow up of these patients is limited, complications may be underreported.

It is thought that the downward motion of the insertion of the tracheotomy tube, which is recommended to avoid tearing the posterior wall, causes inward tearing and the depression of suprastomal anterior tracheal wall. Cadaveric studies support the findings of significant endotracheal mucosal lacerations and multiple comminuted injuries in two or more adjacent cartilage rings.[89] These findings were confirmed in an autopsy study of PDT patients by Van Heurn and colleagues,[92] which showed 11 of 12 to have tracheal ring fractures, including 2 patients who had fractured cricoid cartilage. Furthermore, on a histopathologic level, PDT creates a higher degree of acute cartilaginous damage in the anterior tracheal wall than sharp surgical dissection.[93]

Because the tube tract is formed by a percutaneous method, no surgical opening is available to assist with insertion if the tube becomes accidentally displaced from the airway. Although there is no difference in decannulation rates between open surgical and percutaneous tracheotomy, the subsequent collapse of the tract may make tube replacement difficult or impossible. Therefore, the first routine tracheotomy change is often delayed several weeks.[94] The surgeon should consider patient factors including body habitus and neck anatomy for such a scenario before performing PDT.

Pediatric Tracheotomy

Tracheotomy in the pediatric population carries specific risks and pitfalls that merit special attention. Important differences include the small pediatric airway, the various options for pediatric tracheotomy tubes, different indications for a tracheotomy, and the involvement of the parent as a third-party caretaker for long-term cannulation.

The indications for pediatric tracheotomy generally differ from those of adults. Congenital malformations and acute infectious processes play a more prominent role. Diphtheria, which stimulated the historic acceptance of tracheotomy, is fortunately rare now. Positive-pressure oral–nasal ventilation with CPAP and bi-level positive airway pressure helps to avoid intubation in numerous cases. Neonates and infants requiring long-term ventilation via endotracheal tubes are at increased risk for the development of subglottic stenosis and subglottic cysts.[95] However, increased risks associated with pediatric tracheotomy contribute to the practice of maintaining long-term endotracheal intubation in neonatal intensive care units.[96] Therefore the risks of tracheotomy must be carefully weighed against the benefits in these children.

Intraoperative complications of pediatric tracheotomy are relatively rare, yet they are still more likely to occur than complications in adults as a result of the size of the airway and the possibility of congenitally abnormal anatomy. The smaller airway makes the misplacement of the tube into the paratracheal space or the esophagus a possibility. The formation of a tracheoesophageal fistula requires immediate recognition and treatment with tube alimentation and surgical closure. The relatively higher cupula of the lungs in children makes the possibility of pneumothorax more likely. A routine postoperative chest radiograph should be obtained,[97] which is not the case for adults. Pediatric tracheotomies are usually not performed under local anesthesia, so the loss of the airway is less of an issue, because the patient is likely to already be intubated. However, for those cases in which the establishment of an airway is the primary goal of the procedure, this can be a most difficult operation.

The operative technique of tracheotomy is different for the pediatric population. Most surgeons will use stay sutures on the trachea itself to help with reintubation in the event of accidental tube dislodgement. The technique for entering the trachea varies and can differ from a single vertical incision to an H incision or a star-shaped incision.[98] No controlled studies exist comparing these various techniques, so the true advantage of one technique over another has not been demonstrated. Flap techniques show a decreased incidence of decannulation but an increased incidence of tracheocutaneous fistulas.[43,69,99,100]

After the tracheotomy is performed and the tube is in place, most surgeons will use a flexible or rigid bronchoscope to demonstrate the intraluminal placement of the tube. The tube is secured with twill tape. The first tracheotomy tube change is performed after 3 to 7 days, depending on surgeon preference.[101]

Postoperative complications in the pediatric population are similar to those of adults. However, several important differences exist, most of which are related to the size of the airway. To increase the airway size, a majority of pediatric tracheostomy tubes do not have an inner cannula. Thus the plugging of the tube can constitute

an airway emergency that cannot be solved by simply changing an inner cannula. A routine program of hygiene including frequent tube suctioning and saline lavage is necessary with these tubes. Furthermore, frequent suctioning itself can cause granulation tissue to form in response to trauma of the tracheal wall. Therefore the amount of suction tubing allowed into the tube should be limited to the length of the tube itself.

In the event of tracheal plugging, the staff on site must to be prepared to either change the tracheotomy tube or to intubate the patient if the tube obstruction cannot be cleared. In some institutions, this responsibility lies with properly trained nursing staff members. Instructions regarding the patient's airway and whether the patient can be orally intubated need to be available. The authors keep a similar-sized tracheotomy tube, a smaller tube, an endotracheal tube, scissors to cut ties, and new ties at the bedside of all tracheotomy patients. Because a tube change can be difficult even under optimal circumstances, it is imperative to avoid this situation with diligent tracheotomy tube care and hygiene.

Similarly, because the length of the tube is shorter, accidental decannulation is more common in the pediatric population. Again, diligent care and routine inspection of the tube are necessary to avoid this complication. The authors recommend twill tape ties, which are placed snugly around the patient's neck to avoid accidental decannulation. The unadjustable, knotted twill ties prevent the nursing staff or parents from loosening the ties for perceived improved comfort. However, enough laxity should be left in the ties, and the skin of the neck should be monitored to ensure that skin necrosis does not develop.

Care of the tracheotomy tube must be taught to the parents as soon as practically possible so that they are comfortable with the care of the tube and trained for all emergency situations that may arise at home. The authors have instituted a home-care program led by our nursing staff for all parents of tracheotomy patients.

Common late complications of pediatric tracheotomy tubes include granulation formation and a persistent tracheocutaneous fistula. Granulation can be minimized with appropriate tube positioning and sizing as well as proper tube hygiene. A regular tube change has been shown to reduce granulation tissue as well.[102] Fistulas are usually the result of long-term tracheostomy, but they can also be technique dependent. Closure of tracheocutaneous fistulas requires a separate surgical procedure, usually with a multilayer closure that includes an interposed muscle flap.[69]

A devastating late complication of pediatric tracheotomy is a TIF. Avoiding pressure of the tube along the anterior tracheal wall can prevent this complication. A "sentinel bleed" from a tracheostoma requires a bronchoscopy to evaluate for possible anterior erosion. If a bleed occurs, digital pressure in the sternal notch or inserting and inflating a cuffed tube can temporarily control bleeding until operative intervention with ligation of the artery and a muscle interposition flap can be performed.

In summary, the pediatric tracheostomy complication profile is similar to that seen with adults. The smaller airway diameter and length make the tracheotomy tube more susceptible to the obstruction of airflow, with narrowing of the lumen caused by mucus plugging. Therefore diligence with regard to hygiene is necessary to avoid problems. The smaller and more pliable airway requires the surgeon to pay meticulous attention to surgical technique to avoid problems such as accidental decannulation. The early recognition and treatment of complications are necessary. Proper education of the patient's caretakers is mandatory to prevent long-term complications.

TRACHEAL SURGERY

Several surgical interventions of the trachea currently exist, including laryngotracheal segmental or sleeve resection and reanastomosis, laryngotracheal endoluminal or open stenting for stenosis, laryngotracheal separation for aspiration, and endoscopic excision or dilation of limited strictures. Many cases of tracheal stenosis are related to a history of tracheotomy. A full discussion of each of these procedures is beyond the scope of this chapter. Significant complications are discussed, with an emphasis on tracheal stenosis.

Indications for Tracheal Surgery

Causes of tracheal obstruction requiring intervention are postintubation stenosis, TIF, acquired or congenital tracheomalacia, tumor,[103] idiopathic laryngotracheal stenosis, infection, extrinsic compression, trauma, and caustic or thermal injury.[104,105] Laryngotracheal stenosis and tracheal stenosis can affect the entire age spectrum, with variations with regard to cause. The incidence of laryngotracheal stenosis greatly increased after the introduction of intubation in neonates.[106] In young children, mucosal injury may induce a perichondritis that leads to chondritis with subsequent necrosis and the collapse of cartilage. The healing process leads to scar formation with fibrous deposition that can narrow the airway. Risk factors for acquired subglottic stenosis in neonates include prolonged intubation, excessive motion of the endotracheal tube, traumatic or multiple intubations, low birth weight (<1500 gm), the use of nasogastric tubes, the reflux of gastric contents, and a compromised immune status.[104,107] Positive-pressure nasal ventilation with bi-level positive airway pressure and CPAP in neonatal intensive care units has reduced the need for oral intubation and subsequent tracheotomy.

Types of Tracheal Surgery

Tracheal resections may be necessary to manage tracheal stenosis, tracheal tumors, stomal tumor recurrence, tracheomalacia, and congenital deformities. The sites and size of stenosis will vary with the pathology. Alternative methods of establishing airway patency in certain cases include the endoscopic removal of scar with cold or laser techniques, subglottic or cricoid stenting with autologous graft, stenting the obstruction with a T-tube or a tracheal stent, or bypass of the obstruction with a tracheotomy tube.

Surgical Technique of Tracheal Resection

The exact approach to the trachea may vary as a result of patient-related factors such as the pathology and the tracheal location. A well-defined stenosis can be delimited both radiologically (Figure 34-8) and endoscopically. As described by Grillo,[105] the patient is positioned with the head in extension with a rolled sheet or an inflatable bag under the shoulders for the resection. Lower laryngeal lesions and upper tracheal lesions can be accessed through an anterior transcervical approach. A transverse collar incision is placed 1 cm above the clavicular heads. The length is determined by the extent of exposure that is needed superiorly. Subplatysmal flaps are elevated superiorly to the level of the cricoid cartilage and inferiorly to the level of the sternal notch. The anterior jugular veins are divided and raised with the flap superiorly. The anterior border of the sternocleidomastoid muscle is dissected from its attachment to the sternum. The midline is identified, and the strap muscles are dissected in the midline. The pretracheal fat is dissected above the sternal notch. The cricoid ring is identified, and tissue is cleared off of the trachea superior to the thyroid isthmus. The thyroid isthmus is then divided, and the gland is elevated off of the anterior wall of the trachea. Care is taken to preserve the lateral blood supply of the trachea throughout the procedure. For stenosis with a prior tracheotomy, the anterior wall of the trachea just superior to the region of maximal adherence is identified.

If needed, a sternotomy is performed. A vertical skin incision can be made from the prior incision over the sternum to 2 cm below the sternal angle. The anterior tracheal surface is dissected completely from the cricoid cartilage to the carina. The dissection is carried close to the tracheal wall to avoid injury to the recurrent laryngeal nerves. Circumferential dissection is performed at the level of the lower border of the

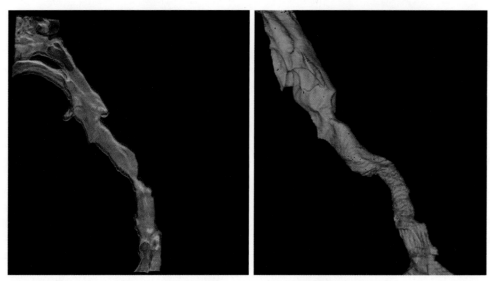

Figure 34-8. Tracheal stenosis before and after stenting. The extent of the stenosis should be mapped out preoperatively with imaging and endoscopically to determine the extent of the defect. Small lesions amenable to stenting can be identified and managed in appropriate cases. (Courtesy of Christine Glastonbury, Department of Neuroradiology, University of California, San Francisco.)

lesion. If possible, the circumferential dissection is carried up along the lesion itself. The trachea is divided inferiorly and intubated beyond the stenosis. The stenotic segment is elevated from the esophagus in a superior direction. The superior tracheal rings are retracted laterally, with heavy sutures placed in the mid-lateral tracheal line at a point one to two rings above the intended line of tracheal division. Lower traction sutures are then placed.

A Penrose drain is passed around the trachea at the lower end of the resection, where the circumferential dissection has been performed. The anesthesiologist is asked to deflate the cuff, and the tracheal ring heavy sutures (i.e., 2.0 Vicryl [Ethicon, Inc., Somerville, NJ]) are placed vertically in the mid-lateral line of the trachea at full thickness around a single ring. The superior trachea is divided above the stenosis (Figure 34-9).

After resection, the remaining tracheal ends are examined to ensure that the tissue is healthy enough for closure. Neck flexion (i.e., 20–35 degrees) can provide 3.4 cm to 6.0 cm of length.[105] Inferior and superior traction sutures are used to bring the trachea together without excessive tension. If more than 4 cm of trachea is resected, it is prudent to perform a laryngeal release procedure.[103] A laryngeal release consists of one of two maneuvers. A thyrohyoid release as described by Dedo and Fishman[108] is a division of the thyrohyoid muscles and the thyrohyoid membrane. A suprahyoid release[109] consists of the division of the muscular attachments from the hyoid and dividing the hyoid bone itself. The anastomosis is commenced, with successive 4.0 Vicryl sutures (5.0 in infants and small children) passed through the tracheal wall and the mucosal lumen. The sutures are spaced about 4 mm apart. After all of the sutures are

placed, the endotracheal tube is removed from the lower trachea, and an oral endotracheal tube is advanced into the field and guided into the distal trachea. The anastomotic sutures are now tightened. The shoulder roll is removed or deflated. The wound is then closed with reapproximation of the thyroid isthmus and the strap muscles over the suction drains. The sternum, if divided, is closed with wires, and the platysma and the skin are closed. A heavy suture can be placed from the skin of the chin to the sternum to keep the patient in flexion postoperatively for 7 days. Extubation can usually be carried out as the patient awakens. Tracheotomy is avoided initially to prevent restenosis.

COMPLICATIONS

Tracheal Resection

Indications for endoscopic dilation and laser vaporization are limited to strictures of less than 1 cm without cartilage support.[110] Larger lesions are best treated with resection and reanastomosis.[111] The application of topical mitomycin C was introduced in 2000 by Rahbar and Shapshay,[112] but its role is controversial, because follow-up animal studies, retrospective studies, and a prospective trial have shown mixed results.[113–115] Furthermore, some authors believe that mitomycin C delays healing and that it may increase obstructing granuloma formation.[114,116] The correction of subglottic stenosis has been described, with laryngotracheal resection and reanastomosis[117,118] and a variety of grafts and stents performed in single or multistage procedures.[119,121]

Tracheal resection is performed for postintubation stenosis, neoplasm, idiopathic laryngotracheal stenosis, or

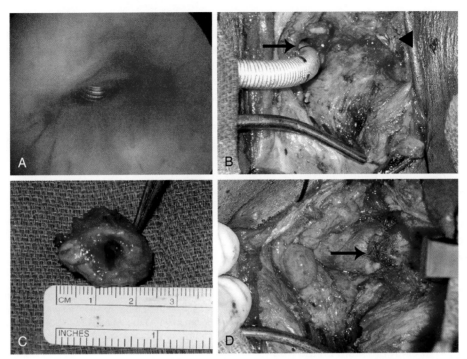

Figure 34-9. Tracheal resection. **A,** An endoscopic view of the subglottis reveals significant acquired stenosis in this adult, who was intubated for 8 weeks before tracheotomy. Note an armored endotracheal tube in the distal airway. **B,** A tracheal resection was performed that involved the removal of approximately 3.0 cm of trachea. The superior cut was made just below the cricoid cartilage *(arrowhead),* and the inferior cut was below the fifth tracheal ring *(arrow).* The transoral endotracheal tube is kept in position so that it may be advanced past the anastomosis on the posterior wall of the trachea, which has been approximated. **C,** The resected segment is depicted in the axial plane, which shows marked narrowing of the lumen. **D,** After a suprahyoid release and an inferior tracheal mobilization, a multilayer anastomosis is performed *(arrow),* which allows for end-to-end approximation. Note that the knots of the sutures are extraluminal.

tracheoesophageal fistula. A recent review of the Massachusetts General Hospital experience by Wright and colleagues[103] included 901 patients from 1975 to 2003. They reported a 9% anastomotic complication rate and a 1% mortality rate. Ninety-five percent of patients had a good result, and 4% required a tracheostomy, which is in agreement with the success rate of 80% to 96% reported in the literature.[122,123] Recurrent laryngeal nerve paralysis is reported to occur at a rate of 2% to 3%.[124,125]

Anastomotic complications can be treated with reoperation, repeated dilation, temporary tracheostomy or T-tube, or permanent tracheostomy. Predictors of anastomotic complications are reoperation, diabetes mellitus, resections that are more than 4 cm long, laryngotracheal resection with anastomosis to the larynx, an age of less than 17 years, and the need for tracheostomy before the operation. Some smaller series have suggested that patients with cardiopulmonary disease and older age may take longer to extubate.[123,126]

Morbidity as a result of tracheal resection includes subcutaneous emphysema, pneumonia, hematoma, and sepsis. Anastomotic complications include granulation tissue or stenosis at the anastomosis site or the separation of the anastomosed segments that required either an airway appliance or reoperation. Granulation tissue likely occurs as a result of partial or complete

separation at the anastomosis. Suture reaction can cause minor granulomas. Variables that were not found to be associated with complications include the use of prednisone (>10 mg/d within the first 7 days after surgery), the year of operation, the incisional approach, and a body mass index of more than 30 kg/m^2. The need for a suprahyoid release is associated with an increased failure rate, but this is obviously related to the greater length of the segment being resected. The effect of steroid use on wound complications is unclear, and its use is frequently minimized.

Anastomotic failure must be diagnosed early, and it is best assessed with computed tomography scanning of the neck and chest to search for extratracheal air. This examination is supplemented by bronchoscopy. In the case of separation with extratracheal infection, the airway should be secured with a tracheostomy or T-tube and the infection drained. The T-tube is preferred in an attempt to reduce stomal irritation. Reoperation should be performed after a minimum interval of 6 to 12 months to allow for the resolution of inflammation.[103]

INTRALUMINAL STENTS

Special note should be made of intraluminal stents, which have gained a prominent role in the management of airway obstruction across the age range. Indications for stent placement vary from infancy to adulthood and are still evolving. Silicone stents have the advantage of being removable after long periods of time, but the expandable metal stents have better internal and external diameter ratios, and they can be placed with flexible bronchoscopy. A survey of the American Association of Bronchology revealed that only 6% of pulmonologists in the United States can perform rigid bronchoscopy,[127] which has thus given rise to the popularity of expandable metal stents. Expandable metal stents exhibit tissue ingrowth and in some cases have been found to become essentially embedded within the tracheal wall. This can lead to difficulties with the removal of the stent if the need should arise. This has prompted surgeons to call for the careful selection of patients receiving an intraluminal stent, especially for patients with benign disease.

Indications in infants and young children include tracheobronchial malacia, postsurgical stricture, and obstruction as a result of extrinsic lesions. Expandable metal stents are designed to expand to preset sizes, and they can continue to exert pressure on the tracheal wall if the lumen is too small. By contrast, the Palmaz balloon-expanded stent (Cordis Corporation, Miami, FL) can be sized at the time of placement. Complications of intraluminal stents include obstructing granulation tissue, stent migration, and tracheal erosion. Granulomas are reported with a frequency of 3% to 36%[128-131] and occur most frequently at the distal and proximal ends of the stent.[128,132] Proper sizing of the stent, avoidance of the subglottis, and avoid placement of the stent in extremely inflamed mucosa are considered important to prevent complications.

Among adults, expandable metal stents are placed for the symptomatic relief of obstructing malignancies, for postsurgical strictures, and for a variety of benign conditions (e.g., tracheomalacia, external tracheal vascular, mass compression). Stents can provide the immediate short-term relief of symptoms, and they allow some patients to discontinue positive-pressure ventilatory support. However, the complications of the long-term use of these stents is unclear.[133] Reported complications in adults with short-term and mid-term follow up occur in up to 50% of patients and include granulomas, mucus plugging, recurrent respiratory infections, stent migration, and metal fatigue/fracture.[133,134] As a result of difficulties with the removal of the stent and the development of significant complications, some authors argue that stents should be reserved for patients with benign conditions who are unable to undergo the surgical repair of their lesions.[133]

Stent removal can be achieved, and it is considered in cases of failing stents or in children who are outgrowing their conditions. Filler and colleagues[128] reported the successful removal of 11 stents from 8 children. They also noted the death of a child during attempted stent removal as a result of the stent's attachment to the tracheal wall. This complication underscores the importance of surgeons being prepared to use all means necessary to relieve a life-threatening airway obstruction during stent removal. Cardiopulmonary bypass should be available on standby during such cases.

REFERENCES

1. American Academy of Otolaryngology: *The history of tracheotomy* (website): www.entlink.net/museum/exhibits/Early-History. (Accessed April, 2007)
2. Montgomery W: Tracheotomy and tracheostomy tubes. In Montgomery W, editor: *Surgery of the larynx, trachea, esophagus, and neck,* Philadelphia, 2002, WB Saunders.
3. Goldenberg D et al: Tracheotomy: Changing indications and a review of 1,130 cases. *J Otolaryngol* 2002;31(4):211–215.
4. Santos PM, Afrassiabi A, Weymuller EA Jr: Risk factors associated with prolonged intubation and laryngeal injury. *Otolaryngol Head Neck Surg* 1994;111(4):453–459.
5. Gaynor EB, Greenberg SB: Untoward sequelae of prolonged intubation. *Laryngoscope* 1985;95(12):1461–1467.
6. Shelden CH, Pudenz RH, Tichy FY: Percutaneous tracheotomy. *J Am Med Assoc* 1957;165(16):2068–2070.
7. Toy FJ, Weinstein JD: A percutaneous tracheostomy device. *Surgery* 1969;65(2):384–389.
8. Ciaglia P, Firsching R, Syniec C: Elective percutaneous dilatational tracheostomy: A new simple bedside procedure: Preliminary report. *Chest* 1985;87(6):715–719.
9. Wang MB et al: Early experience with percutaneous tracheotomy. *Laryngoscope* 1992;102(2):157–162.
10. Cheng E, Fee WE Jr: Dilatational versus standard tracheostomy: A meta-analysis. *Ann Otol Rhinol Laryngol* 2000;109(9):803–807.
11. Freeman BD et al: A meta-analysis of prospective trials comparing percutaneous and surgical tracheostomy in critically ill patients. *Chest* 2000;118(5):1412–1418.
12. Freeman BD et al: A prospective, randomized study comparing percutaneous with surgical tracheostomy in critically ill patients. *Crit Care Med* 2001;29(5):926–930.
13. Delaney A, Bagshaw SM, Nalos M: Percutaneous dilatational tracheostomy versus surgical tracheostomy in critically ill patients: A systematic review and meta-analysis. *Crit Care* 2006;10(2):R55.
14. Kost KM: Endoscopic percutaneous dilatational tracheotomy: A prospective evaluation of 500 consecutive cases. *Laryngoscope* 2005;115(10 Pt 2):1–30.
15. Silvester W et al: Percutaneous versus surgical tracheostomy: A randomized controlled study with long-term follow-up. *Crit Care Med* 2006;34(8):2145–2152.
16. Friedman Y et al: Comparison of percutaneous and surgical tracheostomies. *Chest* 1996;110(2):480–485.
17. Heffner JE: The role of tracheotomy in weaning. *Chest* 2001;120(6 Suppl):477S–481S.
18. Donnelly WH: Histopathology of endotracheal intubation: An autopsy study of 99 cases. *Arch Pathol* 1969;88(5):511–520.
19. Lindholm CE: Prolonged endotracheal intubation. *Acta Anaesthesiol Scand Suppl* 1970;33:1–131.
20. Heffner JE: The technique of tracheotomy and cricothyroidotomy: When to operate—And how to manage complications. *J Crit Illn* 1995;10(8):561–568.
21. Rumbak MJ et al: A prospective, randomized, study comparing early percutaneous dilational tracheotomy to prolonged translaryngeal intubation (delayed tracheotomy) in critically ill medical patients. *Crit Care Med* 2004;32(8):1689–1694.
22. Clum SR, Rumbak MJ: Mobilizing the patient in the intensive care unit: The role of early tracheotomy. *Crit Care Clin* 2007;23(1):71–79.
23. McGill J, Clinton JE, Ruiz E: Cricothyrotomy in the emergency department. *Ann Emerg Med* 1982;11(7):361–364.
24. Goldenberg D et al: Tracheotomy complications: A retrospective study of 1130 cases. *Otolaryngol Head Neck Surg* 2000;123(4):495–500.

25. Reilly H, Sasaki C: Tracheotomy complications. In Krespi YP, editor: *Complications in head and neck surgery,* Philadelphia, 1993, WB Saunders.

26. Cole IE: Elective percutaneous (Rapitrac) tracheotomy: Results of a prospective trial. *Laryngoscope* 1994;104(10):1271–1275.

27. Myers EN, Carrau RL: Early complications of tracheotomy: Incidence and management. *Clin Chest Med* 1991;12(3):589–595.

28. Moore K: *Clinically oriented anatomy,* Baltimore, 1992, Williams and Wilkins.

29. Shima H et al: Anatomy of microvascular anastomosis in the neck. *Plast Reconstr Surg* 1998;101(1):33–41.

30. Toni R et al: Anthropological variations in the anatomy of the human thyroid arteries. *Thyroid* 2003;13(2):183–192.

31. Calhoun KH et al: Management of the thyroid isthmus in tracheostomy: A prospective and retrospective study. *Otolaryngol Head Neck Surg* 1994;111(4):450–452.

32. Kirchner JA: Avoiding problems in tracheotomy. *Laryngoscope* 1986;96(1):55–57.

33. Hilal EY: Management of the thyroid isthmus in tracheostomy: A prospective and retrospective study. *Otolaryngol Head Neck Surg* 1995;113(3):338–339.

34. Ozlugedik S et al: Surgical importance of highly located innominate artery in neck surgery. *Am J Otolaryngol* 2005;26(5):330–332.

35. Rampil I: Anesthesia for laser surgery. In Miller RD, editor: *Miller's anesthesia,* ed 6, St Louis, 2005, Elsevier.

36. Thompson JW et al: Fire in the operating room during tracheostomy. *South Med J* 1998;91(3):243–247.

37. Tykocinski M, Thomson P, Hooper R: Airway fire during tracheotomy. *ANZ J Surg* 2006;76(3):195–197.

38. ECRI, editor: A clinician's guide to surgical fires. *Health Devices* 2003;32:5–24.

39. Shapiro JD, el-Baz NM: N2O has no place during oropharyngeal and laryngotracheal procedures. *Anesthesiology* 1987;66(3):447–448.

40. Weber SM, Hargunani CA, Wax MK: DuraPrep and the risk of fire during tracheostomy. *Head Neck* 2006;28(7):649–652.

41. Smith DK, Grillone GA, Fuleihan N: Use of postoperative chest x-ray after elective adult tracheotomy. *Otolaryngol Head Neck Surg* 1999;120(6):848–851.

42. Bradley P, editor: Management of the obstructed airway and tracheostomy. In Kerr AG, editor: *Scott-Brown's otolaryngology,* London, 1997, Butterworth-Heinemann.

43. Carr MM et al: Complications in pediatric tracheostomies. *Laryngoscope* 2001;111(11 Pt 1):1925–1928.

44. Eliachar I et al: Permanent tracheostomy. *Head Neck Surg* 1984;7(2):99–103.

45. Park SY, Smith RV: Comparison of postoperative cardiopulmonary examinations and chest radiographs to detect pulmonary complications after adult tracheotomy. *Otolaryngol Head Neck Surg* 1999;121(3):274–276.

46. Berg LF et al: Mechanisms of pneumothorax following tracheal intubation. *Ann Otol Rhinol Laryngol* 1988;97(5 Pt 1):500–505.

47. Barlow DW, Weymuller EA Jr, Wood DE: Tracheotomy and the role of postoperative chest radiography in adult patients. *Ann Otol Rhinol Laryngol* 1994;103(9):665–668.

48. Spankus EM et al: Craniocervical necrotizing fasciitis. *Otolaryngol Head Neck Surg* 1984;92(3):261–265.

49. Wang RC, Perlman PW, Parnes SM: Near-fatal complications of tracheotomy infections and their prevention. *Head Neck* 1989;11(6):528–533.

50. Newlands SD, Makielski KH: Cervical osteomyelitis after percutaneous transtracheal ventilation and tracheotomy. *Head Neck* 1996;18(3):295–298.

51. Goldenberg JD et al: Negative-pressure pulmonary edema in the otolaryngology patient. *Otolaryngol Head Neck Surg* 1997;117(1):62–66.

52. Tami TA et al: Pulmonary edema and acute upper airway obstruction. *Laryngoscope* 1986;96(5):506–509.

53. Kollef MH, Pluss J: Noncardiogenic pulmonary edema following upper airway obstruction: 7 cases and a review of the literature. *Medicine (Baltimore)* 1991;70(2):91–98.

54. Holmes JR, Hensinger RN, Wojtys EW: Postoperative pulmonary edema in young, athletic adults. *Am J Sports Med* 1991;19(4):365–371.

55. Bonadio WA, Losek JD: The characteristics of children with epiglottitis who develop the complication of pulmonary edema. *Arch Otolaryngol Head Neck Surg* 1991;117(2):205–207.

56. Esclamado RM et al: Perioperative complications and risk factors in the surgical treatment of obstructive sleep apnea syndrome. *Laryngoscope* 1989;99(11):1125–1129.

57. Wright CD: Management of tracheoinnominate artery fistula. *Chest Surg Clin N Am* 1996;6(4):865–873.

58. Wood DE, Mathisen DJ: Late complications of tracheotomy. *Clin Chest Med* 1991;12(3):597–609.

59. Jones JW et al: Tracheo-innominate artery erosion: Successful surgical management of a devastating complication. *Ann Surg* 1976;184(2):194–204.

60. Oshinsky AE, Rubin JS, Gwozdz CS: The anatomical basis for post-tracheotomy innominate artery rupture. *Laryngoscope* 1988;98(10):1061–1064.

61. Myers WO, Lawton BR, Sautter RD: An operation for tracheal-innominate artery fistula. *Arch Surg* 1972;105(2):269–274.

62. Grillo HC: Surgical approaches to the trachea. *Surg Gynecol Obstet* 1969;129(2):347–352.

63. Utley JR et al: Definitive management of innominate artery hemorrhage complicating tracheostomy. *JAMA* 1972;220(4):577–579.

64. Yang FY et al: Trachea-innominate artery fistula: Retrospective comparison of treatment methods. *South Med J* 1988;81(6):701–706.

65. Sasaki CT, Horiuchi M, Koss N: Tracheostomy-related subglottic stenosis: Bacteriologic pathogenesis. *Laryngoscope* 1979;89(6 Pt 1):857–865.

66. Gianoli GJ, Miller RH, Guarisco JL: Tracheotomy in the first year of life. *Ann Otol Rhinol Laryngol* 1990;99(11):896–901.

67. Werkhaven J, Maddern BR, Stool SE: Posttracheotomy granulation tissue managed by carbon dioxide laser excision. *Ann Otol Rhinol Laryngol* 1989;98(10):828–830.

68. van Heurn LW, van Geffen GJ, Brink PR: Clinical experience with percutaneous dilatational tracheostomy: Report of 150 cases. *Eur J Surg* 1996;162(7):531–535.

69. Sautter NB et al: Closure of persistent tracheocutaneous fistula following "starplasty" tracheostomy in children. *Int J Pediatr Otorhinolaryngol* 2006;70(1):99–105.

70. Eaton DA, Brown OE, Parry D: Simple technique for tracheocutaneous fistula closure in the pediatric population. *Ann Otol Rhinol Laryngol* 2003;112(1):17–19.

71. Keenan JP et al: Management of tracheocutaneous fistula. *Arch Otolaryngol* 1978;104(9):530–531.

72. White AK, Smitheringale AJ: Treatment of tracheocutaneous fistulae in children. *J Otolaryngol* 1989;18(1):49–52.

73. Harley HR: Ulcerative tracheo-oesophageal fistula during treatment by tracheostomy and intermittent positive pressure ventilation. *Thorax* 1972;27(3):338–352.

74. Arola MK: Tracheostomy and its complications: A retrospective study of 794 tracheostomized patients. *Ann Chir Gynaecol* 1981;70(3):96–106.

75. Macchiarini P et al: Evaluation and outcome of different surgical techniques for postintubation tracheoesophageal fistulas. *J Thorac Cardiovasc Surg* 2000;119(2):268–276.

76. Shaari CM, Biller HF: Staged repair of cervical tracheoesophageal fistulae. *Laryngoscope* 1996;106(11):1398–1402.

77. Wolf M et al: Acquired tracheoesophageal fistula in critically ill patients. *Ann Otol Rhinol Laryngol* 2000;109(8 Pt 1):731–735.

78. Arola MK, Inberg MV, Puhakka H: Tracheal stenosis after tracheostomy and after orotracheal cuffed intubation. *Acta Chir Scand* 1981;147(3):183–192.

79. Grillo H: Post intubation stenosis. In Grillo H, editor: *Surgery of the trachea and bronchi,* Hamilton, Ontario, Canada, 1990, BC Decker.

80. Grillo HC et al: Postintubation tracheal stenosis: Treatment and results. *J Thorac Cardiovasc Surg* 1995;109(3):486–493.

81. Dedo HH: Surgery of the larynx and trachea. In: *Segmental resection of the trachea,* Hamilton, Ontario, Canada, 1990, BC Decker.

82. Cooper JD, Grillo HC: The evolution of tracheal injury due to ventilatory assistance through cuffed tubes: A pathologic study. *Ann Surg* 1969;169(3):334–348.

83. Meyer M et al: Repeat bedside percutaneous dilational tracheostomy is a safe procedure. *Crit Care Med* 2002;30(5):986–988.

84. Byhahn C et al: Peri-operative complications during percutaneous tracheostomy in obese patients. *Anaesthesia* 2005;60(1):12–15.

85. Ben Nun A, Altman E, Best LA: Extended indications for percutaneous tracheostomy. *Ann Thorac Surg* 2005;80(4):1276–1279.

86. Hazard P, Jones C, Benitone J: Comparative clinical trial of standard operative tracheostomy with percutaneous tracheostomy. *Crit Care Med* 1991;19(8):1018–1024.

87. Paul A et al: Percutaneous endoscopic tracheostomy. *Ann Thorac Surg* 1989;47(2):314–315.

88. Ho EC, Kapila A, Colquhoun-Flannery W: Tracheal ring fracture and early tracheomalacia following percutaneous dilatational tracheostomy. *BMC Ear Nose Throat Disord* 2005;5:6.

89. Hotchkiss KS, McCaffrey JC: Laryngotracheal injury after percutaneous dilational tracheostomy in cadaver specimens. *Laryngoscope* 2003;113(1):16–20.

90. McFarlane C et al: Laryngotracheal stenosis: A serious complication of percutaneous tracheostomy. *Anaesthesia* 1994;49(1):38–40.

91. Koitschev A et al: Suprastomal tracheal stenosis after dilational and surgical tracheostomy in critically ill patients. *Anaesthesia* 2006;61(9):832–837.

92. van Heurn LW et al: Pathologic changes of the trachea after percutaneous dilatational tracheotomy. *Chest* 1996;109(6):1466–1469.

93. Stoeckli SJ, Breitbach T, Schmid S: A clinical and histologic comparison of percutaneous dilational versus conventional surgical tracheostomy. *Laryngoscope* 1997;107(12 Pt 1):1643–1646.

94. Beiderlinden M et al: Complications of bronchoscopically guided percutaneous dilational tracheostomy: Beyond the learning curve. *Intensive Care Med* 2002;28(1):59–62.

95. Johnson LB et al: Acquired subglottic cysts in preterm infants. *J Otolaryngol* 2005;34(2):75–78.

96. Kadilak PR, Vanasse S, Sheridan RL: Favorable short- and long-term outcomes of prolonged translaryngeal intubation in critically ill children. *J Burn Care Rehabil* 2004;25(3):262–265.

97. Greenberg JS et al: The role of postoperative chest radiography in pediatric tracheotomy. *Int J Pediatr Otorhinolaryngol* 2001;60(1):41–47.

98. Solares CA et al: Starplasty: Revisiting a pediatric tracheostomy technique. *Otolaryngol Head Neck Surg* 2004;131(5):717–722.

99. Park JY et al: Maturation of the pediatric tracheostomy stoma: Effect on complications. *Ann Otol Rhinol Laryngol* 1999;108(12):1115–1119.

100. Rozsasi A et al: A single-center 6-year experience with two types of pediatric tracheostomy. *Int J Pediatr Otorhinolaryngol* 2005;69(5):607–613.

101. Deutsch ES: Early tracheostomy tube change in children. *Arch Otolaryngol Head Neck Surg* 1998;124(11):1237–1238.

102. Yaremchuk K: Regular tracheostomy tube changes to prevent formation of granulation tissue. *Laryngoscope* 2003;113(1):1–10.

103. Wright CD et al: Anastomotic complications after tracheal resection: Prognostic factors and management. *J Thorac Cardiovasc Surg* 2004;128(5):731–739.

104. Younis RT, Lazar RH, Astor F: Posterior cartilage graft in single-stage laryngotracheal reconstruction. *Otolaryngol Head Neck Surg* 2003;129(3):168–175.

105. Grillo H: Surgery of the trachea and bronchi. In Grillo H, editor: *Tracheal reconstruction: Anterior approach and extended resection,* Hamilton, Ontario, Canada, 2004, BC Decker.

106. Cotton R: Management of subglottic stenosis in infancy and childhood: Review of a consecutive series of cases managed by surgical reconstruction. *Ann Otol Rhinol Laryngol* 1978;87(5 Pt 1):649–657.

107. Lusk RP, Gray S, Muntz HR: Single-stage laryngotracheal reconstruction. *Arch Otolaryngol Head Neck Surg* 1991;117(2):171–173.

108. Dedo HH, Fishman NH: The results of laryngeal release, tracheal mobilization and resection for tracheal stenosis in 19 patients. *Laryngoscope* 1973;83(8):1204–1210.

109. Montgomery WW: Suprahyoid release for tracheal anastomosis. *Arch Otolaryngol* 1974;99(4):255–260.

110. Simpson GT et al: Predictive factors of success or failure in the endoscopic management of laryngeal and tracheal stenosis. *Ann Otol Rhinol Laryngol* 1982;91(4 Pt 1):384–388.

111. Grillo HC: The management of tracheal stenosis following assisted respiration. *J Thorac Cardiovasc Surg* 1969;57(1):52–71.

112. Rahbar R, Valdez TA, Shapshay SM: Preliminary results of intraoperative mitomycin-C in the treatment and prevention of glottic and subglottic stenosis. *J Voice* 2000;14(2):282–286.

113. Simpson CB, James JC: The efficacy of mitomycin-C in the treatment of laryngotracheal stenosis. *Laryngoscope* 2006;116(10):1923–1925.

114. Eliashar R et al: Mitomycin does not prevent laryngotracheal repeat stenosis after endoscopic dilation surgery: An animal study. *Laryngoscope* 2004;114(4):743–746.

115. Hartnick CJ et al: Topical mitomycin application after laryngotracheal reconstruction: A randomized, double-blind, placebo-controlled trial. *Arch Otolaryngol Head Neck Surg* 2001;127(10):1260–1264.

116. Hueman EM, Simpson CB: Airway complications from topical mitomycin C. *Otolaryngol Head Neck Surg* 2005;133(6):831–835.

117. Maddaus MA et al: Subglottic tracheal resection and synchronous laryngeal reconstruction. *J Thorac Cardiovasc Surg* 1992;104(5):1443–1450.

118. Pearson FG et al: Primary tracheal anastomosis after resection of the cricoid cartilage with preservation of recurrent laryngeal nerves. *J Thorac Cardiovasc Surg* 1975;70(5):806–816.

119. McCaffrey TV: Management of subglottic stenosis in the adult. *Ann Otol Rhinol Laryngol* 1991;100(2):90–94.

120. Freeland AP: The long-term results of hyoid-sternohyoid grafts in the correction of subglottic stenosis. *J Laryngol Otol* 1986;100(6):665–674.

121. Duncavage JA, Toohill RJ, Isert DR: Composite nasal septal graft reconstruction of the partial laryngectomized canine. *Otolaryngology* 1978;86(2):ORL285–ORL290.

122. Laccourreye O et al: Cricotracheal anastomosis for assisted ventilation-induced stenosis. *Arch Otolaryngol Head Neck Surg* 1997;123(10):1074–1077.

123. Wolf M et al: Laryngotracheal anastomosis: Primary and revised procedures. *Laryngoscope* 2001;111(4 Pt 1):622–627.

124. Laccourreye O et al: Tracheal resection with end-to-end anastomosis for isolated postintubation cervical trachea stenosis: Long-term results. *Ann Otol Rhinol Laryngol* 1996;105(12):944–948.

125. Grillo HC, Zannini P, Michelassi F: Complications of tracheal reconstruction: Incidence, treatment, and prevention. *J Thorac Cardiovasc Surg* 1986;91(3):322–328.

126. Gavilan J, Cerdeira MA, Toledano A: Surgical treatment of laryngotracheal stenosis: A review of 60 cases. *Ann Otol Rhinol Laryngol* 1998;107(7):588–592.

127. Prakash UB, Offord KP, Stubbs SE: Bronchoscopy in North America: The ACCP survey. *Chest* 1991;100(6):1668–1675.

128. Filler RM, Forte V, Chait P: Tracheobronchial stenting for the treatment of airway obstruction. *J Pediatr Surg* 1998;33(2):304–311.

129. Dasgupta A et al: Self-expandable metallic airway stent insertion employing flexible bronchoscopy: Preliminary results. *Chest* 1998;114(1):106–109.

130. Tsang V, Goldstraw P: Self-expanding metal stent for tracheobronchial strictures. *Eur J Cardiothorac Surg* 1992;6(10):555–560.

131. Brichon PY et al: Endovascular stents for bronchial stenosis after lung transplantation. *Transplant Proc* 1992;24(6):2656–2659.

132. Eller RL et al: Expandable tracheal stenting for benign disease: Worth the complications? *Ann Otol Rhinol Laryngol* 2006;115(4):247–252.

133. Madden BP, Loke TK, Sheth AC: Do expandable metallic airway stents have a role in the management of patients with benign tracheobronchial disease? *Ann Thorac Surg* 2006;82:274–278.

134. Saad CP et al: The role of self-expandable metallic stents for the treatment of airway complications after lung transplantation. *Transplantation* 2003;75(9):1532–1538.

CHAPTER 35

Complications of Hypopharyngectomy and Hypopharyngeal Reconstruction

Adam S. Jacobson and Eric M. Genden

Primary carcinoma of the hypopharynx and advanced tumors of the upper aerodigestive tract that extend into the hypopharynx are associated with a poor prognosis. Primary medical therapy consists of external-beam radiation therapy or a combination of radiation and chemotherapy. Chemoradiation can result in laryngeal preservation in many patients.[1-3] Unfortunately, surgical salvage after primary medical therapy is a relatively common event, and it represents a significantly more difficult scenario than surgery as the primary modality of treatment. In general, pharyngectomy with or without a simultaneous laryngectomy is a challenge for the reconstructive surgeon among patients that have undergone radiation or combined chemoradiation. The ablative and reconstructive surgeons must remain focused on minimizing the overall morbidity of the procedure without compromising the functional outcome with regard to swallowing and voice restoration. The ability to swallow and the maintenance of the voice hold a very high value for patients when they are queried about quality of life.[4-6]

The most common indications for laryngopharyngectomy have changed significantly during the past decade. During the 1980s and the early 1990s, laryngopharyngectomy was commonly performed for the primary management of extensive tumors involving the hypopharynx and advanced tumors of the larynx. Since the introduction of laryngeal preservation protocols, laryngopharyngectomy is most commonly performed as a salvage procedure for persistent or recurrent disease. As a result, many of these patients suffer from the all-too-common side effects of chemotherapy and radiation, including malnutrition, cachexia, anemia, immunosuppression, and impaired wound healing. These conditions place patients undergoing salvage surgery at a high risk for both intraoperative and postoperative complications.

A classic laryngopharyngectomy implies the resection of the entire pharynx, the larynx, and the cervical esophagus. The preoperative assessment of the tumor is essential to rule out invasion of the carotid artery, the mediastinal structures, or the prevertebral musculature, all of which represent relatively strong contraindications to surgery. Although tumor ablation can be a challenge (especially with regard to the prevention of vascular injury

and chylous leak), most of the potential complications are related to the reconstructive component of the procedure. The variety of complications that can result from a laryngopharyngectomy and the subsequent reconstruction can be categorized into intraoperative, early postoperative, and late postoperative complications (Box 35-1).

INTRAOPERATIVE COMPLICATIONS

Vascular Injury

Intraoperative injury of one of the great vessels can result in a cerebrovascular accident and death. Therefore careful preoperative evaluation to assess the likelihood of great-vessel involvement and the safety of temporary or permanent ligation of the carotid artery must be determined. In cases in which tumor appears to be adjacent to the common carotid artery or to extend into the mediastinum, it is recommended that a preoperative angiogram with a balloon-occlusion test be performed. The information gained from these tests empowers the surgeon with the knowledge that the patient will be able to tolerate the ligation of the carotid artery without neurologic sequelae. If the patient can tolerate a balloon-occlusion test without neurologic changes, then the surgeon can make the decision to resect the involved portion of the carotid artery and to reconstruct the artery appropriately. Preoperative consultation with a vascular surgeon and thoughtful planning are essential. It is recommended that the reconstruction of the carotid artery occur at the time of the initial resection rather than the ligation.

Similarly, tumors that invade the mediastinal structures or the anterior mediastinum should be carefully assessed with preoperative imaging, including computed tomography scanning, magnetic resonance imaging, and angiography. One must be fully informed of the extent of mediastinal extension before undertaking an ablative procedure. If mediastinal extension is present on preoperative imaging, coordination with the thoracic surgical team is essential to performing a well-planned and well-executed ablation. The thoracic team can provide safe access to the mediastinum to enable the head and neck surgeon to have control of the mediastinal vascular structures. This thoughtful preparation can prevent disastrous complications such as an inadvertent laceration of the innominate vessels.

When vascular injury occurs during a hypopharyngectomy, it is essential to have access to and control of the proximal and distal carotid artery. With this in mind, for cases in which vascular invasion is suspected, the proximal and distal carotid artery should be isolated with elastic loops before tumor ablation. This control of the artery allows the well-prepared head and neck surgeon to have both time and options. In the event that the carotid artery is injured during the course of surgery or if the surgeon elects to resect a portion of the carotid artery, he or she can keep control of the situation by using the proximal and distal vessel loops. After the bleeding has been controlled, the site of injury can be isolated and inspected. The stump pressure of the distal vessel may be tested; if it is more than 50% of the mean arterial pressure, the risk of stroke is significantly decreased.[7,8] With the bleeding under control, the vascular team can be mobilized, and a temporary shunt can be placed while the repair of the vessel is performed. In the setting of a patient who has passed a balloon-occlusion test preoperatively, the surgeon can elect to ligate the carotid artery and to proceed with anticoagulation.

Anticoagulation is considered when a permanent carotid ligation or a carotid repair is performed because there is a risk of anterograde and retrograde thrombosis propagation, which can result in emboli, stroke, and death.[9] Because this risk of thrombosis propagations exists, it is essential to closely monitor the neurologic status of the patient during the immediate postoperative period.

Distal Extension

Although preoperative imaging is essential in delineating the extent of the tumor, it is not uncommon for tumors of the hypopharynx to have spread submucosally more extensively than is suggested by the preoperative imaging.[10] As a result, one complication of laryngopharyngectomy includes the distal extension of tumor into the thoracic esophagus and possibly the mediastinum. Because of the high propensity for submucosal spread, it is essential to perform a frozen-section examination of the distal margins to ensure that they are clear of tumor cells. If the margins are positive, one must continue the resection until there are negative margins obtained (Figure 35-1). If necessary, a total esophagectomy should be performed to prevent a marginal recurrence. With this in mind, it is important to discuss with each patient the possibility of a total esophagectomy and a gastric pull-up reconstruction. Although the rate of submucosal spread has been documented to be as high as 58%, the requirement for an unplanned total esophagectomy and gastric pull up is rare.[10]

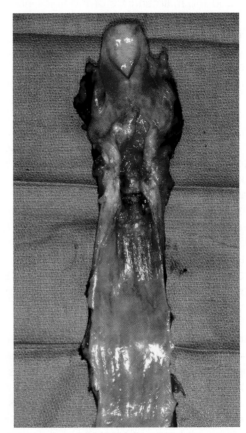

Figure 35-1. Pharyngoesophagectomy specimen performed for submucosal extension.

Chyle Leak

A tear in the cervical thoracic duct will lead to an almost immediate extravasation of chylous fluid into the neck wound. In the normal adult, the thoracic duct transports up to 4 L of chyle per day, allowing for a rapid accumulation of fluid within the neck.[11] This conditions occurs in 1% to 2.5% of radical neck dissections, with the majority (75%–92%) being on the left side.[12] An uncontrolled chyle leak can impair nutrition, compromise and delay wound healing, and prolong hospitalization. A loss of chyle from the body will rapidly deplete the body of its stores of fluid, proteins, and electrolytes. The careful postoperative monitoring of serum electrolytes and proteins with the accurate repletion of these substances is essential.

A chyle leak is usually noted intraoperatively when clear or turbid fluid accumulates in the root of the neck. If there is a question about the presence of a chyle leak, the patient can be placed in the Trendelenburg position, and a prolonged positive-pressure breath can be applied to observe for a leak. Chyle fistulas can generally be prevented by ligating the lymphatic pedicle at the base of the neck during the dissection. If a tear in the thoracic duct occurs, surgical clips or a figure-eight stitch are used to ligate the lymphatic pedicle until there is no evidence of chyle reaccumulating during a Valsalva maneuver. Meticulous technique must be used during this repair to prevent damage to the phrenic and vagus nerves and to prevent a persistent chyle leak postoperatively. Even with a meticulous intraoperative repair, these patients are at high risk for a postoperative chylous fistula.[13–15]

Invasion of the Prevertebral Fascia

Invasion of the prevertebral fascia is a contraindication to the surgical resection of an advanced hypopharyngeal lesion. The careful evaluation of preoperative computed tomography scanning or magnetic resonance imaging is essential for determining the resectability of squamous cell carcinoma of the upper aerodigestive tract. When prevertebral invasion is unexpectedly identified intraoperatively, the prevertebral fascia and musculature can be resected; however, extension into this area has been associated with a poor prognosis. When tumors invade laterally, they may involve the vertebral artery. Injury to this portion of the vascular system can result in Wallenberg syndrome (Box 35-2).

POSTOPERATIVE COMPLICATIONS

The postoperative complications of laryngopharyngectomy and hypopharyngeal reconstruction can be divided into early complications and late complications.

BOX 35-2 Signs and Symptoms of Wallenberg Syndrome

Wallenberg syndrome is caused by the occlusion of the posterior inferior cerebellar artery or the vertebral artery.

ON THE IPSILATERAL SIDE

Horner syndrome, hypohidrosis, and vasodilation of the face

Limb ataxia and asynergia

Ataxia and muscle hypotonia

Loss of the sensation of pain and temperature in the face and a reduced corneal reflex

Nystagmus

Hypacusis

Dysarthria and dysphagia (i.e., paralysis of the palatal elevation pharyngeal constrictors and the vocal cord)

Tachycardia and dyspnea

Dysgeusia

Palatal myoclonus

ON THE CONTRALATERAL SIDE

Loss of the sensation of pain and temperature in the body and the extremities

---

Early complications include deep venous thrombosis (DVT), pulmonary embolism (PE), wound infection, salivary leak and fistula, chyle leak, wound breakdown, great vessel rupture, hypocalcemia, and flap failure. Late complications include pharyngoesophageal stenosis, dysphagia, permanent feeding-tube dependence, and marginal recurrence.

Because hypopharyngeal reconstruction often follows a total laryngopharyngectomy, many of the patients undergoing this procedure will have received combined chemoradiation. Radiation causes small-vessel intimal fibrosis that compromises wound healing and that may lead to a higher rate of wound healing failure. Free flap reconstruction of the pharyngoesophageal segment has become the most popular method for reconstructing patients after total laryngopharyngectomy. The reconstruction may be accomplished using either a fasciocutaneous free flap or an enteric free flap. The most common fasciocutaneous flaps include the radial forearm free flap (Figure 35-2) and the anterolateral thigh free flap (Figures 35-3 and 35-4). The commonly used enteric free flaps include the jejunum free flap and the gastroomental free flap (Figure 35-5).

Although there is significant debate regarding the optimal donor site, each patient must be evaluated as an individual, and the donor site must be chosen on the basis of a variety of factors, including age, performance status, and history of prior surgery. The radial forearm free flap offers an excellent donor site because of its

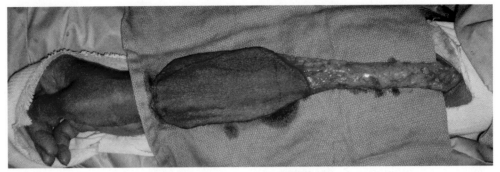

Figure 35-2. Radial forearm free flap.

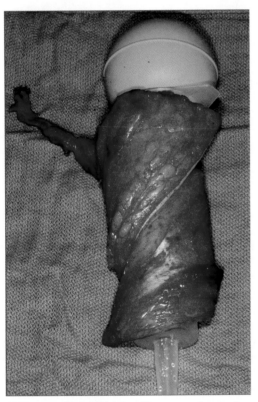

Figure 35-3. Anterolateral thigh free flap wrapped around an irrigation bulb to form a neopharynx.

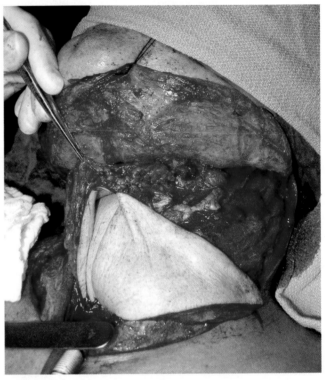

Figure 35-4. Anterolateral thigh inset for pharyngoesophageal reconstruction.

easy accessibility, allowing for a two-team ablation and reconstruction, a long vascular pedicle, and general reliability.[16] Similarly, the anterolateral thigh free flap provides a fasciocutaneous flap with a long vascular pedicle, high reliability, the ability to perform a two-team approach, and minimal donor-site morbidity.[16]

With respect to enteric flaps, for many years the jejunum has been the donor site of choice, largely because of its tubed design. The jejunum is harvested through a midline laparotomy, and, as a result, it may be complicated by the inherent issues associated with a laparotomy. Although the jejunum has been used successfully for many years, during recent years, the gastroomental free flap has become popularized as a result of the omentum

that accompanies the free flap. Unlike the jejunal free flap, the gastroomental free flap provides an extremely well-vascularized omentum that is ideal for protecting the mediastinal contents in cases that require combined pharyngoesophagectomy and mediastinal dissection.

EARLY POSTOPERATIVE COMPLICATIONS

Flap-Related Complications

Early complications related to hypopharyngeal reconstruction are most commonly related to the failure of the free flap. Although the rates of free flap failure are less than 5% in most tertiary care institutions, many of the patients undergoing this procedure have had prior

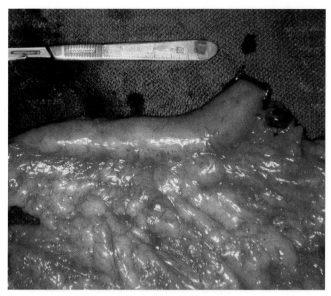

Figure 35-5. Gastroomental free flap.

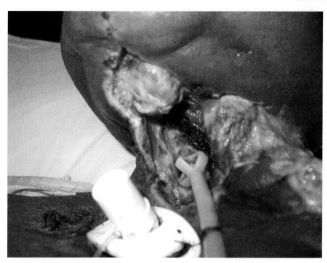

Figure 35-6. Wound breakdown after chemotherapy and/or radiation therapy failure and salvage total laryngopharyngectomy.

surgery, chemotherapy, or radiation.[17] As a result, the vessels in the neck are commonly destroyed by a previous ablation or compromised by radiation changes. The lack of nonirradiated, healthy recipient vessels in the neck can significantly complicate and lengthen the reconstructive portion of the surgery.[18] If less-than-healthy vessels are used, the chance of flap failure will increase. If healthy vessels can be located but they do not provide the optimal geometry for the flap pedicle, the chance of flap failure will rise.

In addition to flap failure being a constant concern, the dehiscence of the suture lines of the neopharynx and the neoesophagus is also a significant risk. A well-planned reconstruction starts with an appropriately chosen donor site and ends with a well-executed reconstruction on a technical basis. If the donor site that is chosen results in a flap that is too bulky, there will be excessive stress on the suture lines, thereby putting the patient at risk for flap dehiscence. Poorly executed sutures during the closure of the proximal and distal anastomosis of the neopharynx will undoubtedly lead to a salivary leak.

The most significant risk of free flap failure in the hypopharyngectomy patient relates to salivary leak. A small dehiscence in the reconstruction's suture line can lead to a significant enough salivary leak that the flap pedicle will become infected and thrombose. When a free flap fails, every effort should be made to salvage it immediately. In rare cases, the revision and salvage of the free flap is not possible. In such situations, the patient is commonly left with an exposed carotid artery, jugular vein, or mediastinal vascular structures (Figure 35-6). The dissemination of saliva in these areas can lead to infection and vascular blowout. As a result, it is imperative to prevent the salivary contamination of the vascular compartment. In a desperate situation such as this, a second free or pedicled flap should be performed immediately, whenever possible.[17]

Chyle Leak

A chyle leak is usually detected in the postoperative setting when there is milky drainage from the neck drains. These patients can be treated conservatively or with surgical intervention.[14] Common to both forms of treatment are drainage of the fluid from the neck space using a suction or passive drain, decreasing chyle production, and providing appropriate fluid and nutritional replacement. Conservative management is usually instituted initially (if it is a low-volume leak), because there is a relatively high rate of spontaneous resolution.[19] Conservative management consists of interventions that reduce chylous flow. Included within this management are adequate drainage, a nutritional intake that is high in medium-chain triglycerides, and a pressure dressing over the base of the neck to prevent the reaccumulation of chyle. Medium-chain triglycerides are helpful because they are absorbed directly into the portal circulation, bypassing the lymphatic system. Volume status and electrolyte, hemoglobin, and albumin levels should be checked regularly. Lucente and colleagues[20] reported that all of their chyle fistulas resolved within 7 days when the patient was placed on a diet high in medium-chain triglycerides. Interestingly, all of their fistulas had a peak 24-hour drainage of less than 500 ml.[20]

If conservative management fails after 2 weeks or if there is a high-volume leak (i.e., ≥1 L of chyle per day), surgical therapy should be instituted.[13,19] Additionally, nutritional or metabolic complications such as electrolyte depletion and immunosuppression are strong indications for instituting a surgical repair of the injured thoracic duct.

Because the injury to the thoracic duct is within a neck that has been previously operated on, a neck exploration can be performed to localize the injured lymphatic pedicle, and the ligation of the pedicle is performed. A few hours before the procedure, the patient can be fed a diet high in fat (e.g., cream) in an attempt to increase the lymphatic flow for the intraoperative localization of the leak. If the origin of the leak is very low in the neck or upper chest and cannot be localized, a thoracic duct ligation can be performed via an open lateral thoracotomy or a closed thoracoscopy.[21,22]

Salivary Fistula

As previously discussed, one of the more common complications after hypopharyngeal reconstruction is the formation of a pharyngocutaneous fistula. This situation is a result of dehiscence at either the proximal, distal, or vertical suture lines. In most cases, because the proximal pharynx and the distal esophagus have been compromised by chemoradiation, this is the location where a dehiscence will most likely occur. The early identification of a salivary fistula is essential to prevent extensive complications. Pharyngocutaneous fistulas rates after hypopharyngectomy have been reported to be as high as 31%.[23] Signs such as edema of the skin flaps, a rise in the white blood cell count, erythema of the overlying skin flaps, or tenderness should quickly raise the suspicion of a salivary leak. Some authors have advocated using a salivary bypass tube during the acute healing process to decrease the rate of fistula.[24,25] The intent is to minimize stress on the suture lines by reducing the direct contact of saliva with the healing suture lines. It is unclear whether this prophylactic measure decreases the incidence of salivary leaks, but it remains a technique that is used throughout the community.

A pharyngocutaneous fistula may occur as a result of a technical error during reconstruction, impaired wound healing, or persistent distal obstruction to flow. In general, fistulae that occur within the first 3 days of the postoperative course are commonly the result of a technical error in wound closure or a persistent distal obstruction to salivary flow. The most common technical error is an errant stitch that results in a gap in the pharyngeal suture line or the incomplete imbrication of the mucosal lining. Factors such as the type of suture used during closure have been demonstrated to affect the rate of fistula formation. Verma and colleagues[26] found that the use of Vicryl suture during the pharyngeal closure resulted in a lower fistula rate than was seen with the use of chromic catgut.

A distal obstruction to salivary flow is not common, but a distal stricture as a result of a tight mucosal closure or an undiscovered distal esophageal lesion can occur. In this predicament, the path of least resistance is no longer via the distal esophagus but rather into the neck through a weakness in the pharyngeal suture line. Additionally, a tight mucosal closure in the distal pharynx may result in increased pharyngeal pressures. Wang and colleagues[27] reported that leaving the pharyngeal constrictor muscles open may reduce the pressures in the newly reconstructed pharyngoesophageal segment and ultimately reduce the chance of fistula formation. As an additional measure to reduce intraluminal pressure, a cricopharyngeal myotomy can be performed to decrease the distal narrowing of the esophageal inlet caused by the constant tonic contraction of the cricopharyngeus muscle.

Although a variety of additional factors—including the choice of antibiotic,[28] intraoperative transfusion,[29] and the presence of systemic disease[30]—have been linked to the incidence of fistula formation, it has been universally accepted that radiation exposure significantly increases the risk of fistula formation. The effects of radiation therapy on tissue (e.g., fibrosis, hypoxia, impaired leukocyte migration, delayed wound healing) are largely dose dependant.[31] High-dose radiation (i.e., >50 Gy) leads to a cascade of events in which the fibroblast population becomes dysfunctional and depleted, thereby resulting in hypovascularity. Furthermore, atherosclerosis is aggravated by the induction of myointimal fibrosis.[31,32] Mendelsohn and Bridger[33] reviewed 100 consecutive patients with postoperative fistulae and found that radiation therapy was the most significant predictor of fistula. McCombe and Jones[34] later reported a larger series of 357 patients and found that preoperative radiotherapy had a significant impact on the development of a postoperative fistula. In their study, they found that pharyngocutaneous fistulas developed in 39% of the radiated patients and in only in 4% of the nonirradiated patient population.[34] Furthermore, they noted that radiation-related fistulae occurred earlier (day 7), than nonradiation-related fistulae (28 days) and more often led to significant wound-related morbidity as well as death in 6 cases.[34]

When a fistula is identified, it is imperative to direct the saliva away from the mediastinal and vascular compartments. Failure to achieve a medial pharyngocutaneous pathway may lead to the dissemination of saliva into the peripheral neck, which results in the elevation of the skin flaps, wound breakdown, the necrosis of the skin flaps, and, in extreme cases, carotid exposure. The technique used by the authors is the creation of a controlled midline fistula. This allows for the lateral skin flaps to heal, and it prevents the salivary contamination of the great vessels.

In some cases, the creation of a controlled fistula can be performed at the bedside by inserting a Penrose drain through the cervical skin suture line. The drain is then directed to the point of maximum collection and brought out through a midline location in the neck. In other cases, the creation of a diverting fistula requires a trip to the operating room. Operative management consists of a neck exploration with the goal of identifying the site of dehiscence in the neopharynx and advancing cervical skin flaps down to the origin of the salivary leak. This technique essentially matures the fistula and diverts the saliva away from the vascular compartment. After the fistula has matured and the patient has healed appropriately, the fistula is closed secondarily by performing a Wookey procedure.[35,36] A variety of local and regional flaps—including the sternocleidomastoid flap, the deltopectoral flap, the latissimus dorsi flap, and the pectoralis flap[37–39]—have been described for the secondary closure of pharyngocutaneous fistulas.

Free-tissue transfer offers an excellent mechanism for closing extensive pharyngocutaneous fistulas that are not amenable to local or regional flap closure. Microvascular techniques allow for the introduction of healthy vascularized tissue and also for the ability to reliably reconstruct the pharyngoesophageal segment in a single stage. The jejunum is a common donor site, because its tubular structure lends itself to circumferential defects, or it can be divided at the antimesenteric border to serve as a patch graft. De Vries and colleagues[40] examined 18 patients who were treated with a jejunal free flaps for stricture after a pharyngocutaneous fistula, and they found this technique to be both reliable and effective. There are several alternative approaches to the jejunal reconstruction, including a fasciocutaneous free flap. Fasciocutaneous free flaps have been well established as a reliable method of pharyngocutaneous reconstruction. However, among patients who have been irradiated, wound healing and great-vessel exposure are significant risks. The gastroomental free flap offers the unique advantage of an enteric tube with a vascularized omentum. The authors have found that the omentum is ideal for the protection of the great vessels for cases in which wound breakdown and great-vessel exposure are risks after multimodality therapy.[41]

Deep Venous Thrombosis and Pulmonary Embolism

DVT is a relatively common complication of head and neck cancer and its treatment. Unfortunately, head and neck cancer patients are already at a higher risk for DVT as a result of their underlying carcinoma and the associated hypercoagulable state. Performing a large ablative procedure with a reconstruction can further increase the risk of DVT for these patients as a result of the stasis associated with the excessive length of the surgical procedure and the iatrogenic trauma from the procedure.

One should be on high alert for this dreaded complication and workup any patient that has signs of a DVT, such as lower-extremity tenderness, erythema, palpable cord, or pain on dorsiflexion of the foot. The standard workup includes a lower-extremity duplex scan or a venogram. If there is any clinical suspicion (i.e., dyspnea, tachypnea, tachycardia, or electrocardiogram changes) that a DVT has already advanced to become a PE, one should rapidly obtain a ventilation perfusion scan or a computed tomography angiogram and treat the patient accordingly.

To reduce the incidence and risk of DVT and possible PE in patients with head and neck cancer who undergo surgical therapy, the authors often start DVT prophylaxis during the immediate postoperative period. Currently the standard protocol consists of 5000 U of subcutaneous heparin every 8 hours. Patients who undergo a free flap reconstruction are additionally treated with 81 mg of aspirin daily. Early ambulation and the use of Venodyne (Vasopress, Eatontown, NJ) boots or compression stockings are secondary measures that can help to minimize the risk of stasis leading to DVT formation.[42]

The treatment of DVT consists of immediate anticoagulation with intravenous heparin for 5 to 7 days followed by warfarin to a goal international normalized ratio of 2.0 to 3.0 for a minimum of 3 months postoperatively. Currently some advocate the use of low-molecular-weight heparin as therapy because of its ease of use (i.e., twice-daily dosing subcutaneously) and proven efficacy. Thrombolytic therapy is reserved for massive PE in an attempt to salvage a very difficult situation. The placement of a vena cava filter is usually considered for patients with a high risk of bleeding or for those with objectively diagnosed recurrent PE despite adequate anticoagulation.

Wound Infection

Uncomplicated wound infections are relatively uncommon after a hypopharyngectomy and hypopharyngeal reconstruction, considering the fact that the operative field is contaminated with saliva throughout the procedure. Prophylactically, the authors commonly administer 1 g of cefazolin and 500 mg of metronidazole intraoperatively as well as postoperatively for three doses over a 24-hour period. Although a wound infection in the neck is relatively uncommon, one must be vigilant when examining these patients for the development of erythema, warmth, and tenderness of the cervical skin. If these signs of cellulitis manifest, one must treat the patient without hesitation. If a wound infection is allowed to progress, the suture lines will quickly dehisce, and a free flap pedicle will thrombose, leaving the patient with an outcome that is less than optimal. Additionally, one must remain highly suspicious that a salivary leak is the cause of a wound infection until proven otherwise.

Wound Breakdown

Generally wound breakdown is the result of an uncontrolled wound infection or a salivary leak. If a salivary leak is allowed to progress and to contaminate the entire neck, the neovascularization that should take place during the healing process is impaired. This can lead to ischemia of the reconstruction itself (i.e., thrombosis of a free flap pedicle) or to the failure of the cervical skin flaps to seat and, ultimately, to wound breakdown.

Another possible cause of wound breakdown is excessive tension on the suture lines caused by a tight closure. One must carefully consider how much tension is being placed on the cervical skin suture lines during the closure, because, during the postoperative period, the flap tends to engorge and swell, thus increasing the tension placed on the already tight closure. If the closure is too tight, one must strongly consider the use of a split-thickness skin graft to release the tension on the suture lines of the cervical skin closure. After a wound breakdown begins, it is often difficult to regain control of the wound. Doing so can require a tremendous amount of local wound care and possibly revision surgery and a prolonged hospital course (see Figure 35-6).

Major Vessel Rupture

Rupture of the great vessels is most commonly the result of an unrecognized salivary leak. Human saliva contains not only oral flora but also digestive enzymes that, when combined, can be extremely dangerous if allowed to bathe the great vessels. One must quickly recognize that a salivary leak is present and divert the saliva away from the great vessels using either a Penrose drain at the bedside or by creating a controlled pharyngostome. Less commonly, wound breakdown can lead to the exposure of the great vessels to air. This situation can quickly lead to the desiccation of the walls of the great vessels, resulting in rupture. Exposure of the great vessels must be recognized early and treated aggressively with local wound care or, if necessary, local, regional, or free-tissue transfer to prevent a disastrous event.

Regardless of the cause, if there is a rupture of the great vessels, immediate action is necessary to salvage this catastrophic situation. First, pressure must be applied to the ipsilateral neck to attempt to slow and control the hemorrhage. Second, two large-bore intravenous lines must be inserted, and fluids must be run into the patient, wide open. Third, packed red blood cells must be called for immediately. Fourth, the

patient must be transported to the operating room for an emergency neck exploration and for control of the ruptured vessel. The vascular team should be present in the operating room, and a repair must be performed. If a repair is not possible for technical reasons, ligation of the ruptured vessel is indicated. Without the information from a preoperative balloon-occlusion test to guide this decision, the operative surgeon takes the risk of a catastrophic cerebrovascular accident occurring in an attempt to prevent exsanguination.

Cardiopulmonary Issues

As with any major surgical procedure, patients undergoing hypopharyngectomy and a reconstruction are at risk for a myocardial infarction or a new-onset arrhythmia. Additionally, because hypopharyngectomy and hypopharyngeal reconstruction require the extensive manipulation of the airway, these patients are at an increased risk of aspiration pneumonia. Often these patients have a fresh tracheotomy that can be used to protect the airway intraoperatively and that can be used for pulmonary toilet during the postoperative period.

Hypocalcemia

Permanent and transient hypocalcemia can result from extensive dissection at the base of the neck and in the mediastinum. An extensive dissection in these regions can lead to ablation of the parathyroid glands or ischemia of these glands with either permanent or transient hypocalcemia. Clark and colleagues[23] found that postoperative hypocalcemia occurred in 44% of their patients who underwent surgery for hypopharyngeal carcinoma. This serious complication must be recognized during the immediate postoperative period so that the known complications of hypocalcemia can be avoided (Box 35-3).

Sudden changes in levels of ionized serum calcium result in perioral and distal-extremity paresthesias as the first signs. If the calcium levels continue to decline, patients can experience tetany, bronchospasm, mental status changes, seizures, laryngospasm, and cardiac arrhythmias. Chvostek sign and Trousseau sign often develop as

---

BOX 35-3 Acute Physiologic Effects of Hypocalcemia

Perioral and distal-extremity paresthesias
Tetany
Bronchospasm
Mental status changes
Seizures
Laryngospasm
Cardiac arrhythmias
Positive Chvostek and Trousseau signs as a result
of neuromuscular irritability

a result of increased neuromuscular irritability when serum calcium levels drop to less than 8 mg/dl.

Treatment for hypocalcemia is initiated if the patient is symptomatic or if serum calcium levels drop to less than 7 mg/dl. The intravenous repletion of calcium can be performed during the short term (i.e., titrated to symptom resolution) with a transition to enteral repletion with calcium carbonate and vitamin D for the long term. These adjustments should be performed in consultation with an endocrinologist. When these patients return to the outpatient setting, an endocrinologist must closely monitor them for the return of parathyroid gland function and the stability of serum calcium levels. Unfortunately, permanent enteral calcium carbonate and vitamin D may be necessary for some patients, which will increase the number of medications that they must remember to take on a daily basis.

LATE POSTOPERATIVE COMPLICATIONS

Late complications of hypopharyngectomy and hypopharyngeal reconstruction include pharyngoesophageal stenosis, dysphagia, and marginal recurrence.

Pharyngoesophageal Stenosis

Pharyngoesophageal stenosis represents the most common complication after total laryngopharyngectomy, and it has been reported to occur in up to 15% of the patients undergoing hypopharyngecotomy[23] (Figure 35-7). This may occur either because the tissue used for reconstruction was poorly designed or, more commonly, because of

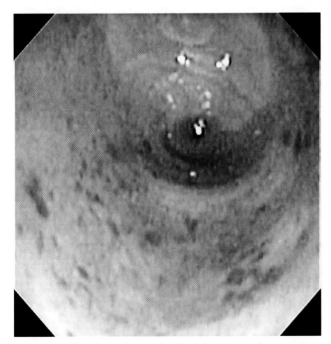

Figure 35-7. Esophageal stenosis after total laryngopharyngectomy and chemoradiation.

the natural forces associated with contraction and healing. Strictures occur most commonly at the distal suture line and result from ischemia at the distal flap or the proximal esophagus. When stenosis is identified, it may be managed conservatively with routine esophageal dilatation. Unfortunately, in most cases, dilatation of pharyngoesophageal stenosis represents a temporizing measure. Most commonly, a revision procedure is required. Revision usually includes the interposition of an epithelial segment to widen the anastomosis, which is usually the site of stenosis. Although a multitude of reconstructive options exist for the repair of a pharyngoesophageal stricture, currently only four different techniques are used: (1) free jejunal transfer; (2) radial forearm free flap; (3) pedicled pectoralis major flap; and (4) gastric pull up. The difficult choice is between the complete revision of the reconstruction and widening the area of stenosis with a patch graft.

Dysphagia

The hypopharynx and the cervical esophagus are dynamic tubular structures that provide a continuum from the oral cavity to the thoracic esophagus. They act in a coordinated fashion to facilitate the transit of the food bolus and secretions. Coordinated contraction and passive relaxation of the pharyngeal musculature in combination with lubrication from salivary and mucosal secretions allow for the smooth passage of the food bolus. It has been shown that the major contributor to the propagation of the food bolus is the action of the tongue rather than the constrictor muscles. This finding is an advantage for the reconstructive surgeon, because all current reconstructive techniques focus on the restoration of the structure of the pharynx as a passive conduit.

Defects of the hypopharynx can be classified broadly as partial (i.e., involving only a portion of the wall of the pharynx) or circumferential. The reconstructive requirement for each type is distinct. Partial defects usually have residual functional anatomy; therefore reconstruction requires simply patching the defect while limiting the disruption of the normal function of the native surrounding tissue. The reconstruction of circumferential defects is a far more difficult challenge. The reconstruction must replace the entire circumference of the pharynx and allow for the unimpeded passage of food and liquid to avoid dysphagia. Unfortunately, the coordinated peristaltic activity of the native pharynx is lost, and the patient must rely on the tongue to propel the bolus and on the reconstructed segment to act as a resistance-free conduit to retain the ability to eat and drink.[43]

The creation of an adynamic segment in such a dynamic region of the upper aerodigestive tract often leaves patients complaining of dysphagia. Although they are able to perform the initial steps in swallowing, including the oral and pharyngeal phases, they have difficulty with transporting the food bolus down the neopharynx and the neoesophagus. The adynamic reconstructed segment often represents an obstruction of the swallowing mechanism. As a result, patients are encouraged to drink abundant amounts of fluid while eating to lubricate the food bolus and to facilitate swallowing. In rare cases, this can represent an insurmountable problem for the patient who ultimately requires a permanent gastrostomy or jejunostomy tube for supplemental (if not complete) enteral feeding.

Marginal Recurrence

Recurrence at the site of the hypopharyngeal reconstruction is always a concern. A rigid surveillance program including computed tomography and positron emission tomography scanning should be initiated immediately after surgical reconstruction. Although secondary malignancy always represents a risk, recurrence at the margin of the resection site is always a concern. Surveillance should be performed not only with imaging techniques but with direct physical examination using transnasal pharyngoscopy, laryngoscopy, and esophagoscopy. A barium swallow and periodic diagnostic operative esophagoscopies will often be helpful to rule out recurrence at a location that is difficult to visualize in the office setting.

CONCLUSION

The risks associated with hypopharyngectomy and hypopharyngeal reconstruction can be broken down into intraoperative, early postoperative, and late postoperative. The intraoperative complications are generally avoided by careful preoperative evaluation and meticulous surgical technique. The early and late postoperative complications must be identified quickly and managed aggressively to prevent the evolution of a small complication into a disastrous one.

REFERENCES

1. Urba S, Wolf GT: Organ preservation in multimodality therapy of head and neck cancer. *Hematol Oncol Clin North Am* 1991;5(4):713–724.
2. Wolf GT, Urba S, Hazuka M: Induction chemotherapy for organ preservation in advanced squamous cell carcinoma of the oral cavity and oropharynx. *Recent Results Cancer Res* 1994;134:133–143.
3. Gilbert J, Forastiere AA: Organ preservation trials for laryngeal cancer. *Otolaryngol Clin North Am* 2002;35(5):vi, 1035–1054.
4. Sherman AC, Simonton S, Adams DC, et al: Assessing quality of life in patients with head and neck cancer: Cross-validation of the European Organization for Research and Treatment of Cancer (EORTC) Quality of Life Head and Neck module (QLQ-H&N35): *Arch Otolaryngol Head Neck Surg* 2000;126(4):459–467.
5. Hanna E, Sherman AC: Quality-of-life issues in head and neck cancer. *Curr Oncol Rep* 1999;1(2):124–128.
6. Fung K, Lyden TH, Lee J, et al: Voice and swallowing outcomes of an organ-preservation trial for advanced laryngeal cancer. *Int J Radiat Oncol Biol Phys* 2005;63(5):1395–1399.
7. Morishima H, Kurata A, Miyasaka Y, et al: Efficacy of the stump pressure ratio as a guide to the safety of permanent occlusion of the internal carotid artery. *Neurol Res* 1998;20(8):732–736.
8. Kato K, Tomura N, Takahashi S, et al: Balloon occlusion test of the internal carotid artery: Correlation with stump pressure and 99mTc-HMPAO SPECT. *Acta Radiol* 2006;47(10):1073–1078.
9. Heros RC: Thromboembolic complications after combined internal carotid ligation and extra- to intracranial bypass. *Surg Neurol* 1984;21(1):75–79.
10. Ho CM, Ng WF, Lam KH, et al: Submucosal tumor extension in hypopharyngeal cancer. *Arch Otolaryngol Head Neck Surg* 1997;123(9):959–965.
11. Tilney NL, Murray JE: Chronic thoracic duct fistula: Operative technic and physiologic effects in man. *Ann Surg* 1968;167(1):1–8.
12. de Gier HH, Balm AJ, Bruning PF, et al: Systematic approach to the treatment of chylous leakage after neck dissection. *Head Neck* 1996;18(4):347–351.
13. Crumley RL, Smith JD: Postoperative chylous fistula prevention and management. *Laryngoscope* 1976;86(6):804–813.
14. Spiro JD, Spiro RH, Strong EW: The management of chyle fistula. *Laryngoscope* 1990;100(7):771–774.
15. Myers EN, Dinerman WS: Management of chylous fistulas. *Laryngoscope* 1975;85(5):835–840.
16. Genden EM, Jacobson AS: The role of the anterolateral thigh flap for pharyngoesophageal reconstruction. *Arch Otolaryngol Head Neck Surg* 2005;131(9):796–799.
17. Varvares MA, Lin D, Hadlock T, et al: Success of multiple, sequential, free tissue transfers to the head and neck. *Laryngoscope* 2005;115(1):101–104.
18. Urken ML, Higgins KM, Lee B, et al: Internal mammary artery and vein: Recipient vessels for free tissue transfer to the head and neck in the vessel-depleted neck. *Head Neck* 2006;28(9):797–801.
19. Nussenbaum B, Liu JH, Sinard RJ: Systematic management of chyle fistula: The Southwestern experience and review of the literature. *Otolaryngol Head Neck Surg* 2000;122(1):31–38.
20. Lucente FE, Diktaban T, Lawson W, et al: Chyle fistula management. *Otolaryngol Head Neck Surg* 1981;89(4):575–578.
21. Gunnlaugsson CB, Iannettoni MD, Yu B, et al: Management of chyle fistula utilizing thoracoscopic ligation of the thoracic duct. *ORL J Otorhinolaryngol Relat Spec* 2004;66(3):148–154.
22. Hayden JD, Sue-Ling HM, Sarela AI, et al: Minimally invasive management of chylous fistula after esophagectomy. *Dis Esophagus* 2007;20(3):251–255.
23. Clark JR, de Almeida J, Gilbert R, et al: Primary and salvage (hypo)pharyngectomy: Analysis and outcome. *Head Neck* 2006;28(8):671–677.
24. Murray DJ, Gilbert RW, Vesely MJ, et al: Functional outcomes and donor site morbidity following circumferential pharyngoesophageal reconstruction using an anterolateral thigh flap and salivary bypass tube. *Head Neck* 2007;29(2):147–154.
25. Varvares MA, Cheney ML, Gliklich RE, et al: Use of the radial forearm fasciocutaneous free flap and montgomery salivary bypass tube for pharyngoesophageal reconstruction. *Head Neck* 2000;22(5):463–468.
26. Verma A, Panda NK, Mehta S, et al: Post laryngectomy complications and their mode of management: An analysis of 203 cases. *Indian J Cancer* 1989;2 6(4):247–254.
27. Wang CP, Tseng TC, Lee RC, et al: The techniques of nonmuscular closure of hypopharyngeal defect following total laryngectomy: The assessment of complication and pharyngoesophageal segment. *J Laryngol Otol* 1997;111(11):1060–1063.
28. Horgan EC, Dedo HH: Prevention of major and minor fistulae after laryngectomy. *Laryngoscope* 1979;89(2 Pt 1):250–260.
29. Hier M, Black MJ, Lafond G: Pharyngo-cutaneous fistulas after total laryngectomy: Incidence, etiology and outcome analysis. *J Otolaryngol* 1993;22(3):164–166.
30. Dedo DD, Alonso WA, Ogura JH: Incidence, predisposing factors and outcome of pharyngocutaneous fistulas complicating head

and neck cancer surgery. *Ann Otol Rhinol Laryngol* 1975;84(6): 833–840.

31. Konings AW, Smit Sibinga CT, Aarnoudse MW, et al: Initial events in radiation-induced atheromatosis. II: Damage to intimal cells. *Strahlentherapie* 1978;154(11):795–800.

32. Kirkpatrick JB: Pathogenesis of foam cell lesions in irradiated arteries. *Am J Pathol* 1967;50(2):291–309.

33. Mendelsohn MS, Bridger GP: Pharyngocutaneous fistulae following laryngectomy. *Aust N Z J Surg* 1985;55(2):177–179.

34. McCombe AW, Jones AS: Radiotherapy and complications of laryngectomy. *J Laryngol Otol* 1993;107(2):130–132.

35. Silver CE, Som ML: Reconstruction of the cervical esophagus after total pharyngolaryngectomy: A modified Wookey operation. *Ann Surg* 1967;165(2):239–243.

36. Wookey H: The surgical treatment of carcinoma of the pharynx and upper esophagus. *Surg Gynecol Obstet* 1942;75:499–506.

37. Gupta AK, Bhasin D, Shah R: Closure of post laryngectomy pharyngocutaneous fistula with sternocleidomastoid muscle flap. *Ann Acad Med Singapore* 1983;12(2 Suppl):407–410.

38. Liu R, Gullane P, Brown D, et al: Pectoralis major myocutaneous pedicled flap in head and neck reconstruction: Retrospective review of indications and results in 244 consecutive cases at the Toronto General Hospital. *J Otolaryngol* 2001;30(1):34–40.

39. Kimura Y, Tojima H, Nakamura T, et al: Deltopectral flap for one-stage reconstruction of pharyngocutaneous fistulae following total laryngectomy. *Acta Otolaryngol Suppl* 1994;511:175–178.

40. de Vries EJ, Myers EN, Johnson JT, et al: Jejunal interposition for repair of stricture or fistula after laryngectomy. *Ann Otol Rhinol Laryngol* 1990;99(6 Pt 1):496–498.

41. Genden EM, Kaufman MR, Katz B, et al: Tubed gastro-omental free flap for pharyngoesophageal reconstruction. *Arch Otolaryngol Head Neck Surg* 2001;127(7):847–853.

42. Moreano EH, Hutchison JL, McCulloch TM, et al: Incidence of deep venous thrombosis and pulmonary embolism in otolaryngology—head and neck surgery. *Otolaryngol Head Neck Surg* 1998;118(6):777–784.

43. Clayman GL, Weber RS, Guillamondegui O, et al: Laryngeal preservation for advanced laryngeal and hypopharyngeal cancers. *Arch Otolaryngol Head Neck Surg* 1995;121(2):219–223.

PART 4

Neck, Thyroid, and Parathyroid

CHAPTER 36

Complications of Surgery of the Neck

Wayne M. Koch

Surgery limited to the neck is less risky than more complex head and neck surgical procedures, such as composite resection, in which the upper aerodigestive tract is entered. Although still a major surgical procedure, cervical nodal dissection may seem safe for this reason, and the surgeon may minimize the potential for complications. However, the neck is located in a strategic position, encompassing all of the vital lines of communication and supply between the head and the body. Important functions including speech, deglutition, respiration, and the movement of the head and upper extremities are dependent on the cervical nerves and muscles. The intricate and compact organization of neural, vascular, muscular, and skeletal structures in the neck invoke a sense of awe for the genius and beauty of its design and a wholesome respect for the peril that awaits the unprepared surgeon who ventures therein.

It is the surgeon's responsibility to do all in his or her power to reduce the risk of complications. Preoperative assessment of the patient must be thorough, with the surgeon gathering information about factors that may predispose the patient to complications and allowing for precise planning of the procedure. Contingency plans can then be made for anticipated possibilities. Precise attention to anatomic detail and surgical technique helps the surgeon to avoid intraoperative mishaps and to reduce the risk of postoperative complication. A team of health-care providers with experience in the recognition and management of postoperative head and neck complications must vigilantly monitor the patient after surgery.

The predominant changes in the management of cervical nodal metastases during the past decade have been the result of the following:

1. The increasing frequency of primary chemoradiation for head and neck squamous cell carcinoma, even in cases with bulky nodal disease

2. Efforts to reduce surgical morbidity with the use of selective dissection

Until recently, most organ-preservation protocols contained plans for scheduled postradiation neck dissection for all patients with N2 or N3 disease. In a substantial number of cases, however, there is no viable tumor detected in the resected neck specimen. Improved response rates combined with dense scarring make the preoperative assessment of viability of residual tumor bulk difficult. Performing a procedure with increased risk of complication only to find no viable tumor on the pathology report is a thorny endeavor. As a result, many clinicians are now challenging the dogma of the planned posttherapy neck dissection. Efforts to determine when a neck dissection is needed using computerized imaging, positron emission tomography scanning, ultrasonography, and fine-needle aspiration (FNA) have been used to try to determine when a residual mass with viable tumor cells is present. The accuracy of these methods to identify residual viable tumor remains limited.[1]

Performing a neck dissection after chemoradiation is technically challenging, particularly in the area of previous bulky disease that has received a boost of focused radiation therapy. Reports of complications as a result of planned neck dissection after chemoradiotherapy range from 0% to 17%, and chyle leak and wound breakdown are especially common.[2–4]

PROCEDURES OTHER THAN NECK DISSECTION

Minor surgery of the neck may be regarded as less likely to be associated with complications. However, it is deceptive to think that a lesser procedure portends less risk. The exposure of structures is more limited, and so the definite identification of key nerves is actually more difficult. Because occasional neck surgeons may feel that small procedures (e.g., deep cervical node biopsy) are within their range of expertise, a disproportionate number of complications may occur during these procedures. The surgeon must be very familiar with the anatomy and exercise heightened alertness and caution. Nerves that are known to be near a lesion should be positively identified and protected before the excision of the lesion.

This chapter parallels the experience of the surgeon managing a patient undergoing neck dissection. Preoperative planning and preventive considerations are discussed first. Potential pitfalls of the operative procedure are then reviewed. Technical measures designed to avoid later complications are spelled out, and a discussion of postoperative complications follows. As a result of this organization, certain topics (e.g., carotid hemorrhage) are considered at several separate points in the text.

PREOPERATIVE CONSIDERATIONS: PREVENTION OF COMPLICATIONS

History

A careful history begins any thorough surgical evaluation. The surgeon should inquire about prior surgery and tumor therapy. Previous neck surgery may have an impact on incision design and alerts the surgeon to the potential presence of iatrogenic anatomic alterations. Previous incisional biopsy of a metastatic malignant node dictates the incorporation of the old scar into the specimen to be excised to ensure the complete eradication of tumor.

Radiation therapy causes subdermal fibrosis and scar, which makes surgery more difficult. Prior radiation therapy also slows healing, thus heightening the risk of postoperative complication. Current symptoms should be noted, because they may alert the surgeon to the aggressiveness of disease. For example, perineural invasion by metastatic tumor may result in cervical pain or referred otalgia. Handedness should be noted, because nerve injury on the patient's dominant side may impair upper-extremity function and have a profound impact on the patient's ability to perform his or her usual occupation and activities.

Aspects of the general medical history may raise concerns about wound healing and overall surgical and anesthetic risk. Most head and neck cancer patients have used alcohol and tobacco excessively. These habits are associated with chronic obstructive pulmonary disease, liver dysfunction, and atherosclerosis. Questions should address the systems affected by these processes. Impaired pulmonary function will adversely affect a patient's ability to tolerate the respiratory insult of phrenic nerve injury, chylothorax, or pneumothorax. A history of cerebrovascular accident or transient ischemic attack should alert the surgeon to the likely presence of atherosclerotic plaques in the carotid arteries. Particular care would then be warranted when working near these vessels.

Previous thyroid or laryngeal surgery with neck irradiation may be associated with hypothyroidism,[5] and appropriate thyroid function studies should be obtained. Untreated hypothyroidism may cause delayed wound healing and postpone the return to normal activities postoperatively. Diabetes mellitus is similarly associated with impaired wound healing. Peripheral neuropathy as a result of diabetes may contribute to suboptimal results after nerve injury and repair.

Patients should be encouraged to cease smoking as long before surgery as possible. Continued tobacco use during the perioperative period exacerbates pulmonary dysfunction and may impair vascular perfusion, resulting in flap loss. Wound healing and recovery are closely associated with nutritional balance.[6] In the severely malnourished patient with head and neck cancer, the delay of surgery for several weeks for nutritional support with nasogastric or gastrostomy tube, or parenteral feedings, is advisable. The history may disclose an underlying swallowing problem that may be further compromised by surgery. Edema of the aerodigestive tract after neck dissection or injury to the superior laryngeal nerve could render a patient with marginal swallowing tube dependent. Preoperative evaluation by a speech–language pathologist trained in swallowing rehabilitation methods is valuable in cases where difficulty with swallowing is anticipated.

Physical Examination

Physical characteristics such as neck flexibility, length, and thickness affect the ease of surgical access and may influence plans for the incision and positioning. Careful study of the lesion to be excised is of great importance. Its precise location, size, firmness, and mobility with respect to surrounding structures should be noted (Figures 36-1 and 36-2). Consideration is given to important structures near the mass, and plans must be made for their preservation. Any metastatic node with a dimension of more than 3 cm is most likely a group of matted nodes. Together with decreased mobility of the mass, large size is a harbinger of spread of tumor outside of the capsule of the lymph node, which is a poor prognostic indicator.[7] Magnetic resonance imaging (MRI) can also discern extracapsular spread.[8] Efforts to search for distant metastatic disease in these patients should be greater and should include imaging studies of the lungs and liver. Reduced mobility of the mass may be caused by the extension of disease into the sternocleidomastoid muscle (SCM), the jugular vein, the skin, or another nearby structure.

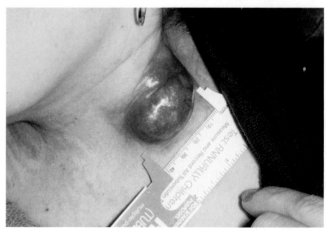

Figure 36-1. Measuring a lesion.

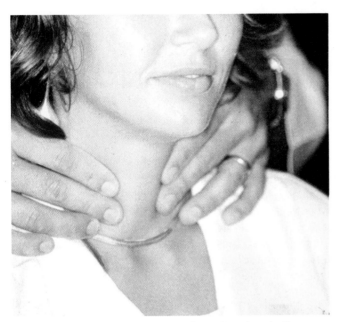

Figure 36-2. Proper hand positioning for neck node palpation.

Fixation of the mass is indicative of extension into deeper structures such as the carotid artery, the skeletal structures, or the deep cervical musculature. Carotid invasion typically causes the fixation of superoinferior but not anteroposterior movement. Fixation does not mean that the carotid wall is definitely invaded, but it should raise concern and cause the surgeon to plan for that possibility. Computed tomography (CT) scanning and arteriography may or may not help to confirm such involvement when it is suspected.

Inspection of the neck skin is useful. The location of surgical scars must be noted to plan incisions. The extent of ports used in radiation therapy can sometimes be discerned by observing the area of beard loss in males. Fixation of a neck mass to the skin indicates the extension of tumor into the dermis. The affected skin must be excised, and plans for flap coverage must be considered. Of course, the physical examination must include a full head and neck evaluation to assess the primary tumor and the upper airway before general anesthesia is administered. These considerations are beyond the scope of this chapter.

Radiographic Evaluation

Computer-assisted imaging methods (i.e., CT, MRI, PET) are useful for the preoperative evaluation of the neck. These modalities are used for the assessment of the extent of palpable disease and the detection of clinically inapparent nodes.[9] Intravenous contrast (diatrizoate meglumine and diatrizoate sodium [Hypaque] and gadolinium for CT and MRI, respectively) helps to distinguish tumor from vessels. Contrast is also useful

to assess tumor vascularity, the relationship of tumor to the great vessels, and vessel patency. CT scans are able to detect cortical bone and cartilage erosion, which are important concerns when a mass approaches the base of the skull, the vertebral bodies, the laryngeal skeleton, the hyoid, or the mandible.

The radiographic detection of suspicious nodes may provide the impetus for more extensive dissection than would otherwise be contemplated. Nodes that are more than 1.5 cm in diameter and that demonstrate the radiographic features of central necrosis and peripheral contrast enhancement have a high likelihood of containing metastatic tumor.[10] On the basis of radiologic studies, a comprehensive ipsilateral dissection or even bilateral surgery may be indicated rather than regional nodal dissection.

When a suspicious node is detected by one of these imaging modalities but is not clinically palpable, CT scanning or ultrasound may be used to guide FNA biopsy. Radiologic guidance of FNA can also help avoid trauma to the great vessels when a node is intimately associated with them. The use of ultrasound guidance to sample the sentinel node identified by lymphoscintigraphy has recently been described as a method to gauge the need for neck dissection.[11]

Evaluation Before Carotid Resection

If the physical examination or radiographic studies indicate possible carotid artery invasion by tumor, the surgeon may consider the option of carotid resection. Tumor invasion of deep structures is associated with a very poor prognosis. Atkinson and colleagues[12] performed carotid resection on 12 patients with head and neck cancer, 7 (58%) of whom died or had recurrent disease within 1 year. Of those who were free of disease at the time of writing, most had been followed for less than 2 years. Fee and colleagues[13] reported a mean survival of 15 months in a group of 29 patients with large masses attached to the carotid. These patients were treated with the debulking of tumor and radioactive seed implantation. Distant metastases were subsequently discovered in 45% of these patients, whereas 38% had recurrence in the neck. Kennedy and Krause[14] presented a retrospective series of 28 patients with similar outcomes but with an even higher incidence of distant metastasis (67%). They concluded that the five patients who developed recurrent neck disease without distant spread may have benefited from a more aggressive surgical approach to the neck. In the light of the very limited survival despite aggressive therapy in this situation, the therapeutic goal may appropriately be considered to be effective palliation. If the tumor has already failed to respond to radiation, chemotherapy, or both, surgical resection is the only remaining therapeutic option. Surgical debulking of the mass may prevent further erosion into the carotid with hemorrhage or skin breakdown with bleeding, pain, and infection.

Carotid resection is also controversial because of a risk of perioperative neurologic sequelae and death. During the first half of this century, carotid ligation carried with it a 45% risk of cerebral complication and a 30% chance of death as reported by Moore and Baker[15] when reviewing a series of 88 patients. A more recent but much smaller series ($N = 18$) attested to the value of preoperative planning for the resection of the vessel. When carotid resection was done emergently as a result of acute hemorrhage, 7 of 11 patients (64%) died within 2 weeks of surgery. Patients undergoing elective resection fared much better, with 6 of 7 (86%) surviving the perioperative period.[16] Within the past decade, Atkinson and colleagues[12] reported only one perioperative death and two central nervous system (CNS) injuries in a series of 12 cancer patients undergoing elective carotid resection, owing in part to careful preoperative evaluation and case selection.

CT or MRI scanning and arteriography may detect carotid encasement by tumor, but they are rarely accurate predictors of the invasion of the vessel wall. Thus arterial wall invasion may only be confirmed at surgery. When carotid involvement is suspected by physical examination and radiographic studies, further preoperative evaluation of the cerebral blood supply is indicated to decide what will be done if invasion is present. The adequacy of collateral cerebral circulation must be assessed to determine the risk of carotid ligation. In 1980, Enzmann and colleagues[17] described a method using angiography with temporary balloon occlusion and the measurement of carotid back pressure. Clinical or electroencephalographic evaluation of CNS function is performed during occlusion.

A later modification of the temporary balloon-occlusion test with the measurement of cerebral blood flow using stable xenon-enhanced CT was described by DeVries and colleagues.[18] The method involves four-vessel angiography with pressure monitoring in the distal internal carotid artery (ICA). Occlusion of the ICA for 15 minutes is performed with continuous electroencephalographic or clinical monitoring of the patient. After this period of occlusion, the patient breathes a mixture of air and xenon while in position for a cerebral CT scan. Scans are performed first with the balloon inflated and again 20 minutes after the restoration of normal blood flow. Cerebral blood-flow measurements are determined by subtracting the values obtained during occlusion from those measured with unimpeded flow to determine the adequacy of collateral circulation. This approach attempts to identify patients who are at

high and low risk for complications after carotid resection. Of 136 patients studied with this technique, 11 were determined to be at very high risk for stroke if the ICA was ligated, whereas 96 were predicted to have minimal risk. None of the high-risk patients underwent carotid ligation.

Temporary occlusion intraoperatively in high-risk patients caused neurologic sequelae on the two occasions when it was performed. Twenty-one of the low-risk patients had ligation or permanent balloon occlusion of the ICA with no CNS change. Patients who tolerated only short periods of occlusion of the ICA were considered to require bypass grafting at the time of carotid resection (described later in this chapter). Other studies demonstrate that balloon-occlusion test results are less-than-perfect predictors of neurologic risk.[19] High-risk patients may be managed conservatively with chemotherapy and radiation or with surgical debulking, peeling tumor from the carotid, and radioactive seed implantation. Even the latter is risky in this group, because the carotid may be weakened by tumor and thus result in rupture. Among patients with marked atherosclerotic narrowing of the contralateral carotid, endarterectomy may improve cerebral blood flow, thus permitting the subsequent resection of the artery that has been invaded by tumor.

Recent series of carotid resection and ligation or occlusion testing demonstrate no substantial advances as compared with decades-old studies. A risk of stroke of nearly 25% and a median survival of 12 months remain the rule when the carotid artery involved with tumor is addressed surgically. Occasional long-term survival is achieved.[20–22]

Fine-Needle Aspiration Biopsy

When a patient presents with a neck mass without an obvious cause, the surgeon is faced with a diagnostic dilemma. A careful history and physical examination should raise suspicion of neoplasm in certain patients. To verify these suspicions, it may be necessary to obtain a specimen from the neck mass for histologic study. In 1930, Martin and Ellis[23] drew attention to the danger of tumor spillage and seeding at the time of the open biopsy of neck masses. Since that time, FNA with cytopathologic evaluation has become the method of choice for initial attempts to obtain a diagnostic specimen from a neck mass. In addition to the workup of neck masses of uncertain cause, FNA may be useful for judging the need for neck dissection when physical examination or radiographic study identifies small nodes in patients with a known primary malignancy.

The risk associated with FNA is low. Most series simply report no complications, but bleeding is the principal concern. The recommended needle gauge (i.e., 22–25) is small, and bleeding is easily controlled with firm pressure (Figure 36-3). When the neck mass lies in close proximity to the great vessels or has physical characteristics that are suggestive of a vascular lesion, however, the surgeon should give careful thought before proceeding with FNA. The presence of a bruit should alert the clinician to the possible diagnosis of paraganglioma, whereas a soft, compressible mass may be a hemangioma or a lymphangioma. Radiographic analysis including CT scanning or MRI with intravenous contrast or selective angiography is useful to confirm the vascular nature of a mass and to further characterize its extent, growth pattern, and vessel of origin. The radiographic evaluation may make the diagnosis obvious and thus preclude the need for FNA.

FNA of carotid body tumors is controversial. Engzell and colleagues[24] have reported a death as a result of carotid thrombus and cerebral embolism after FNA of a carotid body tumor. Others report no problems after the FNA of paragangliomas.[25] Still, the advice of Engzell and colleagues to reserve FNA for patients in whom the workup is not conclusive is wise. Nerve injury has not been reported after FNA in the head and neck. If FNA is performed in the immediate path of a nerve, an in-and-out movement along a single needle trajectory should be used rather than changing angles between passes.

Reports of tumor seeding along the FNA track have occasionally appeared for malignancies in sites outside of the head and neck.[26] Considering the vast number of neck FNA procedures performed without tumor spread, seeding is only a hypothetical consideration. It has been recommended that the needle gauge be limited to 22 or smaller and that the number of passes through normal parenchyma be kept to a minimum.[27] Others advocate the excision of the aspiration tract at the time of definitive surgery.[28] The latter would seem to be unnecessary given the preponderance of experience in the literature indicating the

safety of using FNA. Batsakis and colleagues[29] have raised concern regarding the effect of FNA on the ability to render an accurate tissue diagnosis of salivary-gland tumors that have been studied by FNA and that later undergo resection. These adverse effects of FNA are unusual in the authors' experience.

OPERATIVE TECHNIQUE: INTRAOPERATIVE COMPLICATIONS

Preparation for Surgery

The surgeon should prepare to execute a carefully constructed plan that has been designed to minimize the need for last-minute intraoperative changes. Thought must be given to patient positioning to optimize surgical exposure. Plans for intraoperative monitoring are discussed beforehand with the anesthesiologist to determine line placement and airway management. Central venous pressure (CVP) catheters should not be placed on the ipsilateral side, if possible. Even long-line CVP catheters placed in the antecubital vein may enter the internal jugular (IJ) vein, thus risking surgical encounter (this is described later in this chapter). The surgeon should discuss intraoperative fluid management with the anesthesiologist before beginning the case. The injudicious replacement of fluids greatly increases postoperative edema and adds to the risk of the syndrome of inappropriate antidiuretic hormone (SIADH; also described later in this chapter). Communication between the surgeon and the anesthesiologist should be maintained throughout the case with regard to anticipated blood loss and the need for blood replacement.

Careful attention to detail with regard to preparation of the skin, draping, and maintaining sterility throughout the procedure should make postoperative wound infection extremely uncommon. The value of prophylactic antibiotics for neck surgery that does not involve entry into the upper aerodigestive tract is limited. In a retrospective study of 192 patients undergoing uncontaminated neck dissection, Carrau and colleagues[30] were unable to show a statistically significant impact of the use of prophylactic antibiotics for reducing the incidence of postoperative wound infection. There were 10 patients in a group of 99 (10%) that did not receive antibiotics who developed a wound infection. Of the 93 patients who did receive antibiotics, there were only 3 cases (3.3%) of wound infection. The failure of these results to reach statistical significance may be the result of the low overall incidence of infection and the relatively small number of patients studied. The use of prophylactic antibiotics (particularly a single agent or a first-generation cephalosporin) involves a low risk of complication. The benefits of prophylactic antibiotics may therefore outweigh the risks.

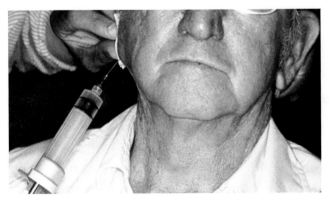

Figure 36-3. Fine-needle aspiration.

Current demand for evidence-based medicine is driving a reexamination of this issue. The use of prophylactic antibiotics for surgical cases is the only criteria pertinent to surgeons included in the initial "pay-for-performance" list endorsed by the Centers for Medicare and Medicaid Services. There have been no prospective randomized trials providing level II evidence of the effectiveness of prophylactic antibiotics. Existing evidence does support limiting the use of antibiotics to the immediate perioperative period only, thus reducing the risk of selection of resistant microorganisms. Slattery and colleagues[31] demonstrated in a retrospective analysis of 120 patients that 24 hours of antibiotic coverage was equally effective to longer courses.

Plans should be made for all potentially important contingencies. For example, when tumor resection may necessitate carotid ligation in patients without adequate collateral circulation, arrangements must be made for vascular bypass grafting, including the availability of a vascular surgeon. If radioactive implants may be needed as a result of possible sites of unresectable invasion into deep structures, consultation with a radiation oncologist must be obtained. Vein, nerve, and skin graft or flap sites are prepared and draped if the use of such grafts is contemplated. The neck is prepared and draped so that the mastoid tip, the clavicles, and the anterior border of the trapezius are exposed at the boundaries of the dissection.

Incision

The design of the incision for neck dissection has definite cosmetic and safety ramifications. Flap necrosis with tissue loss as a result of poorly designed incisions may result in wound infection, fistula, or vessel exposure and hemorrhage (Figure 36-4). Insofar as is possible, incisions should be placed in skin creases or along lines of relaxed skin tension. When a portion of an incision must violate this rule, cosmesis is enhanced by using a curved line to prevent linear scar contracture (Figure 36-5). Scars from previous neck surgery must be taken into account when designing the incision. When an incisional biopsy of a malignant mass has been performed before neck dissection, the scar and tract should be excised with the dissected specimen. Scars from other types of procedures may be incorporated into the incision or crossed at right angles by the new incision. Skin that is fixed to tumor should be encompassed and removed with the specimen. Inadequate surgical exposure, which is a potential contributor to a host of complications, is avoided when incisions are well conceived. A long, gently curving "hockeystick" or L-shaped incision provides good exposure and excellent cosmesis in many cases (Figure 36-6, A). The horizontal portion extends anteriorly, crossing the midline to the contralateral SCM at a height of 3 cm to 5 cm above the clavicle. Exposure of the posterior triangle may be inadequate with this approach when the neck is thick, thereby necessitating a vertical limb extension.

When the oral cavity or the submental region must be reached, the horizontal portion of the incision must be placed more superiorly; however, it is best kept at least two fingerbreadths below the mandibular body to avoid injury to the marginal mandibular branch of the facial nerve. Parallel horizontal (i.e., MacFee) incisions (Figure 36-6, B) are the choice of some surgeons because of superior cosmetic results. Adequate exposure can be attained with this approach, but the discontinuous view of the operative field makes it a less-than-optimal choice for the inexperienced surgeon. Alternatively, a vertical limb may be extended from a curvilinear submandibular incision (Figure 36-6, C). With a complex incision with trifurcation, the limb should be begun at right angles to the main incision to avoid compromising the vascular supply to the corners of the flaps. The trifurcation should be placed where the external jugular vein crosses the posterior border of the SCM rather than over the carotid artery. This position reduces the risk of vessel exposure should flap necrosis occur at the trifurcation. The vertical limb

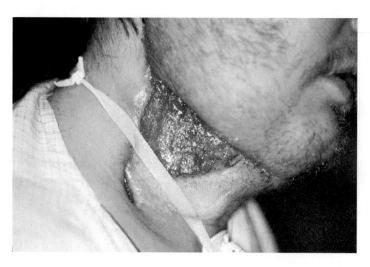

Figure 36-4. Flap loss.

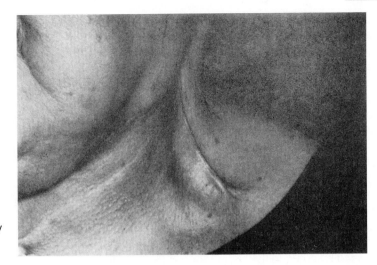

Figure 36-5. Poor cosmetic results with scar hypertrophy and webbing as a result of the linear design of the perpendicular limb of the neck incision.

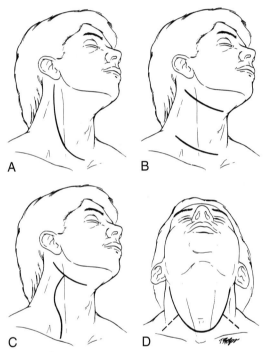

Figure 36-6. Recommended incisions for neck dissection. **A,** "Hockey-stick" curvilinear incision. **B,** MacFee incision. **C,** Modified Schobinger incision. **D,** Large apron flap for bilateral neck dissection.

may form a hypertrophic scar as it crosses the concave area in the neck contour at the level of the hyoid bone. For this reason, the vertical limb describes a broad, gentle S curve to lengthen it and break up the straight line. When bilateral neck dissections are required, a large, superiorly based apron flap is a good option (Figure 36-6, *D*). Lengthy, complex incisions are marked with superficial crosshatch scratches or methylene blue tattoos to facilitate accurate apposition at closure. Injection along the planned incision with a vasoconstrictor such as 1:100,000 epinephrine solution reduces skin bleeding at the time of incision. To be effective, injection should be performed at least 7 to 10 minutes before the incision.

Elevation of Skin Flaps

Sensory Branches of the Cervical Plexus

As the skin flaps are elevated in a subplatysmal plane, several branches of the cervical plexus are immediately encountered overlying the SCM. The division of the branches of the cervical plexus will result in a sensory deficit that extends from the pinna to the chest wall below the clavicle. Most of this sensory deficit will spontaneously resolve postoperatively over a period of months. The earlobe is one area that often remains permanently insensate. In addition, the cut nerve endings may become trigger points for postoperative pain as a result of disordered neuronal repair, scar entrapment, and neuroma formation.[32]

For these reasons, some have advocated the preservation of the cervical plexus in functional neck dissection.[33] This adds to the complexity of the surgical dissection, particularly in the region where the nerves cross the SCM at the Erb point. It may be unwise to preserve the cutaneous branches of the cervical plexus in the setting of bulky pathologic nodes. An oncologically sound resection of the tumor is the first priority. The greater auricular nerve serves as an excellent landmark for the proper plane for elevation of the superior skin flap, because it lies lateral to the SCM. The nerve should be kept down on the SCM during flap elevation, and the decision of whether to preserve it can be made later. The preservation of the supraclavicular nerves requires dissection through the posterior triangle fat pad. Care must be exercised here, because these nerves may be confused with the spinal accessory nerve.

Preservation of the great auricular nerve improves quality of life in that the earlobe receives no other sensory input, and permanent hypoesthesia here has esthetic as well as practical detrimental effects. Other branches also may be preserved, thereby reducing hypoesthesia from the superior chest wall to the mandible. The preservation of these branches makes the dissection of the posterior and inferior regions much more tedious. If the surgeon is unfamiliar with techniques of watching both beneath and behind the SCM, this could result in inadvertent injury to cranial nerve XI or incomplete clearance of nodal bearing tissue. In one study, the quality of life was judged to be significantly better in terms of reduced neck and shoulder pain in a group of patients in whom the cervical sensory nerves were preserved.[34]

If a tracheotomy is performed as a part of the procedure, however, care should be taken to avoid the connection of the elevated skin flap with the tracheotomy dissection. If such a connection occurs inadvertently, it should be closed by suturing the subcutaneous tissue of the flap to strap muscles before wound closure to avoid air leakage from the tracheotomy site to the surgical drains. Such an air leak may otherwise contribute to the risk of postoperative wound infection.

Marginal Mandibular Branch of the Facial Nerve

As the superior neck flap is elevated, attention should be turned to preserving the marginal mandibular (MM) branch of the facial nerve. Injury to this nerve causes an obvious cosmetic deformity with asymmetry of the motion of the corner of the mouth (Figure 36-7). It may also contribute to drooling and difficulty with swallowing because of an inability to maintain labial closure during the oral preparatory phase.

In thin patients, the MM may be easily identified, cascading from the parotid fascia over the fibrovascular tissue that connects the submandibular gland to the mandibular body (Figure 36-8). If it is not immediately visible, the nerve may be located by careful dissection. Although the nerve can usually be identified by its anatomic location, it is advisable to withhold muscle relaxants until both the MM and the spinal accessory nerves have been identified. The use of a nerve stimulator should be kept to a minimum with the power at the

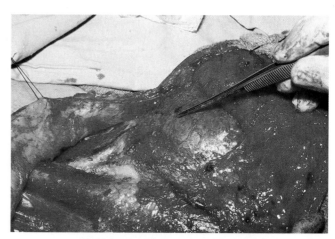

Figure 36-8. Cervical branch in fascia.

lowest (i.e., 0.5 mAmp) setting, because the repeated stimulation of the nerve can result in neurapraxia. The cervical branch of the facial nerve is located more inferiorly on the submandibular gland fascia. It may have arborizations reconnecting with the MM branch. In addition, the cervical branch innervation of the platysma contributes to the downward motion of the lip. The cervical branch may be confused with the MM branch. When both branches have been identified, it may be necessary to sacrifice the cervical branch; this may be done without permanent functional deficit. Note that, since the platysma muscle contributes to the downward movement of the lower lip, any anterolateral incision going through platysma will cause some degree of lip motion impairment.

The approach to the preservation of this nerve varies depending on the presence or suspicion of pathologic lymph nodes along the external facial vein. When such nodes are likely, the nerve should be preserved by identifying it as it passes over the vein and carefully dissecting it free of the surrounding tissue that is to be included in the surgical specimen. If the nerve must be mobilized to preserve it, the technique used in dissection should avoid injury to the nerve by direct contact with instruments or lifting and stretching the nerve as much as possible. The mobilized nerve then can be protected during further dissection by the fixation of perineural tissue to the elevated superior skin flap.

When concern about the presence of pathologic facial lymph nodes is low, the MM branch of the facial nerve can be preserved by incising the fascia of the submandibular gland low on the gland and elevating this fascia with the superior neck flap (Figure 36-9). The external facial vein is also ligated inferiorly as it emerges from the fatty tissue in the submandibular triangle, and the superior stump of the vein is retracted with the skin flap. The MM branch is thus rolled up with the elevated skin and kept away from further surgical dissection. If the MM branch is inadvertently cut during dissection,

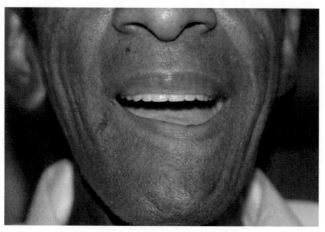

Figure 36-7. Marginal nerve weakness.

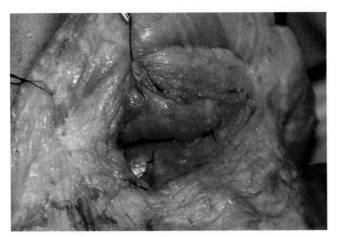

Figure 36-9. Submandibular fascia elevation.

immediate neurorrhaphy should be performed. This can be done with magnification using 8-0 to 10-0 monofilament nylon suture placed in the epineurium.

Lingual Nerve

The lingual branch of the trigeminal nerve (cranial nerve VIII) is located under the deep cervical fascia beneath the submandibular gland. Level I neck dissection incorporating submandibular gland excision puts this nerve at risk for injury. The lingual and hypoglossal nerves should be visualized beneath the gland before sharp dissection in this region. The anterior retraction of the mylohyoid muscle facilitates the needed exposure. The lingual nerve traces a downward loop as it gives off its branch to the submandibular ganglion. The main body of the nerve must be appreciated before the dissection and division of the branch to the ganglion. Control of the nerve branch and its accompanying vessels before dividing this structure prevents the need to cauterize near the main trunk of the nerve. Failure to protect the lingual nerve leads to annoying hypoesthesia or paresthesias of the hemitongue with resultant difficulty with speech and deglutition.

Spinal Accessory Nerve

Pain and weakness of the shoulder are among the most common postoperative complications of neck dissection. Sacrifice of or damage to the spinal accessory nerve (cranial nerve XI) is a major contributing factor to complaints related to the shoulder. Many surgeons routinely modify the standard radical neck dissection by isolating and preserving this nerve in an effort to prevent shoulder dysfunction. Alternatively, the posterior triangle may be left untouched in a selective or regional neck dissection (e.g., supraomohyoid dissection).[35]

The primary concern of the surgeon caring for a cancer patient must be the complete extirpation of malignancy. A growing number of reports in the literature advocate the routine use of selective anterior neck dissection because of the rarity of posterior triangle nodal involvement by metastatic disease.[36–38]

Schuller and colleagues[39] point out that cranial nerve XI is much more likely to be close to pathologic nodes along its course in the upper jugular region (i.e., level II) than in the posterior triangle. Of 50 neck specimens from patients with a variety of primary sites, 21 had nodes along this nerve, and 19 of these (90.5%) had involvement only in the superior portion of the nerve's path. With this in mind, Eisele and colleagues[40] advocate the examination of the anterosuperior portion of cranial nerve XI early during the procedure. They dissect under the anterior edge of the SCM to identify the nerve overlying the jugular vein high in the neck, inspecting for suspicious nodes. If nodal disease is encountered intimately related to the nerve, cranial nerve XI preservation is abandoned, thereby saving further time and effort. In the authors' experience, however, cranial nerve XI can be preserved in many cases, even when it is surrounded by suspicious nodes. Often an escape route between nodes can be identified, sometimes posterior and deep to the nerve, where blunt dissection can free the nerve without directly violating nodal tissue.

No careful prospective randomized study of survival or recurrence exists comparing the results of nerve-sparing and radical neck dissection. Retrospective series that report the outcomes of nerve-sparing procedures as being equal to or better than radical surgery are subject to criticism about bias introduced by the criteria used to select one type of surgery rather than another. These reports at least serve to demonstrate that sparing cranial nerve XI can be accomplished without greatly compromising the oncologic result, even in the face of clinically involved nodes.[41–43]

Whether the preservation of cranial nerve XI substantially improves shoulder function continues to be debated. The degree of trauma to the nerve likely depends on how much of its length is exposed (i.e., proximal, intra, and distal to SCM) and how it is handled. Wide variabilities in outcome from both radical and nerve-sparing surgeries are reported in studies that cite subjective assessment of pain and functionality by patients. Questionnaires used by several investigators failed to demonstrate a statistically significant benefit of nerve-sparing surgery.[44,45] Indeed, in one study, 40% of radical neck dissection patients reported no significant postoperative shoulder pain or dysfunction.[46] Other reports indicate a higher incidence of shoulder complaints among patients who have undergone radical surgery.[47] It is likely the case that, the more carefully one investigates shoulder dysfunction, the more evidence one finds. Muscle strength testing and electromyography consistently show a greater level of function among patients in whom cranial nerve XI has been spared.[44,45,48,49]

The contribution of the cervical plexus to trapezius innervation has been invoked as a factor in the variability of shoulder function after the sacrifice of cranial nerve XI and as a rationale for sparing these fibers during neck dissection (Figure 36-10). Weitz and colleagues[50] claim good shoulder function results among 12 patients in whom the C2 through C4 roots were spared and proximal cranial nerve XI was cut as it entered the SCM. They do not state how shoulder function was assessed, however. Alternatively, when cranial nerve XI is left intact, the sacrifice of the cervical contribution does not seem to have a significant negative impact on shoulder function, according to Soo and colleagues.[51] Their electromyography findings, however, serve as evidence for minor motor input from the cervical plexus to cranial nerve XI, especially going to the lower two thirds of the trapezius. This is in contrast with Weisberger's[52] conclusions from a study of the stimulation of the ventral rami of the cervical spinal nerves in cats and humans. He states that there is rarely any evidence of motor input from the cervical plexus. According to Weisberger, motor potentials recorded in the trapezius instead are caused by the spread of current to contiguous tissues. Still, the temporary but significant shoulder dysfunction noted by Remmler and colleagues[49] may be caused in part by the sacrifice of the cervical roots as well as by the neurapraxia caused by the surgical stretching and irritation of cranial nerve XI. Not surprisingly, patients

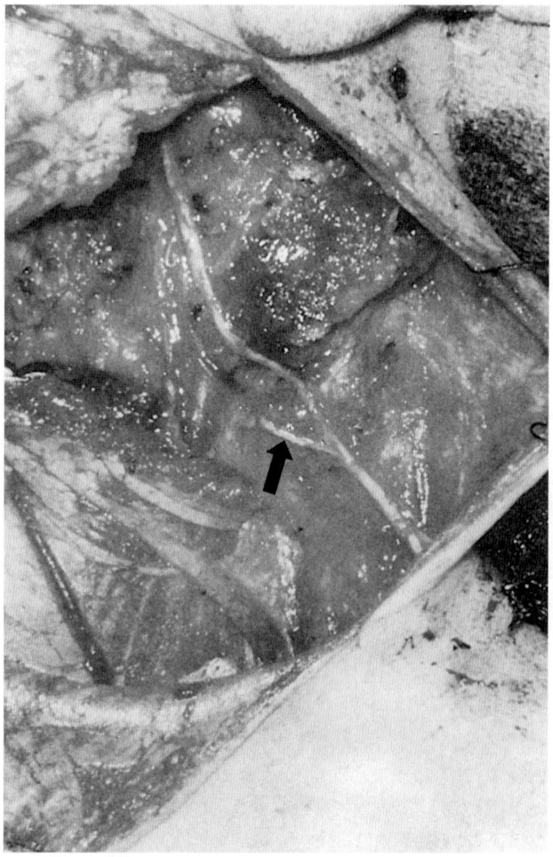

Figure 36-10. Contribution of the cervical plexus to the spinal accessory nerve *(arrow)*. The presence of motor-nerve contributions to the spinal accessory nerve is controversial.

undergoing supraomohyoid dissection have shoulder function that is superior to those who have had a full dissection sparing cranial nerve XI, probably because of the complete lack of surgical manipulation of the posterior triangle in the selective procedure.[45]

If the decision has been made to preserve the spinal accessory nerve, then the surgeon must identify it carefully in each region along its course. In some individuals, the nerve is very superficial in the posterior triangle, and it can be inadvertently injured during flap elevation. The platysma, which is a reliable landmark for depth of flap elevation in the anterior neck, splays out and eventually ends in the posterior triangle. Experienced surgeons note a virtual plane extrapolated from the level of the platysma posteriorly in which no substantial vessels are encountered. Care must be taken to not perforate the skin during this portion of flap elevation. Considerable individual variation exists with regard to the amount of fibrofatty tissue surrounding the nerve, thus adding to the difficulty of finding and preserving it.

The spinal accessory nerve follows a reasonably constant path through the posterior triangle. It extends from a point one fingerbreadth (i.e., 2 cm) above the Erb point (where the cervical plexus branches cross the posterior border of the SCM) and courses inferiorly and posteriorly, disappearing under the trapezius muscle at a point approximately two fingerbreadths above the clavicle. Occasionally there may be difficulty distinguishing cranial nerve XI from the supraclavicular sensory branches of the cervical plexus. Tracing the candidate nerve superiorly under the SCM and toward the jugular vein confirms its identity as the spinal accessory nerve. If necessary, a single low-amperage impulse by a nerve stimulator can be used to confirm the identity of the nerve, but this type of stimulation should be kept to a minimum. As dissection continues superiorly, the surgeon must be aware that the nerve can course through the body of the SCM or merely send branches to that muscle as it passes beneath it. The location of the nerve as it courses away from the muscle adjacent to the internal jugular vein toward the jugular foramen should be confirmed before further dissection in the superior jugular region (Figure 36-11). Once again, gentle handling of the nerve to avoid stretching and repeated stimulation by the instrumentation is important to minimize postsurgical neurapraxia.

When cranial nerve XI is injured or must be sacrificed because of tumor along its course, some authors have reported good success with cable grafting of the nerve from the skull base to the distal stump.[47,53] Objective postoperative assessment of shoulder function after cable grafting has demonstrated a level of function that is intermediate between that seen with sacrifice or preservation of the nerve.[53]

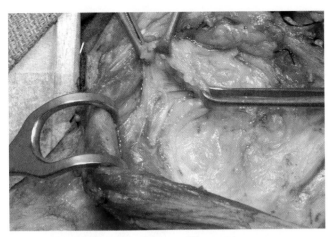

Figure 36-11. Cranial nerve XI's superior course.

Dissection of the Inferior Neck

Vagus Nerve

Whether the surgeon plans to sacrifice or preserve the IJ vein, it is necessary to first identify all of the structures in the carotid sheath. Inadvertent injury to the vagus nerve may occur during the process of ligating the vein. Particularly treacherous is the large IJ vein. One may see cranial nerve X on one side of the IJ vein and then include it in isolated tissue destined for clamping while working from the other side. The surgeon and his or her assistant must make a positive identification of the nerve from both anterior and posterior approaches before setting the clamps or ties. Injury to the vagus nerve at this location will result in ipsilateral laryngeal and pharyngeal paralysis and a loss of sensation in the larynx at the level of the true vocal cord and below. A breathy voice, an inefficient cough, and a subjective sense of dyspnea result. Dysphagia may also occur as a result of inefficient pharyngeal peristalsis together with a tendency for laryngeal penetration during swallowing, especially of thin liquids. The loss of more distal vagal innervation has little clinical effect.

Immediate neurorrhaphy of the transected vagus nerve is generally not considered to be useful. Experimental evidence from canine studies indicates good recovery of the neuronal count and of the diameter of recurrent laryngeal nerves repaired immediately after transection. However, neither abduction nor adduction of the vocal cords was restored in these animals.[54] Still, immediate neurorrhaphy may allow for the preservation of some muscle tone with the prevention of atrophy despite misdirected reinnervation and synkinesis.[55] Techniques such as nerve-muscle pedicle grafting[56] remain controversial and are not recommended for use at the time of intraoperative vagal injury. Consideration may be given to immediate intraoperative vocal-cord augmentation. Micronized AlloDerm (Cymetra) injection provides temporary vocal-cord medialization that lasts for more than 12 months. The need

and desirability of permanent cord medialization can be discussed with the patient later.[57] If the possible need to sacrifice the vagus nerve has been anticipated (e.g., schwannoma or paraganglioma of the vagus nerve in the parapharyngeal space), vocal-cord augmentation may be included in the operative consent. If not, vocal-cord injection can easily be done postoperatively, after the situation has been explained to the patient.

Venous Injury

The IJ vein often has small, thin-walled branches, and rough dissection can result in hemorrhage with significant blood loss and the obfuscation of important structures. Dissection around the vein should be performed with a blunt clamp making spreading motions perpendicular to the wall of the vein to avoid injury to these branches. Alternatively, sharp-knife dissection and feathering over the edge of the vein exposes the branches. Injury to the venous system low in the neck may also occur because of an unusually high position of the subclavian vein. When hemorrhage from the inferior IJ or the subclavian vein cannot be controlled from the cervical exposure, it may be necessary to resect the head of the clavicle to obtain exposure and control of the injured vessel. The necessary bone instruments for this emergency must be available during every neck dissection. If the subclavian vein is cross-clamped and ligated, swelling of the upper extremity will complicate the postoperative course.

Any uncontrolled rent in a vein located above the level of the heart carries a risk for venous air embolism. Air embolism is a potentially fatal (albeit uncommon) occurrence. It must be suspected whenever cardiovascular collapse occurs during neck dissection, especially when it is temporally related to dissection near the internal or external jugular, subclavian, and transverse cervical veins. After air enters the vein, it travels to the heart and mixes with blood to form foam that is compressed during systole and that expands during diastole. This prevents adequate output from the right ventricle. The anesthesiologist will hear a loud churning sound on auscultation that is caused by the heart beating against the air–blood mixture as the pulmonary arterial pressure rises. Right heart failure ensues with increased CVP. Decreased filling pressure for the left heart results in systemic circulatory collapse with diminished cardiac output, cyanosis, arrhythmias, and tachycardia.[58]

When massive venous air embolism is suspected, the patient must immediately be placed in a left lateral decubitus position with the head tilted down (i.e., Trendelenburg). This causes the air bubbles to shift away from the outflow tract of the right ventricle, thereby allowing for the resumption of adequate cardiac output. Cardiac resuscitative measures including closed-heart massage, vasopressors, and 100% oxygen ventilation under positive pressure are continued until circulation is restored.

Nitrous oxide should be discontinued, because it increases the size of air bubbles within the circulatory system. Positive-pressure ventilation is used, because the gradients that cause air-bubble entry into the venous system are increased by the fall in thoracic pressure that occurs with active inspiration. Resuscitation may be successful without the aspiration of air from the right ventricle in most cases.[59] If cardiac collapse persists, however, aspiration of the air may be required. This may be possible via the CVP line if there is one present, and it can be passed into the right ventricle. If not, percutaneous needle aspiration can be performed.[60] Ericsson and colleages[59] reported 68 fatalities (73%) in 93 cases of venous air embolism. Six of these occurred during head and neck operations.[61] In one case report,[62] as little as 100 ml of air was shown to be lethal. Smaller air emboli may proceed to the small pulmonary arterioles and capillaries. Here microthrombi form as a result of platelet activation at the bubble–blood interface. Subsequently inflammatory vasoactive mediators are released, resulting in pulmonary vasoconstriction, increased lung flow resistance, decreased compliance, and areas of ventilation–perfusion mismatch. Air may also pass to the left heart either through a probe-patent foramen ovale in the septum or through the pulmonary microcirculation. Gas bubbles then proceed to the cerebral circulation, where they can cause cerebral ischemia and edema with neurologic sequelae. These neurologic problems may appear postoperatively with a progressive decline in the level of consciousness. If this occurs, hyperbaric oxygen therapy should be administered immediately.[63]

Venous air embolism may be prevented by avoiding operative positioning with the head elevated and by the careful dissection and ligation of veins during neck surgery. The negative pressure within the venous system that predisposes a patient to air embolus increases when the patient is positioned with the head elevated. If vascular control is lost, the vein should be immediately digitally compressed below the site of injury while repair or ligation is accomplished. The surgical and anesthesia team must be alert to the possibility and signs of air embolism and prepared to take the emergency measures previously outlined.

When the IJ vein is ligated, a misdirected longline CVP catheter may be found within the vein's lumen (Figure 36-12). Although the antecubital vein site is an easy, safe route of CVP insertion that is out of the field of neck dissection, proper threading of the catheter into the superior vena cava is difficult from this position. The incidence of placement of the CVP tip into the IJ vein is about 15%.[64] If the misplacement is not detected and corrected when the vein is ligated, it can result in catheter-tip embolism, thrombophlebitis, and septicemia. When positioning or constraints on venous access dictate that the ipsilateral antecubital or femoral vein be used for CVP placement, the

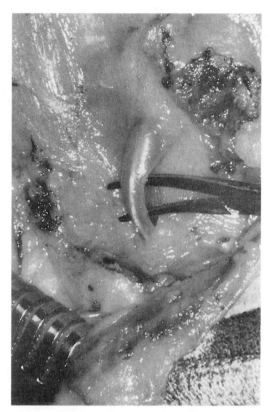

Figure 36-12. A central venous pressure line visible within the internal jugular vein at the time of neck dissection.

surgeon should palpate the IJ vein before cross-clamping. If the catheter is malpositioned, it can be withdrawn and rethreaded by the anesthesiologist. If the catheter is inadvertently divided with the vein, it is important to retrieve the distal tip. Usually this is possible by allowing for the free flow of blood for a few seconds or by grasping the catheter with a clamp to remove or secure it until the distal vein is ligated.

Posterior Triangle Floor

When the posterior triangle is to be dissected, the floor of the triangle must be identified inferiorly. The phrenic nerve and brachial plexus are located beneath the deep cervical fascia. The transverse cervical artery and vein course through the posterior triangle parallel to the clavicle. In a functional neck dissection, these vessels may be isolated and preserved. This allows for their potential use as recipient vessels for vascularized free-tissue transfer or for an inferior trapezius flap at some time in the future. The apex of the pleura may be encountered in the root of the neck. It is located deep to the deep cervical fascia and need not be exposed. If it is violated, pneumothorax may result. An abrupt change in oxygenation and a lack of breath sounds on auscultation should alert the anesthesiologist to this problem. An intraoperative chest radiograph may confirm the need for a chest tube. Repair of the pleural rent is also required.

Lymphatic Ducts

The cervical lymphatic ducts and, on the left side, the thoracic duct are located inferomedially in the neck. As with many complications, the best way to manage a lymphatic leak is to prevent it from occurring. The intraoperative identification of all lymphatic ducts followed by gentle and effective ligation with nonabsorbable suture is the best way to prevent a leak. The thoracic duct usually emerges in the left neck, bringing chyle from the abdomen and the thorax. It arches deep to the great vessels but superficial to the thyrocervical trunk, the vertebral artery, the phrenic nerve, and the anterior scalene muscle, looping from medial to lateral and then back to the IJ vein.[65] Before entering the venous system, it is joined by the left cervical lymphatic vessels. The right neck also has a lymphatic duct that drains the right head, neck, lung, and upper extremity and the convex surface of the liver. The cervical lymphatic ducts are formed by the confluence of jugular, subclavian, and bronchomediastinal trunks. The ducts enter the great veins of the neck near the junction of the IJ and the subclavian veins. The pattern and location of entry is widely variable and possibly multiple, although entry into the distal IJ vein is the usual course[66] (Figure 36-13). Because of the multiple branches, the ligation of one structure does not guarantee the control of all potential sites of leakage. It is classically taught that the thoracic duct is a right-sided structure in fewer than 5% of individuals.[67] In Crumley and Smith's[65] series, 25% of lymphatic drainage occurred in the right neck. Profuse lymphatic fluid often collects after neck dissection in cases with bulky and diffuse metastatic disease. Thus a vigilant search for lymphatic structures is warranted when dissecting either side.

One effective approach to the floor of the posterior triangle is to score the superficial cervical fascia with a knife or scissors just superior to the clavicle in a horizontal fashion beginning several centimeters lateral to the carotid sheath after the contents of the sheath have been identified. Firm blunt dissection sweeping the fibrofatty tissue superiorly and using bipolar cautery or clamps to control small vessels found in this region allows for the precise identification of the important structures in the floor of the posterior triangle. The thoracic duct is sometimes located immediately, but at times the lymphatic structures are very small or inapparent. As the surgeon moves medially from the phrenic nerve and laterally from the vagus, all lymphatic vascular structures should be doubly clamped and ligated. Every effort should be made to avoid tearing these thin-walled structures. In the left neck, the entrance of the cervical lymphatics into the thoracic duct from above and the site of emergence of the duct from behind the carotid artery several centimeters above the clavicle are often forgotten sites of potential lymphatic leakage.

Chyle leakage is usually easily recognized intraoperatively by the pooling of characteristically milky fluid in the inferomedial corner of the neck. Flow can be increased by having the anesthesiologist hyperinflate the lungs to identify the site of ductal injury. Efforts to identify and ligate the lymphatics must be made cautiously, avoiding inadvertent injury to the vagus nerve or the phrenic nerve. When a single point of leakage cannot be identified, figure-of-8 ligatures in the region of greatest lymphatic collection may be effective. For situations in which there is a persistent but very slow rate of chyle flow despite exhaustive efforts to ligate the duct, a local pedicle of fibromuscular tissue may be rotated over the site and mattressed to surrounding tissue. A layer of fibrin glue may be useful as a sealant over the repair.[68,69] The area should be inspected again just before the wound is closed. As the patient emerges from deep levels of anesthesia, the intrathoracic pressure increases, and chyle may appear. In Crumley and Smith's[65] series, 75% of postoperative chylous leaks had first been noted during surgery. Under no circumstances should the neck be closed while chylous drainage persists.

Brachial Plexus

Lateral to the phrenic nerve beneath the fascial floor of the posterior triangle is the brachial plexus, which is wedged between the scalenus muscles. This structure, like the phrenic nerve, is deep to the deep cervical fascia, and it should be easily preserved when gentle blunt dissection of the fat overlying the fascia is performed. Occasionally the upper trunk of the brachial plexus or

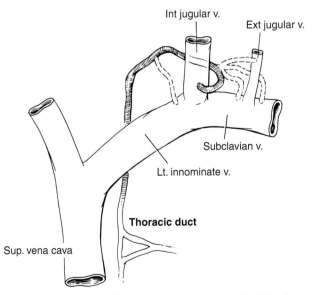

Figure 36-13. Anatomy of the thoracic duct. In most individuals, the duct enters the internal jugular vein (*solid lines*), but a number of possible anatomic variations exist (*dashed lines*).

the anterior division of the cervical nerves (i.e., C5 and C6) that form it may lie within a sheath of fat and could be mistakenly included in the dissection in an effort to thoroughly clean the posterior triangle.[70] In addition, the presence of supraclavicular sensory nerves that may be safely sacrificed can make dissection in this area somewhat confusing. Injury to the upper trunk affects the function of the supraspinatus, the infraspinatus, the biceps muscles, and the triceps muscles as a result of the complex pattern of nerve branching and anastomosis in the trunks and cords of the brachial plexus. Any fat that does not come away from the floor of the posterior triangle with gentle blunt dissection must be cautiously examined to be certain that there is no nerve running within. If a nerve is present, the surgeon must decide whether to dissect it free of the surrounding fat or to leave the fat at the floor of the dissection; this will depend on the presence of bulky level V nodal disease.

Cervical Plexus Contributions to the Phrenic Nerve

As elevation of the contents of the posterior triangle proceeds from the trapezius toward the carotid sheath, the cervical plexus contributions to the phrenic nerve or to a loop of the phrenic nerve itself may be injured. Although not life-threatening, phrenic injury results in the paralysis of the ipsilateral diaphragm, and it may contribute to postoperative pulmonary complications. The ability to compensate for aspiration, atelectasis, pneumothorax, chylothorax, or other pulmonary insult may be seriously compromised by the loss of innervation to the diaphragm, thus prolonging the need for ventilatory support. Fluoroscopic examination postoperatively confirms the diagnosis of phrenic injury with the paralysis of the injured diaphragm (Figure 36-14). The phrenic

nerve is formed by the anterior division branches of C3 through C5. These cervical nerves also contribute to the sensory nerves that proceed from behind the SCM at the Erb point. Because the sensory branches are encountered running up in the reflected specimen, care must be taken to cut them high on the specimen and to sweep the proximal stump downward to the muscle floor. This avoids injury to the phrenic contributions, which may tent upward with traction on the surgical specimen.

Jugular Vein Dissection

It is important to clear the upper jugular nodes thoroughly, because they are common sites for tumor recurrence (Figure 36-15). Cranial nerve XI, if it is being preserved, must be cleared of surrounding fibrofatty tissue and kept in view during this procedure. Exposure of the digastric muscle and the upward elevation of it allows for the thorough removal of underlying lymphatic tissue. If the IJ vein is to be ligated, it should first be thoroughly exposed, with the position of the vagus and hypoglossal nerves being noted. A loss of control of the upper jugular stump is managed by packing the skull base with microfibrillar collagen hemostat (i.e., Avitene), oxidized regenerated cellulose (i.e., Surgicel), or fat. A flap of levator scapulae or splenius cervicis muscle can be rotated into the site, if necessary. In functional neck surgery, the ansa cervicalis and hypoglossi may be preserved as dissection proceeds over the IJ vein, taking the superficial carotid fascia. Maintenance of the functional integrity of the innervation to the strap muscles assists with deglutition. The loss of this muscle function may contribute to multifactorial postoperative dysphagia. The IJ vein has several large tributaries that enter it anterosuperiorly. If it is to be spared, care must be taken to ligate these branches well away from the wall

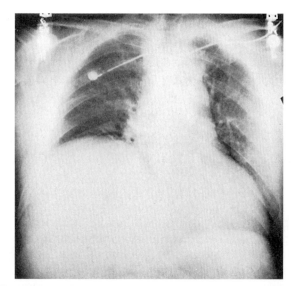

Figure 36-14. Elevation of the right hemidiaphragm as a result of phrenic nerve injury in the neck.

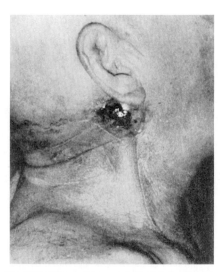

Figure 36-15. Recurrence of tumor at the mastoid tip 6 months after radical neck dissection.

of the preserved vein. Narrowing of the vein probably contributes to the postoperative thrombosis and occlusion that are reported to occur in 15% of preserved jugular veins.[71] Facial edema, increased intracranial pressure (ICP), and the sequelae of radical neck surgery follow.

Sympathetic Trunk

As the dissection of the carotid sheath is completed, a transition must be made between the deep cervical (i.e., prevertebral) fascia and the fascia of the carotid sheath. Failure to recognize and accomplish this may result in injury to the cervical sympathetic chain that lies deep to the carotid artery. There is rarely any reason to enter this area during tumor removal, but, when tumor is adherent to the deep cervical musculature posterior to the artery, the surgeon may stray as a cuff of muscle is taken in an effort to remove all of the tumor. The fusiform superior cervical ganglion located from the level of the atlas to C2 and C3 must not be mistaken for a retropharyngeal lymph node. Unlike these nodes, the ganglion should be deep to the deep cervical fascia.

The neurologic deficit caused by injury to the cervical sympathetic nerves depends on the site of injury. A full Horner syndrome consists of the following ipsilateral conditions (Figure 36-16):

1. Miosis (pupillary constriction as a result of unopposed constrictor input from cranial nerve III when sympathetic input to the dilator pupillae muscle is lost)

2. Ptosis (as a result of the paralysis of the smooth muscle of Horner)

3. Transient blush (the loss of vasoconstrictor tone that returns in a matter of days)

4. Anhidrosis (the loss of the sympathetic innervation of the sweat glands)

5. Nasal congestion

No Horner syndrome will result from an injury below the stellate ganglion located behind the vertebral artery in the root of the neck. If preganglionic fibers at the C8 through T1 level are injured, pupillociliary signs without anhidrosis are seen. Injury to the intracranial ICA or the cavernous sinus may also produce a partial Horner syndrome without anhidrosis, because sweat fibers leave the oculopupillary fibers after synapsing in the superior cervical ganglion. Anhidrosis alone may result from a lesion below the first thoracic ganglion.[72]

Carotid Artery Injury and Resection

Tumor invasion of the carotid artery is a relatively uncommon event of advanced aggressive disease or revision surgery for a recurrent neck mass. Even large neck masses with decreased mobility can often be carefully dissected free of the vessel. However, this may thin the vessel wall and raise the chances for carotid rupture, particularly in the setting of prior neck irradiation. Thus, when tumor does not approach the carotid sheath, the adventitia should not be violated. When tumor cannot be cleared from the carotid, the surgeon must make a difficult choice. The procedure can be aborted, leaving bulk disease in the neck. Alternatively, the tumor can be shaved from the carotid, or the vessel can be resected. If the carotid is resected, a decision about bypass grafting must also be made. Ideally the potential for tumor invading the carotid will have been foreseen preoperatively and a contingency plan made ready. It is unlikely that carotid involvement will be found intraoperatively when physical and radiographic warnings are absent. More likely is that the finding of carotid invasion, which

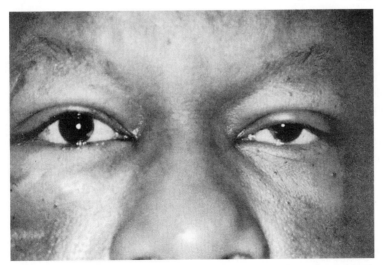

Figure 36-16. Left-sided Horner syndrome as a result of the injury of the cervical sympathetic trunk, resulting in ptosis, miosis, and anhidrosis.

was present in 5.5% of neck dissections in one series, will merely confirm preoperative suspicions.[14]

Moore and Baker[15] reported an 11.4% mortality rate and a 31.4% incidence of cerebral complication in the latter half of their series of carotid ligation in patients who had no preoperative assessment of collateral flow. This indicates that proceeding with carotid resection when vessel invasion has not been suspected and worked up carries a risk that is inordinately high. This is particularly true given the small potential benefit to patients with that extent of disease who have poor long-term prognoses. If faced with unanticipated carotid artery invasion, the intraoperative estimation of a patient's ability to withstand ligation is possible by measuring carotid stump pressure.[73] After the vessel is exposed, a 22-gauge needle attached to a pressure transducer is inserted into the artery distal to an occluding clamp. Stump pressures of 50 mm Hg to 70 mm Hg are reported to be indicative of adequate collateral flow, thus allowing for ligation without reconstruction. However, intraoperative stump pressures may be unreliable. A more conservative recommendation by Hibbert[74] is to resect without reconstruction when stump pressures exceed 70 mm Hg, to resect with reconstruction for pressures from 55 mm Hg to 70 mm Hg, and to not only replace the vessel but to use a temporary shunt intraoperatively for pressures below 55 mm Hg.

The use of systematic anticoagulants (i.e., heparin 5000 U subcutaneously) among patients who undergo carotid ligation may be beneficial. The rationale for this practice is the prevention of delayed neurologic sequelae as a result of thrombosis in the vessel stump with subsequent clot embolism. For the same reason, it is usually recommended that the internal carotid be tied off as close to the skull base as possible. Doing so prevents the formation of a pouch where a clot can propagate. Autopsies of patients in the series reported by Moore and Baker[15] do not support an important role of thromboembolic events in the fatalities of patients after carotid ligation. Instead, abnormalities in the brain were usually the result of low perfusion and subsequent infarction.

A major contributing factor to mortality associated with carotid ligation is transient hypotension. Moore and Baker[15] attribute the improved results in the later part of their series to the anticipation of the transient hypotensive episode that follows vessel cross-clamping and the aggressive maintenance of blood pressure during that time.

Care must be taken to ensure the secure ligation of the vessel. The walls of an atherosclerotic carotid artery may tear easily. The site of ligation must be distant from tissue weakened by tumor, dissection, infection, or radiation.

Reconstruction of a resected carotid artery can be achieved with an autogenous vein (saphenous) or a Gore-Tex or Dacron graft. Alloplastic graft material is not recommended by some as a result of the contaminated, irradiated nature of many of these cases.[66] Alternatively, scarring and fibrosis may occlude vein grafts, which has led others to advocate the use of prosthetic grafts.[75]

An alternative to carotid resection is to debulk the tumor, peeling it from the vessel and separating the adventitia from the tunica media. External-beam therapy or radioactive ^{125}iodine implants (i.e., brachytherapy) can be used in an effort to control residual cancer. This approach was reported by Fee and colleagues[13] to have good early results.

The risk of the delayed rupture of the carotid may be reduced by ensuring good coverage of the weakened vessel. If the skin has been resected over the carotid, a myocutaneous flap is recommended. The muscle pedicle can be sutured to tissue around the carotid to ensure that muscle will adhere to the vessel wall. The use of dermal grafts and rotated muscle pedicle flaps (e.g., levator scapulae) has been advocated for high-risk cases.[76] However, the value of these tissues to cover the carotid has been questioned. The use of dermal grafts is associated with a 7% incidence of minor complications. At the same time, they have not been shown to reduce the rate of carotid catastrophe. They are no substitute for tight mucosal closure and coverage achieved with healthy tissue, particularly a healthy myocutaneous flap.

Even when tumor is not adherent to the vessel wall, dissection around the carotid can be hazardous. Atherosclerotic plaque may be dislodged and cause embolic damage if a diseased carotid is handled roughly. Bradyarrhythmia and hypotension are commonly seen during the manipulation of the carotid. Undue pressure on the carotid sinus may result in ventricular fibrillation, particularly when a patient is digitalized. The instillation of 1% xylocaine without epinephrine into the subadventitial tissue with a 25- or 27-gauge needle blunts the carotid sinus reflex temporarily as dissection continues. Intravenous atropine is also effective. If bradycardia occurs, the surgical team should stop the manipulation of the vessel until preventive measures take effect.

Anterior Dissection

The hypoglossal (cranial nerve XII) and superior laryngeal nerves lie on the floor of the anterior dissection and should be preserved whenever possible. The hypoglossal is more superficial, but it lies beneath a layer of fascia, usually accompanied by complex venae comitantes. Injury to these veins should be avoided. The

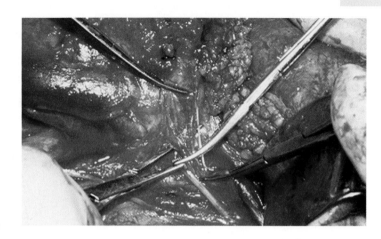

Figure 36-17. Cranial nerve XII dissection.

area just anterior and superior to the carotid bifurcation is a common site of soft-tissue invasion by metastatic tumor with extracapsular spread. The external carotid artery can be sacrificed without significant sequelae, but cranial nerve XII should be preserved when possible or repaired with cable graft, if necessary (Figure 36-17). The internal branch of the superior laryngeal nerve passes under the carotid, coursing over the pharyngeal constrictor muscle to enter the thyrohyoid membrane and provide sensory innervation to the supraglottic larynx. Injury to the superior laryngeal nerve contributes to the risk of postoperative aspiration. Unless it is involved with tumor, the fascia encasing the visceral neck structures should not be violated, with the superior laryngeal nerve kept out of harm's way. The ansa hypoglossi descends from cranial nerve XII as it turns superiorly, running just anterior to the IJ and the common carotid artery immediately superficial to the superior thyroid artery and the superior laryngeal nerve. Dissection beneath the plane of the ansa is rarely needed.

Concomitant Bilateral Neck Dissections

Bilateral neck dissections may be indicated when clinical disease is present bilaterally or when a large midline primary tumor (i.e., the base of the tongue, the supraglottis, the floor of the mouth) is present with an associated high incidence of bilateral occult metastases. Bilateral radical neck dissection has been considered ill advised because of an increase in postoperative complications related to the interruption of venous return, including facial edema, blindness, increased ICP, and even death.[77] A number of alternatives to simultaneous bilateral radical neck dissection exist, including the use of postoperative radiotherapy for stage N0 or N1 necks, staged surgery delaying the ligation of the IJ vein on the less-involved side by 6 to 8 weeks, and simultaneous surgery that spares the IJ vein on at least one side. If the last option is chosen, the possibility of postoperative thrombosis and the occlusion of the preserved IJ vein must be considered.[71] With

careful intraoperative fluid management and postoperative vigilance for signs of increased ICP, bilateral radical neck dissection is well tolerated in selected cases. General physical disability, prior radiation, and the need for extensive surgery to extricate the primary tumor are concurrent risk factors that must be weighed against the decision to perform bilateral radical neck dissections.

POSTOPERATIVE MANAGEMENT: IMMEDIATE AND DELAYED POSTOPERATIVE COMPLICATIONS

A trend in neck dissection over the past decade has been a tendency to release patients after a short stay or even to do the procedure as an outpatient surgery. Patients with stable home environments can be taught to maintain suction drain catheters and bulbs and to measure and record output. The drain can be removed when the output falls to a target volume during a certain time interval (i.e., 25 cc in 24 hours). The author and colleagues recently reported the clinical course of 23 patients at their institution who were discharged after an overnight hospital stay after neck dissection. There were no unusual complications or problems encountered with this practice. Two patients developed seromas at a later time after drain removal, but this was not felt to be related to early discharge.[78]

IMMEDIATE COMPLICATIONS

Air Leakage

Suction drains are placed beneath the flaps at the time of closure to evacuate any persistent drainage that distends the flaps and that serves as a medium for wound infection. Skin closure must be airtight for the drains to function properly. As previously discussed, a tracheotomy site is one potential source of air leak, so it must be kept separate or sealed off from the rest of the wound. The patient should not be awakened until drains are functioning well with no evidence of air leakage. Leakage noted in the recovery room may sometimes be corrected with one or two additional stitches placed at the bedside or with the placement of ointment or tissue glue. Failing this, the patient may be returned to the operating room to revise the closure. If the surgery involved oral or pharyngeal entry, the problem is compounded. Air leak may be the result of incomplete mucosal closure. Revision is required to prevent the development of an orocutaneous fistula. Such a fistula is exacerbated by active suction from the drains pulling air and saliva through the dehiscence.

Hemorrhage

As the patient emerges from anesthesia, maintaining firm pressure over the dissected neck may help reduce the likelihood of hemorrhage, because the elevated venous pressure that occurs during coughing or struggling may open a sealed vessel. Suction drains are capable of evacuating small amounts of persistent bleeding and of preventing hematoma and related flap necrosis, wound infection, or airway compromise. When the drain system malfunctions or is overwhelmed by a high rate of bleeding, the neck flaps become distended and eventually ecchymotic. At times, the manipulation of the drains may correct the problem if it is relatively minor and detected early. Large amounts of bleeding necessitate wound reexploration, clot evacuation, irrigation, the identification and ligation of uncontrolled vessels, and the placement of new drains. Small arteries (e.g., facial, thyroid, thyrocervical trunk, transverse cervical) or veins are often the cause of bleeding that is sufficient to require surgical control. The undersurface of the SCM, if it is spared, should be inspected, and the provision of the Valsalva maneuver should be requested of the anesthesiologist. However, the identification of a specific bleeding vessel is not always successfully accomplished at reexploration. Still, reexploration may shorten the hospital stay and improve the course recovery simply through the removal of clot and the replacement of functioning drains.[79]

Pulmonary Complications

A chest radiograph is obtained in the recovery room during the immediate postoperative period. Problems with focal atelectasis and fluid overload are common after lengthy surgical procedures. Diuretics and aggressive pulmonary physiotherapy should be initiated as indicated. Pneumothorax is an unusual complication of head and neck surgery, but it may result from CVP line placement or the dissection in the root of the neck. Small pneumothoraces (i.e., <20%) with no evidence of respiratory insufficiency may be managed expectantly with repeated chest radiographs to confirm resolution. More extreme collapse requires the placement of a chest tube.

DELAYED COMPLICATIONS

Problems Associated With Interrupted Venous and Lymphatic Return

Facial edema is common after neck dissection. Although this is most marked with bilateral surgery (Figure 36-18), it may occur with unilateral and even with vein-sparing procedures. High volumes of fluid replacement intraoperatively can exacerbate the problem. The fibrosis of collateral lymphatics results in a greater degree of postoperative edema after surgery in a previously irradiated neck. Massive edema with further venous congestion may contribute to flap necrosis. Chemosis may also accompany severe facial edema.

Of greater concern is increased ICP with various accompanying problems. CVP increases after IJ vein ligation, thus impairing the rate of cerebrospinal fluid absorption. Headache and nausea may herald impaired neurologic function with visual changes and eventual coma. SIADH is a rare sequela of radical neck dissection, but it is more common in the setting of bilateral surgery or prior radiation therapy. In the small series of cases of SIADH after unilateral neck dissection presented by Wenig and Heller,[80] two thirds (4 of 6) of the patients had had radiation during the past, and one had had the contralateral neck operated on previously. SIADH is manifested by a low serum sodium level and a urine osmolality that is more than the serum osmolality.

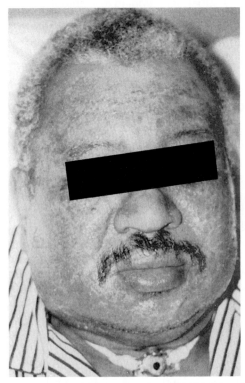

Figure 36-18. Patient with severe facial edema after left radical and right modified neck dissection.

Renal function is normal. Hyponatremia may result in further neurologic sequelae, including weakness, lethargy, mental confusion, convulsion, and coma.

Wenig and Heller[80] stress stringent intraoperative fluid management for high-risk patients to prevent postoperative SIADH. SIADH is managed by restricting the amount of free water that is administered to less than I L per day until serum sodium levels return to normal. More severe cases may require infusions of intravenous saline and the use of furosemide.

Blindness has been reported after bilateral neck dissection. In one case, Balm and colleagues[81] noted bilateral papilledema, distention of the superior orbital veins, and elevated cerebrospinal fluid pressure, thus linking the blindness with elevated ICP. Although most discussions of severe complications caused by increased ICP focus on bilateral neck surgery, such problems can follow unilateral neck dissection, particularly among patients with anomalous intracranial venous drainage.[82]

Head and neck patients are usually positioned with the head of the bed elevated during the immediate postoperative period. If renal function and nutritional status are good, there should be prompt mobilization and the cessation of fluids given intraoperatively. When headache, visual disturbance, or other evidence of increased ICP is noted, diuretics, carbonic anhydrase inhibitors (i.e., acetazolamide), and steroids may be helpful. Continuous lumbar drainage or serial lumbar puncture has been advocated, as has optic nerve decompression in the event of the loss of vision.[81,82]

Excessive Drainage and Chylous Fistula

Within 2 to 3 days postoperatively, the fluid evacuated from a neck dissection wound should become serous, and the volume should decline dramatically. When drainage volume instead begins to increase, the source of the problem must be determined. Chyle may be clear during the postoperative period, when the patient has not yet been fed, and it may be indistinguishable from lymphatic fluid or saliva. When the tail of the parotid gland has been amputated during dissection, a large volume of saliva may collect in the drains. The measurement of the triglycerides and amylase in the fluid will identify its source. If the fluid is saliva (i.e., with a high amylase level and a low triglyceride content), drains may be taken off of wall suction but maintained as a closed system as long as necessary until drainage eventually stops.

Chyle in the suction drains presents a more difficult problem. When the patient begins to eat, the volume increases, and the characteristic milky appearance makes the diagnosis unmistakable (Figure 36-19). A chyle leak may cause physiologic problems in addition

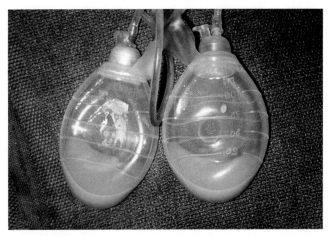

Figure 36-19. Chyle in suction drain bulbs from a patient with postoperative chyle leak.

to problems with wound healing and infection. Chyle is made up of lymph and emulsified fat absorbed in the intestine. It has a high protein content (2%–4%) with electrolytes that are similar to those found in plasma. Seventy percent of ingested fat passes through the thoracic duct, giving chyle a fat content of 1% to 3%.[65] Because chyle flow rates may exceed 2 L per day and because volumes exceeding 500 ml per day are common, severe imbalances of electrolytes, protein, fat, and fat-soluble vitamins and the loss of circulating lymphocytes may occur. The electrolyte and nutritional problems are proportional to the rate of leakage.

The incidence of chylous fistula after radical neck dissection has been reported to be 1% to 2%.[65,83] Prior radiation therapy may be a contributing factor to the development of a postoperative leak. The leak is suspected because of increased wound drainage on the second or third postoperative day in the majority of cases. However, chyle leak can occur later. A case of delayed lymphocele appearing 3 weeks postoperatively has been reported.[84]

The initial management strategy of chyle leak is usually conservative. Nutritional support is modified to minimize the volume of chyle produced, and mechanical means are employed to halt the extravasation. The patient is kept on bed rest with the head elevated. Drains are taken off suction but left in place to allow for the passive egress of fluid, and a pressure dressing is applied. Adequate fluid and electrolyte replacement are directed by strict records of intake and output. The replacement of losses from chyle leakage must be added to maintenance fluids. Parenteral nutrition or enteral feeding with medium-chain triglycerides is begun. Long-chain triglycerides found in fatty meals are broken down into fatty acids that are incorporated into chyle, thus increasing the flow in the thoracic duct. Medium-chain triglycerides are absorbed directly into the portal system, bypassing the thoracic duct.[83] When drainage falls to less than 20 ml per day, drains are removed. The subsequent reaccumulation of a small amount of chyle can be managed by repeated aspiration.

Conservative management can be safely maintained for prolonged periods of time. The expense of prolonged hospitalization and specialized nutritional support, the increased risk of further complications such as wound infection or flap loss, and the need to begin radiation therapy in a timely fashion make it desirable to move on to the surgical management of the leak when conservative therapy is unlikely to succeed. In the series by Spiro and colleagues,[83] conservative management succeeded in 4 of 16 cases, all of which involved a leakage rate of less than 600 ml per day. Six other patients were treated by opening the wound and packing. In these cases, the leak resolved after 11 to 28 days. Crumley and Smith[65] recommended surgical intervention when leakage exceeds 500 ml per day for 4 or 5 consecutive days. Patients with a very high flow rate (i.e., several liters per day) should undergo surgical exploration as soon as possible.

Patients undergoing reexploration are given 4 oz to 6 oz of cream 3 to 24 hours before surgery. Local anesthesia is sufficient in most cases. Patients are placed in the Trendelenburg position, and the wound is opened and filled with saline. Creamy chyle rising from the site of the leak is easily identified in the saline pool, especially when the patient performs a Valsalva maneuver. If necessary, an operating microscope is used to identify the leak. The defect is suture ligated with nonabsorbable material. Fibrin glue,[68,69] Gelfoam, or Surgicel is applied, and the wound is closed over a Penrose drain. Pressure dressings are applied for several days. The success of reexploration is generally excellent.[65,83] Resultant soft-tissue defects may later be filled with an axial muscle or a myocutaneous flap.

Two patients in the series of Spiro and colleagues[83] had chyle leaks that presented with a pleural effusion without significant drainage via neck drains. Chylothorax is a rare event after neck dissection. The site of injury to the thoracic duct in these cases is unclear. The duct has a complex system of branches within the posterior mediastinum.[85] It is theorized that back pressure after the ligation of the main duct may cause the nontraumatic extravasation of chyle in the chest.[86] The amount of chyle leakage may be much greater (i.e., 4500 ml/day in one case) in patients with chylothorax as compared with those with cervical chyle leak. Massive pleural effusion may cause cardiorespiratory compromise as a result of mechanical compression on the lung and the great vessels. Treatment initially may be by repeated thoracentesis or closed thoracostomy drainage. Effusion resolved in one of the cases of Spiro and colleagues[83] when the neck wound was opened and packed;

the other patient required thoracotomy with ligation of the thoracic duct and subtotal pleurectomy.

Wound Infection and Flap Loss

As previously discussed, the incidence of wound infection after surgery of the neck without entry into the aerodigestive tract should be very low. Prophylactic antibiotics may be continued during the first 24 to 72 postoperative hours. Constant suction should be maintained on the drains and sterile technique used when disconnecting and emptying the bulb. Erythema and induration appear before wound dehiscence and the release of purulent drainage. If these early signs are present when the output has abated, thus allowing for drain removal, the tips of the drain from under the flap may be sent for bacterial culture when removed.

Wound infection is a contributing factor to dehiscence and flap skin loss. Others include poor nutrition, prior radiation therapy with damage to small dermal blood vessels, poor incision and flap design producing inferiorly based skin flaps with acutely angled tips, and continued smoking during the perioperative period. Flap elevation superficial to the platysma adds to the problem of skin loss. Leakage from a mucosal closure suture line markedly increases the risk of skin wound breakdown and fistula.

Skin flap loss may be treated conservatively with wet-to-dry sterile dressings changed two to three times daily if the great vessels are not exposed in the wound. Granulation tissue will form given time and nutritional support. Hyperbaric oxygen therapy may speed wound healing, especially among patients who have been heavily irradiated.[87] When a good bed of granulation tissue has formed, the defect can be repaired easily using a split-thickness skin graft or a myocutaneous flap. Topical negative-pressure devices (e.g., vacuum-assisted wound closure [wound VAC]) may be useful, particularly in complicated wounds with pharyngeal fistulas. The hypothetical benefit of wound VAC is the removal of infected secretions and edema with the improvement of microcirculation and the direct stimulation of reparative cellular proliferation to encourage granulation formation.[88–90]

Rupture of the Great Vessels

When wound dehiscence results in the exposure of the carotid artery, it is more ominous, and its management more critical (Figure 36-20). The rupture of the carotid artery is perhaps the most feared complication of head and neck surgery, and its incidence is as high as 3% to 4% in some series.[76,91–93] In 1965, Ketcham and Hoye's[92] series showed that the timing of rupture varied from 6 to 81 postoperative days, with a mean of 16 days. With

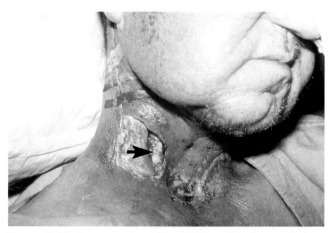

Figure 36-20. Exposure of carotid artery wound dehiscence and flap necrosis.

modern perioperative care, the incidence may now be somewhat lower. Alternatively, postoperative rupture of the internal jugular vein may be more common in this era of structure-sparing surgery. The thin wall of the IJ renders it more susceptible to the erosive action of infection, salivary digestion, and drying.

Risk factors that contribute to great-vessel rupture are similar to those for wound breakdown. Massive tumor with persistence at or near the carotid artery and the violation of the adventitia while peeling disease off of the carotid artery are additional factors. Wound breakdown preceded rupture in 15 of 17 patients reported by Maran and colleagues,[91] whereas 7 had recurrent tumor demonstrated at the time of surgery. The surgery preceding most cases of carotid artery rupture involved the en bloc resection of primary tumor with nodal dissection, but, in some of the cases reviewed by Shumrick,[76] neck dissection alone had been performed. When wound infection and dehiscence occur after neck dissection, the possibility of carotid complications must be anticipated. "Carotid precautions" are initiated, including the maintenance of a blood sample in the blood bank at all times, the communication of concern to all personnel involved in the patient's care, and meticulous wound care. Any loculated purulent material in the wound is drained completely, thereby avoiding the excessive disruption of suture lines. The gentle packing of the wound with moist gauze is replaced frequently to keep tissues clean and moist. The adventitia of the carotid is very susceptible to drying. Because the adventitia brings the blood supply to the rest of the carotid wall, keeping it moist and healthy is critical to preventing blowout. A moderately firm cover dressing with several large bolster sutures, if needed, helps to promote flap adherence to the floor of the dehiscent cavity and halts flap retraction with further vessel exposure. Antibiotics and hyperbaric oxygen therapy may be given to help minimize infection and to promote the formation of granulation tissue. If the

wound is clean, Shumrick[76] advocates immediate coverage of the exposed artery with a vascularized flap. The following doctrine is pertinent: "Don't let the sun set on an exposed carotid artery." However, infected or necrotic wounds may not be successfully covered in this manner. Flaps rotated into an infected bed have less chance of survival. The vessel must be kept clean and moist while preparing the wound for reliable coverage with vascularized tissue. Saliva from a fistula, if present, must be diverted away from the vessel with wound VAC or via a separate direct tract created iatrogenically, if necessary.

Daily inspection of the exposed vessel provides a warning of impending rupture. Morbidity and mortality rates are much lower with planned carotid ligation than when surgery is performed in response to acute hemorrhage. Decay of the carotid wall requires 6 to 10 days to occur, during which a brown eschar forms on deeper and deeper portions of the wall and is debrided with successive dressing changes. During this time, intensive nutritional support, aggressive wound care, and hyperbaric oxygen therapy may render the wound ready for flap coverage. As the media is sloughed, however, the vessel may become aneurysmal. A "sentinel bleed" may herald catastrophic rupture by several days.

As soon as this sequence of events is recognized as being inevitable, plans to manage the vessel either through ligation or endovascular embolization should be undertaken. The patient and family are counseled regarding the serious nature of the step to be taken. The greater risk of complications in the event of spontaneous rupture is made clear during the discussion. Of course, in the presence of recurrent or persistent unresectable disease, the decision to withhold surgical intervention in favor of supportive care alone is a valid alternative.

Selective endovascular embolization performed under sedation or general anesthesia in an interventional radiology suite has been increasingly popular as a less-invasive means of preventing carotid rupture or managing lesser head and neck bleeding. Balloons, platinum coils, and microparticles are available for use in appropriate circumstances. In several series, angiographic vascular control has been shown to have intermediate-term benefit with occasional resultant transient or permanent neurologic deficits.[94,95]

The most important factor to be considered intraoperatively during surgical carotid ligation is the maintenance of adequate blood pressure to ensure cerebral blood flow. Moore and Baker[15] report an 87% incidence of death and a 63% incidence of stroke when hypotension occurred after vessel cross-clamping as compared with 28% and 16%, respectively, when pressure was maintained.

Carotid rupture on the hospital ward is a dramatic and anxiety-inducing event for all concerned. The first care provider on the scene must apply direct digital pressure to stop the hemorrhage. This must be held constant while others ensure a safe airway, place several large intravenous lines, and establish fluid support to maintain blood pressure. Albumin or O-negative whole blood can be given immediately while awaiting cross-matched blood from the blood bank. No effort to find and clamp the vessel should be made on the ward. Two of three deaths in Ketcham and Hoye's[92] series occurred as a result of this ill-advised activity. Instead, the stabilized patient is transported to the operating room with digital pressure maintained on the artery. At this point, another care provider in surgical uniform and sterile gloves assumes the responsibility for control of the vessel; his or her hand is prepared in the field. Flaps are opened, and incisions are extended as needed to expose the vessel wall above and below the site of bleeding. The healthy vessel is clamped and ligated with size 0 silk ties and suture ligature. It may be necessary to resect the clavicular head to achieve proximal vessel control. Every effort should be made to ligate beyond any residual tumor. Because this was not done, a second blowout below the initial ligature occurred in 3 patients in Ketcham and Hoye's series.[92]

Postoperatively, neurologic complications may be immediately obvious or delayed for hours to weeks. Leikensohn and colleagues[93] report 5 deaths (25%) and 10 strokes (50%) in 20 patients undergoing carotid ligation. Six of the ten strokes occurred at least 8 hours after ligation. The authors advocate 5000 U of subcutaneous heparin sulfate every 12 hours after surgery. There was only one death and no strokes in the seven patients who were treated this way in their series.

Pseudoaneurysm of the carotid artery is a very rare complication after head and neck surgery. Conley[96] reported 3 cases from more than 3000 major head and neck surgical procedures. The false aneurysm is actually a late controlled rupture of the carotid with blood dissecting into the surrounding tissues to form a pulsatile mass. It may present up to several years after surgery. Arteriography confirms the suspicion of pseudoaneurysm. Consideration must then be given to surgical or angiographic management.

Local Recurrence of Tumor

Local recurrence of carcinoma is a serious complication that is difficult to manage. The violation of surgical planes and the exposure of the great vessels allow for the spread and deep invasion of recurrent tumor beyond natural barriers. The recognition of recurrence is delayed by the swelling and subdermal scar formation that follows surgery and postoperative radiation therapy.

Recurrence may be the result of incomplete dissection. This may be more common during this era of selective neck dissection; however, in many series, the site of recurrence is most often within the previously dissected region. One area that is particularly susceptible to this is the superiormost portion of the dissection. Level II nodes are common, and dissection in this area must be fastidious. The extracapsular spread of tumor also predisposes patients to recurrence. Attention to intraoperative measures such as irrigation of the wound with sterile water and the changing of gloves and instruments after the tumor has been removed may help to reduce the incidence of tumor recurrence. However, biologic aggressiveness related to factors that are currently poorly understood is probably more important.

Recurrence as a result of tumor spillage may present as a small blister at the suture line that grows to an obvious fungating or ulcerative mass or as a diffuse and poorly demarcated mass beneath normal skin flaps (Figure 36-21). In many cases, radiation therapy has already been used, so further therapeutic options are limited. Surgical resection is feasible in some cases when recurrence has been detected early. This should be considered palliative therapy, with the ultimate prognosis in such cases being poor. Areas of skin involvement by tumor are resected together with bulk disease. Radioactive [125]iodine seeds or catheters for subsequent iridium seed loading may be placed in the residual tumor bed and covered with a healthy vascularized flap (Figure 36-22). Skin breakdown with bleeding, infection, and pain may thus be prevented or postponed. In one series, 77% of 220 cases treated with interstitial brachytherapy achieved local control of recurrent tumor at 6 months.[97] Newer technologies for limited reirradiation such as frameless stereotactic radiosurgery (i.e., CyberKnife [Accuray, Sunnyvale, CA]) are increasingly being applied with similarly promising (if limited) results.[98]

Reexploration of the neck for recurrent tumor (i.e., intraluminal or regional nodal) carries a greatly elevated risk of complication. If the jugular vein or other major venous structures were preserved during the original surgery, these structures will now be encased in scar. The scarring will be even more dense if postoperative radiation therapy has also been delivered. The identification of the vein under these circumstances can be quite difficult, and the control of venous bleeding elevates the risk to nearby neural structures, particularly to cranial nerves X, XI, and XII. Venous entry with troublesome hemorrhage can occur even during initial flap elevation. The surgical and anesthesia team must be prepared for this possibility. Sufficient time must be allotted to the case, recognizing that simple flap elevation and the identification of initial landmarks may consume many minutes. Wide exposure with the initial identification and control of structures in regions that are less affected by scarring is recommended.

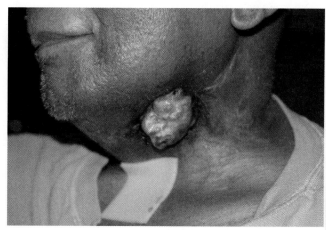

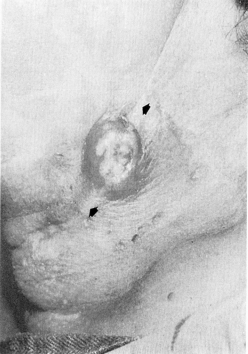

Figure 36-21 A, Fungating tumor in the incision line. **B,** Tumor recurrence presenting as an ulceration in the suture line *(arrows)* of a previous neck dissection.

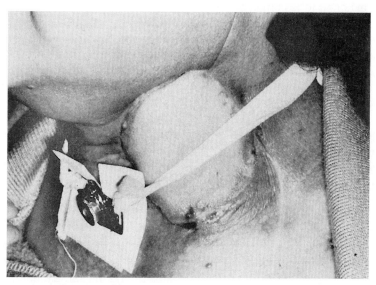

Figure 36-22. Postoperative appearance after the resection of tumor involving the skin and the carotid artery, the placement of ^{125}iodine seeds, and a pectoralis major flap.

Shoulder Pain and Dysfunction

Symptomatic problems with upper-extremity function after neck dissection are common and may occur after radical or modified comprehensive procedures that spare cranial nerve XI (described previously) and, to a lesser degree, after selective neck dissection. Postoperative physical therapy to assist with the mobilization and strengthening of the shoulder is recommended for all neck dissection patients, regardless of the status of the spinal accessory nerve.[99] The loss of stability of the scapula with "winging" as a result of trapezius paralysis

is made worse by the compensatory stretching of the rhomboid and levator scapulae muscles. Shoulder droop is also seen, and periarthritis of the scapulohumeral joint can occur (Figure 36-23). The dull aching pain that results is the most common complaint. The trapezius serves a supportive function when the arm is resting. Its major rotatory activity is seen when the arm is elevated from 35 degrees to 140 degrees in a coronal plain moving laterally. At more than 140 degrees, it again has a supportive role.[100] Thus, after neck dissection, shoulder elevation but not abduction is limited; the passive range

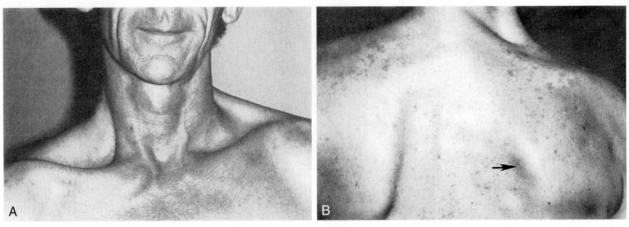

Figure 36-23. A, Right shoulder droop as a result of the spinal accessory nerve. **B,** The prominence of the scapular spine and the medial border *(arrow)* are the result of the rotation of the scapula and the loss of trapezius muscle bulk.

of motion is full. Physical therapy consultation is obtained on postoperative day 1 or 2, and exercise is advanced as soon as wound healing is adequate. Therapy includes heat, massage, and active and passive exercise to strengthen the shoulder musculature.

Modified and selective neck dissection in which cranial nerve XI is preserved and exposed to less manipulation should result in improved shoulder function and comfort. The assessment of this potential benefit may be accomplished with the use of electrical neurophysiologic measurements, with objective assessments of range of motion and strength, or with quality-of-life tools. Using all of these approaches, investigators in Brescia, Italy, recently reported superior results among patients who did not have level V dissected. Only a few patients in the group undergoing level V dissection had disability that affected their daily activities, but some subclinical impairment was observed in the group that underwent only level II through IV dissection, ostensibly as a result of the dissection of the submuscular proximal course of cranial nerve XI.[101] Other investigators report similar results, with a consistently better quality of life documented after selective nerve dissection that does not skeletonize cranial nerve XI in level V, as compared with cases involving comprehensive sparing but dissection of cranial nerve XI.[102,103] In general, time and physical therapy help to mitigate the pain and dysfunction.

Neuroma

Another cause of postoperative pain after neck surgery is the development of a traumatic neuroma. Traumatic neuromas are small, firm nodules that form at the cut end of sensory nerves as a result of disorganized neural regenerative growth. They may be mistaken for recurrent tumor when they are first discovered. However, neuromas rarely exceed 1 cm in diameter. They serve as trigger points for shooting pain, paresthesias, and unpleasant tingling. Typically a small (i.e., 2–3 mm), firm

nodule is palpable at the point of pain. The injection of local anesthetic agents provides temporary pain relief. If this injection has no untoward side effects, it may be followed with ethanol for permanent effect. Burying the nerve endings into muscle may prevent neuroma formation, and this can be done secondarily if a neuroma forms.

Gustatory Sweating

Frey syndrome (gustatory sweating) may occur after radical neck dissection.[104] It may be present over the bed of the submandibular gland or the parotid tail.

First-Bite Syndrome

First-bite syndrome is a distinctive pain phenomenon that occurs after surgery that involves tissues around the carotid artery, the cervical sympathetic trunk, the vagus nerve, the parapharyngeal space, and the parotid gland. It is described as a sharp, aggravating, or griping pain in the neck or jaw that occurs with the first bite of any meal and at times when salivating as a result of olfactory or other gustatory stimulation. Subsequent bites during the same meal are not painful. The problem is typically reported within weeks of surgery. It may resolve spontaneously months later, or it may persist. No effective therapy has been reported. The cause is postulated to be an imbalance between parasympathetic and sympathetic discharge to the parotid gland at the moment of major secretory stimulatory activity.[105–107]

CONCLUSION

Surgery of the neck requires a high level of expertise and familiarity with the complex anatomy of the region. Attention to detail during the workup, the preoperative planning, and the procedure itself will prevent most complications. Factors outside of the surgeon's control—including the aggressiveness of underlying disease, prior therapy, and the nutritional and immune statuses of the patient—must be taken into account. The anticipation of common postoperative problems (e.g., shoulder dysfunction) with the appropriate use of available treatment modalities will help patients to return to an optimal quality of life.

REFERENCES

1. Goguen LA, Posner MR, Tishler RB, et al: Examining the need for neck dissection in the era of chemoradiation therapy for advanced head and neck cancer. *Arch Otolaryngol Head Neck Surg* 2006;132:526–531.
2. Frank DK, Hu KS, Culliney BE, et al: Planned neck dissection after concomitant radiochemotherapy for advanced head and neck cancer. *Laryngoscope* 2005;115(6):1015–1020.
3. Stenson KM, Huo D, Blair E, et al: Planned post-chemoradiation neck dissection: Significance of radiation dose. *Laryngoscope* 2006;116(1):33–36.
4. Narayan K, Crane CH, Kleid S, et al: Planned neck dissection as an adjunct to the management of patients with advanced neck disease treated with definitive radiotherapy: For some or for all? *Head Neck* 1999;21:606–613.
5. Alexander MV, Zajtchuk JT, Henderson RL: Hypothyroidism and wound healing: Occurrence after head and neck radiation and surgery. *Arch Otolaryngol* 1982;108:289–291.
6. Hooley R, Levine H, Flores TC, et al: Predicting postoperative head and neck complications using nutritional assessment: The prognostic nutritional index. *Arch Otolaryngol* 1983;109:83–85.
7. Johnson JT, Barnes EL, Myers EN, et al: The extracapsular spread of tumors in cervical neck metastasis. *Arch Otolaryngol* 1981;107:725–729.
8. Gor DM, Langer JE, Loevner LA: Imaging of cervical lymph nodes in head and neck cancer: The basics. *Radiol Clin North Am* Jan 2006;44(1):viii, 101–110.
9. Hillsamer PJ, Schuller DE, McGhee RB, et al: Improving diagnostic accuracy of cervical metastasis with computed tomography and magnetic resonance imaging. *Arch Otolaryngol Head Neck Surg* 1990;116:1297–1301.
10. Gussack GS, Hodgins PA: Imaging modalities in recurrent head and neck tumors. *Laryngoscope* 1991;101:119–124.
11. Nieuwenhuis EJ, Castelijns JA, Pijpers R, et al: Wait-and-see policy for the N0 neck in early-stage oral and oropharyngeal squamous cell carcinoma using ultrasonography-guided cytology: Is there a role for identification of the sentinel node? *Head Neck* 2002;24(3):282–289.
12. Atkinson DP, Jacobs LA, Weaver AW: Elective carotid resection for squamous cell carcinoma of the head and neck. *Am J Surg* 1984;148:483–488.
13. Fee WE, Goffinet DR, Paryani S, et al: Intraoperative iodine 125 implants: Their use in large tumors in the neck attached to the carotid artery. *Arch Otolaryngol* 983;109:727–730.
14. Kennedy JT, Krause CJ, Loevy S: The importance of tumor attachment to the carotid artery. *Arch Otolaryngol* 1977;103:70–73.
15. Moore O, Baker HW: Carotid-artery ligation in surgery of the head and neck. *Cancer* 1955;8:712–726.
16. Martinez SA, Oller DW, Gee W, et al: Elective carotid artery resection. *Arch Otolaryngol* 1975;101:744–747.
17. Enzmann DR, Miller DC, Olcott C, et al: Carotid back pressures in conjunction with cerebral angiography. *Neuroradiology* 1980;134:415–419.
18. deVries EJ, Sekhar LN, Horton JA, et al: A new method to predict safe resection of the internal carotid. *Laryngoscope* 1990;100:85–88.
19. Chazono H, Okamoto Y, Matsuzaki Z, et al: Carotid artery resection: Preoperative temporary occlusion is not always an accurate predictor of collateral blood flow. *Acta Otolaryngol* 2005;125(2):196–200.
20. Aslan I, Hafiz G, Baserer N, et al: Management of carotid artery invasion in advanced malignancies of head and neck:
comparison of techniques. *Ann Otol Rhinol Laryngol* 2002;111(9):772–777.
21. Freeman SB, Hamaker RC, Borrowdale RB, et al: Management of neck metastasis with carotid artery involvement. *Laryngoscope* 2004;114(1):20–24.
22. Dare AO, Gibbons KJ, Gillihan MD, et al: Hypotensive endovascular test occlusion of the carotid artery in head and neck surgery. *Neurosurg Focus* 2003;14(3):e5.
23. Martin HE, Ellis EB: Biopsy by needle puncture and aspiration. *Ann Surg* 1930;92:169–181.
24. Engzell U, Franzen S, Zajicek J: Aspiration biopsy of tumors of the neck. II: Cytologic findings in 13 cases of carotid body tumors. *Acta Cytol* 1971;15:25–30.
25. Qizilbash Ah, Young JEM: Carotid body tumors and other paragangliomas. In Kline TS, editor: *Guidelines to clinical aspiration biopsy of head and neck*, ed 1, New York, 1988, Igaku-Shoin.
26. Seyfer AE, Walsh DS, Graeber GM, et al: Chest wall implantation of lung cancer after thin-needle aspiration biopsy. *Ann Thorac Surg* 1989;48:284–286.
27. Roussel F: Risk of metastasis during fine needle aspiration. *J Clin Pathol* 1990;43:878.
28. Young JEM, Archibald SD, Shier KJ: Needle aspiration cytologic biopsy in head and neck masses. *Am J Surg* 1981;142:484–489.
29. Batsakis JG, Sneige N, El-Naggar AK: Fine-needle aspiration of salivary glands: Its utility and tissue effects. *Ann Otol Rhinol Laryngol* 1992;101:185–188.
30. Carrau RL, Byzakis J, Wagner RL, et al: Role of prophylactic antibiotics in uncontaminated neck dissections. *Arch Otolaryngol Head Neck Surg* 1991;117:194–195.
31. Slattery WH, Stringer SP, Cassisi NJ: Prophylactic antibiotic use in clean, uncontaminated neck dissection. *Laryngoscope* 1995;105(3 Pt 1):244–246.
32. Brown H, Burns, S, Kaiser W: The spinal accessory nerve plexus, the trapezius muscle, and shoulder stabilization after radical cancer surgery. *Ann Surg* 1988;208:654–661.
33. Bocca E, Pignataro O, Sasaki CT: Functional neck dissection: A description of operative technique. *Arch Otolaryngol* 1980;106:524–527.
34. Roh JL, Yoon YH, Kim SY, et al: Cervical sensory preservation during neck dissection. *Oral Oncol* 2007;43(5):491–498.
35. Robbins KT, Medina JE, Wolfe GT, et al: Standardizing neck dissection terminology. *Arch Otolaryngol Head Neck Surg* 1991;117:601–605.
36. Candela FC, Shah J, Jaques DP, et al: Patterns of cervical node metastasis from squamous carcinoma of the larynx. *Arch Otolaryngol Head Neck Surg* 1990;116:432–435.
37. Skolnik EM, Yee KF, Friedman M, et al: The posterior triangle in radical neck surgery. *Arch Otolaryngol* 1976;102:1–4.
38. McGavran MH, Bauer WC, Ogura JH: The incidence of cervical lymph node metastases from epidermoid carcinoma of the larynx and their relationship to certain characteristics of the primary tumor. *Cancer* 1961;14:55–66.
39. Schuller DE, Platz CE, Krause CJ: Spinal accessory lymph nodes: A prospective study of metastatic involvement. *Laryngoscope* 1978;88:439–450.
40. Eisele DW, Weymuller EA, Price JP: Spinal accessory nerve preservation during neck dissection. *Laryngoscope* 1991;101:433–435.
41. Brandenburg JH, Lee CYS: The eleventh nerve in radical neck surgery. *Laryngoscope* 1981;91:1851–1859.
42. Jesse RH, Ballantyne AJ, Larson D: Radical or modified neck dissection: A therapeutic dilemma. *Am J Surg* 1978;136:516–519.
43. Molinari R, Chiesa F, Cantu G, et al: Retrospective comparison of conservative and radical neck dissection in laryngeal cancer. *Ann Otol* 1980;89:578–581.
44. Schuller DE, Reichis NA, Hamaker RC, et al: Analysis of disability resulting from treatment including radical neck dissection or modified neck dissection. *Head Neck Surg* 1983;6:551–558.
45. Sobol S, Jensen C, Sawyer W, et al: Objective comparison of physical dysfunction after neck dissection. *Am J Surg* 1985;150:503–509.

46. Leipzig B, Suen JY, English JL, et al: Functional evaluation of the spinal accessory nerve after neck dissection. *Am J Surg* 1983;146:526–530.

47. Saunders JR, Hirata RM, Jacques DA: Considering the spinal accessory nerve in head and neck surgery. *Am J Surg* 1985;150:491–494.

48. Zibordi F, Biaocco F, Bini A, et al: Spinal accessory nerve function following neck dissection. *Ann Otol Rhinol Laryngol* 1988;97:83–86.

49. Remmler D, Byers R, Scheetz J, et al: A prospective study of shoulder disability resulting from radical and modified neck dissections. *Head Neck Surg* 1986;8:280–286.

50. Weitz JW, Weitz SL, McElhinney AJ: A technique for preservation of spinal accessory nerve function in radical neck dissection. *Head Neck Surg* 1982;5:75–78.

51. Soo KC, Guiloff RJ, Oh A, et al: Innervation of the trapezius muscle: A study in patients undergoing neck dissections. *Head Neck* 1990;12:488–495.

52. Weisberger EC: The efferent supply of the trapezius muscle: A neuroanatomic basis for the preservation of shoulder function during neck dissection. *Laryngoscope* 1987;97:435–445.

53. Weisberger EC, Lingeman RE: Cable grafting of the spinal accessory nerve for rehabilitation of shoulder function after radical neck dissection. *Laryngoscope* 1987;97:915–918.

54. Tashiro T: Experimental studies in the reinnervation of larynx after accurate neurorrhaphy. *Laryngoscope* 1972;82:225–236.

55. Sato F, Ogura JH: Neurorrhaphy of the recurrent laryngeal nerve. *Laryngoscope* 1978;88:1034–1041.

56. Maniglia AJ, Dodds B, Sorensen K, et al: Newer techniques of laryngeal reinnervation. *Ann Otol Rhinol Laryngol* 1989;98:8–14.

57. Milstein CF, Akst LM, Hicks MD, et al: Long-term effects of micronized Alloderm injection for unilateral vocal fold paralysis. *Laryngoscope* 2005;115(9):1691–1696.

58. Adams VI, Hirsch CS: Venous air embolism from head and neck wounds. *Arch Pathol Lab Med* 1989;113:498–502.

59. Ericsson JA, Gottlieb JD, Sweet RB: Closed-chest cardiac massage in the treatment of venous air embolism. *N Engl J Med* 1964;270:1353–1354.

60. Stallworth JM, Martin JB, Postlethwait RW: Aspiration of the heart in air embolism. *JAMA* 1950;143:1250–1251.

61. Longenecker CG: Venous air embolism during operations on the head and neck. *Plast Reconst Surg* 1965;36:619–621.

62. Yeakel AE: Lethal air embolism from plastic blood storage container. *JAMA* 1968;204:267–269.

63. Dunbar EM, Fox R, Watson B, et al: Successful late treatment of venous air embolism with hyperbaric oxygen. *Post Grad Med J* 1990;66:469–470.

64. Camilleri AE, Davies FW: Aberrant central venous catheter complicating radical neck dissection. *J Laryngol Otol* 1991;105:491–492.

65. Crumley RL, Smith JD: Postoperative chylous fistula prevention and management. *Laryngoscope* 1976;86:804–813.

66. Greenfield J, Gottlieb MI: Variations in the terminal portion of the human thoracic duct. *Arch Surg* 1956;73:955–959.

67. David HK: A statistical study of the thoracic duct in man. *Am J Anat* 1915;17:211–214.

68. Gregor RT. Management of chyle fistulization in association with neck dissection. *Otolaryngol Head Neck Surg* 2000;122:434–439.

69. Velegrakis GA, Prokopakis EP, Papadakis CE, et al: Management of chylous fistula using the fibrin adhesive set. *ORL J Otorhinolaryngol Relat Spec* 1998;60:230–232.

70. Gacek RR: Neck dissection injury of a brachial plexus anatomical variant. *Arch Otolaryngol Head Neck Surg* 1990;116:356–358.

71. Fisher CB, Mattox DE, Zinreich JS: Patency of the internal jugular vein after functional neck dissection. *Laryngoscope* 1988;98:923–927.

72. Collins SL: Cervical sympathetic nerves in surgery of the neck. *Otolaryngol Head Neck Surg* 1991;105:544–555.

73. Ehrenfield WK, Stoney RJ, Wylie RJ: Relation of carotid stump pressure to safety of carotid artery ligation. *Surgery* 1983;93:299–305.

74. Hibbert J: The compromised carotid artery. In Cummings CW, Frederickson JM, Harker LA, et al, editors: *Otolaryngology–head and neck surgery update 1,* St Louis, 1989, Mosby-Year Book.

75. Lore JM, Boulos EJ: Resection and reconstruction of the carotid artery in metastatic squamous cell carcinoma. *Am J Surg* 1981;142:437–442.

76. Shumrick DA: Carotid artery rupture. *Laryngoscope* 1973;83:1051–1060.

77. Ahn C, Sindelar WF: Bilateral radical neck dissection: Report of results in 55 patients. *J Surg Oncol* 1989;40:252–255.

78. Ha PK, Couch ME, Tufano RP, et al: Short stay after neck dissection. *Otolaryngol Head Neck Surgery* 2005;133:677–680.

79. Matory YL, Spiro RH: Wound bleeding after head and neck surgery. *J Surg Oncol* 1993;53(1):17–19.

80. Wenig BL, Heller KS: The syndrome of inappropriate secretion of antidiuretic hormone (SIADH) following neck dissection. *Laryngoscope* 1987;97:467–470.

81. Balm AJM, Brown DH, DeVries WAEJ, et al: Blindness: A potential complication of bilateral neck dissection. *J Laryngol Otol* 1990;104:154–156.

82. Lydiatt DD, Ogren FP, Lydiatt WM, et al: Increased intracranial pressure as a complication of unilateral neck dissection in a patient with congenital absence of the transverse sinus. *Head Neck* 1991;13:359–362.

83. Spiro JD, Spiro RH, Strong EW: The management of chyle fistula. *Laryngoscope* 1990;100:771–774.

84. Chantarasak DN, Groon MF: Delayed lymphocele following neck dissection. *Br J Plast Surg* 1989;42:339–340.

85. Saraceno CA, Farrior RT: Bilateral chylothorax: Rare complication of neck dissection. *Arch Otolaryngol* 1981;107:497–499.

86. Har-El G, Segal K, Sidi J: Bilateral chylothorax complicating radical neck dissection: Report of a case with no concurrent external chylous leakage. *Head Neck Surg* 1985;7:225–230.

87. Grim PS, Gottlieb LJ, Boddie A, et al: Hyperbaric oxygen therapy. *JAMA* 1990;263:2216–2220.

88. Deva AK, Buckland GH, Fisher E, et al: Topical negative pressure in wound management. *Med J Aust* 2000;173(3):128–131.

89. Schuster R, Moradzadeh A, Waxman K: The use of vacuum-assisted closure therapy for the treatment of a large infected facial wound. *Am Surg* 2006;72(2):129–131.

90. Webb LX: New techniques in wound management: Vacuum-assisted wound closure. *J Am Acad Orthop Surg* 2002;10(5):303–311.

91. Maran AGD, Amin M, Wilson JA: Radical neck dissection: A 19-year experience. *J Laryngol Otol* 1989;103:760–764.

92. Ketcham AS, Hoye RC: Spontaneous carotid artery hemorrhage after head and neck surgery. *Am J Surg* 1965;110:649–655.

93. Leikensohn J, Milko D, Cotton R: Carotid artery rupture: Management and prevention of delayed neurological sequelae with low dose heparin. *Arch Otolaryngol* 1978;104:307–310.

94. Morrissey DD, Andersen PE, Nesbit GM, et al: Endovascular management of hemorrhage in patients with head and neck cancer. *Arch Otolaryngol Head Neck Surg* 1997;123(1):15–19.

95. Chaloupka JC, Putnam CM, Citardi MJ, et al: Endovascular therapy for the carotid blowout syndrome in head and neck surgical patients: Diagnostic and managerial considerations. *AJNR Am J Neuroradiol* 1996;17(5):843–852.

96. Conley JT: *Complications of head and neck surgery,* Philadelphia, 1979, WB Saunders.

97. Puthawala A, Nisar Syed AM, Gamie S, et al: Interstitial low-dose-rate brachytherapy as a salvage treatment for recurrent head and neck cancers: Long-term results. *Int J Radiat Oncol Biol Phys* 2001;51(2):354–362.

98. Voynov G, Heron DE, Burton S, et al: Frameless stereotactic radiosurgery for recurrent head and neck carcinoma. *Technol Cancer Res Treat* 2006;5(5):529–535.

99. Gluckman JL, Myer CM, Aseff JN, et al: Rehabilitation following radical neck dissection. *Laryngoscope* 1983;93:1083–1085.

100. Nahum AM, Mullally W, Marmor L: A syndrome resulting from radical neck dissection. *Arch Otolaryngol* 1961;74:82–86.

101. Cappiello J, Piazza C, Giudice M, et al: Shoulder disability after different selective neck dissections (levels II-IV versus levels II-V): A comparative study. *Laryngoscope* 2005;115(2): 259–263.
102. Chepeha DB, Taylor RJ, Chepeha JC, et al: Functional assessment using Constant's Shoulder Scale after modified radical and selective neck dissection. *Head Neck* 2002;24(5):432–436.
103. Kuntz AL, Weymuller EA Jr: Impact of neck dissection on quality of life. *Laryngoscope* 1999;109(8):1334–1338.
104. Myers EN, Conley J: Gustatory sweating after radical neck dissection. *Arch Otolaryngol* 1970;91:534–542.
105. Chiu AG, Cohen JI, Burningham AR, et al: First bite syndrome: A complication of surgery involving the parapharyngeal space. *Head Neck* 2002;24(11):996–999.
106. Truax BT: Gustatory pain: A complication of carotid endarterectomy. *Neurology* 1989;39(9):1258–1260.
107. Wax MK, Shiley SG, Robinson JL, et al: Cervical sympathetic chain schwannoma. *Laryngoscope* 2004;114(12):2210–2213.

CHAPTER 37

Complications of Endoscopic Neck Surgery

Susan K. Anderson and David J. Terris

Endoscopic neck surgery remains in its infancy. The vast majority of the applications have been for endocrine diseases (thyroid and parathyroid surgery) and will therefore occupy most of the attention in this chapter. Endoscopic thyroid surgery may be divided into two basic techniques: endoscopic thyroidectomy and video-assisted thyroidectomy. Purely endoscopic procedures usually involve the use of low-pressure carbon-dioxide insufflation to maintain an operative pocket. As with endoscopic surgery at other anatomic sites, trocars are introduced to provide access for the endoscopes and instrumentation. Incision location for endoscopic thyroidectomy has included chest, breast, axilla, and cervical incisions. Totally endoscopic insufflation-based lateral neck procedures have been implemented clinically on a very limited basis, but a brief discussion of complications known to be associated with this approach is included.

Video-assisted neck surgery parallels conventional neck surgery; portions of the procedure are performed under direct visualization, and the endoscope is used for visualization and magnification, thus allowing the procedure to be performed through a small skin incision. The operative pocket is maintained by retraction rather than insufflation.

COMPLICATIONS UNIQUE TO ENDOSCOPIC INSUFFLATION-BASED NECK SURGERY

Endoscopic surgical techniques that employ carbon dioxide insufflation to create or maintain an intraoperative pocket incur potential complications that are unique to this approach. These include subcutaneous emphysema, hypercarbia, metabolic acidosis, and venous or arterial compression.[1,2]

Subcutaneous Emphysema

Subcutaneous emphysema limited to the surgical area is an expected and acceptable consequence of endoscopic neck procedures that involve the use of gas insufflation. The operative pocket is created within the potential spaces of the neck and maintained with carbon-dioxide insufflation. At the conclusion of the procedure, residual carbon dioxide in the operative pocket and carbon dioxide that has diffused into surrounding tissue will result in subcutaneous emphysema. In animal studies, the degree of subcutaneous emphysema was greater among those subjects who were operated on with higher insufflation

pressures (i.e., ≥ 15 mm Hg), and it may have been the result of pneumomediastinum or simply the result of a greater passage of carbon dioxide into the subcutaneous tissues.[3]

Acidosis and Hypercarbia

The insufflation of extraperitoneal spaces with carbon dioxide for laparoscopic preperitoneal inguinal hernia repair has been shown to cause a more rapid and severe hypercarbia and acidosis as compared with insufflation of the peritoneum.[4] This phenomenon is believed to result from more extensive carbon-dioxide absorption in the preperitoneal space than in the intraperitoneal space. The peritoneum represents a natural barrier to the diffusion of carbon dioxide; in addition, the intraperitoneal pressures equilibrate and stabilize during procedures, which tamponades small capillaries, thus further decreasing the diffusion area.[4] By contrast, the absence of a natural barrier allows carbon dioxide to diffuse into and between the subcutaneous tissues of the neck.

Hypercarbia and acidosis can cause hemodynamic changes by direct action on the cardiovascular system and by indirect action through sympathetic stimulation.[5] The direct effect of carbon dioxide and acidosis can lead to decreased cardiac contractility, the sensitization of the myocardium to the arrhythmogenic effects of catecholamines, and systemic vasodilation. Centrally mediated autonomic effects of hypercarbia may lead to a widespread sympathetic stimulation that results in tachycardia and vasoconstriction, thus reducing the effect of direct vasodilation.[6]

Animal studies evaluating the effects of carbon dioxide insufflation of the neck have shown that, at low insufflation pressures (i.e., ≤ 10 mm Hg), the animals did not develop acidosis or statistically significant hypercarbia.[3] However, with insufflation at high pressures (i.e., ≥ 15 mm Hg), hypercarbia developed, the degree of which was related to the duration of insufflation; the severity of acidosis correlated with the level of pressure used.[3] A case of supraventricular tachycardia, severe subcutaneous emphysema, hypercarbia, and acidosis during endoscopic parathyroidectomy was reported. During this procedure, carbon dioxide was insufflated at 20 mm Hg during a surgical period of 7 hours. The patient developed acidosis (i.e., an arterial pH of 7.19), hypercarbia (i.e., a partial pressure of carbon dioxide in arterial blood level of 63 mm), and severe subcutaneous emphysema that resolved without sequalae.[7] Clinically relevant acidosis and hypercarbia have not been reported when low-pressure carbon-dioxide insufflation has been used.[8,9] Communication with anesthesia providers regarding potential metabolic complications during thyroidectomy involving the use of carbon-dioxide insufflation is appropriate.

ENDOSCOPIC-ASSISTED THYROID SURGERY

Complications associated with endoscopic-assisted thyroid and parathyroid surgery are similar to those encountered during conventional thyroid surgery. Morbidity rates are relatively low, and mortality is rare. Serious complications occur in fewer than 2% of endoscopic thyroid surgeries (Table 37-1).

Recurrent Laryngeal Nerve Injury

Injury to the recurrent laryngeal nerve is a well-recognized complication of thyroid surgery. Injury may occur as a result of partial or complete transection, thermal trauma, traction, compression, or compromised vascular supply. Even in the hands of the most experienced surgeons, a number of patients will suffer from temporary laryngeal paralysis or paresis, which may prove to be permanent. The incidence of permanent paralysis after endoscopic thyroid surgery is 0% to 1.3%, and the incidence of transient paralysis has been reported to be 0% to 3% (see Table 37-1). Permanent paralysis after conventional thyroid surgery occurs in 0.5% to 2.4% of patients, and temporary paralysis occurs in 2.6% to 5.9% of patients.[10] It is important to note that only a subset of patients requiring thyroidectomy are eligible for an endoscopic approach. These patients have smaller thyroid nodules than most patients who undergo conventional surgery, thyroid volumes within the normal range, and no history of thyroiditis, previous neck surgery, or irradiation.[1,11]

Injury to the recurrent laryngeal nerve is often not recognized during the surgery; however, if the nerve is found to have partial or complete transection, a microsurgical repair should be performed. The vocal cords would not be expected to regain normal movement after repair, and they usually assume a paramedian position as a result of misdirected regeneration among the abductor and adductor nerves.[12,13] Nevertheless, neurorrhaphy of the recurrent laryngeal nerve is effective for improving voice quality, aspiration, and maximum phonation time by preventing atrophy of the affected vocal cord.[14]

Routine mirror or flexible fiberoptic laryngoscopy should be performed on all patents before thyroidectomy, and the procedure should be repeated early during the postoperative period. The abnormal function of a vocal cord before surgery is rare; however, the documentation of such a finding is imperative.

UNILATERAL RECURRENT LARYNGEAL NERVE INJURY

Presentation

Unilateral recurrent laryngeal nerve paralysis is frequently well tolerated. Patients typically present during the postoperative period with hoarseness, decreased vocal projection, variation in vocal quality, or breathiness. In a small number of patients, unilateral vocal-cord paralysis can be life-threatening, usually as a consequence of aspiration pneumonia and especially among older patients or those with impaired pulmonary function preoperatively.[15] Permanent unilateral vocal-cord paralysis may cause a decrease in the quality of life as a result of poor voice quality, increased vocal effort, and decreased exercise tolerance.[16]

Treatment

When unilateral recurrent laryngeal nerve paresis becomes apparent, a treatment plan must be defined by the surgeon and the patient. If the patient is tolerating the deficit, a waiting period is recommended. Often a favorable spontaneous recovery occurs, but it may take 6 to 12 months.[17] Patients may benefit from speech therapy during this time. Speech therapy rehabilitation can assist patients with breath support, swallowing exercises, and psychological support.[17] In some patients, the voice outcomes obtained during speech therapy are sufficient to render further intervention unnecessary.

There is a subset of patients that is unable to compensate for unilateral recurrent laryngeal nerve paresis during the period before spontaneous recovery. These patients present with aspiration, dyspnea on exertion, increased vocal effort, and displeasure with their altered voice quality.[17] In these patients, intervention is necessary even if the surgeon believes that a satisfactory recovery will occur. Injection laryngoplasty using resorbable materials is an excellent procedure in this group. The injection of Gelfoam, collagen, Cymetra, and Radiesse voice gel can achieve glottic competence that will last for 6 weeks to 9 months, depending on the material injected.[18–21] These procedures do not interfere with spontaneous recovery; the injection can be repeated, if necessary, and it will not compromise future medialization procedures should they be necessary.

Recurrent laryngeal nerve paralysis that persists for more than 12 months is considered permanent. If poor vocal quality continues, definitive treatment is recommended.

TABLE 37-1 Complications of Endoscopic Thyroidectomy

Recurrent Laryngeal Nerve Paralysis				Hypocalcemia				Postoperative Hematoma	Wound Infection	Type of Procedure	Author, Year
Transient		Permanent		Transient		Permanent					
0/30	0%	0/30	0%	0/30	0%	0/30	0%	0/30	0/30	Endoscopic	Ikeda, 2002*
3/100	3%	1/100	1%	0/100	0%	0/100	0%	0/100	0/100	Endoscopic	Park, 2003†
10/579	1.7%	8/579	1.3%	10/579	1.7%	2/579	0.3%	4/579	0/579	VAT	Miccoli, 2004‡
8/467	1.7%	0/467	0%	64/467	13.7%	3/467	0.6%	1/467	2/467	VAT	Lombardi, 2006§

VAT, Video-assisted thyroidectomy.

*Ikeda Y, Takami H, Sasaki Y, et al: Comparative study of thyroidectomies: Endoscopic surgery versus conventional open surgery. *Surg Endosc* 2002;16(12):1741–1745.

†Park YL, Han WK, Bae WG: 100 cases of endoscopic thyroidectomy: Breast approach. *Surg Laparosc Endosc Percutan Tech* 2003;13(1):20–25.

‡Miccoli P, Berti P, Materazzi G, et al: Minimally invasive video-assisted thyroidectomy: Five years of experience. *J Am Coll Surg* 2004;199(2):243–248.

§Lombardi CP, Raffaelli M, Princi P, et al: Video-assisted thyroidectomy: Report on the experience of a single center in more than four hundred cases. *World J Surg* 2006;30(5):794–801.

Surgical interventions for unilateral vocal-cord paralysis are aimed at medializing the paralyzed cord, improving contact with the opposing normal cord, and reestablishing vocal quality by restoring glottal competence. Vocal-cord medialization is usually accomplished by injection laryngoplasty or medialization laryngoplasty.[17,18]

Injection laryngoplasty can be performed under local or general anesthesia. The chosen material is injected lateral to the vocal ligament via a transoral or percutaneous technique.[19,21] When the vocal deficit is deemed to be permanent, a correspondingly long-term injection material should be selected. Calcium hydroxylapatite and hyaluronic acid have duration of up to 2 years or more. Injections of autologous fat and fascia have the potential to provide permanent augmentation. However, early resorption may lead to incomplete glottic closure, thus prompting the need for repeated procedures.[19–22]

Medialization thyroplasty is performed through a small incision at the lower border of the thyroid cartilage. A window is created in the thyroid cartilage to preserve the inner perichondrium. The thyroarytenoid muscle is medialized using one of several materials, including a Gore-Tex strip, hydroxylapatite, or Silastic blocks placed approximately at the middle third of the vocal cord.[13,17] The procedure is best performed under local anesthesia to allow for patient phonation when evaluating the size and placement of the implant.

BILATERAL RECURRENT LARYNGEAL NERVE INJURY

Presentation

Injury to both recurrent laryngeal nerves during thyroidectomy is a rare event, and its occurrence in endoscopic thyroidectomy has not yet been reported.[1,8,9,23–25] Bilateral recurrent laryngeal nerve injury is usually evident immediately after extubation or during the immediate postoperative period. Airway obstruction occurs because both vocal cords assume the paramedian position. Individuals with this condition usually have biphasic stridor, respiratory distress, or both. Rarely the airway consequences of bilateral vocal-fold paralysis may manifest in a delayed fashion, up to several hours or even days after surgery. Initially some abduction function of the vocal cords is preserved; as the vocal cords medialize, however, the airway becomes compromised, and the patient develops dyspnea and stridor.[18]

Patients who are stridorous as a result of bilateral true vocal-cord paresis should be reintubated. A course of corticosteroid therapy may be initiated to decrease airway edema and to hasten the recovery of nerve function.[18,26] Extubation is usually attempted in the operating room after 24 to 48 hours, and flexible fiberoptic laryngoscopy is performed. If the airway is adequate, the patient may remain extubated and under close surveillance. If there is no improvement in the airway, a tracheostomy is recommended. When bilateral recurrent laryngeal nerve paralysis is determined to be permanent, procedures to improve the airway diameter (e.g., arytenoidectomy, laser cordotomy) are considered.[18,27] Individual needs must be considered with these procedures, because, as the airway caliber is improved, there is a tradeoff with a decrease in vocal quality and an increased risk of aspiration.

Prevention

A thorough understanding of the complex anatomy of the recurrent laryngeal nerve and its relationship with other structures in the neck is necessary for any surgeon who is performing a thyroidectomy. This knowledge is particularly important in endoscopic thyroid surgery, because the endoscope allows for the visualization of these critical anatomic structures from angles and vantage points that are inaccessible in conventional thyroid surgery. The endoscopic thyroid surgeon must be able to identify structures and their relationships with one another with the novel perspectives afforded by the endoscope.

The recurrent laryngeal nerve is routinely identified during endoscopic thyroid surgery and carefully dissected under direct visualization, thereby diminishing the likelihood of injury from the previously discussed mechanisms.[1,8,23,24] Risk to the nerve during thyroid surgery increases when the nerve is not identified.[28] A bloodless surgical field facilitates the identification of the recurrent laryngeal nerve, and the Harmonic Scalpel (Ethicon ENDO-SURGERY, Inc, Cincinnati, Ohio) is a useful tool during endoscopic thyroidectomy for achieving minimal blood loss.[1,11,29] In addition to providing excellent hemostasis, this device generates only modest heat, thereby resulting in much lower lateral thermal damage than is encountered with monopolar or bipolar cautery. The lateral zone of injury for the Harmonic Scalpel has been shown in the porcine model to be 0 m to 1 mm as compared with 240 μm to 15 mm for monopolar electrocautery.[30] The decreased thermal dispersion is particularly important when operating near the recurrent laryngeal nerve.

Intraoperative monitoring of the laryngeal nerves has been described as a means to reduce the risk of nerve injury and to assist with positive nerve identification during conventional thyroid surgery.[31–33] Noninvasive continuous monitoring of the laryngeal nerves can be provided by commercially available products, including an electrode-embedded endotracheal tube (Medtronic Xomed, Jacksonville, Fla) or a postcricoid laryngeal surface electrode. The role of continuous electrophysiologic monitoring of the recurrent laryngeal nerve during endoscopic thyroid surgery has not yet been studied.

SUPERIOR LARYNGEAL NERVE INJURY

The superior laryngeal nerve consists of two branches: the internal laryngeal nerve (sensory), which supplies sensory fibers to the pharynx, and the external laryngeal nerve (motor), which innervates the crico-thyroid muscle. During thyroidectomy, the external branch of the superior laryngeal nerve is at risk for injury, because it descends in close proximity to the superior thyroid artery. Superior laryngeal nerve injury has not been reported during endoscopic thyroid surgery.[1,9,23–25]

Presentation

When the external superior laryngeal nerve is damaged, it results in the paralysis of the cricothyroid muscle, which functions to lengthen, stiffen, and thin the true vocal cord. Voice changes resulting from damage to this nerve may include hoarseness, voice fatigue, poor vocal volume and projection, and decreased vocal register.[18,27] These changes are often well tolerated, and they have a minimal impact on the patient's life. However, this injury may be devastating for a professional singer or a public speaker.

A larynx with a superior laryngeal nerve injury will appear normal at rest during mirror or flexible fiber-optic laryngoscopy. With high-pitch phonation, the vocal cord on the affected side appears to be shorter, and it may have a height difference as compared with the normal side. The posterior glottis may also be observed to rotate toward the affected side.[34] If injury occurs to both superior laryngeal nerves, the vocal cords will appear normal or bowed at rest, but they will not elongate, thus preventing the patient from attaining high-pitch voicing.[18] Videostroboscopy may be a useful tool for diagnosing this injury.

Treatment

The treatment of superior laryngeal nerve paralysis centers on voice therapy. The therapy is particularly useful for eliminating the muscular tension dysphonia that may develop during compensation for the deficit. If it is not corrected, the muscular tension dysphonia can lead to prolonged or permanent voice impairment and structural lesions associated with voice abuse.[34]

Prevention

The superior laryngeal nerve is at risk during the sectioning of the vessels of the superior thyroid pole. Under endoscope visualization, these vessels are selectively ligated either with surgical clips or the Harmonic Scalpel, or the superior pole is sequentially ligated and mobilized without vascular identification. Endoscopic magnification facilitates the identification of small structures in the neck, and the superior laryngeal nerve is commonly identified during endoscopic thyroidectomy.[1,8,24]

HYPOPARATHYROIDISM

Transient and permanent hypoparathyroidism are known complications that are associated with thyroidectomy and that result in hypocalcemia. Even when the surgeon is confident that the parathyroid glands are intact and viable at the completion of the procedure, hypocalcemia may occur. The mechanism of hypoparathyroidism after thyroidectomy is not entirely understood, but the manipulation of the parathyroid glands producing transient parathyroid insufficiency or reversible ischemia is commonly cited.[18]

Hypocalcemia after thyroidectomy is usually temporary. Rates of temporary hypocalcemia associated with endoscopic thyroidectomy are reported to range from 0% to 13.7%, with permanent hypocalcemia occurring with an incidence of 0% to 0.6% (see Table 37-1). These rates compare with those for conventional thyroidectomy, for which a widely varying incidence is reported, ranging from 1.6% to 50%. However, most surgeons who have experience with thyroidectomy report a 2% to 3.8% incidence of permanent dysfunction.[27,35,36]

Presentation

The postoperative monitoring of calcium will often reveal a drop in calcium levels, even with unilateral thyroid procedures.[37] Early symptoms are numbness and tingling in the perioral area and the extremities. If these symptoms are not recognized and calcium levels continue to fall, spasm and the tetany of muscles in the extremities may occur. A positive Chvostek sign (i.e., tapping over the main trunk of the facial nerve near the tragus resulting in facial spasm) or Trousseau sign (i.e., carpal spasm elicited with the occlusion of the arm's arterial supply) indicates clinically significant hypocalcemia. If hypocalcemia remains untreated, laryngeal involvement, generalized seizures, and cardiac arrhythmias may occur.

Treatment

The management of asymptomatic hypocalcemia remains controversial.[18] Most authors recommend treatment when the serum calcium level falls below 8.0 mg/dl (normal, 8.6–10.2 mg/dl) with the oral supplementation of 2 g to 3 g daily of calcium carbonate started before discharge with education regarding the signs and symptoms of hypocalcemia. For symptomatic patients and when serum calcium levels fall below 7.5 mg/dl, both daily calcium carbonate and the rapid-acting vitamin-D analog calcitriol (0.25–0.5 µg daily) are given.[27,35] Serum calcium levels should be corrected for low albumin levels, and magnesium should be replaced if necessary before beginning calcium replacement. Among patients who fail to respond to oral supplementation measures, intravenous calcium gluconate may be necessary.

The authors routinely start total thyroidectomy patients on oral calcium carbonate in a tapering-dose fashion over a period of 3 weeks.[38] This has allowed these patients to be discharged to home the day of surgery, with comprehensive instructions regarding the signs and symptoms of hypocalcemia. If hypocalcemia after thyroidectomy is permanent or refractory to preliminary intervention, consultation with an endocrinologist is recommended.

Prevention

Detailed knowledge of the anatomy of the parathyroid glands is important to enable identification and preservation during thyroidectomy. The vascular supply to both the superior and inferior parathyroid glands is usually from the inferior thyroid artery. The identification of the glands and the preservation of their vascular supply by control distal to the glands decreases the likelihood of hypoparathyroidism. If a parathyroid gland is inadvertently resected or devascularized during thyroidectomy, the gland should be minced into small pieces and transplanted into the sternocleidomastoid muscle or the strap muscles.[39]

BLEEDING

Intraoperative bleeding may compromise endoscopic thyroid surgery by compromising or eliminating the surgical view afforded by the endoscope. Bleeding also stains the surgical field, thereby making the identification of vital structures, including the laryngeal nerves, more tedious. Meticulous hemostasis is therefore of particular importance when undertaking endoscopic thyroid surgery.

In part because of the need for absolute intraoperative hemostasis, postoperative hemorrhage in endoscopic thyroidectomy is rare, with a reported incidence of less than 0.2% (see Table 37-1). The reduced dissection involved, the avoidance of subplatysmal flaps, and the use of Harmonic Scalpel technology also all probably contribute to the low incidence. Nevertheless, vigilance for significant postoperative hemorrhage is appropriate, because, in rare cases, it may result in airway compromise and even death.

Presentation

Patients with postoperative hematoma may present with neck swelling or neck pain and in advanced stages with stridor, dyspnea, or hypoxia. Patients with these complaints or findings should be evaluated expeditiously.

Treatment

An expanding hematoma is an emergency that requires immediate attention. It usually occurs in the operating room after extubation or in the recovery room during the early postoperative period. If airway obstruction occurs, the hematoma should be evacuated promptly (at the bedside, if necessary). The wound should then be explored in the operating room after securing the airway. If a hematoma is recognized and does not pose an immediate threat to the airway, a more graduated approach may be pursued. If it is stable, limited, or both, conservative management may be considered.

Conversion to an open procedure should be considered during endoscopic procedures if intraoperative bleeding cannot be adequately controlled or if the surgical field has become obscured, thereby putting vital structures at risk. In a study involving a porcine model evaluating endoscopic approaches for thyroidectomy, conversion from an endoscopic to an open procedure was able to performed in 60 seconds.[21] Therefore the time to convert to an open procedure should not significantly affect vessel control and blood loss.

Prevention

Postoperative hemorrhage is best prevented by pursuing compulsive intraoperative hemostasis. As previously noted, endoscopic techniques require an operative field that is essentially bloodless. The Harmonic Scalpel is an essential instrument for accomplishing endoscopic thyroidectomy.[1,11,29] It denatures protein by using ultrasonic vibrations to transfer mechanical energy that is sufficient to break tertiary hydrogen bonds. The denatured protein coagulum coapts and seals the blood vessels, thereby providing robust hemostasis.[40]

A thorough preoperative history should alert the surgeon to previously unidentified coagulopathy or a family history of a bleeding disorder. If a coagulopathy is identified by the history or with routine laboratory studies, a nonendoscopic minimally invasive or conventional approach to thyroidectomy should be considered.

Routine drainage of the thyroid bed in thyroid surgery remains controversial. A multitude of investigators have found that routine drainage is not effective for decreasing the rate of postoperative complications (particularly hematoma) and that it may contribute to a prolonged hospital stay and surgical site infection.[41,42] Drains are virtually never used in the minimally invasive video-assisted thyroidectomy; however, they are recommended with the axillary endoscopic approach.[1,8,23,24] The decision to drain the thyroid bed is left to the discretion of the surgeon, with the understanding that postoperative hematoma is not prevented by the presence of a drain and that it is not a substitute for adequate intraoperative hemostasis.

WOUND INFECTION

Wound infection is a rare complication after endoscopic thyroid surgery, with a reported incidence of less than 0.4 % (see Table 37-1). If a wound infection occurs, oral antibiotics covering *Streptococcus* and *Staphylococcus* species are typically sufficient to control the process. A single dose of intravenous antibiotics covering the same species before the skin incision and the observation of sterile techniques during surgery are usually effective for achieving a low incidence of postoperative infection.

ENDOSCOPIC PARATHYROIDECTOMY

Endoscopic neck surgery had its origins with Gagner's[43] first endoscopic parathyroidectomy in 1996, which was expanded to thyroidectomy and other procedures. Endoscopic parathyroidectomy has morbidity rates that are low, and mortality has not been reported. Serious complications occur in fewer than 10% of endoscopic parathyroid surgeries, the majority of which are associated with hypocalcemia (Table 37-2). Other complications (e.g., permanent injury to the recurrent laryngeal nerve) occur in less than 1% of cases, and the rate of persistent hyperparathyroidism in endoscopic parathyroidectomy is less than 1.6% (see Table 37-2).

Patient selection is an integral step in successful endoscopic parathyroidectomy. Patients who are eligible for minimally invasive procedures have sporadic hyperparathyroidism, preoperative localization of at least one affected parathyroid gland that is less than 3 cm in its largest dimension, no suspicion of parathyroid carcinoma, and the absence of bulky thyroid disease.[44] As experience with endoscopic techniques grows, the criteria of eligibility for an endoscopic parathyroidectomy may expand to include more patients. A midline approach affords the surgeon access to both neck compartments, thereby allowing for bilateral endoscopic cervical exploration and the opportunity to address concomitant thyroid disease.[44,45]

Intraoperative parathyroid hormone testing is complimentary to endoscopic parathyroidectomy. The Miami criteria (i.e., a drop of $\geq 50\%$ from the highest of either preoperative baseline or pre-excision levels at 10 minutes after gland excision) are used by many surgeons to assess the adequacy of surgery.[46,47] Endoscopic parathyroidectomy starts as a directed unilateral procedure, and the results of intraoperative parathyroid hormone testing provide insight to determine whether if adequate excision has been completed or further exploration in needed. Either bilateral endoscopic exploration or conversion to an open procedure can be pursued. Complications associated with endoscopic parathyroidectomy mirror those associated with endoscopic thyroidectomy, and the treatment of any complication is the same as that outlined for thyroidectomy.

CONCLUSION

Although endoscopic neck surgery remains in its infancy, a significant role for it in thyroidectomy and parathyroidectomy is emerging. Complications associated with endoscopic thyroidectomy and parathyroidectomy mirror those associated with conventional open approaches, and the rates are comparable. As experience with these procedures grow, innovators in the field will undoubtedly expand their endoscopic repertoire to include other commonly performed neck surgeries. As endoscopic neck surgery becomes more widely adopted, continuous evaluation of its efficiency and complications will be necessary.

TABLE 37-2 Complications of Endoscopic Parathyroidectomy

Author, Year	Type of Procedure	Persistent Hyperparathyroidism		Postoperative Hematoma		Conversion to Open Procedure		Hypocalcemia		Recurrent Laryngeal Nerve Paralysis — Permanent		Recurrent Laryngeal Nerve Paralysis — Transient	
Miccoli, 2000[*]	MIVAP	0.7%	1/137	0%	0/137	8.8%	12/137	7.3%	10/137	0.7%	1/137	0%	0/137
Lo, 2003[†]	MIVAP	0%	0/66	0%	0/66	6%	4/66	9.1%	6/66	0%	0/66	3%	2/66
Miccoli, 2004[‡]	MIVAP	1.7%	6/359	0.3%	1/359	6.4%	23/359	2.8%	10/359	0.8%	3/359	NR	NR
Henry, 2004[§]	MIVAP	0.8%	3/365	0.5%	2/365	13.4%	49/365	NR	NR	0.3%	1/365	0%	0/365
Barczynski, 2006[¶]	MIVAP	0%	0/30	0%	0/30	0%	0/30	10%	3/30	0%	0/30	0%	0/30

MIVAP, Minimally invasive video-assisted parathyroidectomy; NR, not reported.

[*]Miccoli P, Berti P, Conte M, et al: Minimally invasive video-assisted parathyroidectomy: Lesson learned from 137 cases. *J Am Coll Surg* 2000;191(6):613–618.
[†]Lo CY, Chan WF, Luk JM: Minimally invasive endoscopic-assisted parathyroidectomy for primary hyperparathyroidism. *Surg Endosc* 2003;17(12):1932–1936.
[‡]Miccoli P, Berti P, Materazzi G, et al: Results of video-assisted parathyroidectomy: Single institution's six-year experience. *World J Surg* 2004;28(12):1216–1218.
[§]Henry JF, Sebag F, Tamagnini P, et al: Endoscopic parathyroid surgery: Results of 365 consecutive procedures. *World J Surg* 2004;28(12):1219–1223.
[¶]Barczynski M, Cichon S, Konturek A, et al: Minimally invasive video-assisted parathyroidectomy versus open minimally invasive parathyroidectomy for a solitary parathyroid adenoma: A prospective, randomized, blinded trial. *World J Surg* 2006;30(5):721–731.

REFERENCES

1. Lombardi CP, Raffaelli M, Princi P, et al: Video-assisted thyroidectomy: Report on the experience of a single center in more than four hundred cases. *World J Surg* 2006;30(5):794–801.
2. Ochiai R, Takeda J, Noguchi J, et al: Subcutaneous carbon dioxide insufflation does not cause hypercarbia during endoscopic thyroidectomy. *Anesth Analg* 2000;90(3):760–762.
3. Bellantone R, Lombardi CP, Rubino F, et al: Arterial PCO2 and cardiovascular function during endoscopic neck surgery with carbon dioxide insufflation. *Arch Surg* 2001;136(7):822–827.
4. Liem MS, Kallewaard JW, de Smet AM, et al: Does hypercarbia develop faster during laparoscopic herniorrhaphy than during laparoscopic cholecystectomy? Assessment with continuous blood gas monitoring. *Anesth Analg* 1995;81(6):1243–1249.
5. Neudecker J, Sauerland S, Neugebauer E, et al: The European Association for Endoscopic Surgery clinical practice guideline on the pneumoperitoneum for laparoscopic surgery. *Surg Endosc* 2002;16(7):1121–1143.
6. Gutt CN, Oniu T, Mehrabi A, et al: Circulatory and respiratory complications of carbon dioxide insufflation. *Dig Surg* 2004;21(2):95–105.
7. Gottlieb A, Sprung J, Zheng XM, et al: Massive subcutaneous emphysema and severe hypercarbia in a patient during endoscopic transcervical parathyroidectomy using carbon dioxide insufflation. *Anesth Analg* 1997;84(5):1154–1156.
8. Ikeda Y, Takami H, Niimi M, et al: Endoscopic thyroidectomy and parathyroidectomy by the axillary approach: A preliminary report. *Surg Endosc* 2002;16(1):92–95.
9. Ikeda Y, Takami H, Sasaki Y, et al: Comparative study of thyroidectomies: Endoscopic surgery versus conventional open surgery. *Surg Endosc* 2002;16(12):1741–1745.
10. Myssiorek D. Recurrent laryngeal nerve paralysis: Anatomy and etiology. *Otolaryngol Clin North Am* 2004;37(1):v, 25–44.
11. Ikeda Y, Takami H, Sasaki Y, et al: Are there significant benefits of minimally invasive endoscopic thyroidectomy? *World J Surg* 2004;28(11):1075–1078.
12. Miyauchi A, Matsusaka K, Kihara M, et al: The role of ansa-to-recurrent-laryngeal nerve anastomosis in operations for thyroid cancer. *Eur J Surg* 1998;164(12):927–933.
13. Siribodhi C, Sundmaker W, Atkins JP, et al: Electromyographic studies of laryngeal paralysis and regeneration of laryngeal motor nerves in dogs. *Laryngoscope* 1963;73:148–164.
14. Chou FF, Su CY, Jeng SF, et al: Neurorrhaphy of the recurrent laryngeal nerve. *J Am Coll Surg* 2003;197(1):52–57.
15. Laccourreye O, Paczona R, Ageel M, et al: Intracordal autologous fat injection for aspiration after recurrent laryngeal nerve paralysis. *Eur Arch Otorhinolaryngol* 1999;256(9):458–461.
16. Spector BC, Netterville JL, Billante C, et al: Quality-of-life assessment in patients with unilateral vocal cord paralysis. *Otolaryngol Head Neck Surg* 2001;125(3):176–182.
17. Hartl DM, Travagli JP, Leboulleux S, et al: Clinical review: Current concepts in the management of unilateral recurrent laryngeal nerve paralysis after thyroid surgery. *J Clin Endocrinol Metab* 2005;90(5):3084–3088.
18. Fewins J, Simpson CB, Miller FR: Complications of thyroid and parathyroid surgery. *Otolaryngol Clin North Am* 2003;36(1):x, 189–206.
19. O'Leary MA, Grillone GA: Injection laryngoplasty. *Otolaryngol Clin North Am* 2006;39(1):43–54.
20. Kwon TK, Buckmire R: Injection laryngoplasty for management of unilateral vocal fold paralysis. *Curr Opin Otolaryngol Head Neck Surg* 2004;12(6):538–542.
21. Terris DJ, Haus BM, Nettar K, et al: Prospective evaluation of endoscopic approaches to the thyroid compartment. *Laryngoscope* 2004;114(8):1377–1382.
22. Belafsky PC, Postma GN: Vocal fold augmentation with calcium hydroxylapatite. *Otolaryngol Head Neck Surg* 2004;131(4):351–354.
23. Miccoli P, Materazzi G: Minimally invasive, video-assisted thyroidectomy (MIVAT). *Surg Clin North Am* 2004;84(3):735–741.
24. Miccoli P, Berti P, Materazzi G, et al: Minimally invasive video-assisted thyroidectomy: Five years of experience. *J Am Coll Surg* 2004;199(2):243–248.
25. Spinelli C, Bertocchini A, Donatini G, et al: Minimally invasive video-assisted thyroidectomy: Report of 16 cases in children older than 10 years. *J Pediatr Surg* 2004;39(9):1312–1315.
26. Wang LF, Lee KW, Kuo WR, et al: The efficacy of intraoperative corticosteroids in recurrent laryngeal nerve palsy after thyroid surgery. *World J Surg* 2006;30(3):299–303.
27. Zarnegar R, Brunaud L, Clark OH: Prevention, evaluation, and management of complications following thyroidectomy for thyroid carcinoma. *Endocrinol Metab Clin North Am* 2003;32(2):483–502.
28. Thomusch O, Machens A, Sekulla C, et al: Multivariate analysis of risk factors for postoperative complications in benign goiter surgery: Prospective multicenter study in Germany. *World J Surg* 2000;24(11):1335–1341.
29. Terris DJ, Seybt MW, Gourin CG, et al: Ultrasonic technology facilitates minimal access thyroid surgery. *Laryngoscope* 2006;116(6):851–854.
30. McCarus SD: Physiologic mechanism of the ultrasonically activated scalpel. *J Am Assoc Gynecol Laparosc* 1996;3(4):601–608.
31. Affleck BD, Swartz K, Brennan J: Surgical considerations and controversies in thyroid and parathyroid surgery. *Otolaryngol Clin North Am* 2003;36(1):x, 159–187.
32. Marcus B, Edwards B, Yoo S, et al: Recurrent laryngeal nerve monitoring in thyroid and parathyroid surgery: The University of Michigan experience. *Laryngoscope* 2003;113(2):356–361.
33. Snyder SK, Hendricks JC: Intraoperative neurophysiology testing of the recurrent laryngeal nerve: Plaudits and pitfalls. *Surgery* 2005;138(6):1183–1192.
34. Dursun G, Sataloff RT, Spiegel JR, et al: Superior laryngeal nerve paresis and paralysis. *J Voice* 1996;10(2):206–211.
35. Reeve T, Thompson NW: Complications of thyroid surgery: How to avoid them, how to manage them, and observations on their possible effect on the whole patient. *World J Surg* 2000;24(8):971–975.
36. Bergamaschi R, Becouarn G, Ronceray J, et al: Morbidity of thyroid surgery. *Am J Surg* 1998;176(1):71–75.
37. Falk SA, Birken EA, Baran DT: Temporary postthyroidectomy hypocalcemia. *Arch Otolaryngol Head Neck Surg* 1988;114(2):168–174.
38. Terris DJ, Moister B, Seybt MW, et al: Outpatient thyroid surgery is desirable and safe. *Otolaryngol Head Neck Surg* 2007;136(4):556–559.
39. Olson JA, Jr, DeBenedetti MK, Baumann DS, et al: Parathyroid autotransplantation during thyroidectomy: Results of long-term follow-up. *Ann Surg* 1996;223(5):472–480.
40. Walker RA, Syed ZA: Harmonic scalpel tonsillectomy versus electrocautery tonsillectomy: A comparative pilot study. *Otolaryngol Head Neck Surg* 2001;125(5):449–455.
41. Ozlem N, Ozdogan M, Gurer A, et al: Should the thyroid bed be drained after thyroidectomy? *Langenbecks Arch Surg* 2006;391(3):228–230.
42. Suslu N, Vural S, Oncel M, et al: Is the insertion of drains after uncomplicated thyroid surgery always necessary? *Surg Today* 2006;36(3):215–218.
43. Gagner M: Endoscopic subtotal parathyroidectomy in patients with primary hyperparathyroidism. *Br J Surg* 1996;83(6):875.
44. Miccoli P, Berti P, Materazzi G, et al: Results of video-assisted parathyroidectomy: Single institution's six-year experience. *World J Surg* 2004;28(12):1216–1218.
45. Barczynski M, Cichon S, Konturek A, et al: Minimally invasive video-assisted parathyroidectomy versus open minimally invasive parathyroidectomy for a solitary parathyroid adenoma: A prospective, randomized, blinded trial. *World J Surg* 2006;30(5):721–731.
46. Carneiro DM, Solorzano CC, Nader MC, et al: Comparison of intraoperative iPTH assay (QPTH) criteria in guiding parathyroidectomy: Which criterion is the most accurate? *Surgery* 2003;134(6):973–981.
47. Irvin GL 3rd, Solorzano CC, Carneiro DM: Quick intraoperative parathyroid hormone assay: Surgical adjunct to allow limited parathyroidectomy, improve success rate, and predict outcome. *World J Surg* 2004;28(12):1287–1292.

CHAPTER 38

Complications of Surgery of the Carotid Artery

Bruce A. Perler

CAROTID ENDARTERECTOMY

Since its introduction during the early 1950s, carotid endarterectomy (CEA) has become the most commonly performed peripheral vascular operation in the United States. Although there have been fluctuations in the overall volume of operations carried out from year to year, most recently at least 130,000 procedures have been performed annually in the United States.[1]

The introduction of carotid angioplasty and stenting (CAS) may begin to affect carotid surgery caseload in the future (vida infra). The growth of the surgical treatment of extracranial carotid atherosclerosis is understandable, because stroke is the third leading cause of death in the United States. At least 70% of fatal strokes are nonhemorrhagic, and carotid disease is responsible for the majority of them. Furthermore, a voluminous literature has documented that CEA effectively reduces the risk of stroke among patients with significant extracranial carotid disease, and it may be performed with acceptable morbidity in the hands of experienced vascular surgeons.

The safety and efficacy of CEA and its superiority as compared with the optimal medical therapy of patients with symptomatic and asymptomatic carotid disease was confirmed by the completion of two critical multicenter prospective randomized clinical trials: the North American Symptomatic Carotid Endarterectomy Trial (NASCET) and the Asymptomatic Carotid Atherosclerosis Study (ACAS), respectively.[2–4] The ACAS findings were recently confirmed by the completion of the Asymptomatic Carotid Surgery Trial in Europe.[5]

This chapter documents the spectrum of potential complications of CEA, from minor to potentially life-threatening, including the incidence, the causes, the methods of prevention, and the appropriate treatments. Attention is also directed at the complications of CAS and the resection of carotid body tumors.

CARDIAC COMPLICATIONS

Incidence

Although perioperative stroke is the most feared complication of CEA, it in fact occurs much less often than cardiac complications. Myocardial infarction is responsible for 25% to 50% of all perioperative deaths after CEA, and, among patients with symptomatic coronary artery disease (CAD), cardiac morbidity is responsible for approximately 75% of all perioperative deaths.[6–8] Furthermore, more late deaths are caused by myocardial infarction than by stroke or other causes.[6,7,9,10] These observations reflect the systemic nature of arteriosclerosis in general and specifically the prevalence of CAD among patients with significant carotid lesions. At least 40% to 50% of patients who undergo CEA have symptomatic CAD.[11–13] In a prospective angiographic study, severe surgically correctable CAD was identified in 20% of patients presenting for the treatment of carotid disease.[14]

Despite the prevalence of CAD among patients undergoing CEA, operative mortality has declined significantly during the past two decades, with an incidence of 0% to 3% in several large series in both university[15–21] and community hospitals.[22–26] In an analysis of 23,237 CEAs performed in the state of Maryland from 1994 to 2003 that included 47 hospitals and more than 400 surgeons, the perioperative mortality rate was 0.54%.[26] In California, 51,231 CEAs were performed from 1999 to 2003, with a statewide perioperative mortality rate of 0.48%.[26] This is consistent with the results of an analysis of the outcomes of CEA in a national database, in which an operative mortality rate of 0.61% was found for 35,821 CEAs.[27] The improvement in outcome during the past two decades in large measure reflects the increasing performance of CEA by surgeons who have relatively high surgical volumes.[26–28] In addition, there has been a significant reduction in cardiac morbidity, which historically was a major contributor to perioperative mortality. In an analysis of the outcomes of CEAs performed over a 10-year period, including 1440 cases, the incidence of perioperative myocardial infarction was 1.5%.[29] In another recent individual institutional study, the incidence of perioperative cardiac complications was 0.5%.[30]

Prevention

These favorable results reflect improvements in the preoperative cardiac evaluation of patients scheduled for CEA as well as aggressive intraoperative and postoperative hemodynamic monitoring and treatment. Several clinical findings have been found to be highly predictive of cardiac morbidity after CEA, including Q waves on the electrocardiogram, exertional angina, recent myocardial infarction, history of ventricular arrhythmias, congestive heart failure, diabetes mellitus, and an age of more than 70 years. If one or more of these markers are present, the patient should undergo stress thallium scintigraphy or intravenous dipyridamole–thallium scanning. If the radionuclide scan is positive, coronary angiography is indicated. If moderate to severe CAD is identified, the patient with stable carotid disease should undergo percutaneous transluminal coronary angioplasty or coronary artery bypass before CEA, which significantly reduces the risk of cardiac morbidity associated with that procedure. A small minority of patients with critical carotid artery disease and severe CAD may be candidates for combined CEA and coronary artery bypass.[31,32] Alternatively, patients with one or more of these clinical signs but with negative radionuclide studies or with modest disease documented on coronary angiography can undergo CEA with minimal cardiac risk, as long as rigorous hemodynamic monitoring and appropriate pharmacologic management are employed intraoperatively and after surgery.

Furthermore, in addition to the more sensitive screening of patients for significant CAD, perioperative cardiac morbidity has been reduced by the more effective medical management of this patient population, including the administration of β-blockers during the perioperative period.[33,34] In addition, there is growing evidence to support the benefits of statin drugs for the peripheral vascular disease patient population, including those undergoing CEA. In a recent analysis of 1566 patients undergoing CEA that included 1440 isolated CEA procedures, the incidence of perioperative myocardial infarction was 1.2% among patients receiving statins as compared with 2.1% among those not taking statins at the time of surgery ($P = .191$). Perioperative mortality was 0.3% and 2.1% among those taking and those not taking statin drugs ($P = .002$), respectively.[29]

STROKE AND TRANSIENT ISCHEMIC ATTACKS

The sole purpose of CEA is the prevention of stroke. Therefore the incidence of this complication perioperatively and during long-term follow up is a paramount determinant of its efficacy. Considerable clinical experience was reported during the last three decades that indicated that CEA substantially reduced the risk of subsequent stroke among patients with significant symptomatic as well as asymptomatic extracranial carotid atherosclerotic lesions who underwent successful endarterectomy.[35–41] The preponderance of the data supporting the role of CEA for patients with significant carotid artery disease was derived from retrospective and typically individual institutional series. The safety and efficacy of CEA, however, has now been confirmed

with the completion of several multicenter randomized prospective clinical trials.

Symptomatic Disease

NASCET, which was funded by the National Institutes of Health, included both high-grade and moderate-grade stenosis investigations. In the NASCET high-grade stenosis investigation, 659 patients with symptomatic internal carotid stenosis (70%–99%) were randomized to optimal medical management or CEA and optimal medical management. At the 2-year follow up, there was a highly significant reduction in ipsilateral stroke incidence (9% vs. 26%) among patients who underwent CEA.[2] This benefit became apparent within 3 months of randomization, and it persisted through 8 years of follow up. In the moderate stenosis limb of the investigation, 865 patients with a 50% to 69% internal carotid stenosis were randomized. At the 5-year follow up, the ipsilateral stroke incidence was 22.2% among medical patients and 16.7% for surgical patients ($P = .045$), and this benefit persisted through 8 years of follow up.[3] On the basis of these data, it is now widely accepted that CEA is the treatment of choice for patients with symptomatic disease and 50% internal carotid stenoses and who are appropriate surgical candidates.

Asymptomatic Disease

The management of asymptomatic carotid disease has been more controversial, because the long-term risk of stroke is not as great among asymptomatic patients as compared with symptomatic patients. In ACAS, which was also funded by the National Institutes of Health, 1600 patients with an asymptomatic stenosis of 60% or more were randomized to optimal medical management or CEA and optimal medical management. At the 5-year follow up, the stroke and death rates were 5.1% in the CEA group and 11% in the medical management group ($P = .004$).[4] The Asymptomatic Carotid Surgery Trial was recently concluded in Europe. This trial involved the randomization of 3200 patients with a 60% or more asymptomatic internal carotid stenosis, and it had an outcome that was comparable to that of ACAS. The 5-year stroke and death rates were 6.4% for CEA patients and 11.8% for medically managed patients ($P < .0001$).[5] Although these trials suggest that CEA is indicated for patients with an asymptomatic internal carotid stenosis of 60% of more, close examination of the data indicates that the benefit of CEA in terms of stroke reduction was 1% to 2% per year. Therefore many clinicians today will reserve operative intervention for patients with a greater asymptomatic stenosis of 80% or more, and they will use clinical judgment to individualize this decision. This threshold may be lower in the setting of an ulcerated plaque, bilateral carotid disease, a history of progression in the degree of stenosis while under medical management, a strong family history of stroke, or other confounding factors.

Perioperative Stroke: Cause and Management

The incidence of perioperative stroke has also been shown to be inversely proportional to the practice volume and level of training of the surgeon.[42] More recent studies have confirmed the close relationship of operator volume and clinical outcome after CEA.[26,28] For example, in a statewide analysis of 23,237 CEAs performed by more than 400 surgeons in 47 Maryland hospitals from 1994 to 2003, there was a highly significant difference between in-hospital stroke incidence among surgeons with low volume (i.e., <15) as compared with those with moderate volume (i.e., between 15 and 74) and high volume (i.e., >75) annual CEA caseloads.[26]

Perioperative stroke and transient ischemic attacks may result from a variety of causes (Box 38-1). Clinical variables associated with an increased incidence of perioperative stroke include the presence of plaque ulceration, the degree of disease in the contralateral internal carotid artery, the status of intracerebral collaterals, and the integrity of the cerebral autoregulatory mechanism.[43] Symptomatic status is also strongly correlated with the incidence of perioperative stroke. The risk of stroke is lowest among patients who undergo surgery for asymptomatic disease; it is higher among patients undergoing operation after experiencing one or more transient ischemic attacks, and it is highest among those who have already experienced an ischemic stroke.[44] In a detailed study of the causes of perioperative stroke associated with CEA among patients in all clinical classes, more than 20 mechanisms were delineated. In general, however, these can be grouped in decreasing order of frequency as postoperative arterial thrombosis and embolization, cerebral ischemia during carotid clamping, and intracerebral hemorrhage.[44] Perioperative carotid arterial thrombosis most often results from technical imperfections in the performance of the operation, such as intimal disruption during the placement of the intraluminal shunt, residual intimal flaps or atheromatous disease, or residual luminal thrombus.[44] Completion imaging studies such as duplex scanning or arteriography may be performed to confirm the technical adequacy of the reconstruction.

BOX 38-1 Causes of Perioperative Stroke and Transient Ischemic Attack

Ischemia during carotid clamping
Thrombosis of the operative site
Embolization
Intracerebral hemorrhage
Unknown mechanisms

Auscultation with a continuous wave Doppler, although more subjective, will also identify some cases of abnormal flow after the unclamping of the carotid artery.

Maximizing the chance for neurologic recovery is mostly dependent on the early recognition of the deficit and the immediate institution of proper therapy. Because not all deficits result from causes that are surgically correctable, an accurate diagnosis is critical to implementing appropriate therapy. Establishing the correct diagnosis depends on the time of the onset of symptoms with respect to the operative procedure in conjunction with selected noninvasive vascular laboratory or radiologic studies.

The patient undergoing CEA under general anesthesia should be awakened in the operating room immediately after closing the wound so that a neurologic examination can be performed. If a new focal central neurologic deficit is identified, the artery should be immediately reexplored. If acute thrombosis of the endarterectomy site is identified, a meticulous search for a technical defect (e.g., a distal intimal ledge) should be performed. Extending the endarterectomy, performing a patch angioplasty (if one was not initially carried out), or resecting the vessel and replacing it with a bypass graft are possible options, depending on the operative findings.

If at reexploration the vessel is found to be patent, the most likely explanation for the defect is either ischemia during carotid clamping or, much more likely, intraoperative embolization. The risk of intraoperative embolization can be minimized by the administration of aspirin preoperatively, minimizing vessel manipulation before clamping, and instituting an intravenous low-molecular-weight dextran drip at the completion of the procedure. Nevertheless, in a small minority of patients, excessive platelet deposition may occur acutely on the endarterectomized artery, thus predisposing the patient to distal embolization or even acute thrombosis of the vessel. In either case, the author would favor the resection of the endarterectomy segment and graft replacement. Conversely, if the vessel appears normal at reexploration, which suggests that the patient experienced either embolization during vessel dissection before clamping or ischemia during clamping, the treatment is medical: close attention must be paid to hemodynamic monitoring and blood pressure stability postoperatively.

The likelihood of the patient sustaining a neurologic insult as a result of ischemia during carotid clamping may be minimized with the placement of an intraluminal shunt during the endarterectomy procedure. It is the author's personal bias to perform the operation with the routine use of a shunt, although others advocate selective shunting. Some perform the operation under local anesthesia so that the patient's neurologic course may be monitored in the awake state and thus help determine the need for shunt placement.[45] Others advocate using continuous electroencephalographic monitoring intraoperatively to determine the need for shunt placement.[46] Alternatively, the level of internal carotid artery back pressure is a reasonable measure of collateral cerebral blood flow during carotid clamping. A minimum back pressure of 25 mm Hg in the patient without prior ipsilateral cerebral infarction is considered sufficient to obviate the need for shunt placement.[43]

If the patient awakens neurologically intact in the operating room and then develops a new deficit in the recovery room or later postoperatively, the differential diagnosis is more complex. Initially the patient should undergo noninvasive vascular laboratory testing with duplex ultrasound if it can be rapidly obtained. If this testing indicates an occlusion of the vessel or abnormal flow velocities that are suggestive of an intimal flap or of another anatomic deficit, the patient should be immediately taken to the operating room for reexploration. Timing is crucial, because most neurologic deficits are significantly reversible if flow is restored within 1 to 2 hours after vessel thrombosis. If the noninvasive studies are negative, which suggests a patent vessel, a head computed tomography (CT) scan should be immediately performed to rule out a cerebral hemorrhage. If this is also negative, carotid angiography should be performed to identify any technical defect requiring revision at the operative site.

The availability of intracerebral catheter-directed thrombolysis has provided another option for neurologic salvage in the patient who experiences an embolic event associated with carotid endarterectomy. A report from the Johns Hopkins Hospital documented the first successful case of immediate postoperative thrombolytic therapy using urokinase for a patient who underwent CEA for a high-grade stenosis with an angiographically documented fresh intraluminal thrombus and who awakened with hemiplegia and aphasia.[47] An embolus to the middle cerebral artery was confirmed on postoperative arteriography, and the patient underwent lysis with catheter-directed administration of 500,000 units of urokinase, with complete neurologic recovery. Others have reported the administration of thrombolytic therapy intraoperatively for CEA complicated by cerebral embolism.[48,49]

Although a head CT scan may not have sufficient sensitivity to identify a very early stroke, it should be performed to rule out an intracerebral hemorrhage. This cause of postoperative stroke usually occurs several days after CEA. It is often associated with severe hypertension, and the acute neurologic deficit is often preceded by severe headache. In essence, intracerebral hemorrhage represents the most devastating manifestation of the hyperperfusion syndrome that can occur after CEA, and it is clearly the most devastating cause of stroke. The

reported incidence of cerebral hyperperfusion syndrome ranges from 0.4% to 7.7% after CEA.[50,51] This complication is now also being recognized after CAS procedures.[52,53] Symptoms include a migraine-like headache that progresses to seizures and that, in its most severe manifestation, results in an intracerebral hemorrhagic stroke. Although this is an uncommon complication of CEA and CAS, it conveys a very high mortality rate that approaches 75% to 100% in some series.[54,55] The cause of the hyperperfusion syndrome appears to be increased regional cerebral blood flow after the relief of a high-grade carotid stenosis in the setting of severe contralateral carotid disease caused by disordered intracerebral autoregulation.[52] The recognition of the patient who is at increased risk of intracerebral hemorrhage after CEA is much easier than its prevention. Systemic hypertension appears to be an important risk factor. Therefore strict attention to postoperative blood pressure control, especially in the patient who undergoes CEA of a high-grade stenosis contralateral to a compete internal carotid artery occlusion or severe stenosis, is paramount. There may be some association with the use of anticoagulants and antiplatelet agents, but this evidence is speculative at best. If a cerebral hemorrhage is diagnosed, neurosurgical consultation is required to determine the necessity of craniotomy.

Despite the increased sensitivity of diagnostic modalities in contemporary practice, in at least 20% of patients who experience stroke, the precise cause may not be identified (see Box 37-1). In many of these cases, even if the CT scan does not confirm a cerebral infarct, embolization from a cardiac source or another source may be responsible. In this situation, even if a cardiac ultrasound does not reveal thrombus, formal anticoagulation is indicated. In most cases, excellent neurologic recovery can be anticipated.

BLOOD-PRESSURE INSTABILITY

Incidence and Cause

The most common medical problem seen after carotid surgery is systemic blood-pressure instability. Sporadic episodes of severe hypotension, hypertension, or both occur in 19% to 66% of patients after CEA,[56–60] and postoperative myocardial infarction and stroke occur much more commonly among patients who experience these blood-pressure fluctuations.[35,58]

Hypotension usually occurs within the first 2 hours after CEA; it is usually associated with a bradycardia, and it most likely results from disordered baroreceptor function.[59–61] The carotid sinus baroreceptors, which are located in the outer muscle layer of the vessel at the carotid bifurcation, transmit impulses through the carotid sinus nerve to the vasomotor center within the medulla. Carotid sinus stimulation inhibits central nervous system sympathetic activity with a subsequent reduction in heart rate and blood pressure.[56,62,63] Considerable evidence suggests that endarterectomy of the fixed atheromatous plaque at the bifurcation, with its chronic dampening effect on the pulse pressure, creates a heightened sensitivity of the baroreceptor mechanism that results in reduced central nervous system sympathetic activity and thus hypotension, bradycardia, or both.[59,61,64,65] This theory is supported by the clinical observation that the injection of the carotid sinus with local anesthetic reduces the incidence of this complication.[61] This reflex hypotension persists until the carotid sinus mechanism has been reset.[56] Others have suggested that preoperative hypovolemia may be responsible in some cases.[64] Recent evidence suggests that patients with significant contralateral carotid disease have a reduced baroreceptor reserve and therefore manifest more pronounced baroreceptor dysfunction and hemodynamic lability after CEA.[65]

Although the development of hypertension after CEA is closely correlated with preoperative (especially poorly controlled) hypertension, its mechanism remains poorly understood.[57] Baroreceptor dysfunction as a result of the enervation of the carotid bulb has commonly been assumed to be responsible,[66] although considerable evidence is accumulating to refute this hypothesis.[57,61] The association between preoperative hypertension and severe hypertensive episodes after CEA suggests that other possible mechanisms, including elevated cerebral norepinerphrine[67] or renin production,[68] may be responsible. In at least 80% of patients, this hypertensive response normalizes within the first 24 hours after surgery; in approximately 60% of patients, it returns to normal within the first 16 hours after surgery.[37]

Treatment

The episodic and generally unpredictable nature of hypotension, hypertension, or both after CEA is one of the more cogent reasons for observing the patient in a monitored unit. This should at least be done initially, with an indwelling radial artery catheter provided for systemic blood-pressure measurement. Hypotension should first be treated with infusions of colloid solutions. When normovolemia has been achieved, if relative hypotension persists, the author favors supporting the blood pressure with an intravenous infusion of neosynephrine, which is an α-adrenergic agent. The dosage should be adjusted to maintain the systolic blood pressure within at least 20 mm Hg of the preoperative level. In almost all cases, the patient may be weaned off of this vasoconstricting agent during the first postoperative day.

Conversely, it is the author's opinion that postoperative hypertension is most effectively and safely treated with intravenous sodium nitroprusside, which is a direct relaxer of arterial smooth muscle. Its effect is immediate, and it is quickly dissipated by stopping the infusion, thus making it an ideal agent to use after CEA, when abrupt blood-pressure fluctuations often occur. The agent should be titrated to maintain the systolic pressure within 20 mm Hg of the preoperative level to avoid sudden marked pressure drops. If myocardial ischemia is associated with these hypertensive episodes, intravenous nitroglycerin should also be administered. Most patients are able to resume their preoperative oral antihypertensive agents on the evening of surgery or within the next 12 hours, and this often obviates the need for further and more prolonged intravenous therapy.

CRANIAL NERVE DYSFUNCTION

Incidence

Cranial nerve dysfunction is the most common neurologic complication of CEA, and it is clearly one of the more troublesome for many patients. The incidence of the postoperative dysfunction of cranial nerves range from 5% to 19.8% in several retrospective series, and a variety of nerves may be affected[12,43,69-79] (Table 38-1). The wide discrepancy in the incidence of this complication is a reflection of how aggressively various authors have attempted to document it in their patients, because many deficits may not be easily discernable on routine physical examinations. In other words, retrospective reviews, which constitute much of the published literature in this area, may significantly underestimate the true incidence of cranial nerve dysfunction after CEA. In a prospective study of patients undergoing 450 CEA procedures who also underwent postoperative otolaryngology examinations, 72 cranial nerve injuries were identified in 60 (13%) patients. Approximately one third of the patients with documented deficits were asymptomatic and would have been missed by cursory clinical examination.[72] In another prospective study of 139 patients who underwent 169 CEA procedures and

TABLE 38-1 Incidence of Cranial Nerve Dysfunction After Carotid Endarterectomy[12,70-77]

Nerve	Reported Incidence (%)
Hypoglossal	4.4–17.5
Recurrent laryngeal	1.5–15
Superior laryngeal	1.8–4.5
Marginal mandibular	1.1–3.1
Glossopharyngeal	0.2–1.5
Spinal accessory	<1.0

in which formal evaluations were performed preoperatively and postoperatively, cranial nerve injury was documented after 19.8% of the operations. This reflected a much higher incidence of nerve injury as compared with the results of a retrospective analysis from this institution.[73] In a more recent prospective study of 183 consecutive CEAs, 26 (14.2%) cranial nerve injuries were identified in 26 patients.[74] In another prospective study of this problem, Evans and colleagues[75] reported a 16% incidence of cranial nerve dysfunction after 128 CEA procedures performed on 116 patients on the basis of clinical examinations. When the patients underwent formal testing and examination by speech–language pathologists, however, the incidence of deficits rose to 39%. Most of these deficits were uncovered by a more detailed evaluation of laryngeal nerve function.

Anatomic and Clinical Considerations

Iatrogenic injury to the cranial nerves and their branches results from the close anatomic proximity of these structures to the carotid bifurcation (Figure 38-1). Most deficits are caused by direct blunt injury during the dissection, stretch trauma from excessive retraction, electrocoagulation damage, inexact ligature placement, or pressure injury as a result of postoperative hematoma

formation. Cranial nerve injury is much more likely during reoperative surgery as a result of excessive scar formation.[43] In one recent detailed analysis, the incidence of cranial nerve dysfunction correlated with the duration of operation. Specifically, there was a significantly higher incidence of nerve injury when the duration of the CEA exceeded 2 hours.[76]

In the vast majority of cases, the clinical deficit is transient, with complete resolution noted within weeks to months after the procedure. In one prospective study, all injuries resolved within 5 months.[76] In another prospective study, almost all nerve deficits resolved with 12 months after CEA, although it was noted that two patients with recurrent laryngeal nerve dysfunction regained normal function at 20 and 50 months after the CEA, respectively.[74] On the basis of a review of the outcomes of the European Carotid Surgery Trial randomized prospective investigation, it was noted that the risk of permanent nerve injury was 0.5%.[76] In another report, the incidence of permanent cranial nerve injury was only 1.1%.[74]

The disability resulting from cranial nerve injury varies from minimal to severe, depending on the nerve involved and the mechanism of operative insult. Hypoglossal

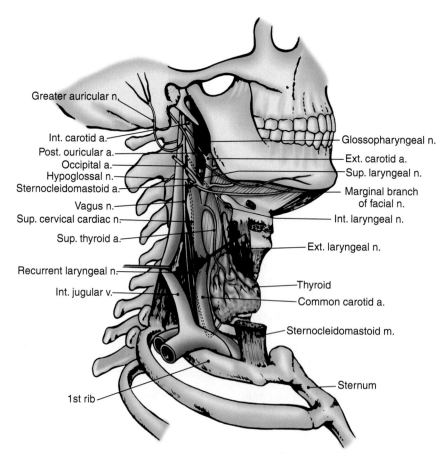

Figure 38-1. The relationship of cranial nerves and their major branches to the common, internal, and external carotid arteries in the neck. (From Bernhard VM, Towne JB, editors: *Complications in vascular surgery,* New York, 1980, Grune & Stratton. Printed with author permission.)

nerve dysfunction, which is manifested by ipsilateral tongue weakness and deviation to the affected side with protrusion and difficulty with mastication, is the most common cranial nerve deficit documented in most reports (see Table 38-1). The structure descends from the hypoglossal canal (anterior condylar foramen) medial to the internal carotid artery and then courses lateral to the external carotid artery, usually several centimeters distal to the carotid bifurcation, although in rare cases it may cross at the carotid bifurcation.[71] In this situation, in the patient with an unusually high carotid bifurcation or if the atheromatous plaque extends well past the origin of the internal carotid artery, cephalad mobilization of the nerve is usually required for adequate operative exposure. In most cases, this mobilization can be safely accomplished by the division of the ansa hypoglossi, without morbidity. In other cases, the division of the tethering branches of the external carotid artery or the internal jugular vein is required, thus increasing the likelihood of transient injury. Although unilateral hypoglossal nerve injury is rarely serious, bilateral deficits have been associated with serious articulation and swallowing difficulties as well as upper-airway obstruction requiring tracheotomy.[70] Therefore it is important to assess the functional integrity of this nerve after CEA in the patient who is scheduled for early contralateral CEA.[36]

The vagus nerve is easily identified within the carotid sheath posterior to the common carotid artery (see Figure 38-1), although, in the occasional patient, it may lie anterior to the carotid and be mistaken for the ansa hypoglossi. Before the division of the latter structure, therefore, the vagus nerve should first be clearly identified. The recurrent laryngeal branch usually originates from the vagus within the mediastinum, looping around the subclavian artery on the right or the aortic arch on the left side and passing cephalad in the tracheoesophageal groove. In most cases, this nerve is not in close proximity to the operative field and not likely to be directly injured. Typically recurrent laryngeal nerve dysfunction results from vagus nerve trauma. In rare cases, the recurrent laryngeal nerve arises from the vagus nerve at the level of the carotid bifurcation (the so-called "nonrecurrent" recurrent laryngeal nerve) and enters the larynx posterior to the common carotid artery. Careful arterial dissection and clamp application should minimize the likelihood of vagus or recurrent laryngeal nerve injury, which results in paralysis of the ipsilateral vocal cord in the paramedian position and is manifested by hoarseness and the loss of an effective cough mechanism. In the occasional patient, the vagus and hypoglossal nerves will be in apposition in the upper portion of the operative field, and no effort should be made to separate these structures to minimize the risk of injury. Every patient undergoing CEA should have a careful examination of vocal-cord function performed, especially if there has been previous contralateral carotid, thyroid, or parathyroid surgery, because

bilateral vocal-cord paralysis may cause postoperative airway obstruction.

The superior laryngeal nerve originates from the vagus near the jugular foramen and passes obliquely to the larynx posterior to the external and internal carotid arteries, where it divides into internal and external branches (see Figure 38-1). It usually is not visualized during routine dissection during CEA, and it may be injured by the injudicious clamping of the internal or external carotid arteries. Injury to the external branch of the superior laryngeal nerve primarily results in a loss of tensioning of the ipsilateral vocal cord, and it may be manifested clinically by the early fatigability of the voice and difficulty with voice modulation in the high registers. Conversely, injury to the internal branch may result in decreased sensation at the laryngeal inlet and mild swallowing difficulty.[74]

Injury to the marginal mandibular branch of the facial nerve causes the impairment of lower-lip depression. This may be cosmetically bothersome to the patient. This nerve courses from the anterior border of the parotid gland between the platysma and the deep cervical fascia across the masseter muscle and the ramus of the mandible. It may be drawn into the operative field as the patient's head is turned to the opposite side and the chin is extended for exposure of the carotid bifurcation. Injury is usually the result of excessive stretch from self-retaining retractors in a transverse cervical incision. When a longitudinal incision is employed for CEA, angling the superior aspect of the incision posteriorly toward the mastoid process below the angle of the mandible will minimize the risk of injury to the nerve.[69]

Injury to the glossopharyngeal and spinal accessory nerves is exceedingly uncommon during CEA as a result of their anatomic location at the upper extent of the operative field (see Figure 38-1). In rare cases in which excessive mobilization or division of the digastric muscle is required for distal internal carotid exposure, however, either nerve may be encountered and traumatized. The glossopharyngeal nerve provides sensory and motor innervation to the larynx. Symptoms of glossopharyngeal nerve injury range from mild dysphasia to recurrent aspiration.[74,77]

The spinal accessory nerve exits the jugular foramen and runs posterior to the stylohoid muscle, and it enters the most cephalad extent of the sternocleidomastoid muscle. Injury is manifested by shoulder droop and pain, scapular winging, and difficulty with abducting the shoulder as a result of weakness of the trapezius muscle.[74,78]

Two important cutaneous sensory nerves that are frequently injured during the performance of CEA are the greater auricular and transverse cervical nerves. In one prospective study, the incidence of greater auricular and transverse cervical nerve injury was 60% and 69%, respectively, 1 week after CEA.[80] The greater auricular nerve courses along the most superior area of the typical CEA longitudinal incision, and the transverse cervical nerve travels along the most inferior area of this incision. Injury to the greater auricular nerve is manifested by numbness of the face near the angle of the mandible and the lower ear.

WOUND COMPLICATIONS

Infections

Unlike most peripheral vascular reconstructive procedures in which chronic ischemia compromises wound healing and predisposes the patient to infection, the vascular supply to the neck is rich, even in the patient with severe atherosclerotic disease. Therefore CEA is rarely associated with infectious complications. Difficulty with primary healing occasionally is seen when this operation is performed in a previously radiated field, but it is almost nonexistent in the absence of this complicating factor.[43] The reported incidence of wound infection (generally cellulitis) ranges from 0.09% to 0.15%.[66,81]

The increasing use of patches and in many cases synthetic materials to repair the arteriotomy after CEA raises concern about an increased incidence of infectious complications. Although the true incidence of patch infection has not been established, it is extremely unusual and essentially a case report type of complication. In several recent studies, not a single case of patch infection was documented.[81-83] In another comprehensive review of the literature, 57 carotid pseudoaneurysms were identified, and 40 were associated with carotid patches. However, only four (10%) carotid pseudoaneurysms were attributed to an infectious cause.[84]

Although the benefit of perioperative antibiotics has not been conclusively demonstrated in the patient population undergoing CEA and although this is typically a relatively short and clean operative procedure, the seriousness of arterial infection in this clinical setting is such that perioperative prophylactic antibiotics should be administered. In a recent review of eight patients who presented with infected carotid patch pseudoaneurysms, it is interesting to note that none had received perioperative antibiotics.[85] Because *Staphylococcus* species have been most often identified in carotid patch infections, a broad-spectrum antibiotic (e.g., cephalosporin) should be administered.[86] The patient should receive a dose before the skin incision, and he or she should receive at least two more doses during the postoperative period. The topical irrigation of the wound with an antibiotic solution is also helpful to remove any devitalized tissue from the operative site before wound closure. Likewise, because these patients are typically systemically anticoagulated with heparin

intraoperatively and in most cases managed with antiplatelet therapy postoperatively, the author favors closure of the incision over a closed suction drain to minimize the likelihood of postoperative hematoma formation, which also can predispose the patient to infection.

The diagnosis of a patch infection or infected pseudoaneurysm should be suspected in the patient who presents with erythema, tenderness, and swelling of the neck after CEA. A carotid duplex ultrasound examination should be performed to assess for the presence of a pseudoaneurysm, fluid or gas around the patch and vessels, and generally poor tissue incorporation. In the elective setting and in the absence of active bleeding, an arteriogram should be performed to plan operative intervention. Adequate proximal and distal exposure should be obtained, and one must be prepared to perform mandibular subluxation to expedite distal vascular control. As in the management of arterial infection at other anatomic sites, the complete excision of the infected patch and the adjacent tissues is mandatory, along with extensive surrounding soft-tissue debridement. Arterial reconstruction should be performed with autogenous tissue, typically with the use of the saphenous vein. Coverage of the repair site with a rotational muscle flap is another adjunct to help eradicate residual pockets of infection and to achieve secure would closure.[87,88] Although the duration of therapy is not well established, at least 3 to 6 weeks of organism-specific antibiotic administration seems reasonable on the basis of reported experience.[89]

Bleeding

Postoperative hemorrhage is a very uncommon yet important complication of CEA. The reported incidence ranges from 0.7% to 3.0%.[11,64,90-93] Most cases result from diffuse capillary oozing caused by the systemic anticoagulation achieved with heparin during the procedure and the concomitant administration of antiplatelet drugs. Although not systematically studied, at least anecdotally this degree of oozing appears to be higher among patients who are taking the antiplatelet agent clopidogrel at the time of surgery. Nevertheless, if there are strong indications for the administration of this agent (e.g., a recent coronary stent procedure, symptomatic carotid disease), the author recommends not stopping the agent before surgery. In general, unless bleeding appears excessive at operation, the author does not favor the reversal of the heparin effect with protamine sulfate at the completion of the procedure. The neck incision should be closed over a suction drain. The acute onset of bright red blood drainage output postoperatively is suggestive of suture line disruption, and it is an indication for urgent reexploration. Similarly, the development of a hematoma in the neck, which is often the result of inadequate function of the drain, may cause airway obstruction, and it is an indication for reexploration of the wound. The gradual development of a neck hematoma usually results from the inadequate ligature of the facial vein or of other muscle arterioles or venules.[43]

RECURRENT CAROTID STENOSIS

One of the more important arterial complications of a CEA is the development of recurrent carotid stenosis. The incidence of this complication depends on the definition of a recurrent stenosis, the method of diagnosis, and the duration of follow up. It has been estimated to occur in 5% to 22% of patients in several published individual institutional series, although only approximately 3% of these lesions are symptomatic.[94–98] In a meta-analysis of 55 reports, the overall incidence of recurrent carotid stenosis after CEA was 6% to 14%, which reflected an annual incidence of restenosis or occlusion of 1.5% to 4.5%.[99] In another analysis of the Medline database, the rate of restenosis was 10% within the first year, 3% during the second year, and 2% during the third year after CEA, which suggests that the rate of restenosis is clearly not a linear process biologically.[100] Within the first 36 months after CEA, recurrent stenosis usually results from intimal hyperplasia. Evidence from serial duplex evaluations suggests that at least some of these lesions regress with time. This may in part be responsible for some variability in the reported rates of recurrent stenosis. An occasional "recurrent" stenosis in fact represents residual arteriosclerotic disease after the endarterectomy. Lesions that develop more than a few years after CEA usually result from progressive or new arteriosclerotic disease.

Recurrent stenoses develop more often among women, patients who continue to smoke, diabetic patients, hypertensive patients, and patients with hypercholesterolemia.[98] Female gender appears to be a particular risk factor for early recurrent stenoses.[94] It has also been suggested that intraoperative injury as a result of arterial clamping, the placement of an intraluminal shunt, or the placement of tacking sutures within the vessel may also predispose patients to early myointimal hyperplasia lesions.[95]

There is growing evidence that the closure of the carotid arteriotomy at the initial operation as a patch angioplasty may reduce the incidence of recurrent stenoses.[101–104] In a randomized prospective clinical trial that included 399 patients, the incidence of long-term recurrent stenosis or occlusion after CEA was 34% with primary closure, 9% with vein patching, and 2% with a polytetrafluoroethylene patch.[105] There is no compelling evidence to support the use of autogenous vein as opposed to synthetic patch material. In a recent Cochrane review, there did not appear to be superiority for one synthetic patch material as compared with another.[106]

The issue of reoperation for recurrent carotid stenosis is unsettled. Although it has been assumed by most that the long-term risk of stroke is lower than it is among patients with primary carotid lesions, at least one recent report has challenged that.[107] There have been no randomized prospective clinical trials assessing conservative medical management as compared with reintervention for patients with recurrent stenoses. Furthermore, the long-term risk of stroke among patients with recurrent stenoses is not well established. Clearly one can reasonably assume that early recurrent stenoses caused by myointimal hyperplasia appear to be much more benign than later lesions caused by atherosclerotic disease. Therefore, in contemporary practice, the indications for reoperation depend on the timing of the presentation and the suspected pathologic lesion. Within the first 2 to 3 years after CEA, when intimal hyperplasia is most likely, patients should be followed with serial duplex scans if they are asymptomatic; operation should be reserved for symptomatic patients. When recurrent disease develops later (usually as a result of arteriosclerosis), reoperation should be performed on symptomatic patients or on those with high-grade (i.e., >80%) asymptomatic stenoses.

If recurrent disease develops in an unpatched vessel, the lesion can usually be treated with patch angioplasty. Alternatively, if recurrent disease develops in an artery that was previously patched, the author favors resecting the disease segment and placing an interposition bypass graft. Recent experience suggests that the risks of perioperative stroke and death among patients undergoing reoperative CEA for recurrent stenoses are comparable with the results of primary operative procedures.[95,108,109] Furthermore, long-term stroke-free survival rates appear to be comparable for operations performed for both primary and recurrent stenoses.[95] For example, in a recent series of 153 reoperative CEAs performed on 145 patients, the perioperative stroke rate was 1.9%, and there was no operative mortality.[110] Alternatively, the incidence of cranial nerve injury appears to be higher among patients undergoing reoperative CEA.[95] At the same time, recurrent carotid stenoses may be treated with endovascular techniques. Early experience suggests acceptable results of percutaneous angioplasty and stenting for recurrent carotid stenoses as compared with reoperative open procedures.[111,112] A major advantage of endovascular therapy is the avoidance of cranial nerve injury, although long-term results are not yet available.

CAROTID ENDARTERECTOMY AFTER RADIATION THERAPY

Experimental studies in a number of animal models have demonstrated that external-beam radiation therapy produces an arterial lesion that is pathologically similar to human arteriosclerosis[113–115] and that, in man, obliterative arterial lesions that result from therapeutic radiation therapy have been described in a variety of anatomic sites.[116,117] Within the extracranial arterial circulation, the carotid artery has been most commonly involved, as a result of either the predisposition of arteriosclerosis to occur at the carotid bifurcation or of the frequency with which radiation therapy is delivered to the jugular chain of lymph nodes.[116,118] Carotid occlusive lesions caused by radiation injury tend to be quite focal; they usually occur in atypical locations, such as in the proximal or mid common carotid artery, and often there is no evidence of occlusive disease in the other vessels. Conversely, classic arteriosclerotic lesions may be more diffuse, and they almost always occur at the carotid bifurcation, with the involvement of the internal and external carotid arteries.[119]

Furthermore, severe periarterial fibrosis is invariably noted at operation in the patient who has previously received radiation therapy. The dissection and mobilization of the involved vessels and the identification of adjacent cranial nerves and their branches is more difficult, thus increasing the risk of iatrogenic nerve injury, although the precise incidence of cranial nerve injury associated with carotid endarterectomy in the previously irradiated patient has not been well defined. Although the relief of the carotid obstruction can be achieved in most patients with radiation-induced carotid lesions by conventional endarterectomy, separation of the plaque from the underlying arterial media is usually more difficult.[116,118,120] When the fibrotic process is so severe that endarterectomy does not appear to be feasible, a patch angioplasty may be performed to restore an adequate arterial lumen. Alternatively, the involved segment of the vessel may be resected and an interposition bypass graft performed, ideally with the proximal and distal anastomoses placed outside of the irradiated field. Because irradiated tissues typically manifest poor healing characteristics, wound breakdown, infection, or both occur at least twice as often than when carotid artery surgery is performed without prior radiation therapy.[43] In the most difficult cases, wound closure with a rotational muscle flap is a reasonable option.

In the light of these anatomic considerations, it has been assumed that CEA is a more risky procedure when it is performed on a patient after previous radiation therapy. Perhaps this patient population would be better served by undergoing CAS. However, recent experience suggests that, in the hands of experienced operators, CEA can be performed with acceptable results in this patient population.[121] For example, in a series of 11 patients undergoing CEA after neck irradiation, there were no perioperative deaths or strokes.[122] In another recent series, 24 patients underwent 26 CEA procedures at a mean follow up of 17 years after neck irradiation, with no perioperative strokes or deaths. However, cranial nerve injury occurred in six patients, and wound infections occurred in two patients.[122] In other words, although perioperative stroke and deaths rates may be comparable to the outcomes of patients undergoing CEA in the absence of previous neck irradiation, local complication rates can be expected to be higher.[121,122] Alternatively, long-term stroke prevention appears to be comparable to what has been reported among patients who have not undergone previous irradiation therapy.[122]

CAROTID ANGIOPLASTY AND STENTING

The treatment of carotid artery disease is clearly evolving with the introduction of CAS. This endovascular approach to the treatment of this patient population is still in the investigational stage, and most studies have assessed the management of patients deemed to be at high risk for CEA. Most attention has been focused on the major complications of CAS: periprocedural stroke and death. In a review of six major industry-sponsored trials and registries of CAS, the periprocedural stroke and death rates ranged from 3.8% to 7.8%.[123] In 2004, the U.S. Food and Drug Administration approved CAS for the management of high-risk CEA patients on the basis of the results of the ACCULINK for Revascularization of Carotids in High Risk patients (ARCHeR) registry. Among the 581 patients enrolled in this investigation, the 30-day combined stroke and death rate was 6.9%, including 5.4% among patients with asymptomatic carotid disease and 11.6% among patients with symptomatic carotid disease.[124] Advanced age appears to be a particular risk factor for periprocedural stroke among patients undergoing CAS, and the rate of complications appears to be especially high among octogenarians. For example, in the Carotid Endarterectomy versus Stent Trial of CAS versus CEA, which was sponsored by the National Institutes of Health, the 30-day stroke rates were as follows[125]:

- 1.7% for patients less than 60 years old
- 1.3% for patients between the ages of 60 and 69 years
- 5.3% for patients between the ages of 70 and 79 years
- 12.1% for patients 80 years old and older

A purported advantage of CAS as compared with CEA is a reduction in the rate of myocardial ischemia in this patient population. However, myocardial ischemia does complicate CAS procedures. For example, in the ARCHeR trial, the 30-day rate of myocardial infarction was 2.5%, and the 30-day combined stroke/death/myocardial infarction rate was 8.3%.[124] In fact, hemodynamic lability occurs often in association with CAS and likely results from the stretching of the carotid sinus and the periadventitial baroreceptors.[126,127] In one recent series of 327 patients undergoing CAS, symptomatic hypotension occurred in 4.9% of patients.[126] In another report, a reduction of systemic blood pressure of at least 40 mm Hg was noted in 50% of patients undergoing CAS.[128] Bradycardia appeared to be a very common problem, at least in the earlier experience with CAS; it was noted in 71% of cases in one report.[129] More recently this has occurred less often as a result of the use of self-expanding stents and the judicious administration of atropine intraprocedurally.[126]

As noted previously, one of the most devastating (albeit uncommon) complications of CEA is intracerebral hemorrhage. This phenomenon is also being seen among patients who undergo CAS. In fact, it has been suggested that the incidence may be greater after CAS than after CEA.[52,53] In the largest series reported to date, the incidence of cerebral hyperperfusion was 1.1% and the incidence of intracranial hemorrhage was 0.67% after CAS.[52] Other reports have documented an incidence of intracranial hemorrhage in 1.4% and 2.3% of cases, respectively.[130,131] The pathophysiologic mechanism and the poor clinical prognosis of intracranial hemorrhage after CAS appear to be the same as after CEA.[52,53]

CAROTID BODY TUMORS

Carotid body tumors are relatively uncommon neoplasms that arise from chemoreceptor tissue located on the posterior aspect of the carotid bifurcation. The natural history of this lesion is one of slow growth with local invasion, potentially causing cranial nerve dysfunction or upper-airway obstruction. This course as well as the difficulty with differentiating malignant from benign lesions, even by histologic examination, mandates complete surgical excision in all patients, unless advanced age or other medical conditions contraindicate treatment. However, the extreme vascularity of these lesions and their dense adherence to the carotid arteries make surgical excision a more demanding technical challenge than routine CEA and are responsible for higher complication rates than are seen after CEA.

The incidence of complications associated with the excision of carotid body tumors is closely correlated with the size of the tumor and the degree of arterial invasion, which is best described by the Shamblin classification.[132-134] A type I tumor is small, localized, and easily separated from the adjacent artery wall. Type II lesions are larger, adherent to the artery, and partially encapsulate the vessel. Type III lesions are densely adherent to and intimately surround the carotid arteries.[133] Whereas type I lesions are easily dissected from the artery, type II lesions usually require so-called subadventitial dissection, and many type III lesions will require arterial excision and reconstruction.[134,135]

In the workup of the patient with a carotid body tumor, arteriography has been the gold standard diagnostic tool. It will provide precise information with respect to tumor size, anatomic location, and encroachment on vascular structures, and it can assess for the presence of atherosclerotic disease, which may complicate vascular reconstruction if this becomes necessary at the time of tumor resection.[136] CT scans have been increasingly used to evaluate carotid body tumors, particularly small lesions. CT scanning with intravenous contrast administration is very helpful for defining the size of the tumor and its anatomic location.[135] Magnetic resonance angiography is a relatively noninvasive alternative to formal contrast angiography for the evaluation of these patients.[136] In the light of these alternative diagnostic modalities, some have reserved contrast arteriography for larger tumors.[137]

The role of preoperative selective tumor embolization remains controversial. It is felt by many that selective embolization reduces intraoperative blood loss and reduces the complexity of the resection.[138-141] Alternatively, others believe that the modest benefit in terms of reduced intraoperative blood loss does not justify the risk of stroke that is associated with angiography.[142,143] In contemporary practice, selective tumor embolization is reserved for patients with large tumors.[137]

The technical details of carotid body tumor resection have clearly been refined during recent years. Although it is often stated that the tumor resection should be carried out in a "subadventitial" plane, in fact the dissection should be carried out along a plane between the tumor and the adventitia to protect the integrity of the underlying artery.[144] Loupe magnification can be very helpful for identifying small feeding blood vessels to minimize blood loss. Likewise, the bipolar cautery should be liberally used to develop the dissection plane.[138]

Improvements in preoperative imaging and the refinement of the technical details of tumor resection have resulted in a dramatic reduction in the risk associated with the operative excision of carotid body tumors. Today almost all carotid body tumors can be excised with negligible operative mortality and with a perioperative stroke rate of less than 3%.[144] In a report from the Johns Hopkins Hospital, 27 patients underwent carotid body tumor resection from 1990 through 2000, with no deaths and 1 stroke (4%).[145] Plukker and colleagues[136] reported a 30-year experience that included 35 patients who underwent the complete resection of 41 carotid body tumors with no operative mortality. In another report of 29 patients who underwent the resection of 34 carotid body tumors during a 30-year interval, there was 1 death (3%) as a result of a pulmonary embolism, and there were no strokes.[135] In a very recent series that included 25 patients who underwent carotid body tumor resection, there were no deaths and no permanent neurologic deficits.[137] The reduction in the incidence of central neurologic deficits during the last decade reflects an aggressive approach to vascular reconstruction in this clinical scenario. In the absence of arterial reconstruction, stroke rates have approached 30%, whereas today the incidence of stroke is approximately 1% with arterial reconstruction.[137]

The most common surgical complication continues to be cranial nerve injury, which occurs in 10% to 56% of patients who undergo surgical excision.[136,145–158] The most commonly involved nerves are the hypoglossal nerve, the superior laryngeal nerve, the vagus nerve, the mandibular branch of the facial nerve, the pharyngeal branch of the vagus nerve, the glossopharyngeal nerve, the spinal accessory nerve, and the sympathetic chain.[136]

Although some of these patients have a preoperative cranial nerve deficit, in the majority of cases neurologic morbidity results from a poor understanding of the anatomic course of neural structures, from the adherence or incorporation of the nerve in the tumor surface, or from suboptimal operative exposure in a bloody field as a result of the extreme vascularity of these lesions.[144] Clearly most cranial nerve injuries occur during the resection of bulky, extremely vascular carotid body tumors (i.e., Shamblin type II and III lesions). As previously noted, preoperative selective tumor embolization may reduce intraoperative blood loss, improve exposure, and lessen the risk of cranial nerve dysfunction in this patient population.[153–158]

QUALITY-OF-LIFE ISSUES

The influence of surgical procedures on the quality of life of patients is becoming an increasingly important concern in surgery, and head and neck surgical procedures are no exception. This is especially true among patients who undergo CEA. In addition to the potentially adverse impact of the procedure—like any surgical intervention—on the overall quality of life related to perioperative complications, pain, and the impact on functional ability, significant attention has been directed to the potential of this procedure to actually improve (or harm) the overall quality of life in this patient population with respect to overall cognitive function.

In a recent study, 109 patients underwent cognitive testing and quality-of-life assessment 1 week before and 6 months after CEA. In addition, transcranial Doppler examinations were carried out during the surgical procedure to detect the cerebral microembolization of atherosclerotic debris. The patients' self-reported health-related quality of life did not significantly deteriorate at 6 months after surgery. A minority of patients (25%) manifested some decline in cognitive functioning, but, surprisingly, this decline did not correlate with the degree of microembolization during surgery.[159] In another study, cognitive testing was performed on 44 patients who underwent CEA and compared with that of 18 medically treated patients at 8 to 11 years after presentation. No significant adverse impact of CEA was identified in the majority of patients. However, patients who underwent operation twice during this period were subjectively worse as compared with other subgroups.[160]

In fact, several investigations have suggested an improvement in quality of life related to improved cognitive functioning among patients who undergo CEA. In one study, 11 patients underwent intelligence and personality tests just before and 6 weeks after CEA, and increases in cognitive performance were documented after CEA.[161] In another report, 25 patients undergoing CEA underwent a series of neuropsychological tests 1 week before and 2 weeks and 8 months after CEA. This study demonstrated that CEA did not impair neuropsychological performance and that it was actually associated with some improvement in performance. There was also a slight improvement in quality of life.[162] In a more recent study, the quality of life was investigated with the Sickness Impact Profile among patients undergoing CEA. Preoperative testing revealed that the Sickness Impact Profile scores of stroke patients and shunted patients were higher than other patient subgroups, which reflects a poorer health-related quality of life, but there was no documented adverse impact of the operation on these patients. Improvement in health-related quality of life was documented only among patients who underwent CEA with a shunt, perhaps indicating more severe carotid disease.[163] Another study did not confirm an improvement in mental status or an increased sense of psychological well-being among patients who underwent CEA.[164] It is clear that there is considerable psychological influence on the perception of health-related quality of life among patients who undergo CEA. In a recent study of 50 patients undergoing CEA for symptomatic disease, there was considerable improvement in the patients' perception of their overall quality of life. Of relevance to the issues in this chapter is that patients who experienced postoperative complications did not manifest an improvement in their postoperative health scores.[165]

REFERENCES

1. Rutkow IM, Ernst CB: An analysis of vascular surgical manpower requirements and vascular surgical rates in the United States. *J Vasc Surg* 1986;3:74–83.
2. North American Symptomatic Carotid Endarterectomy Trial Collaborators: Beneficial effect of carotid endarterectomy in symptomatic patients with high grade carotid stenosis. *N Engl J Med* 1991;325:445–453.
3. Barnett HJ, Taylor DW, Eliasziw M, et al: Beneficial effect of carotid endarterectomy in patients with symptomatic moderate or

severe stenosis: North American symptomatic carotid endarterectomy trial collaborators. *N Engl J Med* 1998;339:1415–1425.

4. Executive Committee for the Asymptomatic Carotid Atherosclerosis Study: Endarterectomy for asymptomatic carotid artery stenosis. *JAMA* 1995;273:1421–1428.

5. MRC Asymptomatic Carotid Surgery Trial (ACST) Collaborative Group: Prevention of disabling and fatal strokes by successful carotid endarterectomy in patients without recent neurologic symptoms: Randomized clinical trial. *Lancet* 2004;363: 1491–1502.

6. Kazmers A, Cerqueira MD, Zierler RE: The role of preoperative radionuclide left ventricular ejection fraction for risk assessment in carotid surgery. *Arch Surg* 1988;416–419.

7. Hertzer NR, Lees CD: Fatal myocardial infarction following carotid endarterectomy. *Ann Surg* 1981;194:212–218.

8. O'Donnell TF, Callow AD, Willet C, et al: The impact of coronary artery disease on carotid endarterectomy. *Ann Surg* 1983;208:705–712.

9. Bernstein EF, Humber PB, Collins GM, et al: Life expectancy and late stroke following carotid endarterectomy. *Ann Surg* 1982;198:80–86.

10. Hertzer NR, Arison R: Cumulative stroke and survival ten years after carotid endarterectomy. *J Vasc Surg* 1985;2:661–668.

11. Nunn DB: Carotid endarterectomy: An analysis of 234 operative cases. *Ann Surg* 1975;182:733–738.

12. Deweese JA, Robb CG, Satran R, et al: Results of carotid endarterectomy of transient ischemic attacks: Five years later. *Ann Surg* 1973;178:258–264.

13. Hertzer NR, Loop FD, Taylor PC, et al: Staged and combined surgical approach for simultaneous carotid and coronary vascular disease. *Surgery* 1978;86:303–811.

14. Hertzer NR, Beven EG, Young JR, et al: Coronary artery disease in peripheral vascular patients: A classification of 1000 coronary angiograms and results of surgical management. *Ann Surg* 1983;199:223–233.

15. Whitney DG, Kahn EM, Estes JW, et al: Carotid artery surgery without an indwelling shunt: 1917 consecutive procedures. *Arch Surg* 1980;115:1393–1399.

16. Cranley JJ: Presidential address: Stroke—A perspective. *Surgery* 1982;91:537–549.

17. Peitzman AB, Webster MW, Loubeau JM, et al: Carotid endarterectomy under regional (conductive) anesthesia. *Ann Surg* 1982;196:59–64.

18. Whittemore AD, Kaufman JL, Kohler TR, et al: Routine electroencephalographic (EEG) monitoring during carotid endarterectomy. *Ann Surg* 1983;197:707–713.

19. Sachs SM, Fulewider JT, Smith RB III, et al: Does contralateral carotid occlusion influence neurologic fate of carotid endarterectomy? *Surgery* 1984;96:839–844.

20. Sundt TM Jr, Sharborough FW, Marsch WR, et al: The risk-benefit ratio of intra-operative shunting during carotid endarterectomy: Relevancy to operative and postoperative results and complications. *Ann Surg* 1986;203:196–204.

21. Hertzer NR, Beven EG, O'Hara PJ, et al: A perspective study of vein angioplasty during carotid endarterectomy: Three-year results for 801 patients and 917 operations. *Ann Surg* 1987;206: 628–635.

22. Brott T, Thalinger K: The practice of carotid endarterectomy in a large metropolitan area. *Stroke* 1984;15:950–955.

23. Slavish LG, Nicholas GG, Gee W: Review of a community hospital experience with carotid endarterectomy. *Stroke* 1984;15:956–959.

24. Caffereata HT, Gainey MD: Carotid endarterectomy in the community hospital: A continuing controversy. *J Cardiovas Surg* 1986;27:557–560.

25. Kempczinski RF, Brott TG, Labutta RJ: The influence of surgical specialty and caseload on the results of carotid endarterectomy. *J Vasc Surg* 1986;3:911–916.

26. Matsen SL, Change DC, Perler BA, et al: Trends in the in-hospital stroke rate following carotid endarterectomy in California and Maryland. *J Vasc Surg* 2006;44:889–895.

27. Cowan JA Jr, Dimick JB, Thompson BG, et al: Surgeon volume as an indicator of outcomes after carotid endarterectomy: An effect independent of specialty practice and hospital volume. *J Am Coll Surg* 2003;196:826–827.

28. Perler BA, Dardik A, Burleyson GP, et al: Influence of age and hospital volume on the results of carotid endarterectomy: A statewide analysis of 9918 cases. *J Vasc Surg* 1998;27:25–31.

29. McGirt MJ, Perler BA, Brooke BS, et al: 3-hydroxy-3-methylglutaryl coenzyme A reductase inhibitors reduce the risk of perioperative stroke and mortality after carotid endarterectomy. *J Vasc Surg* 2005;42:829–836.

30. LaMuraglia GM, Brewster DC, Moncure AC, et al: Carotid endarterectomy at the millennium: What interventional therapy must match. *Ann Surg* 2004;240:535–544.

31. Durand DJ, Perler BA, Roseborough GS et al: Mandatory versus selective preoperative carotid screening: A retrospective analysis. *Ann Thorac Surg* 2004;78:159–166.

32. Naylor R, Cuffe RL, Rothwell PM, et al: A systematic review of outcomes following staged and synchronous carotid endarterectomy and coronary artery bypass. *Eur J Vasc Endovasc Surg* 2003;25:380–389.

33. Poldermans D, Bax JJ, Schouten O, et al: Should major vascular surgery be delayed because of perioperative cardiac testing in intermediate-risk patients receiving beta-blocker therapy with tight heart rate control? *J Am Coll Cardiol* 2006;48:964–969.

34. Kertai MD, Klein J, Bax JJ, et al: Predicting perioperative cardiac risk. *Prog Cardiovasc Dis* 2005;47:240–257.

35. Rubin JR, Goldstone J, McIntyre KE Jr, et al: The value of carotid endarterectomy in reducing the morbidity and mortality of recurrent stroke. *J Vasc Surg* 1986;4:443–449.

36. Takolunder RJ, Bergentz S-E, Ericsson BF: Carotid artery surgery in patients with minor stroke. *Br J Surg* 1983;70:13–16.

37. Thompson JE: Don't throw out the baby with the bathwater: A perspective on carotid endarterectomy. *J Vasc Surg* 1986;4: 542–545.

38. Matsumoto N, Whisnant JP, Karland LT, et al: Natural history of stroke in Rochester, Minnesota, 1955-1969: An extension of a previous study, 1945-1954. *Stroke* 1973;4:20–29.

39. Imparato AM, Ramirez A, Riles T, et al: Cerebral protection in carotid surgery. *Arch Surg* 1982;117:1073–1078.

40. Hertzer NR: Presidential address: Carotid endarterectomy: A crisis in confidence. *J Vasc Surg* 1988;7:611–619.

41. Hertzer NR: Early complications of carotid endarterectomy: Incidence, diagnosis, and management. In More WS, editor: *Surgery for cerebrovascular disease,* New York, 1987, Churchill Livingstone.

42. Hertzer NR, Avellone JC, Farrell CJ, et al: The risk of carotid endarterectomy in a metropolitan community with observation on surgeon's experience and hospital size. *J Vasc Surg* 1984;1: 13–21.

43. Gelebart HA, Moore WS: Carotid endarterectomy: Current status. *Curr Probl Surg* 1991;3:183–192.

44. Riles TS, Imparato AM, Jacobwitz GR, et al: The cause of perioperative stroke after carotid endarterectomy. *J Vasc Surg* 1994;19:206–216.

45. Hafner CD, Evans W: Carotid endarterectomy with local anesthesia: Results and advantages. *J Vasc Surg* 1988;7:232–239.

46. Sundt TM, Sharbrough FW, Piepgras DG, et al: Correlation of cerebral blood flow and electroencephalographic changes during carotid endarterectomy. *Mayo Clinic Proc* 1981;56: 533–543.

47. Perler BA, Murphy K, Sternbach Y, et al: Immediate postoperative thrombolytic therapy: An aggressive strategy for neurologic salvage when cerebral thromboembolism complicates carotid endarterectomy. *J Vasc Surg* 2000;31:1033–1037.

48. Barr JD, Horowitz MB, Mathis JM, et al: Intraoperative urokinase infusion for embolic stroke during carotid endarterectomy. *Neurosurgery* 1995;36:606–611.

49. Comerota AJ, Eze AR: Intraoperative high dose regional urokinase infusion for cerebrovascular occlusion after carotid endarterectomy. *J Vasc Surg* 1996;24:1008–1016.

50. Ascher E, Markevich N, Schutzer RW, et al: Cerebral hyperperfusion syndrome after carotid endarterectomy: Predictive factors and hemodynamic changes. *J Vasc Surg* 2003;37:769–777.

51. Karapanayiotides T, Meuli R, Devuyst G, et al: Postcarotid endarterectomy hyperperfusion or reperfusion syndrome. *Stroke* 2005;36:21–26.

52. Abou-Chebyl A, Yadav JS, Reginelli JP, et al: Intracranial hemorrhage and hyperperfusion syndrome following carotid artery stenting: Risk factors, prevention, and treatment. *J Am Coll Cardiol* 2004;43:1596–1601.

53. Kaku Y, Yoshimura S, Kokuzawa J: Factors predictive of cerebral hyperperfusion after carotid angioplasty and stent placement. *Am J Neuroradiol* 2004;25:1403–1408.

54. Perler BA, Williams GM: Post-carotid endarterectomy intracerebral hemorrhage: A continuing challenge. *Vasc Surg* 1996;30:712–775.

55. Hafner DH, Smith RB, Perdue GD, et al: Massive intracerebral hemorrhage following carotid endarterectomy. *Arch Surg* 1987;122:248–255.

56. Bove EL, Fry WJ, Gross WS, et al: Hypotension and hypertension as consequences of baroreceptor dysfunction following carotid endarterectomy. *Surgery* 1979;25:633–637.

57. Towne JB, Bernard VM: The relationship of postoperative hypertension to complications following carotid endarterectomy. *Surgery* 1980;88:575–580.

58. Cafferata HT, Mercant RF Jr, DePalma RG: Avoidance of post carotid endarterectomy hypertension. *Ann Surg* 1982;196:465–472.

59. Pine R, Avellone JC, Hoffman M, et al: Control of post carotid endarterectomy hypotension with baroreceptor blockage. *Am J Surg* 1984;147:763–765.

60. Levs MS, Salzman WE, Silen W: Hypertension complication carotid endarterectomy. *Stroke* 1970;1:307–313.

61. Angell-James JE, Lumley JSP: The effects of carotid endarterectomy on the mechanical properties of the carotid sinus and carotid sinus nerve activity in atherosclerotic patients. *Br J Surg* 1974;61:805–810.

62. Scher AM: Carotid and aortic regulation of arterial blood pressure. *Circulation* 1977;56:521–527.

63. Wade JG, Larson CP Jr, Hickey RF, et al: Effect of carotid endarterectomy on carotid chemoreceptor and baroreceptor function in man. *N Engl J Med* 1970;282:823–829.

64. Ranson JHC, Imparato AM, Clauss RH, et al: Factors in the mortality and morbidity associated with surgical treatment of cerebrovascular insufficiency. *Circulation* 1969;39(5 Suppl I):I269–I274.

65. Thompson JE: Complications of carotid endarterectomy and their prevention. *J Vasc Surg* 1979;3:155–163.

66. Nouraei SAR, Al-Rawi PG, Sigaudo-Roussel D, et al: Carotid endarterectomy impairs blood pressure homeostasis by reducing the physiologic baroreceptor reserve. *J Vasc Surg* 2005;41:631–637.

67. Ahn SS, Marcus DR, Moore WS: Post-carotid endarterectomy hypertension: Association with elevated cranial norepinephrine. *J Vasc Surg* 1989;9:351–360.

68. Smith BL: Hypertension following carotid endartectomy: The role of cerebral rennin production. *J Vasc Surg* 1989;1:623–627.

69. Verta MJ, Applebaum EL, McCluskey DA, et al: Cranial nerve injury during carotid endarterectomy. *Ann Surg* 1977;185:192–195.

70. Hertzer NR, Felman BJ, Beven EG, et al: A prospective study of the incidence of injury to the cranial nerves during carotid endarterectomy. *Surg Gynecol Obstet* 1980;151:781–784.

71. Hertzer NR: Postoperative management and complications following extracranial carotid reconstruction. In Rutherford RB, editor: *Vascular surgery*, ed 2, Philadelphia, 1984, WB Saunders.

72. Forssell C, Takolander R, Bergqvist D, et al: Cranial nerve injuries associated with carotid endarterectomy: A prospective study. *Acta Chir Scand* 1985;151:595–598.

73. Schauber MD, Fontenelle LJ, Solomon JW, et al: Cranial/cervical nerve dysfunction after carotid endarterectomy. *J Vasc Surg* 1997;25:481–487.

74. Evans WE, Mendelowitz DS, Liapis C, et al: Motor speech deficit following carotid endarterectomy. *Ann Surg* 1982;196:461–469.

75. Cunningham EJ, Bond R, Mayberg MR, et al: Risk of persistent cranial nerve injury after carotid endarterectomy. *J Neurosurg* 2004;101:445–448.

76. Rosenbloom M, Friedman SG, Lamparello PJ, et al: Glossopharyngeal nerve injury complicating carotid endarterectomy. *J Vasc Surg* 1987;5:469–471.

77. Tucker JA, Gee W, Nicholas GG, et al: Accessory nerve injury during carotid endarterectomy. *J Vasc Surg* 1987;5:440–444.

78. Baqeant TE, Tondini D, Lysons D: Bilateral hypoglossal nerve palsy following a second carotid endarterectomy. *Anesthesiology* 1973;43:595–596.

79. Dehn TC, Taylor GW: Cranial and cervical nerve damage associated with carotid endarterectomy. *Br J Surg* 1983;70:365–368.

80. Myers SI, Valentine RJ, Chervu A, et al: Saphenous vein versus primary closure for carotid endarterectomy: Long-term assessment of a randomized prospective study. *J Vasc Surg* 1994;19:15–22.

81. Perler BA, Ursin F, Shanks U, et al: Carotid Dacron patch angioplasty: Immediate and long-term results of a prospective series. *Cardiovasc Surg* 1995;3:631–636.

82. Rosenthal D, Archie JP Jr, Garcia-Rinaldi R, et al: Carotid patch angioplasty: Immediate and long-term results. *J Vasc Surg* 1990;12:326–333.

83. Branch CL, Davis CH Jr: False aneurysm complicating carotid endarterectomy. *Neurosurgery* 1987;19:421–425.

84. Raptis S, Baker SR: Infected false aneurysms of the carotid arteries after carotid endarterectomy. *Eur J Vasc Surg* 1996;11:148–152.

85. Graver LM, Mulcare RJ: Pseudoaneurysms after carotid endarterectomy. *J Cardiovasc Surg* 1986;27:294–297.

86. Perler BA, Vander Kolk CA, Dufreswne CA, et al: Can infected prosthetic grafts be salvaged with rotational muscle flaps? *Surgery* 1991;110:30–34.

87. Leemans CR, Balm AJM, Gregor RT, et al: Management of carotid artery exposure with pectoralis major myofascial flap transfer and split thickness skin coverage. *J Laryngol Otol* 1995;109:1176–1180.

88. Zacharoulis DC, Gupta SK, Seymour P, et al: Use of muscle flap to cover infections of the carotid artery after carotid endarterectomy. *J Vasc Surg* 1997;11:148–152.

89. Hertzer NR: Non-stroke complications of carotid endarterectomy. In Berhard VM, Towne JB, editors: *Complications in vascular surgery*, ed 2, Orlando, Fla, 1985, Grune & Stratton.

90. Rainer WG, Guillen J, Bloomquist CD, et al: Carotid surgery: Morbidity and mortality in 257 operations. *Am J Surg* 1968;116:678–681.

91. Sundt TM, Sandok BA, Whisnant JP: Carotid endarterectomy: Complications and pre-operative assessment of risk. *Mayo Clin Proc* 1975;50:301–306.

92. Kunkel JM, Gomez ER, Spebar MJ, et al: Wound hematomas after carotid endarterectomy. *Am J Surg* 1984;148:844–847.

93. LaMuraglia GM, Stoner MC, Brewster DC, et al: Determinants of carotid endarterectomy anatomic durability: Effects of serum lipids and lipid-lowering drugs. *J Vasc Surg* 2005;41:762–768.

94. Sadideen H, Taylor PR, Padayachee TS: Restenosis after carotid endarterectomy. *Int J Clin Pract* 2006;60:1125–1130.

95. Salvian A, Baker JD, Machleder HI, et al: Cause and noninvasive detection of restenosis after carotid endarterectomy. *Am J Surg* 1983;146:29–34.

96. Zierler RE, Bandyk DF, Thiele BL, et al: Carotid artery stenosis following endartectomy. *Arch Surg* 1982;117:1408–1415.

97. Callow AD, Nitzberg R, Prendville E, et al: Surgical treatment of cerebral ischemia secondary to recurrent carotid stenosis. In Ernst CB, Stanley JC, editors: *Current therapy in vascular surgery*, ed 2, Philadelphia, 1991, BC Decker.

98. Lattimer CR, Burnand KG: Recurrent carotid stenosis after carotid endarterectomy. *Br J Surg* 1997;84:1206–1219.

99. Frericks H, Kievit J, van Baalen JM, et al: Carotid recurrent stenosis and risk of ipsilateral stroke: A systemic review of the literature. *Stroke* 1998;29:244–250.

100. Curley S, Edwards WS, Jacob TP: Recurrent carotid stenosis after autologous tissue patching. *J Vasc Surg* 1987;6:350–354.

101. Das MB, Hertzer NR, Ratliff NB, et al: Recurrent carotid stenosis: A five year series of 65 reoperations. *Ann Surg* 1985;202:28–35.

102. Eikelboom BC, Rob G, Ackerstaff A, et al: Benefits of carotid patching: A randomized study. *J Vasc Surg* 1988;7:240–247.

103. Hertzer NR, Beven EG, O'Hara PJ, et al: A prospective study of vein patch angioplasty during carotid endarterectomy. *Ann Surg* 1987;206:628–635.

104. AbuRahma AF, Robinson PA, Saidy S, et al: Prospective randomized trial of carotid endarterectomy with primary closure and patch angioplasty with saphenous vein, jugular vein, and polytetrafluoroethylene: Long-term follow-up. *J Vasc Surg* 1998;27:222–234.

105. Bond R, Rerkasem K, Naylor R, et al: Patches of different types for carotid patch angioplasty. *Cochrane Database Syst Rev* 2004;(2):CD000071.

106. O'Donnell TF Jr, Rodriguez AA, Fortunato JE, et al: Management of recurrent carotid stenosis: Should asymptomatic lesions be treated surgically? *J Vasc Surg* 1996;24:207–212.

107. AbuRahma AF, Jenings TG, Wulu JT, et al: Redo carotid endarterectomy versus primary carotid endarterectomy. *Stroke* 2001; 32:2782–2792.

108. Archie JP Jr: Reoperations for carotid artery stenosis: Role of primary and secondary reconstructions. *J Vasc Surg* 2001;33: 495–503.

109. Stoner MC, Cambria RP, Brewster DC, et al: Safety and efficacy of reoperative carotid endarterectomy: A 14-year experience. *J Vasc Surg* 2005;41:942–949.

110. Hobson RW, Goldstein JE, Jamil Z, et al: Carotid restenosis: Operative and endovascular management. *J Vasc Surg* 1999;29: 228–238.

111. McDonnell CO, Legge D, Twomey E, et al: Carotid artery angioplasty for restenosis following endarterectomy. *Eur J Vasc Endovasc Surg* 2004;27:163–166.

112. Gold H: Production of arteriosclerosis in the rat: Effect of x-ray and a high-fat diet. *Arch Pathol* 1961;71:268–273.

113. Kirkpatrick JB: Pathogenesis of foam cell lesions in irradiated arteries. *Am J Pathol* 1967;50:291–300.

114. Lindsay S, Entenman C, Ellis E, et al: Aortic arteriosclerosis in the dog after localize aortic irradiation with electrons. *Circ Res* 1962;10:61–67.

115. Silverberg GD, Britt RH, Goffinet DR: Radiation-induced carotid artery disease. *Cancer* 1978;41:130–137.

116. Peters WR, Schlicke CP, Schmutz DD: Peripheral vascular disease following radiation therapy. *Am Surg* 1979;45:700–702.

117. Eldering SC, Fernandez RN, Grotta JC, et al: Carotid artery disease following external cervical irradiation. *Ann Surg* 1981; 194:609–615.

118. Bergqvist D, Jonsson K, Nilsson M, et al: Treatment of arterial lesions after radiation therapy. *Surg Gynecol Obstet* 1987;165: 116–120.

119. McCready RA, Hyde GL, Bivins BA, et al: Radiation-induced arterial injuries. *Surgery* 1983;93:306–312.

120. Friedell ML, Joseph BP, Cohen MJ, et al: Surgery for carotid artery stenosis following neck irradiation. *Ann Vasc Surg* 2001;15:13–18.

121. Kashyap VS, Moore WS, Quinones-Baldrich WJ: Carotid artery repair for radiation-associated atherosclerosis is a safe and durable procedure. *J Vasc Surg* 1999;29:90–99.

122. Cazaban S, Maiza D, Coffin O, et al: Surgical treatment of recurrent carotid artery stenosis and carotid artery stenosis after neck irradiation: Evaluation of operative risk. *Ann Vasc Surg* 2003;17:393–400.

123. Narins C, Illig KA: Patient selection for carotid stenting versus endarterectomy: A systemic review. *J Vasc Surg* 2006;44:661–672.

124. Gray WA, Hopkins LN, Yadav S, et al: Protected carotid artery stenting in high-surgical risk patients: The ARCHeR results. *J Vasc Surg* 2006;44:258–269.

125. Hobson RW II, Howard VJ, Roubin GS, et al: Carotid artery stenting is associated with increased complications in octogenarians: 30-day stroke and death rates in the CREST lead-in phase. *J Vasc Surg* 2004;40:1106–1111.

126. Groschel K, Ernemann U, Rieker A, et al: Incidence and risk factors for medical complications after carotid artery stenting. *J Vasc Surg* 2005;42:1101–1107.

127. Miekusch W, Schillinger M, Sabeti S, et al: Hypotension and bradycardia after elective carotid stenting: Frequency and risk factors. *J Endovasc Ther* 2003;10:851–859.

128. Tan KT, Cleveland TJ, Berczi V, et al: Timing and frequency of complications after carotid artery stenting: What is the optimal period of observation? *J Vasc Surg* 2003;38:236–243.

129. Yadav JS, Rubin GS, Iyer S, et al: Elective stenting of the extracranial carotid arteries. *Circulation* 1997;95:376–381.

130. Schoser BG, Heesen C, Eckert B, et al: Cerebral hyperperfusion injury after percutaneous transluminal angioplasty of extracranial arteries. *J Neurol* 1997;244:101–104.

131. Meyers PM, Higashaida RT, Phatouros CC, et al: Cerebral hyperperfusion syndrome after percutaneous transluminal stenting of the craniocervical arteries. *Neurosurgery* 2000;47:335–343.

132. van Asperen de Boer FR, Terpstra JL, Vink M: Diagnosis, treatment and operative complications of carotid body tumors. *Br J Surg* 1981;68:433–438.

133. Shamblin WR, ReMine WH, Sheps, SG, et al: Carotid body tumor (chemodectoma): A clinicopathologic analysis of ninety cases. *Am J Surg* 1971;122:732–739.

134. Lees CD, Levine HL, Beven EG, et al: Tumors of the carotid body: Experience with 41 operative cases. *Am J Surg* 1981; 142:362–365.

135. Patetsios P, Gable DR, Garrett WV, et al: Management of carotid body paragangliomas and review of a 30-year experience. *Ann Vasc Surg* 2002;16:331–338.

136. Plukker JTM, Brongers EP, Verney A, et al: Outcome of surgical treatment of carotid body paragangliomas. *Br J Surg* 2001;88:1382–1386.

137. Atefi S, Nikeghbalain S, Yarmohammadi H, et al: Surgical management of carotid body tumours: A 24-year surgical experience. *ANZ J Surg* 2006;76:214–217.

138. LaMuraglia GM, Fabian RL, Brewster DC, et al: The current surgical management of carotid body paragangliomas. *J Vasc Surg* 1992;15:1038–1045.

139. Muhm M, Polterauer P, Gstottner W, et al: Diagnostic and therapeutic approaches to carotid body tumors: Review of 24 patients. *Arch Surg* 1997;132:279–284.

140. Little VR, Reilly LN, Romos TK: Preoperative embolization of carotid body tumors: When is it appropriate? *Ann Vasc Surg* 1996;10:464–468.

141. Brackman D, Kiney S, Fu K: Glomus tumor: Diagnosis and management. *Head Neck Surg* 1987;9:306–311.

142. Murphy TP, Brackman DE: Effects of pre-operative embolization on glomus jugulare tumors. *Laryngoscope* 1989;99:1244–1247.

143. Hallett JW Jr, Nora JD, Hollier LH, et al: Trends in neurovascular complications of surgical management experience with 153 tumors. *J Vasc Surg* 1988;7:284–291.

144. Irons GB, Weiland LH, Brown WL: Paragangliomas of the neck: Clinical and pathologic analysis of 110 cases. *Surg Clin North Am* 1977;57:575–583.

145. Dardik A, Eisele DW, Williams GM, et al: A contemporary assessment of carotid body tumor surgery. *Vasc Endovascular Surg* 2002;36:277–283.

146. Krupski WC, Effeney DJ, Ehrenfeld WK, et al: Cervical chemodectoma: Technical considerations and management options. *Am J Surg* 1982;114:215–220.

147. Rosen IB, Palmer JA, Goldberg M, et al: Vascular problems associated with carotid body tumors. *Am J Surg* 1981;142: 459–463.

148. Padberg FT Jr, Cady B, Persson AV: Carotid body tumor: The Lahey clinic experience. *Am J Surg* 1983;145:526–528.

149. Dent TL, Thompson NW, Fry WJ: Carotid body tumors. *Surgery* 1976;80:365–372.

150. Farr HW: Carotid body tumors: A 40-year study. *CA Cancer J Clin* 1980;30:260–265.

151. Gaylis H, Mieny CJ: The incidence of malignancy in carotid body tumors. *Br J Surg* 1977;64:885–889.

152. Smith RF, Shetty PC, Reddy DJ: Surgical treatment of carotid paragangliomas presenting unusual technical difficulties. *J Vasc Surg* 1988;7:631–637.

153. DuBois J, Kelly W, McMenamin P, et al: Bilateral carotid body tumors managed with preoperative embolization: A case report and review. *J Vasc Surg* 1987;5:648–650.

154. Hennessy O, Jamieson CW, Allison DJ: Pre-operation embolization of chemodectoma. *Br J Radiol* 1984;57:845–846.

155. Kumar AJ, Kaufman SL, Patt J, et al: Preoperative embolization of hypervascular head and neck neoplasm using microfibrillar collagen. *AJNR Am J Neuroradiol* 1982;3:163–168.

156. Iaccarino V, Sodano A, Belfiore G, et al: Embolization of glomus tumors of the carotid: Temporary or definitive? *Cardiovasc Intervent Radiol* 1985;8:206–210.

157. Borges LF, Heros RC, DeBrun G: Carotid body tumors managed with preoperative embolization. *J Neurosurg* 1983;59:867–870.

158. Schick PM, Hieshima GB, White RA, et al: Arterial catheter embolization followed by surgery for large chemodectoma. *Surgery* 1980;8:459–464.

159. Lloyd AJ, Hayes PD, London NJM, et al: Does carotid endarterectomy lead to a decline in cognitive function or health related quality of life? *J Clin Exp Neuropsychol* 2004;26:817–825.

160. Sirkka A, Salenius JP, Portin R, et al: Quality of life and cognitive performance after carotid endarterectomy during long-term follow-up. *Acta Neurol Scand* 1992;85:58–62.

161. King GD, Gideon DA, Haynes CD, et al: Intellectual and personality changes associated with carotid endarterectomy. *J Clin Psychol* 1977;33:215–220.

162. De Leo D, Serraiotto L, Pellegrini C, et al: Outcome from carotid endarterectomy: Neuropsychological performances, depressive symptoms and quality of life: 8-months follow-up. *Int J Psychiatry Med* 1987;17:317–325.

163. Vriens EM, Post MW, Jacobs HM, et al: Changes in health-related quality of life after carotid endarterectomy. *Eur J Vasc Endovasc Surg* 1998;16:395–400.

164. Parker JC, Granberg BW, Nichols WK, et al: Mental status outcomes following carotid endarterectomy: A six-month analysis. *J Clin Neuropsychol* 1983;5:345–353.

165. Dardik A, Minor J, Watson C, et al: Improved quality of life among patients with symptomatic carotid artery disease undergoing carotid endarterectomy. *J Vasc Surg* 2001;33:329–333.

CHAPTER 39

Complications of Thyroid Surgery

Christine G. Gourin and David W. Eisele

During the late 1800s and the early 1900s, the majority of complications of thyroid surgery were related to hemorrhage and infection.[1,2] At that time, mortality rates were as high as 50%, and they were largely the result of intraoperative bleeding and sepsis. Theodor Kocher, who was awarded the Nobel Prize for Medicine in 1909, revolutionized the field of thyroid surgery when he perfected the technique of thyroidectomy. Kocher dramatically reduced the rate of complications of thyroidectomy and achieved a reduction in the mortality rate to 0.5% in a series of more than 5000 thyroid operations.[1] Since Kocher's time, many additional refinements in the technique of thyroidectomy have been contributed by other surgeons, and these have resulted in further reductions in the occurrence of complications. This chapter focuses on the present-day complications of thyroid surgery with emphasis on the prevention, frequency, and management of such complications.

RECURRENT LARYNGEAL NERVE

Recurrent Laryngeal Nerve Paralysis

Injury to the recurrent laryngeal nerve (RLN) represents a major and feared complication of thyroidectomy. Reported incidences of this complication in the recent literature vary between 1% and 5% for temporary RLN paralysis and between 0.1% and 1.8% for permanent RLN paralysis[3–13] (Table 39-1).

Factors that are associated with an increased likelihood of postoperative RLN paralysis are the extent of thyroid resection, the surgeon's experience, reoperative surgery, and malignancy.[13–18] Because vocal-fold dysfunction can be present preoperatively as a result of compression from benign or malignant disease, invasion by malignant neoplasm, inflammation, hemorrhage, and idiopathic causes and because it may arise postoperatively from intraoperative nerve injury despite a lack of voice abnormality, formal preoperate and postoperative evaluations of laryngeal function are necessary to accurately assess the incidence and occurrence of this complication. Some series reported in the literature fail to document routine laryngeal function evaluation pre-operatively and postoperatively, and, therefore, these reports may not reflect the true incidence of RLN paralysis.[19,20] Because of the complexity of the assessment of laryngeal function, expertise in laryngeal evaluation is important. Laryngeal videostroboscopy provides the best means of evaluating laryngeal function preoperatively and postoperatively. Videostroboscopy allows

for the detection of subtle functional abnormalities that may be missed with more routine mirror or fiber-optic laryngoscopy.[11,19–22] Direct laryngoscopy performed immediately after the completion of the surgical procedure, while the patient is awakening from anesthesia, is not considered to be an accurate means for the assessment of laryngeal function.

RLN injury may result in ipsilateral vocal-fold immobility. The affected vocal fold lies in the paramedian position during the initial weeks after surgery. Subtle voice changes may be noticed. With inspiration, the vocal fold fails to abduct. With phonation, some vocal-fold adduction may be observed as a result of the action of the interarytenoid muscle, which receives bilateral innervation. Hoarseness becomes more noticeable and problematic as the vocal fold lateralizes further with denervation changes.

Mechanisms of intraoperative RLN injury include division, laceration, stretch or traction, pressure, crush, electrical, ligature entrapment, ischemia, and suction injuries. The surgeon should exercise caution during dissection near the nerve and avoid excessive nerve manipulation. Meticulous hemostasis should be maintained during the operation. Bleeding should be controlled with the judicious use of bipolar electrocautery, the careful placement of ligatures, or the Hemostatix Scalpel (Hemostatix, Memphis, TN). The use of unipolar Bovie electrocautery should be avoided near the nerve. Newer surgical devices for intraoperative vessel sealing such as the LigaSure bipolar electrosealing device (Valleylab, Boulder, CO) and ultrasonically activated shears (i.e., Harmonic Scalpel [Ethicon Endosurgery, Inc., Somerville, NJ]) have been shown to reduce operative time without increasing the risk of injury to the RLN.[23–28] The thyroid gland should be gently manipulated to avoid nerve traction injury. Magnification with operating loupes may improve visualization and aid in the dissection and preservation of the RLN.[29]

The use of perioperative steroids as prophylaxis against nerve injury is controversial. Loré reported a statistically significant reduction of the incidence of temporary vocal-fold paralysis from 9.0% to 2.6% as well as a reduction in the longest duration of temporary paralysis from 9 months to 2 months with a steroid regimen consisting of methylprednisolone (Solu-Medrol; 40 mg) preoperatively and a Medrol Dosepak postoperatively.[30] Other investigators have found no significant effect of perioperative steroids on the incidence of temporary or

TABLE 39-1 Recent Reported Incidences of Vocal-Fold Paralysis after Thyroidectomy

Series*	Temporary		Permanent	
	N	%	*N*	%
Chiang et al. (2005)[3†]	35/678	5.1	5/678	0.9
Ozbas et al. (2005)[4]	11/750	1.5	1/750	0.1
Filho et al. (2005)[5]	14/1020	1.4	4/1,020	0.4
Rosato et al. (2004)[6]	297/14,934	2.0	149/14,934	1.0
Bron and O'Brien (2004)[7]	19/834	2.3	9/834	1.1
Friguglietti et al. (2003)[8]	15/563	2.7	1/563	0.2
Bellantone et al. (2002)[9]	13/526	2.5	4/526	0.8
Hermann et al. (2002)[10†]	809/26,323	3.1	217/26,323	0.8
Prim et al. (2001)[11†]	10/890	1.1	8/890	0.9
Lo et al. (2000)[12]	26/500	5.2	6/500	1.4
Moulton-Barrett et al. (1997)[13]	7/274	2.1	6/274	1.8
Average	**1256/47,292**	**2.7**	**410/47,292**	**0.9**

*All series reported the routine preoperative and postoperative assessment of vocal fold function.
†Reported for nerves at risk.

permanent nerve injury, although a single dose of intra-operative steroids has been shown to reduce the duration of temporary paresis.[31]

Most surgeons advocate the routine identification of the laryngeal nerve during thyroidectomy to visualize and protect the nerve during dissection.[19] The incidence of nerve injury is reduced when routine RLN identification is performed.[32,33] The RLN can be identified superior to the thoracic inlet in the triangular space bound by the trachea and the esophagus medially, the carotid artery laterally, and the thyroid lobe superiorly before glandular mobilization. Alternatively, the nerve can be located laterally near the inferior thyroid artery or superiorly where the nerve enters the larynx. The nerve is usually located in the tracheoesophageal groove, but it may be situated more laterally.[34] The right RLN enters the tracheoesophageal groove more obliquely than does the left.[35] After the nerve is identified by careful dissection, it is followed superiorly. The RLN has a variable relationship with the inferior thyroid artery, so meticulous dissection technique is required to avoided unwanted bleeding.[34]

The use of an esophageal stethoscope may distort the anatomic relationships of this region, thus encumbering RLN identification. Esophageal stethoscopes have also been implicated as a cause of vocal-fold paralysis,[36] and, therefore, some surgeons avoid their use during thyroid surgery.

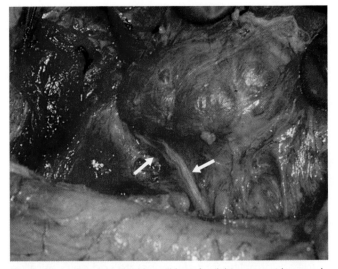

Figure 39-1. Extralaryngeal branching of a right recurrent laryngeal nerve *(arrows)*.

The RLN frequently branches before it enters the larynx (Figure 39-1). As many as 65% of cases may demonstrate an extralaryngeal branching pattern, with two to three terminal branches noted in the majority of cases.[37] Nemiroff and Katz[38] noted branching in 41% of nerves but bilateral nerve branching in only 14% of cases. In most cases (87%), branching occurred less than 3 cm below the inferior border of the cricoid.[38] Branches to the abductor and adductor muscles do not separate extralaryngeally, and, therefore, all RLN branches must be preserved. RLN identification inferiorly as a single nerve trunk (before nerve branching) allows the surgeon to carefully follow the nerve superiorly and to preserve all nerve branches should branching occur.

During thyroidectomy, the surgeon must be aware of the variable relationship of the RLN with the inferior thyroid artery.[37] The RLN can pass anterior or posterior to the inferior thyroid artery, and it has been described as intertwined between the branches of the inferior thyroid artery in as many as 84% of cases.[34,39] The variability of the RLN–inferior thyroid artery relationship makes the inferior thyroid artery an unreliable landmark for RLN identification.

The area in which the RLN is most vulnerable to injury during thyroidectomy is near the posterior suspensory ligament of Berry (Figure 39-2, A). The RLN typically passes deep to this ligament, but it may also pass through or in front of the ligament.[40] Thus, with medial retraction of the lobe, the course of the nerve can be altered, thereby making the nerve susceptible to injury or subjecting the RLN to excessive traction. Sharp division of Berry's ligament without the careful visualization and protection of the RLN puts it at risk for injury.

There is frequently a small laryngeal branch of the inferior thyroid artery in close relationship with the suspensory ligament[37,40] (Figure 39-2, B). This vessel should be anticipated during the division of the ligament and divided and ligated when it is identified. If bleeding from this vessel occurs, it should be carefully controlled. The surgeon should avoid undue sponge pressure, blind clamping, or suction in this region, which is in close proximity to the nerve. The application of microfibrillar collagen hemostat with gentle pressure will usually control troublesome bleeding from this vessel (Figure 39-3).

Nonrecurrent Laryngeal Nerve

The surgeon should be alert to the possibility of a "nonrecurrent" laryngeal nerve. This anatomic anomaly, in which the laryngeal nerve courses from the vagus to the larynx without following a recurrent course around the subclavian artery or the aortic arch, results from abnormal aortic arch development.

A nonrecurrent laryngeal nerve has been reported to occur in approximately 0.5% of patients on the right side, and it is associated with abnormal development of the subclavian artery.[37,41–43] On the right side, this anomaly is associated with the absence of the innominate artery and a right subclavian artery that arises from the aortic arch distal to the left subclavian artery that courses retroesophageally (Figure 39-4).

The nerve in such cases has a cervical origin, without coursing around the subclavian artery. Approximately 25% of patients with this anomaly complain of dysphagia as a result of esophageal compression by the anomalous retroesophageal right subclavian artery.[44] Such vascular esophageal compression can usually be diagnosed with a

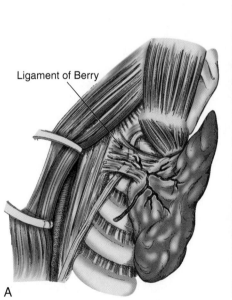
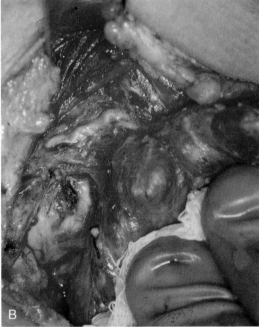
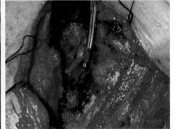

Ligament of Berry

A   B

Figure 39-2. A, The intimate relationship of the recurrent laryngeal nerve with the posterior suspensory ligament of Berry. Glandular retraction can alter the course of the nerve. **B,** The laryngeal branch of the inferior thyroid artery is in close proximity to the ligament, and it can cause troublesome bleeding in this area.

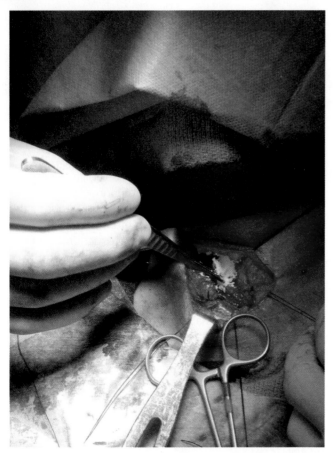

Figure 39-3. The application of microfibrillar collagen hemostat for the control of bleeding in proximity to the recurrent laryngeal nerve.

contrast esophagram. Simultaneous right-sided recurrent and nonrecurrent laryngeal nerves have been reported in approximately 0.2% of cases.[45] In these instances, an unusually small-diameter right RLN was observed to merge with a larger nonrecurrent nerve. The occurrence of a left-sided nonrecurrent laryngeal nerve is rare. Henry and colleagues[44] reported only two left nonrecurrent nerves in 4673 dissections (i.e., 0.04%). This anomaly is associated with a right-sided aortic arch and situs inversus.

Failure to find the RLN in its usual anatomic position or the finding of an unusually small-diameter RLN should alert the surgeon to the possibility of a nonrecurrent laryngeal nerve. In this circumstance, attention should be directed to the laryngeal entry point of the nerve. Alternatively, the vagus nerve can be identified and then the RLN traced from its point of origin from the vagus nerve. This potential anomaly emphasizes the importance of systematic nerve identification during thyroidectomy.

Intraoperative Recurrent Laryngeal Nerve Monitoring

The electrophysiologic identification and monitoring of the integrity of the RLN during thyroidectomy has become more common practice during recent years.[46-57]

Several methods of RLN monitoring have been described, including intraoperative electromyography (EMG) using hook-wire or needle recording electrodes placed endoscopically into the thyroarytenoid or vocalis muscle[48,51,53]; postcricoid surface electrodes that monitor the activity of the posterior cricoarytenoid muscle[46]; posterior cricoarytenoid muscle palpation[47,54]; and endotracheal tubes that incorporate surface electrodes that monitor laryngeal muscle activity, which is the most widely used method[51,52,54-57] (Figure 39-5, *A–D*). The RLN can be stimulated (Figure 39-5, *E*) and evoked EMG activity recorded (Figure 39-6). In addition, EMG activity related to surgical manipulation and nerve stimulation can be monitored during the surgical procedure. With such monitoring, neuromuscular blocking agents must be avoided.

RLN monitoring has been shown to be useful as an aid in the identification of the RLN, but it has not been shown to significantly alter the incidence of RLN injury in most reported series, and it does not uniformly predict postoperative outcome.[48-50,52,53,55] The lack of studies that demonstrate a statistically significant decline in nerve-injury rates with RLN monitoring stems partly from the fact that the incidence of RLN injury is very low, and most published reports originate from high-volume thyroid surgical practices where surgery is performed by or under the guidance of experienced thyroid surgeons. Visual RLN identification remains the "gold standard" in thyroid surgery, and RLN monitoring does not replace a careful visual search for the RLN; rather it is recommended as an adjunct.[48]

RLN monitoring may be useful as a teaching aid, to confirm nerve integrity after dissection (see Figure 39-6), and in cases of advanced neoplasms or reoperation[50,55] (Figure 39-7). An advantage for RLN monitoring has been shown for the less-experienced thyroid surgeon. In a review of 16,448 thyroid operations, Dralle and colleagues[48] found a correlation between thyroid surgery volumes and a benefit from RLN monitoring, with a lower rate of permanent RLN paralysis when RLN monitoring was used by low-volume thyroid surgeons (<45 cases per year). However, no significant difference was found for experienced thyroid surgeons when RLN monitoring was employed as compared with the standard method of visual RLN identification.[48]

Management of the Divided Recurrent Laryngeal Nerve

The management of the injured RLN identified at the time of surgery is controversial. The RLN carries fibers to both the abductor and adductor muscles of the intrinsic larynx. There have been reports of normal laryngeal function after neurorrhaphy of the divided RLN.[58-60] However, most cases of RLN neurorrhaphy result in

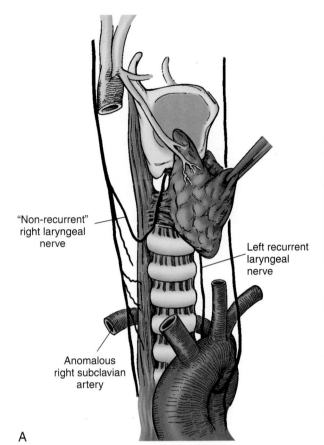

"Non-recurrent" right laryngeal nerve

Left recurrent laryngeal nerve

Anomalous right subclavian artery

A

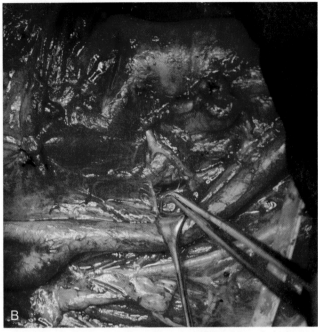

B

Figure 39-4. **A,** Right nonrecurrent laryngeal nerve. Note the vascular anomaly with the retroesophageal course of the right subclavian artery. **B,** Right nonrecurrent laryngeal nerve. (Courtesy of William Gray, MD.)

varying degrees of laryngeal synkinesis, with misdirection of the regenerating inspiratory nerve fibers to the adductor laryngeal muscles and of the expiratory nerve fibers to the abductor laryngeal muscles.[61] Incomplete recovery of vocal-fold motion may also be related to a reduction in the number of reinnervated motor units after nerve repair.[62]

Arguments for immediate neurorrhaphy of the divided RLN include the occasional return of normal laryngeal function and the maintenance of the bulk and tone of the thyroarytenoid muscle, which may otherwise undergo denervation atrophy.[58,63] Arguments against the performance of neurorrhaphy for the divided RLN include the theoretic possibility of synkinetic reinnervation with medial bulging of the ipsilateral vocal fold with inspiration, which results in airway narrowing, and dysphonia caused by synkinetic reinnervation as a result of jerky, uncoordinated vocal-fold movements during phonation related to "fast-twitch" nerve fibers regenerating as normally slower thyroarytenoid fibers.[61,64] In addition, there have been reports of normal laryngeal function after the division of the RLN without nerve repair, which suggests that, in some patients, either complete denervation does not occur or effective regeneration does occur.[65,66]

Spontaneous regeneration has been shown to occur after RLN transection, and this may explain why some patients appear to regain some degree of tone and have EMG activity in the ipsilateral thyroarytenoid muscle.[65-67] This spontaneous reinnervation has been shown to influence vocal-fold position, and may explain why some patients have a relatively adequate voice after RLN injury.[65]

Reinnervation techniques have been reported to be a successful method of managing RLN transection. One method of reinnervation of the divided RLN is the ansa cervicalis–RLN transfer procedure as described by Crumley.[68-70] With this procedure, the ansa hypoglossi branch to the sternothyroid muscle is transected and transferred to the distal (laryngeal) stump of the RLN. Laryngeal reinnervation by the ansa cervicalis provides muscle tone and mass to all of the ipsilateral intrinsic laryngeal muscles, thereby resulting in the restoration of vocal-cord mass, compliance, and tension as well as the stabilization of the arytenoids.[68] Voice quality is reported to be near normal after this procedure.[71] This technique has also been reported to be effective for the management of laryngeal synkinesis caused by RLN injury or as a result of primary neurorrhaphy of a transected RLN.[68]

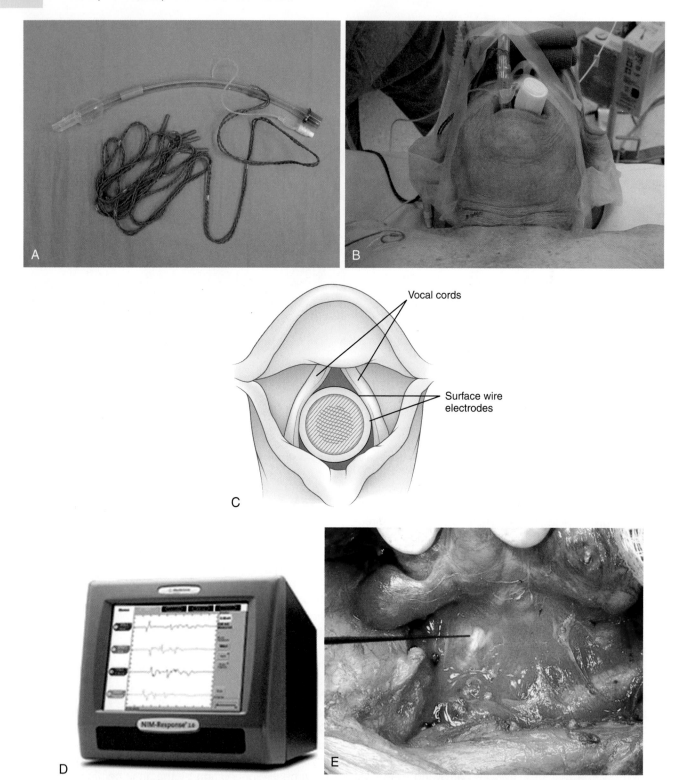

Figure 39-5. A, Electromyography (EMG) endotracheal tube (Xomed [Medtronic Zomed, Jacksonville, FL]). **B,** EMG endotracheal tube secured to ensure proper tube orientation and position. **C,** Diagram of an EMG endotracheal tube positioned at the glottis. **D,** Xomed Nerve Integrity Monitor. **E,** Intraoperative stimulation of the left recurrent laryngeal nerve.

Treatment of Unilateral Vocal-Cord Paralysis

Not all patients with vocal-fold paralysis as a result of RLN injury will complain of significant voice change postoperatively, which emphasizes the importance of the postoperative assessment of vocal-fold function in all patients undergoing thyroidectomy. In some patients with vocal-fold paralysis, edema of the paralyzed vocal fold or hyperadduction of the normal vocal fold may allow for the compensatory closure of the glottis, which results in a near-normal voice. However, most

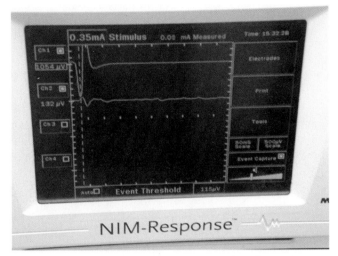

Figure 39-6. Normal electromyography response with recurrent laryngeal nerve stimulation after thyroid lobectomy confirming the integrity of the nerve.

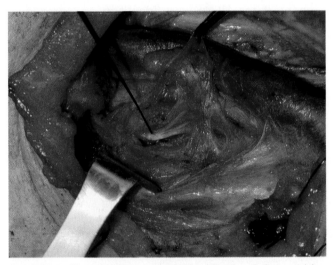

Figure 39-7. Recurrent laryngeal nerve identification during a revision central neck dissection.

patients will have various degrees of voice changes, and symptoms become more prominent weeks to months postoperatively as edema resolves or the denervated vocal fold atrophies.[72]

Some patients with vocal-fold paralysis may benefit from voice therapy under the direction of a speech–language pathologist. In these cases, patients are trained to produce voice under optimal physiologic conditions. Symptomatic patients who fail to improve with voice therapy are considered candidates for vocal-fold medialization procedures, including vocal-fold injection, medialization thyroplasty, and arytenoid adduction procedures.

Injection of the paralyzed vocal fold with temporary materials such as Gelfoam, Cymetra, Radiesse Lite, autologous fat, or collagen provides for temporary vocal-cord medialization, which results in improved

glottic closure.[73,74] All of these substances can be injected via direct laryngoscopy in the operating room or in the clinic transorally or transcervically. These injectables are gradually absorbed over an approximately 1- to 6-month period.[61,73] Repeated injections of these temporary fillers can be performed while waiting for the spontaneous recovery of vocal-fold function. Furthermore, spontaneous reinnervation may allow for the immobile vocal fold to rest in a favorable position and thus allow the patient to compensate without further intervention.

The patient in whom the return of vocal-fold function or compensation may occur should be observed for a period of 6 to 12 months before consideration of a permanent procedure for vocal-fold medialization. A longer waiting period may be warranted for left-sided paralysis as compared with right-sided paralysis as a result of the longer course of the left RLN.

Teflon injection has been used to provide permanent vocal-fold medialization, but, as a result of complications related to granuloma formation and migration, its use has largely been abandoned.[75] It may still have a role in the palliation of terminally ill patients. Calcium hydroxyapatite in the form of microspheres with a gel carrier (i.e., Radiesse) has been approved by the U.S. Food and Drug Administration as a longer-lasting injectable material that appears to have excellent results without the complications related to Teflon.[76,77]

Medialization thyroplasty is an alternative to vocal-fold injection for medialization of the paralyzed vocal fold.[78,79] This procedure medializes the vocal fold with the placement of an appropriately sized implant via a window in the thyroid lamina. This procedure is usually performed with the patient under local anesthesia, which allows for intraoperative vocalization and the assessment of the optimal placement and size of the implant. Medialization thyroplasty is a reversible procedure if vocal-fold function returns. Arytenoid adduction in conjunction with medialization thyroplasty is indicated when a patient does not achieve a near-normal voice from medialization alone.[73,80]

Rarely, a patient with unilateral vocal-fold paralysis will experience inspiratory airway obstruction. The degree of obstruction can be evaluated objectively by flow-volume loop studies. The characteristic flow-volume loop pattern is one of variable extrathoracic obstruction.[81] The proposed cause of glottic insufficiency related to unilateral vocal-fold paralysis is that the flaccid vocal fold behaves as a variable obstruction by narrowing the glottis with inspiration. In this situation, improved inspiratory flow can actually be achieved by vocal-fold injection, which converts the flaccid vocal fold to a more fixed structure with improved inspiratory flow rates.[81]

Laryngeal EMG may provide additional information regarding the return of function after injury to the RLN.[82] Needle electrodes are placed in the intrinsic laryngeal musculature several weeks after injury. Fibrillation potentials, absent or decreased motor unit potentials, and positive waves are EMG findings that indicate denervation and predict a poor potential for recovery. Normal or polyphasic potentials predict recovery for most—but not all—patients.

Bilateral Recurrent Laryngeal Nerve Injury

Injury to both RLNs is a rare complication of thyroidectomy, but it must be considered in all cases that place both RLNs at risk or when there is preexisting dysfunction of one vocal fold and the contralateral functioning nerve is placed at risk from surgery. With bilateral vocal-fold paralysis, airway obstruction may result after extubation as a result of the failure of vocal-fold abduction. Immediately after extubation, there may initially be an adequate airway as a result of a stenting effect of the endotracheal tube or of the flaccidity of the vocal folds. However, as a result of reinnervation, the vocal folds gradually assume paramedian positions with resultant airway compromise.

After total thyroidectomy, patients are preferably extubated in the controlled environment of the operating room. This allows for the assessment of the laryngeal airway, because inspiratory stridor may occur and progress after extubation. Airway compromise requires the immediate establishment of an airway, preferably by reintubation. If both RLNs were identified and preserved intraoperatively, then recovery of function is possible. However, neuropraxic nerve injury usually takes 6 to 12 weeks to recover; therefore a patient may require airway intervention with a tracheotomy. Other acute management options include continuous positive airway pressure,[83] heliox[8] (Figure 39-8), and temporary endoscopic laterofixation of the vocal fold.[85–87]

One option for the treatment of permanent bilateral vocal-fold paralysis is maintenance of a tracheotomy tube with a speaking valve. Vocal quality is usually quite good with this approach, because the position of the paralyzed vocal folds allows for vocal-fold vibration.

Multiple surgical options exist for the treatment of permanent bilateral vocal-fold paralysis to allow for tracheotomy decannulation. These procedures, which include laser cordotomy, endoscopic arytenoidectomy, and extralaryngeal arytenoidectomy with lateralization, sacrifice some vocal quality for the desired improvement in the glottic airway. The timing of treatment depends on the surgeon's experience during the

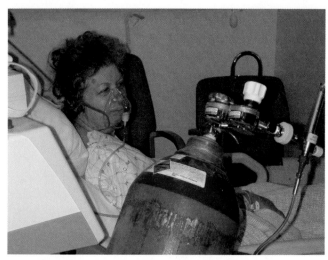

Figure 39-8. Heliox for the acute management of airway obstruction caused by bilateral vocal-fold paresis after thyroidectomy.

surgery. If the RLNs were identified and preserved during surgery, an adequate period of observation (usually 9 to 12 months) for the return of function of either or both vocal folds should be followed before these surgical procedures are considered. A stable interim airway can be provided by tracheotomy, arytenoidopexy, or vocal-fold laterofixation, all of which are reversible.[85,86]

Some patients with permanent bilateral vocal-fold paralysis may be successfully decannulated without airway surgery. Such patients must usually adopt a more sedentary lifestyle, because inspiratory airway obstruction occurs with increased ventilatory demand. Any further narrowing of the glottis (e.g., related to an upper respiratory infection) may precipitate severe airway obstruction in these patients. Therefore decannulation in patients with bilateral vocal-fold paralysis should be performed with caution because of the risk of significant airway compromise after the removal of the tracheotomy tube.

EXTERNAL BRANCH OF THE SUPERIOR LARYNGEAL NERVE INJURY

The external branch of the superior laryngeal nerve (EBSLN), which is supplied by the vagus nerve, innervates the cricothyroid muscle, which lengthens and tenses the vocal cord (Figure 39-9). Damage to this nerve results in an inability to attain the high registers of voice and singing, impaired pitch regulation, and vocal weakness or fatigue, although a normal speaking voice is often present. The incidence of EBSLN injury during thyroid surgery ranges from 0% to 20%, with most studies reporting an incidence of 5% to 10% and permanent paralysis reported in 0% to 5% of cases.[20,22,37,39,88–90] Because the manifestations of EBSLN injury may be

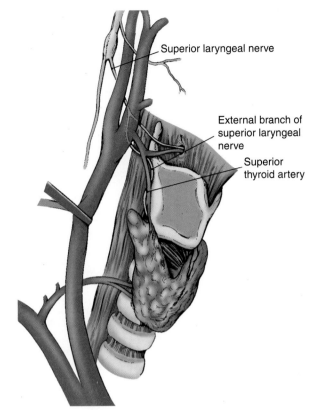

Figure 39-9. The course of the superior laryngeal nerve. As shown, the close proximity of this nerve to the superior pole vessels is possible.

Superior laryngeal nerve

External branch of superior laryngeal nerve

Superior thyroid artery

subtle and because EMG analysis of the cricothyroid muscle is not performed routinely during postoperative follow up, the true incidence of this complication may be underestimated. It has been reported that as many as 87% of patients have subjective changes in vocal loudness, pitch, and singing after uncomplicated thyroidectomy that may be a result of either scarring or unrecognized EBSLN injury.[21]

The visual examination of the larynx with an isolated EBSLN injury is often unrevealing. With attempted supramaximal pitch elevation, the posterior larynx may be observed to rotate toward the contralateral functioning cricothyroid muscle. Laryngeal videostroboscopy may reveal asymmetric vibratory patterns at higher pitches of phonation, and acoustic analysis reveals a decreased frequency and range.[21,91] Cricothyroid muscle EMG evaluation can be used to confirm a suspected EBSLN injury.

Injury to the EBSLN can be a devastating complication for the patient who uses the voice professionally, such as a singer. This problem was dramatically demonstrated when the famous opera coloratura soprano Amelita Galli-Curci sustained this complication during thyroidectomy for an enlarging goiter in 1935, thus contributing to the end of her career.[92]

Because the EBSLN can course between branches of the superior thyroid artery or because it is intimately related to this vessel in approximately one fourth of patients, glandular retraction can stretch this nerve.[93,94] Mass clamping and ligation of the superior thyroid vessels can result in injury to this nerve. In contrast with the RLN, some surgeons do not advocate the routine identification of the EBSLN. Rather, the nerve is avoided by the careful division of the superior pole vessels on the capsule of the upper pole of the thyroid gland.[90,93] The division of the sternothyroid muscle will provide improved operative exposure to this area, if needed.

Some surgeons do advocate the routine identification of the EBSLN.[89,94-96] Cernea and colleagues[89] reported a 0% paralysis rate with routine EBSNL identification as compared with a 12% rate without identification. In a randomized prospective study involving cricothyroid muscle EMG evaluations, Hurtado-Lopez and colleagues[96] demonstrated a diminished rate of EBSLN injury as compared with cases that did not identify the nerve. By contrast, another prospective randomized study by Bellantone and colleagues[97] compared two matched groups. One group had routine EBSLN identification, whereas the other group had EBSLN avoidance. At 6 months postoperatively, the incidence of EBSLN injury was less than 1% in both groups and without a statistical difference in the rates of nerve injury.[97] The intraoperative electrophysiologic monitoring of the superior laryngeal nerve can be used for EBSLN identification and preservation in select cases.[98]

The treatment of EBSLN paralysis usually consists of voice therapy. Selective cricothyroid muscle reinnervation with a muscle–nerve–muscle neurotization technique using an autologous nerve graft between the innervated cricothyroid muscle and the nonfunctional contralateral denervated cricothyroid muscle has been reported to result in EMG evidence of the reinnervation of the cricothyroid muscle.[99]

HYPOPARATHYROIDISM

Hypoparathyroidism is a serious complication of thyroidectomy that is related to the inadvertent removal of the parathyroid glands, damage to the glands, or the interruption of their blood supply. The occurrence of this complication is related to the expertise of the surgeon in preserving vascularized parathyroid tissue.

The incidences of temporary and permanent hypoparathyroidism after thyroidectomy in recently reported series are shown in Table 39-2. Temporary hypoparathyroidism occurs in approximately 10% to 15% of patients, whereas permanent hypoparathyroidism occurs less frequently (1% to 3%).[4-9,11,13,100,101] An increased incidence of

TABLE 39-2 Recent Reported Incidences of Hypoparathyroidism after Thyroid Operations

Series	Temporary		Permanent	
	N	%	N	%
Ozbas et al. (2005)[4]	131/750	17.5	1/750	0.1
Filho et al. (2005)[5]	134/1020	13.1	26/1020	2.5
Rosato et al. (2004)[6]	1240/14,934	6.8	254/14,934	1.7
Bron and O'Brien (2004)[7]	120/834	14.4	20/834	2.4
Friguglietti et al. (2003)[8]	65/563	11.5	3/563	0.5
Bellantone et al. (2002)[9]	41/526	7.8	18/526	3.4
Prim et al. (2001)[11]	51/321	15.9	7/321	2.2
Moulton-Barrett et al. (1997)[13]	10/274	10.5	1/274	1.1
Pattou et al. (1998)[100]	58/1071	5.4	5/1071	0.5
Shaha and Jaffe (1998)[101]	2/600	0.3	0/600	0
Average	**1852/20,892**	**8.9**	**335/20,892**	**1.6**

postoperative hypocalcemia is associated with central compartment neck dissection, reoperation, and surgery for substernal goiter, carcinoma, or Graves disease.[101-104] Temporary hypoparathyroidism is thought to be caused by glandular ischemia from injury or devascularization, and it appears to be inversely related to the extent of surgery, the surgeon's experience, and the number of parathyroid glands preserved with their intact blood supply.[100,105] Calcitonin release after the manipulation of the thyroid gland may result in peripheral insensitivity to parathyroid hormone (PTH), but it has not been consistently demonstrated in cases of hypocalcemia after thyroid surgery.[106,107]

The parathyroid glands are commonly intimately related to the thyroid gland, but ectopic locations of one or more of the glands are possible. The position of the inferior parathyroid gland is more variable than that of the superior parathyroid gland.[108] The parathyroids are surrounded by a thin capsule that is comprised of pretracheal fascia, but they appear to be distinct from the thyroid gland, thus allowing for their separation from thyroid tissue.[101] Intrathyroidal parathyroid glands, however, may infrequently occur.[108] Supernumerary glands may be present in 2% to 8% of patients.[109]

Both the inferior and superior parathyroid glands receive their blood supply from parathyroid arteries that arise primarily as branches of the inferior thyroid artery[101] (Figure 39-10). However, the superior parathyroid glands may be infrequently supplied by the superior thyroid artery or from an anastomosis between the inferior and superior thyroid arteries.[101] The parathyroid glands are dependent on their blood supply from these vessels, and vascular connections between the parathyroid gland and the thyroid gland are unusual. This fact emphasizes the importance of the preservation of the integrity of the parathyroid arteries to maintain a sufficient vascular supply to the parathyroid glands.

During thyroid lobectomy, care must be taken to not divide the inferior thyroid artery before it supplies the parathyroid glands. Instead, the terminal branches of the inferior thyroid artery are ligated near the capsule of the thyroid gland, thus preserving the blood supply to the parathyroid glands (Figure 39-11). Meticulous hemostasis and a dry surgical field are important when identifying and dissecting the parathyroid glands from the thyroid gland. Optical magnification may further aid the surgeon in the identification and preservation of the parathyroid blood supply.

The surgeon must be able to recognize parathyroid tissue and to differentiate a parathyroid gland from adipose tissue, lymph nodes, and thyroid tissue. Parathyroid tissue is characteristically caramel, tan, or brownish; oblong and

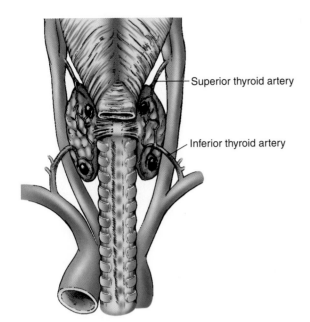

Figure 39-10. Blood supply to the parathyroid glands as viewed posteriorly. Both the inferior and superior parathyroid glands are supplied by parathyroid arteries that originate as branches of the inferior thyroid artery in nearly all cases.

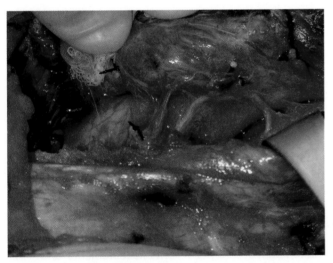

Figure 39-11. Preservation of the left parathyroid gland during thyroidectomy. Branches of the inferior thyroid artery have been ligated near the capsule of the thyroid gland.

flattened; and approximately 6 to 8 mm in size.[101] Adipose tissue is typically more yellow and lymph nodes more gray than parathyroid tissue. Parathyroid glands are usually surrounded by fat, which gives them a characteristic appearance. Adipose tissue floats in saline, whereas parathyroid glands and lymph nodes sink.

The autotransplantation of devascularized parathyroid glands is advocated to reduce the risk of permanent hypoparathyroidism.[101,110–113] The function of an autotransplanted gland is more predictable than that of an injured gland left in situ.[110] Autotransplantation has been recommended for cases in which the viability of

even just one gland is of concern, and it has been shown to result in a lower incidence of permanent postoperative hypoparathyroidism.[101,110–112] Devascularized glands should be confirmed to be parathyroid tissue by frozen section to avoid the transplantation of tumor or other nonparathyroid tissue.[101] The removed thyroid gland should be carefully examined for attached parathyroid glands, and any parathyroid glands that are identified on the removed thyroid gland should be retrieved (Figure 39-12, *A*). Autotransplantation is performed by sectioning the parathyroid gland into small (i.e., ~1 mm) pieces (Figure 39-12, *B*) and placing the tissue into a well-vascularized cervical muscle such as the sternocleidomastoid muscle (Figure 39-12, *C*).[112]

A clinical situation that may be encountered is the need for completion of total thyroidectomy or reoperation after prior thyroid lobectomy, at which time the parathyroid glands and their blood supply may not have been carefully preserved. For this reason, parathyroid preservation should be performed routinely during thyroid lobectomy and extreme care taken to maintain parathyroid viability during reoperation on the basis of the possibility of the compromise of the contralateral parathyroid glands during the prior surgery. The surgical dictum "every parathyroid gland should be treated as if it is the last one" should be followed.

The risk of hypoparathyroidism increases when a central neck dissection or a mediastinal dissection is performed at the time of thyroidectomy for carcinoma.[101–104] This increased risk is probably related to the inadvertent removal of aberrant parathyroid glands and increased surgical dissection with the resultant devascularization of the parathyroid glands.

Patients at risk for hypoparathyroidism include those undergoing total thyroidectomy, lobectomy after previous contralateral lobectomy, or reoperation. Postoperatively these patients should be monitored closely for signs and symptoms of hypocalcemia. Symptoms of hypocalcemia include circumoral paresthesias, paresthesias of the hands and feet, muscle cramps, tetany, seizures, chest pain, laryngeal spasm with stridor, generalized weakness, anxiety, and apprehension.

Signs of hypocalcemia include a positive Chvostek sign, which involves facial twitching elicited by tapping over the facial nerve. It is important to keep in mind that this sign is present in approximately 10% to 20% of normal individuals. Another sign of hypocalcemia is a positive Trousseau sign, which involves ischemia-induced carpal spasm elicited by the inflation of a blood pressure cuff to exceed the systolic blood pressure and occlude the brachial artery. This test is painful to the patient and therefore not commonly performed. Cardiac arrhythmia with a prolonged

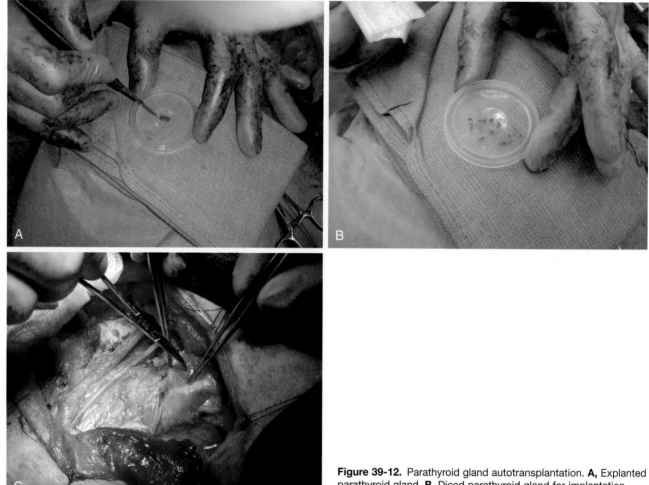

Figure 39-12. Parathyroid gland autotransplantation. **A,** Explanted parathyroid gland. **B,** Diced parathyroid gland for implantation. **C,** Cervical muscle pocket for parathyroid tissue implantation.

QT interval is another possible sign of hypocalcemia. Serum calcium should be closely monitored postoperatively in high-risk patients. The late development of hypocalcemia beyond 48 to 72 hours postoperatively is unusual.

Acute symptomatic hypocalcemia requires immediate calcium replacement. Calcium gluconate 10% (i.e., 10–20 ml) is administered by intravenous infusion over 5 to 10 minutes. A slow infusion of calcium gluconate is instituted (i.e., 1–2 g in 100–200 ml saline over 6 hours). Oral calcium replacement is also begun and consists of calcium carbonate, calcium gluconate, calcium citrate, or calcium lactate in divided doses to provide 2 gm to 10 g per day. Oral calcitriol (i.e., 1, 25-dihydroxyvitamin D_3 at 0.25–0.5 μg/day) is begun if oral calcium replacement alone is inadequate to maintain a normal serum calcium level.

Serum calcium levels are followed weekly in patients who receive calcium replacement therapy until levels have stabilized, and then evaluated every 6 to 8 weeks, with attempts made to wean the patient from calcium.

Temporary hypoparathyroidism will usually resolve within 4 weeks, but it may persist for months,[114] and it is likely to be permanent among patients who require calcium and vitamin D at 1 year postoperatively.

Postoperative serum calcium measurements and PTH levels have been used to predict which patients are at risk for postoperative hypocalcemia.[115–120] Several studies have demonstrated that the slope of the curve of two sequential serum calcium levels during the first 12 hours after surgery, plotted as a function of time, predicts normocalcemia in all patients with positive sloping curves.[115,117] The majority of patients who have negative sloping curves but calcium levels within the low-normal range can be safely discharged with oral calcium supplementation and education regarding the symptoms of hypocalcemia. However, these patients should undergo initial observation for a 24-hour period to monitor for signs and symptoms of hypocalcemia.[115,117,121,122]

The rapid PTH assay has similarly been investigated as a method of predicting the development of significant hypocalcemia. Two studies have demonstrated that, in patients undergoing total thyroidectomy, a 1-hour postoperative PTH level of less than 10 pg/ml was predictive of hypocalcemia.[118,123] In a series of 40 patients, Lam and Kerr[123] reported that a 1-hour postoperative PTH level of 8 pg/ml or less was associated with postoperative hypocalcemia in all patients. In a larger series of 199 patients undergoing total thyroidectomy, Vescan and colleagues[118] reported that a 1-hour postoperative PTH level of less than 10.4 pg/ml predicted hypocalcemia with a 99% specificity and a 95% sensitivity. Because PTH levels may continue to decrease for as long as 4 hours after total thyroidectomy, intraoperative or immediate postoperative PTH may not predict postoperative hypocalcemia in all patients who are at risk.[124] In a prospective study of PTH levels in 103 patients who underwent thyroid and parathyroid surgery, Chia and colleagues[125] found that all patients who required calcium supplementation had PTH levels of less than 15 pg/ml at 8 hours after surgery, resulting in a sensitivity of 100% and a specificity of 91%. The major limitation to the widespread use of the PTH assay is the added financial costs incurred by this test.[116,118–120,126,127]

HYPOTHYROIDISM AND HYPERTHYROIDISM

Hypothyroidism is an expected sequela of total thyroidectomy. For cases in which thyroid suppression therapy is not necessary, thyroid replacement therapy is initiated postoperatively, usually L-thyroxine at 1.8 μg/kg/day. The dose of L-thyroxine is adjusted on the basis of the results of serum thyroid-stimulating hormone (TSH) and thyroxine (T$_4$) levels performed 4 to 6 weeks after the institution of thyroid replacement therapy.

Hypothyroidism can occur after thyroid lobectomy if the remaining thyroid lobe does not produce sufficient thyroid hormone to maintain a euthyroid state. The reported incidence of hypothyroidism after hemithyroidectomy varies from 18% to 50%.[128–131] Patients may have subclinical hypothyroidism. Serum TSH levels should be routinely checked after hemithyroidectomy to detect hypothyroidism. Most patients who are found to have an elevated TSH level after hemithyroidectomy will require thyroid hormone replacement therapy. However, some patients will become euthyroid without intervention.[130]

Hypothyroidism has been implicated as a factor in impaired wound healing. This association emphasizes the importance of adequate thyroid function preoperatively.

Persistent hyperthyroidism is a failure of treatment after thyroidectomy when it is performed for hyperthyroidism (e.g., Graves disease). Medical treatment for persistent hyperthyroidism in this situation is usually preferred to reoperation because of the risks of RLN injury and hypoparathyroidism.

OTHER COMPLICATIONS OF THYROIDECTOMY

Hemorrhage and Hematoma

Hematoma formation after thyroidectomy is a surgical emergency. Hematoma is an unusual postoperative complication that occurs in less than 2% of cases.[4,5,7–9,132–137] This complication is thought to be related to inadequate hemostasis at the time of surgery. Multiple randomized clinical studies have documented that the presence of a drain has no effect on the incidence of hematoma formation.[138–145] Furthermore, a meta-analysis of eight randomized, controlled studies showed no significant difference in the rates of hematoma occurrence with or without drain placement.[146] The identification of patients who are at risk remains obscure. There appears to be no difference in the occurrence of this complication between total versus subtotal thyroidectomy, unilateral versus bilateral surgery, concomitant procedures or pathology such as goiter or the presence of malignancy.[143]

The avoidance of hematoma formation requires meticulous attention to hemostasis intraoperatively. Inadequate wound hemostasis sometimes can be identified with maneuvers that increase venous pressure before wound closure. These include the Valsalva maneuver (Figure 39-13), the placement of the patient in the Trendelenburg position, and suctioning the airway to elicit a cough. Any bleeding noted with these maneuvers should be carefully controlled. A smooth emergence from general anesthesia with the avoidance of bucking and the prevention of postoperative nausea and vomiting with antiemetic medications may help to avoid hematoma formation. Perioperative corticosteroids have been shown to reduce postoperative nausea and vomiting after thyroidectomy.[147,148] Newer

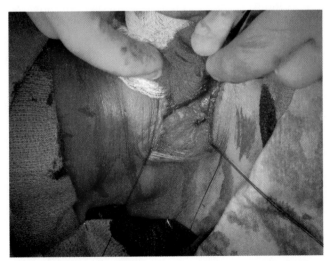

Figure 39-13. Wound bleeding elicited by a Valsalva maneuver after thyroidectomy.

surgical devices for intraoperative vessel sealing, such as the bipolar electrosealing device (LigaSure) and ultrasonically activated shears (i.e., Harmonic Scalpel), have been shown to reduce operative time, but they do not significantly decrease the incidence of hematoma.[23–28]

The majority of hematomas cause clinical signs and symptoms within 24 hours after surgery.[138,143,149] In one large series reported by Burkey and colleagues,[143] the mean time for the development of symptoms of hematoma was 17 hours postoperatively, and 60% of patients had symptoms manifest after 6 hours. Hematoma can cause severe upper-airway obstruction. Airway obstruction may manifest itself with the development of laryngeal edema as a result of venous congestion before there is visible neck swelling. Patients may complain of neck pain or pressure. Alternatively, neck swelling may be obvious, and there may be hemorrhage from the wound and the drain site, if a drain is present. Skin discoloration may also be apparent.

The treatment of a neck hematoma consists of opening the surgical wound immediately to decompress and evacuate the hematoma if there is respiratory distress and to ensure an adequate airway. Intubation may be difficult as a result of upper-airway edema, and an emergent tracheotomy may be necessary. After the airway is controlled, the patient should be returned to the operating room for formal wound exploration and the control of bleeding blood vessels. A readily identifiable bleeding vessel is not identified during wound exploration in all patients.[143,150,151] Bleeding usually occurs deep to the strap muscles. For this reason, the strap muscles should be closed in an interrupted fashion, with gaps left to allow for the anterior decompression of hemorrhage should it occur.[152]

Reoperation for hemorrhage increases the risk of injury to the RLN, and, therefore, extreme care must be taken to avoid this complication.[153] Bulky neck-wound dressings should be avoided after thyroidectomy. This practice allows for the close observation of the patient's neck for swelling, which may indicate postoperative bleeding. Neck pressure dressings do not prevent hematoma formation and may obscure the identification of this complication; they should therefore be avoided.

Mediastinal hemorrhage after the transcervical removal of a substernal goiter is unusual.[154–156] If this complication occurs and cannot be controlled from the cervical approach, median sternotomy may be necessary. The insertion and inflation of a Foley catheter into the mediastinum for the tamponade of hemorrhage has been described as a simple and effective method for controlling mediastinal bleeding.[157]

Seroma

Seroma is reported to occur in between 1% and 6% of cases after thyroidectomy.[4,5,7,9,132,134] Seromas may be evacuated by needle aspiration (Figure 39-14), the placement of a closed-suction drain, drainage through the wound, or management with observation, because the gradual resorption of a seroma will occur. With intervention, care must be taken to avoid bacterial contamination of the wound.

The incidence of seroma formation increases with the extent of surgery, with a higher incidence reported after bilateral procedures or after the removal of large substernal goiters.[138,139,158,159] A trend toward an increased incidence of seroma formation has been shown when neck drains are not used.[139] For this reason, many surgeons advocate the selective use of drains for those cases in which a large dead space results from resection, such as after the removal of a substernal goiter or a large multinodular goiter.[138,139]

Infection

Infection after thyroidectomy is uncommon, and it occurs in less than 2% of cases.[4–7,9,132,134,152] Infection is best prevented by meticulous sterile surgical technique and the gentle handing of tissues. Thyroidectomy is considered to be a clean surgical procedure, and infection occurs as a result of a break in sterile technique. Several studies have shown a higher incidence of wound infection after thyroidectomy among patients who had drain placement as compared with those without drains.[160,161]

Perioperative antibiotics for thyroidectomy have not been shown to alter the incidence of infection; therefore they are not routinely recommended.[162] Wound cellulitis after thyroid surgery is treated with antibiotics and local wound care. The development of a neck abscess

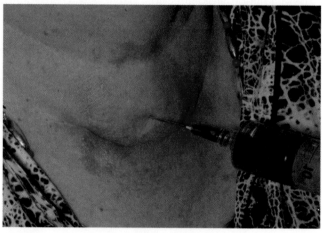

Figure 39-14. Needle aspiration of a neck seroma after thyroidectomy.

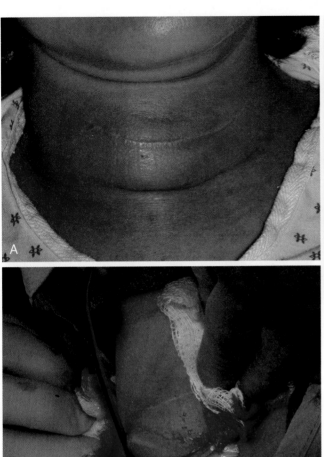

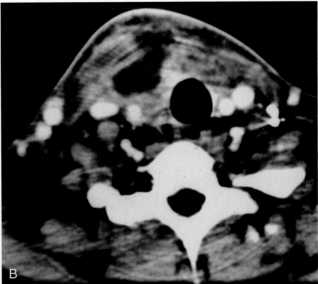

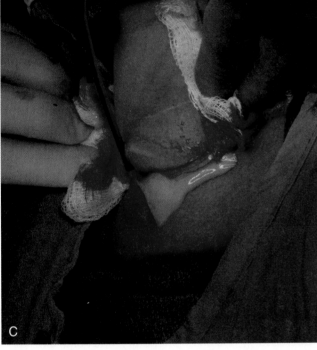

Figure 39-15. A, Neck abscess after secondary thyroidectomy. **B,** Computed tomography scan of same patient shown in **A** demonstrating abscess. **C,** Incision and drainage of the neck abscess.

(Figure 39-15, *A* and *B*) requires incision and drainage (Figure 39-15, *C*) as well as the administration of intravenous antibiotics, which are adjusted according to intraoperative culture results. Deep neck abscess formation after thyroidectomy should raise the suspicion of an aerodigestive tract injury with secondary neck contamination, and the trachea and esophagus should therefore be carefully examined to rule out injury.

Hypertrophic Scar and Keloid

In most cases, thyroidectomy scars heal well, with excellent cosmetic results. Care must be taken during incision planning to place the incision within a skin crease or a relaxed skin tension line. Proper incision placement can be facilitated by the examination of the patient's neck while the patient is sitting upright. This gives the surgeon the proper perspective of the neck anatomy for incision-planning purposes. Planning the incision when the patient is supine with the neck hyperextended may result in the placement of an incision lower in the neck than desired, which is difficult to camouflage. Neck distortion by tumor or goiter may make incision placement difficult. The surgeon should strive to place the incision so that a symmetric scar results postoperatively.

The neck incision should be of sufficient length to allow for adequate operative exposure and to minimize the need for vigorous wound retraction intraoperatively (Figure 39-16). The wound skin edges should be carefully protected from injury from retractors or

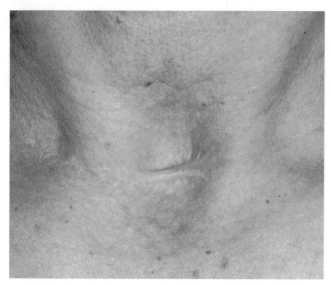

Figure 39-16. Thyroidectomy scar related to wound-edge abrasions resulting from the vigorous intraoperative retraction of a small incision.

electrocautery. Some surgeons prefer to guard the skin edges with a surgical sponge or towel intraoperatively to prevent skin-edge injury. Incision cross-hatch marks should be avoided to prevent additional scarring. Methylene blue tattoos along the incision allow for proper wound realignment without the risk of additional scars.

Proper wound closure is important to obtain optimal healing. Sutures or staples are removed in a timely fashion to avoid permanent marks along the wound. Patients are cautioned to protect the healing wound from sun exposure to prevent scar hyperpigmentation. Breast support is recommended postoperatively.

Hypertrophic scars and keloid formation (Figure 39-17) can occur after thyroidectomy, particularly among susceptible patients. These complications may be related to the proximity of the incision to the manubrium and the sternal area, where such scarring is more common than in other parts of the body. The treatment of hypertrophic scarring and keloid formation consists of steroid injections and scar revision, if necessary. Laser therapy can be used as an adjunct to scar revision in severe cases. Slight edema of the superior flap can occur postoperatively and is related to lymphatic stasis. This problem will resolve gradually with time.

Temporary Voice Change without Laryngeal Nerve Injury

Temporary voice change after thyroidectomy occurs frequently. Temporary laryngeal edema from intubation and surgical manipulation may contribute to mild hoarseness during the immediate postoperative period. This problem usually resolves after several days.

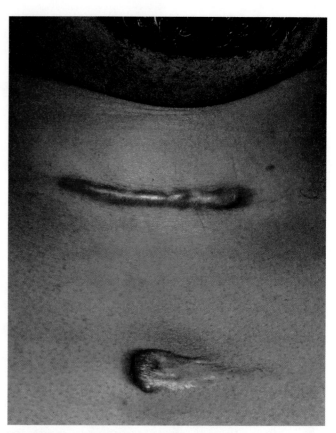

Figure 39-17. Keloid after thyroidectomy. Note the keloid over the sternum from a different operative procedure.

Sinagra and colleagues[21] reported that 87% of patients who underwent total thyroidectomy noted a change in voice postoperatively. Vocal fatigue was the most common complaint. Other symptoms included voice alteration with loud speaking, changes in voice pitch, and singing impairment. Hong and Kim[163] evaluated 57 thyroidectomy patients with normal vocal-cord motion and normal cricothyroid muscle EMGs, and they noted a decrease in speaking phonatory time and diminished vocal range in a significant number of these patients at 1 and 3 months postoperatively. At 6 months, the voice was found to have normalized. Temporary laryngeal fixation and strap muscle impairment are proposed mechanisms for this temporary vocal dysfunction.[163]

Esophageal and Tracheal Injury

Injury to the trachea and esophagus may rarely occur during thyroidectomy. Such injury can result in wound contamination, infection, and fistula if it is not identified and properly treated intraoperatively. Esophageal injuries should be repaired with a meticulous watertight closure technique in an inverted fashion. Closure is performed with absorbable sutures such as polyglactin 910 (i.e., Vicryl). The placement of a strap muscle flap over the repair may provide for additional closure. A drain should be placed in the wound, and perioperative antibiotics should be administered. Oral intake is prohibited for several days postoperatively.

Thyrotoxic Storm

Thyrotoxic storm or crisis is at present a rare but extremely serious complication of thyroid surgery in hyperthyroid patients. In these patients, a sudden decrease in thyroid hormone binding with illness or stress can cause an acute elevation of the free unbound fraction. This problem is largely preventable by the identification of the hyperthyroid patient preoperatively with thyroid function testing. Surgery on a hyperthyroid patient should be delayed until the patient is rendered euthyroid with antithyroid medication such as the thioamides propylthiouracil or methimazole, which inhibit the organification of iodine. Iodine (i.e., Lugol solution) administration is also beneficial to inhibit pre-formed thyroid hormone release from the gland.[164] β-Adrenergic blockers such as atenolol or propranolol may be beneficial for blocking the peripheral sympathetic effects of hyperthyroidism preoperatively. However, β-blockade alone has no effect on thyroid hormone synthesis or release; therefore treatment with β-blockers alone preoperatively is less effective for preventing thyrotoxic storm than simultaneous treatment with thioamides and iodine. Preoperative preparation with iopanoic acid (i.e., 500 mg bid), dexamethasone (i.e., 1 mg bid), propylthiouracil, or methimazole and β-blockade has been shown to be successful among patients with severe hyperthyroidism, with the successful avoidance of thyrotoxic storm.[165] β-Blockade must be continued throughout the perioperative period.[166]

Thyrotoxic storm can occur intraoperatively, and is manifested by extreme signs of thyrotoxicosis, including fever, tachycardia, cardiac arrhythmias, and, in extreme cases, cardiovascular collapse, hepatic failure, and death. These signs should be differentiated from the signs of malignant hyperthermia. When thyrotoxic storm is suspected, thyroid gland manipulation should cease and the operation quickly terminated. β-Blockade and steroid administration are the first-line measures of treatment. Propranolol (4–10 mg/kg) is administered to reduce sympathetic activity, and it also blocks the peripheral conversion of T_4 to triiodothyronine (T_3). Steroids (i.e., hydrocortisone 100–300 mg) ameliorate the toxicity associated with thyrotoxicosis by reducing fever, iodine uptake, thyroid-stimulating hormone levels, and the inhibition of the peripheral conversion of T_4 to T_3. Thioamides and iodides are also used acutely to block thyroid hormone synthesis, and propylthiouracil inhibits the peripheral conversion of T_4 to T_3. In conjunction with steroid administration and β-blockade, the patient is promptly treated with intravenous propylthiouracil (600 mg) and sodium iodine (1.0–2.5 g) to reduce thyroid hormone production and release. The patient is

cooled rapidly with cooling blankets, and appropriate intravenous fluids and glucose are administered. All patients should be monitored in an intensive care unit, because fluid requirements may be significant, and blood-pressure support may be required.

Postoperatively, in the awake patient, thyrotoxic storm frequently presents with altered mental status that includes confusion and agitation in addition to high fever and tachycardia. Similar symptoms may occur with severe infection, which should be excluded. Early recognition and prompt intervention are required to prevent subsequent cardiovascular and hepatic failure. Thyrotoxic storm is a potentially lethal complication, and its successful management depends on prompt recognition and proper therapy.

AIRWAY COMPLICATIONS

Difficult Intubation

Patients with goiters or invasive thyroid carcinomas may pose difficulties during intubation by the anesthesiologist. The surgeon and anesthesiologist should communicate preoperatively and agree on an airway management plan. The surgeon should be present at the time of intubation to assist with airway control, if necessary.

Voyagis and Kyriakis[167] reported a 6.8% incidence of difficult intubation among patients with a goiter. Difficult intubation only occurred in those patients with tracheal deviation. They noted no difficulty with mask ventilation in these patients. Shen and colleagues[154] reported an 8% incidence of difficult intubation in a series of patients with substernal goiter. All patients with difficulty required multiple intubation attempts, and one suffered a pharyngeal tear. Bouaggad and colleagues[168] reported a 5% incidence of difficult intubation in patients with goiter. By multivariate analysis, large goiters and malignant goiters were noted to be independent risk factors for difficult intubation.[168]

Because the site of airway obstruction related to goiters is typically located in the trachea, intubation can usually be accomplished with a standard endotracheal tube. The tube will usually pass the narrowed tracheal segment without difficulty. An endotracheal tube stylet may be helpful, and an array of different-sized endotracheal tubes should be readily available should a smaller-diameter tube be needed.

Tracheomalacia

Tracheomalacia represents the weakness of the cartilaginous trachea related to chronic pressure erosion, usually from longstanding compression by goiter.[158,169] Severe tracheomalacia is rare and can be identified intraoperatively by the observation of a soft and collapsible trachea. Rahim and colleagues[169] reported a 6% incidence of tracheomalacia among patients with large goiters. They noted that tracheomalacia was associated with longstanding goiter, significant retrosternal extension, and difficult intubation.

Significant tracheomalacia can result in tracheal collapse and respiratory obstruction after extubation after thyroidectomy. If such obstruction occurs, the patient should be reintubated. Extubation is then performed 24 to 48 hours later under controlled conditions. Recurrent respiratory obstruction necessitates tracheostomy or reintubation for a longer period of time, with the endotracheal tube serving as a splint until paratracheal fibrosis results in satisfactory tracheal support.[158,169] Bilateral vocal-cord paralysis, which is a much more common cause of postoperative airway distress, should be ruled out. When extubation is not possible as a result of a significant loss of tracheal support, management options include the miniplate fixation of the tracheal cartilages, mesh splinting, or tracheal resection.

Pneumothorax

Pneumothorax is a rare complication after thyroidectomy, but it can occur after the removal of a large substernal goiter.[170] A postoperative chest radiograph is useful for the assessment of possible pneumothorax in such cases, but it is not routinely performed after standard thyroidectomy.

Rare Complications

Rare complications of thyroidectomy include Horner syndrome related to injury to the cervical sympathetic trunk and chylous fistula from injury to the thoracic duct.

COMPLICATIONS OF THYROGLOSSAL DUCT CYST SURGERY

A major complication of thyroglossal duct cyst excision is cyst recurrence as a result of inadequate surgery. Prior infection requiring incision and drainage also has been implicated as a factor that increases the possibility of recurrence.[171-173] Excision by the Sistrunk procedure with the removal of the central portion of the hyoid bone and a core of tissue through the base of tongue to the foramen cecum is necessary to remove the duct, which is intimately related to the hyoid bone, and also to remove the duct or ducts between the hyoid and the foramen cecum.[174] Recurrence rates of approximately 5% have been reported after the Sistrunk procedure.[173] Most recurrences occur within 3 months of surgery, but some may present years later.[173] Risk factors for recurrence are the performance of cystectomy alone (without a formal Sistrunk procedure), a history of recurrent

(i.e., >2) infections before surgery, and incision and drainage procedures before definitive resection.[171-173] Thyroglossal cyst recurrence after surgery requires a more extensive resection of the suprahyoid tissue.[171]

Uncommon complications after thyroglossal duct cyst excision include wound infection, abscess, seroma, and hematoma. Postoperative hemorrhage or infection can result in respiratory obstruction; therefore wound drainage and close observation postoperatively are recommended. The complication rate is increased when surgery is performed in the setting of acute inflammation.[174] Salivary fistula formation is possible if entry into the pharynx occurs during dissection. If the pharynx is opened, adequate closure of the entry site should be performed with absorbable sutures.

Iatrogenic hypothyroidism is a rare potential complication of thyroglossal duct cyst excision. The thyroid gland may be undescended, and therefore the removal of all functioning thyroid tissue may occur with cyst excision. The confirmation of a descended thyroid gland should occur preoperatively by physical examination or with an imaging study such as neck ultrasonography.

Injury to the hypoglossal nerve and the superior laryngeal nerve are rare potential complications, particularly for cysts located lateral to the midline and recurrent cysts. Careful dissection and knowledge of the course of these nerves is important to avoid their injury. Postoperatively, odynophagia and dysphagia can sometimes occur, and these are related to the dissection of the hyoid and the foramen cecum. However, these problems usually gradually resolve within several weeks postoperatively.

OUTPATIENT THYROID SURGERY

Thyroidectomy can be safely performed on an outpatient basis in selected patients. Steckler[175] was the first to report no major complications in 41 patients who underwent thyroid lobectomy and who were discharged home on the day of surgery with close outpatient follow up. LoGerfo and colleagues[176] reported a series of 134 thyroid procedures, 76 of which were performed as outpatient thyroid surgeries. Of the 76 patients who underwent outpatient surgery, 21 had total thyroidectomy, 13 had subtotal thyroidectomy, and 42 had lobectomy. There was no difference in the incidence of complications in the group treated as outpatients as compared with patients observed in the hospital setting. A recent study by Spanknebel and colleagues[152] demonstrated the safety of early (<6 hours) hospital discharge for patients who had thyroidectomy with local anesthesia using a strict patient-selection protocol. Local anesthesia limits barriers to early hospital discharge, such as nausea, vomiting, pain, and urinary retention.[152]

The greatest concerns regarding early discharge after thyroidectomy are the development of postoperative airway obstruction, hemorrhage, or severe hypocalcemia. Postoperative calcium measurements or PTH levels have been used to generate algorithms that predict patients who are at risk for postoperative hypocalcemia.[115–120] The slope of the curve of two sequential serum calcium levels predicts normocalcemia in all patients with positive sloping curves and in the majority of patients with negative sloping curves but levels within the low normal range, who can be safely discharged with oral calcium supplementation and teaching.[115,117] The rapid PTH assay can similarly be used to predict the development of significant hypocalcemia, but its major limitation for wide use is significant added costs.[116,118–120,125–127] Alternatively, routine postoperative supplemental oral calcium administration allows outpatient surgery to be accomplished in the majority of patients undergoing uneventful unilateral or total thyroidectomy without added expense or resource use.[177]

Careful patient selection is mandatory for the safe performance of outpatient thyroid surgery. Total thyroidectomy is not a contraindication for early hospital discharge as long as clinical symptoms of hypocalcemia are not present and patients are provided with adequate teaching regarding the signs and symptoms of hypocalcemia and given prophylactic calcium supplementation. Patients in whom inpatient observation should still be considered include medically infirm patients with comorbid conditions, patients with large substernal goiters with a large dead space who have had drain placement, patients undergoing concomitant procedures that would require hospital admission, and patients with blood dyscrasias.[175] In addition, patients in whom the status of all parathyroid glands is of concern are best monitored in an inpatient setting. Patients must be comfortable with the outpatient approach, knowledgeable about postoperative complications, and remain in proximity to the hospital postoperatively.[176] The close follow up of these patients is important to minimize morbidity.

QUALITY OF LIFE

Several recent studies have evaluated quality of life (QOL) after thyroidectomy. Shah and colleagues.[178] evaluated QOL prospectively for 12 months in patients who had either total thyroidectomy or hemithyroidectomy. Patients who had a total thyroidectomy did not have a significantly different QOL than those who had a hemithyroidectomy, which indicates that QOL is not affected by the extent of thyroid surgery. Patients with thyroid cancer had a diminished QOL during the first 6 months postoperatively as compared with those with benign thyroid disease.

Dagan and colleagues[179] evaluated QOL among patients who underwent total thyroidectomy for well-differentiated thyroid carcinoma. The overall QOL in these patients was good. Some gender and age-related differences in QOL were noted. The QOL was found to be better in young patients. Women rated the distress of thyroid hormone withdrawal more highly than men did.

ACKNOWLEDGMENTS

The authors would like to thank Dr. Mark Courey for his review and edits of the manuscript.

REFERENCES

1. Halsted WS: The operative story of goiter. *Johns Hopkins Hosp Rep* 1920;19:169–257.
2. Becker WF: Pioneers in thyroid surgery. *Ann Surg* 1977;185:493–504.
3. Chiang F, Wang L, Huang Y, et al: Recurrent laryngeal nerve palsy after thyroidectomy with routine identification of the recurrent laryngeal nerve. *Surgery* 2005;137:342–347.
4. Ozbas S, Kocak S, Aydintug S, et al: Comparison of the complications of subtotal, near total and total thyroidectomy in the surgical management of multinodular goitre. *Endocr J* 2005;52:199–205.
5. Filho JG, Kowalski LP: Surgical complications after thyroid surgery performed in a cancer hospital. *Otolaryngol Head Neck Surg* 2005;132:490–494.
6. Rosato L, Avenia N, Bernante P, et al: Complications of thyroid surgery: Analysis of a multicentric study on 14,934 patients operated on in Italy over 5 years. *World J Surg* 2004;28:271–276.
7. Bron LP, O'Brien CJ: Total thyroidectomy for clinically benign disease of the thyroid gland. *Br J Surg* 2004;91:569–574.
8. Friguglietti CU, Lin CS, Kulcsar MA: Total thyroidectomy for benign thyroid disease. *Laryngoscope* 2003;113:1820–1826.
9. Bellantone R, Lombardi CP, Bossola M, et al: Total thyroidectomy for management of benign thyroid disease: Review of 526 cases. *World J Surg* 2002;26:1468–1471.
10. Hermann M, Alk G, Roka R, et al: Laryngeal recurrent nerve injury in surgery for benign thyroid disease: Effect of nerve dissection and impact of individual surgeon in more than 27,000 nerves at risk. *Ann Surg* 2002;235:261–268.
11. Prim MP, De Diego JI, Hardisson D, et al: Factors related to nerve injury and hypocalcemia in thyroid gland surgery. *Otolaryngol Head Neck Surg* 2001;124:111–114.
12. Lo C, Kwok K, Yuen P: A prospective evaluation of recurrent laryngeal nerve paralysis during thyroidectomy. *Arch Surg* 2000;135:204–207.
13. Moulton-Barrett R, Crumley R, Jalilie S, et al: Complications of thyroid surgery. *Int Surg* 1997;82:63–66.
14. Bergamaschi R, Becouarn G, Ronceray J, et al: Morbidity of thyroid surgery. *Am J Surg* 1998;176:71–75.
15. Sosa JA, Bowman HM, Tielsch JM, et al: The importance of surgeon experience for clinical and economic outcomes from thyroidectomy. *Ann Surg* 1998;228:320–330.
16. Harness JK, Fung L, Thompson NW, et al: Total thyroidectomy: Complications and technique. *World J Surg* 1986;10:781–786.
17. Levin KE, Clark AH, Duh Q, et al: Reoperative thyroid surgery. *Surgery* 1992;111:604–609.
18. Falk SA, McCaffrey TV: Management of the recurrent laryngeal nerve in suspected and proven thyroid cancer. *Otolaryngol Head Neck Surg* 1995;113:42–48.
19. Steurer M, Passler C, Denk DM, et al: Advantages of recurrent laryngeal nerve identification in thyroidectomy and parathyroidectomy and the importance of preoperative and postoperative laryngoscopic examination in more than 1000 nerves at risk. *Laryngoscope* 2002;112:124–133.
20. McIvor NP, Flint DJ, Gillibrand J, et al: Thyroid surgery and voice-related outcomes. *ANZ J Surg* 2000;70:179–183.

21. Sinagra DL, Montesinos MR, Tacchi VA, et al: Voice changes after thyroidectomy without recurrent laryngeal nerve injury. *J Am Coll Surg* 2004;199:556–560.

22. Rosato L, Carlevato MT, De Toma G, et al: Recurrent laryngeal nerve damage and phonetic modifications after total thyroidectomy: Surgical malpractice only or predictable sequelae? *World J Surg* 2005;29:780–784.

23. Franko J, Kish KJ, Pezzi CM, et al: Safely increasing the efficacy of thyroidectomy using a new bipolar electrosealing device (LigaSure) versus conventional clamp-and-tie technique. *Am Surg* 2006;72:132–136.

24. Voutilainen PE, Haglund CH: Ultrasonically activated shears in thyroidectomies: A randomized trial. *Ann Surg* 2000;231:322–328.

25. Kiriakopoulos A, Dimitros T, Dimitros L: Use of a diathermy system in thyroid surgery. *Arch Surg* 2004;139:997–1000.

26. Siperstein AE, Berber E, Morkoyun E: The use of the harmonic scalpel vs conventional knot tying for vessel ligation in thyroid surgery. *Arch Surg* 2002;137:137–142.

27. Lachanas VA, Prokopakis EP, Mpenakis AA, et al: The use of Ligasure Vessel Sealing System in thyroid surgery. *Otolaryngol Head Neck Surg* 2005;132:487–489.

28. Shemen L: Thyroidectomy using the harmonic scalpel: Analysis of 105 cases. *Otolaryngol Head Neck Surg* 2002;127:284–288.

29. Testini M, Nacchiero M, Piccinni G, et al : Total thyroidectomy is improved by loupe magnification. *Microsurgery* 2004;24:39–42.

30. Loré JM: Complications of thyroid surgery. In Loré JM, editor: *An atlas of head and neck surgery,* ed 3, Philadelphia, 1988, WB Saunders, 1988.

31. Wang L, Lee K, Kuo W, et al: The efficacy of intraoperative corticosteroids in recurrent laryngeal nerve palsy after thyroid surgery. *World J Surg* 2006;30:299–303.

32. Herranz-Gonzalez J, Gavilan J, Matinez-Vidal J, et al: Complications following thyroid surgery. *Arch Otolaryngol Head Neck Surg* 1991;117:516–518.

33. Riddell V: Thyroidectomy: Prevention of bilateral recurrent nerve palsy: Results of identification of the nerve over 23 consecutive years (1946-69) with description of an additional safety measure. *Br J Surg* 1970;57:1–11.

34. Hisham AN, Lukman MR: Recurrent laryngeal nerve in thyroid surgery: A critical appraisal. *ANZ J Surg* 2002;72:887–889.

35. Wheeler MH: Thyroid surgery and the recurrent laryngeal nerve. *Br J Surg* 1999;86:291–292.

36. Friedman M, Toriumi DM: Esophageal stethoscope: Another possible cause of vocal cord paralysis. *Arch Otolaryngol Head Neck Surg* 1989;115:95–98.

37. Karlan MS, Catz B, Dunkelman D, et al: A safe technique for thyroidectomy with complete nerve dissection and parathyroid preservation. *Head Neck Surg* 1984;6:1014–1019.

38. Nemiroff PM, Katz AD: Extralaryngeal divisions of the recurrent laryngeal nerve: Surgical and clinical significance. *Am J Surg* 1982;144:466–469.

39. Monfared A, Gorti G, Kim D: Microsurgical anatomy of the laryngeal nerves as related to thyroid surgery. *Laryngoscope* 2002;112:386–392.

40. Loré JM: Practical anatomical considerations in thyroid tumor surgery. *Arch Otolaryngol* 1983;109:568–574.

41. Srinivasan V, Premachandra DJ: Non-recurrent laryngeal nerve: Identification during thyroid surgery. *ORL J Otorhinolaryngol Relat Spec* 1997;59:57–59.

42. Toniato A, Mazzarotto R, Piotto A, et al: Identification of the nonrecurrent laryngeal nerve during thyroid surgery: 20 year experience. *World J Surg* 2004;28:659–661.

43. Hermans R, Dewandel P, Debruyne F, et al: Arteria lusoria identified on preoperative CT and nonrecurrent inferior laryngeal nerve during thyroidectomy: A prospective study. *Head Neck* 2003;25:113–117.

44. Henry JF, Audiffret J, Denizot A, et al: The nonrecurrent inferior laryngeal nerve: Review of 33 cases, including two on the left side. *Surgery* 1988;104:977–984.

45. Proye CAG, Carnaille BM, Goropoulos A: Nonrecurrent and recurrent inferior laryngeal nerve: A surgical pitfall in cervical exploration. *Am J Surg* 1991;162:495–496.

46. Marcus B, Edwards B, Yoo S, et al: Recurrent laryngeal nerve monitoring in thyroid and parathyroid surgery: The University of Michigan experience. *Laryngoscope* 2003;113:356–361.

47. Otto RA, Cochran CS: Sensitivity and specificity of intraoperative recurrent laryngeal nerve stimulation in predicting postoperative nerve paralysis. *Ann Otol Rhinol Laryngol* 2002;111:1005–1007.

48. Dralle H, Sekulla C, Haerting J, et al: Risk factors of paralysis and functional outcome after recurrent laryngeal nerve monitoring in thyroid surgery. *Surgery* 2004;136:1310–1322.

49. Hermann M, Hellebart C, Freissmuth M: Neuromonitoring in thyroid surgery: Prospective evaluation of intraoperative electrophysiological responses for the prediction of recurrent laryngeal nerve injury. *Ann Surg* 2004;240:9–17.

50. Witt RL: Recurrent laryngeal nerve electrophysiologic monitoring in thyroid surgery: The standard of care? *J Voice* 2005;19:497–500.

51. Djohan RS, Rodriguez HE, Connolly MM, et al: Intraoperative monitoring of recurrent laryngeal nerve function. *Am Surg* 2000;66:595–597.

52. Beldi G, Kinsbergen T, Schlumpf R: Evaluation of intraoperative recurrent nerve monitoring in thyroid surgery. *World J Surg* 2004;28:589–591.

53. Yarbrough DE, Thompson GB, Kasperbauer JL, et al: Intraoperative electromyographic monitoring of the recurrent laryngeal nerve in reoperative thyroid and parathyroid surgery. *Surgery* 2004;136:1107–1115.

54. Randolph GW, Kobler JB, Wilkins J: Recurrent laryngeal nerve identification and assessment during thyroid surgery: Laryngeal palpation. *World J Surg* 2004;28:755–760.

55. Robertson ML, Steward DL, Gluckman JL, et al: Continuous laryngeal nerve integrity monitoring during thyroidectomy: Does it reduce risk of injury? *Otolaryngol Head Neck Surg* 2004;131:596–600.

56. Eisele DW: Intraoperative electrophysiologic monitoring of the recurrent laryngeal nerve. *Laryngoscope* 1996;106:443–449.

57. Khan A, Pearlman RC, Bianchi DA, et al: Experience with two types of electromyography monitoring electrodes during thyroid surgery. *Am J Otolaryngol* 1997;18:99–102.

58. Green DC, Ward PH: The management of the divided recurrent laryngeal nerve. *Laryngoscope* 1978;88:1034–1041.

59. Horsley J: Suture of the recurrent laryngeal nerve with report of a case. *Trans South Surg Gynecol Assoc* 1909;22:161–167.

60. Lahey FH: Suture of the recurrent laryngeal nerve for bilateral abductor paralysis. *Ann Surg* 1927;87:481–484.

61. Crumley RL: Repair of the recurrent laryngeal nerve. *Otolaryngol Clin North Am* 1990;23:553–563.

62. Mu L, Yang S: Electromyographic study on end-to-end anastomosis of the recurrent laryngeal nerve in dogs. *Laryngoscope* 1990;100:1009–1017.

63. Chou FF, Su CY, Jeng SF, et al: Neurorrhaphy of the recurrent laryngeal nerve. *J Am Coll Surg* 2003;197:52–57.

64. Crumley RL: Current status of laryngeal reinnervation. In Johnson JT, editor: *Instructional courses,* vol 4, St Louis, 1991, Mosby-Year Book.

65. Woodson GE: Configuration of the glottis in laryngeal paralysis: I: Clinical study. *Laryngoscope* 1993;103:1227–1234.

66. Netterville JL, Stone RE, Rainey C, et al: Recurrent laryngeal nerve avulsion for treatment of spasmodic dysphonia. *Ann Otol Rhinol Laryngol* 1991;100:10–14.

67. Crumley RL: Laryngeal synkinesis revisited. *Ann Otol Rhinol Laryngol* 2000;109:365–371.

68. Crumley RL: Update: Ansa cervicalis to recurrent laryngeal nerve anastomosis for unilateral laryngeal paralysis. *Laryngoscope* 1991;101:384–388.

69. Crumley RL: Voice quality following laryngeal reinnervation by ansa hypoglossi transfer. *Laryngoscope* 1986;96:611–616.

70. Crumley RL: Unilateral recurrent laryngeal nerve paralysis. *J Voice* 1994;8:79–83.

71. Maronian N, Waugh P, Robinson L, et al: Electromyographic findings in recurrent laryngeal nerve reinnervation. *Ann Otol Rhinol Laryngol* 2003;112:314–323.

72. Netterville JL, Aly A, Ossoff RH: Evaluation and treatment of complications of thyroid and parathyroid surgery. *Otolaryngol Clin N Am* 1990;23:529–552.

73. Hartl DM, Travagli JP, Leboulleux S, et al: Clinical review: Current concepts in the management of unilateral recurrent laryngeal nerve paralysis after thyroid surgery. *J Clin Endocrinol Metab* 2005;90:3084–3088.

74. Kwon TK, Buckmire R: Injection laryngoplasty for management of unilateral vocal cord paralysis. *Curr Opin Otolaryngol Head Neck Surg* 2004;12:538–542.

75. O'Leary MA, Grillone GA: Injection laryngoplasty. *Otolaryngol Clin North Am* 2006;39:43–54.

76. Belafsky PC, Postma GN: Vocal fold augmentation with calcium hydroxylapatite. *Otolaryngol Head Neck Surg* 2004;131: 351–3544.

77. Rosen CA, Gartner-Schmidt J, Casiano R, et al: Vocal fold augmentation with calcium hydroxylapatite (CaHA). *Otolaryngol Head Neck Surg* 2007;136:198–204.

78. Isshiki N, Taira T, Kojima H, et al: Recent modifications in thyroplasty type I. *Ann Otol Rhinol Laryngol* 1989;98:777–779.

79. Koufman JA: Laryngoplasty for vocal cord medialization: An alternative to Teflon. *Laryngoscope* 1986;96:726–731.

80. Zeitels SM, Mauri M, Dailey SH: Adduction arytenopexy for vocal fold paralysis: Indications and technique. *J Laryngol Otol* 2004;118:508–516.

81. Kashima HK: Documentation of upper airway obstruction in unilateral vocal cord paralysis: Flow-volume loop studies in 43 subjects. *Laryngoscope* 1984;94:923–937.

82. Parnes SM, Satya-Murti S: Predictive value of laryngeal electromyography in patients with vocal cord paralysis of neurogenic origin. *Laryngoscope* 1985;95:1323–1326.

83. Montiel GC, Quadrelli SA, Roncoroni AJ, et al: Treatment of respiratory insufficiency secondary to vocal cord bilateral paralysis with continuous positive pressure. *Medicina (B Aires)* 1994;54:241–244.

84. Christopher K, Arbelaez C, Yodice PC: Bilateral vocal cord dysfunction complicating short-term intubation and the utility of heliox. *Respiration* 2002;69:366–368.

85. Jori J, Rovo L, Czigner J: Vocal cord laterofixation as early treatment for acute bilateral abductor paralysis after thyroid surgery. *Eur Arch Otorhinolaryngol* 1998;255:375–378.

86. Rovo I, Jori J, Ivan L, et al: Early vocal cord laterofixation for the treatment of bilateral vocal cord immobility. *Eur Arch Otorhinolaryngol* 2001;258:509–513.

87. Lichtenberger G: Reversible laterofixation of the paralyzed vocal cord without tracheotomy. *Ann Otol Rhinol Laryngol* 2002;111:21–26.

88. Echeverri A, Flexon PB: Electrophysiologic nerve stimulation for identifying the recurrent laryngeal nerve in thyroid surgery: Review of 70 consecutive thyroid surgeries. *Am Surg* 1998;64:328–333.

89. Cernea CR, Ferraz AR, Furlani J, et al: Identification of the external branch of the superior laryngeal nerve during thyroidectomy. *Am J Surg* 1992;164:634–639.

90. Lore JM Jr, Kokocharov SI, Kaufman S, et al: Thirty-eight–year evaluation of a surgical technique to protect the external branch of the superior laryngeal nerve during thyroidectomy. *Ann Otol Rhinol Laryngol* 1998;107:1015–1022.

91. Robinson JL, Mandel S, Sataloff RT: Objective voice measures in nonsinging patients with unilateral superior laryngeal nerve paralysis. *J Voice* 2005;19:665–667.

92. Crookes PF, Recabaren JA: Injury to the superior laryngeal branch of the vagus during thyroidectomy: Lesson or myth? *Ann Surg* 2001;233:588–593.

93. Shaha AR: Safe ligation of superior thyroid vessels. *J Surg Oncol* 1993;53:208.

94. Cernea CR, Nishio S, Hojaij FC: Identification of the external branch of the superior laryngeal nerve in large goiters. *Am J Otolaryngol* 1995;16:307–311.

95. Friedman M, LoSavio P, Ibrahim H: Superior laryngeal nerve identification and preservation in thyroidectomy. *Arch Otolaryngol Head Neck Surg* 2002;128:296–303.

96. Hurtado-Lopez LM, Pacheco-Alvarez MI, Montes-Castillo MD, et al: Importance of the intraoperative identification of the external branch of the superior laryngeal nerve during thyroidectomy: Electromyographic evaluation. *Thyroid* 2005;15:449–454.

97. Bellantone R, Boscherini M, Lombardi CP, et al: Is the identification of the external branch of the superior laryngeal nerve mandatory in thyroid operation? Results of a prospective randomized study. *Surgery* 2001;130:1055–1059.

98. Jonas J, Bahr R: Neuromonitoring of the external branch of the superior laryngeal nerve during thyroid surgery. *Am J Surg* 2000;179:234–236.

99. El-Kashlan HKJ, Carroll WR, Hogikyan ND, et al: Selective cricothyroid muscle reinnervation by muscle-nerve-muscle neurotization. *Arch Otolaryngol Head Neck Surg* 2001;127:1211–1215.

100. Pattou F, Combemale F, Fabre S, et al: Hypocalcemia following thyroid surgery: Incidence and prediction of outcome. *World J Surg* 1998;22:718–724.

101. Shaha AR, Jaffe BM: Parathyroid preservation during thyroid surgery. *Am J Otolaryngol* 1998;19:113–117.

102. Harness JK, Fung L, Thompson NW, et al: Total thyroidectomy: Complications and technique. *World J Surg* 1986;10:781–786.

103. Wingert DJ, Friesen SR, Pierce GE, et al: Post-thyroidectomy hypocalcemia. Incidence and risk factors. *Am J Surg* 1986;152: 606–610.

104. McHenry CR, Speroff T, Wentworth D, et al: Risk factors for postthyroidectomy hypocalcemia. *Surgery* 1994;116:641–648.

105. Falk SA, Birken EA, Baran DT: Temporary postthyroidectomy hypocalcemia. *Arch Otolaryngol Head Neck Surg* 1988;114: 168–174.

106. Watson CG, Steed DL, Robinson AG, et al: The role of calcitonin and parathyroid hormone in the pathogenesis of postthyroidectomy hypocalcemia. *Metab Clin Exp* 1981;30:588–589.

107. Demeester-Mirkine N, Hooghe L, Van Geertruyden J, et al: Hypocalcemia after thyroidectomy. *Arch Surg* 1992;127:854–858.

108. Shen W, Duren M, Morita E, et al: Reoperation for persistent or recurrent primary hyperparathyroidism. *Arch Surg* 1996;131: 861–869.

109. Rice DH: Surgery of the parathyroid glands. *Otolaryngol Clin N Am* 1996;29:693–699.

110. Lo C, Lam K: Postoperative hypocalcemia in patients who did or did not undergo parathyroid autotransplantation during thyroidectomy: A comparative study. *Surgery* 1998;124:1081–1087.

111. Olson JA Jr, DeBenedetti MK, Baumann DS, et al: Parathyroid autotransplantation during thyroidectomy: Results of long-term follow-up. *Ann Surg* 1996;5:472–480.

112. Shaha AR, Burnett C, Jaffe BM: Parathyroid autotransplantation during thyroid surgery. *J Surg Oncol* 1991;46:21–24.

113. Walker RP, Paloyan E, Kelley TF, et al: Parathyroid autotransplantation in patients undergoing a total thyroidectomy: A review of 261 patients. *Otolaryngol Head Neck Surg* 1994;111:258–264.

114. Szubin L, Kacker A, Kakani R, et al: The management of postthyroidectomy hypocalcemia. *Ear Nose Throat J* 1996;75: 612–616.

115. Nahas ZS, Farrag TY, Lin FR, et al: A safe and cost-effective short hospital stay protocol to identify patients at low risk for the development of significant hypocalcemia after total thyroidectomy. *Laryngoscope* 2006;116:906–910.

116. Higgins KM, Mandell DL, Govindaraj S, et al: The role of intraoperative rapid parathyroid hormone monitoring for predicting thyroidectomy-related hypocalcemia. *Arch Otolaryngol Head Neck Surg* 2004;130:63–67.

117. Adams J, Andersen P, Everts E, et al: Early postoperative calcium levels as predictors of hypocalcemia. *Laryngoscope* 1998;108:1829–1831.

118. Vescan A, Witterick I, Freeman J: Parathyroid hormone as a predictor of hypocalcemia after thyroidectomy. *Laryngoscope* 2005;115:2105–2108.

119. Scurry WC, Beus KS, Hollenbeak CS, et al: Perioperative parathyroid hormone assay for diagnosis and management of postthyroidectomy hypocalcemia. *Laryngoscope* 2005;115: 1362–1366.

120. Warren FM, Andersen P, Wax MK, et al: Perioperative parathyroid hormone levels in thyroid surgery: Preliminary report. *Laryngoscope* 2004;114:689–693.

121. Gulluoglu BM, Manukyan MN, Cingi A, et al: Early prediction of normocalcemia after thyroid surgery. *World J Surg* 2005; 29:1288–1293.

122. Luu Q, Andersen PE, Adams J, et al: The predictive value of perioperative calcium levels after thyroid/parathyroid surgery. *Head Neck* 2002;24:63–67.

123. Lam A, Kerr PD: Parathyroid hormone: an early predictor of postthyroidectomy hypocalcemia. *Laryngoscope* 2003;113: 2196–2200.

124. Lombardi CP, Raffaelli M, Princi P, et al: Early prediction of postthyroidectomy hypocalcemia by one single iPTH measurement. *Surgery* 2004;136:1236–1241.

125. Chia SH, Weisman RA, Tieu D, et al: Prospective study of perioperative factors predicting hypocalcemia after thyroid and parathyroid surgery. *Arch Otolaryngol Head Neck Surg* 2006; 132:41–45.

126. Lindblom P, Westerdagk J, Bergenfelz A: Low parathyroid hormone levels after thyroid surgery: A feasible predictor of hypocalcemia. *Surgery* 2002;131:515–520.

127. Seehofer D, Rayes N, Ulrich F, et al: Intraoperative measurement of intact parathyroid hormone in renal hyperparathyroidism by an inexpensive routine assay. *Langenbecks Arch Surg* 2001;286:440–443.

128. McHenry CR, Slusarczyk SJ: Hypothyroidism following hemithyroidectomy: Incidence, risk factors, and management. *Surgery* 2000;128:994–998.

129. Miller F, Paulson D, Prihoda TJ, et al: Risk factors for the development of hypothyroidism after hemithyroidectomy. *Arch Otolaryngol Head Neck Surg* 2006;132:36–38.

130. Piper HG, Bugis SP, Wilkins GE, et al: Detecting and defining hypothyroidism after hemithyroidectomy. *Am J Surg* 2005;189: 587–591.

131. Farkas EA, King TA, Bolton JS, et al: A comparison of total thyroidectomy and lobectomy in the treatment of dominant thyroid nodules. *Am Surg* 2002;68:678–682.

132. Filho JG, Kowalski LP: Postoperative complications of thyroidectomy for differentiated thyroid carcinoma. *Am J Otolaryngol* 2004;25:225–230.

133. Mittendorf EA, McHenry CR: Thyroidectomy for selected patients with thyrotoxicosis. *Arch Otolaryngol Head Neck Surg* 2001;127:61–65.

134. Bhattacharyya N, Fried MP: Assessment of the morbidity and complications of total thyroidectomy. *Arch Otolaryngol Head Neck Surg* 2002;128:389–392.

135. Abbas G, Dubner S, Keller KS: Re-operation for bleeding after thyroidectomy and parathyroidectomy. *Head Neck* 2001;23:544–546.

136. Matory YL, Spiro RH: Wound bleeding after head and neck surgery. *J Surg Oncol* 1993;53:17–19.

137. Lacoste L, Gineste D, Karayan J, et al: Airway complications in thyroid surgery. *Ann Otol Rhinol Laryngol* 1993;102:441–446.

138. Shaha AR, Jaffe BM: Selective use of drains in thyroid surgery. *J Surg Oncol* 1993;52:241–243.

139. Ayyash K, Khammash M, Tibblin S: Drain vs. no drain in primary thyroid and parathyroid surgery. *Eur J Surg* 1991;157:113–114.

140. Wihlborg O, Bergljung L, Martensson H: To drain or not to drain in thyroid surgery: A controlled clinical study. *Arch Surg* 1988; 123:40–41.

141. Peix JL, Teboul F, Feldman H, et al: Drainage after thyroidectomy: A randomized clinical trial. *Int Surg* 1992;77:122–124.

142. Suslu N, Vural S, Oncel M, et al: Is the insertion of drains after uncomplicated thyroid surgery always necessary? *Surg Today* 2006;36:215–218.

143. Burkey SH, van Heerden JA, Thompson GB, et al: Reexploration for symptomatic hematomas after cervical exploration. *Surgery* 2001;130:914–920.

144. Hurtado-Lopez LM, Lopez-Romero S, Rizzo-Fuentes C, et al: Selective use of drains in thyroid surgery. *Head Neck* 2001;23: 189–193.

145. Lee SW, Choi EC, Lee YM, et al: Is lack of placement of drains after thyroidectomy with central neck dissection safe? A prospective, randomized study. *Laryngoscope* 2006;116: 1632–1635.

146. Corsten M, Johnson S, Alherabi A: Is suction drainage an effective means of preventing hematoma in thyroid surgery? A meta-analysis. *J Otolaryngol* 2005;34:415–417.

147. Fugii Y, Nakayama M: Efficacy of dexamethasone for reducing postoperative nausea and vomiting and analgesic requirements after thyroidectomy. *Otolaryngol Head Neck Surg* 2007; 136:274–277.

148. Wang JJ, Ho ST, Lee SC, et al: The use of dexamethasone for preventing postoperative nausea and vomiting in females undergoing thyroidectomy: A dose-ranging study. *Anesth Analg* 2000;91:1404–1407.

149. Shaha AR, Jaffe BM: Practical management of postthyroidectomy hematoma. *J Surg Oncol* 1994;57:235–238.

150. Shaha A, Jaffe BM: Complications of thyroid surgery performed by residents. *Surgery* 1988;104:1109–1114.

151. Matory YL, Spiro RH: Wound bleeding after head and neck surgery. *J Surg Oncol* 1993;53:17–19.

152. Spanknebel K, Chabot JA, DiGeorgi M, et al: Thyroidectomy using local anesthesia: A report of 1,025 cases over 16 years. *J Am Coll Surg* 2005;201:375–385.

153. Martensson H, Terins J: Recurrent laryngeal nerve palsy in thyroid gland surgery related to operations and nerves at risk. *Arch Surg* 1985;120:475–477.

154. Shen WT, Kebebew E, Duh QY, et al: Predictors of airway complication after thyroidectomy for substernal goiter. *Arch Surg* 2004;138:656–660.

155. Torre G, Borgonovo G, Amato A, et al: Surgical management of substernal goiter: Analysis of 237 patients. *Am Surg* 1995; 61:826–831.

156. Shaha A, Alfonso AE, Jaffe BM: Operative treatment of substernal goiters. *Head Neck* 1989;11:325–330.

157. Clark OH, Lal G: Novel technique for control of mediastinal bleeding during thyroidectomy for substernal goiter. *J Am Coll Surg* 2003;196:818–820.

158. Singh B, Lucente FE, Shaha AR: Substernal goiter: a clinical review. *Am J Otolaryngol* 1994;15:409–416.

159. Sanders LE, Rossi RL, Shahian DM, et al: Mediastinal goiters: The need for an aggressive approach. *Arch Surg* 1992;127: 609–613.

160. Tabaqchali MA, Hanson JM, Proud G. Drains for thyroidectomy/parathyroidectomy: Fact or fiction? *Ann R Coll Surg Engl* 1999; 81:302–305.

161. Karayacin K, Besim H, Ercan F, et al: Thyroidectomy with and without drains. *East Afr Med J* 1997;74:431–432.

162. Johnson JT, Wagner RL: Infection following uncontaminated head and neck surgery. *Otolaryngol Head Neck Surg* 1987; 113:369–369.

163. Hong KH, Kim YK: Phonatory characteristics of patients undergoing thyroidectomy without laryngeal nerve injury. *Otolaryngol Head Neck Surg* 1997;117:399–404.

164. Gourin CG, Johnson JT: Postoperative complications. In Randolph GW, editor: *Surgery of the thyroid and parathyroid glands,* Philadelphia, 2003, Saunders.

165. Panzer C, Beazley R, Braverman L: Rapid preoperative preparation for severe hyperthyroid Graves' disease. *J Clin Endocrinol Metab* 2004;89:2142–2144.

166. Reeve T, Thompson NW: Complications of thyroid surgery: How to avoid them, how to manage them, and observations on their possible effect on the whole patient. *World J Surg* 2000;24:971–975.

167. Voyagis GS, Kyriakos KP: The effect of goiter on endotracheal intubation. *Anesth Analg* 1997;84:611–612.

168. Bouaggad A, Nejmi SE, Bouderka MA, et al: Prediction of difficult tracheal intubation in thyroid surgery. *Anesth Analg* 2004; 99:603–606.

169. Abdel Rahim AA, Ahmed ME, Hassan MA: Respiratory complications after thyroidectomy and the need for tracheostomy in patients with a large goitre. *Br J Surg* 1999;86:88–90.

170. Cho AT, Cohen JP, Som ML: Management of substernal and intrathoracic goiters. *Otolaryngol Head Neck Surg* 1986;94: 282–287.

171. Josephson GD, Spencer WR, Josephson JS: Thyroglossal duct cyst: The New York Eye and Ear Infirmary experience and a literature review. *Ear Nose Throat J* 1998;77:642–651.

172. Kaselas C, Tsikopoulos G, Chortis C, et al: Thyroglossal duct cyst's inflammation: When do we operate? *Pediatr Surg Int* 2005;21:991–993.

173. Marionowski R, Ait Amre JL, Morisseau-Durand MP, et al: Risk factors for thyroglossal duct remnants after Sistrunk procedure in a pediatric population. *Int J Pediatr Otorhinolaryngol* 2003; 67:19–23.

174. Maddalozzo J, Venkatesan TK, Gupta P: Complications associated with the Sistrunk procedure. *Laryngoscope* 2001;111: 119–123.

175. Steckler RM: Outpatient thyroidectomy: A feasibility study. *Am J Surg* 1986;152:417–419.

176. LoGerfo P, Gates R, Gazetas P: Outpatient and short-stay thyroid surgery. *Head Neck* 1991;13:97–101.

177. Moore FD Jr: Oral calcium supplements to enhance early hospital discharge after bilateral surgical treatment of the thyroid gland or exploration of the parathyroid glands. *J Am Coll Surg* 1994;178:11–16.

178. Shah MD, Witterick IJ, Eski SJ, et al: Quality of life in patients undergoing thyroid surgery. *J Otolaryngol* 2006;35:209–215.

179. Dagan T, Bedrin L, Horowitz Z, et al: Quality of life of well-differentiated thyroid carcinoma patients. *J Laryngol Otol* 2004;118:537–542.

CHAPTER 40

Complications
of Parathyroid Surgery

Lisa A. Orloff

The parathyroid glands were only identified as recently as 1850 in an Indian rhinoceros in a London zoo by anatomist Richard Owen. Human parathyroid glands were first recognized by Swedish medical student Ivar Sandström during the 1880s.[1] The first recorded intentional and successful (albeit transiently) parathyroidectomy was performed in 1925 by Felix Mandl of Vienna.[2] The existence of some "factor" that regulated serum calcium homeostasis was suspected, because patients who underwent thyroidectomy had a high incidence of postoperative tetany, as first described by Wölfer in 1879.[1] The French pathologist Gley performed work during the 1890s that led to a true understanding of the parathyroid glands, their function, and the importance of their preservation during thyroid surgery to prevent tetany.[1,2] Surgery directly on the parathyroid glands is almost exclusively performed to correct the endocrinopathy of hyperparathyroidism (HPT) and its associated hypercalcemia. Rarely are nonfunctioning parathyroid cysts or tumors excised purely because of their mass effect. Today parathyroidectomy is a common procedure with indications and surgical techniques that have been and that continue to be refined. The majority of parathyroid surgery is directed at curing primary, idiopathic, or sporadic HPT, but HPT associated with multiple endocrine neoplasia syndromes, familial HPT (i.e., HPT-jaw tumor and other) syndromes, and secondary and tertiary HPT associated with chronic renal failure are also causes for parathyroid surgery. HPT is primarily a surgical disease that can be treated safely and with an exceptionally high overall success rate. However, the potential for significant complications is very real, mainly as a result of the positioning of the parathyroid glands amid anatomy that is complex, convoluted, and camouflaging.

First and foremost, the diagnosis of primary HPT must be accurate for surgery to be appropriate and successful. The diagnoses of secondary and tertiary HPT are usually obvious as a result of the known metabolic complications of chronic renal failure. Alternatively, the differential diagnosis of hypercalcemia is quite broad, and the most common and significant other major cause of hypercalcemia is malignancy, which must be ruled out. Parathyroid surgery performed in patients with hypercalcemia resulting from other causes, including familial hypocalciuric hypercalcemia, lithium therapy, sarcoidosis or other granulomatous diseases, immobilization, vitamin A or D intoxication, milk–alkali

syndrome, acute renal failure, or other endocrinopathies is sure to fail in its effort to correct this metabolic derangement.[3]

QUALITY-OF-LIFE SIGNIFICANCE

After the diagnosis of hyperparathyroidism has been made, the decision of whether to perform surgery generally revolves around current and potential future quality-of-life issues. Both acute and chronic symptoms may prompt surgical intervention. Symptomatic renal calculi are the most common acute cause for the detection of HPT and subsequent intervention. Alternatively, routine serum calcium testing often leads to the incidental detection of hypercalcemia, which is retrospectively associated with vague chronic symptoms such as fatigue, memory and cognitive impairment, gastrointestinal symptoms, bone pain, and depression. These symptoms in combination with the potential for the progressive loss of bone mineral density, the potential for symptomatic nephrolithiasis, and the potential negative influence on the management of hypertension typically prompt consideration of parathyroidectomy. Patients are increasingly seeking treatment armed with information and expectations derived from the Internet about the range of symptoms of HPT and the treatment options. The perceived risks and symptoms of HPT are weighed against the potential risks of surgical intervention on an individual patient basis. Overall, parathyroid surgery is extremely safe; nevertheless, as with thyroid surgery (see Chapter 39), the management of complications that do occasionally occur strongly influences long-term morbidity.

WOUND COMPLICATIONS

Hemorrhage and Hematoma

Life-threatening intraoperative hemorrhage is rarely encountered during parathyroid surgery.[4] However, unrecognized hemorrhage during surgery, even if it is minor, can have dire consequences in the form of postoperative airway-obstructing hematoma. Meticulous hemostasis during parathyroidectomy is required for this reason and for the optimal identification of the adjacent neural structures and the often well-camouflaged parathyroid glands themselves. The pursuit of hemostasis itself must be done in a very precise manner, typically using bipolar cautery, Harmonic technology, or vessel ligation with sutures or clips to avoid nerve damage. Bleeding is more problematic in the presence of recognized or unrecognized coagulopathies or unreversed anticoagulant therapy. Blood loss is also more likely in the setting of coexisting thyroid enlargement that requires dissection and mobilization as well as with venous hypertension, aberrant blood supply, and the substernal or intrathoracic location of an enlarged parathyroid gland.[5–7] The most common vascular anomaly (i.e., in up to 5% of patients on the left side and 2% on the right side)[5] is the absence of an inferior thyroid artery branch of the thyrocervical trunk. In such patients, branches of the thyroid ima artery coming directly from the subclavian artery supply the parathyroid glands, and they can be in an unexpected retrosternal or less accessible location. During the resection of intrathymic or ectopic mediastinal parathyroids, it is critical to control the inferior thyroid vessels in the neck, because the retraction of divided vessels into the mediastinum may require sternotomy to gain vascular control.[8]

Achieving satisfactory hemostasis before wound closure can be facilitated by identifying sources of bleeding through wound irrigation, head flexion, Trendelenberg Positioning, and a positive-pressure Valsalva maneuver. Minor troublesome oozing may be controlled with the application of fibrin glue or similar hemostatic substances if the source is not readily identifiable.[4,9]

The incidence of postoperative hematoma in thyroid and parathyroid surgery combined is 0% to 3%[6,8,10–12]; the reported incidence in parathyroidectomy alone is less than 1%.[13] Hematomas can result from inadequate hemostasis during surgery, from increased arterial and venous pressure at extubation, or emergence from general anesthesia as a result of coughing, a Valsalva maneuver, or pain. Neither pressure dressings nor surgical drains prevent hematoma formation, but drain output has the potential advantage of providing an earlier visual display of postoperative hemorrhage. A number of retrospective and randomized clinical studies have documented that the use of a drain in thyroid and parathyroid surgery has no impact on the incidence of hematoma formation.[14–17] "Queen Anne" or other bulky neck dressings obscure the neck from surveillance and can actually aggravate the symptoms of airway compression if a hematoma does develop. The serial measurement of neck circumference during the early postoperative period is an objective method for detecting an expanding hematoma.

Early recognition and intervention are critical to the management of postoperative neck hematoma. Delayed intervention can lead to airway compression, laryngeal edema, postobstructive pulmonary edema, and even death. Most hematomas are clinically apparent within 2 to 4 hours of surgery, thus justifying the move toward outpatient parathyroidectomy in select cases after a several-hour period of observation during recovery. However, if a hematoma is detected, it should immediately be explored and evacuated, preferably in the operating room. The bedside removal of neck sutures allows for acute airway decompression, but intubation and exploration for the control of hemorrhage are best done with experienced personnel and appropriate lighting and equipment in the operating room setting. Ironically, most explorations fail to identify a specific bleeding vessel[6,10] yet achieve airway decompression and the removal of extravasated blood that can otherwise lead to impaired wound healing.[11,18,19]

Seroma

Seroma associated with thyroid and parathyroid surgery combined has a reported incidence of 0% to 6%.[20] Seroma formation is more common in cases of bilateral dissection, substernal dissection, and concomitant subtotal thyroidectomy, and a trend toward greater seroma formation has been seen when drainage is not used in these settings.[14,21] The selective usage of drains is therefore recommended, and closed drains can also treat seromas, thereby obviating the need for repeated aspiration. In the modern era of minimally invasive and directed parathyroidectomy, drains are less and less commonly employed.

Infection

Wound infections (Figure 40-1) associated with parathyroid surgery are quite rare, occurring in fewer than 2% of cases.[10,12,14,18,22] Prophylactic antibiotics are not indicated, because these are clean procedures of relatively short duration. Neither the use of perioperative antibiotics nor the use of a drain has been shown to alter the

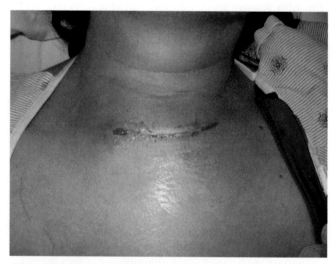

Figure 40-1. Wound infection in a patient who underwent thyroidectomy for massive goiter; similar findings would be expected in an infected parathyroidectomy wound.

incidence of wound infection,[14,23,24] which is attributable to a break in sterile technique or to a violation of the airway, pharynx, or esophagus, a risk that is more likely with thyroidectomy than with parathyroidectomy. Skin or respiratory contaminants would be the offending microorganisms, and targeted antibiotic coverage is indicated if wound infection develops after surgery. The adequate drainage of an infected wound is essential.[24]

Scar

Unfavorable wound healing is a product of patient factors, disease factors, and technical factors. Most parathyroidectomy scars are unobtrusive, being created in the relaxed skin tension lines of the low anterior neck. Directed parathyroidectomy is more commonly associated with smaller incisions and scars than with traditional bilateral parathyroid exploration. The transcervical approach is still standard, although transaxillary thyroidectomy has been described and parathyroidectomy considered, which would leave no neck scar whatsoever.[25] Hypertrophic scar formation varies among individuals, but it can be exacerbated by excessive tension in wound closure, trauma to the wound edges as a result of retraction or thermal injury during instrumentation, or a lack of meticulous alignment of the skin edges during closure. Unfavorable scars are more common in the vertical or sternotomy components of parathyroidectomy scars in the rare instances in which a mediastinal parathyroid cannot be removed through a cervical incision alone (Figure 40-2).

NEUROLOGIC COMPLICATIONS

Recurrent Laryngeal Nerve Injury

As with thyroid surgery, unilateral or especially bilateral recurrent laryngeal nerve (RLN) injuries are among the most feared complications of parathyroid surgery, with

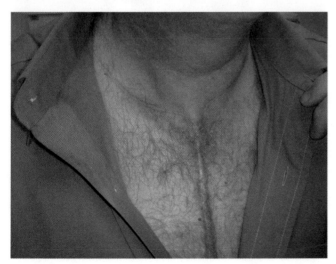

Figure 40-2. Hypertrophic sternotomy scar.

an incidence of 0% to 6%.[8,10,12,18–20,22,26] The recognition of RLN paralysis depends on how avidly it is sought, and the true incidence can only be determined when both preoperative and postoperative laryngoscopy are performed[27] (Figures 40-3, 40-4, and 40-5). Transient RLN paresis reportedly occurs in 1% to 2% of parathyroidectomies on the basis of subjective temporary postoperative voice change. Reoperative parathyroid surgery carries a greatly increased risk of RLN paralysis, with an incidence of up to 17% or more.[28,29]

Knowledge of the anatomic relationships of the RLNs to the parathyroid glands and of variations in nerve location and branching is essential to minimizing the risk of injury. The right RLN normally branches from the vagus nerve and loops around the right subclavian artery to

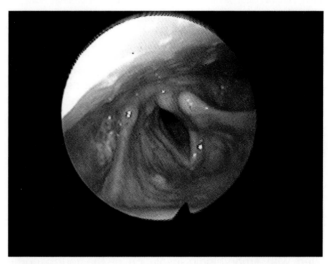

Figure 40-3. Unilateral (left) vocal-fold paralysis. Note the shortening and bowing of the left vocal fold (right) and the anterior position of the arytenoid.

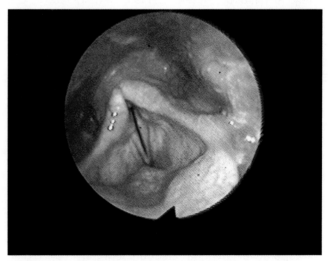

Figure 40-4. Bilateral vocal-fold paralysis after parathyroid exploration (maximum airway). Note the bilaterally medialized vocal folds. The patient had a relatively strong voice but an inadequate airway and required tracheotomy.

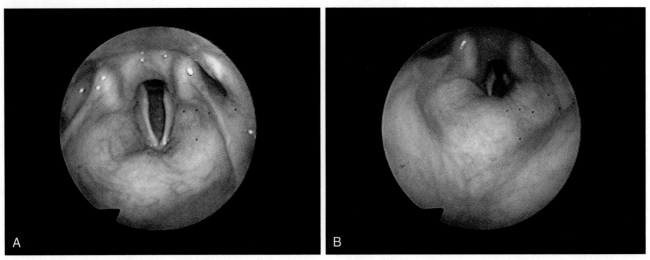

Figure 40-5. Bilateral vocal-fold paralysis with the vocal folds in a lateralized position. This patient had a very breathy voice and aspiration but no airway difficulties. **A,** Respiration view. **B,** Phonation view.

ascend or "recur" in a cephalad and slightly oblique direction to the larynx. The left RLN originates from the intrathoracic left vagus nerve and loops underneath the aortic arch to ascend vertically within the tracheoesophageal groove. The RLN on either side passes over, under, or between the branches of the inferior thyroid artery and through or near the suspensory ligament of Berry of the thyroid, and it enters the larynx beneath the constrictor muscle lateral to the articulation of the cricothyroid joint.[30,31] A nonrecurrent right RLN occurs in 0.5% of cases and has a cervical origin directly from the vagus nerve, without looping around the subclavian artery. This anatomic variation is associated with embryologic involution of the fourth aortic arch, resulting in the right subclavian artery taking origin from the aorta distal to the ligamentum arteriosum,[32,33] but this is usually not suspected preoperatively. A nonrecurrent left RLN is extremely rare, and it is associated with situs inversus and a left-sided retroesophageal subclavian artery.[33,34] The RLN on either side demonstrates extralaryngeal branching in up to 65% of individuals,[32,35] so the identification and protection of what appears to be a single nerve branch in no way ensures a lack of injury.

The inferior parathyroid glands are typically positioned ventral and medial to the RLN, and the superior parathyroid glands are typically dorsal and lateral to the RLN, although parathyroid enlargement can distort this relationship. Medial retraction of the thyroid gland during parathyroid surgery can also alter the orientation of the RLN.

Intraoperative laryngeal electromyography can aid in the identification, preservation, and prognostication of the function of the RLNs. Postcricoid surface electrodes and endotracheal tube-based electrodes are

commercially available for the intraoperative monitoring of the posterior cricoarytenoid and the thyroarytenoid muscles, respectively[36,37] (Figure 40-6). Neuromuscular relaxation must be avoided if nerve monitoring is to be achieved, but otherwise surgery with continuous nerve monitoring is performed in the same way as unmonitored surgery. Direct nerve stimulation that elicits a muscular response confirms the integrity of nerve function, whereas simple visual identification of an intact RLN does not confirm intact function.

The management of the inadvertent transection of the RLN is controversial. Primary reanastomosis can be performed with the hope of recovering some function and preserving some muscle tone, but laryngeal synkinesis can result.[38] Ansa-cervicalis-to-RLN anastomosis can also preserve vocal fold tone and bulk and result in good voice and glottic competence.[39]

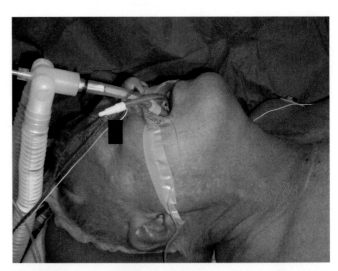

Figure 40-6. Intraoperative laryngeal nerve monitoring with endotracheal tube-based electrodes.

In the absence of routine postoperative laryngoscopy, the recognition of unilateral RLN injury may be delayed by several weeks as a result of initial intubation-related laryngeal edema offsetting the symptoms of vocal fold weakness. Hoarseness, dysphagia, and aspiration may become more pronounced over a period of several weeks as the paralyzed vocal fold lateralizes and its muscles begin to atrophy. If the RLN is known to be anatomically intact and the recovery of function is anticipated, then noninvasive speech therapy alone may be beneficial for promoting compensatory laryngeal behavior. If voice impairment or aspiration is significant, then temporary vocal fold medialization with the injection of Gelfoam or collagen is an appropriate consideration. For permanent vocal fold paralysis, rehabilitative surgical options include medialization laryngoplasty, arytenoid adduction, and reinnervation with an ansa cervicalis-to-RLN anastomosis.[40]

Bilateral RLN injury is a far more serious and less subtle complication of parathyroid surgery. Immediate postoperative respiratory distress despite relatively good voice quality should raise suspicion of bilateral vocal fold motion impairment. The first priority is to secure an airway. Oral intubation and steroid therapy are the preferred initial measures, and a controlled attempt at extubation with the fiber-optic evaluation of vocal fold mobility can be performed within the next few days. The failure of extubation and the confirmation of bilateral vocal fold paralysis then warrant tracheotomy under controlled conditions. The subsequent management of bilateral vocal fold paralysis that fails to recover may include vocal fold laterofixation, arytenoidopexy, reinnervation, cordotomy, or arytenoidectomy. All of these procedures have variable results and may or may not enable decannulation.

The risk of bilateral RLN injury has been reduced by the evolution of the directed approach to parathyroidectomy facilitated by the preoperative parathyroid localization of unilateral parathyroid adenomas. Alternatively, the use of minimally invasive techniques and the narrow exposure of targeted parathyroids reduces the exposure and identification of the RLN. The incidence of RLN injury during thyroid surgery has been shown to be reduced if the nerve is identified and dissected out along its course,[41] which of course is not always feasible in small-incision parathyroid surgery. It is incumbent on the surgeon to realize that an unseen nerve is not necessarily a preserved nerve and that the use of nerve-monitoring techniques may be even more justified in such minimal-access situations. Reports are limited, but the incidence of unilateral recurrent laryngeal nerve injury associated with minimally invasive approaches appears to be similar to that associated with larger-incision parathyroidectomy procedures.[42,43] Similarly, the risk of RLN injury is higher during reoperative parathyroid surgery, whereas the ease with which the RLNs can be identified is reduced as a result of scarring, thus warranting even greater consideration for intraoperative nerve monitoring.

Superior Laryngeal Nerve Injury

The external branch of the superior laryngeal nerve (EBSLN), which innervates the cricothyroid muscle, is also at risk during parathyroid and thyroid surgery, although to a lesser degree during parathyroidectomy than the RLN is. The EBSLN is closely associated with the superior thyroid artery, although in a variable relationship. The nerve is not routinely visualized in 25% or more of thyroid surgeries, and it is positively identified less often than not during parathyroid surgery, so its proximity must be considered even when it is unseen. Careful dissection in the region of the superior thyroid pole on the surface of the gland can help to minimize injury to the EBSLN. The use of a nerve stimulator can also be beneficial to the identification of the EBSLN.[44]

Unilateral injury to the EBSLN causes a loss of pitch elevation and easy vocal fatigability as a result of the loss of cricothyroid muscle tone and function. Laryngoscopic findings, although subtle, include vocal fold bowing, asymmetry of the vocal fold level, and laryngeal tilting toward the unaffected side. Cricothyroid electromyography is the most accurate diagnostic test. Bilateral EBSLN injury results in an even greater lowering of pitch and a breathiness of the voice. Speech therapy is the mainstay of treatment.

Sympathetic Trunk

Although rare, damage to the sympathetic trunk with resultant Horner syndrome can occur as a result of the exploration for ectopic parathyroids. Because ectopic parathyroid glands can reside within the carotid sheath, their dissection may involve the skeletonization of a portion of the common carotid artery. The sympathetic trunk coursing along the posterior aspect of the carotid artery is thereby at risk, and its injury results in ptosis, miosis, anisocoria, and anhidrosis of the face.

ENDOCRINE AND METABOLIC COMPLICATIONS

Hypocalcemia

Postoperative hypocalcemia is one of the most common complications of parathyroid surgery. Temporary hypocalcemia has been reported to occur in 0% to 35% of patients after parathyroidectomy, and permanent hypocalcemia occurs in 0% to 2.2% after traditional (bilateral exploration) parathyroidectomy.[20] When a unilateral or directed surgical approach is used, the risk of permanent hypoparathyroidism is eliminated, unless the patient has undergone previous surgery that may have involved the contralateral parathyroid glands. Alternatively, surgery for parathyroid hyperplasia including subtotal parathyroidectomy or total parathyroidectomy with parathyroid autotransplantation increases the risk of permanent hypoparathyroidism. Permanent hypoparathyroidism is also more likely after reoperative parathyroid surgery.

Transient hypoparathyroidism can occur after successful parathyroidectomy as a result of the "hungry bone syndrome"[45] as well as because of the suppression or atrophy of residual parathyroid glands, which may take days or weeks to regain normal function. HPT is associated with a predominance of osteoclast activity, with increased bone resorption to maintain serum calcium levels. In turn, normal parathyroid gland function is suppressed by increased serum calcium levels that result from bone resorption. An indication of this bone depletion is an elevated preoperative serum alkaline phosphatase level. After parathyroidectomy, active calcium uptake by bone occurs and may necessitate calcium supplementation to maintain serum calcium levels. Hungry bone syndrome may persist for several months after parathyroidectomy.

Acute postoperative hypocalcemia is relatively common and must be anticipated and managed promptly. The monitoring of serial serum calcium levels is the most objective means of detecting hypocalcemia. However, in the current era of short-stay or outpatient parathyroidectomy, hypocalcemia may not have developed by the time that the patient is otherwise ready for discharge from the hospital. Therefore patients must be advised regarding the possibility and physicians must be alert to the possible development of hypocalcemia in patients after departure from the hospital. One approach to the prevention of symptomatic hypocalcemia is to empirically prescribe supplemental calcium with or without vitamin D after surgery, which can be tapered over several weeks' time; the cost-effectiveness of this approach is not known. An alternative approach is to monitor serial serum calcium levels through outpatient testing after discharge. The critical period for serum calcium level measurement with respect to determining the need for calcium supplementation is 24 to 72 hours after surgery.[45–48] Patients with total serum calcium levels below 8.0 mg/dl on two occasions during the first 48 hours after surgery are more likely to require prolonged calcium supplementation.[46–49]

A recent technique for attempting to predict postoperative hypocalcemia after thyroid (but not parathyroid) surgery has been to perform a rapid parathyroid hormone (PTH) assay during the immediate postoperative period.[50–52] However, this approach does not have the same usefulness for patients who start with an abnormally elevated baseline PTH level and with suppressed residual normal parathyroid glands. The best use of the intraoperative PTH assay in patients with primary HPT is during surgery itself to add confidence to the completeness of the removal of hyperfunctioning parathyroid tissue, as discussed later in this chapter.

The following risk factors for severe postoperative hypocalcemia after parathyroidectomy have been identified: markedly elevated preoperative PTH levels (i.e., five times the upper reference value or more), a history of previous surgery, biopsy or excision of more than two parathyroid glands, and concomitant thyroid surgery.[53] Patients with renal HPT are more prone to developing profound postoperative hypocalcemia.[54] Vitamin D deficiency and elevated serum alkaline phosphatase as markers of increased bone turnover are also relative risk factors of unclear significance. Furthermore, hypomagnesemia often accompanies and potentiates the effects of hypocalcemia, and magnesium supplementation may be necessary in addition to calcium supplementation to reverse the metabolic consequences.[55,56]

Symptomatic hypocalcemia relates to the rate and the extent of the decline in serum calcium levels.[57] Symptoms most often correspond to a total serum level of less than 8.0 mg/dl, and they initially involve perioral tingling and numbness in the lips, hands, and feet as well as a feeling of anxiety. Initial signs include a positive Chvostek sign, which consists of the involuntary contraction of the facial muscles (especially the orbicularis oris) upon tapping of the cheek over the facial nerve. Of note is that approximately 15% of normocalcemic patients have a positive Chvostek sign, so a baseline preoperative response should be documented.[40] Progressive hypocalcemia leads to mental status changes, overt tetany, muscle cramps and spasms, hypotension, and prolongation of the QT interval on electrocardiogram.

Symptomatic hypocalcemia warrants prompt correction to arrest the progression of neuromuscular excitability and to avoid the challenge of a greater deficit to correct over time. Immediate intravenous infusion of calcium gluconate over 5 minutes (i.e., 10 ml or 1 ampule of a 10% solution, available on most crash carts) may be repeated as often as necessary to bring the total serum calcium levels to more than 8.0 mg/dl. After initial correction, the most practical maintenance approach is an intravenous drip of calcium gluconate (10 ampoules dissolved in 500 or 1000 ml of sodium chloride and continuously infused at 20–50 ml/hr for 24–48 hours), during which serial calcium measurements are made. Patients are also given oral calcium carbonate (i.e., 500–1500 mg two to four times a day or calcium gluconate or calcium lactate) with or without calcitriol (i.e., 1,25-dihydroxyvitamin D3 0.25–1.0 μg one to three times a day) to enhance the intestinal absorption of calcium. Oral aluminum hydroxide gel and a low-phosphate diet can be prescribed to lower serum phosphate levels, which, when elevated, depress calcium levels; thiazide diuretics can be used to decrease the renal loss of calcium in patients with resistant hypocalcemia. Patients are weaned off of intravenous calcium as their serum levels stabilize, and they are slowly weaned off of oral supplementation over the next 4 to 8 weeks as their residual parathyroid function recovers.

Hypocalcemia should be anticipated during the first weeks to months after total parathyroidectomy and parathyroid autotransplantation. The recovery of parathyroid function is successful with 80% or more of fresh parathyroid autografts[58] within 5 weeks of transplantation.[59] The success rates of cryopreserved autografts are much more variable (17%–83%), and they decrease with the duration of cryopreservation.[58]

Persistent Hypercalcemia

Another dreaded outcome of parathyroidectomy is persistent hypercalcemia or failure of the adequate removal of hyperfunctioning parathyroid tissue. It is difficult to improve on a traditional success rate of 95% to 98% for parathyroid surgery with or without preoperative localization studies.[12,26,60–63] Primary HPT is the result of a single adenoma in 85% to 95% of cases, with double adenomas in 2% to 6% of patients and hyperplasia in 2% to 15% of patients.[20] Most cases of failed parathyroidectomy are the result of a failure to localize and remove an adenomatous parathyroid gland.[28,64] The elusive hyperfunctioning glands at surgical exploration tend to overlap with the subset of parathyroid lesions that are not identified by typical localization studies, and they can present a difficult and at times frustrating challenge, even for experienced surgeons. Nevertheless, preoperative localization studies are very useful (if not essential) in this era of directed and minimally invasive parathyroidectomy,[64–66] especially in cases of persistent or recurrent HPT.[67] In de novo cases, the two most preferred noninvasive localization studies are technetium-99m sestamibi scintigraphy[68–71] (sensitivity, 54%–93%; Figure 40-7) and high-resolution ultrasonography (sensitivity, 57%–93%; Figure 40-8) performed by dedicated sonographers, radiologists, or parathyroid surgeons.[65]

A detailed search for a parathyroid adenoma or residual hyperplastic glands includes, as needed, mobilization of the thyroid gland, a thorough exploration of the right and left tracheoesophageal grooves and the retroesophageal space, exploration within both carotid sheaths up to the angles of the mandible, and cervical thymectomy and cervical mediastinal exploration. It may also be helpful to trace the branches of either inferior thyroid

artery distally, because these may lead to an ectopic gland.[72] If the offending gland remains elusive, a thyroid lobectomy should be performed on the side where the occult gland had been demonstrated on preoperative localization studies or on the basis of where the remaining gland should be after the identification of normal glands on the basis of typical bilateral symmetry. Biopsies should be obtained and clips used to mark all identifiable parathyroids. Median sternotomy is not recommended during the initial unsuccessful exploration unless a localization study clearly indicates the presence of mediastinal disease that is not accessible transcervically, because most occult parathyroids are located in the neck.[64]

Intraoperative PTH monitoring has become commonplace as a result of the development of a rapid immunoradiometric PTH assay. Taking advantage of the very short half-life (2–5 minutes) of PTH, serial peripheral blood samples taken before and after the excision of suspected abnormal parathyroid tissue are assayed with an expectation of a 50% or more drop in PTH from baseline within 10 minutes of single adenoma excision.[73] An insufficient decline in the PTH level prompts additional PTH testing or additional exploration for residual hyperfunctioning parathyroid tissue representing multigland disease.[74] False-negative and false-positive results have been reported, although rates of overall accuracy of 93%, of sensitivity of 94%, of a positive predictive value of 98%, and of a specificity of 79% have been described.[75] The usefulness of intraoperative PTH monitoring in surgery for secondary HPT and for multiple endocrine neoplasia I syndrome has also been described,[76,77] although the decline in PTH level tends to occur in a more stepwise fashion when measured serially after the removal of each parathyroid gland as opposed to a precipitous decline to a level within the normal range.[78]

Recurrent hyperparathyroidism is defined as recurrent hypercalcemia at least 6 months after successful parathyroidectomy and normocalcemia. Although recurrence is rare among patients who undergo the resection of a single adenoma, the recurrence rate is much higher (up to 33% or more[79]) among patients with multiple endocrine neoplasia I or familial HPT. Patients with these syndromes must therefore be followed for the long term, and their initial treatment most often should consist of subtotal (i.e., 3.5 gland) parathyroidectomy or total parathyroidectomy with autotransplantation as well as parathyroid cryopreservation.[79] Recurrent HPT is also more common among patients with renal HPT, occurring in 5% of patients who undergo parathyroidectomy without autotransplantation and in as many as 14% of patients with autotransplantation.[22,80,81] When recurrent HPT does occur, treatment should be preceded by the confirmation of the diagnosis via the review of appropriate laboratory tests, the review of the

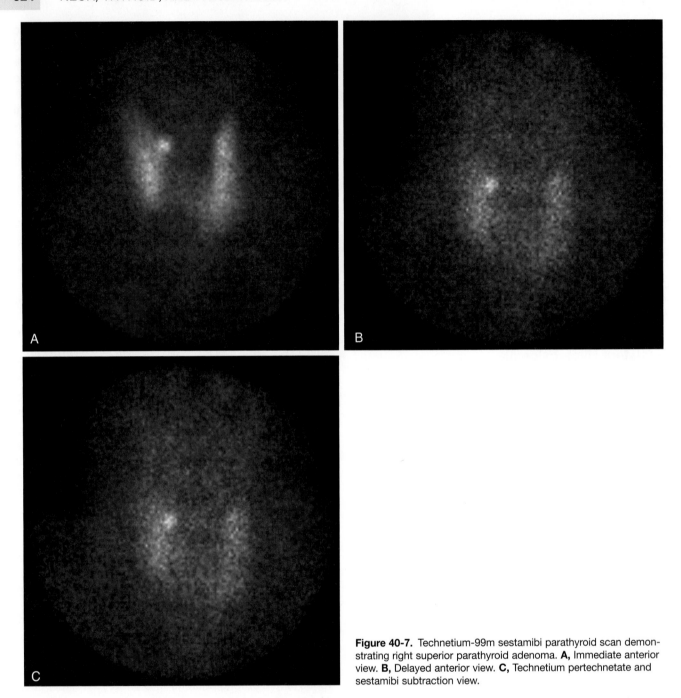

Figure 40-7. Technetium-99m sestamibi parathyroid scan demonstrating right superior parathyroid adenoma. **A,** Immediate anterior view. **B,** Delayed anterior view. **C,** Technetium pertechnetate and sestamibi subtraction view.

original parathyroid operative report (when available), the liberal use of localization studies, the performance of indirect or fiber-optic laryngoscopy (which should in fact be routine among patients with HPT), and a consideration of the use of intraoperative laryngeal nerve monitoring (even if this is not typically used in the de novo parathyroidectomy setting).

In addition to the preoperative localization studies already described (i.e., ultrasonography and technetium-99m sestamibi scintigraphy), other useful studies may include magnetic resonance imaging, single photon emission computed tomography (SPECT) in combina-

tion with technetium-99m sestamibi,[82] ultrasound-guided needle aspiration of suspected lesions for PTH assay and for cytologic analysis,[83] and selective venous sampling for PTH.[84] Potentially useful intraoperative tools include intravenous infusion of methylene blue for parathyroid staining[85] (Figure 40-9), intraoperative PTH assay for the real-time assessment of the surgical correction of HPT, and intraoperative gamma detection of radiation from preoperatively administered technetium-99m sestamibi.[86]

One rare and rarely discussed cause of recurrent hypercalcemia is parathyromatosis, which is composed of

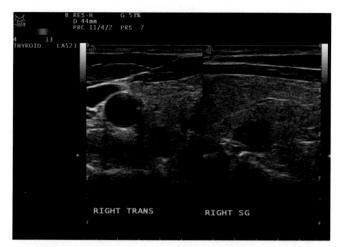

Figure 40-8. High-resolution ultrasonography that demonstrates the right superior parathyroid adenoma of the same patient as seen in Figure 40-7. *Left,* Transverse plane. Note the position of the adenoma posterior to the plane of the carotid artery. *Right,* Sagittal plane. Note the position of the adenoma posterior to the thyroid lobe and superior to its midpoint.

multiple foci of benign hyperfunctioning parathyroid tissue in the neck, in the mediastinum, or within an autograft in the forearm or elsewhere.[87] Parathyromatosis most commonly occurs among patients who have undergone parathyroidectomy, but a few cases of de novo parathyromatosis have been reported. The theories explaining the development of parathyromatosis include the mishandling of parathyroid glands during excision, which results in capsule breakage and the seeding of parathyroid cells into the surgical field, or the activation of parathyroid rests by the potent physiologic stimuli associated with chronic renal failure. The best way to prevent iatrogenic parathyromatosis is through the meticulous handling of parathyroid tissue, with every effort made to not rupture, fracture, or remove tissue in a piecemeal fashion. The treatment of parathyromatosis is to remove all gross disease, which may require thyroid lobectomy or total thyroidectomy, thymectomy, and the removal of all nonvital structures in the paratracheal and paraesophageal regions.

OTHER COMPLICATIONS

Malignant Complications

Parathyroid carcinomas are rare but relentless tumors that can slowly lead to uncontrollable hypercalcemia and death. Parathyroid carcinoma represents less than 1% of all cases of primary HPT in most parts of the world.[88] The initial metabolic manifestations of parathyroid carcinoma—although often more extreme—are similar to those of benign primary HPT, thus making the preoperative distinction from adenomatous or hyperplastic hyperparathyroidism difficult. Physical examination findings in patients with parathyroid carcinoma include a palpable neck mass in up to 69% of cases; up to 20% of patients with parathyroid carcinoma have cervical lymph node metastases, and up to one third have distant metastases to the lung, bone, and liver at the time of diagnosis. A high index of suspicion is required to anticipate the presence of parathyroid carcinoma and to perform the appropriate initial surgical procedure, which is the en bloc resection of the mass and adjacent tissue. It is critical that the capsule of the tumor not be violated during removal so that seeding of the neck is avoided. Inadequate resection as a result of a lack of recognition or suspicion of carcinoma generally leads to locally recurrent carcinoma and recurrent hypercalcemia that ultimately may prove to be fatal.

Life-Threatening Hypercalcemia

Hypercalcemic crisis (i.e., a serum calcium level of >14 mg/dl) as a result of HPT is a medical emergency. Medical therapy includes intravenous fluid resuscitation

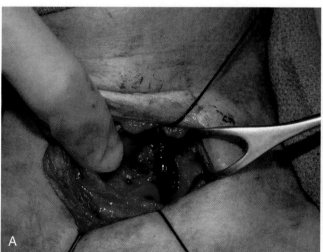

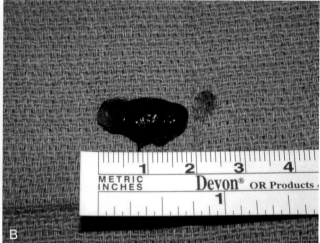

Figure 40-9. Methylene blue staining of a parathyroid adenoma. **A,** In situ left inferior parathyroid. **B,** Ex vivo specimen stained blue.

to restore fluid volume and enhance calcium excretion. Loop-diuretic therapy enhances calciuresis. Short-term calcitonin therapy lowers serum calcium transiently by inhibiting osteoclast-mediated bone resorption; bisphosphonate therapy achieves the same goal for a more protracted period of time. The most useful long-term therapy is with calcimimetic agents such as cinacalcet, which can induce decreased levels of PTH secretion for prolonged periods of time in patients with inoperable disease. However, after a patient is stabilized, parathyroidectomy is the treatment of choice whenever feasible.[88]

Other Complications

Pneumomediastinum, pneumothorax, and hemothorax are uncommon complications that are usually associated with mediastinal dissection during parathyroid surgery.[89] Chyle leaks are also rare, and they are usually associated with concomitant neck dissection.[18] Rare symptoms related to hypocalcemic tetany include diplopia and congestive heart failure.[90,91] Tracheal or esophageal lacerations are rare, and they are treated with primary repair. Anesthetic complications can occur with parathyroid surgery as they can with any surgery (whether it is performed under general or local anesthesia), and they should be handled accordingly.

CONCLUSION

Complication rates associated with parathyroid surgery vary depending on the extent of the procedure, the experience of the surgeon, the underlying pathology, and whether the surgery is revisionary. The incidence of complications can be minimized by careful preoperative planning and meticulous intraoperative surgical technique. The early recognition of complications leads to interventions that can minimize their impact and morbidity.

REFERENCES

1. Organ CH Jr: The history of parathyroid surgery, 1850-1996: The Excelsior Surgical Society 1998 Edward D. Churchill Lecture. *J Am Coll Surg* 2000;191:284.
2. Welbourn RB: *The history of endocrine surgery*, New York, 1990, Praeger Publishers.
3. Strewler GJ: A 64-year-old woman with primary hyperparathyroidism. *JAMA* 2005;293:1772–1779.
4. Matthews TW, Briant TD: The use of fibrin tissue glue in thyroid surgery: Resource utilization implications. *J Otolaryngol* 1991;20:276.
5. Calderelli DD, Holinger LD: Complications and sequelae of thyroid surgery. *Otolaryngol Clin North Am* 1980;13:85.
6. Matory YL, Spiro RH: Wound bleeding after head and neck surgery. *J Surg Oncol* 1993;53:17.
7. Fewins J, Simpson CB, Miller FR: Complications of thyroid and parathyroid surgery. *Otolaryngol Clin North Am* 2003;36:189–206.
8. Singh B, Lucente FE, Shaha AR: Substernal goiter: A clinical review. *Am J Otolaryngol* 1994;15:409.
9. Patel M, Garg R, Rice DH: Fibrin glue in thyroid and parathyroid surgery: Is under-flap suction still necessary? *Ear Nose Throat J* 2006;85:530–532.
10. Shaha A, Jaffe BM: Complications of thyroid surgery performed by residents. *Surgery* 1988;104:1109.
11. Shaha AR, Jaffe BM: Practical management of post-thyroidectomy hematoma. *J Surg Oncol* 1994;57:235.
12. Ryan JA Jr, Lee F: Effectiveness and safety of 100 consecutive parathyroidectomies. *Am J Surg* 1997;173:441.
13. Low RA, Katz AD: Parathyroidectomy via bilateral cervical exploration: A retrospective review of 866 cases. *Head Neck* 1998;20:583–587.
14. Ayyash K, Khammash M, Tibblin S: Drain vs no drain in primary thyroid and parathyroid surgery. *Eur J Surg* 1991;157:113.
15. Wihlborg O, Bergljung L, Martensson H: To drain or not to drain in thyroid surgery: A controlled clinical study. *Arch Surg* 1988;123:40.
16. Kristoffersson A, Sandzen B, Jarhult J: Drainage in uncomplicated thyroid and parathyroid surgery. *Br J Surg* 1986;73:121.
17. Peix JL et al: Drainage after thyroidectomy: A randomized clinical trial. *Int Surg* 1992;77:122.
18. Bergamaschi R et al: Morbidity of thyroid surgery. *Am J Surg* 1998;176:71.
19. Moulton-Barrett R et al: Complications of thyroid surgery. *Int Surg* 1997;82:63.
20. Gourin CG, Johnson JT: Postoperative complications. In Randolph GW, editor: *Surgery of the thyroid and parathyroid glands,* St Louis, 2003, Elsevier.
21. Ruark DS, Abdel-Misih RZ: Thyroid and parathyroid surgery without drains. *Head Neck* 1992;14:285.
22. Punch JD, Thompson NW, Merion RM: Subtotal parathyroidectomy in dialysis and post-renal transplant patients. *Arch Surg* 1995;130:538.
23. Johnson JT, Wagner RL: Infection following uncontaminated head and neck surgery. *Arch Otolaryngol Head Neck Surg* 1987;113:368.
24. Tabet J, Johnson JT: Wound infection in head and neck surgery: Prophylaxis, etiology and management. *J Otolaryngol* 1990;19:197.
25. Lobe TE, Wright SK, Irish MS: Novel uses of surgical robotics in head and neck surgery. *J Laparoendosc Adv Surg Tech A* 2005;15:647–652.
26. Coston SD, Pelton JJ: Success of cervical exploration for patients with asymptomatic primary hyperparathyroidism. *Am J Surg* 1999;177:69.
27. Randolph GW, Kamani D: The importance of preoperative laryngoscopy in patients undergoing thyroidectomy: Voice, vocal cord function, and the preoperative detection of invasive thyroid malignancy. *Surgery* 2006;139:357–362.
28. Shen W et al: Reoperation for persistent or recurrent primary hyperparathyroidism. *Arch Surg* 1996;131:861.
29. Patow CA, Norton JA, Brennan MF: Vocal cord paralysis and reoperative parathyroidectomy: A prospective study. *Ann Surg* 1986;203:282–285.
30. Rustad WH, Morrison LF: Revised anatomy of the recurrent laryngeal nerves: Surgical importance based on the dissection of 100 cadavers. *Laryngoscope* 1952;62:237–249.
31. Shindo ML, Wu JC, Park EE: Surgical anatomy of the recurrent laryngeal nerve revisited. *Otolayrngol Head Neck Surg* 2005;133:514–519.
32. Karlan MS et al: A safe technique for thyroidectomy with complete nerve dissection and parathyroid preservation. *Head Neck Surg* 1984;6:1014.
33. Srinivasan V, Premachandra DJ: Non-recurrent laryngeal nerve: Identification during thyroid surgery. *Otorhinolaryngol* 1997;59:57.
34. Cannon CR: The anomaly of nonrecurrent laryngeal nerve: Identification and management. *Otolaryngol Head Neck Surg* 1999;120:769.
35. Katz AD: Extralaryngeal division of the recurrent laryngeal nerve. *Am J Surg* 1986;152:407–410.
36. Khan A et al: Experience with two types of electromyography monitoring electrodes during thyroid surgery. *Am J Otolaryngol* 1997;18:99.

37. Eisele DW: Intraoperative electrophysiologic monitoring of the recurrent laryngeal nerve. *Laryngoscope* 1996;106:443.

38. Crumley RL: Repair of the recurrent laryngeal nerve. *Otolaryngol Clin North Am* 1990;23:553.

39. Crumley RL: Voice quality following laryngeal reinnervation by ansa hypoglossi transfer. *Laryngoscope* 1986;96:611.

40. Netterville JL, Aly A, Ossoff RH: Evaluation and treatment of complications of thyroid and parathyroid surgery. *Otolaryngol Clin North Am* 1990;23:529.

41. Riddell V: Thyroidectomy: Prevention of bilateral recurrent laryngeal nerve palsy: Results of identification of the nerve over 23 consecutive years (1946-1969) with description of an additional safety measure. *Br J Surg* 1970;57:1.

42. Bergenfelz A, Kanngiesser V, Zielke A, et al: Conventional bilateral cervical explorations versus open minimally invasive parathyroidectomy under local anaesthesia for primary hyperparathyroidism. *Br J Surg* 2005;92:190–197.

43. Inabnet WB, Fulla Y, Richard B, et al: Unilateral neck exploration under local anesthesia: The approach of choice for asymptomatic primary hyperparathyroidism. *Surgery* 1999;126:1004–1010.

44. Cernea CR et al: Identification of the external branch of the superior laryngeal nerve during thyroidectomy. *Am J Surg* 1992;164:634.

45. McHenry CR et al: Risk factors for postthyroidectomy hypocalcemia. *Surgery* 1994;116:641.

46. Pattou F et al: Hypocalcemia following thyroid surgery: Incidence and prediction of outcome. *World J Surg* 1998;22:718.

47. Adams J et al: Early postoperative calcium levels as predictors of hypocalcemia. *Laryngoscope* 1998;108:1829.

48. Moore FD Jr: Oral calcium supplements to enhance early hospital discharge after bilateral surgical treatment of the thyroid gland or exploration of the parathyroid glands. *J Am Coll Surg* 1994;178:11.

49. Szubin L et al: The management of post-thyroidectomy hypocalcemia. *Ear Nose Throat J* 1996;75:612.

50. Roh JL, Park CI: Intraoperative parathyroid hormone assay for management of patients undergoing total thyroidectomy. *Head Neck* 2006;28:990–997.

51. Khafif A, Pivoarov A, Medina JE, et al: Parathyroid hormone: A sensitive predictor of hypocalcemia following total thyroidectomy. *Otolaryngol Head Neck Surg* 2006;134:907–910.

52. Ghareri BA, Liebler SL, Andersen PE, et al: Perioperative parathyroid hormone levels in thyroid surgery. *Laryngoscope* 2006;116:518–521.

53. Kald BA, Heath DI, Lausen I, et al: Risk assessment for severe postoperative hypocalcaemia after neck exploration for primary hyperparathyroidism. *Scand J Surg* 2005;94:216–220.

54. Mittendorf EA, Merlino JI, McHenry CR: Post-parathyroidectomy hypocalcemia: Incidence, risk factors, and management. *Am Surg* 2004;70:114–120.

55. Desport JC, Bregeon Y, Devalois B, et al: Hypomagnesemia associated with hypocalcemia after undetected parathyroidectomy. *Ann Fr Anesth Reanim* 1992;11:470–472.

56. Falko JM, Bush CA, Tzagournis M, et al: Case report: Congestive heart failure complicating the hungry bone syndrome. *Am J Med Sci* 1976;271:85–89.

57. Waldstein SS: Medical complications of thyroid surgery. *Otolaryngol Clin North Am* 1980;13:99.

58. Cohen MS, Dilley WG, Wells SA, et al: Long-term functionality of cryopreserved parathyroid autografts: A 13-year prospective analysis. *Surgery* 2005;138:1033–1041.

59. Echenique-Elizondo M, Diaz-Aguirregoitia FJ, Amondarain JA, et al: Parathyroid graft function after presternal subcutaneous autotransplantation for renal hyperparathyroidism. *Arch Surg* 2006;141:33–38.

60. van Heerdan JA, Grant CS: Surgical treatment of primary hyperparathyroidism: An institutional perspective. *World J Surg* 1991;15:688–692.

61. Molinari AS, Irvin GL 3rd, Deriso GT, et al: Incidence of multiglandular disease in primary hyperparathyroidism determined by parathyroid hormone secretion. *Surgery* 1996;12;934.

62. Sofferman RA, Nathan MH, Fairbank JT, et al: Preoperative technetium Tc 99m sestamibi imaging: Paving the way to minimal-access parathyroid surgery. *Arch Otolayrngol Head Neck Surg* 1996;122:369.

63. Sofferman RA, Standage J, Tang ME: Minimal-access parathyroid surgery using intraoperative parathyroid hormone assay. *Laryngoscope* 1998;108:1497.

64. Rotstein L, Irish J, Gullane P, et al: Reoperative parathyroidectomy in the era of localization technology. *Head Neck* 1998;20:535.

65. Steward DL, Danielson GP, Afman CE, et al: Parathyroid adenoma localization: Surgeon-performed ultrasound versus sestamibi. *Laryngoscope* 2006;116:1380–1384.

66. Solorzano CC, Lee TM, Ramirez MC, et al: Surgeon-performed ultrasound improves localization of abnormal parathyroid glands. *Am Surg* 2005;71:557–563.

67. Udelsman R, Donovan PI: Remedial parathyroid surgery: Changing trends in 130 consecutive cases. *Ann Surg* 2006;244:471–479.

68. Berczi C, Mezosi E, Galuska L, et al: Technetium-99m-sestamibi/pertechnetate subtraction scintigraphy vs. ultrasonography for preoperative localization in primary hyperparathyroidism. *Eur Radiol* 2002;12:605–609.

69. Purcell GP, Dirbas FM, Jeffrey RB, et al: Parathyroid localization with high-resolution ultrasound and technetium Tc 99m sestamibi. *Arch Surg* 1999;134:824–828.

70. Reeder SB, Desser TS, Weigel RJ, et al: Sonography in primary hyperparathyroidism: A review with emphasis on scanning technique. *J Ultrasound Med* 2002;21:539–552.

71. Kebapci M, Entok E, Kebapci N, et al: Preoperative evaluation of parathyroid lesions in patients with concomitant thyroid disease: Role of high resolution ultrasonography and dual phase technetium 99m sestamibi scintigraphy. *J Endocrinol Invest* 2004;27:24–30.

72. Edis AJ: Surgical anatomy and technique of neck exploration for primary hyperparathyroidism. *Surg Clin North Am* 1977;57:495–505.

73. Patel PC, Pellitteri PK, Patel NM, et al: Use of a rapid intraoperative parathyroid hormone assay in the surgical management of parathyroid disease. *Arch Otolaryngol Head Neck Surg* 1998;124:559–562.

74. Chen H, Pruhs Z, Starling JR, Mack E: Intraoperative parathyroid hormone testing improves cure rates in patients undergoing minimally invasive parathyroidectomy. *Surgery* 2005;138:583–590.

75. Westerdahl J, Bergenfelz A: Parathyroid surgical failures with sufficient decline of intraoperative parathyroid hormone levels. *Arch Surg* 2006;141:589–594.

76. Chou FF, Lee CH, Chen JB, et al: Intraoperative parathyroid hormone measurement in patients with secondary hyperparathyroidism. *Arch Surg* 2002;137:341–344.

77. Gioviale MC, Gambino G, Maione C, et al: Intraoperative parathyroid hormone monitoring during parathyroidectomy for hyperparathyroidism in waiting list and kidney transplant patients. *Transplant Proc* 2006;38:1003–1005.

78. Tonelli F, Spini S, Tommasi M, et al: Intraoperative parathormone measurement in patients with multiple endocrine neoplasia type I syndrome and hyperparathyroidism. *World J Surg* 2000;24:556–563.

79. Elaraj DM, Skarulis MC, Libutti SK, et al: Results of initial operation for hyperparathyroidism in patients with multiple endocrine neoplasia type 1. *Surgery* 2003;134:858–865.

80. Stracke S, Jehle PM, Sturm D, et al: Clinical course after total parathyroidectomy without autotransplantation in patients with end-stage renal failure. *Am J Kidney Dis* 1999;33:304.

81. Baker LR, Otieno LS, Brown AL, et al: Pitfalls after total parathyroidectomy and parathyroid autotransplantation in chronic renal failure. *Am J Nephrol* 1991;11:186.

82. Krausz Y, Bettman L, Guralnik L, et al: Technetium-99m-MIBI SPECT/CT in primary hyperparathyroidism. *World J Surg* 2006;30:76–83.

83. Stephen AE, Milas M, Garner CN, et al: Use of surgeon-performed office ultrasound and parathyroid fine needle aspiration for complex parathyroid localization. *Surgery* 2005;138:1143–1151.

84. Eloy JA, Mitty H, Genden EM: Preoperative selective venous sampling for nonlocalizing parathyroid adenomas. *Thyroid* 2006;16:787–790.

85. Orloff LA: Methylene blue and sestamibi: Complementary tools for localizing parathyroids. *Laryngoscope* 2001;111:1901–1904.

86. Chen H, Mack E, Starling JR: A comprehensive evaluation of perioperative adjuncts during minimally invasive parathyroidectomy: Which is most reliable? *Ann Surg* 2005;242:375–383.

87. Lentsch EJ, Withrow KP, Ackermann D, et al: Parathyromatosis and recurrent hyperparathyroidism. *Arch Otolaryngol Head Neck Surg* 2003;129:894–896.

88. Orloff LA, Eisele DW: Surgical management of parathyroid carcinoma. In Tufano R, Weber R, Zeiger M, editors: *Atlas of thyroid and parathyroid surgery,* Philadelphia, Elsevier, in press.

89. Slater B, Inabnet WB: Pneumothorax: An uncommon complication of minimally invasive parathyroidectomy. *Surg Laparosc Endosc Percutan Tech* 2005;15:38–40.

90. Trombetti A, Stoermann C, Martin PY, et al: Transient diplopia after parathyroidectomy for hyperparathyroidism in chronic haemodialysed patients. *Nephrol Dial Transplant* 2005;20:217–219.

91. Iwazu Y, Muto S, Ikeuchi S, et al: Reversible hypocalcemic heart failure with T wave alternans and increased QTc dispersion in a patient with chronic renal failure after parathyroidectomy. *Clin Nephrol* 2006;65:65–70.

PART 5

Nose, Paranasal Sinuses, and Aesthetic Surgery

CHAPTER 41

Complications of Nasal Surgery and Epistaxis Management

Alexis H. Jackman and Marvin P. Fried

The surgical treatments of rhinologic disease and the management of epistaxis are some of the oldest and most common procedures performed by otolaryngologists. These treatments make use of traditional techniques in conjunction with technologic advances such as nasal endoscopes, laser therapies, and innovative medical materials, and their complications are both well established and new. The aim of this chapter is to present current scientific knowledge regarding the complications of epistaxis management and nasal surgery so that such complications can be prevented whenever possible and so that, whenever possible, complications can be prevented, and when they do occur, they can be managed appropriately.

EPISTAXIS

Epistaxis is one of the most common emergencies in otolaryngology. In most cases, bleeding is relatively mild, and effective treatment is promptly administered; however, in some cases, bleeding persists despite simple interventions or is severe from the outset. In rare cases, epistaxis can be a potentially life-threatening event. Regardless of the severity, universal precautions should be strictly followed, because an estimated 69% of medical care staff members are contaminated with blood while treating patients with epistaxis.[1] Gloves, face masks, and gowns should be worn starting with the initial encounter. In the case of severe epistaxis, the physician must remain alert to the signs and symptoms of an actual or impending airway emergency. Intubation or, in rare circumstances, the establishment of a surgical airway may be required. Prior knowledge of equipment and staff member availability assistance can improve the timeliness of intervention and positively affect patient outcome.

In stable patients, evaluation begins with a through history aimed at determining the cause and possible exacerbating factors of the epistaxis as well as the overall health status of the patient. A variety of causes are associated with epistaxis (Box 41-1). Specific questions should be asked regarding medical conditions (e.g., hypertension, arteriosclerosis, coagulopathies, liver disease, vascular abnormalities), prescription and over-the-counter medications (e.g., aspirin, ibuprofen), and herbal supplements (e.g., garlic, gingko, ginseng). Patients with hereditary hemorrhagic telangiectasia (HHT), an autosomal-dominant disorder, make up a special treatment group, because alterations in the elastin and muscular components of vessel walls lead to the formation of mucocutaneous telangiectasias that predispose these patients to chronic, recurrent

nosebleeds. In these patients and others with recurrent or refractory bleeding, a treatment history of prior episodes of epistaxis should be obtained. In addition, patients with severe or recurrent epistaxis should undergo laboratory testing to evaluate their hemodynamic statuses and coagulation profiles.

A careful physical examination is essential to identify the site of the bleeding, which in upward of 90% of cases arise from blood vessels in the anterior septum in a region known as the *Little area*.[2] Here terminal branches of the superior labial branch of the facial artery, the anterior ethmoidal artery, and sphenopalatine artery anastomose to form the Kiesselbach plexus, which, given its anterior location, is susceptible to crusting and digital trauma. Epistaxis arising from the superior aspect of the nose is uncommon, and it is usually the result of facial trauma or sinonasal surgery. The blood supply to this region is from the anterior and posterior ethmoidal arteries. These arteries are derived from the ophthalmic artery, which is a terminal branch of the internal carotid artery. Although both the anterior and posterior ethmoidal arteries are at risk, the anterior ethmoidal artery is more commonly the source of epistaxis.[3] In the posterior aspect of the nose, a network of anastomoses (i.e., Woodruff's plexus) accounts for the majority of the remaining cases of epistaxis. Woodruff's plexus is derived from the posterior septal artery, a branch of the sphenopalatine artery. In addition, crossover between the right and left arterial systems exists, and these collateral vessels from the contralateral side of the nose can also be a source of bleeding.

Traditionally the management of epistaxis is broadly classified according to location; however, factors such as the severity and cause of the bleeding as well as the patient's overall health status also contribute. Recent advances in endoscopic techniques, interventional radiology, and hemostatic devices and materials have added to the myriad of options available, and a simple algorithm no longer exists. Decision making requires thorough knowledge of the advantages and limitations of the various treatment options, clinician expertise, and ancillary resources.

CAUTERIZATION

In mild cases of anterior epistaxis, initial treatment often involves chemical cauterization with silver nitrate. Silver nitrate sticks are readily available in most emergency rooms, outpatient clinics, and hospitals, and they are an effective, well-tolerated treatment for both adults and children.[4] Although more likely used as a second-line

BOX 41-1 Causes of Epistaxis

TRAUMATIC INJURY
- Digital manipulation
- Facial trauma
- Iatrogenic injury: nasal surgery, instrumentation (e.g., nasal packing, suctioning, nasogastric tube placement, nasotracheal intubation)
- Foreign body

NASAL IRRITANTS
- Environmental: dust, smoke
- Pharmacologic: cocaine, topical corticosteroids, decongestants

INFLAMMATORY AND INFECTIOUS DISEASES
- Allergic rhinitis
- Rhinitis medicamentosa
- Rhinosinusitis
- Rhinoscleroma

CONGENITAL AND GENETIC ABNORMALITIES
- Hereditary hemorrhagic telangiectasia (Osler–Weber–Rendu disease)
- Congenital coagulopathies: hemophilia, von Willebrand disease
- Anatomic variations: deviated nasal septum

SYSTEMIC DISEASES
- Atherosclerosis
- Wegener granulomatosis
- Sarcoidosis
- Syphilis

PHARMACOLOGIC THERAPY, INCLUDING HOMEOPATHIC SUPPLEMENTS
- Coumadin
- Aspirin
- Ibuprofen
- Ginkgo Biloba
- Garlic
- Ginseng
- Vitamin E
- Ephedra

IDIOPATHIC CAUSES

therapy, electrocauterization has broad applications. It is used to treat both anterior and posterior bleeds of variable severity that are recurrent or unresponsive to chemical cauterization or nasal packing. Electrocauterization is performed under either local or general anesthesia, and the choice of monopolar versus bipolar cauterization depends on the site and cause of the bleeding. Bipolar cauterization has the distinct advantage of the control of field size, and it is the preferred method for cases in which repeated cauterization is necessary or when cauterization is required in areas that are adjacent to delicate structures such as the orbit and the skull base. In addition, bipolar cauterization has been proven to be an effective treatment for intranasal HHT-associated teleangiectaias.[5]

Complications of Cauterization

Complications of cauterization include accidental burns as well as crusting, mucosal ulceration, and septal perforation. These reactions are attributed to local inflammatory reactions of the blood vessels in the perichondrium, which supply the underlining cartilage.[6] Although the exact incidence of septal perforation is unknown, very few patients develop septal perforations after cauterization despite the large number of patients treated; however, an increased risk among patients with repeated and bilateral cauterization has been postulated. Specific complications associated with silver nitrate include silver tattooing and skin staining.[4,7] Recommended precautions include the careful placement of silver nitrate with adequate visualization and the use of additional therapies such as topical ointments in patients with repeated epistaxis. Furthermore, the application of a saline-soaked pledget after application removes unreacted silver nitrate as it forms a precipitate and limits inadvertent cauterization.[8] Complications associated with both monopolar and bipolar electrocauterization are primarily the result of inadvertent cauterization. A few serious complications, such as cerebrospinal fluid (CSF) leak and ophthalmic injury, have also been reported when intentional cauterization affected nearby critical structures. These complications reflect the close proximity and anatomic variability of the anterior ethmoidal artery, the posterior ethmoidal artery, the optic nerve, and the skull base. In one case, bipolar cauterization of the posterior ethmoidal artery resulted in scotoma and a visual-field deficit caused by the injury of the optic nerve or its related blood supply.[9]

LASER PHOTOCOAGULATION

Use of Laser Photocoagulation

For the management of epistaxis, laser therapy is primarily used for the treatment of HHT-associated telangiectasias, and it is particularly useful for addressing small lesions. A variety of lasers such as argon, potassium–titanyl–phosphate, and neodymium-doped yttrium–aluminum–garnet can be used. Under endoscopic visualization, the laser beam is focused to create a small, discrete spot size that is then repeated around the lesion in the shape of a rosette. This technique is not as useful in larger lesions, because a central high-flow area may persist; if this is addressed directly, it often results in bleeding, thereby hindering further ablation.[4] These larger lesions may require alternative treatment, such as electrocauterization. In some patients with HHT, recurrent bleeding occurs despite multiple interventions including septodermoplasty. In very severe cases, nasal closure should be considered.

Complications of Laser Photocoagulation

Like all laser surgery, special safety precautions need to be taken to avoid complications such as unintentional exposure from directed or reflected laser energy. Eye protection is essential. The patient's eyes should be taped closed and his or her face covered with wet cloth. In addition, the surgeon and all operating room personnel are required to wear protective glasses or goggles. Although in most rhinologic laser surgeries healing is uneventful, synechiae, strictures, and septal perforations may result.

HEMOSTATIC AGENTS

Various biodegradable hemostatic compounds are currently used for the treatment of epistaxis, either alone or in combination with other treatment modalities (Table 41-1). For example, a small piece of Surgicel (Johnson & Johnson Medical, Arlington, Tex), which is a gelatin sponge, can be placed over a cauterization site to facilitate hemostasis by the local compression and contact activation of the clotting cascade. In addition, it acts as a protective covering. FloSeal (Baxter, Deerfield, Ill) is a viscous gel that consists of collagen and bovine thrombin that acts on contact with the bleeding mucosal surface, and it has been shown to be an affective alternative to nasal packing for anterior epistaxis.[10,11] The advantages of these hemostatic agents include their ease of application, which is relatively comfortable and atraumatic to nasal mucosa, and the lack of the need to remove them.

NASAL PACKING

Use of Nasal Packing

Nasal packing is a longstanding treatment for the control of both anterior and posterior epistaxis. A wide variety of packing materials, which act by the compression of local vasculature, are available. In addition to temporizing bleeding, nasal packing ideally should create a moist environment that facilitates healing without causing local irritation or a foreign-body reaction. Traditional nasal packing consisted of ribbon gauze impregnated with a lubricant (e.g., Vaseline Ribbon Gauze and Clauden Nasal Ribbon Gauze, Lohmann Corp, Hebron, Ky) or antibiotic ointment (e.g., Bismuth Iodoform Paraffin Pack, Evans Medical Ltd, Leatherhead, United Kingdom). Although gauze packing can be easily manipulated into position, the mesh framework allows for the significant ingrowth of tissue so that the removal of the gauze causes tissue disruption and bleeding.[12] During the 1970s, an absorbent nonadherent nasal packing that consisted of a cotton fleece covered in a water-repellent, perforated, plastic film was introduced to address the problem of mucosal disruption, and it continues to be a commonly used nasal packing (e.g., Telfa, The Kendall Company, Boston, Mass). More recently, hygroscopic foam packing (e.g., Merocel, Medtronic Xomed, Jacksonville, Fla) has been developed, which is capable of absorbing an amount of liquid of up to 10 to 20 times its own weight.[13] When hydrated, these increasingly popular packing materials act by compressing the local vasculature. Various brands and models are available, some of which have been developed with special applicators and ventilation devices. In the case of finger stalls, the foam is contained in rubber packaging, which can be either individually or commercially fabricated to further minimize mucosal damage.

Complications of Nasal Packing

In general, nasal packing is a safe and effective method of treating epistaxis. However, some important local and systemic complications exist. Minor mucosal damage on insertion is common, and it can occur to varying degrees with all types of nasal packing. Associated mucosal lacerations may worsen bleeding, and they are particularly common in patients with deviated nasal septa. Although rare, more severe complications (e.g., the violation of the skull base and the orbit with nasal packing) have been reported.[14,15] Knowledge of the nasal

TABLE 41-1 Hemostatic Compounds

Compound	Trade Name	Manufacturer	Mechanism of Action
Gelatin sponge	Surgifoam	Johnson & Johnson, Inc	Compression, contact activation of the intrinsic clotting pathway
Oxidized regenerated cellulose	Surgicel	Johnson & Johnson, Inc	Compression, contact activation of the intrinsic clotting pathway
Microfibular collagen	Avitene	Davol, Inc	Contact activation of the intrinsic clotting pathway, directly activates platelets
Fibrin sealant	FloSeal	Baxter, Inc	Contact activation of the common clotting pathway

anatomy, delicate technique, and adequate light for visualization are essential for avoiding insertion trauma. On removal, packing should be well hydrated to limit mucosal disruption and pain.

Infectious Complications

Infectious complications associated with nasal packing are uncommon and, in most cases, local. Rhinosinusitis can develop as a result of the obstruction of the osteomeatal complex or the sphenoethmoidal recess by nasal packing or its associated mucosal edema.[16] Although spontaneous resolution usually occurs after the packing is removed or after a short course of antibiotics, a few patients go on to develop chronic rhinosinusitis, which may require surgery (Figure 41-1). Despite the demonstration of bacteremia in patients with nasal packing, systemic infections that result from hematogenous spread associated with nasal packing are very rare.[17] In one case, a patient developed *Staphylococcus aureus* endocarditis 3 days after nasal packing.[18]

Toxic shock syndrome (TSS) is a rare and potentially fatal infectious complication of epistaxis management. Although more commonly associated with vaginal tampon usage, TSS is also associated with nasal packing. Most cases result from the release of an exotoxin produced by phage 1 *S. aureus*. Diagnostic criteria from the Centers for Disease Control and Prevention include a fever of more than 102°F, diffuse macular erythroderma (i.e., rash), desquamation, and hypotension. In addition, at least three organ systems must be involved. The presentation of TSS usually occurs with 48 hours, and it has been associated with several different types of nasal packing.[19-22] Furthermore, although antibiotics are commonly recommended for the prevention of this and other infectious complications, their efficacy remains a subject of debate.[23-25] Treatment begins with the immediate removal of all nasal packing, nasal culture, and the debridement of any necrotic or infected tissue; however, local wound infections are rare.[26] Management is largely medical, with anti-staphylococcal antibiotics and fluid resuscitation being the keystones of therapy.

Respiratory Complications

The posterior dislocation of the nasal packing is a serious and life-threatening complication. Posterior dislocation has resulted in both the ingestion and aspiration of nasal packing.[27,28] Finger-cot aspiration is particularly worrisome, because acute asphyxiation by complete laryngeal occlusion has been reported. Safety measures include knotting the bilateral packing anterior to the septum and suturing the finger stalls to the septum to prevent posterior dislocation.[13] Other respiratory considerations include the possibility of packing-induced obstructive sleep apnea and the activation of the nasopulmonary reflex. Patients with cardiac and pulmonary disease who undergo bilateral nasal packing should be admitted for observation.

BALLOON TAMPONADE

Use of Balloon Tamponade

The use of nasal balloons to tamponade bleeding dates back to Beck in 1917; however, newer devices have expanded the role of balloon tamponade for the treatment of epistaxis.[29] Rapid Rhino (Applied Therapeutics, Tampa, Fla) is a pneumatic packing that is covered with a carboxymethylcellulose hydrocolloid, a lubricant, and a platelet aggregator that has been reported to be as effective for the treatment of anterior epistaxis as Merocel packing.[30] It has the added benefit of the increased ease of insertion and removal. In addition to the complications of other types of nasal packing, balloon therapy is associated with pressure-related mucosal damage, and higher rates of fibrin accumulation, adhesions, and nasal obstruction have been demonstrated.[31]

For the treatment of posterior epistaxis, Foley catheters are used primarily for the acute management of severe bleeding that is unresponsive to nasal packing. Newer treatment modalities such as endoscopic ligation and angioembolization are becoming increasingly popular for the definitive treatment of posterior bleeding. The balloon is inserted along the floor of the nasal cavity; when it is in the nasopharynx, it is inflated with water. Gauze packing is placed in the nasal cavity, with the balloon acting as the posterior wall. The catheter is then secured externally to prevent distal migration by placing pressure on the nasal ala. After the patient is stabilized, close monitoring of the patient's cardiopulmonary status is necessary, because upper-airway obstruction can occur.

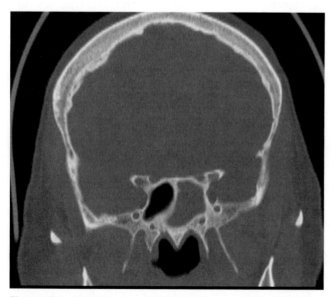

Figure 41-1. Coronal computed tomography scan of a patient who developed left-sided chronic sphenoid sinusitis after nasal packing for epistaxis.

Complications of Balloon Tamponade

Foley catheters are associated with the same complications as nasal packing; however, they are more common (e.g., in the case of respiratory compromise), and they may be more severe. Moreover, patient tolerance is often limited. The intracranial penetration of Foley catheters has been reported with severe neurologic sequelae such as visual loss and mental status changes. Postinsertion computed tomography (CT) scans have demonstrated optic nerve damage and intracranial hemorrhage with pneumocephalic trail.[32] Local mucosal damage can be significant, with the necrosis of the nasal mucosa, the septum, and the ala. Several methods have been described to avoid alar necrosis with gauze packing, the cut port of the Foley catheter, or both.[33,34]

ANGIOEMBOLIZATION

Use of Angioembolization

First described in 1974, angioembolization has become a useful tool for the treatment of posterior epistaxis that is unresponsive to nasal packing in medical centers with skilled interventional radiologists trained in this procedure. An initial angiogram of the internal and external carotid artery systems is performed to demonstrate the site of bleeding; this is optimally performed with the nasal packing removed. Before embolization, vascular abnormalities (e.g., posttraumatic pseudoaneurysm, carotid cavernous fistula) and anastomoses that may allow for the passage of materials used in the embolization into the cerebral or ophthalmic circulation must be excluded. After the targeted vessel has been identified and embolization has been deemed safe, embolization materials such as polyvinyl alcohol microparticles or Gelfoam pledgets are injected along with iodinated contrast via the microcatheter tip in a rapid, targeted fashion to the arteriolar bed. Successful occlusion is demonstrated by a significant decrease in vascular flow on postembolization angiography. In most cases, bleeding has been found to arise from the distal branches of the internal maxillary artery. In a small percentage of patients, the source of bleeding may be from a branch of the facial artery or from the contralateral internal maxillary artery, and embolization may be required. Reported success rates range from 71% to 100%.[35–38] The failure of angioembolization is mostly the result of the involvement of the anterior ethmoid artery, which arises from the ophthalmic branch of the internal carotid artery and therefore cannot be embolized. Other arteries that contribute to nasal bleeding and that have led to the failure of angioembolization include the accessory meningeal artery and the ascending pharyngeal artery.[39]

Complications of Angioembolization

Significant complications, although rare, are associated with angioembolization, including cerebrovascular accidents and other neurologic sequelae such as cranial nerve palsy and visual loss. These complications can occur when anastomotic networks, such as the ethmoidal collaterals and the meningo-hypophyseal arteries between the external carotid system and the brain and eye are present but not identified on preembolization angiography. For example, the failure to identify a faint choroidal blush on selective catheterization of the external carotid artery has resulted in permanent visual loss as a result of the embolization of the central retinal artery via the lacrimal artery.[40] In addition, local ischemia in the distribution of the embolized artery has led to permanent facial scarring as a result of alar necrosis and skin sloughing. These complications, although rare—and, in the case of cerebrovascular accident, occur in less than 1% of cases—should be thoroughly discussed with the patient.[38,39,41]

SURGICAL LIGATION

Use of Surgical Ligation

Surgical ligation is the mainstay of therapy for the treatment of intractable epistaxis arising from the anterior ethmoidal artery (AEA). Traditionally ligation has been performed via an open approach using a Lynch-type incision with the placement of the vascular clip on the AEA between the periorbital fascia and its entrance into the lamina papyracea. Recently limited success via an endoscopic approach has been reported; however, to clip the AEA, it must be suspended from the ethmoidal roof by mesentery of adequate length to fit the clip entirely around the artery. In a cadaver study of 45 nasal cavities, this amount of mesentery was only found to be present in 36% of cavities.[42] Therefore, if an endoscopic approach fails, conversion to an open approach may be required.

For the management of posterior epistaxis, surgical ligation of the sphenopalatine artery, the internal maxillary artery, and the external carotid artery have been described. These ligations involve a variety of approaches, such as transantral, transoral, and transcervical. Because ligation is optimally performed as close as possible to the involved vessel, new endoscopic techniques for sphenopalatine artery ligation are becoming increasingly popular for the treatment of posterior epistaxis. An important endoscopic landmark for the sphenopalatine artery ligation is the crista ethmoidalis, which is a perpendicular crest of bone that abuts the most posteroinferior aspect of the basal lamella.[43] High success rates and low complication rates have been reported. In a pooled series of 127 patients, the endoscopic ligation of the sphenopalatine artery had a success rate of 98%, and no complications were reported.[44] Although uncommon, treatment failures can occur, and they are usually the result of a lack of recognition of the varied branching patterns of the sphenopalatine artery, which often branches proximal to the nasal cavity. In one study, the branches were demonstrated to enter via multiple foramen in up to 12% of patients.[45]

Complications of Surgical Ligation

Both open and endoscopic approaches to AEA ligation require intimate knowledge of the microanatomy of the orbit region, including the anterior and posterior ethmoidal neurovascular bundles, the optic nerve, and the skull base. The violation of these structures can lead to potentially devastating complications, such as visual loss and CSF leak. During endoscopic ligation, intraorbital retraction of the AEA can lead to an orbital hematoma and dangerous increases in intraorbital pressure. In addition, CSF leak has been a reported complication of the intranasal ligation of the AEA, and anatomic studies have demonstrated dural attachments to the AEA mesentery.[46] Complications associated with surgical ligation for posterior epistaxis are uncommon, and they are the result of local ischemia such as inferior turbinate necrosis.[47]

NASAL SURGERY

Nasal disorders are one of the most common problems dealt with by otolaryngologists, and they make up a large percentage of patient visits. Often nasal disorders require surgical treatment and include, among others, septal surgery, turbinoplasty, and the control of epistaxis. Although in general nasal surgeries are safe and effective, a wide variety of complications may result, such as postoperative bleeding, septal hematoma, septal perforation, and CSF rhinorrhea. This section will focus on the causes and management of the surgical complications that are unique to surgery of the nasal cavity.

Postoperative Bleeding

Postoperative bleeding is the most common complication of most nasal surgery, including septoplasty and turbinoplasty.[48,49] A through preoperative history targeted at identifying patients who are predisposed to bleeding (e.g., from bleeding disorders, as a result of over-the-counter or prescribed medications) is an important step in the prevention of postoperative bleeding. Common iatrogenic sources of bleeding in nasal surgery include trauma to the sphenopalatine artery if the lateral attachment of the middle turbinate is violated; the nasal branch of the sphenopalatine artery, which runs across the face of the sphenoid to supply the posterior aspect of the nasal septum; and the anterior ethmoidal artery when the vessel is pedicled from the skull base, although this vessel is more commonly the source of postoperative bleeding after

sinus surgery. In addition, diffuse mucosal bleeding is a common complication of turbinate surgery. It can occur during the immediate or late postoperative period, and it is frequently observed after the removal of nasal packing.[48] The management of postoperative bleeding is similar to that of other causes of epistaxis. However, in the case of immediate postoperative bleeding that is uncontrolled by simple nasal packing, a reasonable alternative is promptly returning the patient to the operating room for diagnostic nasal endoscopy and the control of epistaxis under local or general anesthesia.

Hematoma and Abscess

A septal hematoma is a collection of blood between the cartilaginous and bony septum and its overlying perichondrium and periosteum, which transits the only blood supply to the underlying structures. When the accumulation of blood exerts increasing pressure, blood flow is interrupted. If sustained, avascular necrosis of the cartilage and bone can result, which can be associated with both functional and cosmetic consequences.[50] Septal hematomas are most commonly the result of nasal trauma in which shearing forces disrupt the vasculature of the tightly adherent perichondrium. They have been found to occur in up to 15% of patients with nasal fractures; however, they may occur independent of any external signs of trauma.[51,52] In addition, septal hematomas may be iatrogenic. They are not routinely encountered in septal surgery; however, they can occur any time that the septum is manipulated, such as during the placement of nasal packing as part of epistaxis management. Of note us that bilateral hematomas have been reported in a small percentage of cases, and they can cause significant airway obstruction.

Diagnosis of Septal Hematoma

The diagnosis of septal hematoma is clinical, and it requires both clinical awareness and careful examination. Early symptoms such as pain and nasal obstruction may be nonspecific, and more characteristic symptoms such as severe pain, tenderness to tip palpation, and fever may occur up to 72 hours after injury.[50,52] Careful examination includes visual inspection with illumination and suction. The application of a topical vasoconstrictor such as phenylephrine hydrochloride or oxymetazoline is useful for reducing concomitant mucosal swelling. Key observations include a thickened, discolored mass on the septum.[52–55] Gentle palpation either digitally or with a cotton swab may aid in the diagnosis, with findings ranging from a fluctuant mass to a doughy swelling with a size that does not change with application of topical vasoconstrictors.[51] Although radiographic imaging may be obtained to assess a patient for other maxillofacial fractures, it is not indicated for the diagnosis of septal hematomas, because studies have not shown imaging to be a reliable method for diagnosing septal hematoma.[53]

Treatment of Septal Hematoma

Septal hematomas are treated by incision and drainage as soon as the diagnosis is made and the patient is medically stabilized. This is performed either using a headlight or nasal endoscope, and the nasal cavity is reexamined to determine whether a hematoma is present bilaterally before an incision is made. If so, care must be taken to stagger the incisions so as to not interrupt the entire blood supply of the underlying cartilage. After the incision is made, any purulence noted should be collected for Gram staining and culture. A thorough inspection for any active bleeding is conducted. In addition, all nonviable cartilage or bone should be debrided, and the wound should be well irrigated. The mucosal flaps are reapproximated, and the cavity is packed. The nasal cavity should be reexamined in 2 to 3 days to ensure that the hematoma has not reaccumulated and that an infection has not developed.

Complications of Septal Hematoma

Septal hematomas involve a variety of potential complications such as septal abscess formation, septal perforation, and subsequent saddle-nose deformity. These complications can occur as quickly as 3 days, and, if cartilage necrosis is significant, the loss of the dorsal support may result in a permanent saddle-nose deformity. Infectious complications of septal hematomas, such as meningitis, intracranial abscess, orbital cellulites, and cavernous sinus thrombosis, have been reported. *Staphylococcus aureus*, *Haemophilus influenza*, and *Streptococcus pneumonia* are the most common isolated bacterial species. Patient symptoms such as throbbing pain, spiking fevers, visual loss, and mental status changes should alert the physician to the possibility of these rare but serious complications.[49]

Septal Perforation

Septal perforation is a common clinical finding with many diverse causes, with traumatic injury accounting for a large portion of cases. Other potential causes of septal perforation include infection (e.g., syphilis), systemic diseases such as Wegener granulomatosis and sarcoidosis, and primary and metastatic neoplasms. In other cases, septal perforations may be the result of exposure to mucosal irritants or topical vasoconstrictors, such as topical decongestants and cocaine. Important information can be gained from a thorough history. Specific questions concerning facial trauma, sinonasal surgery, and over-the-counter and prescription medications as well as recreational drug use should be investigated. Nasal endoscopy can be helpful for establishing a differential diagnosis, and findings such as nasal crusting, nodular mucosa, and synechiae can be useful for formulating a differential diagnosis. However, the clinical history and the physical appearance may not accurately predict the histologic diagnosis,

and often further workup including nasal culture, laboratory, and histopathologic evaluation are warranted.[56] Infectious causes such as fungus and mycobacterium species should be considered. In addition to routine Gram staining and culture, special cultures for fungus and mycobacterium should also be sent.

Treatment of Septal Hematoma

Septal perforation is a well-known complication of nasal packing and surgery of the nasal septum. Traditionally techniques of septal surgery have been broadly classified according to the fate of the resected nasal septum. In a submucosal resection (SMR), the resected cartilage and bone are removed, whereas in a septoplasty they are repositioned. Several articles have been published comparing the relative rates of septal perforations with SMR and septoplasty, and, in general, septoplasty has been associated with a slightly reduced rate. In a review article of nine studies with 1408 patients having long-term follow up, Bateman and Woolford[57] reported a slightly increased rate of septal perforation with SMR (range, 3% to 8%) as compared with septoplasty (range, 2% to 5%). However, today most surgeons use a combination of these two methods. In addition, very limited septal surgery under endoscopic visualization is becoming increasingly popular.[58,59] This new technique has been found to be a particularly useful method for addressing isolated septal spurs that tend to occur where the cartilaginous and bony septum widen at the base to attach to the maxillary crest.

Management options for nasal septal perforation include observation as well as medical and surgical therapy. The initial treatment for patients complaining of nasal crusting and mild epistaxis includes nasal saline irrigation and applications of emollient. In select cases, the placement of a nasal obturator may be beneficial. In patients whose symptoms are not adequately controlled with medical therapy, surgical repair can be considered; however, repair can be challenging, and it is associated with a higher rate of reperforation than primary septal surgery.[60] A variety of techniques such as endoscopy-assisted closure, monopedicled or bipedicled mucosal flaps, and interposition grafts have been described in the literature, and the choice of technique depends on the size and location of the perforation as well as the surgeon's preference.[61]

ORBITAL COMPLICATIONS

Orbital complications in nasal surgery are associated with optic neuropathy and include incidents such as the violation of the lamina papyracea, orbital hematoma, and orbital apex syndrome.[62] Optic neuropathy can result from direct trauma to the optic nerve or its blood supply. In addition, intranasal injections of fluid (e.g., corticosteroids, local anesthetics) have resulted in embolic occlusion or vasospasm in branches of the ophthalmic artery and visual loss; however, of the thousands of intranasal injections performed, this complication has resulted in permanent visual loss in only a handful of cases.[63–66]

Direct damage or ischemic injury can result from the inadvertent penetration of the lamina papyracea in nasal surgery. When this occurs, further instrumentation should be terminated. The area is then carefully inspected to determine the extent of injury, and the vision is assessed. However, if the patient is under general anesthesia, the examination of the globe and the pupillary light reflex should suffice. The patient is then monitored for signs of a developing orbital hematoma such as proptosis, ecchymosis, and lid edema. If the injury is limited and surgical landmarks are well established, surgery can be resumed, albeit away from the site of injury. When orbital fat obscures the view, it can be gently lateralized with a Freer elevator. Overpacking of the nasal cavity may lead to increased intraorbital pressure and therefore should be avoided. In addition, the patient is advised to sneeze with the mouth open, if necessary, to prevent the development of the pneumatization of the orbit.

Orbital hematoma is a dreaded complication of nasal surgery, because the compression of the optic nerve can lead to ischemic injury. Orbital hematoma may be sudden or slow in onset, depending on the source of bleeding. Signs and symptoms of orbital hematoma include orbital pressure, pain, ecchymosis, and proptosis. Physical examination should include the assessment of vision, including light perception, visual acuity, color perception, visual fields, papillary light reflex, and a funduscopic examination. Extraocular movement and a resistance to retropulsion should also be assessed. If an orbital hematoma is suspected, all nasal packing should be immediately removed, and an ophthalmologic consult should be obtained. Intraocular pressure can be assessed with the use of a tonometer. For patients with mildly elevated intraocular pressure, medical therapy such as topical timolol and parenteral diuretics may be sufficient; however, in the setting of a rapidly expanding orbital hematoma and deteriorating vision, surgical therapy consisting of lateral canthotomy and cantholysis or endoscopic decompression should be performed.

INTRACRANIAL COMPLICATIONS

Intracranial complications, including CSF fistula, pneumocephalus, and meningitis, can result from blunt or penetrating injuries to the skull base. Although rare, these complications also occur in very rare cases of nasal surgery, and they can be associated with significant morbidity and, in some cases, mortality. The most common site of injury to the skull base is at or medial to the insertion of the vertical portion of the middle turbinate, where the dura is tightly adherent to the cribriform plate. At this site, even minute fractures often result in a CSF leak, particularly at the point of least resistance, where the anterior ethmoidal artery exits the skull base.[67]

Various types of nasal instrumentation have resulted in the inadvertent intracranial penetration of objects such as nasogastric tubes, nasal packing, and esophageal thermometers. For example, Fletcher and colleagues[68] reported a 64% mortality rate associated with inadvertent intracranial nasogastric tube placement. After this emergency has been discovered, imaging of the brain and paranasal sinuses should be obtained immediately, a neurosurgery consult obtained, and antibiotic prophylaxis initiated. Although more common during paranasal sinus surgery, intracranial complications have also been reported during nasal surgery.[49,69] In most cases, the manipulation of the septum and the middle turbinate during nasal surgery can provide the very minimal amount of torque needed to fracture the cribriform plate and produce a CSF leak. In addition, the asymmetry of the skull base can increase the risk of skull-base penetration.[69,70] If this condition is identified immediately and no injury to the dura or the intracranial contents has occurred, the defect can be immediately repaired using an endoscopic approach.

Patient complaints can include clear, nonviscous rhinorrhea that is constant, gushing, or intermittent; a salty or metallic taste; and headache. Fluid should be collected and tested for the presence of β-2 transferrin, which is a protein that is present only in CSF, perilymph, and aqueous humor. In addition, a high-resolution CT scan should be obtained to identify the location and size of the defect. Conservative management that includes strict bed rest, minimal head elevation, and stool softeners has proven to be effective for the treatment of delayed CSF leaks, because 70% of postoperative CSF leaks resolve with conservative measures.[71] However, if conservative measures fail, surgical repair is necessary, and success rates with endoscopic approaches are upward of 90%.[72,73]

Anosmia

Although an improvement in the patient's sense of smell after nasal surgery has been demonstrated in many cases of nasal surgery, olfactory loss can occur.[74,75] Olfactory dysfunction is classified into two broad categories (neuronal or conductive), and both have been associated with loss of smell after nasal surgery. Conductive causes of loss of smell after nasal surgery have been attributed to local factors such as edema, structural changes such as turbinate malposition, and nasal synechiae. Neuronal causes include direct trauma or resulting inflammation of the olfactory neuroepithelium.[76,77] This specialized tissue is located primarily along the cribriform plate, and it extends inferiorly onto the upper aspect of the nasal septum and the superior turbinate. Recently olfactory epithelium has been demonstrated as anterior as the head of the middle turbinate and as inferior as the body of the middle turbinate.[77,78] In addition, disruption anywhere along the olfactory neuronal pathway may lead to olfactory dysfunction; therefore the manipulation of tissue in the area of the olfactory cleft and the cribriform should be avoided to prevent postoperative anosmia.

Smell is essential to the enjoyment of food and beverages as well as to the detection of environmental hazards. Subjective complaints of the loss of smell should be evaluated using objective measures. The most common methods of testing olfactory function are olfactory threshold tests and odor identification tests such as the University of Pennsylvania Smell Identification Test, which is a quick, well-validated, and easy-to-use scratch-and-sniff test.[79] The treatment of postoperative olfactory function depends on the mechanism of loss. In cases of conductive loss caused by obstructive edema, a short course of corticosteroids may be beneficial, whereas for patients with an infectious cause, antibiotic therapy may be added. Neural causes of olfactory loss are more difficult to treat; however, current research into olfactory neuronal apoptosis and its associated pharmacologic targets may provide future treatment possibilities.[80] Moreover, all patients should be warned about the safety issues associated with anosmia, because these patients are at a significantly increased risk of experiencing an olfactory-related hazardous event.[81]

Atrophic Rhinitis and Empty-Nose Syndrome

Atrophic rhinitis and empty-nose syndrome are chronic conditions that can arise as complications of nasal surgery (particularly turbinate surgery). A wide variety of techniques exist to address the turbinates, including submucous turbinectomy, laser ablation, and radiofrequency turbinoplasty. All of these can lead to the excessive removal, destruction, or alteration of functional nasal tissue and impair the ability of the nose to regulate airflow as well as to humidify, heat, and purify inspired air. In addition, techniques that result in bone exposure have been shown to lead to prolonged healing and crusting.[82] From a clinical perspective, preservation of a key area known as the *internal nasal valve* is essential. The internal nasal valve is composed of the lower edge of the upper lateral cartilage, the septum, and the head of the inferior turbinate. The internal valve controls more than 50% of nasal airway resistance. Nasal air temperature and humidity increases are higher in this region and along the entire length of the middle turbinate.[83,84]

In atrophic rhinitis that occurs as a result of nasal surgery, anatomic alterations of the turbinates and the internal nasal valve lead to the destruction, atrophy, and drying of the nasal mucosa. Subsequently the stasis of viscous secretions leads to a characteristic fetid odor referred to as *ozaena*. *Empty-nose syndrome* is named after the characteristic CT findings of an absence of nasal and bone structures, although excessive tissue removal produces a paradoxic perception of nasal obstruction. Some patients experience symptoms of atrophic rhinitis as well as pain and discomfort. Empty-nose syndrome has been associated with both inferior turbinate and middle turbinate resection. Several surgical procedures for the treatment of atrophic rhinitis and empty-nose syndrome have been described, such as the placement of graft materials (e.g., Plastipore [Richards Manufacturing Company, Memphis, TN], hydroxyapatite cement) to rebuild the inferior turbinate and thereby decrease turbulent nasal airflow. In severe cases, the temporary closure of nasal cavities to promote the return of normal mucosal function may be beneficial.[85-88] However, the mainstay of treatment is nasal saline irrigation and culture-directed antibiotics when bacterial suprainfection occurs. Patients should be counseled to avoid mucosal irritants such as smoke, decongestants, and antihistamines, because they may exacerbate symptoms.

REFERENCES

1. Carney AS, Weir J, Baldwin DL: Contamination with blood during management of epistaxis. *BMJ* 1995;311:1064.
2. Chiu T, Dunn JS: An anatomical study of the arteries of the anterior nasal septum. *Otolaryngol Head Neck Surg* 2006;134: 33–36.
3. Singh B: Combined internal maxillary and anterior ethmoidal arterial occlusion: The treatment of choice in intractable epistaxis. *J Laryngol Otol* 1992;106:507–510.
4. Amin M, Glynn F, Phelan S, et al: Silver nitrate cauterization, does concentration matter? *Clin Otolaryngol* 2007;32:197–208.
5. Ghaheri B, Fong K, Hwang P: The utility of bipolar electrocautery in hereditary hemorrhagic telangiectasia. *Otolaryngol Head Neck Surg* 2006;1134:1006–1009.
6. Murthy P, Nilssen EL, Rao S, et al: A randomized clinical trial of antiseptic nasal cream and silver nitrate cautery in the treatment of recurrent anterior epistaxis. *Clin Otolaryngol* 1999;24: 228–231.
7. Mayall F, Wild D: A silver tattoo of the nasal mucosa after silver nitrate cautery. *J Laryngol Otol* 1996;110:609–610.
8. Matria S, Gupta D: A simple technique to avoid staining of the skin around vestibule following cautery. *Clin Otolaryngol* 2007;32:74.
9. Yen, S, Yen M, Foroozan R: Orbital apex syndrome after ethmoidal artery ligation for recurrent epistaxis. *Ophthal Plast Reconstr Surg* 2004;20:392–394.
10. Mathiasen RA, Cruz RM: Prospective, randomized, controlled clinical trial of a novel matrix hemostatic sealant in patients with acute anterior epistaxis. *Laryngoscope* 2005;115:899–902.
11. Vaiman M, Sarfaty S, Shlamkovich N, et al: Fibrin sealant: Alternative to nasal packing in endonasal operations: A prospective randomized study. *Isr Med Assoc J* 2005;7:571–574.
12. Garth RJ, Brightwall AP: A comparison of packing materials used in nasal surgery. *J Laryngol Otol* 1994;108:564–566.
13. Weber R, Keerl R, Hochapfel F, et al: Packing in endonasal surgery. *Am J Otolaryngol* 2001;22:306–320.
14. Hollis GJ: Massive pneumocephalus following Merocel nasal tamponade for epistaxis. *Acad Emerg Med* 2000;7:1073–1074.
15. Oluwole AO, Hanif J: Proptosis following nasal tamponade. *J Laryngol Otol* 1996;110: 265–266.

16. Lanza DC, Kennedy DW: Endoscopic sinus surgery. In Bailey B, editor: *Head and Neck Surgery: Otolaryngology,* vol 1, Philadelphia, 1993, Lippincott.

17. Herzon FS: Bacteremia and local infections with nasal packing. *Arch Otolaryngol* 1971;94:317–320.

18. Jayawardena S, Eisdofer J, Indulkar S, et al: Infective endocarditis of native valve after anterior nasal packing. *Am J Ther* 2006;13:460–462.

19. Allen ST, Liland JB, Nichols CG, et al: Toxic shock syndrome associated with use of latex nasal packing. *Arch Intern Med* 1990;150:2587–2588.

20. Hull HF, Mann JM, Sands CJ, et al: Toxic shock syndrome related with nasal packing. *Arch Otolaryngol* 1983;109:624–629.

21. Mansfield CJ, Peterson MB: Toxic shock syndrome: Associated with nasal packing. *Clin Pediatr* 1989;28:443–445.

22. De Veries N, van der Baan: Toxic shock syndrome after nasal packing: Is prevention possible? A review of the literature. *Rhinology* 1989;27:125–128.

23. Kayguusuz I, Kizirgil A, Karlida T, et al: Bacteremia in septoplasty and septorhinoplasty surgery. *Rhinology* 2003;41:76–79.

24. Finelli PF, Ross JW: Endocarditis following nasal packing: Need for prophylaxis [letter]. *Clin Infect Dis* 1994;19:984–985.

25. Makitie T, Aaltonen A, Hytonen LM, et al: Postoperative infection following nasal septoplasty. *Acta Otolaryngol Suppl* 2000;543: 165–166.

26. Rhee CA, Smith RJ, Jackson IT: Toxic shock syndrome associated with suction-assisted lipectomy. *Aesthetic Plast Surg* 1994;18: 161–163.

27. Oluwole MO, Hanif J: Swallowed nasal pack: A rare but serious complication of the management of epistaxis. *J Laryngol Otol* 2004;118:372–373.

28. Spillman D: [A report of two fatal aspirations of nasal packings (author's transl)]. *Laryngol Rhinol Otol (Stuttg)* 1981;60:56.

29. Beck AL: An inflatable rubber bag for intranasal use: Balloon tamponade. *Am J Surg* 1917;31:77–79.

30. Malik BK, Belloso BA, Timmas MS: Randomized controlled trial comparing Merocel and Rapid Rhino packing in management of anterior epistaxis. *Clin Otolaryngol* 2005;30:333–337.

31. Watson MG, Campbell JB, Shenoi PM: Nasal surgery: Does the type of nasal pack influence the result? *Rhinology* 1989;27:105–111.

32. Espinosa PS, Smith CD, Berger JR: Homonymous hemianopsia complicating treatment of postoperative epistaxis. *Neurology* 2006;67:1305.

33. Thomas L, Karagama YG, Watson C: Avoiding alar necrosis with post-nasal packs. *J Laryngol Otol* 2005;119:727–728.

34. Monem SA, Mann G, Suortamo SH: A method of safely securing Foley's catheter in the management of posterior epistaxis with prevention of alar cartilage necrosis. *Auris Nasus Larynx* 2000;27: 357–358.

35. Sokoloff J, Waskom T, McDonald D, et al: Therapeutic percutaneous embolization to control epistaxis. *Radiology* 1974;111:285–287.

36. Elden L, Montanera W, TerBrugge K, et al: Angiographic embolization for the treatment of epistaxis: A review of 108 cases. *Otolaryngol Head Neck Surg* 1994;111:44–50.

37. Vitek J: Idiopathic intractable epistaxis: Endovascular therapy. *Radiology* 1991;81:113–116.

38. Tseng EY, Narducci CA, Willing SJ, et al: Angiographic embolization for epistaxis: A review of 114 cases. *Laryngoscope* 108: 615–619.

39. Duncan IC, Dos Santos C: Accessory meningeal arterial supply to the posterior nasal cavity: Another reason for failed endovascular treatment of epistaxis. *Cardiovasc Intervent Radiol* 2003;26:488–491.

40. Mames RN, Snady-McCoy L, Guy J: Central retinal and posterior ciliary artery occlusion after particle embolization of the external carotid artery system. *Ophthalmology* 1991;98:527–531.

41. Sadri M, Midwinter K, Ahmed A, et al: Assessment of safety and efficacy of arterial embolisation in the management of intractable epistaxis. *Eur Arch Otol Rhinolaryngol* 2006;263:560–566.

42. Floreani SR, Nair SB, Switajewski MC, et al: Endoscopic anterior ethmoidal artery ligation: A cadaver study. *Laryngoscope* 2006;116:1263–1267.

43. Bolger WE, Borgie RC, Melder P: The role of the crista ethmoidalis in endoscopic sphenopalatine artery ligation. *Am J Rhinology* 1999;13:81–86.

44. Kumar S, Shetty A, Rockey J, et al: Contemporary surgical treatment of epistaxis. What is the evidence for sphenopalatine artery ligation? *Clin Otolaryngol Allied Sci* 2003;23:360–363.

45. Wareing MJ, Padgham ND: Osteologic classification of the sphenopalatine foramen. *Laryngoscope* 1998;108:125–127.

46. Duncan IC, Dos Santos C: Accessory meningeal arterial supply to the posterior nasal cavity: Another reason for failed endovascular treatment of epistaxis. *Cardiovasc Intervent Radiol* 2003;26: 488–491.

47. Moorthy R, Anand R, Prior M, et al: Inferior turbinate necrosis following endoscopic sphenopalatine artery ligation. *Otolaryngol Head Neck Surg* 2003;129:159–160.

48. Goldwyn RM: Unexpected bleeding after elective nasal surgery. *Ann Plast Surg* 1979;2:201–204.

49. Teichgraeber JF, Riley WB, Parks DH: Nasal surgery complications. *Plast Reconstr Surg* 1990;85:527–531.

50. Ginsburg CM, Leach JL: Infected nasal septal hematoma. *Pediatr Infect Dis J* 1995;14:1012–1013.

51. Canty PA, Berkowitz RG: Hematoma and abscess of the nasal septum in children. *Arch Otolaryngol Head Neck Surg* 1996;122: 1373–1376.

52. Lopez MA, Liu JH, Hartley BE, et al: Septal hematoma and abscess after nasal trauma. *Clin Pediatr* 2000;30:609–610.

53. Olsen KD, Carpenter RJ, Kern EB: Nasal septal trauma in children. *Pediatrics* 1979;64:32–35.

54. Nuss RC, Healy GB: Methods of examination. In Bluestone CD, Stool SE, Kenna MA, editors: *Pediatric otolaryngology,* Philadelphia, 1996, WB Saunders, pp 744–758.

55. Olsen KD, Carpenter RJ, Kern EB: Nasal septal injury in children. *Arch Otolaryngol* 1980;106:317–320.

56. Diamantopoulos II, Jones NS: The investigations of nasal septal perforations and ulcers. *J Laryngol Otol* 2001;115:541–544.

57. Bateman ND, Woolford, TJ: Informed consent for septal surgery: The evidence base. *J Laryngol Otol* 2003;117:186–188.

58. Hwang PH, McLaughlin RB, Kennedy DW: Endoscopic septoplasty: Indications, technique, and results. *Otolaryngol Head Neck Surg* 1999;102:678–682.

59. Chung BJ, Batra PS, Citardi MJ, et al: Endoscopic septoplasty: Revisitation of technique, indications, and outcomes. *Am J Rhinol* 2007;21:307–311.

60. Goh AY, Hussian SS: Different surgical treatment for nasal septal perforation and their outcome. *J Laryngol Otol* 2007;121:419–426.

61. Romo T 3rd, Sclafani AP, Falk AN, et al: A graduated approach to the repair of nasal septal perforations. *Plast Reconstr Surg* 1999;103:66–75.

62. Jainson SG, Bhatty SM, Chopra SK, et al: Orbital apex syndrome: A rare complication of septorhinoplasty. *Indian J Ophthalmol* 1994;42:213–214.

63. Whiteman DW, Rosen DA, Pinkerton RM: Retinal and choroidal embolism after intranasal corticosteroid injection. *Am J Ophthalmology* 1980;89:851–853.

64. Savino PJ, Burde RM, Mills RP: Visual loss following intranasal anesthetic injection. *J Clin Neuroophthalmol* 1990;10:140–144.

65. Johns KJ, Chandra SR: Visual loss following intranasal corticosteroid injection. *JAMA* 1989;261:2413.

66. Mabry RL: Intraturbinal steroid injection: Indications, results, and complications. *Southern Med J* 1978;71:789–794.

67. Stankiewicz JA: Cerebrospinal fluid fistula and endoscopic sinus surgery. *Laryngoscope* 1991;101:250–256.

68. Fletcher SA, Henderson LT, Minor ME, et al: The successful surgical removal of intracranial nasogastric tubes. *J Trauma* 1987;2: 948–952.

69. Bolger WE, Maj MC, Borgie RC, et al: The role of the crista ethmoidalis in endoscopic sphenopalatine artery ligation. *Am J Rhinology* 1999;13:81–86.

70. Onerci TM, Ayhan K, Ogretmenoglu O: Two consecutive cases of cerebrospinal fluid rhinorrhea after septoplasty operation. *Am J Otolaryngol* 2004;25:352–356.

71. Mattox DE, Kennedy DW: Endoscopic management of cerebrospinal fluid leaks and cephaloceles. *Laryngoscope* 1990;100:857–862.

72. Lanza DC, O'Brien DA, Kennedy DW: Endoscopic repair of cerebrospinal fluid fistulae and encephaloceles. *Laryngoscope* 1996;106(9 Pt 1):1119–1125.

73. Kirtane MV, Gautham K, Shradddha RU: Endoscopic CSF rhinorrhea closure: Our experience in 267 cases. *Otolaryngol Head Neck Surg* 2005;132:208–212.

74. Kimmelman CP: The risk to olfaction from nasal surgery. *Laryngoscope* 104;98:981–988.

75. Snow JB: Causes of olfactory and gustatory disorders. In Gretchell TV, Bartshuk LM, Doty RL, et al, editors: *Smell and taste in health and disease,* New York, 1991, Raven Press, pp 445–449.

76. Seiden AM, Smith DV: Endoscopic intranasal surgery is an approach to restoring olfactory function. *Chem Senses* 1998;13:735.

77. Leopold DA, Humel T, Schwob JE, et al: Anterior distribution of human olfactory epithelium. *Laryngoscope* 2000;110:417–421.

78. Feron F, Perry C, McGrath JJ, et al: New techniques for biopsy and culture of human olfactory epithelial neurons. *Arch Otolaryngol Head Neck Surg* 1998;124:861–866.

79. Doty RL, Shaman P, Kimmelman CP, et al: University of Pennsylvania Smell Identification Test: A rapid quantitative olfactory function test for clinic. *Laryngoscope* 1984;94:176–178.

80. Kern RC, Haines DB, Robinson AM: Pathology of the olfactory mucosa: Implications for the treatment of olfactory dysfunction. *Laryngoscope* 2004;114:279–285.

81. Santos DV, Reiter ER, DiNardo LJ, et al: Hazardous events associated with impaired olfactory function. *Arch Otolaryngol Head Neck Surg* 2004;130:317–319.

82. Friedman M, Tanyeri H, Lim J, et al: A safe alternative technique for inferior turbinate reduction. *Laryngoscope* 1999;109:1834–1837.

83. Elad D: Analysis of airflow patterns in the human nose. *Med Biol Eng Comput* 1993;31:585–592.

84. Keck T, Leiacker R, Riechmann H, et al: Temperature profile in the nasal cavity. *Laryngoscope* 2000;110:651–654.

85. Houser SM: Empty nose syndrome associated with middle turbinate resection. *Otolaryngol Head Neck Surg* 2006;135:972–973.

86. Rice DH: Rebuilding the inferior turbinate with hydroxyapatite cement. *Ear Nose Throat J* 2000;70:276–277.

87. Goldenberg D, Dnino J, Netzer A, et al: Plastipore implants in the surgical treatment of atrophic rhinitis: Techniques and results. *Otolaryngol Head Neck Surg* 2000;122:794–797.

88. Dutt SN, Kameswaran M: The aetiology and management of atrophic rhinitis. *J Laryngol Otol* 2005;119:843–852.

CHAPTER 42

Complications of Surgery of the Paranasal Sinuses

Amol M. Bhatki and Andrew N. Goldberg

Because of highly variable individual anatomy and the intimate relationships to the orbit, the anterior cranial fossa, and the vascular structures, sinus surgery has many potential complications. In 1929, Harris Mosher, a pioneer of endonasal sinus surgery, believed that ethmoidectomy should be a simple surgery; in practice, however, it "proved to be one of the easiest operations with which to kill a person."[1] Because of serious complications during this era, external surgical approaches were the standard for surgical management, and these centered on the amputation or ablation of the sinus cavity for all causes of sinus pathology.

In the modern era, recent advances in endoscopic technology and instrumentation provide excellent visualization and technical precision. Improved radiographic technology for computed tomography (CT) scanning, magnetic resonance imaging (MRI), and image-guidance systems enable the detailed preoperative and intraoperative analysis of complex anatomy. As a result, diagnostics accurately identify pathology, and surgical therapy addresses disease while preserving normal sinonasal structure and function. Currently the surgical extirpation of the sinuses for inflammatory and infectious causes is not usually necessary; rather, functional drainage procedures are typically favored.

Although the endoscopic technique and superior modern imaging have empowered the otolaryngologist, they have not resulted in a significant reduction in complications.[2] May and colleagues[2] have classified the complications that result from sinus surgery as minor and major (Box 42-1).

Because of its importance in the prevention of complications, a systematic method for preoperative assessment will be reviewed in this chapter. The complications associated with bleeding, orbital injury, intracranial injury, and scarring will next be considered in detail along with preventative strategies. Lastly, complications of open sinus procedures will be discussed.

PREOPERATIVE CONSIDERATIONS

The prevention of complications for all surgical procedures begins with thorough preoperative assessment and planning. With the employment of the following strategies, intraoperative bleeding, violation of the orbit or the skull base, and ocular injury during functional endoscopic sinus surgery (FESS) can typically be prevented.

Preoperative Assessment

Although the nasal and sinus mucosa are highly vascular, sinus surgery need not be a bloody procedure. Because bleeding that obscures visualization appears to be a common cause of intraoperative complications, minimizing intraoperative hemorrhage is essential.

First, the surgeon should ensure preoperatively that the patient's hemostatic system is intact. The history should include liver disease, bleeding after previous surgery, antiplatelet or anticoagulant medication, and a family history of blood dyscrasias or bleeding disorders. Screening laboratory studies can further investigate abnormalities in the patient's history. Patients are typically also restricted from aspirin and nonsteroidal anti-inflammatory drugs for 2 weeks before surgery.

For patients with reactive hypervascular nasal mucosa or nasal polyposis, a course of preoperative steroids may reduce intraoperative bleeding. In a pilot study by Sieskiewicz and colleagues,[3] patients with severe nasal polyposis received 30 mg of prednisone for 5 days before FESS. Steroid patients had less bleeding and significantly better intraoperative visual conditions as compared with matched control subjects. Similarly, when chronic infection is present, a preoperative course of oral antibiotics may help to reduce tissue vascularity and inflammation.

It is also prudent to review the patient's ophthalmologic history and to document gross visual acuity and ocular range of motion. Formal ophthalmologic consultation may be necessary if abnormalities are found. For example, a patient's history is important if that patient has undergone glaucoma surgery, because the use of orbital massage may be contraindicated. A significant change in the patient's baseline visual acuity, new diplopia, or visual field defects may be the earliest signs of evolving orbital complications.

Nasal endoscopy is another fundamental aspect of preoperative assessment. This routine component of the physical examination can be performed with relative comfort using topical anesthetics, and it should be performed before and after decongestion. One can examine the

BOX 42-1 Complications from Sinus Surgery

MINOR COMPLICATIONS

Temporary, requiring no treatment
- Subcutaneous periorbital emphysema
- Periorbital ecchymosis (preseptal)
- Dental or lip pain or numbness

Temporary, corrected with treatment
- Bronchial asthma
- Adhesions
- Epistaxis
- Infection of sinuses

Permanent, not correctable (persist beyond 1 year)
- Dental or lip pain or numbness
- Loss of smell

MAJOR COMPLICATIONS

Corrected with treatment
- Orbital hematoma (retrobulbar)
- Loss of vision
- Diplopia
- Epiphora
- Carotid artery injury
- Hemorrhage requiring transfusion
- Cerebrospinal fluid leak
- Meningitis
- Brain abscess
- Focal brain hemorrhage

Permanent, despite treatment
- Death
- Blindness
- Diplopia
- Stroke
- Central nervous system deficit

Modified from May M, Levine HL, Mester SJ, et al: Complications of endoscopic sinus surgery: Analysis of 2108 patients—Incidence and prevention. *Laryngoscope* 1994;104:1080–1083.

entire septum and determine the need for a concomitant septoplasty for surgical access. Edema, hypervascularity, the presence of purulence, and the extent of polyposis are also documented to define the extent of disease.

Imaging

Another essential aspect of preoperative planning includes a thorough and detailed review of the patient's radiographic scans. Cross-sectional imaging not only provides diagnostic information, but it is also invaluable for exquisitely detailing anatomy that is inherently highly variable among individuals. Plain films occupied a central role only three decades ago, but they are now essentially obsolete.[4,5] They sufficed for cursory maxillary and frontal sinus evaluation, but they lacked the resolution to display the delicate anatomy of the ethmoids, the sphenoids, and their complex relationship with the orbit and the skull base.[5] CT scanning is currently the main modality that is used for diagnostic evaluation and the requisite anatomic assessment before FESS. MRI offers additional information in selected cases, particularly for skull-base dehiscence and when the better soft-tissue definition of intracranial or orbital contents is necessary.

A coronal plane that is within 10 degrees of perpendicular to the hard palate best displays the osteomeatal complex and replicates the working plane during FESS.[6] The compulsory coronal view also allows one to accurately assess anatomic variables such as ethmoid roof height, skull-base integrity, lamina papyracea dehiscence, and the location of the anterior ethmoid artery. Axial and sagittal views supplement the coronal plane and provide additional three-dimensional detail.

CT scanning is the primary modality for assessing sinonasal disease, and it is an essential component of the preoperative evaluation. This type of scanning displays excellent bony anatomic detail, and, with the evolution of helical scanning, it can rapidly acquire thin-slice axial data suitable for three-dimensional and multiplanar reformatting in the sagittal and coronal planes.[7] Although reconstructed images were initially critiqued for stairstep artifact that deformed fine lamellae, modern scanners with ceramic detectors and multidetector arrays offer superb detail.[8] High-resolution axial scanning with coronal reconstructions is fast becoming the standard for imaging. It reduces the problems associated with dental amalgam and motion artifact, and it also eliminates the need for neck extension in patients with cervical spine disease.[9,10] With the introduction of modern spiral scanners, however, radiation exposure has increased, and it is several-fold that of conventional radiographs.[5] It is therefore recommended that screening scans be limited to one to two per year, especially among children and women of childbearing age.[11,12]

Although the requisite delineation of bony detail is limited, MRI is significantly better for establishing disease extension beyond the paranasal sinus, especially into the orbit and the intracranial fossae. Its main advantages include superior soft-tissue resolution and a lack of radiation as compared with CT scanning. The ability to fuse coregistered images from MRI and CT can further improve delineation of disease extent and provide multimodal intraoperative image guidance.[5]

Detailed Review of Computed Tomography Scanning

The inherent variability of paranasal sinus anatomy among individuals provides one of the main challenges to performing safe endoscopic sinus surgery. The systematic study of several key points should be routinely reviewed in a checklist fashion when planning surgery (Box 42-2). Special attention to normal landmarks, such

BOX 42-2 Details of Sinus Computed Tomography Imaging that Should Be Routinely Reviewed

1. Relationship of the uncinate process with the lamina papyracea
2. Integrity and irregularity of the lamina papyracea
3. Configuration of the anterior ethmoid roof
4. Location of the anterior ethmoid artery
5. Height of the posterior ethmoid roof
6. Presence of an Onodi cell
7. Sphenoid sinus pneumatization and bony covering of the internal carotid artery

as the middle turbinate (or remnant), is especially important during revision surgery. Furthermore, a review of the coronal CT scan and the checklist in the operating room just before surgery allows for the reassessment of disease distribution, potential surgical pitfalls, and anatomic anomalies. An ideal time for this review is after the application of a topical vasoconstrictive agent.

The surgeon should first evaluate the relationship of the uncinate process to the lamina papyracea. If the infundibulum is atelectatic and the uncinate is displaced against the lamina papyracea (Figure 42-1), one must exercise caution when incising the lateral nasal wall to prevent inadvertent orbital entry. This is especially crucial in cases of a hypoplastic maxillary sinus, which occurs in 4% to 10% of patients.[13–17] In several large series of maxillary sinus hypoplasia, the uncinate was consistently lateralized, and the medial orbital wall was medially displaced; both of these anomalies predispose a patient to orbital penetration, and preoperative recognition is imperative to avoid orbital complications.[13–17]

The integrity of the lamina papyracea must then be carefully inspected. Orbital wall abnormalities may be related to previous trauma with resultant orbital fractures, previous surgery, or demineralization of the medial orbital wall from chronic sinusitis, typically caused by a pressure effect from polyposis. Congenital defects that cause the protrusion of the orbital contents into the ethmoid sinus are unusual.[15] In one study of 1024 CT scans, dehiscences were seen in as many as 6% of cases.[18] In addition to bony defects and protrusions, a low-window-setting CT image will accentuate soft tissue and reveal the herniation of orbital fat or medial rectus muscle tissue into the ethmoid air cells[15] (Figure 42-2). However, ethmoid opacification as a result of inflammatory disease can limit radiographic sensitivity to lamina papyracea abnormalities; therefore the surgeon should always proceed cautiously while delineating the medial orbital wall during ethmoid dissection.

The shape and irregularities of the ethmoid roof should also be closely examined. Anteriorly the configuration of the fovea ethmoidalis may range from nearly horizontal, in some patients, to almost vertical in others. When measuring the angle formed by the medial orbital wall and the fovea ethmoidalis, a wide range is seen because 12% of patients have an angle of less than 55 degrees, and 2% have an angle of less than 45 degrees.[15] The lateral lamellae of the cribriform plates also varies in height, as described by Keros[19] (Figure 42-3). In 70% of patients, the cribriform plate lies 4 mm to 7 mm below the ethmoid roof, whereas in 18% of patients it is 12 mm to 16 mm below the ethmoid roof.[20] In patients with a Keros class III configuration, the medial aspect of the

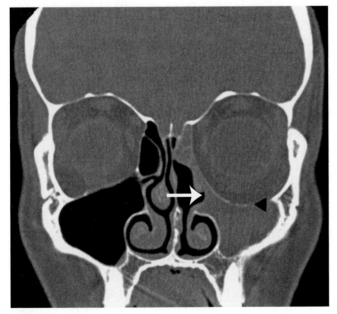

Figure 42-1. Lateralized uncinate process. Atelectatic lateralized uncinate process *(white arrow)* in the setting of silent sinus syndrome. Note the inferiorly displaced orbital floor *(black arrowhead)* with characteristic hypoglobus.

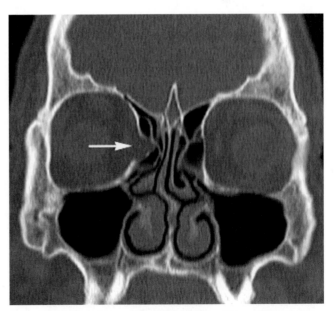

Figure 42-2. Irregular medial orbital contours. This patient has previous trauma and bony orbital dehiscence *(arrow)*, with a protrusion of orbital fat. (Courtesy of Steven D. Pletcher.)

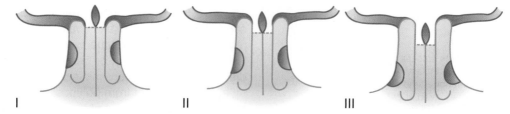

Figure 42-3. Keros classification. Class I: Lamina cribrosa 0 mm to 3 mm inferior to the fovea ethmoidalis. Class II: Lamina cribrosa 4 mm to 7 mm inferior to the fovea ethmoidalis. Class III: Lamina cribrosa more than 8 mm inferior to the fovea ethmoidalis.

ethmoidal roof will be formed mainly by the thin lateral lamellae, which averages only 0.05 mm in thickness.[21] This thin bone provides little resistance, and perforation results in entry into the anterior cranial fossa and cerebrospinal fluid (CSF) leakage. One should also scrutinize for skull-base asymmetry where one lamella of the cribriform is lower than the contralateral side. This may be present in up to 12% of individuals.[22]

The careful evaluation of the integrity and height of the skull base is vital to preventing intracranial complications. As one proceeds posteriorly, the skull base is not parallel to the hard palate; rather, it slopes inferiorly (Figure 42-4). Because pneumatization patterns can vary among individuals, the vertical height from the medial aspect of the antral roof to the posterior skull base (i.e., the planum sphenoidale) should be noted. The surgeon can thus estimate the working distance in this area and accommodate for the naturally sloping skull base.

Extensive posterior ethmoid pneumatization can include the optic nerve in what is termed an *Onodi* (i.e., sphenoethmoid) *cell variant*. The Anatomic Terminology Group defines this as the most posterior ethmoid cell that "pneumatizes laterally and superiorly to the sphenoid

sinus and is intimately associated with the optic nerve."[23] The incidence is estimated to be from 8% to 14%.[23–25] The Onodi cell's relationship with the optic nerve makes its identification paramount. On a coronal CT scan, the Onodi variation is best identified as the superior cell when tiered or stacked sphenoid cells are present[26] (Figure 42-5). Furthermore, the optic nerve and even a portion of the carotid artery may be covered by only a thin layer of bone; alternatively, they may be completely dehiscent or even lie within the posterior ethmoidal sinus itself.[24,27] Special care should be taken during the posterior ethmoid dissection of an Onodi variant, especially when optic nerve or carotid artery dehiscence is present.

The cavernous segment of the internal carotid artery runs in the lateral aspect of the basisphenoid. The thin bone covering the carotid (0.5 mm thick) is often insufficient for protection.[28] In 15% to 22% of cases, the bony wall is completely dehiscent, and the internal carotid artery is separated from the sphenoid sinus by only dura mater and mucosa.[15,27] Moreover, the sphenoid sinus septum is rarely directly in the midline. Its posterior insertion more typically lies laterally adjacent to one of the cavernous carotid arteries. When indicated, the manipulation of this septum should be performed carefully to avoid carotid injury. The optic nerve, which runs in the superolateral aspect of the basisphenoid, can also be dehiscent or have a thinned wall in 1% to 24% of individuals.[15,29–31] Consequently, preoperative imaging of this area should be meticulously reviewed, and special care must be taken when dissecting in this region.

Lastly, the anterior ethmoid artery should be identified in the anterior skull base. On a CT scan, the artery is best identified on coronal sections at the level of the posterior aspect of the globe. This artery branches off of the ophthalmic artery within the retrobulbar space and then normally traverses the skull base through the canalis orbitocranialis. However, in 14% to 40% of cases, the artery may travel in a bony mesentery 1 mm to 3 mm below the skull base[21,32] (Figure 42-6). A pinch in the superior aspect of the medial orbital wall identifies the artery and its relationship with the skull base. Mistaking the artery for a bony ethmoidal septation can

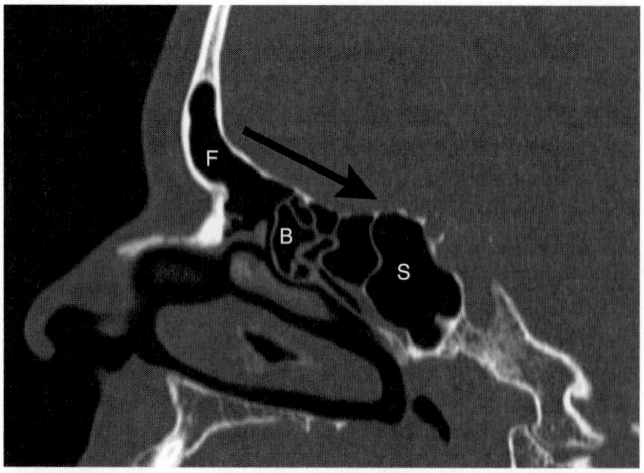

Figure 42-4. Slope of the skull base. This sagittal computed tomography scan depicts the inferior slope of the skull base as one proceeds from the bulla ethmoidalis (B) anteriorly to the sphenoid sinus (S) posteriorly. F, frontal sinus.

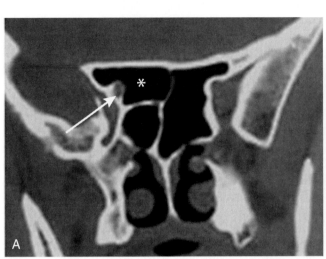

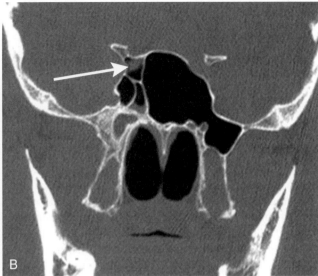

Figure 42-5. The Onodi cell. **A,** The Onodi cell variant is the superior cell on the coronal view (*). It takes the appearance of a vertically stacked sphenoid sinus. **B,** The optic nerve travels in the lateral wall of the Onodi cell, and it is sometimes completely dehiscent *(arrow)*.

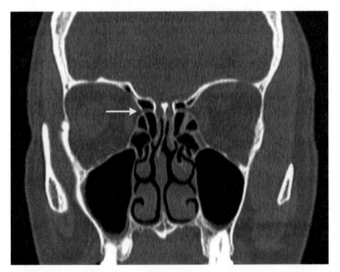

Figure 42-6. Anterior ethmoid artery. The anterior ethmoid artery can be identified as a pinch in the superior aspect of the medial orbital wall in the region of the posterior aspect of the globe *(arrow)*. The artery can hang in a bony mesentery below the skull base, as seen here, where it is at risk for transection.

lead to significant intraoperative epistaxis and the formation of a retrobulbar hematoma.

Informed Consent

Informed consent is the process of explaining a procedure and its risks, benefits, and alternative treatments before instituting therapy. The elements of informed consent include a description of the patient's condition and the treatment being recommended, the risks of the recommended treatment, and the benefits of proposed treatment. Alternative treatments—including the implications of no treatment—should be discussed.[33] It is the surgeon's responsibility to have thorough disclosure so

that a patient may make an appropriately informed decision. Standards vary among states but revolve around what a reasonably prudent physician would disclose to his or her patients and what a reasonable person or layperson in the same situation as the patient would desire to know.[34]

Although the major complications of endoscopic sinus surgery are rare, the devastating impact of visual, intracranial, or cardiopulmonary ramifications necessitate their discussion. In a survey of the members of the American Academy of Otolaryngology–Head and Neck Surgery, nearly 60% of responders believed that a 1% risk of complication warranted discussion, and more than 95% discussed CSF leak and orbital injury routinely.[35] A follow-up survey of patients confirmed that a majority (69%) wished to be informed of complications that occurred as commonly as 1 in 100 cases.[36] However, regardless of frequency, the vast majority of patients wanted to know about specific complications, including orbital injury, CSF leak, the need for revision surgery, smell impairment, myocardial infarction, and cerebrovascular accident.[37] Therefore, despite their infrequency, patients expect an otolaryngologist to discuss all major complications of FESS, because these complications can significantly affect a patient's quality of life.

Surgeon Experience

The experience of the surgeon with endoscopic sinus surgical techniques may be the most crucial factor for determining the risk and type of complication. Two studies nicely illustrate this concept. Stankiewicz,[37] after his first 180 endoscopic ethmoidectomies, initially reported a 29% complication rate, with approximately one third of the cases involving major complications. In a follow-up report, his complication rate had dropped dramatically to 2.2% as his experience grew with the subsequent 180 procedures.[38] Keerl and colleagues[39] expanded this idea after retrospectively evaluating 1500 endoscopic sinus surgery cases. They divided surgeons into three subsets. The beginner, who had performed less than 30 surgeries, had the highest rate of complications, with a propensity for dural injuries. As experience progressed from 30 to 180 procedures, overall complication rates were lower, but there was a tendency for orbital injury. Only after 180 surgeries did a surgeon become expert and exhibit the low complication rates commensurate with published data. The safety of endoscopic techniques is well documented; however, it is clear that the surgeon's experience is critical to achieving successful and safe results.

INTRAOPERATIVE COMPLICATIONS

Bleeding

Significant hemorrhage during endoscopic sinus surgery is an unusual event, and it occurs in only 0.2% to 0.5% of cases.[2,40] As previously noted, the control of intraoperative hemorrhage begins preoperatively with the treatment of mucosal inflammation, typically with antibiotics and oral steroids. Intraoperatively, mucosal bleeding is generally controlled easily with topical vasoconstrictive sponges. Persistent bleeding or arterial bleeding from the sphenopalatine, the anterior ethmoid, or the posterior ethmoid artery or branches may require microfibrillar collagen packing or electrocautery. Bleeding in the region of the anterior ethmoid artery indicates proximity to the skull base; the control of bleeding with bipolar cautery limits the intracranial injury sometimes seen with monopolar current. Posterior bleeding from the branches of the sphenopalatine artery is also often amenable to cautery. However, endoscopic sphenopalatine artery ligation may be necessary in rare situations, and it can easily be performed by surgeons with an endoscopic skill set.[41]

If persistent bleeding interferes with operative visualization, it is safer to terminate the procedure and, if necessary, return at a later time, possibly using an alternative approach. Poor visualization as a result of bleeding appears to be the primary cause of major complications with FESS. Patient safety should not be compromised if the standard maneuvers do not improve surgical conditions.

Cavernous Carotid Injury

Intraoperative injury of the cavernous carotid deserves special mention because the resultant mortality rate approaches 25%; this catastrophic complication is fortunately quite rare.[42] Violation of the internal carotid artery may present as immediate hemorrhage, or it may deceivingly manifest as delayed posterior epistaxis, cavernous-carotid fistula, or an intercavernous arterial aneurysm. In most cases, iatrogenic injury results in immediate and massive hemorrhage, which must be rapidly managed by sphenoid sinus packing and the external compression of bilateral carotid arteries in the neck for a maximum of 2 minutes. When the blood pressure has stabilized, a muscle and fascia graft secured with a tamponade and nasal packing may control bleeding and repair the arterial violation.[42] However, carotid angiography is useful for confirming and identifying the extent of injury and for assessing collateral circulation. The patient should therefore be transferred to a tertiary care facility that has neurointerventional capabilities in case balloon occlusion, selective embolization, or carotid–carotid bypass is required. The abrupt definitive occlusion of the internal carotid artery carries a 17% to 26% risk of stroke and 12% mortality rate.[43,44] After approximately 1 week, nasal packing may be slowly removed in the controlled setting of an operating room, with repacking being necessary for refractory hemorrhage. Immediate and long-term follow up with angiography is mandatory to rule out fistula or aneurysm formation.

Prevention

Persistent minimal bleeding can lead to complications by obscuring the visualization of the surgical field and associated landmarks. Box 42-3 summarizes key strategies to prevent bleeding during FESS. Meticulous dissection, the liberal application of vasoconstrictive agents, and certain anesthetics can minimize bleeding and its ensuing consequences.

The insertion of the endoscope and all instruments must be accomplished in a deliberate, controlled fashion. Direct visualization of instrument introduction, especially in the anterior nasal cavity, precludes mucosal injury and resultant bleeding. Even minimal bleeding

---

BOX 42-3 Strategies for Controlling Bleeding during Functional Endoscopic Sinus Surgery

1. Ensure that the patient has no history of bleeding or blood dyscrasias.
2. Terminate all antiplatelet medication 2 weeks before surgery.
3. Use preoperative oral steroids and antibiotics to minimize mucosal inflammation.
4. Locate the anterior ethmoid artery on a sinus computed tomography scan.
5. Evaluate the sphenoid sinus for carotid dehiscence on a sinus computed tomography scan.
6. Maintain good intraoperative blood pressure control (i.e., a mean arterial pressure of 80 mm Hg, if medically appropriate).
7. Administer topical and injectable vasoconstrictive agents.
8. Handle tissues gently, and dissect sharply.
9. Use the microdebrider to remove polyps.
10. Administer total intravenous anesthesia.

may obscure anatomy and repeatedly soil the endoscope tip. Nasal cavity mucosa should be gently handled with blunt instruments, whereas mucosal cuts should be sharp and deliberate. By decreasing venous pressure, elevation of the head of the bed may also lessen bleeding. If clinically appropriate, it is important to maintain a low blood pressure during the procedure, preferably to a mean arterial pressure of 80 mm Hg. Dialogue with the anesthesiologist is helpful to achieve a low mean blood pressure that is safe for the patient and maintains adequate end-organ perfusion.

Topical agents such as epinephrine, oxymetazoline, and cocaine effectively produce adrenergic vasoconstriction. Systemic absorption, however limited, may produce hypertension and tachycardia in some individuals. Because oxymetazoline is selectively α adrenergic with only minimal β activity, it has the fewest systemic side effects. Typically a combination of agents is used; topical 0.05% oxymetazoline is administered in the preoperative holding area, and epinephrine (1:1000) or cocaine (4%) cottonoids are packed to topically prepare the nose before surgery.

The superimposed vasoconstrictive and tamponade effects of the submucosal infiltration of an anesthetic solution with adrenaline further minimize mucosal bleeding and congestion. Typically a solution of 1% lidocaine with 1:100,000 epinephrine is injected into the lateral nasal wall and sometimes into the vertical lamella of the middle turbinate (Figure 42-7). Although rarely a factor in sinus surgery, the total dose of lidocaine should not exceed

7 mg/kg when adrenaline is used concomitantly.[45] Irrespective of the dose or concentration of adrenaline administered, Yang and colleagues[46,47] observed a transient but statistically significant hypotension within 30 seconds of nasal injection. However, these effects were self-limited and did not require any intervention; complete resolution occurred within 4 minutes. The surgeon should consider the patient's medical history and notify anesthesia personnel before injection so that the hypotension, if present, can be anticipated and observed carefully.

Infiltration of the pterygopalatine fossa via the greater palatine foramen with vasoconstrictive agents has been demonstrated to significantly reduce intraoperative bleeding and to improve surgical field conditions during endoscopic sinus surgery and septorhinoplasty.[48,49] The vasoconstriction of the internal maxillary artery and its branches (mainly the sphenopalatine artery) are hypothesized to produce this effect.[48] Injections should be performed carefully, because complications can include intravascular injection, infraorbital nerve injury, and anesthesia or injury of the orbital nerves.[50] A cadaveric study by Douglas and colleagues[51] revealed the mean length of the greater palatine canal to be 18.9 mm, with an additional palatal soft tissue of 6.9-mm thickness. Other studies in different patient populations show slightly shorter distances.[52,53] To perform this maneuver safely, therefore, the authors bend a 25-gauge needle at a 45-degree angle 20 mm from the tip, insert the needle into the greater palatine canal up to the bend, and inject 2 ml of lidocaine 1% with epinephrine (1:100,000). The bend in the needle identifies the optimal depth of insertion and prevents injury to important structures within the pterygopalatine fossa itself.

Total intravenous anesthesia (TIVA) techniques are superior to inhaled anesthetic agents for limiting intraoperative bleeding. Pavlin and colleagues[54] prospectively demonstrated that propofol, as compared with isoflurane and nitrous oxide, significantly improved subjective operative conditions. Subsequent larger prospective studies confirmed that TIVA with propofol/remifentanil[55,56] or propofol/fentanyl[57] combinations consistently provided superior surgical conditions and decreased blood loss, often by 50%. Of special interest is that the mean arterial blood pressure did not differ between study groups and that a lower heart rate, instead, correlated with improved surgical visualization.[56,58] Furthermore, TIVA provides the added benefits of earlier emergence and a return to cognitive function as compared with inhaled anesthetics.[59,60] However, because of an increased incidence of awareness syndrome and an uncertain depth of anesthesia, some anesthesiologists are reluctant or uncomfortable with the use of this technique.

Because of the potential for neurologic deficit and high mortality, the avoidance of carotid artery injury is

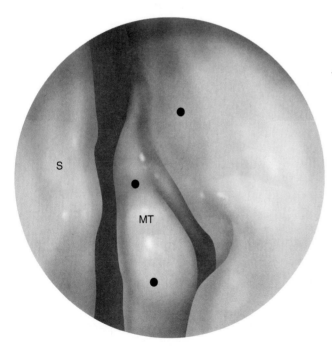

Figure 42-7. Injection sites. This endoscopic view of the middle meatus depicts the typical locations for infiltration with vasoconstrictive agents. *MT,* Middle turbinate; *S,* septum. (Courtesy of Andrew N. Goldberg.)

of paramount importance. Examination of the sphenoid sinus on CT in both the coronal and axial planes should specifically evaluate for carotid and optic nerve dehiscences.

Instrumentation of the sphenoid is performed with special caution in these circumstances. Furthermore, after the sphenoidotomy, the avoidance of dissection or manipulation along the lateral aspects of the sphenoid sinus will prevent inadvertent carotid injury. Similarly, the sphenoid septum should not be manipulated, because it often posteriorly attaches just adjacent to the cavernous carotid. If the removal of the septum is indicated, the bone should be removed sharply without twisting or pulling, because this may lead to carotid artery avulsion or dissection.

ORBITAL COMPLICATIONS

Orbital complications such as orbital entry, retrobulbar hematoma, medial rectus injury, blindness, and nasolacrimal duct injury can occur as a result of endoscopic sinus surgery. Orbital injuries caused by sinus surgery were seen more commonly with the traditional extranasal approaches. May and colleagues[2] reported that the only statistically significant difference between their meta-analysis of traditional versus FESS techniques was orbital complications, especially retrobulbar hematoma. In their series of 2108 patients, they reported minor and major orbital complication rates of 1.7% and 0.05%, respectively.[2] Other authors similarly demonstrate an overall orbital complication rate of 0.3% to 2.7%.[22,61–64]

Medial Orbital Wall Injury

With the more common use of powered instrumentation (specifically the microdebrider), orbital violations can quickly result in injury of the orbital contents and subsequent visual impairment.[65] Applying gentle pressure on the globe may result in the movement or protrusion of the orbital contents into the sinonasal cavity. This maneuver facilitates the identification of subtle orbital wall violations before significant injury has occurred.

If the lamina papyracea and the underlying periorbita are violated, orbital fat will be exposed. Further dissection in this region is immediately terminated, and the surgeon should restrain the urge to manipulate the herniated tissue. The lamina is next positively identified at an adjacent location and widely skeletonized. Careful dissection may proceed provided that the lamina is clearly visualized and no additional injury to the orbital tissue occurs. Signs such as lid edema, ecchymosis, proptosis, and an afferent papillary defect indicating orbital hematoma should be recognized early. In all cases of orbital violation, tight nasal packing and postoperative nose blowing are prohibited.

Retrobulbar Hematoma

Retrobulbar hematomas are the most common cause of major orbital complications.[2] Symptoms include decreased visual acuity and ocular pain. Examination findings may demonstrate ecchymosis or firm proptosis with differential globe compressibility as compared with the contralateral normal eye (Figure 42-8). Furthermore, intraocular pressures of more than 40 mm Hg and an afferent papillary defect with the previously described findings constitute immediate indications for external decompression.[66] Orbital hematomas can have either an arterial or a venous cause.[67] Rapidly expanding hematomas from either the anterior or posterior ethmoidal artery need to be treated immediately, because the increased intraocular and resultant ischemia can lead to blindness within 60 to 90 minutes.[40] Hematomas that progress slowly probably have a venous source (e.g., the veins that line the lamina papyracea). Although these hematomas are frequently unrecognized until the patient is in the recovery room or at home, the same urgency and treatment algorithm apply.

For initial management, nasal packing is removed, vision is checked, and an ophthalmologic consultation is emergently requested while the globe is massaged and the head is elevated. If the intraocular pressure is elevated, topical timolol (0.5%), intravenous acetazolamide (500 mg), and intravenous mannitol (20% solution at a dose of 1–2 mg/kg) are administered.[68] If signs progress and vision continues to deteriorate, a lateral canthotomy and an inferior cantholysis will immediately release orbital pressure by expanding the orbital compartment. To perform this procedure, the lateral canthus is infiltrated with lidocaine solution that contains epinephrine. Iris scissors divide the lateral canthus at its apex. The inferior canthal tendon is identified by

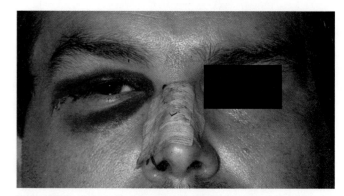

Figure 42-8. Retrobulbar hematoma. Signs of retrobulbar hematoma include proptosis, visual changes, ecchymosis, afferent pupillary defect, and a resistance to globe pressure. The patient shown here experienced vision loss after emerging from anesthesia. A canthotomy and cantholysis were performed to decompress the orbit. The retrobulbar hematoma was drained, and the patient's vision was restored. (Courtesy of Donald C. Lanza.)

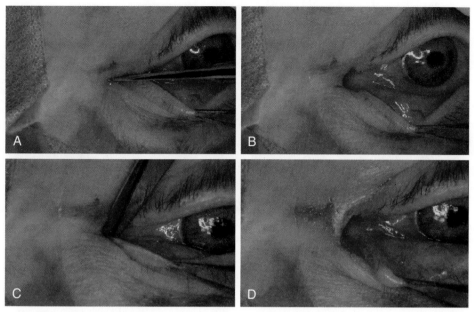

Figure 42-9. Steps for lateral canthotomy and cantholysis. **A,** The lateral canthus is divided at its apex. **B,** The eyelid is retracted inferiorly. **C,** The inferior canthal tendon is then palpated and transected. **D,** The inferior eyelid is completely released. (Courtesy of Roberta E. Gausas.)

palpation as the lower eyelid is retracted inferiorly and divided[69] (Figure 42-9). Frequently these maneuvers lead to a rapid recovery of visual acuity and the reversal of an afferent papillary defect.

Surgical orbital decompression—either endoscopically or via an external approach—may be necessary if active bleeding or visual changes persist.[70] During decompression, the periosteum should be widely incised, but no attempt should be made to find the bleeding vessel within the orbital structures, because this could lead to further intraorbital injury.[40]

Optic Nerve Injury

Optic nerve injury can occur during posterior ethmoidectomy or sphenoid dissection and result in decreased visual acuity and visual field defects.[62] A thorough ophthalmologic evaluation is necessary to precisely document the deficiency and to evaluate for concomitant injuries (e.g., medial rectus dysfunction). Guidelines for the optimal management of optic nerve trauma are lacking. The use of high doses of intravenous steroids remains controversial.[70-71] When optic nerve injury is confirmed, common protocols suggest the administration of intravenous dexamethasone with an initial loading dose of 1 mg/kg followed by 0.5 mg/kg every 6 hours thereafter.[70] If vision improves, therapy is continued for another 5 days. If vision fails to improve within 36 hours or initially improves but then deteriorates, one should strongly consider optic nerve decompression.

However, in a comparative interventional study of 133 patients, the International Optic Nerve Trauma Study failed to demonstrate a difference in outcomes when comparing steroid therapy, surgical optic nerve decompression, and observation in patients with traumatic optic neuropathy.[72] They concluded that neither steroids nor surgical decompression should be considered the standard of care and that, in many cases, no intervention may suffice for the management of a traumatized optic nerve. One should also remember that the extravasation of local anesthesia into the orbit, especially from sphenopalatine injection, can also lead to pupillary dilation, visual disturbance, and reduced globe mobility; however, because the intraocular pressure is normal and these impairments are transient, this phenomenon is easily differentiated from optic nerve injury and retrobulbar hematoma.

Medial Rectus Injury

Medial rectus injury with muscle loss or entrapment results in a characteristic divergent strabismus with almost absent adduction.[73] The muscle is at highest risk where the medial rectus is in closest proximity to the medial orbital wall in the posterior orbit[74] (Figure 42-10). If a patient has diplopia after FESS, forced duction testing is performed to assess entrapment; surgical exploration may be necessary to diagnose and repair this condition. Damage to the nerve or the vascular supply may also limit the function of the medial rectus; some (if not total) recovery can be expected at 9 months in this scenario.[73] If spontaneous improvement in extraocular motion has ceased and strabismus measurements have stabilized, extraocular muscle surgery is indicated to minimize residual strabismus and diplopia.[75]

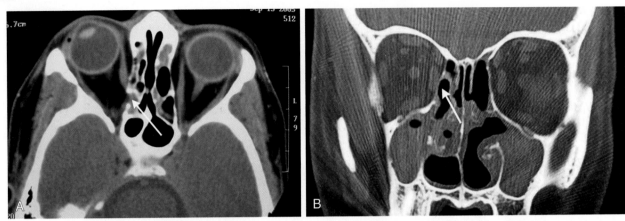

Figure 42-10. Medial rectus injury. Computed tomography scans demonstrate injury to the medial rectus in the **(A)** axial and **(B)** coronal views *(arrows)* as it courses close to the lamina papyracea. Minimal intervening orbital fat is present at the posterior aspect of the medial orbital wall.

Nasolacrimal Duct Injury

Injury to the nasolacrimal duct can occur when the enlargement of the maxillary antrostomy is performed anteriorly. The duct is often within several millimeters of the natural ostium and covered only by thin bone. Inadvertent lacrimal system injuries occur in as many as 15% of FESS cases.[76,77] Despite the frequency, injuries invariably heal spontaneously, often without resultant symptomatic epiphora. If ductal injury is suspected intraoperatively, dissection in that area ceases, and the patient is observed for several months for the development of epiphora. Intubation of the nasolacrimal system can be considered for severe injury, but it is rarely necessary.

Prevention

Given the serious impairments produced by major orbital injuries, surgeons should exercise several strategies to prevent these complications (Box 42-4). Injuries more commonly occur in the right orbit, because the right-handed surgeon is positioned to the right of the

patient.[22] Medial rectus injury occurs more commonly in the posterior ethmoids, where the muscle immediately juxtaposes the lamina papyracea and the intervening retrobulbar fat is absent.[74]

The early identification of the lamina papyracea reduces the potential for orbital penetration. If the infundibulum is atelectatic, endoscopic backbiting forceps can be used to perform the uncinectomy. A laterally directed uncinate incision may result in inadvertent entry into the orbit; this was the most common cause of orbital violation in the large series reported by May and colleagues.[2] Although the creation of a large antrostomy is controversial from a functional perspective, many surgeons routinely open the maxillary sinus widely for orientation. A wide antrostomy allows the surgeon to directly visualize the orbital floor, the medial orbital wall, and the posterior maxillary sinus wall simultaneously. Orbital floor identification provides orientation in the superoinferior dimension, whereas medial orbital wall visualization provides mediolateral orientation. The posterior maxillary wall, in turn, orients the surgeon in an anteroposterior plane.

After a three-dimensional perspective is achieved, the complete skeletonization of the medial orbital wall early in ethmoidectomy will minimize orbital violation. After the lamina papyracea has been identified, bony ethmoid septations are cleared, with the up-biting forceps kept vertically oriented. The vector of powered instrumentation should not be directed into the medial orbital wall, and the opening of the microdebrider blade should always be in sight.[65] Posterior ethmoid dissection should proceed cautiously along the lamina, especially if an Onodi cell is present. Orbital dehiscences can be highlighted when the palpation of the globe produces bulging periorbita or herniating orbital fat. The eyes are routinely examined for lid edema, ecchymosis, or proptosis intraoperatively. Moreover, the anterior ethmoid artery should be identified, both on

---

BOX 42-4 Strategies for Preventing Orbital Injury during Functional Endoscopic Sinus Surgery

1. Study computed tomography scans for orbital integrity and any variations of the medial orbital wall.
2. Assess for lateralized uncinate process or atelectatic infundibulum on sinus computed tomography scans.
3. Do not enlarge the natural maxillary ostium anteriorly (to avoid the nasolacrimal duct).
4. Create a wide medial maxillary antrostomy to gain perspective.
5. Identify and skeletonize the lamina papyracea early during ethmoidectomy.
6. Obtain the complete exposure of the lamina with the removal of all septations.
7. Gently palpate the globe intermittently while observing the medial orbital wall endoscopically.
8. Do not further manipulate the herniated orbital fat.
9. Orient the microdebrider away from the orbital wall, and always keep the blade opening in sight.

imaging and endoscopically, to avoid inadvertent division and ensuing retrobulbar hematoma.

To avoid injury to the nasolacrimal duct, its proximity to the natural ostium of the maxillary sinus and the uncinate process should be noted; the duct lies approximately 9 mm (range, 0.5 mm to 18 mm) from the natural antral ostium.[78] The bony structures of the nasolacrimal duct are thin and often offer little protection from iatrogenic injury. After the natural ostium of the maxillary sinus is identified, it should be opened inferiorly and posteriorly only. This will minimize injury to the duct, and it preserves 180 degrees of unscathed mucosa to maintain effective mucociliary clearance.

CEREBROSPINAL FLUID LEAK

The incidence of skull-base violation during sinus surgery ranges from 0.2% to 0.5%,[2,22,61,63] and iatrogenic injuries constitute 16% of all cases of CSF rhinorrhea.[79] The two most common locations of skull-base breach during FESS are the posterior ethmoid roof and the lateral lamella of the cribriform plate.[79] For the former, the inferior slope of the skull base combined with endoscopic disorientation may result in an inaccurate assessment of skull-base height. Because ethmoid septations and skull-base bone appear similar, an inadvertent superior vector of dissection may lead to skull-base violation. As previously discussed, the lengths of the lateral lamellae of the cribriform plate also vary.[20] Medial dissection during anterior ethmoidectomy, frontal recess exploration, or middle turbinate resection may unintentionally injure this very thin bone and breach the skull base, thus exposing the dura over the gyrus recti.

Skull-base and dural violation often may not be recognized during surgery and appear as CSF rhinorrhea during the postoperative period. In such a case, the exact site of injury may be unknown. When using powered instrumentation, however, skull-base injury occurs quickly and results in a large bony and dural defect that is often visualized immediately after the fact. Injury to the brain parenchyma, intracranial bleeding, and ascending infection are serious ensuing complications.

With occult skull-base defects, studies to diagnose and localize the lesion must be performed; detailed nasal endoscopy is helpful to accomplish this. However, in the setting of postoperative inflammation or infection, detailed anatomy may not be clearly discernable. If nasal fluid can be collected, a β-2 transferrin test is an excellent study to identify CSF leakage and differentiate it from rhinitis or residual saline from nasal irrigation. The β isoform of transferrin, which is found only in CSF, aqueous humor, and perilymph, separates and is identified during electrophoresis.[80] Now considered the gold standard, the β-2 transferrin assay has specificity and

sensitivity that exceed 92% and a positive predictive value of 100% as described in a retrospective review of 68 patients at the University of Pittsburgh.[81] This test is limited by the fact that the patient must have active rhinorrhea, because 1 ml of specimen is necessary to run the assay. Furthermore, although the presence of CSF leakage can be determined with high accuracy, this test cannot localize the defect within the skull base.

In addition to nasal endoscopy, high-resolution CT scanning is the initial radiographic study of choice. Concomitant sinus disease or head trauma can limit the sensitivity, and the study has a higher rate of false positives. With the addition of cisternography, CT scanning has an increased sensitivity. However, this improvement is predicated on the presence of an active leak. Furthermore, intrathecal contrast administration and the invasiveness of this procedure limit its widespread use. MRI is useful to differentiate inflammatory disease from brain tissue and to delineate the extent of concomitant encephalocele (Figure 42-11). MRI cisternography has a sensitivity that is comparable with that of CT cisternography, but it is noninvasive and easily obtained.[82] Because bony detail is limited, this study is usually performed as an adjunct to high-resolution CT.[83]

Lastly, the intrathecal administration of fluorescein may help to identify occult skull-base defects during surgical endoscopy. After the subarachnoid space has been cannulated by lumbar puncture, 10 ml of CSF is mixed with 0.1 ml of 10% fluorescein (i.e., 10 mg), and this solution is injected slowly over 5 to 10 minutes. It is important to note that fluorescein contains a black-box warning that prohibits intrathecal injection because of concerns for grand mal seizures. However, adverse events occur only when more than 100 mg are injected.[84] At smaller doses, the incidence of adverse events is quite remote, and the safety of intrathecal fluorescein is well established. Alternatively, intrathecal injection of a radioisotope tracer can be used to diagnose CSF leaks. The poor ability of this study to localize the site of leak in combination with high false-positive and false-negative rates limits its use.[85]

The conservative treatment of CSF leaks with bed rest and lumbar drainage has limited effectiveness for surgical defects that are identified postoperatively, and operative management is usually required. The technique for surgical repair is identical for leaks that are identified intraoperatively or postoperatively. Endoscopic repair is usually possible, with success rates of more than 90%.[86,87]

After a rim of surrounding mucosa has been removed and the dura is circumferentially elevated off of the intracranial aspect of the defect, a free cartilage graft can be placed intracranially (but extradurally) in an underlay fashion[79] (Figure 42-12). A larger free mucosal graft can then be

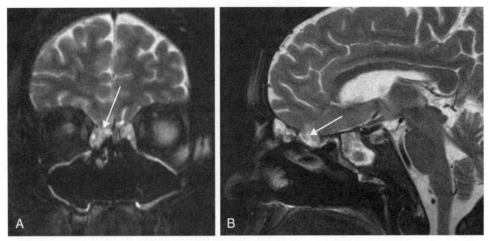

Figure 42-11. Skull-base injury with encephalocele. Skull-base injuries frequently occur at the lateral lamella of the cribriform plate. Large defects can result in encephalocele formation *(arrows)* in addition to cerebrospinal fluid leaks, as demonstrated by these T2 coronal **(A)** and sagittal **(B)** magnetic resonance images.

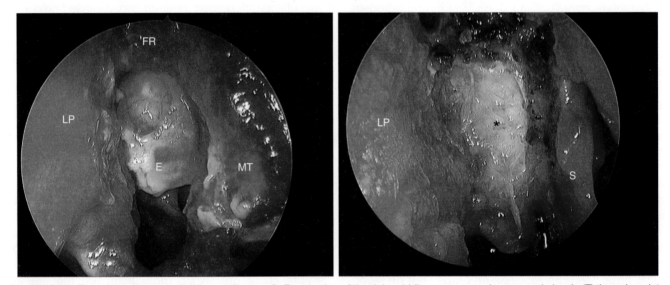

Figure 42-12. Encephalocele repaired with a cartilage graft. Examination of the right middle meatus reveals an encephalocele *(E)* through an iatrogenic skull-base defect posterior to the frontal recess *(FR)* and medial to the orbital wall and lamina papyrecea. A preexisting septal perforation is also present in the septum *(S)*. The middle turbinate *(MT)* was resected to gain exposure, and the encephalocele was cauterized and reduced. After the dura was elevated, a cartilage underlay graft *(*)* was placed intracranially but extradurally *(right)*. A free mucosal overlay graft reinforced the repair.

placed below the defect as an overlay. Fibrin glue holds the graft in place, while the nose is packed with Gelfoam and Gelfilm. A Merocel pack is finally placed inferiorly to buttress the repair.[79] The patient is maintained on bed rest for 3 days with a lumbar drain in place. The drain is clamped on postoperative day 3 and removed on the subsequent day if the patient is without symptoms. The packing is removed on postoperative day 5, and the patient is instructed to refrain from straining, bending, or heavy lifting.

Prevention

Several key strategies to avoid skull-base injury are summarized in Box 42-5. First, the early identification of the ethmoid roof is recommended. A 0-degree

nasal endoscope is used to penetrate the basal lamella of the middle turbinate inferiorly and medially, the posterior ethmoidal cells are entered, and the skull base is confirmed anterior to the sphenoid face. The roof of the ethmoid, however, can easily be mistaken for a bony septation of a posterior ethmoid cell. Therefore meticulous dissection and maintaining orientation are critical. After the skull base is identified in the posterior ethmoids, a 30-degree angled endoscope allows for dissection to be continued along the skull base from posterior to anterior in a retrograde fashion.[88] Along with direct visualization, gentle palpation anterior and posterior to the residual septa helps to establish a plane of dissection and maintains the safe resection of tissue while avoiding skull-base penetration.

BOX 42-5 Strategies for Preventing Skull-Base Injury during Functional Endoscopic Sinus Surgery

1. Assess the integrity of the skull base on a coronal computed tomography (CT) scan.
2. Identify the Keros class of the medial skull base on a coronal CT scan.
3. Estimate the posterior ethmoid height and the slope of skull base on coronal and sagittal CT scans.
4. Avoid medial and superior dissection during ethmoidectomy.
5. Penetrate the basal lamella medially and inferiorly.
6. Identify the skull base at the sphenoid face, and then dissect the skull base retrograde.
7. Use a 0-degree scope for ethmoid dissection and a 30-degree scope for skull-base dissection.
8. Palpate behind all septations before removal.

Caution should also be exercised when clearing tissue from the medial aspect of the ethmoid roof. The bone of the lateral lamella of the cribriform is 0.05 mm, which is 10 times thinner than the more lateral ethmoid roof.[21] Because this is the most frequent area of skull-base violation during FESS, it is imperative that dissection instruments be directed laterally.

SCARRING AND SYNECHIA

Adhesions and synechia formation are among the more common minor complications of sinus surgery. As a result of underreporting, the rates of synechia in the literature likely underestimate its actual incidence. Depending on the location, synechia may be asymptomatic and only impair endoscopic surveillance. However, ostial narrowing and drainage obstruction can occur if adhesions are located in the middle meatus. Meticulous and sharp dissection along with gentle tissue handling and limited collateral mucosal injury are key elements in the prevention of scar formation. Mucosal stripping should be avoided, because the ensuing osteitis of the underlying bone and granulation tissue predispose the patient to ostial narrowing and synechia formation. The use of powered instruments does not significantly affect adhesion formation.[89] Furthermore, absorbable packing and mitomycin C may not have significant benefits.[90–92] Thorough postoperative debridement may reduce scarring, but no standard frequency or interval has been shown to be superior.

Scarring of the middle turbinate to the lateral nasal wall can occur, thereby obliterating the middle meatus. Regardless of the adequacy of the surgical sinusotomies, drainage becomes impossible in this setting. Again, the mucous membranes along the lateral aspect of the middle turbinate should not be traumatized by instrument insertion or during tissue dissection. At the termination of the case, the stability of the middle turbinate should be assessed. If it is flaccid or prone to lateral collapse, it should be medialized. This can be accomplished by attaching the middle turbinate to the septum using an absorbable suture of 4-0 plain gut or Vicryl. Alternatively, the mucosa along the medial aspect of the middle turbinate and the adjacent septal mucosa can be abraded after the turbinate is medialized; this will allow for scarring of the turbinate preferentially in the medial direction, thus maintaining the patency of the middle meatus. Middle turbinate excision is considered for cases in which the aforementioned maneuvers are unsuccessful.

COMPLICATIONS OF EXTERNAL APPROACHES FOR SINUS SURGERY

External Ethmoidectomy

The external approach for ethmoidectomy has been widely used for decades and has proven to be successful. In the modern era of endoscopic sinus surgery, the external approach is still applicable for specific problems such as anterior ethmoid artery ligation, the drainage of subperiosteal or orbital abscesses, and sinonasal tumors invading the ethmoid labyrinth.[93] Many of the aforementioned complications may occur with this approach, including bleeding, orbital or skull-base injury, and synechia formation. Complications specific to the external approach are scarring of the facial skin, medial canthal displacement, and diplopia from superior oblique injury.

Typically a curvilinear incision is made midway between the nasion and the medial canthus. This Lynch incision often heals well, leaving an inconspicuous scar. In some patients, especially people of Asian decent, hypertrophy or webbing of the scar can occur.[94] Gentle tissue handling and meticulous closure can minimize scar formation. A running W-plasty or a single W-plasty incorporated into the center of the incision will also help to further camouflage the facial scar.[93] The canthal ligament should next be elevated cleanly off of the underlying bone and returned to its native site at the conclusion of the procedure to restore aesthetic facial symmetry. To avoid damage to the trochlea with its resultant diplopia, the periosteum in this region must be elevated cleanly off of the bone. Furthermore, during this procedure, globe retraction should be gentle and released on occasion to prevent ischemia to the retina. The identification of the frontoethmoid suture line, the identification of the anterior and posterior ethmoid arteries, and the careful elevation of the periorbita will prevent skull-base violation, excessive bleeding, and injury to the intraorbital contents, respectively.

Caldwell–Luc Procedure and Maxillary Inferior Meatal Antrostomy

Although intraoperative complications from the Caldwell–Luc operation are uncommon, several minor and moderate complications that are troublesome to the patient may occur.[95] These include tooth numbness, infraorbital nerve paresthesia or dysesthesia, and oral antral fistula. To prevent these complications, bone removal should be sufficiently wide to allow for adequate surgical access (particularly anteromedially), but care should be taken to not fracture or remove any bone from the infraorbital foramen or too closely to the roots of the maxillary teeth. The formation of an inferior meatal nasoantral window is rarely performed for chronic sinusitis, because it is not a physiologic opening for mucociliary clearance. In addition to the tendency for spontaneous closure and the recidivism of this disease, the creation of a nasoantral window may also cause nasolacrimal duct injury and epiphora. The area of the nasolacrimal duct close to the anterior end of the turbinate should therefore be avoided if a nasoantral window is necessary.

Frontal Sinus Trephine

Potential complications include supraorbital hypoesthesia, trochlea damage, intracranial entry, fistula, and osteomyelitis. Because the dimensions of the frontal sinus are highly variable, the mandatory review of preoperative CT imaging is essential. The incision should terminate medial to the supraorbital notch to obviate the potential for supraorbital nerve injury. After elevating the periosteum, the side of a round burr provides better control and a safer entry into the sinus as compared with a perforating burr. Theoretically, entry through the floor of the sinus carries less risk of osteomyelitis than entry through the diploic bone of the anterior wall.

Frontal Sinus Osteoplastic Flap

The osteoplastic flap approach carries a risk of complications including intracranial entry, supraorbital nerve injury, infection, delayed mucocele formation, and headache. The dimensions of the frontal sinus must be carefully measured by CT scanning, Caldwell plain views in the posteroanterior orientation, or image-guidance systems.

The most frequent intraoperative complication is intracranial entry when incising the anterior wall of the sinus, and the rate of CSF leak is approximately 3%. This cut should be beveled, within the boundaries of the frontal sinus, and carefully controlled. When doubt exists, making several burr holes, transillumination, and passing a wire through a trephine are helpful confirmatory techniques.[96]

Long-term success depends not only on the removal of all mucoperiosteum from the frontal sinus but also on the careful exenteration of any frontal recess cells. After obliteration has been completed, the bone flap is fixed using sutures or microplates to avoid any mobility and frontal bossing. A recent study of serial MRI scans for the long-term follow up (i.e., 1–12 years) of 51 patients detected mucocele formation in 10%, and a significant decrease in the fat content of the sinus over time.[97] Persistent symptoms caused by late infection or residual disease are difficult to assess both clinically and radiographically after this procedure. MRI findings are often nonspecific, and they do not correlate well with clinical findings, thus making the assessment of persistent postoperative symptoms difficult.[98]

Transeptal Approach to the Sphenoid Sinus

The transeptal approach provides wide exposure of the sphenoid sinus bilaterally. This makes it ideal for the transsphenoid resection of skull-base and pituitary tumors. Intraoperative complications include many outlined earlier in the chapter, including inadvertent intracranial entry and carotid artery injury. Tooth numbness, septal perforation, and the loss of nasal tip support are the most common postoperative complications specific to this procedure; however, they are relatively infrequent.[99] The careful elevation and preservation of the mucoperichondrial flaps and the protection of septal cartilage will minimize these complications.

CONCLUSION

The anatomy of the paranasal sinuses is variable, with important anatomic structures in close proximity to areas of surgical interest. An intimate knowledge of the anatomy of the region and imaging studies before and during surgery provide the surgeon with the tools needed to proceed in a safe manner. Despite proper training and careful technique, inadvertent injury may occur during surgery. It is incumbent on the surgeon to remain vigilant during the preoperative and intraoperative exercise of sinus surgery and to recognize operative misadventures at the earliest juncture. Knowledge of techniques for the assessment and management of the complications of sinus surgery will assist the surgeon with minimizing unwanted operative sequelae.

REFERENCES

1. Mosher HP: The surgical anatomy of the ethmoid labyrinth. *Trans Am Acad Opthalmol Otolaryngol* 1929;31:376–410.
2. May M, Levine HL, Mester SJ, et al: Complications of endoscopic sinus surgery: Analysis of 2108 patients—Incidence and prevention. *Laryngoscope* 1994;104:1080–1083.
3. Sieskiewicz A, Olszewska E, Rogowski M, et al: Preoperative corticosteroid oral therapy and intraoperative bleeding during functional endoscopic sinus surgery in patients with severe nasal polyposis: A preliminary investigation. *Ann Otol Rhinol Laryngol* 2006;115:490–494.
4. Goldstein J, Phillips C: Current indications and techniques in evaluating inflammatory disease and neoplasia of the sinonasal cavities. *Curr Probl Diagn Radiol* 1998;27:41–71.
5. Zinreich SJ: Progress in sinonasal imaging. *Ann Otol Rhinol Laryngol Suppl* 2006;196:61–65.
6. Melhem E, Olivero P, Benson M, et al: Optimal CT evaluation for functional endoscopic sinus surgery. *AJNR Am J Neuroradiol* 1996;17:181–188.

7. Bernhardt TM, Rapp-Bernhardt U, Fessel A, et al: CT scanning of the paranasal sinuses: Axial helical CT with reconstruction in the coronal direction versus coronal helical CT. *Br J Radiol* 1998;71:846–851.

8. Berland LL, Smith JK: Multidetector-array CT: Once again, technology creates new opportunities. *Radiology* 1998;209:327–329.

9. Aygun N, Zinreich SJ: Imaging for functional endoscopic sinus surgery. *Otolaryngol Clin North Am* 2006;39:403–416.

10. Klevansky A: The efficacy of multiplanar reconstructions of helical CT of the paranasal sinuses. *AJR Am J Roentgenol* 1999;173:493–495.

11. Slovis TL: Children, computed tomography radiation dose, and the As Low As Reasonably Achievable (ALARA) concept. *Pediatrics* 2003;112:971–972.

12. Frush DP, Donnelly LF, Rosen NS: Computed tomography and radiation risks: What pediatric health care providers should know. *Pediatrics* 2003;112:951–957.

13. Bolger WE, Woodruff WW, Morehead J, et al: Maxillary sinus hypoplasia: Classification and description of associated uncinate hypoplasia. *Otolaryngol Head Neck Surg* 1990;103:759–765.

14. Furin MJ, Zinreich SJ, Kennedy DW: The atelectatic maxillary sinus. *Am J Rhinol* 1991;5:79–83.

15. Meyers RM, Valvassori G: Interpretation of anatomic variations of computed tomography scans of the sinuses: A surgeon's perspective. *Laryngoscope* 1998;108:422–425.

16. Sirikci A, Bayazit Y, Gumusburun E, et al: A new approach to the classification of maxillary sinus hypoplasia with relevant clinical implications. *Surg Radiol Anat* 2001;22:243–247.

17. Kantarci M, Karasen RM, Alper F, et al: Remarkable anatomic variations in paranasal sinus region and their clinical importance. *Eur J Radiol* 2004;50:296–302.

18. Moon HH, Kee HC, Yang GM, et al: Nontraumatic prolapse of the orbital contents into the ethmoid sinus: Evaluation with screening sinus CT. *Am J Otolaryngol* 1966;17:184–189.

19. Keros P: On the practical value of differences in the level of the lamina cribrosa of the ethmoid. *Z Laryngol Rhinol Otol* 1962;41:809–813.

20. Keros P: Uber die praktische bedeutung der niveau-unterscheide der lamina cribrosa des ethmoids. In Naumann HH, editor: *Head and neck surgery. Volume 1. Face and facial skull,* Philadelphia, 1980, WB Saunders.

21. Kainz J, Stammberger H: The roof of the anterior ethmoid: A place of least resistance in the skull base. *Am J Rhinol* 1989;3:191–199.

22. Dessi P, Castro F, Triglia JM, et al: Major complications of sinus surgery: A review of 1192 procedures. *J Laryngol Otol* 1994;108:212–215.

23. Stammberger HR, Kennedy DW: Paranasal sinuses: Anatomic terminology and nomenclature: The Anatomic Terminology Group. *Ann Otol Rhinol Laryngol Suppl* 1995;167:7–16.

24. Banssberg SF, Narner SG, Forbes G: Relationship of the optic nerve to the paranasal sinuses as shown by computed tomography. *Otolaryngol Head Neck Surg* 1987;96:331–335.

25. Yanagisawa E, Weaver EM, Ashikawa R: The Onodi (sphenoethmoid) cell. *Ear Nose Throat J* 1998;77:578–580.

26. Allmond L, Murr AH: Clinical problem solving: Radiology: Radiology quiz case 1: Opacified Onodi cell. *Arch Otolaryngol Head Neck Surg* 2002;128:596, 598–599.

27. Kennedy DW, Zinreich SJ, Hassab MH: The internal carotid artery as it relates to endonasal sphenoethmoidectomy. *Am J Rhinol* 1990;4:7–12.

28. Fujii K, Chambers SM, Rhoton AL Jr: Neurovascular relationships of the sphenoid sinus: A microsurgical study. *J Neurosurg* 1979;50:31–39.

29. Unal B, Bademci G, Bilgili YK, et al: Risky anatomic variations of sphenoid sinus for surgery. *Surg Radiol Anat* 2006;28:195–201.

30. Sapci T, Derin E, Almac S, et al: The relationship between the sphenoid and the posterior ethmoid sinuses and the optic nerves in Turkish patients. *Rhinology* 2004;42:30–34.

31. DeLano MC, Fun FY, Zinreich SJ: Relationship of the optic nerve to the posterior paranasal sinuses: A CT anatomic study. *AJNR Am J Neuroradiol* 1996;17:669–675.

32. Moon HJ, Kim HU, Lee JG, et al: Surgical anatomy of the anterior ethmoidal canal in ethmoid roof. *Laryngoscope* 2001;111:900–904.

33. Baker CH: Comment: Informed consent, obligation or opportunity? *J Health Hosp Law* 1993;26:214–215.

34. Bowden MT, Church CA, Chiu AG, et al: Informed consent in functional endoscopic sinus surgery: The patient's perspective. *Otolaryngol Head Neck Surg* 2004;131:126–132.

35. Wolf JS, Malekzadeh S, Berry JA, et al: Informed consent in functional endoscopic sinus surgery. *Laryngoscope* 2002;112:774–778.

36. Wolf JS, Chiu AG, Palmer JN, et al: Informed consent in endoscopic sinus surgery: The patient perspective. *Laryngoscope* 2005;115:492–494.

37. Stankiewicz JA: Complications of endoscopic intranasal ethmoidectomy. *Laryngoscope* 1987;97:1270–1273.

38. Stankiewicz JA: Complications in endoscopic intranasal ethmoidectomy: An update. *Laryngoscope* 1989;99:686–690.

39. Keerl R, Stankiewicz J, Weber R, et al: Surgical experience and complications during endonasal sinus surgery. *Laryngoscope* 1999;109:546–550.

40. Lund VJ, Wright A, Yiotakis J: Complications and medicolegal aspects of endoscopic sinus surgery. *J Royal Soc Med* 1997;90: 422–428.

41. Snyderman CH, Goldman SA, Carrau RL, et al: Endoscopic sphenopalatine artery ligation is an effective method of treatment for posterior epistaxis. *Am J Rhinol* 1999;13:137–140.

42. Weidenbecher M, Huk WJ, Iro H: Internal carotid artery injury during functional endoscopic sinus surgery and its management. *Eur Arch Otorhinolaryngol* 2005;262:640–645.

43. Linskey ME, Jungreis CA, Yonas H, et al: Stroke risk after abrupt internal carotid artery sacrifice: Accuracy of preoperative assessment with balloon test occlusion and stable xenon-enhanced CT. *AJNR Am J Neuroradiol* 1994;15:829–843.

44. Roski RA, Spetzler RF, Nulsen FE: Late complications of carotid ligation in the treatment of intracranial aneurysms. *J Neurosurg* 1981;54:583–587.

45. Lidocaine hydrochloride package insert. Westborough, Mass, 1995, Astra Pharmaceutical Products.

46. Yang JJ, Zheng J, Liu HJ, et al: Epinephrine infiltration on nasal field causes significant hemodynamic changes: Hypotension episode monitored by impedance—Cardiography under general anesthesia. *J Pharm Pharm Sci* 2006;9:190–197.

47. Yang JJ, Wang QP, Wang TY, et al: Marked hypotension induced by adrenaline contained in local anesthetic. *Laryngoscope* 2005;115:348–352.

48. Wormald PJ, Athanasiadis T, Rees G, et al: An evaluation of effect of pterygopalatine fossa injection with local anesthetic and adrenalin in the control of nasal bleeding during endoscopic sinus surgery. *Am J Rhinol* 2005;19:288–292.

49. Williams WT, Ghorayeb BY: Incisive canal and pterygopalatine fossa injection for hemostasis in septorhinoplasty. *Laryngoscope* 1990;100:1245–1247.

50. Mercuri LG: Intraoral second division nerve block. *Oral Surg Oral Med Oral Pathol* 1979;47:109–113.

51. Douglas R, Wormald PJ: Pterygopalatine fossa infiltration through the greater palatine foramen: Where to bend the needle. *Laryngoscope* 2006;116:1255–1257.

52. Methathrathip D, Apinhasmit W, Chompoopong S, et al: Anatomy of the greater palatine foramen and canal and pterygopalatine fossa in Thais: Considerations for maxillary nerve block. *Surg Radiol Anat* 2005;27:511–516.

53. Hassmann H: Form, maβe und verläufe der schädelkanäle. In Lang J, editor: *Clinical anatomy of the nose, nasal cavity and paranasal sinuses,* New York, 1989, Thieme Medical Publishers.

54. Pavlin JD, Colley PS, Weymuller EA Jr, et al: Propofol versus isoflurane for endoscopic sinus surgery. *Am J Otolaryngol* 1999;20:96–101.

55. Wormald PJ, van Renen G, Perks J, et al: The effect of the total intravenous anesthesia compared with inhalational anesthesia on the surgical field during endoscopic sinus surgery. *Am J Rhinol* 2005;19:514–520.

56. Eberhart LH, Folz BJ, Wulf H, et al: Intravenous anesthesia provides optimal surgical conditions during microscopic and endoscopic sinus surgery. *Laryngoscope* 2003;113:1369–1373.

57. Sivaci R, Yilmaz MD, Balci C, et al: Comparison of propofol and sevoflurane anesthesia by means of blood loss during endoscopic sinus surgery. *Saudi Med J* 2004;25:1995–1998.

58. Nair S, Collins M, Hung P, et al: The effect of beta-blocker premedication on the surgical field during endoscopic sinus surgery. *Laryngoscope* 2004;114:1042–1046.

59. Loop T, Priebe HJ: Recovery after anesthesia with remifentanyl combined with propofol, desflurane, or seroflurane for otorhinolaryngeal surgery. *Anesth Analg* 2000;91:123–129.

60. Larsen B, Seitz A, Larsen R: Recovery of cognitive function after remifentanil-propofol anesthesia: A comparison with desflurane and sevoflurane anesthesia. *Anesth Analg* 2000;90:168–174.

61. Vleming M, Middelweerd RJ, de Vries N: Complications of endoscopic sinus surgery. *Arch Otolaryngol Head Neck Surg* 1992;118:617–623.

62. Corey JP, Bumsted R, Panje W, et al: Orbital complications in functional endoscopic sinus surgery. *Otolaryngol Head Neck Surg* 1993;109:814–820.

63. Dursun E, Bayiz U, Korkmaz H, et al: Follow-up results of 415 patients after endoscopic sinus surgery. *Eur Arch Otorhinolaryngol* 1998;255:504–510.

64. Dunya IM, Salman SD, Shore JW: Ophthalmic complications of endoscopic ethmoid surgery and their management. *Am J Otolaryngol* 1996;17:322–331.

65. Graham SM, Nerad JA: Orbital complications in endoscopic sinus surgery using powered instrumentation. *Laryngoscope* 2003;113:874–878.

66. McInnes G, Howes DW: Lateral canthotomy and cantholysis: A simple, vision-saving procedure. *CJEM* 2002;4:49–52.

67. Stankiewicz JA, Chow JM: Two faces of orbital hematoma in intranasal (endoscopic) sinus surgery. *Otolaryngol Head Neck Surg* 1999;120:841–847.

68. Bolger WE, Kennedy DW: Surgical complications and postoperative care. In Kennedy DW, Bolger WE, Zinreich SJ, editors: *Diseases of the sinuses: Diagnosis and management,* Hamilton, Ontario, Canada, 2001, BC Decker.

69. Vassallo S, Hartstein M, Howard D, et al: Traumatic retrobulbar hemorrhage: Emergent decompression by lateral canthotomy and cantholysis. *J Emerg Med* 2002;22:251–256.

70. Levine HL: Ophthalmologic complications of endoscopic sinus surgery. In Levine HL, Clemente MP, editor: *Sinus surgery: Endoscopic and microscopic approaches,* New York, 2005, Thieme.

71. Rajiniganth MG, Gupta AK, Gupta A, et al: Traumatic optic neuropathy: Visual outcome following combined therapy protocol. *Arch Otolaryngol Head Neck Surg* 2003;129:1203–1206.

72. Levin LA, Beck RW, Joseph MP, et al: The treatment of traumatic optic neuropathy: The International Optic Nerve Trauma Study. *Ophthalmology* 1999;106:1268–1277.

73. Rene C, Rose GE, Lenthall R, et al: Major orbital complications of endoscopic sinus surgery. *Br J Ophthalmol* 2001;85:598–603.

74. Penne RB, Flanagan JC, Stefanyszyn MA, et al: Ocular motility disorders secondary to sinus surgery. *Ophthal Plast Reconstr Surg* 1993;9:53–61.

75. Neuhaus RW: Orbital complications secondary to endoscopic sinus surgery. *Ophthalmology* 1990;97:1512–1518.

76. Bolger WE, Parsons DS, Mair EA, et al: Lacrimal drainage system injury in functional endoscopic sinus surgery: Incidence, analysis, and prevention. *Arch Otolaryngol Head Neck Surg* 1992;118:1179–1184.

77. Unlu HH, Goktan C, Aslan A, et al: Injury to the lacrimal apparatus after endoscopic sinus surgery: Surgical implications from active transport dacryocystography. *Otolaryngol Head Neck Surg* 2001;124:308–312.

78. Calhoun K, Waggenspack GA, Simpson CB, et al: CT evaluation of the paranasal sinuses in symptomatic and asymptomatic populations. *Otolaryngol Head Neck Surg* 1991;104:480–483.

79. Schlosser RJ, Bolger WE: Nasal cerebrospinal fluid leaks: Critical review and surgical considerations. *Laryngoscope* 2004;114:255–265.

80. Rauch SD: Transferrin microheterogeneity in human perilymph. *Laryngoscope* 2000;110:545–552.

81. Skedros DG, Cass SP, Hirsch BE, et al: Beta-2 transferrin assay in clinical management of cerebral spinal fluid and perilymphatic fluid leaks. *J Otolaryngol* 1993;22:341–344.

82. Eljamel MS, Pidgeon CN, Toland J, et al: MRI cisternography and the localization of CSF fistulae. *Br J Neurosurg* 1994;8:433–437.

83. Zapalac JS, Marple BF, Schwade ND: Skull base cerebrospinal fluid fistulas: A comprehensive diagnostic algorithm. *Otolaryngol Head Neck Surg* 2002;126:669–676.

84. Keerl R, Weber RK, Draf W, et al: Use of sodium fluorescein solution for detection of cerebrospinal fluid fistulas: An analysis of 420 administrations and reported complications in Europe and the United States. *Laryngoscope* 2004;114:266–272.

85. Stone JA, Castillo M, Neelon B, et al: Evaluation of CSF leaks: High-resolution CT compared with contrast-enhanced CT and radionuclide cisternography. *AJNR Am J Neuroradiol* 1999;20:706–712.

86. Lanza DC, O'Brien DA, Kennedy DW: Endoscopic repair of cerebrospinal fluid fistulae and encephaloceles. *Laryngoscope* 1996;106:1119–1125.

87. Senior BA, Jafri K, Benninger M: Safety and efficacy of endoscopic repair of CSF leaks and encephaloceles: A survey of the members of the American Rhinologic Society. *Am J Rhinol* 2001;15:21–25.

88. Wigand ME: *Endoscopic surgery of the paranasal sinuses and anterior skull base,* New York, 1990, Thieme.

89. Selivanova O, Kuehnemund M, Mann WJ, et al: Comparison of conventional instruments and mechanical debriders for surgery of patients with chronic sinusitis. *Am J Rhinol* 2003;17:197–202.

90. Wormald PJ, Boustred RN, Le T, et al: A prospective single-blind randomized controlled study of use of hyaluronic acid nasal packs in patients after endoscopic sinus surgery. *Am J Rhinol* 2006;20:7–10.

91. Anand VK, Tabaee A, Kacker A, et al: The role of mitomycin C in preventing synechia and stenosis after endoscopic sinus surgery. *Am J Rhinol* 2004;18:311–314.

92. Miller RS, Steward DL, Tami TA, et al: The clinical effects of hyaluronic acid ester nasal dressing (Merogel) on intranasal wound healing after functional endoscopic sinus surgery. *Otolaryngol Head Neck Surg* 2003;128:862–869.

93. Murr AH: Contemporary indications for external approaches to the paranasal sinuses. *Otolaryngol Clin North Am* 2004;37:423–434.

94. Bhatki AM, Kim DW: Upper blepharoplasty in the Asian eyelid. *Facial Plast Surg Clin North Am* 2005;13:525–532.

95. Murray JP: Complications after treatment of chronic maxillary sinus disease with Caldwell-Luc procedure. *Laryngoscope* 1983;93:282–284.

96. Salamone FN, Seiden AM: Modern techniques in osteoplastic flap surgery of the frontal sinus. *Oper Tech Otolaryngol Head Neck Surg* 2004;15:61–66.

97. Weber R, Draf W, Keerl R, et al: Osteoplastic frontal sinus surgery with fat obliteration: Technique and long-term results using magnetic resonance imaging in 82 operations. *Laryngoscope* 2000;110:1037–1044.

98. Loevner LA, Yousem DM, Lanza DC, et al: MR evaluation of frontal sinus osteoplastic flaps with autogenous fat grafts. *AJNR Am J Neuroradiol* 1995;16:1721–1726.

99. Kennedy DW, Cohn ES, Papel ID, et al: Transsphenoidal approach to the sella: The Johns Hopkins experience. *Laryngoscope* 1984;94:1066–1073.

CHAPTER 43

Complications of Rhinoplasty

David W. Kim and M. Jafer Ali

Rhinoplasty is one of the most challenging operations in facial plastic surgery. The anatomy is intricate, three dimensional, and highly variable. Airway function depends on multiple factors, which are modulated with every surgical maneuver. Postoperative scar contracture and healing may alter surgical structural modifications over the lifetime of the patient, affecting both function and cosmesis. For this reason, complications in rhinoplasty are not uncommon. It is estimated that 8% to 15% of primary rhinoplasty patients eventually undergo revision surgery.[1]

PREVENTION OF COMPLICATIONS

The most important means of avoiding complications is to anticipate pitfalls in advance. This is facilitated with an adequate preoperative evaluation that starts with the patient interview, photo documentation, and the physical examination. Adjunct technologies such as computer imaging may also be used for surgical planning as well as to further educate patients and to provide them with realistic expectations.

Patient Interview

The surgeon should list and prioritize patient complaints and gauge the feasibility of surgically addressing specific requests. Functional airway problems that result from anatomic disturbances are surgically correctable. Intermittent obstruction is more likely to be attributable to mucosal inflammatory problems and should not represent the main impetus for surgery. Cosmetic problems should be discussed in detail with the aid of photographs and computer imaging. Each aesthetic complaint should be discussed with regard to its possible cause and the prospects for repair.

Physical Examination

Cosmetic nasal analysis begins with a global assessment of the nasal deformity. Often one or two problem areas are immediately noticeable to the surgeon. These may include an asymmetric tip, dorsal irregularities, or a narrowed base. It is important to prioritize these deformities during surgery, because surgery on each subunit of the nose affects the appearance of the others. The surgeon must modify a given structure on the basis of the status of adjacent structures. Knowing that one aspect of the nose is particularly problematic allows the surgeon to focus on it and to modify the rest of the nose around those corrections. For example, for a patient with an overly foreshortened nose, the surgeon may first choose to correct nasal length and tip projection by resetting the medial crura onto a caudal extension graft. The dorsal height may then be modified in relation to the newly restored tip position.

The systematic assessment of each view of the nose is critical. Quality preoperative photographs allow for detailed preoperative planning that complements analysis performed in the office setting. On the frontal view, symmetry and width should be assessed in each of the vertical thirds of the nose. If the brow–tip aesthetic lines are irregular or asymmetric, the anatomic cause of the problem should be noted. Middle-vault collapse may be visible as pinching in the middle third of the nose or as an inverted-V deformity. The base view provides information about the shape and size of the columella, the alar base, the nostrils, and lobule. On the lateral view, the dorsum is assessed for smoothness, the vertical position of the nasal starting point, convexity or concavity, and the presence of a supratip break. A polybeak may be present as a result of relative supratip excess (i.e., soft tissue or cartilaginous) or because of a deficiency in tip projection. In the lower third, the overall projection and rotation of the nasal tip must be assessed. Using the Goode method, nasal tip projection as defined from the alar crease to the tip defining point should be just over half (i.e., 0.55) of the length of the nose.[2,3] The ideal length should be based on a nasal starting point near the superior palpebral fold and a tip-defining point determined by the ideal degree of tip rotation. One measure of rotation is the nasolabial angle, which in men should be between 90 and 95 degrees and in women between 95 and 105 degrees. In cases of relative tissue excess or deficiency at the premaxilla, this angle may not reflect the degree of rotation at the tip and the infratip lobule.

The surgeon must note the thickness and sebaceous quality of the nasal skin–soft-tissue envelope (SSTE). Particularly in thick-skinned individuals, a reduction of the underlying skeletal framework may cause significant scarring in the dead space. This can cause the SSTE to be exceptionally thick and inelastic. An advantage of such thick SSTE is that irregularities of the underlying nasal skeleton and grafts are camouflaged.

Although patients with thin skin may not have injury to the SSTE, it is important to remember that there is the added risk of contour irregularities becoming visible or palpable. Care must therefore be taken to ensure that all existing bony and cartilaginous structures, grafts, and implants are precisely positioned and smoothly contoured. The benefit of thin skin is that leaving a small amount of dead space will have a greater tendency to contract over time and thus allow for greater degrees of reduction[4] (Figure 43-1).

It is critical to assess nasal airflow, and this should be done both before and after decongestion of the nasal mucosa. The surgeon must note the external stigmata of an obstructed nose or one that is prone to the development of postoperative problems. These characteristics include a thin SSTE, a narrow or collapsed middle vault, short nasal bones, supra-alar pinching, a prominent supra-alar crease, narrow nostrils, and thin lateral nasal walls. An intranasal examination may reveal a narrowed internal valve angle, a dynamic lateral wall collapse, septal deviation, inferior turbinate hypertrophy, mucosal synechiae, or a shortage of lining from a prior excision. The assessment of dynamic function should be performed by observing the lateral wall of the nose with inhalation. Obvious collapse indicates lateral wall weakness. Significant improvement of breathing by supporting the lateral wall with a cotton swab may predict airway improvement with the placement of a supporting graft to the lateral wall. All of these factors must be considered when formulating a surgical plan to restore or preserve a functional airway.

The palpation of the nose is important to determine the shape, position, and strength of the nasal structure. Dorsal irregularities may not be visible beneath a thick SSTE, and they may require digital palpation to be detected. An attempt should be made to trace the lower lateral cartilages to assess position and stability. The resistance and recoil of the nasal tip to digital pressure will provide information about tip support. Finally, the palpation of the caudal nasal septum will help to determine the position and integrity of the caudal septal strut.[5]

Computer Imaging

Computer image modification programs are commercially available, and they are becoming increasingly popular for consultation with cosmetic patients. In secondary rhinoplasty, these programs are particularly valuable, because the patient may have unrealistic goals for surgery or not understand the limitations of the correction of certain deformities. The limitations of surgery that result from soft-tissue considerations, grafting materials, or existing structural damage can be visually demonstrated to the patient to facilitate a mutual understanding between the patient and the surgeon. The physician should provide an image that reflects a reasonable goal for the patient to anticipate. Computer imaging that leads to unrealistic expectations will inevitably lead to an unhappy patient. It is therefore prudent that the surgeon perform the computer imaging in a fashion that portrays an outcome within his or her level of skill and experience.

GENERAL CONSIDERATIONS

Rhinoplasty complications may present as any number of functional and cosmetic complaints. Small asymmetries, malposition, and irregularities may occur as a result

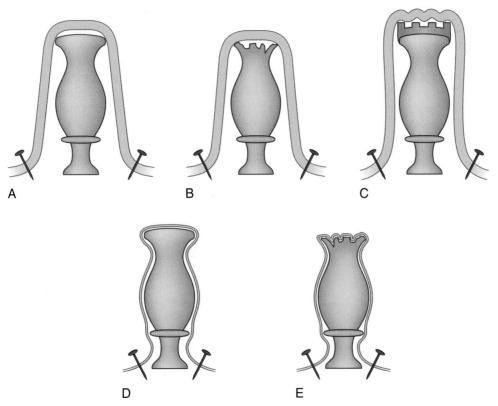

Figure 43-1. Changing nasal form during rhinoplasty is analogous to changing the shape of a sculpture beneath a covering of variable thickness. **A,** A thick blanket covering a fine sculpture like a vase. **B,** With a thick blanket, reductive changes to the shape of the vase (including imperfections) are poorly transmitted through the covering. **C,** Augmentative changes to the vase are necessary to push into a thick covering in order to create appreciable contour changes. **D,** With a thin sheet covering the same vase, the shape of the underlying structure is easily discernible. **E,** Reductive changes made to the vase (including imperfections) are readily discernible through a thin sheet.

of minor errors of technique. These problems are generally straightforward and easily corrected. Significant asymmetries, functional obstruction, and gross deformities are more likely to result from errors of judgment. In such cases, the primary surgeon may have been overly aggressive in excisional or reductive maneuvers or failed to resupport destabilized structures. These problems may not become apparent for years, and they may therefore escape the awareness of the original surgeon. The goal of analysis for secondary rhinoplasty is not only for the diagnosis of these problems but also to determine the limitations and strategies for treatment.

There are several categories of complications, each of which result from different types of surgical errors. The identification, diagnosis, and correction of these problems depend on a thorough understanding of surgical pitfalls and postoperative processes.

A common type of problem encountered is one of subtle asymmetry or the malposition of existing structures, grafts, or implants as a result of minor errors in technique. In thin-skinned patients, suboptimal graft placement or the unequal excision of cartilage may lead to slight cosmetic imperfections. In some cases, skeletal modifications may lead to subtle abnormalities of the nasal pyramid. The imprecise closure of the columellar incision may result in a visible scar. These complications are typically minor and relatively easy to correct. An exception to this is the case of migrating or traumatized alloplastic implants that become infected. Although such a problem may be remedied by removing the implant, if left untreated, the infection may become serious and lead to permanent damage to the nose. Even after an appropriate and technically sound operation, the forces of scar contracture, mechanical trauma, and edema may result in an imperfect outcome.

Errors of omission will result in variable degrees of postoperative problems, depending on the severity and nature of the original problem. This type of error, which is often committed by an inexperienced or overly conservative surgeon, will be evident in photographs before the original operation. Common examples include a persistent caudal septal deviation, a twisted nose, an asymmetric middle vault, and various tip deformities. Because the structures are left relatively undisturbed, these problems are readily corrected with the application of the proper techniques.

A third type of error involves a failure to reconstruct destabilized structures. Many maneuvers in primary rhinoplasty require disassembling the structures of the nose. Left unsupported, these destabilized areas become more susceptible to the forces of scar contracture, gravity, and facial mimetic function. The most common problems of this type include the failure to stabilize the nasal tip at the base after compromising tip-support mechanisms, the failure to resupport the upper lateral cartilages

onto the dorsal nasal septum after cartilaginous hump removal, and the failure to support the lateral nasal wall in patients with a lateral wall deficiency. The correction of such problems usually requires structural grafting techniques to restore strength to the nasal framework.

A more problematic type of error is one of excessive reduction and excision. Excessive caudal septal resection, lateral crural cephalic trim, dorsal hump reduction, alar cartilage division, and alar base reduction may result in an assortment of cosmetic and functional problems. The type and severity of deformity partially depends on the quality of the SSTE. Many of these problems are challenging to repair, because there is a deficiency of tissue that may be difficult to replace. This is particularly true when a portion of the internal lining of the nose has been excised.

The final category of surgical error represents those deformities that stem from gross errors of judgment. Although the problems outlined previously may result from the poor execution of a reasonable surgical strategy, this last class of deformity usually results from a fundamentally flawed plan. These problems may be catastrophic, and it may not be possible to correct them. These mistakes may stem from faulty analysis, a disregard for basic principles of rhinoplasty, or the use of improper techniques for a given problem. The inexperienced but aggressive surgeon is most likely to commit such an error. These problems are varied and typically cause an unnatural appearance. In some cases, they may result in serious cosmetic and functional deformities. Some of the most difficult cases involve situations in which large areas of soft tissue have been excised or violated (Table 43-1).

GENERAL COMPLICATIONS OF NASAL SURGERY

As with all surgery, bleeding and infection are complications that are encountered by the nasal surgeon. Bleeding is best avoided with adequate preoperative local vasoconstricting agents.

Remarkably, the rate of infection in nasal surgery is quite low. In a 5-year study of 1040 patients undergoing septal surgery without prophylactic antibiotics, Yoder and colleagues[6] reported that only 5 patients developed minor nasal infections postoperatively. This is particularly interesting given the high rate of bacterial colonization among nonhospitalized patients. It is estimated that 40% of healthy adults are chronic nasal carriers of *Staphylococcus aureus*.[7] Furthermore, controversy remains regarding the benefit of antibiotics for preventing infection during the postoperative period.[8,9]

The most dreaded infectious complication of nasal surgery is toxic shock syndrome caused by *Staphylococcus*

TABLE 43-1 Common Categories of Rhinoplasty Complications

Class of Surgical Error	Common Examples	Resulting Deformities
Minor error of technique	• Asymmetric skeletal modification (e.g., osteotomies, dome sutures) • Malpositioned graft • Malpositioned implant • Poor closure of the columellar incision	• Asymmetric nasal skeletal deformity • Palpable or visible graft • Palpable or visible implant (possible infection) • Columellar scar
Error of omission	• Various	• Persistent primary deformity
Failure to restabilize	• Failure to stabilize the nasal base • Failure to stabilize the middle vault • Failure to stabilize the lateral wall	• Tip ptosis and underprojection • Pinched middle third, collapse of the ULC, inverted-V deformity, internal valve obstruction • Supra-alar and alar pinching, dynamic external valve obstruction
Excessive excision	• Caudal septum • Cephalic trim of LLC • Dorsal hump reduction • Alar cartilage division • Alar base reduction	• Short nose, wide nasolabial angle, retracted columella • Lateral wall weakness, supra-alar and alar pinching, alar retraction • Scooped dorsum, saddle deformity, bony open roof, middle vault collapse • Palpable or visible graft • Overly narrow alar base; narrow, slit-like nostrils
Gross error of judgment	• Various	• Possible severe deformity

LLC, Lower lateral cartilage; *ULC,* upper lateral cartilage.

enterotoxins. The estimated incidence of this syndrome is 16.5 per 100,000 nasal surgeries, and it is attributed to the use of postoperative nasal packing.[7] Unfortunately antibiotics may not be effective for preventing this complication. In reported cases, the use of antibiotic ointment on nasal packs did not prevent the onset of this syndrome, and most patients had been given prophylactic antibiotics.[10] The primary means of avoiding this potentially deadly complication is minimizing the use of nasal packing and splints.

SPECIFIC DEFORMITIES AND TREATMENTS

The common complications of nasal surgery are outlined in this section, along with their revision strategies. For any given deformity, the thickness of the SSTE will determine how likely it is to be detected and diagnosed before revision surgery. In some cases, it is nearly impossible to determine the structural deficiencies beneath the SSTE. In these situations, the surgeon must be prepared for any number of structural problems that may be encountered intraoperatively. Endonasal approaches may be feasible in some secondary rhinoplasty patients in whom subtle deformities or errors of omission need to be addressed. However, the wider exposure and access afforded by the external rhinoplasty approach are needed to thoroughly correct the deformities encountered in most of these cases.

Dorsal Profile

Dorsal Irregularity

Osseous hump reduction and osteotomies may lead to palpable or visible edges of bone. These deformities must be smoothed or camouflaged to prevent an undesirable aesthetic outcome. Minor postoperative irregularities that are visible can be rasped for revision purposes. Those abnormalities that are palpable may only be treated conservatively, and they often disappear on their own.

A more significant complication of osseous hump reduction is the open-roof deformity. The failure to reappose the nasal bones in the midline after osseous hump reduction will lead to this problem. A large open roof will be visible as two parallel linear vertical grooves near the midline of the upper vault of the nose. A smaller open roof may be palpable but not visible. Complete lateral osteotomies after hump removal will allow for the infracture of the nasal bones and the prevention of this complication.

When a cartilaginous component of a dorsal hump is removed, the dorsal aspect of the upper lateral cartilages and the septal cartilage become separated at the middle vault of the nose. If these relationships are not reestablished, the upper lateral cartilages may undergo gradual postoperative inferomedial contracture and collapse, which results in a pinched appearance of the middle third of the nose. This deformity is exaggerated in a patient with short nasal bones. In thin-skinned individuals, the caudal margin of the nasal bones may be skeletonized and visible externally, thus creating an inverted-V deformity. After cartilaginous hump removal, spreader grafts should be placed between the upper lateral cartilages and the dorsal septum to restore the horizontal and coplanar relationships between these structures (Figure 43-2).

Persistent osseous deformities may be addressed by re-mobilizing the nasal bones through previous osteotomy lines. Often digital manipulation is sufficient to reposition the bones into a symmetric midline position. Alternatively, an osteotome may be used to perform the osteotomies. The leading edge of the instrument will tend to follow the path of the previous osseous cuts. Therefore, if the prior osteotomies were poorly placed, extra caution should be exercised to redirect the revision osteotomies in a proper orientation. For cases in which the cartilaginous dorsum is slightly decreased, onlay grafting may be used to correct irregularities. Small irregularities may be excised to restore a smooth contour.

On the other end of the spectrum is the overly narrowed nasal dorsum. In this case, treatment involves outfracture osteotomies, the placement of spreader grafts, or onlay grafting.

For cases in which the lateral osteotomy is placed too high, a stairstep deformity may result. This can be prevented by taking care to place the osteotomy deep in the maxillary groove and passing through the nasofrontal process of the maxilla. Treatment of the stairstep deformity can involve simply rasping the resultant ridge, or it may necessitate the performance of a lower lateral osteotomy.

Low Dorsum and Saddle Deformities

More dramatic dorsal abnormalities may result from the creation of improper height at the upper or middle third. An inexperienced surgeon may fail to recognize that

dorsal alignment can be balanced by elevating a low radix to match the height of the rest of the dorsum rather than by lowering a relative convexity at the middle vault to the level of a low radix. The projection and rotation of the tip are also critical for determining the ideal dorsal height. If the reduction of the dorsum leaves the tip projected significantly beyond the height of the bridge, the nose may appear scooped, with an illusion of over-rotation on the lateral view. Conversely, if the tip projection falls short of the dorsal line, a polybeak will result. If overaggressive dorsal reduction of the middle vault results in inadequate dorsal septal support, a saddle-nose deformity may ensue. A saddle nose will also result from the disruption of the dorsal strut of the cartilaginous septum. Overly aggressive cartilage resection during septoplasty or cartilage harvest may lead to this dreaded complication. To prevent this problem, the surgeon should try to leave at least a 1-cm to 1.5-cm width of cartilage at both the dorsal and caudal components of the septal L-strut. The dislocation of the cephalic aspect of the dorsal strut from the osseous septum and the nasal bones may also lead to the saddle deformity. Thus, during septal work, the surgeon must take great care to preserve the integrity of the osseocartilaginous junction at this keystone area (Figure 43-3).

In general, a low dorsum causes less shadowing of the nose and creates an illusion of increased width on the frontal view. At the upper third of the nose, this may create an appearance of pseudohypertelorism. The washed-out frontal view makes the brow–tip aesthetic lines indistinct and the general appearance of the upper two thirds amorphous. The ideal lateral profile should be straight or slightly concave at the rhinion for women and straight to slightly convex for men. The overall height of the bridge should be determined by the projection of the tip, which should equal just over one half the nasal length.

Restoring proper bridge height usually calls for onlay material. When a mild to moderate degree of dorsal augmentation is needed for a nose in which some dorsal septal support remains, in which the airway is open,

Figure 43-2. A, Cross-section of the nasal middle vault. **B,** The resection of cartilaginous septum results in the separation of the upper lateral cartilage and the septum. **C,** Inferomedial collapse of the upper lateral cartilages is likely to occur unless the middle vault is restabilized.

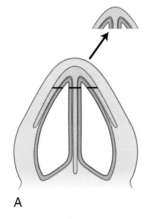

A

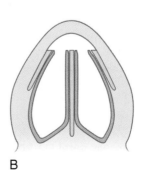

B

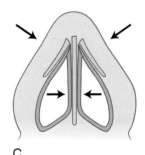

C

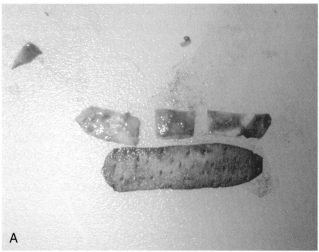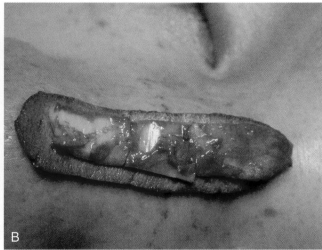

Figure 43-3. **A,** Segments of auricular conchal cartilage cut into small rectangular segments. **B,** Segments sutured onto porcine dermal matrix (ENDURAGen) for implantation and dorsal augmentation.

and in which no soft-tissue limitations exist, dorsal onlay grafts may be appropriate. Using either an endonasal or an open approach, the graft is placed through a tight subperiosteal pocket created at the midline bony dorsum.

The grafting material used depends on the amount of deficiency caused by the saddle deformity. If less than 3 mm to 4 mm of dorsal projection is required, septal or auricular cartilage may be used. Unfortunately, septal cartilage is often compromised or deficient in many saddle-nose deformities. When creating the onlay graft with auricular cartilage, multiple segments may need to be sutured together to achieve the proper overall shape and orientation. If septal and auricular cartilage are available, the septal cartilage can be used to splint the auricular cartilage and minimize the chance of deformity. The septal cartilage should be placed closest to the dorsal skin and sutured firmly to the auricular cartilage. Alternatively, multiple segments of cartilage may be suture stabilized onto an implantable dermal filler matrix. The senior author employs ENDURAGen (Porex, Atlanta, Ga), an acellular porcine collagen implant, for this purpose (see Figure 43-3).

After the graft is secured in favorable position, the SSTE should be redraped to check for external dorsal irregularities. Thinning of the graft may be performed to reduce dorsal height. If augmentation is needed, a layer of acellular dermis or temporalis fascia may be used to provide increased height. The added soft tissue may also be used to camouflage any mild dorsal irregularities.

For situations in which septal or auricular cartilage is insufficiently thick to correct a relatively large dorsal deficiency, costal cartilage may be harvested and carved into an onlay graft. Typically cartilage from the sixth, seventh, eighth, or ninth rib is obtained. After the

costal cartilage onlay graft is obtained and shaped appropriately, it is positioned and secured onto the dorsum as described for septal cartilage onlay grafts. Rib onlay grafting requires that the underlying native L-strut retains its strength and that it can provide some support to the dorsum and the nasal tip. Because the dorsal onlay graft provides minimal inherent support, it will collapse with the rest of the dorsum and tip unless it is supported below by the septum. In more severe cases, the septum may be so compromised that this support is lacking. The degree of the saddling is typically greater, and it may be associated with an underprojected tip. Patients that have suffered a loss of caudal septal support and scar contracture often have a foreshortened nose that requires structurally integrating the dorsal graft to an extended costal cartilage columellar strut, thereby reconstituting an L-shaped support system. The extended columellar strut stabilized posteriorly on the nasal spine and premaxilla and anteriorly by the dorsal graft provides robust tip support. Nasal support becomes independent of the native nasal septum. This technique may be employed to restore nasal support in cases of the total absence of the septum.

The extended columellar strut is based on the concept that, as a columellar strut extends closer to the nasal spine, a theoretic increase in tip support is gained. However, the strut must be strong enough to withstand the downward tension of the tip, particularly if there is minimal support provided by the existing caudal septum. When used in the integrated graft technique, the extended columellar strut must also bear the additional downward pressure exerted by the dorsal graft. Consequently, a very strong, straight segment of rib cartilage is required. Typically each medial crus is completely separated from the nasal septum, and the premaxilla and nasal spine are exposed. The base of the strut is then suture fixated to the periosteum of the nasal spine between the medial crura. A notch in the undersurface of the strut may be made to articulate with the spine and thus prevent migration from the midline.

The dorsal graft is fashioned in the same way as previously described, but it must be made long enough to reach the columellar strut. Again, the cephalic end is snugly placed into a tight subperiosteal pocket in the dorsal bony vault. If the superior aspect of the pocket is too high, the dorsal graft will migrate superiorly and create a blunted nasofrontal angle. A notch is made in the caudal aspect of the dorsal graft in which the tip of the columellar strut will fit. This articulation is suture stabilized with 4.0 polydroxase (Ethicon, Inc., Somerville, NJ) or clear nylon mattress sutures. The angle formed by these grafts will function as the new anterior septal angle. This should be in a favorable midline position, because suture stabilization of the medial and intermediate cartilages onto this structure will determine tip position (Figure 43-4). Dome sutures, shield grafts, and other onlay grafts may provide refinements and camouflage to the reconstructed tip and dorsum. If the saddle deformity involves significant internal lining deficiency or stenosis, auricular composite grafts may need to be used to expand the internal lining.

Nasal Starting Point and Radix

A large or improperly placed radix graft or an inadequate hump reduction may result in excessive dorsal height. A radix graft that is positioned too cephalically will elevate and blunt the nasofrontal angle, thus creating an illusion of a longer nose. If it is placed too caudally, the graft may appear as an unnatural, high dorsal hump. On analysis, the nasal starting point should be at or just below the level of the superior palpebral fissure. The nasofrontal angle should be roughly 120 degrees (although this may vary, depending on the plane of the forehead). The degree of radix projection should be harmonious with the rest of the nasal dorsum and tip projection. Byrd[1] proposes that the ideal radix proportion measured from the junction of the nasal bone to the orbit be one third of the overall nasal length. Repositioning or replacing an existing radix graft may restore the correct nasal starting point and the nasofrontal angle. Such a graft is often created from crushed or bruised cartilage obtained from the nasal septum or from the auricle. Preserving some perichondrium on an auricular cartilage graft will help to preserve some form of the segment after morselization, and it will also aid in the camouflage of the graft. Because these grafts are placed into tight subperichondrial pockets to prevent their migration, it is critical to limit the elevation of the dorsal perichondrium of the bony vault within a narrow space.

Polybeak

The term *polybeak* refers to an abnormality in which the supratip projects beyond the tip. This causes a rounded appearance to the tip with a lack of definition and an absence of a supratip break and a columellar–lobular break. Although the deformity creates the appearance of supratip fullness, the problem may be caused by one of several processes. One possibility is the failure to reduce an overly elevated middle vault and supratip dorsum. In a primary tension nose deformity, the anterior septal angle represents the most projecting point of the nose, with the tip structures "hanging" from this point. Therefore the dorsum at the level of the anterior septal angle must be reduced or the tip brought out beyond this point to establish a proper tip–supratip relationship. The failure to establish this relationship is an error of omission that leads to postoperative polybeak. Paradoxically, a second cause of polybeak is the excessive excision of the dorsal septal cartilage. Particularly in patients with thick, inelastic skin, the SSTE cannot redrape into the area of skeletal reduction. The tissue void fills with scar tissue and fibrosis, which results in a soft-tissue polybeak. Lastly, polybeak may ensue if tip support is compromised and not reconstituted, and the resultant tip ptosis leads to deprojection at the tip with an appearance of supratip fullness[11] (Figure 43-5).

These three types of polybeak deformity require individualized methods of treatment. The correction of the untreated tension nose requires completing the dorsal cartilage reduction and ensuring the presence of a stable nasal base to maintain tip position relative to the dorsum. The correction of the soft-tissue polybeak requires projecting the tip into the thick SSTE beyond the level of the supratip and dorsum. The polybeak caused by tip ptosis mandates reestablishing tip support and returning the tip into its appropriate projection. A variety of methods exist to stabilize the nasal base and restore tip position (these are described later in this chapter). Because these strategies are quite different from each other, it is crucial to understand the cause of the problem before surgery. Palpation is critical to differentiate between soft-tissue fullness and cartilaginous excess. An acute nasolabial angle and a weak tip with little recoil will indicate the presence of tip ptosis as a result of the loss of tip support.

Middle Vault

The middle vault poses one of the most difficult challenges in rhinoplasty. The separation of the upper lateral cartilages from the septum requires suture restabilization to restore the structural relationship, which may include the use of spreader grafts. Failure to do this will result in the inferomedial collapse of the upper lateral cartilages, the pinching of the middle vault, and internal valve airflow obstruction. Particularly in thin-skinned patients with short nasal bones, the collapse and separation of the upper lateral cartilages from the bony vault will result in a visible and palpable inverted-V deformity. Restoring symmetry to a crooked middle vault is extremely difficult and

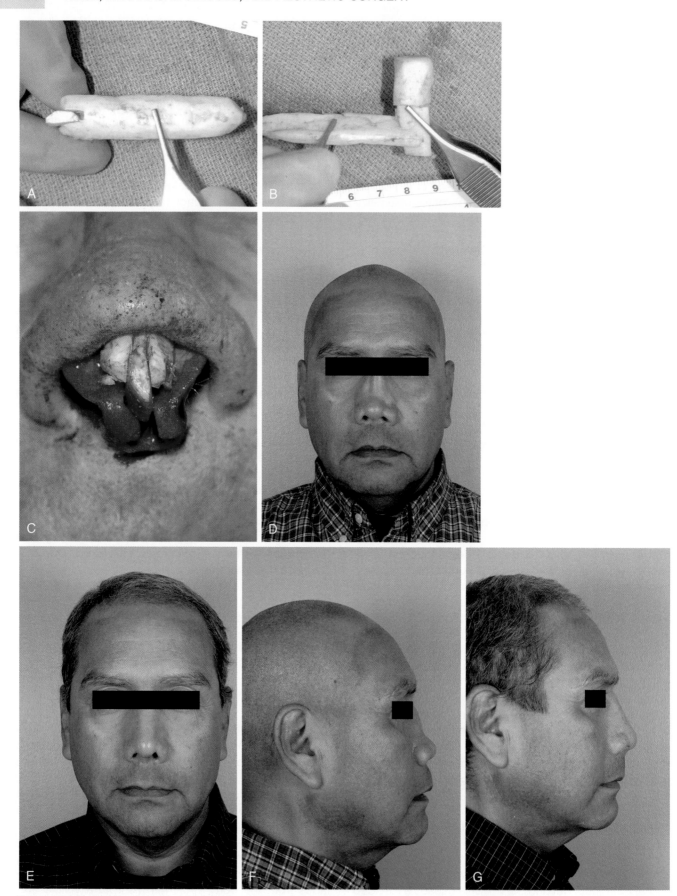

Figure 43-4. A, Typical orientation of a dorsal–caudal integrated costal cartilage graft for severe saddle deformity with absent tip support. **B,** Side view. **C,** In place in nose. **D,** Preoperative frontal view of severe saddle nose from trauma. **E,** Postoperative frontal view. **F,** Preoperative lateral view. **G,** Postoperative lateral view.

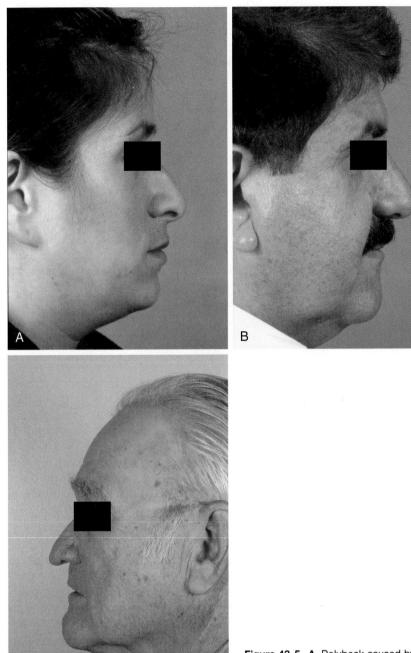

Figure 43-5. A, Polybeak caused by residual high dorsal cartilage. **B,** Polybeak caused by persistent soft-tissue fullness in a thick-skinned patient after dorsal reduction. **C,** Polybeak caused by a loss of support and the descent of the nasal tip.

requires the precise placement of asymmetric spreader grafts stabilized between the dorsal septum and the upper lateral cartilages. Small irregularities or asymmetries are apparent on frontal view as a result of linear shadowing on the nasal sidewalls. These discrepancies often do not become evident until months or years after surgery.

To identify and diagnose these deformities, the revision rhinoplasty surgeon must perform a meticulous examination and analysis of the middle vault. On the frontal

view, the symmetry and width of the nose should be visualized and palpated. The dimensions of the brow–tip aesthetic line should follow a pattern of relative width at the bony vault, slight narrowness at the middle vault, and width again at the tip. This curve should be subtle. Exaggeration of the curvature may indicate middle vault pinching or excessive width at the bony vault or tip. Asymmetry at the middle vault is best determined by visualizing and palpating from above the head of the patient; small areas of irregularity may be appreciated in this manner. Intranasal inspection of the internal valve area should be performed with a speculum and a light source. The internal angle between in the septum and upper lateral cartilage should be at least 15 degrees. Inspection with the patient inspiring may reveal dynamic collapse of the upper lateral cartilages. This dynamic examination is very important, because it can reveal functional problems that otherwise would be missed.[4,12,13]

In almost all cases, the middle vault width and stability are restored through the placement of spreader grafts. As in primary rhinoplasty, these rectangular grafts are suture stabilized between the dorsal septum and the upper lateral cartilages. However, in revision cases, a greater degree of collapse or asymmetry may be present. The surgeon must therefore be prepared to insert wider or more numerous spreader grafts than would be done during standard primary rhinoplasty. In severe cases, the upper lateral cartilages may be collapsed into the nasal airway. In these situations, it is critical that the upper lateral cartilages are grasped and pulled into the proper dorsal position in alignment with the dorsal margin of the septum before the placement of the spreader grafts.

Lateral Nasal Wall

Some of the most common complaints of patients who have undergone rhinoplasty are related to weak, unsupported lateral nasal walls leading to collapse and subsequent nasal obstruction. There are five common causes of lateral nasal wall weakness. Aggressive cephalic trim of the lower lateral crura and the division or resection of the alar cartilages are two potential causes. Failure to correct preexisting lateral wall weakness and supra-alar pinching as well as failure to support the alar lobule and margin in patients with inherently weak cartilage or cephalically positioned lateral crura may also lead to lateral wall problems.

Supra-Alar and External Valve Collapse

Exaggeration of the supralobular crease may represent an inherent deficiency of the cartilage and support of the lateral wall of the nose. This deformity can also develop as a result of scar contracture on the tissue void caused by the excision of the lower lateral crura. Aggressive cephalic trim and the interruption of the lateral crus will decrease the support of the lateral wall and contribute to eventual collapse, which is best detected on frontal and oblique views. Inspiration may lead to further dynamic collapse of the weakened external valve. Intranasal inspection may reveal the fixed or dynamic inspiratory medialization of the alar lobule. The improvement of breathing achieved by supporting the lateral wall with a narrow instrument such as a cotton-tip applicator or a cerumen loop confirms the diagnosis. The degree of collapse may vary in severity, and it will require appropriately sized alar batten grafts for correction[14,15] (Figure 43-6).

These grafts are curved cartilaginous supports placed into the area of maximal lateral wall weakness. Through the external approach, the grafts are placed into tight pockets that overlap and extend lateral to the lateral crura. The curvature of the graft should be oriented to lateralize the supra-alar area with the concave surface medial. The lateral aspect of the graft is usually caudal to the lateral crura, depending on the area of maximal pinching. In severe cases, the grafts may extend all the way to the pyriform aperture to add support. For cases in which the lateral recurvature of the native lateral crura impinges on the nostril width, the lateral crura may be sutured to the alar batten grafts for lateral stabilization. Internal vestibular stents may be placed during the postoperative period to prevent the postoperative medialization of the lateral wall. These stents may be constructed with pliable plastic stents, and they may be maintained in the nasal vestibules while the patient sleeps for a period of 3 to 12 weeks, depending on the severity of the initial problem.[11,16]

Alar Pinching and Retraction

Excisional techniques on the lateral crura may cause weakness and contracture at the alar margin. Cephalic retraction may cause alar elevation, which, on the lateral view, reveals excessive columellar show (unless the columella itself is also retracted).[17] The retracted alar margin may be notched at the apex in cases in which the internal vestibular skin has become scarred from a poorly healed incision. On the lateral view, there should ideally be a columellar show of 2 mm to 4 mm. A distance that exceeds this range suggests the presence of either a retracted ala or a hanging columella. An imaginary line through the long axis of the nostril on the lateral view serves as a marker to help with differentiating these possibilities. Normally the top and bottom of the nostril should be equidistant to this line. If the distance from the top of the nostril to this line significantly exceeds the distance from the bottom of the nostril to this line, alar retraction is present. The converse is true for a hanging columella. This comparison may be applied in cases of decreased columellar show to differentiate between a hooded ala and a retracted columella.[18] Alar retraction on the frontal view creates excessively visible nostrils. Normally the infratip lobule and the alar margins create the shape of a gently curving gull in flight. With retracted ala, the wings of the gull are overly arched as compared with the body.

Contracture from a previous reduction of the lower lateral cartilage may also be evident on the base view as alar pinching. Particularly in cases in which the lower lateral cartilage is weak or cephalically positioned, excisional techniques may lead to the destabilization of an inherently weak alar margin. This pinching can also occur if the tip cartilages have been previously narrowed excessively

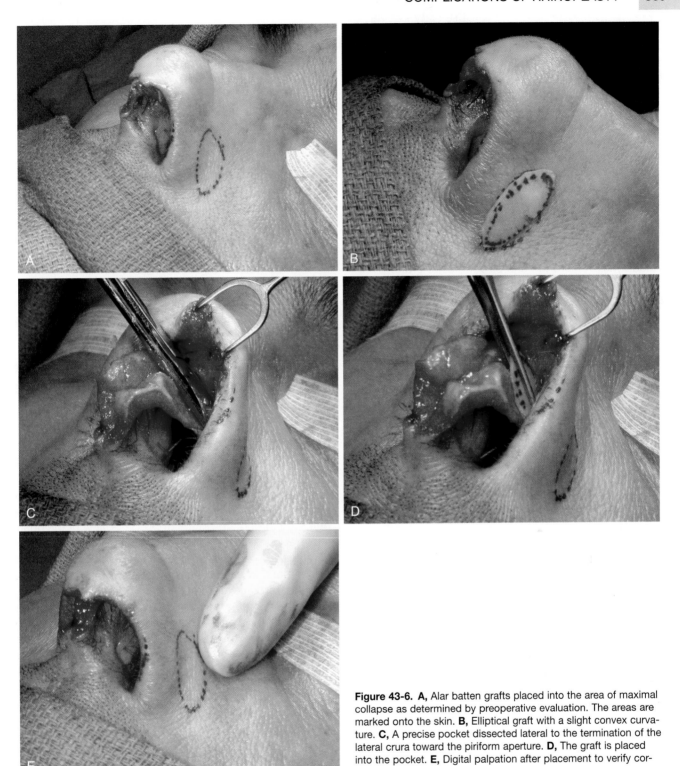

Figure 43-6. A, Alar batten grafts placed into the area of maximal collapse as determined by preoperative evaluation. The areas are marked onto the skin. **B,** Elliptical graft with a slight convex curvature. **C,** A precise pocket dissected lateral to the termination of the lateral crura toward the piriform aperture. **D,** The graft is placed into the pocket. **E,** Digital palpation after placement to verify correct placement.

using a vertical dome division, a lateral crural flap, or the excessive tightening of dome sutures. The concavity of the lateral nostril walls may create an illusion of relative tip width. The nostrils may be thin and slit-like, and they may become more prone to collapse with inspiration. Cephalically positioned lower lateral cartilages may be detected before surgery by palpation of the tip and

supratip areas. When curved and prominent, this anatomic variation will manifest as a parenthesis deformity on the frontal view in which the tip is seemingly enclosed between two curved parentheses (that correspond with the caudal borders of the alar cartilages). If the SSTE is thick and the cartilages are flat, however, this variation may go undetected until surgery.

The placement of alar rim grafts may restore support and create a more triangular nasal base. These grafts are long, narrow cartilaginous grafts that are placed into precise pockets along the alar rim just caudal to the marginal incision. They measure 2 mm to 3 mm in thickness and width and 5 mm to 8 mm in length. Softer material (e.g., cartilage harvested from the ear or from the cephalic trim of the lower lateral cartilage) is preferable. The medial aspect of these grafts may be gently bruised to aid in camouflage. They may be stabilized to the surrounding soft tissue or to the lateral aspect of a shield graft with 6.0 polydroxase suture. These grafts will improve the concave or "knock-kneed" appearance of the rim on the base view and create a more triangular appearance on the basal view. Severe cases of alar retraction may require the use of composite grafts of ear cartilage and skin placed into the marginal incisions to reposition the alar margins in a more caudal position.

Nasal Tip

Some of the most noticeable deformities during secondary rhinoplasty occur in the nasal tip. The challenge lies in modulating the tip position and shape and then maintaining the modifications against the forces of scar contracture. Tip deformities in secondary rhinoplasty patients come in all forms, and they may result from any of the classes of surgical errors that have been previously described. The external rhinoplasty approach to the revision of the nasal tip allows for the unparalleled ability to correct asymmetries.

Irregularities and Bossae

Asymmetry of the tip may result from problems of unequal excision, suture modification, or grafting. Subtle discrepancies may not become evident for several months until the edema resolves. Bossae may form as a result of knuckling or angulation of the lower lateral cartilage and tip grafts as the SSTE contracts. Patients with thin skin and strong cartilage are particularly susceptible to this problem. These palpable and visible irregularities may result from the buckling of weakened or reduced alar cartilage under contractile SSTE forces, or they may result simply from the insufficiently contoured edges of cartilage or grafts under thin skin. Usually the patient is acutely aware of such abnormalities. Conservative cartilage trimming, revising suture modification of the domal cartilage, and onlay camouflaging may correct such problems[5,15,19] (Figure 43-7). In cases of severe structural compromise, the entire tip structure must be reconstructed (this is described later in this chapter).

Persistently Wide or Bulbous Tip

A persistently wide tip after primary rhinoplasty may be the result of the failure of the surgeon to account for a thick, inelastic SSTE when modifying the dome region. In these patients, the addition of dome-binding sutures alone may improve the shape of the alar cartilages

themselves, but this change will not necessarily transmit through the thick SSTE. The failure to project the tip into the skin envelope and to effectively stretch it to conform with the underlying tip shape will lead to this problem. A study of the overall projection and rotation of the tip, the nasolabial angle, and the nasal length should be performed to determine how to best project the tip and restore the optimal tip shape. A shield-shaped tip graft may be sutured to the intermediate and medial crura to provide the desired augmentation to the infratip lobule and tip. Although the nasal base remains unchanged, the leading edge of the shield graft may project beyond the domes by as much as 8 mm. A buttress or cap graft may be placed cephalad to the leading edge of the graft to support the graft and to camouflage the transition to the supratip. Lateral crural grafts are placed on the existing lateral crura and sutured to the lateral edge of the shield graft when the tip graft projects more than 3 mm above the existing domes. These also provide additional support and camouflage to the shield graft. In addition, lateral crural grafts bolster lateral alar support in cases in which the native lateral crura have been weakened or removed.

Another common error of omission that leads to a persistently wide tip is the failure to straighten a convex lateral crura. Domal narrowing will not result in a defined triangular tip appearance if the lateral walls of the triangle are curving outward. Unless the curvature is straightened with suture technique or lateral crural struts, persistent tip width will be present. These problems may be detected through the study of the base view of the nose. If lateral crural struts will be needed, strong segments of cartilage are required to overcome the curvature of the existing alar cartilage. These grafts are placed between the undersurface of the lateral crura and the vestibular skin, which should be carefully elevated. The caudal attachment of the lateral crus and skin should remain intact to prevent the caudal migration of the graft. The graft should extend from just lateral to the domes to the lateral aspect of the lateral crura. The lateral crural strut graft may be stabilized with a full-thickness chromic suture, but it should be finally secured to the lower lateral crura with a 5.0 clear nylon suture (Figure 43-8).

Over-Rotated (Short Nose)

A short-nose deformity is most frequently the result of a loss of support of the caudal septum. The aggressive excision of the caudal margin of the nasal septum results in a loss of tip support, which can then cause upward rotation. The foreshortening or over-rotation of the nasal tip can result in the same deformity as aggressive cephalic trim of the lateral crura. In these situations, the over-rotation and underprojection results from a deformity of the tip rather than of the nasal base. Thus the nasolabial angle may be appropriate despite the appearance of a foreshortened nose. However, if the lower lateral cartilages have been destabilized from the caudal

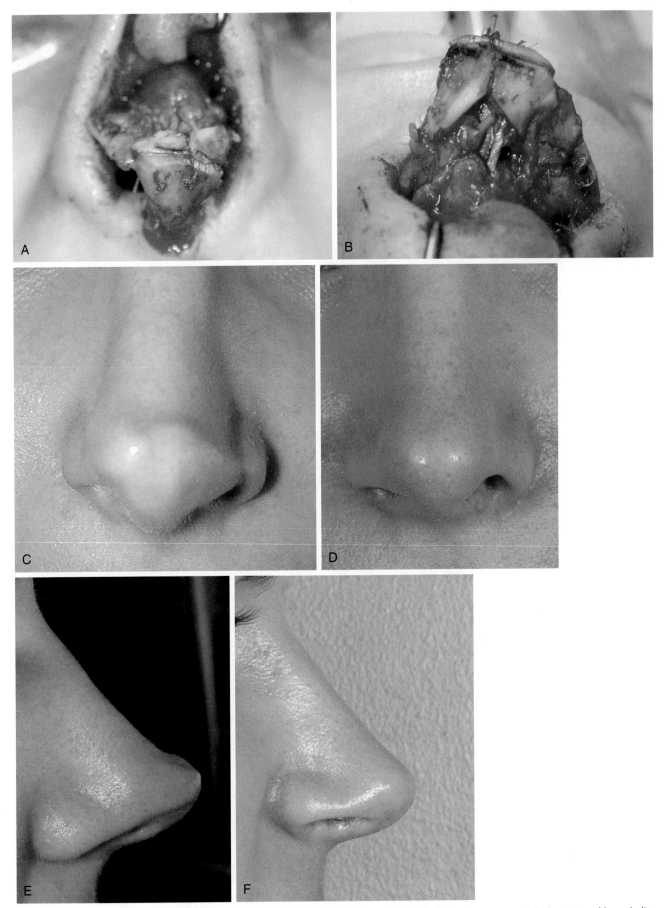

Figure 43-7. A, Shield graft, lateral crural grafts, and multiple crushed cartilage onlay grafts to treat severe nasal tip bossae and irregularity. **B,** Frontal view. **C,** Preoperative frontal view. **D,** Postoperative frontal view. **E,** Preoperative lateral view. **F,** Postoperative lateral view.

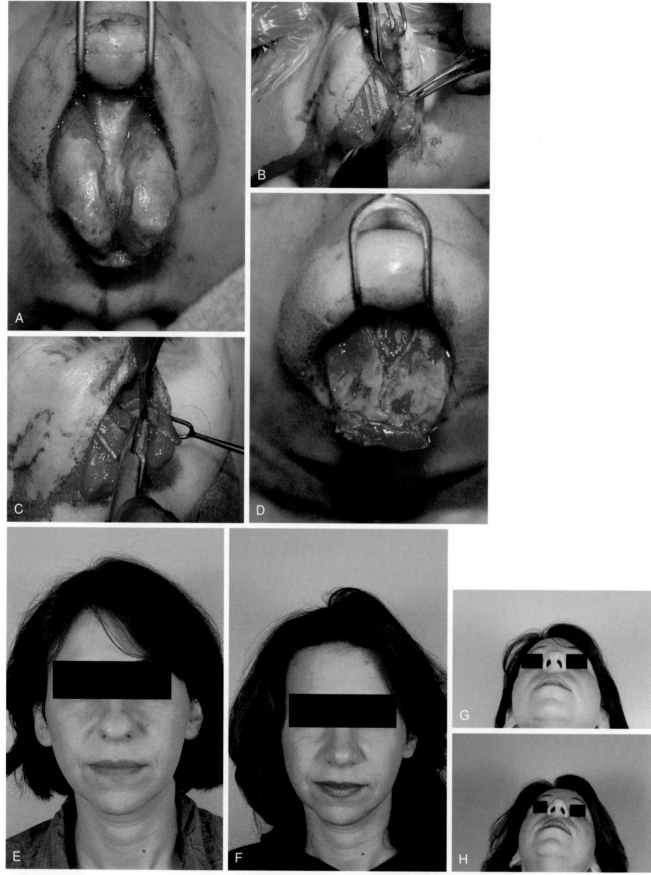

Figure 43-8. A, Overly curved and strong lateral crura causing bulbous tip. **B,** Vestibular mucosa dissected from the undersurface of the lateral crus through a cephalic trim incision. **C,** Long, straight, lateral crural strut placed beneath the native lateral crus. **D,** Lateral crural strut and intradomal sutures force the lateral crus into a straighter orientation. **E,** Preoperative frontal view. **F,** Postoperative frontal view. **G,** Preoperative base view. **H,** Postoperative base view.

septum, scar contracture may pull the entire tripod cephalically. This results in true rotation at the nasal base and tip, causing an obtuse nasolabial angle. In severe cases, the tip may appear rounded or amputated. During analysis, it is important to differentiate this problem from a short nose caused by a truncated caudal septum (described later in this chapter). By palpating the position of the septum and noting the nasolabial angle and the status of the nasal base, this distinction may be made.

The correction of this deformity may require revising or repositioning the domal sutures or rebuilding the tripod structure with a shield graft and lateral crural grafts on the existing domes. This situation is distinct from the short nose caused by prior septal truncation, which may require lengthening the overshortened septum with a caudal extension graft. Decreasing the nasal tip projection will also help to create the illusion of the counterrotation of the nasal tip.

Pinched Tip

A pinched nasal tip results from excessive narrowing of the domes from excisional techniques, dome division, or excessive transdomal sutures. The narrowness of the tip may be further complicated by lateral wall collapse and alar pinching. This unnatural, operated appearance is a sure sign of prior surgery. The normal width of the tip is created by the inherent curvature of the individual domes as well as the normal divergence of the interdomal angle. This divergence creates a natural infratip lobule width, which should be evident from both the base view and the frontal view. The lobule should be wider for men than for women. Restoring a natural tip appearance may require the reconstruction of the tip with a shield graft[19] (Figure 43-9).

Ptotic Tip

Maintaining the tip position after rhinoplasty depends on restoring any tip support mechanisms that are weak or that have been surgically violated. Separating the lower lateral cartilages from the upper lateral cartilages, freeing the medial crura from the caudal septum, and excising or weakening the lower lateral cartilages are common maneuvers in primary rhinoplasty that compromise major tip-support mechanisms. Stabilizing the tip tripod framework at the nasal base can help to prevent the eventual ptosis of the unsupported tip and the subsequent elongation of the nose. Methods of base stabilization include suture stabilization of the medial crura onto a long caudal septum, a caudal extension graft, a columellar strut, and an extended columellar strut.[4] The failure to take such measures may lead to a gradual loss of tip support, a hanging tip and an infratip lobule, an overly acute nasolabial angle, and an underprojected long nose. In addition to the obvious appearance on the lateral view, poor tip strength and recoil on palpation confirm the diagnosis. By using one of the base-stabilizing techniques, the tip position and its support may be restored.

Nasal Septum

Caudal Septum Deviation

The persistence of a caudal septal deviation is one of the most common causes of a significant postoperative deviated tip. Left uncorrected, such a deformity will cause nasal obstruction as well as an obvious cosmetic problem. Intranasal examination should focus on the shape of the caudal septal margin. It may be tilted, C-shaped, fractured, or dislocated from the nasal spine. The nasal spine itself and the posterior septal angle must be examined for position and symmetry. The remainder of the septum must also be thoroughly visualized to check for persistent bony spurs or cartilaginous deviation obstructing the airway. The strength and the caudal–cephalic position of the caudal margin must be assessed to determine the ideal method of correction. A severely weakened or retracted septum may require reconstruction with a large caudal extension graft. A strong, severely deviated caudal septum may need to be removed and replaced with a straight segment of cartilage.

Caudal Septal Excision (Short Nose)

Excessive caudal septal excision may result in the rotation of the tip and a shortened nose. Thus the entire tip tripod is cephalically rotated, which widens the nasolabial angle and leads to a retracted columella. Careful analysis of the nasal base, tip projection and rotation, and palpation of the caudal margin of the septum are critical. The internal vestibular lining should be inspected for previous resection, because redundancy of the skin and mucosa would ensue after septal truncation.

Correction requires restoring septal length with a caudal extension graft and fixating the tip cartilages onto the new caudal septum. Minor deformities may be addressed with plumping grafts at the premaxilla for posterior caudal septal deficiency or columellar onlay grafts. If there is a shortage of vestibular lining, an assessment must be made regarding whether the compromised SSTE will tolerate expansion with such grafts. If not, a skin graft or a composite graft must be considered.

Alar Base

One of the most difficult rhinoplasty complications to correct is the overly narrowed alar base. Alar base reduction should be performed conservatively, with the aim of achieving 60% to 70% of an idealized reduction at the time of primary surgery. Unfortunately, excessive or asymmetric reduction is a common mistake during primary rhinoplasty. On the frontal or base view, the alar insertion should approximate the intercanthal width, and a slight amount of alar flare is acceptable, particularly in men. Ethnic variations allow for a greater degree of interalar width and alar flare, especially in patients of African and Asian descent. Poorly placed incisions or uneven closure may make this problem more conspicuous. Nostril size

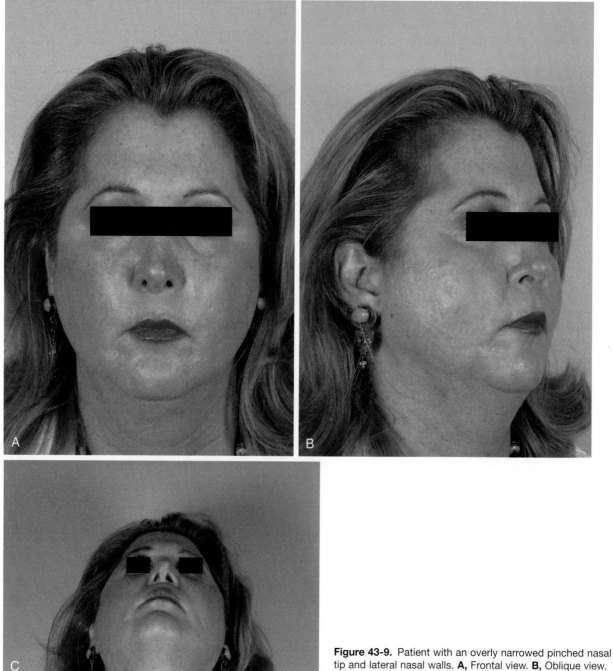

Figure 43-9. Patient with an overly narrowed pinched nasal tip and lateral nasal walls. **A,** Frontal view. **B,** Oblique view. **C,** Base view.

and shape must be noted on the base view. Meticulous measurements should be made of the width of the columellar pedestal, the width of the nasal sill, and the distance of the outer aspect of the alar insertion to the midline. Repositioning the alar base is a three-dimensional process. The horizontal position of the ala may result in the vertical migration of the alar insertion, which can lead to asymmetry. The comparison of the nose with preoperative photos can help with determining which portion of the alar base was previously removed. A significant reduction in the width of the nostril floor and the interalar distance suggests resection primarily of the sill. A reduction of alar

flare suggests resection of the alar sidewall. The reduction of both flare and interalar width suggests excision at the junction of the sill and the alar sidewall, possibly through the use of a sliding alar flap. This analysis will help to determine the shape and size of the tissue needed to replace the previous excision.[16]

Composite grafts harvested from the cymba concha work well to correct such deformities. These grafts may be interposed into incisions placed at the areas of maximal narrowing. A common deformity after overreduction is the overly narrowed or absent nasal sill. In these cases, a composite graft is placed into an incision at the nostril floor, which results in the widening of the sill and interalar distance. Transposition flaps using a superiorly pedicled cheek flap should be avoided, because they tend to cause more distortion, vertical alar malposition, and an unsightly scar (Figure 43-10).

Skin–Soft-Tissue Envelope

If the skin has been significantly damaged, the revision rhinoplasty surgeon must be exceedingly cautious when manipulating or undermining the SSTE. If there is any doubt regarding the integrity of the SSTE, surgery

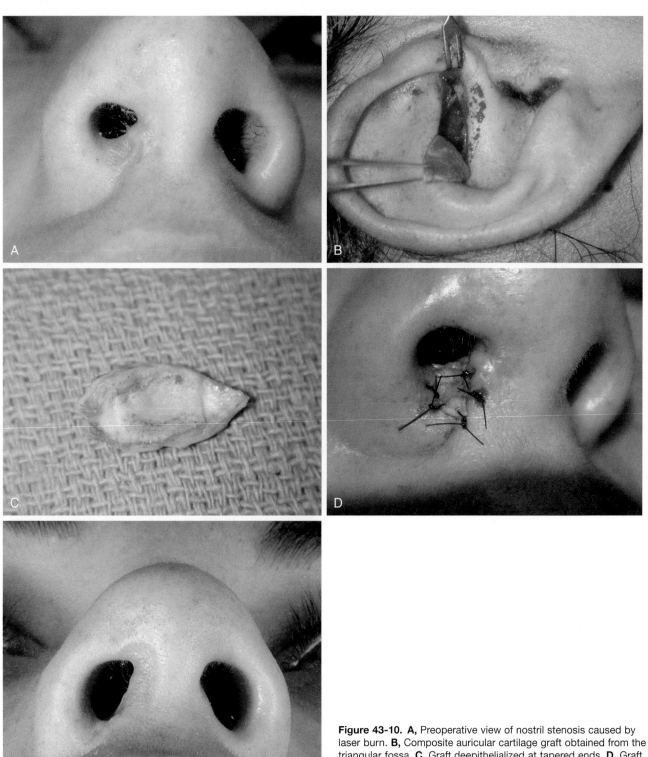

Figure 43-10. A, Preoperative view of nostril stenosis caused by laser burn. **B,** Composite auricular cartilage graft obtained from the triangular fossa. **C,** Graft deepithelialized at tapered ends. **D,** Graft sutured into incision at the scar bed; cartilaginous flanges placed into the deep pockets and skin/cartilage island used to expand the nostril floor. **E,** Postoperative view.

should be delayed to allow for full recovery. Blue discoloration or cutaneous telangiectasias signify damage and an added risk for skin complications. For catastrophic cases in which the soft-tissue envelope has already been severely compromised, one should consider the staged preliminary repair of the SSTE with skin grafts or local or regional flaps before performing any structural nasal surgery.

CONCLUSION

Secondary rhinoplasty may pose the most difficult challenges of facial plastic surgery. Many of the tools of analysis are the same as for primary rhinoplasty. However, these methods must be focused toward the problems and deformities most commonly found during secondary rhinoplasty. The ability to correct these problems is limited by the integrity of the existing structures, the availability of grafting material, and the severity of the individual deformities. In many cases, secondary rhinoplasty becomes an operation of reconstruction more than one of simple refinement. Thus the goal of analysis in secondary rhinoplasty is not only to diagnose these problems but also to determine the limitations and strategies of treatment.

The examples cited represent only a fraction of the multitude of potential problems that the surgeon may encounter. In some cases, the cause of the problem may not become clear until surgery. In the face of compromised nasal structures, scarred soft tissue, and a lack of autogenous grafting material, the revision surgeon must be prepared for the worst of scenarios. Even more than in primary rhinoplasty, this requires meticulous attention to detail during the preoperative analysis. Thoughtful planning based on this analysis as well as a thorough understanding of the problems commonly encountered during revision rhinoplasty will maximize the chances of a favorable outcome.

REFERENCES

1. Byrd HS, Hobar PC: Rhinoplasty: A practical guide for surgical planning. *Plast Reconstr Surg* 1993;91:642–656.
2. Orten SS, Hilger PA: Facial analysis of the rhinoplasty patient. In Papel ID, editor: *Facial plastic and reconstructive surgery,* ed 2, New York, 2002, Thieme Medical Publishers.
3. Tardy ME, Walter MA, Patt BS: The overprojecting nose: Anatomic component analysis and repair. *Facial Plast Surg* 1993;9:306–316.
4. Toriumi DM: Structure approach in rhinoplasty. *Facial Plast Surg Clin North Am* 2000;8:515–537.
5. Tardy ME: *Rhinoplasty: The art and science,* Philadelphia, 1997, WB Saunders.
6. Yoder MG, Weimert TA: Antibiotics and topical surgical preparation solution in septal surgery. *Otolaryngol Head Neck Surg* 1992;106:243–244.
7. Mansfield CJ, Peterson MB: Toxic shock syndrome associated with nasal packing. *Clin Pediatr* 1989;28:443–445.
8. Meyers AD: Prophylactic antibiotics in nasal surgery. *Arch Otolaryngol Head Neck Surg* 1990;116:1125–1126.
9. Jacobson JA, Stevens MH, Kasworm EM: Evaluation of single-dose cefazolin prophylaxis for toxic shock syndrome. *Arch Otolaryngol Head Neck Surg* 1988;114:326–327.
10. Papel ID, Scott JC, Fairbanks DNF: Complications of nasal surgery and epistaxis management. In Eisele DW, editor: *Complications in head and neck surgery,* St Louis, 1993, Mosby.
11. Tardy ME, Kron TK, Younger R, et al: The cartilaginous polybeak: Etiology, prevention, and treatment. *Facial Plast Surg* 1989;6: 113–120.
12. Park SS: Treatment of the internal nasal valve. *Facial Plast Surg Clin North Am* 1999;7:333–346.
13. Toriumi DM: Management of the middle nasal vault. *Op Tech Plast Reconstruct Surg* 1995;2:16–30.
14. Chand MS, Toriumi DM: Treatment of the external nasal valve. *Facial Plast Surg Clin North Am* 1999;7:347–356.
15. Toriumi DM, Josen J, Weinberger M, et al: Use of alar batten grafts for correction of nasal valve collapse. *Arch Otolaryngol Head Neck Surg* 1997;123:802–808.
16. Becker DG, Weinberger MS, Greene BA, Tardy ME: Clinical study of alar anatomy and surgery of the alar base. *Arch Otolaryngol Head Neck Surg* 1997;123:789–795.
17. Tardy ME, Toriumi D: Alar retraction: Composite graft correction. *Facial Plast Surg* 1989;6:101–107.
18. Gunter JP, Rohrich RJ, Friedman RM: Classification and correction of alar-columellar discrepancies in rhinoplasty. *Plast Reconstr Surg* 1996;97:643–648.
19. Toriumi DM, Becker DG: *Rhinoplasty dissection manual,* Philadelphia, 1999, Lippincott.

CHAPTER 44

Complications of Maxillectomy

Jarrod Little and Jeffrey M. Bumpous

A thorough discussion with the patient regarding the potential risks of maxillectomy is essential. These risks can be divided into the following categories: complications of the approach, perioperative and postoperative complications, and complications related to the reconstructive methods used.

COMPLICATIONS OF APPROACH

Aesthetic complications arise from the method of approach, the amount of skin excised, the degree of bony orbital resection, and the method of reconstruction. The Weber–Fergusson incision (Figure 44-1) gives adequate exposure to the maxilla, particularly laterally; however, the subciliary incision predisposes the patient to eyelid complications, including middle lamellar contracture syndrome, ectropion, and prolonged eyelid edema. The extended rhinotomy obviates the lower-eyelid complications by extending the lateral aspect of the incision over the medial canthal region and into the hairline of the brow.[1] This also allows for the maintenance of intact vascularized tissue over the inferior orbital rim, which may be beneficial for reducing the extrusion of inferior orbital hardware. The careful placement and closure of the rhinotomy is essential. As transitions are made in the direction of the skin incision, sharp angles are preferred to gentle curves. A Z-plasty may be incorporated if the rhinotomy incision crosses the medial canthus to prevent postoperative webbing. If lip splitting is required for access, a triangular notch at the vermillion border may lead to easier approximation, decreased scar contracture, and improved aesthetic outcome.

Rhinotomy and maxillectomy may also affect the nasal pyramid, which has been associated with cosmetic complications in 10% of patients.[2] Common nasal complications include ipsilateral nasal collapse, saddle deformity, columellar collapse, and alar retraction. Bony nasal complications may be decreased by placing the medial vertical osteotomy low across the maxillary face to preserve as much nasal bone as possible. If partial septectomy is required, the maintenance or reconstruction of adequate dorsal and caudal struts is required to decrease the incidence of saddle deformity.

PERIOPERATIVE COMPLICATIONS

Hemorrhage

Significant blood loss can be expected during maxillectomy. Leong and colleagues[3] reported an average blood loss of 616 ml. The degree of blood loss increases as dissection proceeds in an anteroposterior direction. Posteriorly, the final aspect of maxillectomy requires osteotomy of the posterior maxillary wall. This osteotomy often violates the pterygoid plexus and results in substantial blood loss. Bipolar cautery of the venous plexus and the ligation of the branches of the internal maxillary artery may be required for hemostasis. Blood loss can be limited by performing the exposure of all osteotomy sites to the degree possible before actually making the osteotomies. Performing the pterygoid osteotomies last is also helpful, because it is often not until the specimen is delivered that access for hemostasis is adequate posteriorly.

Airway

Airway complications after maxillectomy are rare. In a large retrospective review of maxillectomies, Lin and colleagues[4] reported that only 7.7% of patients required simultaneous tracheostomy as a result of bulky flap reconstruction. Of the remaining patients, approximately 1% required postoperative tracheostomy. When maxillectomies are extended to involve the resection of the anterior cranial base, tracheostomy should be considered to decrease the possibility of tension pneumocephalus.

Cerebrospinal Fluid Leak

The leakage of cerebrospinal fluid (CSF) is an uncommon complication of maxillectomy. It occurs most commonly after combination procedures requiring craniotomy and in previously irradiated fields.[2] The majority of CSF leaks may be repaired intraoperatively with primary dural repair, local flaps, or synthetic sealants. During the postoperative period, CSF leakage is best treated with measures to reduce intracranial pressures, such as elevation of the head, bed rest, the introduction of stool softeners, and possible lumbar drainage. The postoperative surgical repair of CSF leakage is reserved for truly refractory cases and often requires the use of vascularized soft tissue, such as microvascular free flaps.

Reconstruction

The resection of the orbital floor in maxillectomy surgery mandates either orbital exenteration or reconstruction to maintain orbital function. Orbital exenteration may be reserved for those tumors that encroach on the intraorbital contents in which more conservative surgery would violate oncologic margins or yield a nonfunctional eye. A variety of methods are available for reconstruction, including skin grafting, obturator prosthetic placement, regional flap reconstruction, and free-tissue transfer.

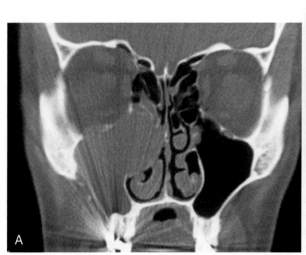

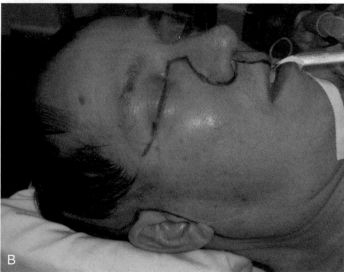

Figure 44-1. Patient with squamous cell carcinoma of the maxillary sinus. Preoperative markings demonstrate the Weber–Fergusson incision using a transconjunctival incision rather than the classically described subciliary component.

Okay and colleagues[5] proposed a classification system on the basis of the extent of resection with guidelines for reconstructive strategies. Defects limited to the palate, the premaxilla, or any portion of the maxillary alveolus and the dentition posterior to the canines may be adequately reconstructed with soft-tissue coverage and/or prosthetic obturation. Defects involving any portion of the hard palate and the tooth-bearing maxillary alveolus and only one canine will generally require prosthetic obturation, free-tissue transfer, or both. More extensive defects are best suited to free-tissue transfer reconstruction, especially when sufficient bony landmarks are not present for the anchoring of the maxillary prostheses.

The reconstruction of total maxillectomy defects requires the reconstruction of the orbital floor and soft-tissue coverage. Nonvascularized bone grafts to the orbital floor in combination with temporalis or free rectus abdominus flap reconstruction results in the more consistent preservation of functional vision and a low incidence of postoperative diplopia or enophthalmos. Previously irradiated beds are poorly receptive to nonvascularized bone grafts. In these cases, a radial forearm osteocutaneous flap or a split iliac crest flap may be more appropriate. Ectropion is the most common complication, occurring to some degree in upward of 77% of patients.[6] Secondary surgical procedures to correct ectropion, which consist of canthopexy, skin grafting, or both, can be successful in a majority of patients.

POSTOPERATIVE COMPLICATIONS

Vascular

Carotid-cavernous fistula may result from the down fracture of the maxilla or the pterygoid osteotomy, thus injuring the internal carotid artery.[7] Patients with a preexisting internal carotid artery aneurysm are at an increased risk. Signs and symptoms are related to the compression of structures within the cavernous sinus, including the oculomotor, trochlear, ophthalmic, and maxillary divisions of the trigeminal nerve. However, abducens nerve palsy may be the earliest neurologic sign, because this is the only nerve that is not covered by dura and that runs free through the sinus. Increased cavernous sinus pressures can lead to venous outflow obstruction from the ophthalmic veins, thus draining the extraocular muscles and the retinal vein. Definitive diagnosis requires angiography; however, computed tomography scanning and magnetic resonance imaging may play a role. Treatment consists of endovascular embolization procedures.

Orbital

Postoperative orbital complications are common with maxillectomy. Perioperative orbital complications can include optic nerve trauma during resection or optic ischemia as a result of the overzealous packing of the maxillary cavity.[8] Imola and colleagues[9] studied patients undergoing surgical management for sinonasal malignancies. Of the patients with orbital preservation, more than 90% retained a functional eye, but 41% had one or more ocular sequelae.[9] Approximately 13% of patients demonstrated mild enophthalmos, if partial wall resection was performed. This increased to 96% in nonreconstructed total floor and multiple wall resections. The rigid fixation of these defects yielded a 52% incidence of minimal to moderate enophthalmos. Diplopia was common during the postoperative period, but it was permanent in only 6% of patients after reconstruction. Damage or disruption of the trochlea in the medial superior orbital wall may also cause diplopia.[2] This is seen when osteotomy extends to the superomedial orbital rim. Trochlear disruption is repaired by the reapproximation of the orbital periosteum. Other ocular sequelae include ectropion, blepharitis, conjunctivitis, exposure keratopathy, epiphora, and optic atrophy. The rates of other ocular sequelae depend on the presence of postoperative radiotherapy.[9] Considering patients with postoperative radiotherapy, without, and combined, the overall incidence of ectropion was 23%, 13%, and 20%, respectively; the incidence of blepharitis and conjunctivitis was 38%, 20%, and 33%, respectively; the incidence of exposure keratopathy was 13%, 7%, and 11%, respectively; and the incidence of epiphora was 5%, 33%, and 13%, respectively. Dryness, optic atrophy, and cataract formation occurred only among those patients receiving radiotherapy, and it developed in 13%, 5%, and 10%, respectively. Epiphora may be prevented by the marsupialization of the lacrimal sac during surgery or by dacryocystorhinostomy with the placement of lacrimal drainage stents. Diba and colleagues[10] demonstrated the resolution of epiphora in 83% of patients treated with postoperative dacryocystorhinostomy.

Reconstruction

Palatal repair may restore oral competency. However, the placement of a dental prosthesis is frequently needed for dental restoration. The placement of a dental prosthesis relies on fixation to the margins of the palatal resection. Fixation and adequate dental restoration may therefore be compromised by extensive palatal reconstruction. Thus reconstructive efforts should be focused toward the orbit and the bony maxilla.[6] Osseous integrated implants may be required for the fixation of an obturator prosthesis. Implants may be subject to infection, mobility, and implant-site bone loss. Implants to the anterior and posterior maxilla are successful in 86% and 57% of patients, respectively.[11] Postoperative radiotherapy reduces success by 2% to 5%.

Diet

Swallowing function may be compromised after maxillectomy as a result of the loss of oral competency, oronasal continuity, altered anatomy after reconstruction, and sensory deficits. Despite this, swallowing function is acceptable in most patients. In those who underwent regional or free flap reconstruction, 44% to 64% were able to eat an unrestricted diet, 36% to 47% could eat a soft diet, and 0% to 8.3% could take only liquids.[12,13]

Speech

Changes in speech are inherent to maxillectomy as a result of the loss of palatal competence and the resulting oronasal continuity. The resulting oronasal cavity increases speech resonance, decreases the frequency of vowels,[14] and alters speech intelligibility. Standardized measures demonstrate a 65% loss of speech intelligibility among patients without palatal prosthesis after maxillectomy. The placement of a palatal prosthesis restores oronasal separation and results in the loss of only 15% of speech intelligibility.[15] When reconstruction is performed with regional or free flaps, speech has been reported to be subjectively normal in 38.9% of patients, near normal in 41.7%, intelligible in 16.7%, and unintelligible in 2.8%.[12]

Infection

Maxillectomy exposes the native microbial flora of the upper aerodigestive tract. This flora may be altered by previous antibiotic use, preoperative radiotherapy, or community-acquired pathogens. Therefore all reconstructive solutions are subject to a relatively heavily contaminated environment. Postoperative packing of the sinonasal cavity in association with skin grafting is best achieved with antimicrobial-impregnated gauze for 5 to 10 days.[16] Postoperative antibiotic prophylaxis is useful to decrease odor, purulent drainage, and possibly the risk of toxic shock syndrome. Muneuchi[17] reported postoperative infection and subsequent fistula formation in 23% of patients who received free flap reconstruction.

Neurologic

Multiple cranial nerve palsies are possible after maxillectomy. The optic nerve is at risk during resection and reconstruction. The maxillary branch of the trigeminal nerve is frequently sacrificed during resection, and the sphenopalatine nerve in the pterygomaxillary fossa is at risk during resection. Trauma to the sphenopalatine nerve can lead to aberrant regeneration and innervation of the nasal mucosa, thereby resulting in gustatory rhinorrhea.[18]

Daily Care

Nasal crusting is common after maxillectomy and requires thorough nasal hygiene and frequent nasal debridements. This complication is reduced with maxillary reconstruction. The maxillary cavity may be obliterated with regional flaps or free-tissue transfer. Alternatively, crusting can be prevented and nasal competency may be preserved by lining the cavity with split-thickness skin grafts.[19] Frequent gentle saline irrigations and controlled endoscopic debridements in the office are helpful for the management of nasal crusting.

Radiation

Radiation-induced cataracts are a traditional complication of radiotherapy directed to the sinonasal region. Early radiation techniques yielded radiation-induced cataracts in the vast majority of patients and a loss of visual acuity in the contralateral eye in one third of patients.[20] More recent techniques using globe and optic-nerve shielding resulted in more than 90% of patients retaining a functional eye but with 41% having one or more ocular sequelae.[9] Postoperative radiotherapy directed to the sinonasal region commonly causes edema of the nasopharyngeal mucosa and the obstruction of the Eustachian tubes. This results in Eustachian-tube dysfunction and serous otitis media in 20% to 25% of patients.[20] This can often be managed with the placement of ventilation tubes. Radiotherapy may also induce pterygoid fibrosis, which results in trismus. After adequate healing, trismus can usually be managed with passive or active jaw-opening methods. Refractory trismus may eventually require brisement procedures or surgical release and reconstruction.[21] Radiotherapy directed to the orbit and paranasal sinuses has also been associated with blindness, brain necrosis, pituitary insufficiency, and hearing loss.[22]

Other Postoperative Complications

Although infrequent, frontal sinus mucocele formation has been reported after maxillectomy.[2] This is likely caused by the disruption or stenosis of the nasofrontal recess. Mucocele may often be prevented intraoperatively with stents and treated postoperatively with endonasal or extracranial methods.

REFERENCES

1. Vural E, Hanna E: Extended lateral rhinotomy incision for total maxillectomy. *Otolaryngol Head Neck Surg* 2000;123(4):512–513.
2. Bernard PJ, Biller HF, Lawson W, et al: Complications following rhinotomy: Review of 148 patients. *Ann Otol Rhinol Laryngol* 1989;98(9):684–692.
3. Leong HK, Chew CT: Blood loss and transfusion in head and neck tumour surgery. *Ann Acad Med Singapore* 1991;20(5):604–609.
4. Lin HS, Wang D, Fee WE, et al: Airway management after maxillectomy: Routine tracheostomy is unnecessary. *Laryngoscope* 2003;113(6):929–932.
5. Okay DJ, Genden E, Buchbinder D, et al: Prosthodontic guidelines for surgical reconstruction of the maxilla: A classification system of defects. *J Prosthet Dent* 2001;86(4):352–363.
6. Cordeiro PG, Santamaria E, Kraus DH, et al: Reconstruction of total maxillectomy defects with preservation of the orbital contents. *Plast Reconstr Surg* 1998;102(6):1874–1887.
7. Holmes JD, Dierks EJ: Carotid-cavernous fistula after partial maxillectomy: Case report. *J Oral Maxillofac Surg* 2001;59(1):102–105.
8. McGuirt WF: Maxillectomy. *Otolaryngol Clin North Am* 1995;28(6):1175–1189.
9. Imola MJ, Schramm VL Jr: Orbital preservation in surgical management of sinonasal malignancy. *Laryngoscope* 2002;112 (8 Pt 1):1357–1365.
10. Diba R, Saadati H, Esmaeli B: Outcomes of dacryocystorhinostomy in patients with head and neck tumors. *Head Neck* 2005;27(1):72–75.
11. Lorant JA, Roumanas E, Nishimura R, et al: Restoration of oral function after maxillectomy with osseous integrated implant retained maxillary obturators. *Am J Surg* 1994;168(5):412–414.
12. Cordeiro PG, Santamaria E: A classification system and algorithm for reconstruction of maxillectomy and midfacial defects. *Plast Reconstr Surg* 2000;105(7):2331–2348.
13. Futran ND: Primary reconstruction of the maxilla following maxillectomy with or without sacrifice of the orbit. *J Oral Maxillofac Surg* 2005;63(12):1765–1769.
14. Sumita YI, Ozawa S, Mukohyama H, et al: Digital acoustic analysis of five vowels in maxillectomy patients. *J Oral Rehabil* 2002;29(7):649–656.
15. Umino S, Masuda G, Ono S, et al: Speech intelligibility following maxillectomy with and without a prosthesis: An analysis of 54 cases. *J Oral Rehabil* 1998;25(2):153–158.
16. Weissler MA, Pillsbury HA: *Complications of head and neck surgery,* New York, 1995, Theime Medical Publishers.
17. Muneuchi G, Miyabe K, Hoshikawa H, et al: Postoperative complications and long-term prognosis of microsurgical reconstruction after total maxillectomy. *Microsurgery* 2006;26(3):171–176.
18. Sadeghi HM, Siciliano S, Reychler H: Gustatory rhinorrhea after maxillectomy: Two case reports and considerations on etiology and pathophysiology. *Int J Oral Maxillofac Surg* 1997;26(2):124–126.
19. Andhoga MA, Wilson GR, McLaughlin W, et al: Split-thickness skin grafted stent for upper airway patency after medial maxillectomy. *Br J Oral Maxillofac Surg* 1993;31(6):385–387.
20. Sakai S, Kubo T, Mori N, et al: A study of the late effects of radiotherapy and operation on patients with maxillary cancer: A survey more than 10 years after initial treatment. *Cancer* 1988;62(10):2114–2117.
21. Mardini S, Chang YM, Tsai CY, et al: Release and free flap reconstruction for trismus that develops after previous intraoral reconstruction. *Plast Reconstr Surg* 2006;118(1):102–107.
22. Jiang GL, Ang KK, Peters LJ, et al: Maxillary sinus carcinomas: Natural history and results of postoperative radiotherapy. *Radiother Oncol* 1991;21(3):193–200.

CHAPTER 45

Complications of Transsphenoidal Hypophysectomy

Karen A. Kölln and Brent A. Senior

Pituitary surgery has evolved greatly during the past 100 years, and otolaryngologists have played a large role in this evolution, which includes recent advances in minimally invasive approaches. Early during the 1900s, a sublabial transseptal approach to the sella was described; however, this was quickly abandoned for a traditional craniotomy as a result of poor visualization, inadequate instrumentation, high mortality, and a concern regarding a higher risk of tumor recurrence.[1] With the advent of antibiotics, intraoperative fluoroscopy, and the operating microscope, the sublabial approach once again gained acceptance during the 1960s.[1] In 1992, Jankowski and colleagues[2] reported the successful exclusive use of 0- and 30-degree endoscopes in three patients with pituitary adenomas; since that time, this strategy has continued to evolve and to come into favor. Numerous procedural reports outlining the surgical technique have been published.[3–5]

The aim of this chapter is to outline the complications of transsphenoidal hypophysectomy and their management. Most studies reporting the morbidity and mortality rates of pituitary surgery are retrospective in nature and employ a spectrum of surgical techniques, including sublabial transseptal and endonasal transsphenoidal approaches that make use of either the operating microscope or straight and angled endoscopes. All transsphenoidal approaches were considered valid for a review of the morbidity and mortality rates of transsphenoidal hypophysectomy presented here.

PITUITARY ANATOMY AND PHYSIOLOGY

The pituitary gland (also known as the *hypophysis cerebri*) is the central regulatory endocrine gland, and it consists of the adenohypophysis (the anterior lobe) and the neurohypophysis (the posterior lobe, also known as the *pars nervosa*). The anterior lobe produces five hormones: (1) thyroid-stimulating hormone; (2) adreno-corticotropic hormone; (3) follicle-stimulating hormone; (4) growth hormone; and (5) prolactin; and (6) proopio-melanocortin (POMC). This last hormone, POMC, is a precursor to numerous physiologically active derivatives, including corticotropin-like intermediate lobe peptide and α- and β-melanocyte stimulating hormones. The posterior lobe consists of axon endings that originate in the hypothalamus. The hormones secreted by the posterior pituitary are oxytocin and vasopressin (also known as *antidiuretic hormone* [ADH]),

which are produced in the hypothalamus and then transferred down the axons and stored in the neurohypophysis, where they are eventually released into the bloodstream.

The pituitary fossa contains the pituitary gland, and it is limited anteriorly, posteriorly, and inferiorly by the sella turcica, which is a depression in the sphenoid bone. The floor of the pituitary fossa lies directly above the roof of the sphenoid sinus; when the sphenoid is more pneumatized, it accounts for a larger amount of the floor. A fold in the dura called the *diaphragma sellae* forms an incomplete roof above the sella that allows for the transmission of the pituitary stalk and its blood supply. The diaphragma also protects the anterior lobe of the pituitary from the overlying optic chiasm. In some instances, the diaphragma allows for the extensive herniation of the arachnoid into the sella, which causes cerebrospinal fluid (CSF) to partially fill the space and flatten the pituitary gland for a condition known as *empty sella*. Lateral to the hypophyseal fossa lay the cavernous sinuses, which contain venous channels separated by fibrous trabeculae as well as the oculomotor nerve, the trochlear nerve, the first and second divisions of the trigeminal nerve, the abducens nerve, and the internal carotid artery. Key landmarks from within the sphenoid sinus include the optic chiasm, which courses anterosuperiorly, and the curve of the internal carotid artery, which sits posterolaterally[6] (Figure 45-1). A firm understanding of the anatomy and physiology of the hypophysis is vital for the preoperative, intraoperative, and postoperative management of pituitary pathology.

PREOPERATIVE EVALUATION

Before a transsphenoidal hypophysectomy, the patient should be evaluated by a multidisciplinary team that includes a neuro-ophthalmologist and an endocrinologist in addition to the neurosurgeon and otolaryngologist who will be performing the procedure. The history should address sinonasal complaints including facial pressure and pain, nasal congestion or obstruction, hyposmia/anosmia, rhinorrhea, postnasal drip, previous nasal trauma, headache, and any other illnesses. A thorough physical examination should be performed specifically to evaluate for visual field loss, decreased visual acuity, stigmata of endocrine dysfunction, and cranial nerve palsies. Sinonasal endoscopy should be performed to evaluate for septal deviation, nasal polyposis, and sinusitis. Imaging is used

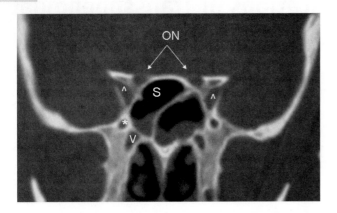

Figure 45-1. Coronal computed tomography scan illustrating sphenoid sinus anatomy. *, Foramen rotundum; ^, internal carotid artery; *ON,* optic nerve; *S,* sphenoid; *V,* vidian canal.

during preoperative evaluation for surgical planning as well as intraoperatively for stereotactic guidance. Imaging should include a noncontrast computed tomography (CT) scan of the paranasal sinuses (to better define the bony anatomy, the pneumatization of the sphenoid, the location of the intersinus septum, the position and possible dehiscence of the internal carotid artery, and the presence of Onodi cells) and magnetic resonance imaging (MRI) of the brain, with special focus on the pituitary gland (to define the extent and location of the tumor, any vascular abnormalities, the involvement of the cavernous sinus, or impingement on the optic nerve or chiasm). Laboratory data including a complete blood cell count and a comprehensive metabolic panel to evaluate for hyponatremia, hypokalemia, hypercalcemia, and hyperglycemia as well as other metabolic abnormalities should be obtained. Coagulation studies including partial thromboplastin time, prothrombin time, and the international normalized ratio should be obtained if there is a family history of bleeding disorders. In addition, endocrine evaluation with prolactin, insulin-like growth factor 1, adrenocorticotropic hormone, thyroid-stimulating hormone, thyroxine, follicle-stimulating hormone, luteinizing hormone, testosterone, morning cortisol, 24-hour urine-free cortisol, and 24-hour urine-free cortisol with a low-dose dexamethasone suppression test should occur as indicated by the clinical scenario.[7]

MORTALITY

Before 1940, mortality rates for transsphenoidal approaches to the pituitary were 5.1% to 10.8%.[8] However, modern series have shown the procedure to be remarkably safe, with overall mortality rates falling to 0% to 1.03% (Table 45-1). Ciric and colleagues[9] surveyed 958 neurosurgeons throughout the United States and reported a mean operative mortality rate of 0.9%; in their own series of 638 patients, they found a

TABLE 45-1   Surgical Mortality of Transsphenoidal Hypophysectomy*

Study	Sample Size	Mortality†	Cause of Death
Jho et al, 1997[39]	50	0.00%	N/A
Ciric et al, 1997[9]	638	0.31%	Pulmonary embolus
Ciric et al, 1997[9]	Survey results	0.90%	Not detailed
Semple et al, 1999[33‡]	105	0.09%	Central pontine myelinolysis after the rapid correction of hyponatremia
Woollons et al, 2000[20]	185	0.00%	N/A
Jho, 2001[40]	160	0.62%	Occlusion of the bilateral internal carotid arteries
Cappabianca et al, 2002[11]	146	0.68%	Postoperative edema of residual lesion leading to the compression of the brainstem and the third ventricle
Kawamata et al, 2002[44]	215	0.00%	N/A
Zada et al, 2003[41]	100	0.00%	N/A
Hammer et al, 2004[12‡]	289	1.03%	Myocardial infarction and/or cardiac failure
White et al, 2004[25]	50	0.00%	N/A
Dusick et al, 2006[37]	259	0.00%	N/A
Netea-Maier et al, 2006[42†]	35	0.00%	N/A

*Surgical mortality listed for all major studies from 1997 to present, with the cause of death listed whenever applicable.
†Defined as death within 30 days of transsphenoidal hypophysectomy.
‡All patients with Cushing disease.

mortality rate of 0.38%. This compares favorably with the reported mortality rate before 1990 of 0% to 1.75%.[10] In Ciric's review, the majority of instances of mortality were found to be the result of medical complications, including pulmonary embolus and cardiac events. The only mortality that was directly related to surgery was caused by the incomplete resection of a macroadenoma with subsequent edema and irreversible neurologic insult.[11] This stresses the importance of the complete resection of pituitary lesions whenever possible, particularly those that expand beyond the confines of the sella, to avoid postoperative hemorrhage or adjacent brain edema. Lesions at the highest risk for this complication are those with a large suprasellar component. Operative experience is positively correlated with decreasing mortality, with surgeons who perform more than 500 cases per year reporting the lowest mortality rate.[9]

Another risk factor for perioperative mortality is Cushing disease. The associated obesity and relative immobility of these patients leads to an increased risk for deep vein thrombosis and subsequent pulmonary embolus. These patients also have significant hypertension and cardiovascular disease, which also contribute to increased perioperative mortality.[12] This should be recognized during the preoperative assessment, and there should be a low threshold for cardiology consultation and evaluation. Vascular injury, meningitis, hypothalamic injury, intracranial abscess or hematoma, and tension pneumocephalus can also lead to perioperative mortality.[10] Overall, however, transsphenoidal hypophysectomy is a safe procedure, especially in the hands of experienced surgeons.

MORBIDITY

Infectious Complications

Infectious complications include sinusitis, meningitis, and intracranial abscess. Meningitis occurs with an incidence of 0.15% to 1.2% (Table 45-2), and it is most commonly associated with sphenoid sinusitis or a postoperative CSF leak. The most common organisms associated with postoperative meningitis are gram-positive species (i.e., staphylococcal and streptococcal species), gram-negative organisms (e.g., *Escherichia coli, Haemophilus influenzae, Klebsiella*), and anaerobes (e.g., *Bacteroides fragilis, Propionibacterium*). The retrograde migration of organisms into the cranial vault is thought to be the cause of postoperative meningitis.[13–15] Van Aken and colleagues[13,14] evaluated the risk factors associated with meningitis after transsphenoidal surgery, specifically assessing the benefits of lumbar drainage in the presence of CSF leak as well as the aggressive medical management of rhinosinusitis in those found to have this disease. The results of their 2004 study were compared with a previous study performed by the same group in 1997. In the 2004 cohort of 278 operations, only 2 patients managed with postoperative lumbar drainage developed meningitis (0.7% of all procedures), which compared favorably with the previous rate of 7 of 228 procedures (3.1%) managed without lumbar drains. In the more recent study, all patients with radiographic evidence of sinusitis were treated preoperatively until the sinusitis was resolved, and all patients with an intraoperative CSF leak were treated with a lumbar drain. None of the patients who had been treated for sinusitis developed meningitis, whereas in the previous study 2 of 3 patients with sinusitis developed meningitis, because they were not aggressively treated preoperatively. When independently evaluated, 1 of 70 individuals with intraoperative CSF leak developed meningitis, and 2 of 3 patients with postoperative rhinorrhea developed meningitis (66%). Also of note is that none of the patients without a CSF leak developed meningitis ($P < 0.0001$).[13,14] Although meningitis can occur independently of these factors, it is clear from this study that both sinusitis and CSF leak should be recognized as important risk factors for the development of meningitis postoperatively. Acute rhinosinusitis diagnosed preoperatively should be treated aggressively, and, if the pituitary procedure is considered nonemergent, it should be delayed until the sinusitis is resolved.

Sinusitis following transsphenoidal hypophysectomy can be caused by gram-positive organisms (e.g., *Staphylococcus aureus, Propionibacterium acnes*), fungal organisms (e.g., *Pseudallescheria boydii*), and gram-negative organisms (i.e., *E. coli, Pseudomonas aeruginosa*). The incidence of sinusitis was reported by Ciric and colleagues[9] in their national survey to be 8.5%, and historically the incidence is reported as being between 1% and 15%. In 2005, Batra and colleagues[16] found a 7.5% incidence of postoperative sinusitis at their institution, and they reported about the nature of sinusitis after transsphenoidal hypophysectomy. Of their cohort of ten patients, seven were referred within the institution, and three additional patients were referred from outside institutions. Interestingly, 90% of these patients had isolated sinusitis, with medical management failing for five of them; these patients ultimately required endoscopic sphenoidotomy. Intraoperative findings included an infected fat graft in one patient, a mucocele in one patient, and a sphenoid fungus ball in three patients.[16] This study underscores the fact that traditionally the long-term follow up of patients after pituitary surgery has not been performed by otolaryngologists. The true incidence of this complication may in fact be underestimated in the literature. Sinusitis should be suspected among patients presenting with sinonasal complaints after pituitary surgery, and it should be aggressively treated. Endoscopic drainage is indicated if medical management does not control the signs and symptoms of sinusitis.

TABLE 45-2 Major Surgical Morbidity*

Study	Procedures	CSF leak[†]	Hematoma	ICA Injury	Meningitis	Stroke	Ophthalmoplegia	Loss of vision[‡]	Epistaxis
Jho et al, 1997[39]	50	2 (0.4%)	0	0	0	0	0	0	0
Ciric et al, 1997[9]	638	7 (1.09%)	4 (0.62%)	0 (0%)	1 (0.15%)	0	2 (0.31%)	3 (0.47%)	10 (0.15%)
Ciric et al, 1997[9]	Survey results	590 (3.9%)	186 (2.9%)	114 (1.1%)	192 (1.5%)	83 (1.3%)	86 (1.4%)	179 (1.8%)	98 (3.4%)
Semple et al, 1999[33§]	105	1 (0.95%)	0	0	0	0	1 (0.95%)	1 (0.95%)	1 (0.95%)
Woollons et al, 2000[20]	185	4.30%	1.60%	0	0.50%	0	1.10%	1.10%	1.10%
Jho, 2001[40]	160	6.00%	0	0	1.20%	0	0	0	0
Cappabianca et al, 2002[11]	146	3 (2.05%)	1 (0.68%)	1 (0.68%)	1 (0.68%)	0	1 (0.68%)	1 (0.68%)	2 (1.36%)
Zada et al, 2003[41]	100	3 (3%)	1 (1%)	1 (1%)	2 (2%)	1 (1%)	0	0	0
Hammer et al, 2004[12§]	289	11 (3.8%)	2 (0.69%)	0	2 (0.69%)	0	0	3 (1.03%)	0
Dusick et al, 2006[37]	259	8 (3.1%)	2 (0.77%)	0	1 (0.38%)	0	0	0	3 (1.15%)

CSF, Cerebrospinal fluid; CN, cranial nerve; ICA, internal carotid artery.
*Surgical morbidity listed for all major studies from 1997 to present.
[†]Defined CSF leak requiring lumbar drain or surgical repair.
[‡]Temporary and permanent loss of vision.
[§]All patients with Cushing disease.

Vascular Complications

Direct vascular injury is a rare but potentially fatal complication during transsphenoidal hypophysectomy. Numerous factors put the carotid artery at risk intraoperatively. As previously described, the carotid artery has a tortuous course within the cavernous sinus; it lies a variable distance from the midline, and it is dehiscent in the sphenoid sinus in 4% of individuals[6] (Figure 45-2). Additionally, the possible extension of pituitary pathology into the cavernous sinus can place the artery at even greater risk. If the preoperative MRI shows a vascular abnormality, some authors suggest obtaining a magnetic resonance angiogram or a traditional angiogram to better define the abnormality and to counsel the patient regarding the risk of surgery.[17]

Intraoperative damage to the carotid artery occurs with an incidence of 0.78% to 1.16%.[17,18] Of the 28 vascular complications reported in a series of 3061 procedures, 7 were fatal, thus leading to an associated mortality rate of 29%.[17] The rate of vascular complications is increased among patients with acromegaly and large invasive adenomas (particularly those with cavernous sinus involvement). In addition, patients who have received prior radiation therapy or who have had a prior transsphenoidal surgery, radiosurgery, or craniotomy are also at increased risk. As such, these patients are particularly benefited by the imaging of the carotids preoperatively. In fact, some surgeons believe that prior transsphenoidal surgery and craniotomy are contraindications to minimally invasive pituitary surgery, although the authors do not feel that this is the case.

If carotid injury does occur, it is recommended to pack the area with resorbable materials (Gelfoam [Pfizer, Belgium] or Surgicel [Johnson and Johnson, Arlington, TX], muscle, fat, or Cottonoid patties to control the hemorrhage but, if possible, not so tightly as to occlude the vessel. An angiogram should be emergently performed to evaluate the extent of injury to the carotid artery. If the injury is significant, balloon occlusion is usually performed, or, alternatively, control of the carotid in the neck may be performed. If the angiogram is initially normal, it should be repeated on postoperative day 6 to 10 to ensure that the patient is not discharged only to have a catastrophic hemorrhagic event. It is important to stress that delayed life-threatening epistaxis can occur 2 to 10 years postoperatively as a result of the rupture of a false aneurysm or an internal carotid–cavernous sinus fistula[18,19] (Figure 45-3). If there is any suspicion of carotid injury, vessel imaging must be performed.

Cavernous sinus thrombosis can occur during the immediate postoperative period or in a delayed fashion (Figure 45-4). This complication can present with cranial neuropathy as a result of impingement on the abducens, oculomotor, trochlear, or trigeminal nerves. Abducens nerve palsy is the most common because it is the most medial neural structure within the cavernous sinus. When this occurs during the immediate postoperative period, overaggressive packing should be suspected, and consideration should be given to packing removal or

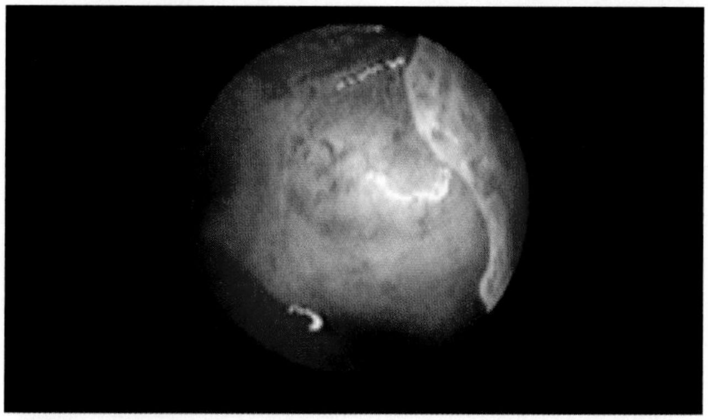

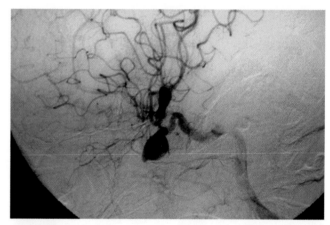

Figure 45-3. Angiogram depicting a carotid artery pseudoaneurysm.

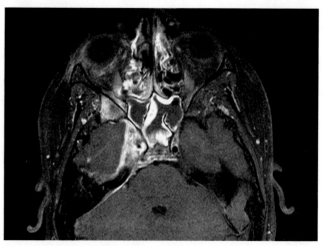

Figure 45-4. Magnetic resonance image displaying cavernous sinus thrombosis on the right.

Figure 45-2. Endoscopic view demonstrating a dehiscent carotid artery within the left sphenoid sinus.

reduction. When cavernous sinus thrombosis occurs in a delayed fashion, it can be caused by an expanding clot within the sinus or an inflammatory reaction to the packing material. Again, packing removal should be considered, and steroids are also prescribed with close observation. These individuals require imaging of the cavernous carotid as well to rule out a false aneurysm or the early development of a carotid–cavernous fistula.[17]

Intracranial vascular morbidity includes subdural hemorrhage, subarachnoid hemorrhage, vasospasm, and intrasellar or suprasellar hemorrhage. Woollons and colleagues[20] reported three instances of intracranial hemorrhage in their series of 165 patients, which led to significant comorbidity, including 2 individuals who experienced visual loss as a result of the hemorrhage. In each of these cases, hemorrhage occurred in the presence of the subtotal resection of a macroadenoma, thereby stressing the need for the meticulous and complete removal of tumor. Change in neurologic status or any new cranial neuropathy should alert the practitioner to this potential complication. A CT scan or an MRI should be obtained, and the patient may require an emergent craniotomy (Figure 45-5).

Early postoperative epistaxis occurs with an incidence of 0.15% to 3.4% (see Table 45-2), and it is usually caused by bleeding from the sphenopalatine artery itself or, more commonly, from the mucosal branches, including the posterior septal artery that crosses the inferior face of the sphenoid sinus. Often the vessel goes into vasospasm during the procedure as a result of topical or injected vasoconstricting agents, but care should be taken to definitively control the bleeding vessel with cautery to prevent postoperative hemorrhage when the agents wear off (Figure 45-6). Intraoperative bleeding from the cavernous sinuses is usually easily controlled by packing and the placement of hemostatic materials. As previously noted, early postoperative epistaxis usually occurs as a result of a nasal vessel such as the posterior septal artery. However, delayed hemorrhage may result from the rupture of a false aneurysm of the carotid or a carotid–cavernous fistula; therefore all patients who present with delayed massive epistaxis should be evaluated with vessel imaging.

Neurologic Complications

Tension pneumocephalus occurs with an estimated incidence of 0.42%.[21] Patients often present with a change in mental status, headache, and cranial nerve deficits. Conservative management with 100% oxygen and strict bed rest can often be sufficient; however, craniotomy may be required to decompress the cranial vault. Pneumosella (i.e., air confined to the sella) can also rarely occur, and it presents uniquely as progressive bitemporal hemianopsia, a change in vision, and with variably occurring headache 2 to 4 weeks after surgery. Yorgason and colleagues[22] reported a patient with increasing visual symptoms 6 months after the resection of a nonsecreting benign pituitary adenoma with suprasellar extension. The endoscopic decompression of the pneumosella was performed. Intraoperatively, a small defect was noted in the floor of the sella, and, after adequate decompression, the sella was not packed, and the floor was repaired with a hemostatic agent and fibrin glue and then bolstered into place with nasal packs. The pneumosella recurred, and the patient was subsequently successfully reconstructed with a fat graft.[22] The avoidance of heavy lifting, straining, and nose blowing after transsphenoidal surgery are imperative to prevent pneumocephalus and pneumosella.

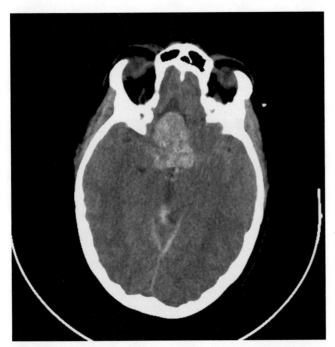

Figure 45-5. Axial computed tomography scan showing an intracranial hemorrhage in the setting of a subtotally resected pituitary adenoma.

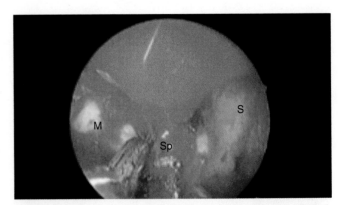

Figure 45-6. Endoscopic view of the sphenopalatine artery during cauterization. *M*, Maxillary sinus; *S*, sphenoid sinus; *SP*, sphenopalatine artery.

Other neurologic sequelae including stroke and seizure occur in up to 1% of transsphenoidal procedures (see Table 45-2). Vasospasm occurs rarely, with only a few case reports in the literature. Blood in the subarachnoid space as a result of surgery may cause cerebral vasospasm leading to infarction in the distribution of a specific vessel. Treatment is usually controlled hypertension and observation.[23]

Sinonasal Complications

Sinonasal morbidity is considered morbidity caused by the surgical approach, and it includes upper-lip numbness, septal deviation, synechiae, septal perforation, anosmia, and mucocele. Results of the national survey by Ciric and colleagues[9] found that one third of surgeons observed nasal septal perforation, with an incidence of 3.3% to 7.6% (Figure 45-7). The specifics regarding approach were not included, and therefore it is unknown if the sublabial or endonasal approach was used. A retrospective investigation of endonasal complications after sublabial and endonasal pituitary surgery was performed in 1999.[24] Patients undergoing the endoscopic procedure overall had fewer endonasal complications. For example, in the endonasal endoscopic group, there were two septal perforations that were posterior in nature and not symptomatic as compared with the sublabial group, in which the septal perforations were larger and symptomatic. At the authors' institution, White and colleagues[25] compared the first 50 minimally invasive pituitary surgeries with the last 50 pituitary procedures performed via the sublabial transseptal approach at the institution. There was a significant decrease in sinonasal complications in the endonasal endoscopic group, including epistaxis ($P = .031$), upper-lip anesthesia ($P = .013$), and septal deviation ($P = .028$). The use of minimally invasive endoscopic techniques instead of traditional translabial approaches eliminates the complications of poorly fitting dentures, facial pain, the loss of tip projection, and upper-lip anesthesia. Wider application of the endoscopic technique with the minimization of mucosal trauma in the sinonasal cavity should continue to decrease the incidence of endonasal complications. However, in all cases, care should continue to be taken to not create mucosal tears on opposing mucosal surfaces.

Cerebrospinal Fluid Rhinorrhea and Fistula

Although the hypophysis is extradural, CSF leak is the most common major surgical morbidity associated with minimally invasive pituitary surgery. This can occur as a result of the arachnoid collapsing through the diaphragma intraoperatively or postoperatively, a large suprasellar extent of tumors that necessitate extensive dissection, an inadvertent dural tear, or an incompetent diaphragma. CSF leaks can occur intraoperatively, or they can present days after surgery, which allows them to be categorized as either intraoperative or postoperative. The incidence of intraoperative CSF leak is 0.2% to 58.0%, and the incidence of postoperative CSF leak that requires extended treatment, including lumbar draining or surgical repair, is 0.4% to 6.0% (Table 45-3).

When CSF leaks are visualized intraoperatively, they should be immediately repaired, because meningitis or tension pneumocephalus can occur if the leak is not initially recognized. However, it has been questioned whether every procedure requires sellar reconstruction. Cappabianca and colleagues[26] recommend the following strategy:

1. Do not repair in the setting of microadenomas, macroadenomas without suprasellar extension, or macroadenomas with suprasellar extension that is incompletely removed.

2. Pack the sella if there is prolapse of suprasellar cistern toward sellar floor or bleeding from the medial wall of the cavernous sinus or the internal carotid artery injury.

3. Pack the sella with or without packing the sphenoid sinus in patients with paninvasive macroadenoma and intraoperative CSF leak.

At the authors' institution, Sonnenburg and colleagues[27] recommended sellar reconstruction only with evidence of intraoperative CSF leak. There was a comparable rate of postoperative CSF leak if no intraoperative leak was identified in the presence or absence of sellar repair. In addition, donor-site morbidity was decreased as a result of the decreased need to harvest fat for sellar reconstruction.

No prospective studies have compared the various techniques of sellar reconstruction to determine whether one technique results in the superior prevention of postoperative CSF leaks and meningitis after transsphenoidal surgery. A risk factor for the inability to control a CSF

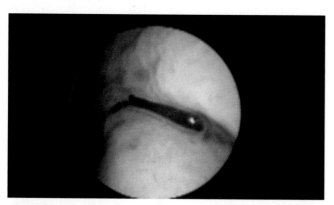

Figure 45-7. Endoscopic view of septal perforation after transsphenoidal hypophysectomy.

TABLE 45-3 Cerebrospinal Fluid Leak and CSF Leak and MIPS*

Study	Procedures	Intraoperative Leak	Postoperative Leak†	Meningitis in Those with Postoperative Leak
Jho et al, 1997[39]	50	1 (0.2%)	2 (0.4%)	Not reported
Ciric et al, 1997[9]	638	Not reported	7 (1.09%)	Not reported
Ciric et al, 1997[9]	Survey results	Not reported	590 (3.9%)	Not reported
Semple et al, 1999[33‡]	105	Not reported	1 (0.95%)	Not reported
Woollons et al, 2000[20]	185	Not reported	4.30%	Not reported
Jho, 2001[40]	160	Not reported	6.00%	Not reported
Cappabianca et al, 2002[11]	146	Not reported	3 (2.05%)	Not reported
Zada et al, 2003[41]	100	57 (57%)	3 (3%)	Not reported
Shiley et al, 2003[28]	217	70 (32.7%)	13 (6.0%)	1 (7.69%)
Sonnenburg et al, 2003[27]	45	8 (17.78%)	1 (3.5%)	0
Hammer et al, 2004[12‡]	289	Not reported	11 (3.8%)	Not reported
van Aken et al, 2004[14]	278	70 (25.2%)	3 (1.1 %)	2 (66%)
Sade et al, 2006[30]	129	43 (33.3%)	2 (1.6%)	2 (100%)
Dusick et al, 2006[37]	259	150 (58%)	8 (3.1%)	Not reported

*Intraoperative and postoperative cerebrospinal fluid leak after transsphenoidal hypophysectomy with associated meningitis, when reported.
†Defined cerebrospinal leak requiring lumbar drain or surgical repair.
‡All patients with Cushing disease.

leak is hydrocephalus, and these patients may ultimately require a ventriculoperitoneal shunt to relieve the CSF leak.[28] Numerous substances have been used for sellar repair, including mucosal and fascial grafts, cartilage and bone fragments, Surgicel, Avitene, lypophilized pericardial bovine graft, dural graft, fibrin glue, muscle, and fat. The authors favor microfibrillar collagen and abdominal fat bolstered with a small resorbable reconstruction miniplate cut to fit under the bone edges of the sella (Figure 45-8). In 2000, a retrospective review of 53 CSF fistulas did not demonstrate any correlation between the success of the repair with the grafting material used.[29] The choice of material is most often made on the basis of surgeon preference and the availability of grafting material rather than an improved outcome of the repair. Some advocate against using fat, because this can impede postoperative tumor surveillance with MRI.[30] Other groups, including the authors' group, find fat resorption appropriate and have not found the fat to interfere with postoperative surveillance.[27]

Postoperative leaks can be treated conservatively with bed rest and head elevation or with repeated lumbar puncture, the placement of a lumbar drain, or surgical reexploration with repair if the leak continues to persist. No studies comparing the nonoperative and operative management of postoperative CSF leak have been performed to date. When placed, the lumbar drain is usually left in place for 3 to 5 days, and drainage is performed at 8 cm³ to 10 cm³ of CSF per hour to allow the defect to heal. Potential advantages of early surgical intervention for postoperative CSF leak include a decreased hospital stay, a decreased risk of developing meningitis for those patients who fail conservative management (lumbar drain) and ultimately require surgical intervention, and possibly avoiding the risk associated with lumbar drain.[28] In 2004, van Aken and colleagues[13] argued for the placement of a lumbar drain in all patients who experience an intraoperative CSF leak. However, lumbar drains do carry their own risks, including meningitis, the overdrainage of CSF, pneumocephalus, temporary blindness and weakness, and cerebellar herniation. Therefore other groups advocate for the placement of lumbar drains only in those individuals at high risk for postoperative CSF leak. The authors do not perform routine lumbar drainage, instead placing lumbar drains only in selected patients who are at high risk for postoperative CSF leak.

There are a few risk factors associated with an increased risk of CSF leak that may guide the surgeon with regard to the decision of whether to perform sellar reconstruction

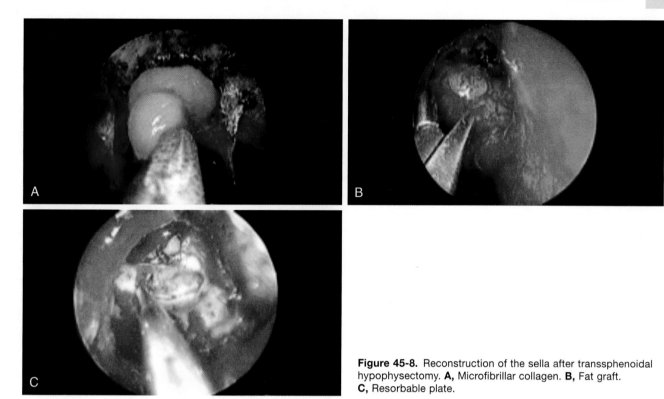

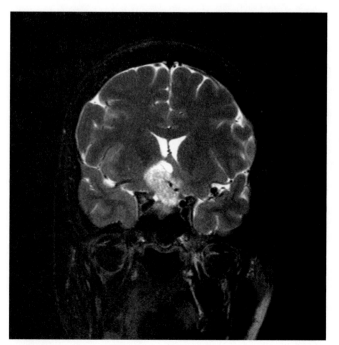

Figure 45-8. Reconstruction of the sella after transsphenoidal hypophysectomy. **A,** Microfibrillar collagen. **B,** Fat graft. **C,** Resorbable plate.

intraoperatively. In 2006, Sade and colleagues[30] determined that, if there is suprasellar extension of the tumor, there is a much increased risk of postoperative CSF leak ($P = .007$; Figures 45-9 and 45-10). Pituitary adenomas were also found to be a risk factor in this study ($P = .48$). By contrast, in a similar study by Shiley and colleagues,[28]

nonadenomatous disease was a risk factor on univariate analysis. On multivariate analysis, however, those authors found intraoperative CSF leak ($P = .004$), revision surgery ($P = .0096$), and closure of the sella ($P = .031$) to be independent risk factors for postoperative CSF leak rather than the tumor type (i.e., adenoma vs. nonadenoma). Prior

Figure 45-9. Coronal magnetic resonance image depicting a dumbbell-shaped tumor with suprasellar extension and compression of the lateral ventricle.

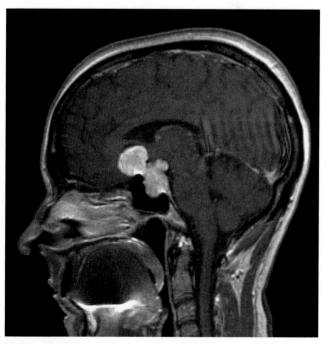

Figure 45-10. Sagittal magnetic resonance image of a dumbbell-shaped tumor.

surgery leads to scarring and altered anatomy that results in a more difficult dissection than primary surgery. Revision surgery is also often performed for a tumor that was not easily visualized or resected at the time of the initial procedure that then necessitates more aggressive dissection along the diaphragma at the time of the repeat procedure, thus creating an increased risk for CSF leak. In addition, Cushing (adrenocorticotropic hormone) adenomas are often not well localized on preoperative scanning, which leads to more aggressive dissection and an up to 80% chance of CSF leak.[28]

During the postoperative period, all patients should be questioned regarding persistent salty rhinorrhea or postnasal drip, and the reservoir test can be performed (i.e., the patient is asked to lean forward and, with the head in a downward tilted position, observed for the leakage of clear fluid). Fluid can be sent for evaluation in the laboratory with β-2 transferrin if there is any question regarding the nature of the rhinorrhea. A CSF leak can occur after patients are discharged, so all patients should be instructed to return with any suspicious symptoms to avoid the risk of meningitis.

Endocrine Complications

Anterior and posterior pituitary dysfunction can complicate the postoperative course after transsphenoidal hypophysectomy. Most frequently, posterior pituitary dysfunction occurs in the form of diabetes insipidus (DI) and rarely as the syndrome of inappropriate ADH (SIADH) secretion. The adenohypophysis is less commonly affected, and usually only one axis is involved.

DI arises as a result of a deficiency of ADH causing poorly concentrated polyuria and increased serum osmolality. This is usually defined as urine output of more than 300 ml per hour for 3 hours with a urine specific gravity of less than 1.005. A serum sodium level of more than 145 mEq/L is particularly suggestive of DI. As a result of the half-life of ADH, DI does not usually begin until several hours postoperatively. Most commonly, DI is transient, occurring during the first 24 to 72 hours, but it complicates up to 31% of pituitary surgery. Permanent DI occurs in 0.25% to 9.0% of cases (Table 45-4). The cause of postoperative DI is thought to be threefold. It is primarily thought to result from the interruption of ADH transport from the hypothalamus as well as from the impairment of ADH release from the neurohypophysis and retrograde damage to cell bodies in the paraventricular and supraventricular nuclei in the hypothalamus. Factors associated with an increased risk of the development of transient DI postoperatively include microadenoma, Rathke cleft cyst, craniopharyngioma, and the occurrence of intraoperative CSF leak.[31] In the authors' series, the greatest risk of DI was found to be the presence of Rathke cleft cysts.[32] It is thought that macroadenomas tend to displace the stalk and the posterior lobe, thus leading to a relatively infrequent incidence of permanent postoperative DI in this patient population.[9]

TABLE 45-4   Postoperative Endocrine Dysfunction*

Study	Procedures	Postoperative DI	Permanent DI	Anterior Pituitary Dysfunction
Jho et al, 1997[39]	50	2 (1.0%)	1 (0.05%)	6 (0.05%)
Ciric et al, 1997[9]	638	22 (3.44%)	Not reported	Not reported
Ciric et al, 1997[9]	Survey results	748 (17.8%)	Not reported	563 (19.4%)
Semple et al, 1999[34†]	105	12 (11.4%)	1 (0.95%)	1 (0.95%)
Hensen J, 1999[43]	1571	487 (31.0%)	4 (0.25%)	37 (2.4%)
Woollons et al, 2000[20]	185	9 (4.9%)	7 (3.8%)	Not reported
Jho, 2001[40]	160	6.4 (4%)	4 (3%)	17 (11.0%)
Cappabianca et al, 2002[11]	146	13 (8.9%)	5 (3.4%)	20 (13.6%)
Zada et al, 2003[41]	100	25 (25.0%)	9 (9.0%)	6 (6.0%)
Dusick et al, 2006[37]	259	Not reported	10 (3.9%)	4 (1.5%)
Nemergut et al, 2005[31]	857	157 (18.3%)	17 (2.0%)	Not reported

DI, Diabetes insipidus.
*Postoperative transient and permanent DI listed with anterior pituitary dysfunction after transsphenoidal pituitary surgery.
†All patients with Cushing disease.

Most authors advocate for minimal intervention with close monitoring when polyuria occurs in the postoperative setting, because most cases will resolve spontaneously within days. In addition, most postoperative patients are awake, alert, and able to tolerate adequate oral intake to match their high urine output. However, these patients do need to be monitored, because if DI becomes severe, decreased mental status, seizures, coma, hypotension, acute renal tubular necrosis, and renal failure can occur. Desmopressin, which is a synthetic analog of vasopressin, is given if the patient's oral intake is significantly less than their output, if the serum sodium level rises to more than 145 mEq/L, or if excessive urine output interferes with sleep.

Damage to the neurohypophysis can also result in SIADH. This occurs in a euvolemic state with a serum sodium concentration of less than 135 mEq/L, a plasma osmolality of less than 280 mOsm/kg, a urine concentration of more than 100 mOsm/kg, and an elevated urine sodium concentration of more than 20 mEq/L. SIADH occurs approximately 7 days postoperatively, when most patients have already been discharged to home. The main treatment for SIADH is fluid restriction, and the dysfunction is usually transient in nature. Olson and colleagues[33] found that the severity and type of posterior pituitary dysfunction after pituitary surgery is related to the degree of surgical manipulation of the pituitary stalk, with SIADH related to less aggressive dissection. Unlike DI, SIADH occurs in a slightly delayed fashion after pituitary surgery; therefore all patients and their families should be counseled regarding the risks of hyponatremia.

The adenohypophysis is damaged with much less frequency than the neurohypophysis. As shown in Table 45-4, the incidence is found to be between 0.05% and 13.6%. Any of the hormonal axes may be aberrant after surgery, although most frequently only one axis is involved. The resection of large macroadenomas increases the risk of damaging the anterior pituitary, and therefore extra caution should be taken to preserve any residual normal tissue during the procedure. In addition, postoperative dysfunction is more likely to occur if hormone dysfunction was present preoperatively.[19]

Particularly concerning during the postoperative period is the disruption of endogenous steroid production, which leads to the routine administration of supplemental steroids during the postoperative period. In addition, patients should undergo thyroid function testing during the postoperative period with appropriate supplementation if deficits are seen. In all cases, the authors recommend close follow up by an endocrinologist for the care of these patients given the range of endocrine complications that can ensue postoperatively.

Ophthalmologic Complications

Loss of vision and ophthalmoplegia are rare complications of transsphenoidal hypophysectomy, with an incidence of 0.3% to 1.4% (see Table 45-2). Visual changes can be the result of optic nerve trauma, infarction, compression from hematoma, or herniation into an empty sella. Damage to the nerves coursing through the cavernous sinuses can lead to ophthalmoplegia, with damage to the abducens being more common than that of the oculomotor nerve as a result of its more medial course. Direct injury to the optic nerve or chiasm can occur during tumor resection or with the aggressive manipulation of the diaphragma. If this occurs, glucocorticosteroids may help to reduce the associated inflammation and protect any viable optic tissue. Infarction of the optic nerves or tract can occur during dissection if there is adherence of the tumor capsule to the optic apparatus. This occurs most commonly in macroadenomas and when the tumor is compromising the optic apparatus preoperatively. Postoperative hematoma may cause compression on the optic nerve or chiasm, which can often be reversible if the area is evacuated expeditiously. When a Hardy speculum is used for exposure, the force can dissipate through the orbit, thereby causing fracture of the optic foramen or orbit; applying the technique of the endoscopic endonasal procedure can avoid this complication altogether. During reconstruction of the sella, overzealous packing may result in the compression of the optic nerves and subsequent visual impairment, which should be seen on a CT scan or an MRI. Cerebral vasospasm leading to infarction of the optic nerve tract has also been shown to cause postoperative visual changes. Potential risk factors for postoperative visual impairment include suprasellar extension, a history of surgery or radiation, and a dumbbell-shaped tumor (i.e., when there is suprasellar extension of the tumor but it is separated from the intrasellar portion by a tight constriction at the diaphragma).[23] Preventive measures include careful dissection, intraoperative stereotactic guidance, and the avoidance of monopolar cautery to prevent heat injury to the optic nerve.

Medical Complications

Medical complications after minimally invasive hypophysectomy are similar to complications found among patients undergoing general anesthesia for other surgical procedures. It is important to note that the majority of mortality reported during the last decade after transsphenoidal hypophysectomy has been the result of deep vein thrombosis or pulmonary embolism. The risk of deep vein thrombosis is even higher among patients with Cushing disease, and these patients should receive aggressive prophylaxis; some facilities are even using empiric aspirin therapy starting on postoperative day 2. It has been hypothesized that, in addition to the routine postoperative immobility and hypercoagulability, the obesity associated with Cushing disease places these patients at increased risk for medical complications.[34] Other medical complications, including pneumonia and urinary tract infection, do not occur with increased incidence among this population.

Anesthesia-Related Complications

Many patients with pituitary pathology have an increased anesthesia risk as a result of hypertension, obesity, electrolyte abnormalities, and cardiac disease. In addition, excessive growth hormone in acromegaly affects the heart, thus leading to cardiac myopathy and pharyngeal tissue; this leads to hypertrophy of the base of the tongue and redundant mucosa, thereby creating a potentially difficult intubation. The evaluation of the airway with flexible fiber-optic nasopharyngolaryngoscopy is preferred preoperatively to assess the amount of pharyngeal involvement in the disease process. Nasotracheal intubation is not possible, because the nasal cavities should remain accessible to the surgeon to perform the procedure. Flexible fiber-optic orotracheal intubation may be necessary if the patient cannot be intubated in the standard fashion. Individuals with Cushing disease and acromegaly are also at increased risk of obstructive sleep apnea, thus further increasing the risk of anesthesia in this population.[35]

Nausea and vomiting should be avoided to decrease the risk of exacerbating electrolyte imbalances and thus increasing intracranial pressure and the possible creation of CSF leak. Aggressive prophylaxis continues to be suggested even though a review of 877 of patients undergoing endonasal transsphenoidal hypophyseal surgery demonstrated an incidence of postoperative emesis of 7.5% irrespective of prophylaxis. Risk factors for postoperative nausea and vomiting were the placement of a fat graft ($P = .001$) and the placement of a lumbar drain ($P = .001$).[7,36] However, it is unclear whether these conditions are independent risk factors or whether they are simply markers of more aggressive dissection and manipulation of the hypophysis and intraoperative CSF leak.

QUALITY OF LIFE

Overall, minimally invasive surgery of the pituitary is safe and effective, and the majority of patients have a superb outcome and postoperative quality of life as a result of the short duration of the hospital stay and no need for nasal packing. Patients who had a revision endonasal hypophysectomy after having a prior sublabial approach stated that the endonasal procedure overall had an easier recovery, less pain, and better nasal airflow. In addition, patients who had nasal packing placed postoperatively had a significantly worse postoperative experience than those who did not ($P = .001$). Patients'

recovery is relatively rapid, with 61% returning to work or school by 1 month postoperatively and 74% returning by 2 months.[37] However, serious complications can arise that can greatly affect an individual's quality of life. These include death, diabetes insipidus, ophthalmoplegia, visual loss, meningitis, and CSF leak, and they need to be discussed with the patient preoperatively.

FUTURE DIRECTIONS

The continued improvement of optics, improved image guidance with real-time updating capabilities, and intraoperative MRI will continue to advance the surgical technique and increase patient safety. Image guidance has helped to advance the field of minimally invasive approaches to the hypophysis by increasing physician comfort and decreasing operative time without any true change in mortality and morbidity rates.[38] However, this will continue to evolve, with possibilities including increased accuracy, increased quality of images, and dynamic image guidance systems becoming available to help assist the surgeon intraoperatively.

REFERENCES

1. Couldwell WT: Transsphenoidal and transcranial surgery for pituitary adenomas. *J Neurooncol* 2004;69:237–256.
2. Jankowski R, Auque J, Simon C, et al: Endoscopic pituitary surgery. *Laryngoscope* 1992;102:198–202.
3. Cappabianca P, Cavallo LM, de Divitiis E: Endoscopic endonasal transsphenoidal surgery. *Neurosurgery* 2004;55:933–941.
4. Rosen MR, Saigal K, Evans J, et al: A review of the endoscopic approach to the pituitary through the sphenoid sinus. *Curr Opin Otolaryngol Head Neck Surg* 2006;14:6–13.
5. Jho HD, Carrau RL, Ko Y, et al: Endoscopic pituitary surgery: An early experience. *Surg Neurol* 1997;47:213–223.
6. Renn WH, Rhoton AL Jr: Microsurgical anatomy of sellar region. *J Neurosurg* 1975;43:288–298.
7. Nemergut EC, Dumont AS, Barry UT, et al: Perioperative management of patients undergoing transsphenoidal pituitary surgery. *Anesth Analg* 2005;101:1170–1181.
8. Kennedy DW, Cohn ES, Papel ID, et al: Transsphenoidal approach to the sella: The Johns Hopkins experience. *Laryngoscope* 1984;94:1066–1074.
9. Ciric I, Ragin A, Baumgartner C, et al: Complications of transsphenoidal surgery: Results of a national survey, review of the literature, and personal experience. *Neurosurgery* 1997;40(2):225–237.
10. Onesti ST, Post KD: Complications of transsphenoidal microsurgery. In Post KD, Friedman E, McCormick P, editors: *Postoperative complications in intracranial neurosurgery,* New York, 1993, Thieme Medical Publishers.
11. Cappabianca P, Cavallo LM, Colao AM, et al: Surgical complications associated with the endoscopic endonasal transsphenoidal approach for pituitary adenomas. *J Neurosurg* 2002;97:293–298.
12. Hammer GD, Tyrrell JB, Lamborn KR, et al: Transsphenoidal microsurgery for Cushing's disease: Initial outcome and long-term results. *J Clin Endocrinol Metab* 2004;89:6348–6357.
13. Van Aken MO, Feelders RA, de Marie S, et al: Cerebrospinal fluid leakage during transsphenoidal surgery: Postoperative external lumbar drainage reduces the risk for meningitis. *Pituitary* 2004;7:89–93.
14. Van Aken MO, de Marie S, van der Lely AJ, et al: Risk factors for meningitis alter transsphenoidal surgery. *Clin Infect Dis* 1997;25:852–856.
15. Romanowski B, Tyrrell DLJ, Weir DKA, et al: Meningitis complicating transsphenoidal hypophysectomy. *Can Med Assoc J* 1981;124:1172–1175.

16. Batra PS, Citardi MJ, Lanza DC: Isolated sphenoid sinusitis after transsphenoidal hypophysectomy. *Am J Rhinol* 2005;19(2):185–189.
17. Laws ER: Vascular complications of transsphenoidal surgery. *Pituitary* 1999;2:163–170.
18. Raymond J, Hardy J, Czepko R, et al: Arterial injuries in transsphenoidal surgery for pituitary adenoma: The role of angiography and endovascular treatment. *Am J Neuroradiol* 1997;18:655–665.
19. Ahuja A, Guterman L, Hopkins LN: Carotid cavernous fistula and false aneurysm of the cavernous carotid artery: Complications of transsphenoidal surgery. *Neurosurgery* 1992;31(4):774–779.
20. Woollons AC, Balakrishnan V, Hunn MK, et al: Complications of transsphenoidal surgery: The Wellington experience. *ANZ J Surg* 2000;70:405–401.
21. Satyarthee GD, Mahapatra: Tension pneumocephalus following transsphenoidal hypophysectomy. *Am J Rhinol* 2005;19(2):185–189.
22. Yorgason JG, Arthur AS, Orlandi RR, et al: Endoscopic decompression of tension pneumosella following transsphenoidal pituitary tumor resection. *Pituitary* 2004;7:171–177.
23. Barrow DL, Tindall GT: Loss of vision after transsphenoidal surgery. *Neurosurgery* 1990;27(1):60–68.
24. Korean I, Hadar T, Rappaport Z, et al: Endoscopic transnasal transsphenoidal microsurgery versus the sublabial approach for treatment of pituitary tumors: Endonasal complications. *Laryngoscope* 1999;109(11):1838–1840.
25. White DR, Sonnenburg RE, Ewend MG, et al: Safety of minimally invasive pituitary surgery (MIPS) compared with a traditional approach. *Laryngoscope* 2004;114:1945–1948.
26. Cappabianca P, Cavallo LM, Esposito F, et al: Sellar repair in endoscopic endonasal transsphenoidal surgery: Results of 170 cases. *Neurosurgery* 2002;51(6):1365–1372.
27. Sonnenburg RE, White D, Ewend MG, et al: Sellar reconstruction: Is it necessary? *Am J Rhinol* 2003;17:343–346.
28. Shiley SG, Limonadi F, Delashaw JB, et al: Incidence, etiology and management of cerebrospinal fluid leaks following transsphenoidal surgery. *Laryngoscope* 2003;113:1283–1288.
29. Zweig JL, Carrau RL, Celin SE, et al: Endoscopic repair of cerebrospinal fluid leaks to the sinonasal tract: Predictors of success. *Otolaryngol Head Neck Surg* 2000;123:195–201.
30. Sade B, Mohr G, Frenkiel S: Management of intra-operative cerebrospinal fluid leak in transnasal transsphenoidal pituitary microsurgery: Use of post-operative lumbar drain and sellar reconstruction without fat packing. *Acta Neurochir (Wien)* 2006;148:13–19.
31. Nemergut EC, Zuo Z, Jane JA, et al: Predictors of diabetes insipidus after transsphenoidal surgery: A review of 881 patients. *J Neurosurg* 2005;103:448–454.
32. Sigounas DG, Sharpless JL, Cheng DM, et al: Predictors and incidence of central diabetes insipidus after endoscopic pituitary surgery. *Neurosurgery* 2008;62:71–78.
33. Olson BR, Gumowski J, Rubino D, et al: Pathophysiology of hyponatremia after transsphenoidal pituitary surgery. *J Neurosurg* 1997;87:499–507.
34. Semple PL, Laws ER Jr: Complications in a contemporary series of patients who underwent transsphenoidal surgery for Cushing's disease. *J Neurosurg* 1999;91(2):175–179.
35. Mickelson S, Rosenthal L, Rock J, et al: Obstructive sleep apnea syndrome and acromegaly. *Otolaryngol Head Neck Surg* 1994;111:25–30.
36. Flynn BC, Nemergut EC: Postoperative nausea and vomiting and pain after transsphenoidal surgery: A review of 877 patients. *Anesth Analg* 2006;103:162–167.
37. Dusick JR, Esposito F, Mattozo CA, et al: Endonasal transsphenoidal surgery: The patient's perspective—Survey results from 259 patients. *Surg Neurol* 2006;65:332–342.
38. Lasio G, Ferroli P, Felisati G, et al: Image-guided endoscopic transnasal removal of recurrent pituitary adenomas. *Neurosurgery* 2002;51(1):132–137.
39. Jho HD, Carrau RL: Endoscopic endonasal transsphenoidal surgery: Experience with 50 patients. *J Neurosurg* 1997;87:44–51.
40. Jho HD: Endoscopic transsphenoidal surgery. *J Neurooncol* 2001;54:187–195.
41. Zada G, Kelly DF, Cohan P, et al: Endonasal transsphenoidal approach for pituitary adenomas and other sellar lesions: An assessment of efficacy, safety and patient impressions. *J Neurosurg* 2003;98:350–358.
42. Netea-Maier RT, van Lindert EJ, den Heijer M, et al: Transsphenoidal pituitary surgery via the endoscopic technique: Results in 35 consecutive patients with Cushing's disease. *Eur J Endocrinol* 2006;154:675–684.
43. Hensen J, Henig A, Fahlbusch R, et al: Prevalence, predictors and patterns of postoperative polyuria and hyponatraemia in the immediate course after transsphenoidal surgery for pituitary adenomas. *Clin Endocrinol (Oxf)* 1999;50:431–439.
44. Kawamata T, Iseki H, Ishizaki R, et al: Minimally invasive endoscope-assisted endonasal trans-sphenoidal microsurgery for pituitary tumors: Experience with 215 cases comparing with sublabial trans-sphenoidal approach. *Neurol Res* 2002;24:259–265.

CHAPTER 46

Complications of Maxillofacial Trauma Surgery

David M. Saito and Andrew H. Murr

GENERAL CONSIDERATIONS

The most critical factors in the care of the trauma patient are the initial evaluation and resuscitation performed in the emergency department setting. A systematic approach to the trauma victim allows for an orderly assessment designed to identify life-threatening injuries while essential resuscitative efforts are put into motion. Victims of maxillofacial trauma are subject to immediate and potentially fatal complications related to these injuries and associated conditions. In a series of 151 patients with maxillofacial fractures, Alvi and colleagues[1] found high rates of concomitant cerebral hematoma (44%), pulmonary contusion (18%), pneumothorax (14%), intraabdominal injury (14%), and cervical spine injury (7%). Therefore it is imperative that a thorough and orderly trauma evaluation be accomplished whenever the diagnosis of maxillofacial trauma is encountered.

Advance Trauma Life Support: The International Standard for Trauma Management

The American College of Surgeons algorithm (i.e., Advanced Trauma Life Support [ATLS]) is now the international standard for trauma management. The correct application of ATLS principles reduces the mortality of trauma victims during the critical first "golden hour" after presentation.[2] ATLS emphasizes a protocol divided into a primary survey, resuscitation, a secondary survey, and definitive care. The primary survey hinges on the serial assessment of the "ABCs": airway, breathing, and circulation. Resuscitation occurs simultaneously with the primary survey as necessary. The secondary survey is performed immediately afterward and consists of a meticulous physical examination of the disrobed patient. Elements of the secondary survey include phlebotomy (for early blood counts, chemistries, arterial blood gasses, and typing with cross-matching) and expedited imaging studies of the cervical spine, chest, and pelvis.

The investigation of possible cervical spine injuries plays a key part in the secondary survey. Radiographic imaging is mandatory except for cases in which clinical clearance of the spine is possible; this requires a fully alert patient who is free of intoxicating agents, who has no neurologic complaints or deficits and a completely pain-free neck and back, and who has no distracting painful injuries elsewhere. When indicated, the radiographic evaluation should include a true lateral cervical spine view (i.e., visualizing the occipitocervical junction and the C7-T1 disk space), an anteroposterior view, and open-mouth views. One study demonstrated that up to 99% of injuries can be detected by using these three views.[3] If the radiographs are inadequate or an injury is found, the trauma victim must then undergo a computed tomography (CT) scan of the cervical spine with coronal and sagittal reconstructions.[4]

Evaluation and Stabilization of the Airway

The evaluation and stabilization of the airway are the foundations of successful trauma management. Supplemental oxygen should be administered to all trauma patients.[5] Airway obstruction may be subtle, delayed, and easily overlooked in a patient with multiple injuries. Providers should have a high index of suspicion for airway compromise with maxillofacial trauma victims, and they need to frequently reassess the airway during the secondary survey and afterward. Blood, secretions, and foreign bodies can obstruct the airway in the oropharynx, the larynx, the hypopharynx, and the trachea. The oropharyngeal airway can be lost as a result of severe facial fractures, gross soft-tissue swelling, or diminished mental status as a result of intoxication or cerebral trauma. Direct laryngotracheal injury must also be considered. In a series of 27 patients with laryngeal fractures, Verschueren and colleagues[6] found that 96% also had maxillofacial injuries and that 74% required advanced airway interventions such as intubation, tracheotomy, or cricothyrotomy.

Initial maneuvers to clear the airway must not distort the patient's neck, and a concomitant cervical spine injury should be assumed until it can be excluded. A member of the trauma team must provide "in-line" stabilization by holding the cervical spine with the hands while immobilizing the head between the forearms. The jaw-thrust and chin-lift maneuvers can be used to prevent pharyngeal collapse, but they may be difficult to perform if there are severely comminuted mandibular fractures. High-volume suction must be available to evacuate blood and secretions. Posteriorly displaced midface fractures may be reduced by grasping the maxilla and pulling anteriorly, thereby improving the airway and slowing hemorrhage.[7] An oropharyngeal airway can be used in the unconscious patient. Another option is the laryngeal mask airway (LMA). Although it is cuffed to maintain its position and an air seal, it cannot protect the airway against regurgitation and aspiration. The LMA can be introduced into the pharynx through a narrow oral cavity while maintaining neck alignment, and the intubating version of the LMA can serve as a guide for tracheal intubation.[8]

Generally the use of nasopharyngeal airways, nasogastric tubes, and nasotracheal tubes is contraindicated for patients with severe midface injury as a result of the concern for iatrogenic intracranial penetration via a concomitant skull-base fracture. The intracranial placement of nasogastric tubes is most frequently reported,[9-12] likely because of their finer diameter and the associated poorer control over direction. Goodisson and colleagues[13] noted that three cases of the intracranial placement of nasotracheal tubes have been reported in the literature.[14-16] The authors also mention that only central anterior skull-base fractures could allow for the passage of an errant nasotracheal tube. In addition, a series of 82 patients with facial fractures who underwent blind nasotracheal intubation resulted in no cases of intracranial placement.[17] These studies suggest that nasotracheal intubation is a safe option for the patient with a maxillofacial injury. Nasotracheal intubation is the preferred route of intubation in the conscious patient, because it does not require neck extension or necessitate sedation or muscle relaxants.

Establishment of the Definitive Airway

The establishment of the "definitive airway" enables the control of ventilation, the administration of high levels of oxygen, and protection against aspiration.[18] This is best achieved with a cuffed tube in the trachea. The technique of choice is usually orotracheal intubation with in-line cervical spine immobilization. Although studies have shown that some movement of the cervical spine still occurs,[19] this method is generally safe in the presence of an unstable cervical spine injury.[20] Other options include blind nasotracheal intubation or fiber-optic assisted intubation. Fiber-optic assistance can be severely limited by bleeding, and the procedure requires trained personnel and expensive equipment. Retrograde intubation with a cricothyroid puncture and a guide wire has been described, but this is potentially time-consuming, and it is not well-established for the emergency setting.[21]

If the patient's anatomy or injuries (e.g., laryngeal trauma, massive facial distortion) make the timely insertion of an endotracheal tube impossible, it will be necessary to create a surgical airway. Repeated attempts at laryngoscopy can add further injury to the airway. Needle cricothyroidotomy is the best option for children, and it can be used as a temporizing measure in an adult patient while preparing for a surgical cricothyroidotomy. A 14-gauge needle with a plastic sheath is inserted through the cricothyroid membrane into the trachea. Oxygen is provided at 15 L per minute via a jet injector, a ventilating bag, or a wall outlet. Ventilation is attempted by giving 1-second injections of oxygen followed by 4-second exhalations. Complications of this approach include aspiration, esophageal injury, subcutaneous emphysema, pneumothorax, and progressive hypercarbia.[18]

Surgical cricothyroidotomy or tracheotomy is the preferred method for urgent surgical airway control. In a series of 5603 adult trauma patients, 66 required a cricothyroidotomy, and there were no complications reported as a result of the procedure.[22] The procedure is performed quickly, but it does require the identification of the cricothyroid membrane in a potentially distorted neck. It should not be attempted in children who are less than 12 years old and in the setting of complete laryngotracheal disruption.[5] Potential complications of cricothyroidotomy are vocal-cord damage, extratracheal tube placement, subcutaneous emphysema, and the later development of subglottic or tracheal stenosis.[23] Wound bleeding from the anterior jugular veins can occur during the attempt to obtain a surgical airway in an emergent situation. This hemorrhage is controlled after the airway is secured.

Emergency tracheotomy is another option for airway control. However, some regard it as a second choice for nonsurgeons or for those practitioners who are not well versed in tracheotomy as a result of its time requirement, difficulty, and potential complications.[7,18,24] A tracheotomy may be needed if a cricothyrotomy is unsafe, as is the case with laryngotracheal disruption or in the presence of an obstructing laryngeal tumor. In a series of 52 trauma patients with penetrating laryngotracheal injury, 3 patients required emergent tracheotomies, and 2 patients underwent cricothyroidotomy.[24]

Attending to the Circulatory System

After the airway has been secured and respiration problems addressed, attention should be paid to the circulatory system. The abdomen and pelvis must be evaluated with chest and pelvic radiographs along with diagnostic peritoneal lavage and bedside ultrasound examination. Facial hemorrhage has been reported in about 1 in 10 serious facial injuries.[25] Actively bleeding wounds (e.g., scalp lacerations) can be quickly and effectively addressed with a temporary suture closure in a running fashion. Severe epistaxis occurs in 2% to 4% of maxillofacial trauma victims,[26] and anterior and posterior nasal packing must be placed as necessary. If a urinary catheter is used as a posterior pack, there is the possibility of exacerbating fracture displacement by balloon inflation.[7]

All displaced facial fractures will bleed, and this bleeding may be unrecognized, because the patient often swallows the blood. Obvious midface and mandible fractures should be manually reduced. Frequent reassessments of the oropharynx for fresh blood should be conducted by the trauma team. Serial arterial blood gas assays may reveal a base deficit, which suggests lactic acidosis from continued hemorrhage.

Life-threatening bleeding can occur with major midface and panfacial injuries. In a series of 912 patients with facial injuries, the incidence of life-threatening hemorrhage among patients with Le Fort fractures was 5.5%.[27] There is extensive collateral blood supply to the midface from both the internal and external carotid arteries. If bleeding persists despite packing and pressure, angiography should be performed to detect the involved vessels. Selective transcatheter arterial embolization, as described by Bynoe and colleagues,[27] is an alternative to surgical neck exploration for uncontrollable bleeding.

Complications That Result from Alcohol and Illicit Drug Intoxication

Alcohol and illicit drug intoxication is intimately associated with maxillofacial trauma and complicates its management. A series of 6114 cases involving facial injuries in the United Kingdom revealed that at least 22% were associated with alcohol consumption.[28] Another study of trauma victims with operative mandible fractures found that 32% admitted to illicit drug use.[29] Alcohol and drug intoxication hampers the history taking and the physical examination of patients with facial injuries, and it complicates the administration of anesthesia for necessary surgical intervention (Figure 46-1). In addition, there is evidence that substance abuse leads to a higher rate of complications with maxillofacial trauma. In a series of 86 patients who underwent the surgical repair of mandible fractures, the rate of infectious complications was 20% among chronic substance abusers as compared with only 6% among nonabusers.[29] Likely reasons for this discrepancy include malnourishment, poor healing capacity, decreased compliance with postoperative instructions and medications, and neglected oral care among substance abusers.

Other Factors to Consider

After the initial assessment and resuscitation of the trauma patient has taken place, several other factors must be taken into account before the definitive management of maxillofacial injuries is attempted. The complete ATLS protocol must be carried out, with concomitant thoracic, abdominal, extremity, and pelvic injuries evaluated and managed by the trauma surgeons.

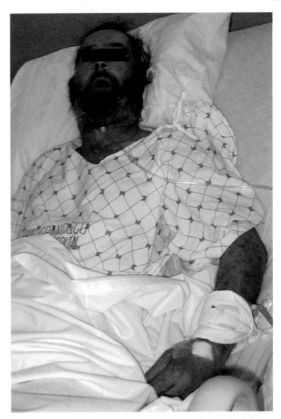

Figure 46-1. Belligerent abuser of many substances who required restraint when initially admitted for a mandible fracture. He became hypoxic when medicated and was intubated shortly after this picture was taken.

Central Nervous System Injuries

A high percentage of facial injury patients (i.e., 82% in the Alvi and colleagues[1] series) also have central nervous system injuries, such as cerebral hemorrhage (i.e., subdural and subarachnoid hemorrhage), cerebral contusions, and pneumocephalus. A full neurosurgical consultation and workup for such conditions must take priority over the treatment of maxillofacial injuries.

Open Wounds

The appropriate deferral of definitive facial reconstruction is possible with initial soft-tissue wound care and closure. Open wounds require thorough saline irrigation followed by debridement with the conservative removal of nonviable tissues and all foreign materials. Normal saline remains the preferred irrigant, because it does not interfere with normal wound healing as many antiseptic solutions do.[30] Debridement of wound edges should be minimal, because facial soft tissue can survive on small pedicles. Minor lacerations can be repaired in the emergency department. In Ong and Dudley's[31] study of facial soft-tissue injuries in 1000 adult trauma patients, most open wounds of the lower face required wound closure with sutures, whereas the upper facial wounds were more amenable to closure with Steri-Strips or glue. The main pitfall of techniques that do not involve the use of local anesthesia (i.e., glue or Steri-Strips [3M, St. Paul, MN]) is inadequate wound exploration and debridement. Although the emergency department staff can repair most lacerations, the facial trauma surgical team should be available for the suture closure of complex facial wounds (Figure 46-2).

Animal and Human Bite Wounds

Animal and human bite wounds frequently occur on the face. Irrigation with normal saline followed by soft-tissue debridement is the mainstay of initial treatment. Fortunately, the head and neck have a lower risk of infection (i.e., <6%) than other areas of the body. [32] Facial dog bite wounds can be safely closed after exploration and cleaning.[33,34] Generally, human bites can also be primarily closed up to 24 hours after the injury.[34,35] High-risk wounds, such as injuries that are more than 24 hours old and nose or ear avulsions with exposed cartilage, should be repaired with delayed primary closure after 3 to 5 days of moist gauze dressing changes.[35] Most authorities recommend the prescription of prophylactic antibiotics after primary wound closure, despite the low rate of infection (i.e., ≈1%) reported in some series.[36] The administration of amoxicillin clavulanate for 3 to 5 days is appropriate for this purpose. Antibiotics must be given for 7 to 14 days for an already infected facial bite wound. Intravenous antibiotic coverage with ticarcillin clavulanate and hospitalization are indicated for immunodeficient patients, badly infected wounds, or deep injuries with exposed cartilage.[32]

Contaminated Wounds

Patients with wounds that have been crushed, devitalized, or contaminated with dirt or rust are believed to be prone to tetanus.[37] All bite wounds are also considered tetanus-prone injuries.[34] The standard of care for tetanus-prone wounds includes the administration of tetanus

toxoid if a booster injection has not been given within the prior 10 years. Furthermore, if the history of tetanus immunization of the victim is unknown or if the primary tetanus immunization was never completed during childhood, tetanus immunoglobulin should be administered along with a toxoid booster.[37] However, in an urban study of five U.S. emergency rooms, none of the 504 patients with tetanus-prone wounds and a history of inadequate primary immunization received tetanus immunoglobulin.[38] Because many trauma victims are unable to communicate their tetanus immunization status, routine toxoid boosters are often given in the emergency department if a wound exists. If practical, a diligent effort to define the patient's primary immunization history should be undertaken, and tetanus immunoglobulin should be administered if doubt regarding the patient's status exists.

IMAGING OF MAXILLOFACIAL TRAUMA PATIENTS

To evaluate a suspected facial fracture, the evaluation of choice is the dedicated CT scan with fine (i.e., 1 mm) cuts in both the axial and coronal dimensions. In the multisystem trauma patient, it is often necessary to rely on physical signs alone to decide when to order a facial CT scan. A study of 777 trauma patients suggested that a higher percentage of facial fractures occur with lip lacerations, intraoral lacerations, periorbital contusions, subconjunctival hemorrhages, and nasal lacerations.[39] Another decision point is the timing of a facial CT scan. Trauma patients are often urgently sent to the CT scanner for the evaluation of the head, the chest, the abdomen, and the pelvis. It may be unsafe to consume valuable time with a facial CT scan at this point. In addition, the victim's cervical spine must be "cleared" before he or she undergoes direct coronal CT imaging.

The thin-section axial CT scan images can be reformatted to generate high-quality coronal images. A study on cadaver heads by Rosenthal and colleagues[40] found that an experienced neuroradiologist can diagnose 97% of facial fractures (i.e., those found on direct axial CT images) by examining reformatted coronal images. By using these reformatted images, the time that an unstable patient must spend in the CT scanner can be reduced, and this also involves a decrease in exposure to ionizing radiation as well as the avoidance of the delay in imaging caused by cervical spine clearance issues. Other advantages of reformatted coronals include the elimination of dental amalgam streak artifacts and their orientation in a true coronal plane, which facilitates the sequential examination of sections.

Axial CT images of the facial bones can also be reconstructed by computer software to generate three-dimensional depictions. This technology allows for the easy visualization of complex fracture patterns and the

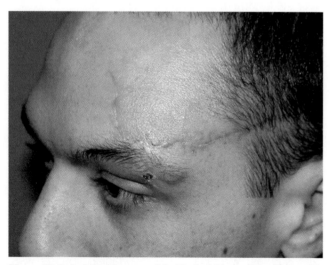

Figure 46-2. Left facial scars related to facial lacerations. Even with meticulous wound closure at the time of the accident, facial scars may require time and revision to achieve optimal camouflage.

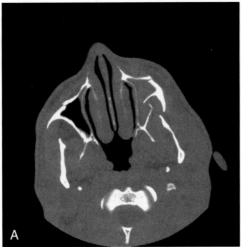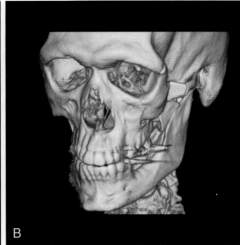

Figure 46-3. Left zygomaticomaxillary complex fracture as shown by an axial computed tomography scan **(A)** and its three-dimensional reconstruction **(B)**.

manipulation of the image to permit unobstructed viewing of any anatomic structure, and it has implications for accurate measurements for prosthesis design. By examining three-dimensional reconstructions of fractured cadaver skulls, radiologists were more accurate in defining the spatial relationship of fractures than they were when examining two-dimensional axial images.[41] This advantage was most pronounced with fractures of the zygomatic and orbital regions (Figure 46-3).

COMPLICATIONS

Nasal Fracture Surgery

The force needed to fracture the nasal bones is less than that needed for any other facial bone.[42] Nasal fractures are therefore the most common type of facial fractures and the third most common fracture of the human skeleton.[43] The initial evaluation must include the cause and time of the trauma, any history of previous facial injuries, any previous nasal deformities, and any history of nasal obstruction or nasal surgery. This should be followed by a careful physical examination that particularly addresses the degree of bony deformity, the presence of cartilaginous deformity, and the character of the soft-tissue injury and swelling. Many authors now advocate a rigid nasal endoscopy to fully explore any nasal septal injury.[42,44] An accurate examination during the acute postinjury phase is handicapped by ecchymoses, edema, and blood. Epistaxis should be treated with firm handheld pressure and, if necessary, directed cautery and nasal packing. The nose is supplied with arterial blood from both the internal and external carotid systems, and injury causing substantial blood loss and requiring transfusion is possible.

Septal Hematoma

The existence of a septal hematoma must be considered and treated emergently to avoid septal necrosis and subsequent saddle-nose deformity (Figure 46-4). A septal

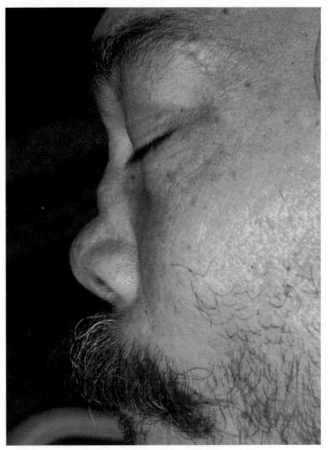

Figure 46-4. Saddle-nose deformity. This deformity can be a complication of septal hematoma or of untreated nasal and septal fracture.

hematoma occurs when blood collects between the perichondrium of the quadrangular cartilage and the cartilage itself. The blood supply to the quadrangular cartilage is tenuous, and the hematoma can cause an interruption in the blood supply, which can lead to the loss of the cartilage and septal perforation. If extensive, a loss of nasal support can result in cosmetic deformity.

If possible, the surgeon should obtain a good-quality photograph of the patient that was taken before the injury. A driver's license photograph may suffice if no other images are available. In addition, seven-view photographs (i.e., anteroposterior and/or right, left laterals and/or right, left obliques and/or low and high basals) of the injured nose should be taken for surgical planning, medicolegal purposes, and as a gauge of treatment success.

Nasal Fracture Reduction

There is controversy regarding the most optimal timing of nasal fracture reduction. It may be possible, if the patient is seen during the first 3 to 6 hours after injury, to reduce the fracture before distorting edema occurs.[43] Otherwise, the patient must be reevaluated in 3 to 5 days, after the swelling has resolved and when possible deformities or obstruction have been unmasked. Patients should be released with instructions to rest, apply ice, and maintain head elevation. Upon return, the degree of posttraumatic deformity (aided by photographs), asymmetry, and airway obstruction drives the decision to attempt reduction. There are instances in which substantial initial edema causes a bothersome cosmetic deformity, but, as it resolves, the patient may be satisfied with both the physical appearance and the functional status, thereby negating the need for surgical intervention. Surgical variables include local versus general anesthesia, closed versus open approaches, and the choice of setting (i.e., clinic treatment room vs. operating room). A delayed rhinoplasty as either a primary or secondary treatment option is a procedure that may be considered about 6 months after injury.

The incidence of nasal deformities after initial reduction that require subsequent rhinoplasty or septorhinoplasty ranges from 14% to 50%.[45–47] The technique of the simple closed reduction of the nasal bones and septum has existed since the time of Hippocrates. The inconsistent results of this seemingly intuitive procedure, however, have prompted surgeons to explore other techniques. In his series of 105 nasal fractures, Staffel[48] compared the results of closed reduction with those of a stepwise protocol that began with closed reduction and progressed to include septoplasty, osteotomies, upper lateral cartilage release, perpendicular ethmoid plate fracture, camouflage with septal cartilage grafts, and hump removal as needed to achieve a straight and pleasing appearance. The patients in the open-reduction protocol group fared significantly better, with 71% achieving an excellent result as compared with only 40% achieving this in the closed reduction group. Despite this, it should be noted that only 13% of the closed-reduction cases showed an obvious deformity on casual observation. More complex surgery may yield a higher percentage of outstanding results, but a simple and timely closed reduction is often an adequate intervention.

Unrecognized and Untreated Injuries of the Nasal Septum

Many sources cite unrecognized and untreated injuries of the nasal septum as a culprit in cases of persistent deformity and dysfunction.[42,43] Verwoerd[49] noted that trauma to the nasal dorsum leads to lesions of the posterior septal cartilage and that the nasal bones tend to unite in the direction of the deviated septum. Murray and colleagues[50] found that patients with nasal bones deviated by more than half of the width of the nasal bridge had a concomitant, C-shaped fracture of the bony and cartilaginous septum. The attempted closed reduction of these fractures resulted in high rates of persistent deformity. Rohrich and Adams[42] developed an algorithm for nasal fracture management over 11 years that yielded a low 9% revision rate. They recommend that, at the time of nasal bone reduction, the base of the fractured nasal septum be replaced into the vomerine groove with either the Asch forceps or the blunt Boies elevator. For nonreducible posteroinferior or anterior septal fractures, they advised acute limited septal reconstruction and/or repositioning at the time of bony reduction (i.e., 5–7 days postinjury).

Infection

Infection is an uncommon complication of nasal fractures. Antibiotic prophylaxis is indicated if the individual is immunocompromised, has a dorsal and/or septal hematoma, or has undergone nasal packing or internal splinting. A potentially serious complication is toxic shock syndrome (TSS), a multisystem disease caused by exotoxin-producing *Staphylococcus aureus* in the nasal mucus membranes. Certain types of nasal packing seem to provide a supportive environment that encourages this syndrome, which has a mortality rate of 10%. A case report from Keller and colleagues[51] describes a child who contracted TSS after a closed nasal fracture reduction in which a single piece of Gelfoam was used for a postreduction pack. Prophylactic antibiotics seem to be ineffective for the prevention of TSS.[52] Treatment should focus on early recognition, the removal of the contaminated foreign body, and debridement as necessary.

Naso-Orbito-Ethmoid Fracture Surgery

A naso-orbito-ethmoid (NOE) fracture involves the nasal bones, the frontal processes of the maxillae, and the ethmoid bones. The classic NOE fracture leaves the patient with a short and retruded nasal bridge, traumatic telecanthus, enophthalmos, and shortened palpebral fissures. The intricate anatomy and difficult exposure of the anatomy makes these fractures among the most difficult of facial injuries to repair successfully. In addition, the resulting deformities of these fractures are extremely difficult to treat.

The highly challenging anatomy of the NOE complex demands excellent surgical exposure. When planning the approach, the surgeon must keep in mind that the major reason for treating NOE fractures is cosmetic deformity. Therefore, the approach should be as aesthetically pleasing as possible. The fractured bones may be exposed with the use of existing lacerations, local incisions (i.e., the "open-sky" approach), or a combination of coronal and lower-lid incisions. Although not described as a primary approach to NOE fractures, the midfacial degloving approach has been used in a small series to approach upper-facial fractures without any skin incisions.[53]

The open-sky technique consists of bilateral Lynch incisions linked by a horizontal incision below the glabella. This approach exposes the NOE complex but precludes the adequate exposure of the inferior orbital rim. Patients may develop scarring and contracture from the skin incisions as well as webbing that may be obvious cosmetically and that may ultimately impair eyelid function.

The coronal approach offers excellent exposure of the upper face and limited cosmetic deformity in patients without a receding hairline, and it can be used to harvest cranial bone for grafts via the same incision. The incision is hidden behind the patient's hairline and carried down to the root of the helix on either side. In patients with male pattern baldness, the trajectory of the incision must be carefully planned or an alternate approach used. The dissection must be carried out in a plane that runs deep to the hair follicles, or else incisional alopecia may occur. In one study, the most common complication of the coronal approach was transient anesthesia of the supraorbital region.[54] This problem is thought to result from manipulation of and traction on the flap, because the supraorbital neurovascular bundles were preserved in this series. In all cases, these complaints were mild and resolved within 6 weeks.

The frontal branch of the facial nerve may be injured despite meticulous technique. If it is not divided, function would be expected to return and improve over weeks to months. It is critical to keep the facial nerve branches superficial to the level of dissection in the temporal region. Other reported complications of the coronal approach include hematoma under the flap, trismus, ptosis, and epiphora. However, these signs and symptoms may be linked to the primary injury rather than the approach.

The medial canthal tendon (MCT) and the fragment of bone on which it inserts (i.e., the "central" fragment) are the key parameters of the evaluation and management of NOE fractures. The frontal process of the maxilla provides the anchoring point of the medial canthal tendon. A clinically useful classification system is built around the fracture patterns of this area: type I, single-segment central fragment; type II, comminuted central fragment with fractures external to the MCT insertion; and type III, comminution of the portion of bone bearing the MCT insertion.

The adequate transnasal reduction of the canthal-bearing central fragment is the most crucial step in NOE fracture repair, and it must be done correctly to prevent the lateral migration of the medial orbital wall as well as postoperative telecanthus.[55,56] In simple NOE fractures with a large, intact central fragment, reduction and fixation with a small plate or wire is sufficient. If the medial orbital rims are comminuted, a 25- or 26-gauge wire is used to fix the frontal processes of the maxillae to each other. The wire must be passed through a hole drilled posterior to the lacrimal fossa, or else the posterior aspects of the fragments will splay outward and cause telecanthus.[57] Ellis[56] notes that the wire should be tightened vigorously in an attempt to "over-reduce" the medial orbital rims, because under-reduction will lead to telecanthus and a widened nasal dorsum. In the rare case of complete canthal disruption from bone, a medial canthopexy is performed that secures the tendon to the contralateral supraorbital rim. The canthus must be positioned correctly by careful manipulation to avoid postoperative asymmetry. Malposition also prevents the lids from adapting to the globe, and it encourages epiphora by keeping the nasolacrimal punctum from contacting the globe surface.[56]

Prevention of Enophthalmos and Preservation of Normal Orbital Volume

Reconstruction of the orbit must be performed to prevent enophthalmos and to preserve normal orbital volume. Markowitz and colleagues[55] note that primary bone grafts to the medial and inferior orbital wall are "almost always" indicated. In Ellis's[56] series, 12 of 26 patients had at least one medial wall deformity that warranted a bone graft reconstruction. Bone grafts are also frequently needed for nasal dorsal augmentation and reconstruction or for significant nasal deformities such as a loss of projection and the shortening of nasal length. In addition, saddle-nose deformity may result from the loss of dorsal support. All 10 patients in the Herford and colleagues[57] study of type III fractures received dorsal nasal bone grafts. One must remember that there is an illusion of decreased intercanthal distance with a greater dorsal nasal projection.[56] Therefore it is important for the surgeon to strive for an excellent dorsal nasal projection to counter any perception of telecanthus from the original insult.

Cerebrospinal Fluid Rhinorrhea

Cerebrospinal fluid (CSF) rhinorrhea is common after NOE fractures as a result of the compromise of the thin fovea ethmoidalis. The incidence of CSF rhinorrhea ranges from 40% to 50% in NOE fracture series.[56,58]

The vast majority of CSF leakage stops spontaneously within 10 days of NOE fracture reduction, and there is a very low incidence of meningitis. It is thought that reducing fracture fragments may indirectly restore dural integrity and halt CSF leakage. In a series of 34 patients with CSF leakage after any craniomaxillofacial trauma, 85% of CSF leaks resolved in 2 to 10 days with the simple regimen of bed rest, head elevation, and strict sinus precautions (e.g., the avoidance of nose blowing, the Valsalva maneuver).[58] A small percentage of patients with persistent leakage will require CSF diversion with lumbar drainage or surgical correction. Prophylactic antibiotics do not seem to prevent meningitis among patients with CSF leakage, and they are therefore not routinely prescribed.[59]

Posttraumatic Dacryostenosis and Epiphora

Posttraumatic dacryostenosis and epiphora are observed in 5% to 47% of patients with NOE fractures.[60,61] Temporary epiphora is probably caused by lacrimal pathway compression from resolving posttraumatic edema. Permanent lacrimal dysfunction results from lacerations of the nasolacrimal duct or rupture of the medial canthal tendon with subsequent lacrimal sac compression. In one analysis, 17 of 58 patients (29%) presented with permanent epiphora after NOE trauma.[61] These patients were remarkable for a longer delay (i.e., ≈20 days) in fracture reduction and a loss of bone from the lacrimal area. Lacrimal dysfunction can be effectively treated with a dacryocystorhinostomy timed about 6 months after trauma, when edema and soft-tissue injuries have stabilized.

Orbital Fracture Surgery

Fractures of the orbit are a common result of maxillofacial trauma, and they are potentially associated with vision-threatening complications that demand urgent intervention. Unilateral blinding injuries have an estimated annual incidence of 500,000 cases, making trauma one of the leading causes of unilateral loss of sight.[7] Therefore an expedient ophthalmology consultation must be obtained during the initial management of these patients. Loss of sight occurs in 3% to 12% of maxillofacial trauma victims,[62] and it may result from direct injury to the globe or the optic nerve, an ischemic injury to the optic nerve, or the loss of eyelid integrity. The most accurate tests to document the loss of vision are visual acuity testing and color perception,[63] but often these determinations are impractical for unconscious and critically ill patients. Clinical examination may be limited to assessments of pupillary size and reactions, globe tension on gentle palpation, and forced duction testing. Funduscopy is challenging without pupil dilation, but it can detect intraocular hemorrhage, retinal edema, retinal detachment, or optic disc swelling. Exophthalmometry is employed to measure globe position,[64] and

slit-lamp examination can diagnose corneal abrasion, hyphema, iritis, lens dislocation, vitreous hemorrhage, or globe rupture. Additionally, a coronal CT scan is essential to evaluate the soft tissues of the orbital space.

Retrobulbar Hemorrhage

As a complication of facial trauma, retrobulbar hemorrhage has been reported to occur in 0.6% of patients before surgery.[65] It usually accompanies nondisplaced fractures of the orbital walls.[66] It can be thought of as a "compartment syndrome" within the rigid space of the orbital septum that leads to ischemic damage of the retina and optic nerve. The diagnosis hinges on orbital pain, proptosis, visual loss, and a loss of pupillary reflexes. A CT scan will reveal severe proptosis, stretching of the optic nerve, and a tented posterior sclera. Irreversible damage to the patient's vision can occur after only 60 minutes of ischemia,[7] and delayed retrobulbar hemorrhage may occur hours to days after injury. Therefore trauma victims with visual complaints must be given a regimen of regular eye observation to avoid complications. On the basis of a survey of practices around the United Kingdom, Bater[67] suggests that eye checks be performed hourly throughout the first 16 hours or during the first night. The treatment of retrobulbar hemorrhage begins with high-dose steroid therapy before surgery to decompress the orbit. If visual loss is already advanced or occurs rapidly, however, the recovery of sight is very unlikely.

Traumatic Optic Neuropathy

Traumatic optic neuropathy occurs when injuring forces damage the optic nerve as it passes through the optic canal. It occurs in 0.5% to 5% of closed head injuries, with visual loss occurring among half of these patients.[68] Displaced orbital fractures or the associated edema may injure the nerve directly. Visual loss is usually profound and instantaneous. Examination reveals an afferent pupillary defect, and imaging will reveal optic canal fractures, soft-tissue swelling, and nerve sheath hematoma. Treatment is controversial and includes early steroid administration followed by surgical decompression in nonresponders. If a complete transection occurs, no treatment is possible, and blindness is a certainty.

Orbital Fractures That Require Surgical Intervention

There are several scenarios in patients with orbital fractures that merit urgent surgical intervention. In the case of clinical diplopia occurring with CT scan evidence of an entrapped muscle or soft tissue, an oculocardiac reflex may develop from increased efferent vagal tone as a result of a damaged trigeminal pathway.[69] The resultant bradycardia and heart block may be fatal, and it demands urgent surgical intervention. In young patients (i.e., <18 years old), the softer orbital bones may form a trapdoor that entraps soft tissue and rapidly leads to muscle or fat ischemia. This causes a "white-eyed" appearance with severe extraocular mobility restriction.[70]

Okinaka and colleagues[71] reported the case of an 8-year-old patient with a minimally displaced floor fracture who exhibited persistent diplopia after surgery on postinjury day 13. There was early and untreatable scar formation between the inferior rectus muscle and the orbital periosteum that was found during surgery. In addition, significant facial asymmetry with enophthalmos in large orbital floor fractures warrants early intervention, especially if the orbital defect is more than one half of the total area of the floor.[72] Even with a small orbital floor defect, the blockage of the maxillary sinus ostium by orbital contents should raise concern for the generation of negative pressure in the sinus and delayed "implosion" of the orbital floor.[73] Finally, severe infraorbital hypesthesia and pain can result from the entrapment of the infraorbital nerve. Several authors suggest that these problems are better managed with early surgical repair.[74,75]

For fractures that do not fall into the aforementioned scenarios, usually a 2-week window of observation is appropriate in the absence of urgent surgical indications. Some of the initial globe displacement and ocular dysmotility become less bothersome with the resolution of muscle edema and hemorrhage and the recovery of motor nerve palsies. With a prolonged delay, however, progressive fibrosis in the orbit and fat atrophy make late repair unsatisfactory (Figure 46-5). The degree of diplopia and the globe position can be followed objectively in the clinic by measures such as the Maddox rod test and the use of a Hertel exophthalmometer.[64] The surgeon must consider each patient with orbital fractures individually and weigh the potential complications of fracture repair against the morbidity of accepting some degree of enophthalmos or diplopia to arrive at the best recommendation for a given patient.

When deciding how to approach an orbital wall fracture, surgeons must consider several discrete approaches, all with inherent advantages and potential complications. The transconjunctival approach has become increasingly popular, because it leaves no visible scar and provides excellent exposure of the inferior orbit. In a review of 400 patients who underwent transconjunctival approaches to the orbit, Mullins and colleagues[76] reported 8 cases of conjunctival granuloma, 2 cases of entropion, and 1 case each of hematoma, ectropion, and lower eyelid laceration. Other series confirm very low rates of ectropion or scleral show, ranging from 0% to 3%.[77,78] In addition to the transconjunctival approach, Suga and colleagues[79] found that a lateral paracanthal incision is often needed to expose the lateral orbital wall and to avoid the lower eyelid laceration caused by excessive retraction. Because this incision results in a visible scar, they concluded that the transconjunctival approach is the most useful for limited repairs of the medial orbital wall.

Transcutaneous approaches to the orbital wall include the subciliary skin-only or the skin-and-muscle approach and its variation, the subtarsal approach. The subciliary incision is placed in a skin crease below the lash line, and this results in a superior aesthetic scar[80] (Figure 46-6).

Unfortunately the subciliary approach disrupts the skin, the muscle, and the septal planes, and it can lead to vertical shortening of the eyelid as the wound heals. The incidence of postoperative ectropion is reported to be between 12% and 42%,[78,81] and permanent scleral show occurs at a rate of 28%.[78] The subtarsal approach causes fewer problems with ectropion or scleral show, but it causes more postoperative edema and a more noticeable scar.[82] Nevertheless, lid suspension techniques and the careful handling of tissue planes

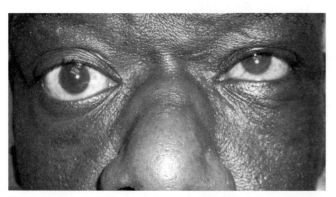

Figure 46-5. Left-sided dystopia as a result of inferior rectus dysfunction from an orbital floor fracture.

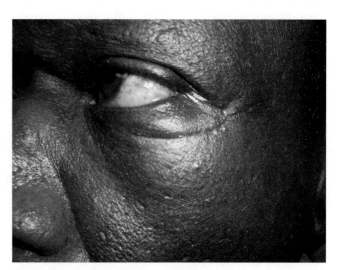

Figure 46-6. Resulting scar 1 month after a subciliary approach to the repair of a left orbital floor fracture.

with subciliary approaches can provide excellent exposure and minimal postoperative lid position problems.

Blindness

Blindness is the gravest complication that can occur after the repair of orbital fractures, and it is fortunately very rare. In a series of 1240 patients who underwent the operative repair of orbital fractures, only 3 patients (0.2%) experienced a complete loss of vision.[83] Other series show similar rates of blindness occurring after the repair of orbital and midface fractures.[84] Postoperative blindness occurs most often after the repair of orbital floor fractures. The cause of blindness is usually an increase in intraorbital pressure caused by hemorrhage or edema. Rarer causes of blindness include central retinal artery occlusion and direct injury of the optic nerve by implanted grafts.[85]

Other Common Complications

The frequency of long-term sequelae after orbital fracture repair has been reported to be as high as 83%,[86] irrespective of the method or the material employed. One of the most common complications (i.e., ≈40%) is numbness of the ipsilateral infraorbital nerve, which can persist for years after surgery. Another common problem is persistent or new-onset diplopia. One study showed a persistence rate of diplopia in 17% of patients who experienced double vision preoperatively[87] (Figure 46-7). This complication primarily affected patients of advanced age or those whose repair was delayed beyond 2 weeks after the injury. Another series of 107 patients revealed a 17% rate of new-onset diplopia and a 7% rate of enophthalmos after orbital floor repair.[86] These problems were disproportionately the result of the use of a Foley catheter or gauze as a maxillary antral packing for the support of the orbital floor. Other reported complaints include blurred vision, increased tear flow, infraorbital nerve hyperesthesia, light sensitivity, and eyelid tics. Transient mydriasis is unusual, but it may be caused if the inferior oblique muscle (along which travel the parasympathetic pupillomotor fibers) is extensively manipulated.[88]

Different materials (e.g., autogenous and alloplastic grafts) are available to reconstruct the orbital floor, and they all have different complication profiles. The most common autogenous donor sites include the split calvarial bone, the iliac crest, and the rib. There is a significant rate of donor site morbidity (i.e., 5%–9%) from the harvest of bone grafts. Complications of harvest include dural tears, pneumothorax, hematoma, and nerve injury.[89] Bone grafts can be misplaced into an intraconal position during floor repair, or they may migrate over time if rigid fixation is not used. This can result in blindness if the bone graft directly impinges on the optic nerve or its blood supply, or it may cause persistent diplopia if the extraocular musculature is compromised by the scar response to the graft. Conchal cartilage from the auricle is also a suitable autogenous material for the repair of orbital floor fractures. Harvest of this material has few donor site complications. The cartilage itself is thin and pliable for relining the orbital floor with minimal potential for the foreign body reaction or future infection, which is a potential concern when using all alloplastic materials.

However, some surgeons prefer alloplastic orbital floor implants constructed from such materials as methylmethacrylate, Teflon, silicone, porous polyethylene, hydroxyapatite, Gelfilm, and others. The ideal implant material should be biocompatible, easily kept in position, easily handled, and free of complications. Bioabsorbable implants created from poly-L-lactic acid, polyglycolic acid, or both have been reported to cause a foreign-body reaction that manifests as intermittent swelling and chronic pain for up to 3 years after surgery.[90] A large comparison of medial wall and floor fracture repairs using porous polyethylene or hydroxyapatite implants resulted in a total complication rate of 7.4% without any significant difference in implant choice.[91] Postoperative enophthalmos (5%), infraorbital paresthesia (2.2%), and

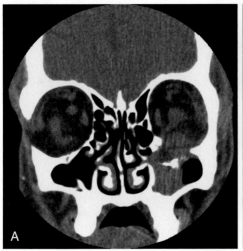

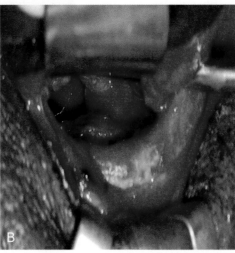

Figure 46-7. A, Computed tomography scan of the left orbit of a patient who complained of persistent diplopia and a limitation of the downward gaze after undergoing the repair of a left orbital floor fracture with an alloplastic sheet implant. This scan revealed an enlarged inferior rectus muscle that was suggestive of hematoma or infarction. Intraoperative findings included confirmation that the alloplastic sheet did not contact the medial extent of the fracture, with adherent muscle in the gap **(B).**

persistent diplopia (1.2%) were the most common sequelae, without any reports of implant removal or infection. However, because inherent complications may develop many years after fracture repair, the complication rate may be under-reported. Jordan and colleagues[92] reported on three patients who presented with alloplastic implant migration anteriorly through the skin or interiorly within the orbit up to 5 years after repair. This study also described six patients who developed fistulae from the orbit to the skin or sinuses and four patients with local infections necessitating implant removal up to 20 years later. Silicone implants specifically have a tendency toward late extrusion or infection years after placement.

Zygomatic Complex Fracture Surgery

The zygomatic complex is the second most injured region of the upper face (after the nasal bones). Because the zygomatic bone comprises the aesthetically important malar prominence, fractures often result in deformity of the middle third of the face (Figure 46-8). In addition, displacement of the zygomatic body and arch may interfere with the movement of the coronoid process of the mandible and cause trismus. Involvement of the orbit can lead to entrapment or restriction of the extraocular muscles, with resulting diplopia.

Various approaches to the zygomatic complex include traditional closed techniques as well as local or coronal scalp incisions. Some surgeons use facial incisions, which leave a visible scar. In addition, an approach through a local incision may be inadequate for complete and uninterrupted visualization of the whole zygomatic complex, including the frontozygomatic and zygomaticotemporal sutures. Zhang and colleagues[93] reported a series of 69 zygomatic complex fractures that were approached with a coronal incision. In their series,

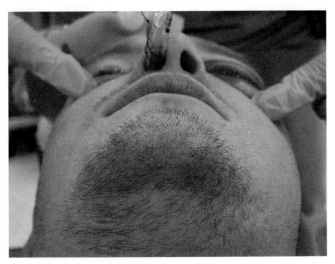

Figure 46-8. Depressed left malar prominence. Depression of the zygomatic complex can lead to facial deformity and enophthalmos in a patient after zygomatic complex fracture.

24 patients reported supraorbital paresthesias, and 6 patients exhibited facial nerve weakness (with most resolving in 1 year), whereas 6 patients had permanent visible scalp scarring with alopecia. The coronal approach should be considered in the settings of comminuted, multiple, late, or bilateral zygomatic fractures.

Paresthesias of the Infraorbital Nerve Distribution

Paresthesias of the infraorbital nerve distribution have been reported in a large percentage of zygomatic complex fractures, with rates ranging from 35% to 94% in published series.[94] The incidence appears to be higher with displaced fractures. Specific symptoms include hypoesthesia, dysesthesia, paresthesia, and anesthesia of the upper lip, the cheek, the lower eyelid, the skin of the nose, the anterior gingiva, and the ipsilateral teeth. De Man and Bax[95] reported that fracture repair with miniplates resulted in a lower incidence of persistent infraorbital paresthesia as compared with interosseous wiring (i.e., 22% vs. 50%). It appears that patients with alterations of both thermal and tactile sensation usually require more than 6 months for the recovery of nerve function, whereas patients with only tactile deficits can expect recovery within 3 months.[94] Patients with debilitating and prolonged intraorbital nerve dysfunction are candidates for neurolysis of the infraorbital nerve.

Aesthetic Complaints

The advent of rigid internal fixation has significantly improved aesthetic complaints after zygomatic complex fracture repair. Becelli and colleagues[96] looked at 14 patients with malar flattening whose fractures were repaired with wire osteosynthesis in which only 1 patient (7%) was "very satisfied" with the cosmetic result. By contrast, 11 patients with the same complaint were treated with osteotomy and rigid internal fixation, and 6 of these patients (55%) were "very satisfied" afterward. Wire stabilization of the fracture fragments often fails to stabilize the necessary angles between the bone ends to restore the malar projection. Rigid fixation with microplates allows for an immediate, firm stabilization of the osseous segments in three dimensions.

Plate Removal

The use of titanium plates for facial fracture reduction is widely accepted. Authors report plate removal rates between 12% and 18%,[97] most often for infection. Recently, more attention has been given to biodegradable materials (e.g., copolymers of poly-L-lactic acid/polyglycolic acid) for the fixation of fractures. These materials have several advantages over titanium plates. In particular, they do not need to be removed as often, they are not sensitive to temperature changes, and they cause less interference with craniofacial growth among children and with postoperative radiography. Biodegradable hardware cannot be used for cases of poor stability of fixation or in the presence of small comminuted bone fragments.[98] They may be especially well-suited for fractures of the zygomatic complex, because this region is a low load-bearing region of the facial skeleton. Wittwer and colleagues[98] found an equivalent 20% complication rate (i.e., infection, dehiscence, tissue reaction, unspecific pain) between biodegradable hardware and titanium plate fixation of zygomatic complex fractures. In the biodegradable study group, 50% of cases were complicated by an implant-related tissue reaction with recurrent pain and swelling around the implant site. All but one of these reactions resolved within 2 years after repair.

Le Fort Fracture Surgery

Maxillary fractures are associated with a relatively high rate of complications, probably as a result of the high-energy nature of the trauma causing these injuries. Motor vehicle injuries and assault are frequently the mechanisms of injury, and there is a high rate of associated facial bone fractures.[99] In a prospective study of 100 adult patients with displaced fractures of the Le Fort type, O'Sullivan and colleagues[99] found an overall complication rate of 36% after operative repair. Most of these complications occurred in the orbital region (i.e., enophthalmos, orbital dystopia) as a result of the dissipation of high-energy forces. Wound problems (e.g., infection, exposed or painful fixation plates) were seen in 9% of the series. Postoperative malocclusion, which is commonly thought of as the most significant complication in these patients, was encountered relatively infrequently (8%). Few patients (3%) were unhappy with their facial contour and requested revision surgery for correction. Concomitant injuries of the maxillary sinuses predispose some patients to sinusitis because of the disturbance of the sinus anatomy and physiology. One series revealed a 60% incidence of sinusitis up to 47 months after fracture repair in 15 patients treated for maxillary sinus fractures.[100]

The surgical approach to Le Fort fractures often involves the selection of a coronal approach, especially when addressing Le Fort II and III fractures. The complications of paresthesia, alopecia, scarring, and facial nerve weakness (especially of the frontal branch) were discussed earlier in this chapter and must be taken into consideration. An alternative approach is the midfacial degloving approach, which offers good exposure of the midface and leaves no external scar.[101] This approach can rarely result in nasal vestibule stenosis, which can be minimized with the exact suturing of nasal incisions. Transient dysfunction of the infraorbital nerve has also been reported after this approach.[102]

Malocclusion After the Treatment of Maxillary Fractures

The incidence of malocclusion after the treatment of maxillary fractures ranges from 8% to 20%.[103] This may result from several mechanisms: improper occlusal reduction during surgery, postsurgical relapse of maxillary position, or a lack of correct passive repositioning of the maxilla during surgery. During the course of Le Fort fracture repair, the maxilla is mobilized and then placed into maxillomandibular fixation (Figure 46-9). The maxillomandibular complex is then rotated superiorly until the midface bony fragments are appropriately reduced and fixated with plates and screws. According to Ellis,[103] however, it may be impossible to passively mobilize the maxilla as a result of posteriorly directed forces from the pterygoid muscles. Rather, he argues that Le Fort I osteotomies are sometimes necessary to achieve the adequate mobility of the maxilla and to provide stable repositioning to match the mandibular dentition. In his series of 24 patients with maxillary osteotomies at the time of initial midface fracture repair, only 1 patient failed to regain pretrauma occlusion.[103]

Complications Related to Internal Fixation Plates

The recovery from maxillary fracture repair is also marked by complications related to internal fixation plates. The reported rates of titanium plate removal in craniofacial surgery range from 12% to 33%.[97] In about half of these cases, the reason for removal is infection of the plate.[104] The next most common complication is usually exposure of the plate (15%–18%). Other cited reasons are persistent pain at the plate site, cold sensitivity of the plate metal, and plate palpability. Fracture malunion and broken hardware may rarely necessitate nonelective plate removal.

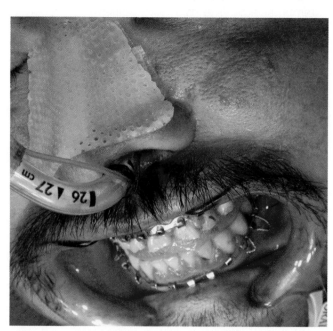

Figure 46-9. Stable maxillomandibular fixation and nasotracheal intubation are necessary to achieve optimal results with open reduction and the internal fixation of midface fractures.

Frontal Sinus Fracture Surgery

The anterior table of the frontal sinus requires a tremendous application of force before a fracture will occur (i.e., 800–2200 pounds of force),[105] and this is typically linked to motor vehicle accidents or instrument-aided assaults. The unique anatomy and position of the frontal sinus lead to well-defined complications in the management of fractures. Posteriorly, the cribriform plate, the dura mater, and the frontal lobes are closely apposed to each other and to the posterior wall of the sinus. The foramina of Breschet are sites of venous drainage in the frontal sinus walls that can serve as routes for the intracranial spread of infection. The frontal sinus is drained exclusively by the variably shaped nasofrontal channel or recess. If the patency of this recess is compromised by fractures, the resultant lack of frontal sinus ventilation can trigger a mucocele formation. In addition, the anterior table of the frontal sinus is the foundation of the aesthetically prominent contour of the forehead. The failure to reduce fracture components adequately using low-profile hardware and with minimal scarring will result in an obvious cosmetic deformity.

The principal route of approach to the frontal sinus is via a coronal incision. Again, the hairline incision may cause a visible scar or associated alopecia. In addition, the approach involves dissection near the supraorbital and supratrochlear nerve, thereby placing the patient at risk for postoperative forehead paresthesias or pain. In fact, chronic forehead pain and headache are the most common complications (14%–39%) reported after frontal sinus fracture repair in some large series.[106,107] The supraorbital nerve must be carefully preserved during both the approach and the reduction and fixation of the fracture fragments. The mid-forehead incision has been proposed as an alternative to the coronal incision for access to the frontal sinus,[108] especially for patients with deep forehead creases, hairline recession, or both.

Cerebrospinal Fluid Leak

The most significant early complication of frontal sinus repair is a CSF leak. CSF rhinorrhea is typically reported after the treatment of severe posterior table fractures with a cranialization procedure.[107] There is lack of consensus regarding the subject of prophylactic antibiotics for this scenario. Treatment options include a lumbar drainage and the administration of acetazolamide. Most CSF leaks will resolve spontaneously within 10 days, after which surgical reexploration should be considered. Meningitis may occur with or without a CSF leak. Meningitis is surely the most hazardous early complication of frontal sinus fracture repairs, and the incidence has been reported to be as high as 6% postoperatively.[109] The condition must be suspected in the context of altered mental status, fever of unknown origin, and neck rigidity. Broad-spectrum antibiotics with excellent CSF penetration must be started as soon as possible.

Mucoceles of the Frontal Sinus

Mucoceles of the frontal sinus are cysts that are made up of mucoperiosteal walls with respiratory epithelium and that are filled with mucus. They exhibit the signs of a sterile chronic infection, and they have the capacity to expand and erode into surrounding structures. When infected, they are called *mucopyoceles,* and they pose a risk for sepsis and meningitis. The basic problem that encourages mucocele formation is a disturbance in sinus ventilation. Many processes (e.g., inflammation, allergy, polyps, tumors, surgery) can compromise ventilation by blocking the nasofrontal outflow tract or by irritating the sinus mucosa. Traumatic fractures can entrap mucosa within the fracture lines or directly injure the nasofrontal recess, and trauma accounts for 9% to 28% of frontal sinus mucocele formation.[110] For this reason, fractures that injure the nasofrontal recess must be treated with the complete and meticulous removal of all of the sinus mucous tissue, and great care must be taken to burr away mucosa that has invaginated into the foramina of Breschet. In the case of cranialization surgery for severe posterior table fractures, the residual sinus mucosa must also be removed to avoid mucocele formation in the now-unventilated sinus space. Recently endoscopic approaches to the frontal sinus have entered the algorithm for the care of these patients; these may be used to avoid obliteration or possibly cranialization.

The detection of mucoceles requires long-term follow up by the surgeon. After a review of the literature, one study reported posttraumatic mucoceles being detected from 1 to 35 years after trauma; a follow-up period of 16 years would identify only 50% of these complications.[110] Regular follow-up evaluations for life are necessary to examine the patient's injury site and to query for the most frequent symptoms of mucocele formation, including frontal headache, proptosis, diplopia, nasal congestion, fluid leakage from the nose, and swelling over the forehead.[111,112] When detected, the mucocele must be evaluated by CT scan to evaluate the amount of bone erosion and magnetic resonance imaging to identify relationships with the brain and orbit. Total surgical extirpation of the mucocele or endoscopic marsupialization must be performed for this problem, and a 7% risk of the recurrence of mucocele after removal still exists[110] (Figure 46-10).

Infectious Complications

Infectious complications may be seen long after the initial trauma and repair. In Gossman and colleagues' review of 96 frontal sinus fractures,[107] 4 patients developed frontal sinusitis 6 to 18 months after their injuries. All of these patients were treated successfully with antibiotic therapy. Wilson and colleagues' study of 64 patients[106] featured a long mean follow-up duration of more than

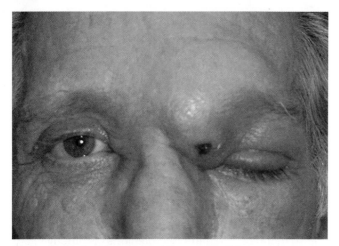

Figure 46-10. Left frontoethmoid mucocele. This may present as a bulge in the medial orbital region many years after the initial trauma.

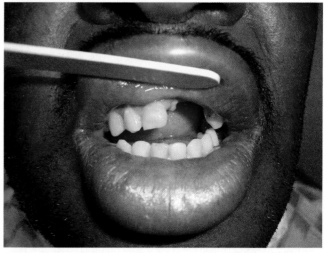

Figure 46-11. "Open-bite" deformity in a patient 1 month after the open reduction of a left parasymphyseal fracture via a transoral approach and the open reduction of a right body fracture via a transcervical approach.

3 years and reported frontal sinusitis complication rates of 28% and 15% in patients treated with open reduction/internal fixation and sinus obliteration, respectively. Brain abscess is a rare but potentially fatal complication of frontal sinus infection. The foramina of Breschet may allow for the passage of low-grade infections within the sinus space into the intracranial space. Brain abscess can present with insidious symptoms such as a loss of appetite, fatigue, and lethargy.[109] A high index of suspicion is needed to diagnose the condition, and a neurosurgical intervention is needed for therapy.

Disfigurement

Historic approaches to the frontal sinus (e.g., the Reidel and Killian procedures) left patients with substantially disfigured appearances. This is much more rare today as a result of the development of microplate internal fixation and the use of split-thickness calvarial bone grafts for the correction of extensive bone loss from the anterior table. In one series, 48 patients with frontal sinus fractures were repaired with open reduction and internal fixation, and only 1 patient complained of forehead asymmetry.[107] Other complications associated with microplate use that require the removal of hardware include plate palpability, visibility, and nonspecific pain around the internal fixation site.

Mandible Fracture Surgery

The various options for managing mandible fractures and the subsequent complications of repair have been relatively well studied in the medical literature. However, there is still a wide variety of opinions regarding the optimal treatment of any given fracture pattern. Reported complications include infection, malunion, delayed union, nonunion, disturbances of sensation, malocclusion (Figure 46-11), and facial deformity. Overall rates of complication range from 7% to 29%.[113] A recent study

by Alpert and colleagues[114] summarized the four types of complications as follows:

1. Those arising during the course of proper treatment
2. Those caused by inadequate/inappropriate treatment
3. Those caused by surgical failure
4. Those that result from no treatment

In general, indications for the closed reduction of mandibular fractures with maxillomandibular fixation include nondisplaced or grossly comminuted fractures, fractures in patients with mixed dentition or atrophic mandibles, and fractures of the coronoid or condyle. Open reduction and internal fixation are commonly employed for most symphyseal and parasymphyseal fractures, displaced body and angle fractures, and some condylar fractures.

Many studies have attempted to discern the most important factors leading to complications after mandible fracture repair. In terms of patient-based characteristics, one of the surest predictors of a complication is the coexistence of substance abuse. Patients with this characteristic are primarily young male victims of interpersonal assault, and alcohol or illicit drug use rates are very common. Passeri and colleagues[115] found a postsurgical complication rate of only 6.2% among patients who did not abuse drugs of any kind. By contrast, the postsurgical complication rates for patients who chronically abused alcohol, nonintravenous drugs, and intravenous drugs were 15.5%, 19.2%, and 30%, respectively. In 2005, Biller and colleagues[29] found that a treatment delay beyond 3 days from the time of injury was not associated with infectious complications. In this series, 20% of patients who admitted to chronic substance use (i.e., the use of alcohol, illicit drugs, and tobacco) developed an infectious postsurgical complication, whereas none of the substance-free individuals did. This association is likely multifactorial, because substance abusers may have poorer healing capacities, they may be more malnourished, and they likely have worse oral hygiene. They also tend to be less compliant with postoperative instructions, less likely to take oral antibiotics as instructed, and more likely to neglect the prescribed oral care required for healing.

The open reduction of a mandible fracture may be achieved via an extraoral or a transoral approach. Although the extraoral approach theoretically preserves a clean field by separating the fixation hardware from the contaminated oral cavity, there is the risk of cosmetically unappealing facial scars and injury to the marginal mandibular branch of the facial nerve. Transoral approaches also allow for the easier removal of teeth or fragments in the fracture line and for the simultaneous control of the occlusion and repositioning of the fragments during the operation. Toma and colleagues'[116] retrospective comparison of the two approaches found no significant difference in complication rates, but 7 of 227 patients needed to be converted from the transoral to the extraoral approach to expose posterior fractures or severely comminuted fractures.

Postoperative Infection

Postoperative infection continues to be a major problem after mandible fracture repair. Although most infections are of minor consequence, they have the potential to develop into osteomyelitis, debilitating pain, skeletal deformities, and the malunion or nonunion of fracture segments. Ellis[117] proposed that fibrous union is a common complication of infection that is caused by the lack of osseous tissue formation in an induced hypoxic environment. Some studies suggest that the rate of wound infection is higher in fractures that are treated by open reduction and internal fixation. A study of 594 mandible fractures treated at an urban teaching center yielded a 5.7% incidence of infection.[118] Closed reduction resulted in fewer postoperative infections than did open techniques, but this difference may be explained by the fact that less complicated fractures are more often treated with this method. Stone and colleagues[119] found that delays in treatment, age, gender, and the number of fractures had no impact on postoperative infection rates. In addition, there does not seem to be any association between the timing of antibiotics (i.e., at the time of injury, perioperatively, or postoperatively) and the development of infection.[120]

Nonunion of Fracture Segments

Of all the possible complications after mandible fracture repair, the most challenging is probably that of nonunion of fracture segments. The normal bony union of the mandible takes place over 4 to 8 weeks. A nonunion occurs when radiographic bony union has not taken place by this time.

Patients suffer from infection, pain, trismus, malnutrition, and deformity, and they require multiple courses of medical treatment and surgery. In Mathog and colleagues'[121] review of 906 patients treated for mandible fractures, the incidence of nonunion was 2.8% (25 patients). In 8 of these patients, unfavorable angle, body, or parasymphyseal fractures were treated inadequately with maxillomandibular fixation alone. As previously discussed, infection at the fracture site can lead to nonunion, and this was seen in 17 of this group's patients.[121] Other predisposing factors likely include malnourishment, generalized disease states, poor patient compliance with postoperative care, and tissue or foreign bodies between the segments. In Mathog and colleagues' series, 24 of 25 nonunion patients required debridement and either internal or external rigid fixation, with 10 patients receiving bone grafts (Figure 46-12).

Techniques to Reduce Postsurgical Complications

The use of locking reconstruction plates offers several advantages as compared with other plating systems. They do not require intimate contact with the mandible, and, therefore, they are easier to adapt and less sensitive to technique. Because the screws lock to the plate, there is no need for bone compression, which may disrupt the cortical bone blood supply and lead to cortical bony resorption. Screws are less likely to loosen from the plate (Figure 46-13) as a result of the locking threading mechanism, thereby avoiding inflammation caused by the mobility of hardware. However, studies have shown similar postoperative rates of complications with the use of locking plates. A review of 56 locking plates used to repair mandibular fractures revealed an infection rate of 6.4%,[122] which is similar to the infection rates reported in other series of internal fixation.

Another technique that may reduce postsurgical complications is the use of noncompression monocortical miniplates along the "ideal line" of osteosynthesis as described by Michelet and Champy.[123] These plates are placed via an intraoral approach, thereby minimizing the need for a large external scar and limiting risk to the

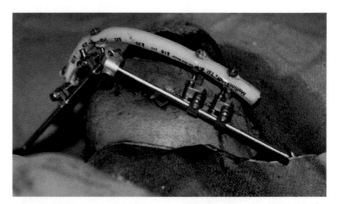

Figure 46-12. External fixation for a mandible fracture. Meticulous attention to anatomic reduction and adherence to principles of internal fixation can promote early mandibular healing and the avoidance of osteomyelitis.

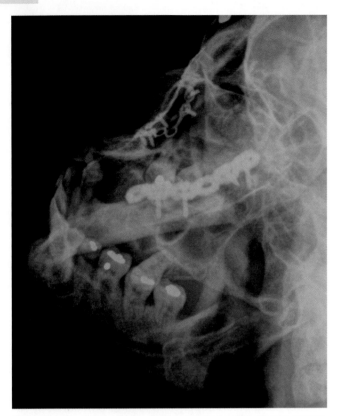

Figure 46-13. Plain radiograph view of the mandible demonstrating loose hardware and missing screws.

inferior alveolar nerve and the marginal mandibular branch. In addition, they require less stripping of the periosteum at the fracture site, and they may lessen the disruption of blood flow to the fracture site. This may be especially important for the management of the mandibular angle fracture, where the thin cross-sectional bone area leads to a higher rate of complications. In an analysis of 68 patients treated with the two-miniplate fixation of angle fractures, Fox and Kellman[124] reported only a 2.9% rate of postoperative infection without any incidence of malunion, nonunion, or osteomyelitis.

Points of Controversy and Discussion

A major point of controversy in the management of mandibular fractures involves the management of a tooth in the fracture line. Such a tooth may act as a portal of infection, and it is generally removed if it is mobile, if it is fractured, if it has periodontal or periapical pathology, or if it is carious.[121] Some authors propose leaving viable teeth in place, because extraction may make the fracture site unstable and thus make reduction more difficult. Thaller and Mabourakh[125] reported a very high rate of infection (30%) if teeth were left in the fracture line, and they performed extraction when there was a tooth root fracture, a markedly denuded root, or poor oral hygiene (Figure 46-14).

Another discussion point concerns the management of condyle fractures. Unless absolute indications for open reduction internal fixation exist (i.e., the displacement of the condyle into the middle cranial fossa, the impossibility of achieving occlusion with closed reduction, or the presence of a foreign body), many surgeons opt to use closed reduction techniques for this fracture. Worsaae and Thorn[126] cited a 39% complication rate with the closed reduction of condylar fractures, including asymmetry, malocclusion, trismus, headaches, and pain. Ellis and Throckmorton[127] found a malocclusion incidence of 28.6% among patients who underwent closed reduction as compared with 0% of patients who experienced open reduction. Of note is the fact that the surgical approach to the condylar process is difficult, and complications such as facial nerve palsy, auriculotemporal nerve dysfunction, Frey syndrome, and notable facial scar have been reported. In a study by Ellis and colleagues,[128] there were few complications after the open reduction internal fixation of condylar fractures using a retromandibular approach. The most common problem was the development of a hypertrophic surgical scar, which affected 7.5% of patients. A palsy of the marginal mandibular branch was noted in 17% of patients at the 6-week follow-up appointment, but none persisted at 6 months. There were no postsurgical infections, but 3 of 93 patients developed

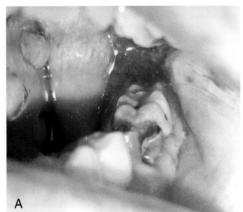
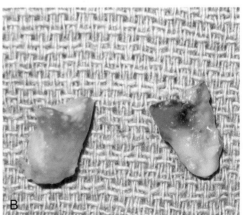

Figure 46-14. A, Decayed and cracked premolar just anterior to a left mandibular angle fracture. **B,** This tooth was extracted in the operating room just before the internal fixation of the fracture.

salivary fistulae that resolved within 3 weeks with pressure dressings and antisialagogues.

CONCLUSION

The nature of maxillofacial trauma provides many challenges to the practitioner who strives to avoid suboptimal or morbid outcomes. Victims arrive to the hospital at unexpected times, often with concurrent serious injuries, and they are typically unable to describe symptoms or cooperate with a detailed physical examination. If an operative intervention is required, the surgeon may need to compromise on the ideal timing or extent of surgery, depending on the patient's condition. Cooperation with emergency physicians, hospitalists, trauma surgeons, and other surgical subspecialties is essential.

When designing the surgical plan, the maxillofacial team must consider the functional, structural, and cosmetic consequences of each procedure. A variety of surgical approaches and techniques for the treatment of facial injuries exists, and the surgeon must choose one on the basis of personal experience and a comprehensive evaluation of the patient. An ever-expanding selection of equipment and prostheses also challenges the surgeon to remain fluent with regard to new developments and to adapt them in practice when deemed appropriate.

Although especially challenging in this patient population, a careful postoperative evaluation and long-term outpatient follow up will help to ensure adequate recovery and to identify complications at an earlier stage. Undesirable outcomes will still occur, despite the best efforts of the surgical team, and it is imperative to recognize, treat, and report these complications. Through vigilant documentation and discussion, this surgical discipline will recognize complications more reliably and work to develop improvements in treatment algorithms where they are needed most.

REFERENCES

1. Alvi A, Doherty T, Lewen G: Facial fractures and concomitant injuries in trauma patients. *Laryngoscope* 2003;113:102–106.
2. Van Olden GD et al: Clinical impact of advanced trauma life support. *Am J Emerg Med* 2004;22(7):522–525.
3. MacDonald RL et al: Diagnosis of cervical spine injury in motor vehicle crash victims: How many x-rays are enough? *J Trauma* 1990;30:392–397.
4. France JC, Bono CM, Vaccaro AR: Initial radiographic evaluation of the spine after trauma: When, what, where, and how to image the acutely traumatized spine. *J Orthop Trauma* 2005; 19:640–649.
5. American College of Surgeons: *Advanced Trauma Life Support for Doctors*, ed 6, Chicago: American College & Surgeons, 1997.
6. Verschueren DS et al: Management of laryngo-tracheal injuries associated with craniomaxillofacial trauma. *J Oral Maxillofac Surg* 2006;64:203–214.
7. Perry M et al: Emergency care in facial trauma: A maxillofacial and ophthalmic perspective. *Injury* 2005;36:875–896.
8. Mason AM: Use of the intubating laryngeal mask airway in pre-hospital care: A case report. *Resuscitation* 2001;51:1–95.
9. Fremstad JD, Martin SH: Lethal complication from insertion of nasogastric tube after severe basilar skull fracture. *J Trauma* 1978;18:820–822.
10. Fletcher SA, Henderson LT, Miner ME, et al: The successful surgical removal of intracranial nasogastric tubes. *J Trauma* 1987;27:948–952.
11. Gregory JA, Turner PT, Reynolds AF: A complication of nasogastric intubation: Intracranial penetration. *J Trauma* 1978;18:823–824.
12. Bouzarth WF: Intracranial nasogastric tube intubation. *J Trauma* 1978;18:818–819.
13. Goodisson DW, Shaw GM, Snape L: Intracranial intubation in patients with maxillofacial injuries associated with base of skull fractures? *J Trauma* 2001;50:363–366.
14. Horellou MF, Mathe D, Feiss P: A hazard of naso-tracheal intubation. *Anaesthesia* 1978;33:73–74.
15. Marlow TJ, Goltra DD Jr, Schabel SI: Intracranial placement of a nasotracheal tube after facial fracture: A rare complication. *J Emerg Med* 1997;15:187–191.
16. Cameron D, Lupton BA: Inadvertent brain penetration during neonatal nasotracheal intubation. *Arch Dis Child* 1993;69:79–80.
17. Rosen CL, Wolfe RE, Chew SE, et al: Blind nasotracheal intubation in the presence of facial trauma. *J Emerg Med* 1997;15: 141–145.
18. Rodricks MB, Deutschman CS: Emergent airway management: Indications and methods in the face of confounding conditions. *Crit Care Clin* 2000;16:389–409.
19. Lennarson PJ et al: Segmental cervical spine motion during orotracheal intubation of the intact and injured spine with and without external stabilization. *J Neurosurg* 2000;92:201–206.
20. Rhee KJ, Green W, Holcroft JW, et al: Oral intubation in the multiply injured patient: The risk of exacerbating spinal cord damage. *Ann Emerg Med* 1990;19:45–48.
21. Barriot P, Riou B: Retrograde technique for tracheal intubation in trauma patients. *Crit Care Med* 1988;16:712–713.
22. Hawkins ML, Shapiro MB, Cue JI, et al: Emergency cricothyroidotomy: A reassessment. *Am Surg* 1995;61:52–55.
23. DeLaurier GA, Hawkins ML, Treat RC, et al: Acute airway management: Role of cricothyroidotomy. *Am Surg* 1990;56:12–15.
24. Bhojani RA et al: Contemporary assessment of laryngotracheal trauma. *J Thorac Cardiovasc Surg* 2005;130:426–432.
25. Frable MA, El-Roman N, Lenis A, et al: Hemorrhagic complications of facial fractures. *Laryngoscope* 1974;84:2051–2057.
26. Buchanan R, Holtman B: Severe epistaxis in facial fractures. *Plast Reconstr Surg* 1983;71:768–770.
27. Bynoe RP et al: Maxillofacial injuries and life-threatening hemorrhage: Treatment with transcatheter arterial embolization. *J Trauma* 2003;55:74–79.
28. Hutchison IL, Magennis P, Shepherd JP, et al: The BAOMS United Kingdom survey of facial injuries—Part 1: Aetiology and the association with alcohol consumption. *Br J Oral Maxillofac Surg* 1998;36:3–13.
29. Biller JA, Pletcher SD, Goldberg AN, et al: Complications and the time to repair of mandible fractures. *Laryngoscope* 2005; 115:769–772.
30. Armstrong BD: Lacerations of the mouth. *Emerg Med Clin North Am* 2000;18:471–480.
31. Ong TK, Dudley M: Craniofacial trauma presenting at an adult accident and emergency department with an emphasis on soft tissue injuries. *Injury* 1999;30:357–363.
32. Stefanopoulos PK, Tarantzopoulou AD: Facial bite wounds: Management update. *Int J Oral Maxillofac Surg* 2005;34:464–472.
33. Chaudhry MA, Macnamara AF, Clark S: Is the management of dog bite wounds evidence based? A postal survey and review of the literature. *Eur J Emerg Med* 2004;11:313–317.
34. Fleisher GR: The management of bite wounds (editorial). *N Engl J Med* 1999;340:138–140.
35. Lieblich SE, Topazian RG: Infection in the patient with maxillofacial trauma. In Fonseca RJ, Walker RV, editors: *Oral and maxillofacial trauma*, ed 2, Philadelphia, 1997, WB Saunders.

36. Guy JR, Zook EG: Successful treatment of acute head and neck dog bite wounds without antibiotics. *Ann Plast Surg* 1986;17: 45–48.

37. Rhee P et al: Tetanus and trauma: A review and recommendations. *J Trauma* 2005;58:1082–1088.

38. Talan DA et al: Tetanus immunity and physician compliance with tetanus prophylaxis practices among emergency department patients presenting with wounds. *Ann Emerg Med* 2004;43: 305–314.

39. Holmgren EP et al: Facial soft tissue injuries as an aid to ordering a combination head and facial computed tomography in trauma patients. *J Oral Maxillofac Surg* 2005;63:651–654.

40. Rosenthal E et al: Diagnostic maxillofacial coronal images reformatted from helically acquired thin-section axial CT data. *Am J Roentgenol* 2000;175:1177–1181.

41. Fox LA et al: Diagnostic performance of CT, MPR and 3DCT imaging in maxillofacial trauma. *Comput Med Imaging Graph* 1995;19:385–395.

42. Rohrich RJ, Adams WP Jr: Nasal fracture management: Minimizing secondary nasal deformities. *Plast Reconstr Surg* 2000;106: 266–273.

43. Mondin V, Rinaldo A, Ferlito A: Management of nasal bone fractures. *Am J Otolaryngol* 2005;26:181–185.

44. Fernandes SV: Nasal fractures: The taming of the shrewd. *Laryngoscope* 2004;114:587–592.

45. Murray J, Maran A: The treatment of nasal injuries by manipulation. *J Laryngol Otol* 1980;94:1405–1410.

46. Crowther JA, O'Donoghue GM: The broken nose: Does familiarity breed neglect? *Ann R Coll Surg Engl* 1987;69: 259–260.

47. Waldron J, Mitchell DB, Ford G: Reduction of fractures nasal bones: Local versus general anesthesia. *Clin Otolaryngol* 1989;14:357–359.

48. Staffel JG: Optimizing treatment of nasal fractures. *Laryngoscope* 2002;112:1709–1719.

49. Verwoerd C: Present day treatment of nasal fractures: Closed versus open reduction. *Facial Plast Surg* 1992;8:220–223.

50. Murray JA, Maran AG, Mackenzie IJ, et al: Open versus closed reduction of the fractured nose. *Arch Otolaryngol* 1984;110: 797–802.

51. Keller JL, Evan KE, Wetmore RF: Toxic shock syndrome after closed reduction of a nasal fracture. *Otolaryngol Head Neck Surg* 1999;120:569–570.

52. Jacobson JA, Stevens MH, Kasworm EM: Evaluation of single dose cefazolin prophylaxis for toxic shock syndrome. *Arch Otolaryngol Head Neck Surg* 1988;114:326–327.

53. Cultrara A, Turk JB, Har-El G: Midfacial degloving approach for repair of naso-orbital-ethmoid and midfacial fractures. *Arch Facial Plast Surg* 2004;6:133–135.

54. Abubaker AO, Sotereanos G, Patterson GT: Use of the coronal surgical incision for reconstruction of severe craniomaxillofacial injuries. *J Oral Maxillofac Surg* 1990;48:579–586.

55. Markowitz BL et al: Management of the medial canthal tendon in nasoethmoid orbital fractures: The importance of the central fragment in classification and treatment. *Plast Reconstr Surg* 1991;87:843–853.

56. Ellis E 3rd: Sequencing treatment for naso-orbito-ethmoid fractures. *J Oral Maxillofac Surg* 1993;51:543–558.

57. Herford AS, Ying T, Brown B: Outcomes of severely comminuted (type III) nasoorbitoethmoid fractures. *J Oral Maxillofac Surg* 2005;63:1266–1277.

58. Bell RB, Dierks EJ, Homer L, et al: Management of cerebrospinal fluid leak associated with craniomaxillofacial trauma. *J Oral Maxillofac Surg* 2004;62:676–684.

59. Clemenza JW, Kaltman SI, Diamond DL: Craniofacial trauma and cerebrospinal leakage: A retrospective clinical study. *J Oral Maxillofac Surg* 1995;53:1004–1007.

60. Gruss JS, Hurwitz JJ, Nik NA, et al: The pattern and incidence of nasolacrimal injury in naso-orbital-ethmoid fractures: The role of delayed assessment and dacryocystorhinostomy. *Br J Plast Surg* 1985;38:116–121.

61. Becelli R et al: Posttraumatic obstruction of lacrimal pathways: A retrospective analysis of 58 consecutive naso-orbitoethmoid fractures. *J Craniofac Surg* 2004;15:29–33.

62. Ioannides C, Freihofer HPM, Bruaset I: Trauma of the upper third of the face. *J Maxillofac Surg* 1984;12:255–261.

63. Al-Qurainy A et al: The characteristics of midfacial fractures and the association with ocular injury: A prospective study. *Br J Oral Maxillofac Surg* 1991;29:291–301.

64. Mazock JB, Schow SR, Triplett RG: Evaluation of ocular changes secondary to blowout fractures. *J Oral Maxillofac Surg* 2004;62:1298–1302.

65. Hislop WS, Dutton GN, Duglas PS: Treatment of retrobulbar hemorrhage in accident and emergency departments. *Br J Oral Maxillofac Surg* 1996;34:289–292.

66. Gerbino G, Ramieri, GA, Nasi A: Diagnosis and treatment of retrobulbar hematomas following blunt orbital trauma: A description of eight cases. *Int J Oral Maxillofac Surg* 2005;34:127–131.

67. Bater MC, Ramchandani PL, Brennan PA: Post-traumatic eye observations. *Br J Oral Maxillofac Surg* 2005;43:410–416.

68. Steinsapir KD, Goldberg RA: Traumatic optic neuropathy. *Surv Ophthalmol* 1994;38:487–518.

69. Burnstine MA: Clinical recommendations for repair of orbital facial fractures. *Curr Opin Ophthalmol* 2003;14:236–240.

70. Bansagi ZC, Meyer DR: Internal orbital fractures in the pediatric age group: Characterization and management. *Ophthalmology* 2000;107:829–836.

71. Okinaka Y, Hara J, Takahashi M: Orbital blowout fracture with persistent mobility deficit due to fibrosis of the inferior rectus muscle and perimuscular tissue. *Ann Otol Rhinol Laryngol* 1999;108:1174–1176.

72. Hawes MJ, Dortzbach RK: Surgery on orbital floor fractures: Influence of time of repair and fracture size. *Ophthalmology* 1983;90:1066–1070.

73. Gagnon MR, Yeatts RP, Williams Z, et al: Delayed enophthalmos following a minimally displaced orbital floor fracture. *Ophthal Plast Reconstr Surg* 2004;20:241–243.

74. Boush GA, Lemke BN: Progressive infraorbital nerve hypesthesia as a primary indication for blow-out fracture repair. *Ophthal Plast Reconstr Surg* 1994;10:271–275.

75. Tengtrisorn S, McNab AA, Elder JE: Persistent infra-orbital nerve hyperaesthesia after blunt orbital trauma. *Aust N Z J Ophthalmol* 1998;26:259–260.

76. Mullins JB, Holds JB, Branham GH, et al: Complications of the transconjunctival approach: A review of 400 cases. *Arch Otolaryngol Head Neck Surg* 1997;123:385–388.

77. Wray RC et al: A comparison of conjunctival and subciliary incisions for orbital fractures. *Br J Plast Surg* 1977;30:142–150.

78. Appling WD, Patrinely JR, Salzer TA: Transconjunctival approach vs subciliary skin-muscle flap approach for orbital fracture repair. *Arch Otolaryngol Head Neck Surg* 1993;119:1000–1007.

79. Suga H, Sugawara Y, Uda H, et al: The Transconjunctival approach for orbital bony surgery: In which cases should it be used? *J Craniofac Surg* 2004;15:454–457.

80. Heckler FR, Songcharoen S, Sultani FA: Subciliary incision and skin-muscle eyelid flap for orbital fractures. *Ann Plast Surg* 1983;10:309–313.

81. Holtmann B, Wray RC, Little AG: A randomized comparison of four incisions for orbital fractures. *Plast Reconstr Surg* 1981;67:731–737.

82. Rohrich RJ, Janis JE, Adams WP: Subciliary versus subtarsal approaches to orbitozygomatic fractures. *Plast Reconstr Surg* 2003;111:1708–1713.

83. Girotto JA et al: Blindness after reduction of facial fractures. *Plast Reconstr Surg* 1998;102:1821–1833.

84. Ord RA: Post-operative retrobulbar hemorrhage and blindness complicating trauma surgery. *Br J Oral Surg* 1981;19:202–207.

85. Converse JM, Smith B, Obear MF, et al: Orbital blowout fractures: A ten-year survey. *Plast Reconstr Surg* 1967;39:20–36.

86. Folkestad L, Westin T: Long-term sequelae after surgery for orbital floor fractures. *Otolaryngol Head Neck Surg* 1999;120: 914–921.

87. Hossal BM, Beatty RL: Diplopia and enophthalmos after surgical repair of blowout fracture. *Orbit* 2002;21:27–33.
88. Bodker FS, Cytryn AS, Putterman AM, et al: Postoperative mydriasis after repair of orbital floor fracture. *Am J Ophthalmol* 1993;115:372–375.
89. Marin PC et al: Complications of orbital reconstruction: Misplacement of bone grafts within the intramuscular cone. *Plast Reconstr Surg* 1998;101:1323–1327.
90. Ng JD, Huynh TH, Burgett R: Complications of bioabsorbable orbital implants and fixation plates. *Ophthal Plast Reconstr Surg* 2004;20:85–86.
91. Nam SB, Bae YC, Moon JS, et al: Analysis of the postoperative outcome in 405 cases of orbital fracture using 2 synthetic orbital implants. *Ann Plast Surg* 2006;56:263–267.
92. Jordan DR et al: Complications associated with alloplastic implants used in orbital fracture repair. *Ophthalmology* 1992;99:1600–1608.
93. Zhang QB, Dong YJ, Li ZB, et al: Coronal incision for treating zygomatic complex fractures. *J Craniomaxillofac Surg* 2006;34:182–185.
94. Pedemonte C, Basili A: Predictive factors in infraorbital sensitivity disturbances following zygomaticomaxillary fractures. *Int J Oral Maxillofac Surg* 2005;34:503–506.
95. De Man K, Bax WA: The influence of the mode of treatment of zygomatic bone fractures on the healing process of the infraorbital nerve. *Br J Oral Maxillofac Surg* 1988;26:419–425.
96. Becelli R et al: Delayed and inadequately treated malar fractures: Evolution in the treatment, presentation of 77 cases, and review of the literature. *Aesthetic Plast Surg* 2002;26:134–138.
97. Nagase DY, Courtemanche DJ, Peters DA: Plate removal in traumatic facial fractures. *Ann Plast Surg* 2005;55:608–611.
98. Wittwer G, Yerit K, Watzinger F: Complications after zygoma fracture fixation: Is there a difference between biodegradable materials and how do they compare with titanium osteosynthesis? *Oral Surg Oral Med Oral Pathol Oral Radiol Endod* 2006;101:419–425.
99. O'Sullivan ST, Snyder BJ, Moore MH, et al: Outcome measurement of the treatment of maxillary fractures: A prospective analysis of 100 consecutive cases. *Br J Plast Surg* 1999;52:519–523.
100. Top H et al: Evaluation of maxillary sinus after treatment of midfacial fractures. *J Oral Maxillofac Surg* 2004;62:1229–1236.
101. Baumann A, Ewers R: Midfacial degloving: An alternative approach for traumatic corrections in the midface. *Int J Oral Maxillofac Surg* 2001;30:272–277.
102. Lenarz T, Keiner S: [Midfacial degloving: An alternative approach to the frontobasal area, the nasal cavity and the paranasal sinuses]. *Laryngorhinootologie* 1992;71:381–387. German.
103. Ellis E: Passive repositioning of maxillary fractures: An occasional impossibility without osteotomy. *J Oral Maxillofac Surg* 2004;62:1477–1485.
104. Francel TJ, Birely BC, Ringelman PR, et al: The fate of plates and screws after facial fracture reconstruction. *Plast Reconstr Surg* 1992;90:568–573.
105. Nahum AM: The biomechanics of maxillofacial trauma. *Clin Plast Surg* 1975;2:59–64.
106. Wilson BC, Davidson B, Corey JP, et al: Comparison of complications following frontal sinus fractures managed with exploration with or without obliteration over 10 years. *Laryngoscope* 1998;98:516–520.
107. Gossman, DG, Archer SM, Arosarena O: Management of frontal sinus fractures: A review of 96 cases. *Laryngoscope* 2006;116:1357–1362.
108. Cheney ML et al: Midforehead incision: An approach to the frontal sinus and upper face. *J Craniofac Surg* 1995;6:408–411.
109. Wallis A, Donald PJ: Frontal sinus fractures: A review of 72 cases. *Laryngoscope* 1988;98:593.
110. Koudstaal MJ et al: Post-trauma mucocele formation in the frontal sinus: A rationale of follow-up. *Int J Oral Maxillofac Surg* 2004;33:751–754.
111. Constantinitis J et al: Therapy of invasive mucoceles of the frontal sinus. *Rhinology* 2001;39:33–38.
112. Sailer HF, Gratz KW, Kalavrezos ND: Frontal sinus fractures: Principles of treatment and long-term results after sinus obliteration with the use of lyophilized cartilage. *J Craniomaxillofac Surg* 1998;26:235–242.
113. Stacey DH et al: Management of mandible fractures. *Plast Reconstr Surg* 2006;117:48e–60e.
114. Alpert B, Engelstad M, Kushner GM: Invited review: Small versus large plate fixation of mandibular fractures. *J Craniomaxillofac Trauma* 1999;5:33–39.
115. Passeri LA, Ellis E 3rd, Sinn DP: Relationship of substance abuse to complications with mandibular fractures. *J Oral Maxillofac Surg* 1993;51:22–25.
116. Toma VS, Mathog RH, Toma RS, et al: Transoral versus extraoral reduction of mandible fractures: A comparison of complication rates and other factors. *Otolaryngol Head Neck Surg* 2003;128:215–219.
117. Ellis E 3rd: Complications of rigid internal fixation for mandibular fractures. *J Craniomaxillofac Trauma* 1996;2:32–39.
118. Lamphier J, Ziccardii V, Ruvo A, et al: Complications of mandibular fractures in an urban teaching center. *J Oral Maxillofac Surg* 2003;61:745–749.
119. Stone I, Dodson T, Bays R: Risk factors for infection following operative treatment of mandibular fractures: A multivariate analysis. *Plast Reconstr Surg* 1993;91:64.
120. Furr AM, Schweinfurth JM, May WL: Factors associated with long-term complications after repair of mandibular fractures. *Laryngoscope* 2006;116:427–430.
121. Mathog RH, Toma V, Clayman L, et al: Nonunion of the mandible: An analysis of contributing factors. *J Oral Maxillofac Surg* 2000;58:746–752.
122. Kirkpatrick D, Gandhi R, Van Sickels JE: Infections associated with locking reconstruction plates: A retrospective review. *J Oral Maxillofac Surg* 2003;61:462–466.
123. Champy M, Lodde JP, Jaeger JH, Wilk A: Biomechanical basis of mandibular osteosynthesis according to the F. X. Michelet method. *Rev Stomatol Chir Maxillofac* 1976;77:248–251.
124. Fox AJ, Kellman RM: Mandibular angle fractures: Two-miniplate fixation and complications. *Arch Facial Plast Surg* 2003;5:464–469.
125. Thaller SR, Mabourakh S: Teeth located in the line of mandibular fracture. *J Craniofac Surg* 1994;5:16.
126. Worsaae N, Thorn JJ: Surgical versus nonsurgical treatment of unilateral dislocated low subcondylar fractures: A clinical study of 52 cases. *J Oral Maxillofac Surg* 1994;52:353–360.
127. Ellis E 3rd, Throckmorton G: Facial symmetry after closed and open reduction of fractures of the mandibular condylar process. *J Oral Maxillofac Surg* 2000;58:719–730.
128. Ellis E 3rd, McFadden D, Simon P, et al: Surgical complications with open treatment of mandibular condylar process fractures. *J Oral Maxillofac Surg* 2000;58:950–958.

CHAPTER 47

Complications of Facial Rejuvenation Surgery

Corinne Elisabeth Horn and J. Regan Thomas

Although complications of any surgery are extremely disappointing for both the surgeon and the patient, because of the elective nature of cosmetic surgery, these complications are especially distressing. No cosmetic procedures should be undertaken lightly, and it is the obligation of the surgeon to thoroughly inform patients of the risks, benefits, and alternatives to cosmetic surgery. The surgeon also has the obligation to ensure that the patient has no medical contraindications to the proposed surgery, including hypertension, bleeding diatheses, cardiac conditions, or pulmonary problems. This is especially true in the older population, who typically seek facial rejuvenation. Furthermore, the surgeon must make an educated assessment of the patient's psychologic stability and ability to comply with the postoperative regimen, including dressings, activity restrictions, and follow up. The goal of this chapter is to describe the complications of the commonly performed cosmetic procedures of rhytidectomy, browlift, and blepharoplasty as well as the techniques to use to avoid them.

RHYTIDECTOMY

Complications of rhytidectomy are typically considered early, when they occur within the first week after surgery, or late, when they occur more than 1 week postoperatively (Table 47-1).

Early Complications

Hematoma

Hematoma is the most common complication of rhytidectomy, with reported rates in larger series ranging from 1% to 15%.[1-6] The severity of hematomas varies widely, from a small-volume seroma to a large, tense, expanding bleed that threatens the viability of the skin flap. Fortunately, the incidence of hematomas requiring surgical intervention and drainage is relatively low, between 1.9% and 3.6%.[3,7]

Most hematomas occur during the first 24 hours after surgery; however, for the first postoperative week, the surgeon should maintain a high index of suspicion. Although hematomas are most commonly unilateral, they can be bilateral. Furthermore, patients should be educated preoperatively about the hallmark symptoms of hematoma, including severe or increasing pain (especially if unilateral or of sudden onset) and pain that is sometimes described as "ear pain" or a "toothache."

Other telltale signs include copious blood on the dressing, extreme swelling and discoloration that extends to the perioral and periocular regions beyond the dressing, a sensation of extreme tightness of the skin, a "hard" quality of the skin, trismus, dyspnea, and anxiety[8] (Figure 47-1). A patient who reports of any of these symptoms during the week after a facelift should be considered to have a hematoma until it is proven otherwise. These symptoms warrant immediate reexamination with the removal of the dressing and the close inspection of the flaps for possible hematoma.

The management of a hematoma after rhytidectomy depends on its volume and severity. A small-volume liquefied seroma (i.e., <10 cc) may be asymptomatic and discovered at the first dressing change. The most common location is the infraauricular and postauricular area.[8] Larger seromas should be evacuated, milked through the suture line, or aspirated transcutaneously with a syringe and a large-gauge needle. This can be done in the office under sterile conditions, and it is fairly comfortable for the patient as a result of the sensory denervation that occurs during flap elevation. Reaccumulation is common; thus these patients should have a pressure dressing placed and be closely monitored until the seroma has completely resolved.

Large, expanding hematomas (i.e., >10 cc or creating obvious skin tension and skin compromise) mandate immediate operative exploration. General anesthesia in the operating room setting is preferred to relieve patient anxiety, to provide adequate lighting, and to maintain sterility. If no operating room is immediately available, then the incision should be opened, and as much hematoma as possible should be evacuated before reexploration. Because large hematomas are typically the result of a bleeding vessel surrounded by copious clotted blood, wide opening and re-elevation of the flap are necessary to evacuate the clot with gentle suction. Irrigation under the flaps allows for the adequate visualization of critical neurovascular structures. Control of the bleeding vessel or vessels with bipolar cautery or ligation with small sutures minimizes potentially devastating sequelae to the surrounding facial nerve branches. Prolonged pressure of more than a few hours on the skin flap can result in venous engorgement and vascular compromise. If skin necrosis results, it can lead to permanent scarring as a result of contracture during wound healing. Like seromas, hematomas can recur.

TABLE 47-1 Early and Delayed Complications of Rhytidectomy

Early (<1 week postoperatively)	Late (>1 week postoperatively)
Hematoma	Hematoma
Flap necrosis	Hypertrophic scars, keloids
Facial nerve injury	Alopecia
Infection	Earlobe distortion
Suture-line dehiscence	Hypesthesia
Hairline alteration	Facial asymmetry
Postoperative depression	Liposuction and contour deformaties

Modified from Shumrick KA: Complications of rhytidectomy. In Eisele DW, editor: *Complications in head and neck surgery,* ed 1, St. Louis, 1993, Mosby.

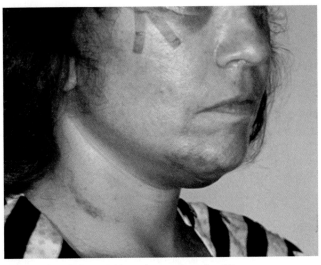

Figure 47-1. Submental hematoma after a facelift.

Therefore a pressure dressing should be placed, and the patient should be monitored daily until the hematoma is definitively resolved.

Although large retrospective studies have identified numerous risk factors for hematoma, perioperative hypertension is probably the most common. Grover and colleagues[2] reported a statistically significant correlation between anterior platysmaplasty, a preoperative systolic blood pressure of more than 150 mm Hg, male gender, aspirin and nonsteroidal anti-inflammatory drug (NSAID) use, and smoking with hematoma formation in a series of 1078 rhytidectomy patients. Another series by Straith and colleagues[9] of 500 facelift patients found that preoperative systolic pressures of more than 150 mm Hg were associated with a 9.2% rate of hematoma as compared

with 2.4% among patients with systolic pressures of less than 150 mm Hg. Berner and colleagues[10] studied 202 facelift patients and found that systolic pressures were maximally elevated 3 hours postoperatively. During this period of "reactive hypertension," preoperative and intraoperative medications became less effective as a result of the adrenergic response to anxiety and pain, and patients with preexisting hypertension had more exaggerated responses postoperatively. Some evidence suggests that perioperative benzodiazepines may counteract this "reactive hypertenstion."[8] Hypertension is an extremely common medical condition among older patients who are typically undergoing facial rejuvenation surgery. Prevention requires preoperative diagnosis and control by the patient's internist, medication to be taken the morning of surgery, postoperative monitoring in the recovery room before discharge, and the continuation of the regimen after surgery.

Antiplatelet medications such as aspirin and NSAIDs have also been linked to hematoma and ecchymoses after rhytidectomy (Figure 47-2). Grover and colleagues[2] found that taking these medications within 2 weeks of rhytidectomy had a statistically higher rate of hematoma formation. Other supplements and over-the-counter medications (e.g., ginseng, garlic, ginkgo biloba, vitamin E) have also been found to inhibit clotting.[11] Thus, to decrease the risk of hematoma, patients should be advised to stop all such medications 2 weeks before surgery.

Increased pressure in the head and neck from coughing, vomiting, bending, or straining can also initiate bleeding and hematoma formation. Gentle emersion from anesthesia, antinausea medications, stool softeners, and activity restriction are an integral part of the intraoperative and postoperative regimen.

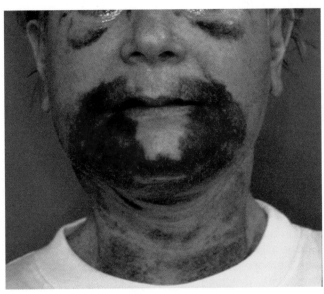

Figure 47-2. Diffuse ecchymoses in a facelift patient who took preoperative aspirin.

Several studies have identified males to be at higher risk of hematoma formation than females. Baker and colleagues[12] studied 137 male patients undergoing facelifts and reported a hematoma rate of 8.7% as compared with 3.3% in large series composed of mostly females. Another study by Lawson and Naidu[13] of 115 male facelift patients described a hematoma rate of 9.6%. Grover and colleagues[14] reported a 12.9% hematoma rate in a study of 62 male facelift patients as compared with a rate of 3.6% in 1016 female patients. These data are consistent with most surgeons' subjective experience of more bleeding during male facelift surgery. Hypotheses to explain this phenomenon include increased vascularity of the subdermal plexus supplying the hair follicles and sebaceous glands and denser connections between the dermis and subcutaneous tissue.[12]

Other factors have also been examined. Although some smaller studies have reported trends toward decreased rate of hematoma with the use of fibrin glue,[15] larger series have not reproduced these results.[2] However, other less quantifiable benefits, such as decreased bruising and edema, have been reported with the use of fibrin glue.[16] The type of anesthesia has not been consistently associated with an increased incidence of hematoma. Rees and colleagues[3] studied 1236 consecutive facelift patients and found a hematoma rate of 1.1% with general anesthesia as compared with 0.9% with monitored intravenous sedation. Other risk factors (e.g., patient age, primary vs. secondary surgery, type of dissection) have also been studied and not found to be associated with hematoma formation.[2]

Flap Necrosis

Skin-flap necrosis is a result of ischemia and compromised vasculature. Rates of skin necrosis ranging from 1.1% to 3.0% have been reported in the literature, and the condition is most commonly the result of local factors.[1,17] Excessive tension on wound closure, unrecognized large hematoma, and poor surgical technique that damages the subdermal plexus can result in vascular congestion and flap necrosis (Figure 47-3). However, skin necrosis may also be the result of systemic factors. Smoking and tobacco products have been associated with a 12-fold increase the risk of flap necrosis.[18] Nicotine patches and smokeless tobacco products are equally problematic, and thus all tobacco products must be stopped a minimum of 2 weeks preoperatively and not used again for 2 weeks postoperatively. Small-vessel disease caused by diabetes, atherosclerosis, collagen vascular diseases such as Raynaud syndrome, or vasculitis may also result in ischemia. These conditions should be identified during the preoperative consultation, and they are typically absolute contraindications to rhytidectomy. Occasionally such patients may be candidates for a "short-flap" facelift, which is a technique that

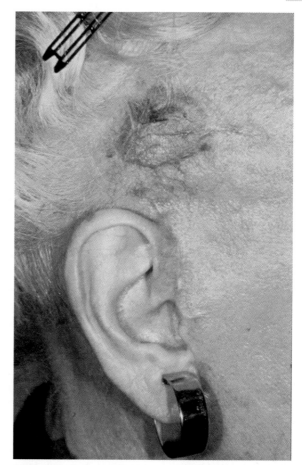

Figure 47-3. Skin-flap necrosis and full-thickness sloughing after a facelift in a patient who had too much tension on the skin-flap closure.

involves minimal undermining, thus preserving a thick vascular flap.

Rhytidectomy flaps are typically broad-based random flaps based on the subdermal and subcutaneous plexuses. Flaps are typically adequately supplied by the excellent blood supply to the head and neck, and their survival is not usually jeopardized, even with extensive distal undermining. The most common site of skin necrosis is the posterosuperior aspect of the postauricular flap at the most distal portion. This area is farthest from the random blood supply and under the most tension from closure. If necrosis occurs, it is typically minor and self-limited. However, necrosis can occur anywhere along the flap where the vasculature is compromised as a result of local surgical trauma or systemic factors.

The management of flap necrosis requires conservative wound care and serial examination. Limited debridement of obviously necrotic tissue is indicated; however, eschars should otherwise not be removed because of their value as a biologic dressing. Antibiotic ointment is applied twice daily to keep the sloughing area moist until reepithelialization and healing by secondary intention is complete. Oral antibiotics may also be indicated, especially if signs of infection develop (e.g., erythema, pain, warmth). If the depth of necrosis is full thickness, healing is likely to result in hypertrophic scarring and possible hyperpigmentation or hypopigmentation. The cautious use of steroid injections may improve the final result of the scar. If necrosis is only partial thickness, scarring and pigmentary changes are much less likely. Hypertrophic scarring usually becomes evident within the first 12 weeks, and the consideration of surgical excision should be delayed for at least 6 months after surgery.[19]

Facial Nerve Injury

Facial nerve injury is a devastating rhytidectomy complication, and it should always be addressed during the preoperative consent process. Fortunately the incidence of motor nerve paralysis reported in the literature is low, ranging from 0.3% to 2.6%.[20] In a series of more than 7000 rhytidectomies analyzed by Baker,[7] 55 complications of facial nerve paralysis (0.7%) were identified, of which 7 cases (0.1%) were permanent. The marginal mandibular branch was most commonly injured (22 of 55), followed by the temporal (18 of 55) and buccal (7 of 55) branches. Another series of 1188 patients reported by McCollough and colleagues[21] described 0% permanent injury and 0.084% temporary facial nerve paresis. These results suggest that facial nerve injury is most commonly the result of neuropraxia from traction, thermal damage from cautery, or needle trauma. Permanent facial nerve injury is likely the result of nerve transection caused by improper surgical planes or injudicious deep dissection.

Infection

Given the excellent blood supply to the head and neck, infection is a rare complication of rhytidectomy. Incidence has been reported as less than 1%, and it typically involves a *Staphylococcus* or *Streptococcus* organism.[22] Most infections occur during the week after surgery, and they can develop despite prophylactic oral antibiotics. Treatment includes intravenous antibiotics and the incision and drainage of any abscesses. Incisions should be very small and along relaxed skin tension lines for optimal camouflage. After infection resolves, patients should be followed for scar formation, which may respond to steroid injections.

Suture-Line Dehiscence

Separation of the wound edges is rare, but, if this condition is not managed appropriately, it can eventually lead to significant scarring. The postauricular area is the most common site of dehiscence because of its site of maximal tension. Most contemporary surgical techniques use a two-layered closure that places all tension on the deeper superficial musculoaponeurotic system (SMAS) layer, which leaves the superficial skin layer free of tension. However, a tight closure may still result in dehiscence.

Conservative management is best for small areas of separation and should include the use of dry wound precautions, peroxide cleanings, and antibiotic ointment application. The area will typically heal by secondary intention within a few weeks. If a larger dehiscence is present, primary closure should be reestablished by excising the edges and resuturing the wound under minimal tension. Steri-Strips (3M, St. Paul, MN) or other mechanisms of wound support may be used. If primary closure is not achieved or if the wound is under significant tension, scarring may result.

Hairline Alteration

All rhytidectomy patients should be counseled that some hairline change will occur. Preoperative analysis will identify patients with a high temporal tuft, especially patients who are undergoing secondary rhytidectomy. In these patients, care should be taken to not raise the hairline further, because this is one of the stigmas of cosmetic surgery (Figure 47-4). In an attempt to preserve the hairline, some surgeons advocate temporal incisions in the non–hair-bearing skin, along the border of the hairline. However, these incisions are often visible, especially among patients with shorter hairstyles, lighter hair colors, and thinning hair. Postauricular step-off deformities result from the improper alignment of the posterior hairline, and

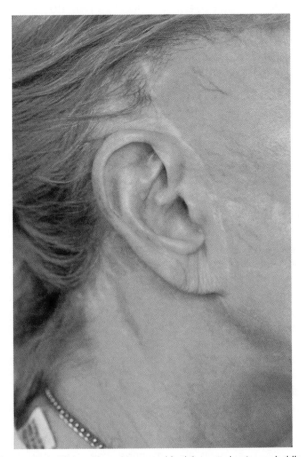

Figure 47-4. Malpositioned temporal incisions and extreme hairline shifts in one patient undergoing secondary rhytidectomy.

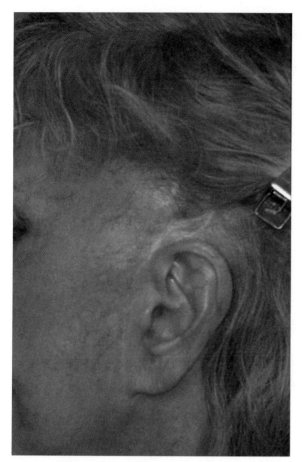

Figure 47-5. Malpositioned incisions with a step-off deformity after the improper alignment of the postauricular hairline.

they may be especially visible in male patients and those with short hairstyles (Figure 47-5).

The management of hairline alteration involves either scar revision techniques or hair transplantation. After waiting a minimum of 3 months, multiple Z-plasties can be used to transpose hair-bearing skin over the area of scar to irregularize and camouflage it. For extreme elevations on hairline, follicular unit grafting can be used to advance the hairline over the scars, but the scar bed is often a poor host for transplanted follicles.

Postoperative Depression

Despite counseling, postoperative depression develops in about 30% of patients during the month after surgery.[23] This is usually short-term and results from relieving the anxiety and stress of surgery as well as the expectations of results. Patients often have disfiguring edema and ecchymoses for several weeks, and they are socially isolated until it resolves. The management of depression includes reassurance by the surgeon and emotional support until the condition resolves. Patients should be seen frequently to monitor the course of depression, and a short course of antidepressants and psychiatric consultation may be considered for extreme cases.

Delayed Complications

Hypertrophic Scars and Keloids

Hypertrophic scars usually develop a few months after surgery (Figure 47-6). They are most common in the retroauricular area, where the thin skin of the postauricular sulcus meets the scalp. The preauricular area is the second most common site. Wound closure tension is often the cause of adverse scarring, although the inappropriate placement of incisions can make these scars more obvious. For this reason, postauricular incisions are optimally placed on the posterior aspect of the conchal bowl, 2 mm to 3 mm beyond the crease. Preauricular incisions should be placed directly in the preauricular crease, and they should pass behind the tragus in women. Retrotragal incisions should not be performed in men to avoid hair-bearing skin on the tragus. Patients who are prone to keloids should be identified; they are not ideal operative candidates.

The management of hypertrophic scars or keloids involves the injection of triamcinolone. A low concentration (i.e., 10 mg/mL) should be used at first, with higher concentrations (i.e., 20–40 mg/mL) reserved for refractory scars. Steroids can result in secondary complications such as telangiectasias and hypopigmentation, so cautious serial injection and observation are appropriate.

Alopecia

Rates of permanent hair loss reported in the literature range from 1% to 3%, although transient hair loss after rhytidectomy is more common.[1] The most common site of hair loss is the temporal area, followed by the postauricular area.[8] Direct trauma to the follicles can be caused by transection, cautery, forceps, tension, or staples along the incision line. Thickened scars may also prevent normal regrowth and result in apparent hair loss. However, even in optimal circumstances, telogen effluvium (i.e., the natural involution of the hair follicle) can result from surgical stress and cause hair loss at and beyond the incision sites.

To minimize the chance of hair loss, temporal flaps should be elevated deep to the hair follicles, and closure tension should be minimized. If alopecia develops, management depends on the cause. Telogen should be managed conservatively, with reassurance that hair growth will return. Thickened scars should be injected with triamcinolone. If alopecia persists beyond a few months, affected areas can be excised, and hair-bearing skin can be reapproximated. Alternatively, follicular unit hair grafts may be transplanted into areas of alopecia. A recent study suggested that there may be a role for minoxidil in the prevention of postoperative alopecia.[24]

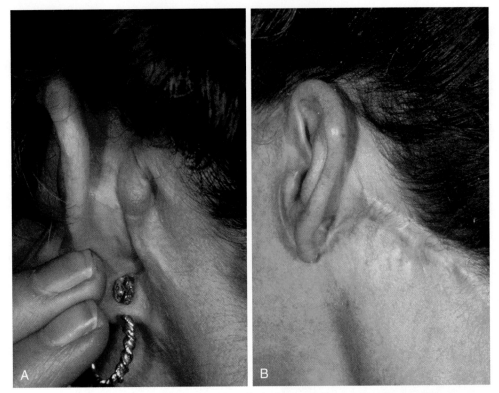

Figure 47-6. Two patients with postauricular hypertrophic scarring after facelift.

Earlobe Malposition and Malpositioned Incisions

The free-hanging earlobe is especially prone to malposition as a result of intraoperative tension or postoperative scar contracture. "Pixie ear" or "satyr ear" results from unopposed downward pull on the flap, and it is an undesirable hallmark of rhytidectomy (Figure 47-7). The prevention of this deformity involves a two-layered closure that places all tension on the SMAS, thus resulting in a slight superior pull on the earlobe during skin closure.

Malpositioned incisions are commonly found anterior to the preauricular sulcus, and they are an unsightly hallmark of cosmetic surgery (Figure 47-8). The revision of poorly placed incisions and earlobe malposition is quite challenging, and the result may never appear completely natural. It is best accomplished by waiting at least 6 months for wound healing and further skin laxity and then performing a V-to-Y advancement into the inferior sulcus of the earlobe.

Hypesthesia

Patients should be counseled that decreased sensation is normal and expected for 4 to 6 weeks after rhytidectomy as a result of the severing of sensory nerve endings during flap elevation. Patients should be warned to avoid extremes of temperature (e.g., frostbite during winter activities, curling iron, hairdryer) and other sources of trauma (e.g., razor shaving) until sensation returns. Raising the flap over the sternocleidomastoid muscle deep to the fascia can result in the severance of

the greater auricular nerve and permanent numbness. If this is recognized in the operating room, the two ends of the nerve should be coapted in a tension-free fashion with 9-0 nylon sutures to allow for regeneration. A transected nerve can also develop a painful neuroma a few months after surgery. The management of a neuroma requires the identification and excision of the mass with the ligation of the stump. If both the proximal and distal ends can be identified, they should be mobilized and reanastomosed.

Facial Asymmetry

Facial asymmetries are common and should be addressed with the patient during preoperative counseling. These are not likely to resolve with rhytidectomy, and they may become more pronounced. Asymmetry may be especially evident in the setting of acute postoperative edema, and it typically resolves spontaneously. Prevention is the best strategy, with intraoperative attention to symmetric flap advancement, SMAS suture placement, and skin redraping. If obvious asymmetries persist for several months, flaps can be elevated and repositioned.

Liposuction and Contour Deformities

Contour deformities typically result from the asymmetric or overzealous liposuction of the jowl and the submental area. Puckering and other irregularities can also result from localized hematomas that are not evacuated and that heal with scar contracture. Initial management should include gentle massage and triamcinolone injection. The

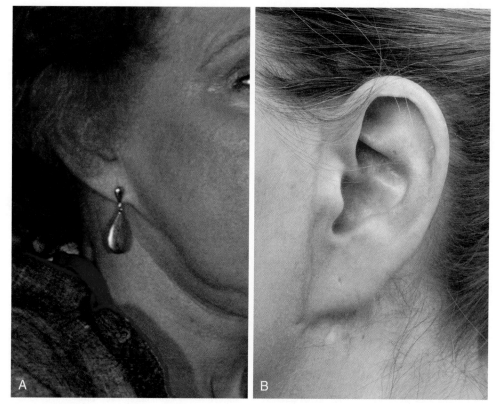

Figure 47-7. A, "Pixie ear" deformity as a result of an unopposed inferior pull of the skin flap. **B,** Another example of "pixie ear" deformity and a malpositioned preauricular incision.

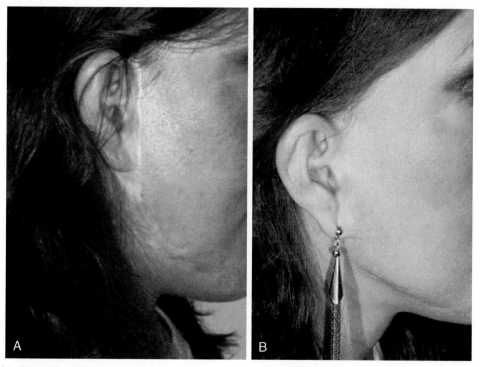

Figure 47-8. A, Malpositioned facelift incision anterior to the preauricular crease. **B,** After revision, with the placement of incisions in a more favorable, less visible location in the preauricular crease and the posttragal area.

management of substantial deformities that do not resolve can include fat or AlloDerm grafting or injection with other soft-tissue fillers.

If a disproportionate quantity of submental or subplatysmal fat is excised, a hollow area of "cobra deformity" results above the hyoid at the cervicomental angle. This is more likely to occur if the platysma has not been plicated. Avoiding excessive liposuction can prevent the deformity, and management typically involves fat augmentation to fill in the defect.

BROWLIFT

The analysis of the upper third of the face is critical in managing the aging face. The evaluation of forehead furrows, the height and shape of the hairline, brow position and symmetry, and upper-lid dermatochalasis are routinely performed. In particular, brow position must be analyzed in patients who are requesting blepharoplasty to decide the degree to which brow ptosis is contributing to dermatochalasis. Normal brow position lies at the orbital rim in males and just above the orbital rim in females. If the brow lies substantially below that, brow repositioning should be performed before addressing the eyelids, because the resuspension of the brow will decrease the amount of eyelid skin to be excised.

Depending on the specific problem, different methods of browlifting may be appropriate (Figure 47-9). These include coronal, trichophytic, endoscopic, mid-forehead, direct brow, and transblepharoplasty browlift. Potential complications vary on the basis of the method of the browlift. Traditionally the coronal browlift was the method of choice for women, especially for those with a low hairline, because incisions can be hidden in the hair, and distal brow structures are accessible as a result of wide exposure. However, the endoscopic approach is currently the gold standard, offering smaller incisions, less disruption of the sensory nerves of the scalp, less potential for alopecia, and equal access to suspend the brow structures. The mid-forehead lift is traditionally used for men with deep horizontal forehead furrows, because incisions can be well masked. As a result of male pattern baldness and the risk of visible incisions, males are generally not considered candidates for coronal or endoscopic procedures. The direct browlift is often used for patients with facial paralysis with atonic frontalis muscles. In a relatively simple procedure, a predictable and dramatic brow elevation (i.e., 1:1) can be achieved, but it is usually only performed for lateral brow elevation, and it does not elevate the entire forehead. The transblepharoplasty approach is an option for patients who are undergoing both upper-lid blepharoplasty and browlift simultaneously, although the elevation that can be achieved is relatively minimal as compared with other techniques. Furthermore, if excessive skin is removed during the

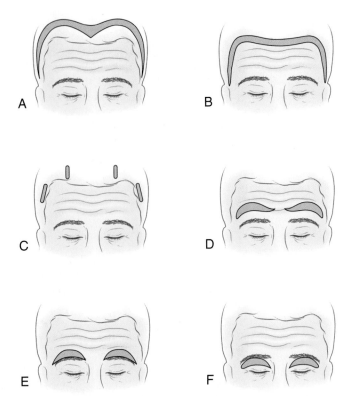

Figure 47-9. Commonly used browlift incisions. **A,** Coronal. **B,** Trichophytic. **C,** Endoscopic. **D,** Mid forehead. **E,** Direct. **F,** Transblepharoplasty.

upper blepharoplasty, suspending the brow further can result in lagophthalmos and corneal exposure.

Although complications can develop with any of these browlift methods, some complications are more commonly associated with specific techniques. Table 47-2 lists the early and delayed (i.e., >1 week) complications of browlifting. A review of forehead and brow anatomy confirms that many of these structures are vulnerable with the use of several techniques (Figure 47-10).

TABLE 47-2 Early and Late Complications of Browlift Surgery

Early (<1 week postoperatively)	Late (>1 week postoperatively)
Hematoma	Alopecia
Temporal nerve injury	Asymmetry
Infection and skin necrosis	Overelevation
Skin irregularities	Scarring
Incision-line dehiscence and irregularities	Hypesthesia

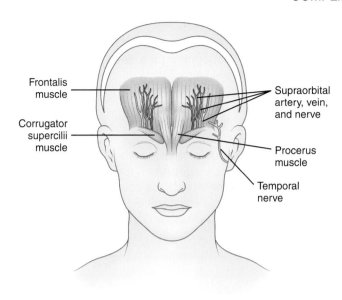

Figure 47-10. Forehead anatomy for browlifting.

Frontalis muscle

Corrugator supercilii muscle

Supraorbital artery, vein, and nerve

Procerus muscle

Temporal nerve

Early Complications

Hematoma

Despite the copious blood supply to the scalp, hematoma is a relatively rare complication of browlifting. The coronal technique creates the largest area of potential space by elevating the subgaleal plane from the bicoronal incision to the brows. However, after it has been identified, this plane is relatively avascular. The skin edges should be conservatively addressed with bipolar cautery, with special care taken in the area of the temporal branch of the facial nerve and in the supraorbital and supratrochlear neurovascular bundles. A suction drain is frequently used to evacuate serosanguineous fluid, and it may be pulled in the office after the output has tapered. Drains are not typically used with the other browlift techniques.

If the suction drain is insufficient or clogged and a large hematoma develops, management involves returning to the operating room for evacuation and hemostasis. However, localized hematoma can occur, and it should be monitored and aspirated with a needle, if necessary. Special care should be taken with the transblepharoplasty technique, because even small quantities of blood can result in an orbital hematoma and compromise vision (see the Blepharoplasty section of this chapter).

Temporal Nerve Injury

The coronal, trichophytic, and endoscopic methods put the temporal branches of the facial nerve at risk during the elevation of the temporal pocket. Although there are many variants of nerve anatomy, the most common is the branching of the main trunk into four or five rami when it exits the parotid; these rami subsequently pass very superficially over the zygomatic arch.[20] The rami travel in the temporoparietal fascia until they reach the undersurface of the frontalis muscle, which is approximately 1 cm lateral to the brow. If either the main trunk or any of the rami are transected, frontalis motor function will be compromised (Figure 47-11).

To prevent damage to the temporal nerve, temporal incisions should be made down to the superficial layer of the deep temporal fascia. This plane can be identified as the layer that is directly adherent to the temporalis muscle and that resists movement; a small cut through this dense white fascia will reveal the temporalis muscle immediately below. This plane is exposed with coronal and trichophytic techniques, but, during endoscopic surgery, visualization is not necessary for temporal elevation as long as the dissector is advanced directly along the deep temporal fascia and glides without resistance. After the cavity is defined to the temporal line, the

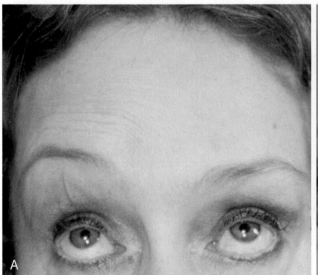
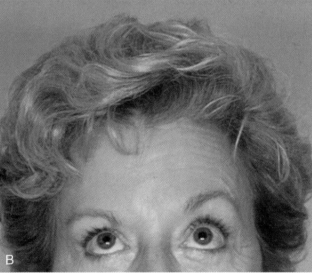

Figure 47-11. A, Left, and **B,** right temporal nerve injury after a browlift.

temporal pocket is connected to the central pocket by taking down the consolidation of the temporalis fascia. This is done under direct visualization to maintain the correct plane and to avoid damage to the temporal nerve. Neuropraxia may also result from excessive tension tenting the temporal and forehead flaps with the coronal, trichophytic, or endoscopic techniques.

Skin Infection and Necrosis

Skin necrosis and infection are rare complications of browlift surgery as a result of the thickness of the musculocutaneous flap and the excellent vascular supply of the supraorbital and supratrochlear vessels. However, with the endoscopic technique, care must be taken to not tent up the frontal skin with the sheathed camera, because localized areas of skin sloughing and necrosis can occur. The management of these areas involves antibiotic ointment and close observation.

Incision-Line Dehiscence

Wound closure under tension is most likely to lead to incision-line dehiscence with the coronal technique. Prevention is aimed at adequate wound support with multiple deep absorbable sutures in the galea followed by skin staples or the use of another strong, nonabsorbable material that should be left in place for 1 week. The management of actual dehiscence involves freshening the edges and reapproximating the hair-bearing skin. Healing by secondary intention will likely result in a patch of

alopecia. If dehiscence occurs after mid-forehead or direct browlift, the same approach should be used, with attention paid to resupporting the deep layer and eliminating tension on the skin.

Irregularities

Although the transection of the corregator and frontalis during browlift was once the method of choice to eliminate glabellar and frontal rhytids, this has for many surgeons been replaced by botulinum toxin A. Less aggressive muscle resection avoids the potential complication of glabellar and frontal irregularities, especially because muscle function has been noted to return over time.[25]

Delayed Complications

Alopecia

Temporary hair loss is common at the incision site and in the surrounding centimeter. However, permanent alopecia can also occur, either from trauma to the follicles or in areas of widened non–hair-bearing scar tissue (Figure 47-12). The coronal browlift involves the most substantial risk of hair loss given the long bicoronal incision that transects numerous follicles as well as the trauma from resuturing and stapling the hair-bearing skin. Furthermore, the highly vascular scalp often requires cauterization for hemostasis, which can further damage hair follicles. Although alopecia can certainly occur with the endoscopic technique, these incisions

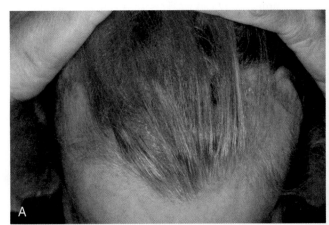

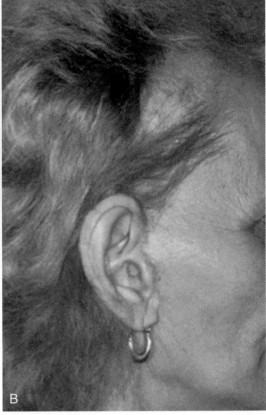

Figure 47-12. Two patients with severe alopecia around the coronal browlift incision sites.

are much smaller; thus hair loss is less likely. Surprisingly, similar alopecia rates between coronal (4%) and endoscopic (2.9%) browlifts were found in one survey, despite the common perception that endoscopic approaches avoid alopecia complications.[26]

Alopecia is prevented by beveling the scalpel blade in the direction of the hair follicles while making the bicoronal incision. The flap edges should be conservatively bipolared (i.e., instead of monopolar cautery) to minimize thermal damage. The flap should be elevated in the avascular subgaleal plane deep to the hair follicles.

Asymmetry

A careful analysis must be performed to determine the cause of postoperative brow asymmetry. Generally a hyperkinetic frontalis or depressor supercilii muscle is the source. Some cases are iatrogenic and result from asymmetric intraoperative elevation or edema that results in the misjudgment of one brow relative to the other. Occasionally neuropraxia of one or more branches of the temporal nerve can cause an asymmetry. Management is targeted at the cause of asymmetry. Hyperkinetic muscles should be treated conservatively with botulinum toxin on the side of the overactivity. Iatrogenic asymmetry can be treated initially with massage and observation, but it may eventually be treated with botulinum toxin. With severe nonresolving asymmetries, surgical options can be considered. For cases of neuropraxia, conservative watchful waiting is required to see if function will recover.

The ideal candidate for a direct browlift requires only the lateral elevation of the brow (e.g., facial paralysis). To elevate the entire structure would require the extension of the incision across the entire eyebrow and result in unacceptable scarring. Elevation depends on the size and shape of the elliptical skin excision, so special care should be taken to maintain symmetry.

Overelevation

Brow overelevation can be a complication of any of the above techniques (Figure 47-13). Both patients and surgeons are also now aware of the potential overcorrection of the brow, which is characterized by the "surprised" look. These results are unnatural and distort the rest of the face. The best prevention is the conservative intraoperative elevation of the brow. Surgical corrections for lowering the brow have been described using tissue expanders and resuspending the brow in a new, lower position.[25]

Scarring

Hypertrophic or keloid scars can occur with any browlift technique. The consequences of the coronal approach are alopecia and widened scars at the incision site in hair-bearing skin. These may be fairly easy to disguise

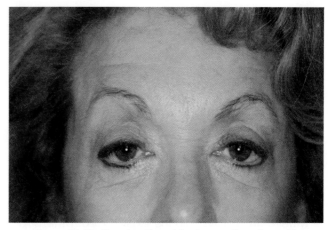

Figure 47-13. Overelevation of the brows after a brow-lift.

with a hairstyle, or they may be extremely bothersome to the patient. Scar tissue can either be excised after waiting at least 6 months, or less dense scars may be transplanted with hair grafts.

The potential for visible scars is especially high with the trichophytic technique as a result of incisions at the hairline. Traditionally these incisions are made just anterior to the hairline and can be camouflaged with irregular geometric incisions. This method has also been described to lower the hairline.[27] Alternatively, reverse-beveling incisions just posterior to the first rows of hair have been described as allowing hairs to grow back through the incision.

With the mid-forehead and direct browlift techniques, incisions cannot be camouflaged by the hair at all. Patients should be informed that healing may take several months, and thick sebaceous skin may be especially prone to poor scarring. Standard wound-closure techniques with careful approximation and slight eversion help ensure ideal scars.

Hypesthesia

All browlift techniques have the potential complication of temporary or permanent hypesthesia. Patients undergoing coronal and trichophytic techniques should be counseled to expect hypesthesia posterior to the incision that may last for several months. The supraorbital and supratrochlear sensory nerves are also at risk where they exit from the foramina in the mediosuperior orbit during the mobilization of the arcus marginalis. The nerves must be directly visualized by turning down the coronal or trichophytic flaps or indirectly visualized with the endoscope to avoid trauma with blunt elevation instruments, and the arcus must be completely released to elevate the brow. However, in up to 10% of patients, these nerves may arise from a foramen 1 cm to 2 cm superior to the supraorbital rim, and they can thus be injured without visualization.[28] Surprisingly, one survey found permanent sensory loss was actually reported to be lower with the coronal approach (0.1%) as compared with endoscopic browlifts (0.57%), despite the subperiosteal "safer plane."[26]

BLEPHAROPLASTY

Blepharoplasty is the third most commonly requested aesthetic procedure, and it is performed by surgeons involved in multiple specialties, including otolaryngology, ophthalmology, and plastic surgery. Complications of upper-lid blepharoplasty are different from those of lower-lid blepharoplasty, and they vary from inconsequential milia to devastating visual loss (Table 47-3). A wide variety of techniques exist for both the upper and the lower lids (e.g., transconjunctival, transcutaneous, pinch), and these techniques are associated with different risks. This chapter summarizes early and late (i.e., >1 week postoperative) complications, their prevention, and their management.

Early Complications

Lower Eyelid Malposition

Lower-lid malposition is the most common complication of blepharoplasty. Severity ranges from mild scleral show (0.5%[29] to between 15% and 20%[30]) to severe ectropion or entropion (1%[30]), depending on the site of contraction (Figure 47-14). As with any surgical procedure, prevention begins by identifying preexisting lid asymmetries, performing careful preoperative analysis, and choosing appropriate surgical candidates. Senile lids with substantial horizontal lid laxity will be unable to resist the forces of inferior contraction after surgery. A lid-shortening procedure (i.e., lateral canthal imbrication, lateral tarsal strip, or full-thickness resection of the lower lid at the lateral canthus) should be considered at the time of blepharoplasty.

TABLE 47-3 Early and Late Complications of Blepharoplasty

Early (<1 week postoperatively)	Late (>1 week postoperatively)
Eyelid malposition	Eyelid contour asymmetry and hollowing
Lagophthalmos	Hypesthesia
Ptosis	Hooding or webbing
Diplopia	Hypertrophic scars
Blindness, visual loss	
Orbital hematoma	
Infection	

Postoperative scleral show describes the downward bowing of the lower lid inferiorly and laterally, which results in more visible conjunctiva and sclera. This is usually mild and transient, and it results from a loss of tone in the orbicularis oculi or lid edema during the immediate postoperative period.[31] Management includes adequate ocular lubrication, taping, and gentle upward massage of the lower lid. The persistence of symptoms may indicate unrecognized horizontal lid laxity as the source of scleral show. This can be addressed with a lid-shortening procedure such as a lateral tarsal strip or a full-thickness lid excision. For borderline cases of lid laxity, a skin–muscle suspension suture may prevent further descent.[29]

Preexisting upper lid ptosis and retraction should also be identified before cosmetic blepharoplasty. Ptosis may be repaired simultaneously with conservative upper-lid blepharoplasty.[32] Unrecognized ptosis can be more obvious after blepharoplasty, when less skin is available to mask the ptotic lid. Alternatively, lid retraction can result from anatomically shallow orbits, thyroid disease, or high myopia, and it should also be recognized before blepharoplasty. These patients may not be surgical candidates at all, but they should at least be counseled that lid retraction may be worsened postoperatively, and they should undergo an extremely conservative surgery or a concurrent midface lift.

True ectropion involves the vertical shortening of the lower lid with the outward rotation of the lid margin away from the globe (see Figures 47-14 and 47-15). Ectropion typically results from the excessive excision of the anterior lamellar skin during transcutaneous blepharoplasty. Other sources include scarring as a result of fat excision, excessive dissection, or bleeding as well as the inadvertent closure of the orbital septum.[33] The unsightly inferior lid position also disrupts the tear film meniscus and the lacrimal drainage apparatus through punctual eversion, which results in epiphora. Prevention lies in conservative skin excision, and there are many methods to test these limits. Some surgeons sit patients up intraoperatively or gently pull down on the cheek to test the effect of gravity on the flap. Patients under minimal sedation can be asked to look up and purse their lips to assess the effect of cheek-tissue mobility.[29] Other management strategies include Frost sutures or the taping of the lower lid superiorly for 24 to 48 hours to help minimize inferior displacement and potential tissue adherence in an abnormal position.[33] If severe ectropion is noted within the first 48 hours and skin from either the upper or lower lids has been banked, then these skin grafts can be replaced. After 48 hours, however, skin grafts are unlikely to heal, and definitive repair should be deferred for 4 to 6 months.[34] Although skin grafts may provide adequate functional repair, the grafted skin may look unnatural.

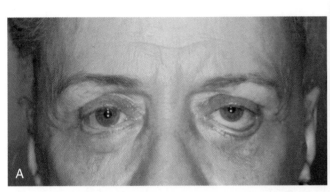
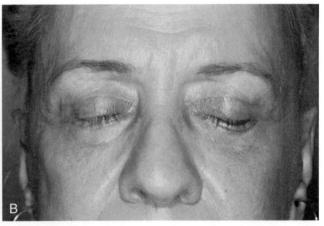

Figure 47-14. A, Right-sided scleral show and left-sided ectropion after transcutaneous blepharoplasty. **B,** Postoperative lagophthalmos that is worse on the left.

Entropion results from the vertical shortening of the posterior lamella, and it may coexist with lower-lid retraction caused by septal scarring. During the early postoperative period, management may be conservative; however, eventual surgical correction with the lysis of adhesions and the placement of spacer grafts is inevitable. Spacer grafts for the posterior and middle lamellae have been described involving the use of the oral mucosa, the hard palate, Hughes tarsoconjunctival grafts, free tarsal conjunctival grafts, AlloDerm, and ear cartilage. In severe cases of vertical lid shortening, simultaneous repair of the posterior, middle, and anterior lamella may also be necessary, and a midface lift may also be required.[35–37] The patient shown in Figures 47-15 through 47-17 with severe ectropion was ultimately repaired with a Hughes tarsoconjunctival graft for the posterior lamella and a skin graft for the anterior lamella.

Lagophthalmos

Incomplete upper-lid closure suggests either a restriction of lid excursion or a paralysis. Prolonged exposure of the ocular surface can result in irritation, tearing, ulceration,

and, ultimately, scarring. The most common cause is the overexcision of the upper-lid skin, but other causes include the shortening of the orbital septum or the imbrication of the orbital septum, the Whitnall ligament, or both.

Patients with dry eyes should be identified preoperatively, and, depending on the severity, they may not be blepharoplasty candidates. However, patients with borderline dry eyes may not yet have symptoms, but compensation can be disrupted with only subtle changes in lid position or minor lagophthalmos. Identifying patients at risk for ocular surface exposure before surgery requires specific inquiries for such conditions as foreign-body sensation, light sensitivity, or worsening symptoms in smoky or air-conditioned rooms. Patients with cranial nerve VII dysfunction and orbicularis weakness, corneal anesthesia from cranial nerve V dysfunction, previous blepharoplasty, or keratoconjunctivitis sicca may have impaired tear-film formation or an impaired blink. Schirmer testing confirms deficient tearing in some patients, but it may not identify all patients who eventually develop dry eyes.[38] All patients should be counseled that dry eyes can develop postoperatively and that they may require lubricating drops.

The prevention of lagophthalmos begins by pinching redundant upper-lid skin with a smooth forceps while the patient is awake and in the seated position and conservatively marking the skin to be excised. The intraoperative pinching of the excess upper-lid tissues with a von Graefe forceps is a trial of the shortening effect on the lid margin. There should be minimal change in lid position and the rotation of the lashes while the skin is pinched. Skin edges should be closed in a single layer, with care taken to not catch the orbital septum or the Whitnall ligament.

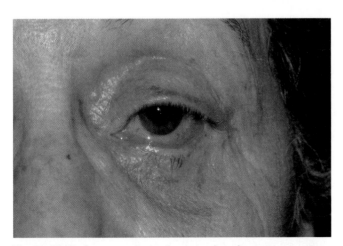

Figure 47-15. Severe postoperative ectropion after transcutaneous blepharoplasty.

Management depends on the severity and cause of the lagophthalmos. All patients should be treated with artificial tear drops 4 to 6 times per day as well as lubricating

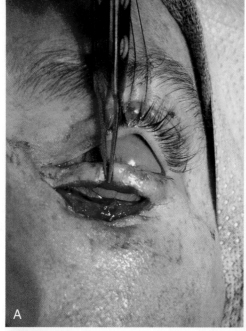

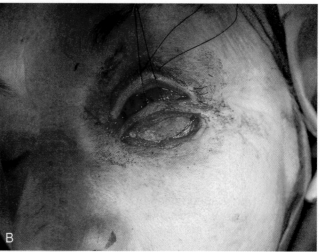

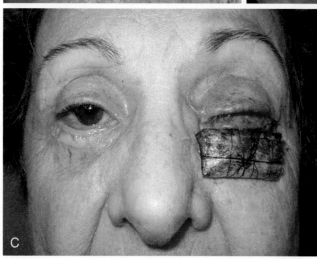

Figure 47-16. Same patient as shown in Figure 47-15. **A,** Intraoperative view of a repair with an incision 4 mm below the lid margin. **B,** A Hughes tarsoconjunctival graft from the upper lid was used to re-create the posterior lamella. The anterior lamella was grafted from postauricular skin. **C,** A postoperative bolster is used to hold these grafts in place during the critical stages of healing.

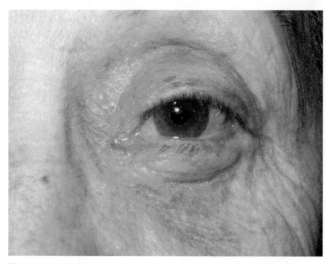

Figure 47-17. Postoperative view of the same patient shown in Figure 47-16, with improved lid position and the resolution of epiphora. Fluoroscene now drains normally through the well-approximated punctum.

ointment, with consideration given to nocturnal moisture chamber or taping. If the orbital septum or the Whitnall ligament has been sutured, the incision must be opened and released. For the overexcision of skin, mild cases often resolve spontaneously as the orbicularis strengthens and the skin stretches by blinking. Gentle finger massage and forced blinking exercises may also be used. More severe cases require skin grafting either from the initial excision (i.e., if <48 hours old and skin has been banked) or from a postauricular donor site.

Ptosis

Transient ptosis can result from hematoma, lid edema, local anesthetic effects, allergy to medications or tape, or reaction to absorbable suture material (Figure 47-18). A hemorrhage involving the levator muscle will compromise elevating function. Persistent ptosis is an infrequent complication, and it is usually the result of levator injury during dissection, fat manipulation, or cautery.

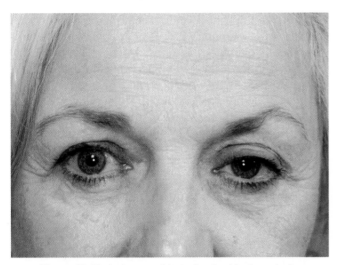

Figure 47-18. Left upper-lid ptosis after blepharoplasty.

Alternatively, the removal of redundant upper-lid skin may make a previously undiagnosed ptosis more obvious. Especially among older patients, preoperative ptosis should be identified, and it can be repaired during the blepharoplasty.[39]

Edema or hemorrhage that results in ptosis should resolve within a few weeks, and it can be managed with ice packs and head elevation. If there is poor levator function, entrapment of the aponeurosis is the most likely, and it should be surgically corrected by the release of the suture before significant fibrosis or scarring occurs.[40] Levator dehiscence is associated with a high lid crease, a translucent upper lid, and good levator function. These conditions may be repaired within a few months with levator advancement and repair onto the tarsus.

All surgeons performing blepharoplasty should have an excellent knowledge of orbital anatomy. The superior tarsal border is the condensation site of the orbicularis muscle and the levator aponeurosis with the orbital septum, and it lacks an intervening fat pad. Thus the septum should be opened more superiorly, where that fat pad is thicker. Traction on the fat pad may tent the aponeurosis into the tissues being excised or stretch an attenuated levator, thereby causing dehiscence. If a dehiscent levator is recognized intraoperatively, it should be repaired.

Diplopia

Diplopia is a rare but serious complication of blepharoplasty, with a frequency of 3 of 920 cases in one review.[41] The causes are either transient or permanent. Temporary causes include hematomas (i.e., as a result of mass effect), local anesthetic toxicity, or the ischemic contracture of the extraocular muscles. Permanent diplopia implies either restrictive or paretic causes. Restrictive mechanisms include structural damage to the extraocular muscles during dissection, the incarceration of a tendon, or scar tissue. Paretic causes can be

the result of excessive cautery deep in the orbit.[42] Reports in the literature most commonly involve the inferior oblique, because it lies between the medial and the middle fat pat. However, the inferior rectus[43] and superior oblique[44] have also been implicated.

As with other complications, preventing diplopia requires a detailed knowledge of orbital anatomy and careful hemostasis. The inferior oblique muscle runs horizontally between the medial and middle fat pads. Some surgeons routinely identify it for protection during surgery, whereas others strategically open the orbital septum directly over the fat pads and minimize pulling on fat. Special care should be taken with secondary blepharoplasty, where scar tissue or more friable tissue could possibly distort anatomic structures. Furthermore, during hemostasis, the surgeon should recognize the possibility of damage to the deeper structures.

If hematoma is the source, diplopia will resolve when the blood resorbs or is surgically drained, and the mass effect disappears. If stitch incarceration of an extraocular muscle during the closure of the septum is a possible source, the wound should be reexplored to release the muscle or tendon.[45] Otherwise, the management of permanent diplopia includes watchful waiting; Hayworth and colleagues[41] report improvement over 6 to 15 months.

Orbital Hematoma, Retrobulbar Hemorrhage, and Blindness

Blindness is a rare but devastating complication of blepharoplasty, with an incidence of 0.0044% to 0.04%.[46,47] Although the exact mechanism of visual loss is controversial, it is likely that either orbital hemorrhage or vasospasm is the culprit. Retrobulbar hemorrhage increases intraorbital and intraocular pressures, which results in retinal ischemic changes, ischemic optic neuropathy, or acute-angle closure glaucoma.[33] Although hemorrhage involving a delay of up to 9 days has been reported, the immediate postoperative period is more common.[48] The presentation is the sudden onset of significant and usually unilateral orbital pain that is associated with proptosis, chemosis, ophthalmoplegia, and a firm globe. Ophthalmologic examination may also show afferent papillary defect, optic nerve ischemia, or central retinal artery occlusion. When no hemorrhage is evident, vasospasm has been implicated, possibly as a result of epinephrine injection.[49]

A medical history should try to elicit any increased risk of bleeding, such as anticoagulants, aspirin, or NSAID use; homeopathic and dietary supplements (e.g., vitamin E, ginseng, garlic, ginkgo biloba); bleeding diatheses; hypertension; and systemic steroid use. If medically feasible, aspirin should not be taken for a minimum of 2 weeks before and after surgery. Warfarin should be stopped 4 to 7 days before surgery, and heparin can be used until the perioperative period. Patients with Graves ophthalmopathy have been associated with increased bleeding as a result of the engorgement of the orbit. Patients with monocular vision or orbital complications of systemic disease (e.g., diabetic retinopathy, severe retinovascular disease) are typically not candidates for cosmetic blepharoplasty.

Direct trauma to the intraorbital vessels during local injection with local anesthesia is another potential source of hemorrhage. Furthermore, the systemic absorption of epinephrine during the injection of local anesthetic has been attributed to hypertensive crisis, aggravated bleeding, and even one case of bilateral blindness.[50] Thus the injection of local anesthesia posterior to the orbital septum should always take place under direct visualization.

Intraoperative technique should always maintain meticulous hemostasis. After fat excision, a clamp should remain on the stump until adequate bipolar cautery is achieved, because small vessels can retract into the orbit and continue to bleed. Excessive traction on the orbital fat should also be avoided to prevent the rupture of deeper vessels, which are more difficult to access. If there is any question about whether a cauterized vessel is likely to bleed, it should be carefully observed and tested with a Valsalva maneuver.

However, even with optimal technique, postoperative circumstances may still result in hemorrhage. Patients should be extubated deep from general anesthesia to avoid coughing and bucking that raise intracranial pressure. Postoperative nausea and vomiting as well as rebound vasodilation during the hours after surgery when the epinephrine wears off can also result in hemorrhage. Opaque dressings are avoided so that the eyes can be continuously observed for the first few hours after surgery, and patients are sent home with a companion. Strict postoperative instructions usually include avoiding active exertion, bending, straining, or nose blowing for the first week. Patients are asked to sleep with 30- to 45-degree head-of-bed elevation and to use ice packs intermittently for the first 24 hours.

The management of acute orbital hemorrhage is a true emergency, and assessing vision is the priority. An emergency ophthalmology consult should be obtained, and a visual examination and intraocular pressure should be documented. If an orbital hemorrhage has occurred and stabilized and the vision is not declining, then close observation is acceptable. In one series of 2750 retrobulbar hemorrhages resulting from all causes, only 2 patients had permanent blindness.[51] If intraocular pressure has risen high enough that vision is compromised, then the retinal vessels are occluded; there is a 60- to 90-minute window during which blood supply

can be reestablished and vision restored. Although medical management with pressure-lowering diuretics (e.g., acetazolamide, mannitol) can be attempted, any decline in vision warrants immediate return to the operative setting. The wound should be reopened, and any clot or hematoma should be evacuated. If vision is not improved or pressure is not relieved, immediate surgical decompression via lateral canthotomy and cantholysis should be performed. In extreme cases, when pressure is still not relieved, endoscopic medial and inferior wall bony decompression of the orbit or anterior-chamber paracentesis can be attempted.[46]

Infection

Infection after blepharoplasty is relatively uncommon because of the excellent vascularity of the eyelids. Typically preoperative antibiotics are given, and topical antibiotic ointment is usually adequate postoperative prophylaxis. Localized stitch abscesses can be drained in the office with the removal of the stitch; however, wound dehiscence may result. Oral antibiotics and warm compresses may speed the resolution of localized infections. However, there have been reports in the literature of orbital cellulitis and abscesses[52] as well as necrotizing fasciitis after blepharoplasty.[53] Morgan[54] described three cases of orbital cellulitis resulting in blindness.

Rapid diagnosis and treatment are critical. The presentation is typically pain, lid edema, erythema, chemosis, and, in more advanced cases, proptosis, ophthalmoplegia, and visual changes. Patients may also have fevers and leukocytosis. A computed tomography scan with contrast of the orbit should reveal the presence of an abscess, which requires immediate surgical drainage and intravenous antibiotics. If only a phlegmon is present, intravenous antibiotics and close monitoring are acceptable.

Delayed Complications

Eyelid Contour Asymmetry and Hollowing

Differences in eyelid contour may be the result of overzealous or inadequate fat excision, asymmetric edema resolution, or lacrimal gland prolapse. Careful analysis and the preoperative marking of prominent fat pads in the preoperative area with the patient in the seated position can be used to identify the appropriate pockets. Three fat compartments exist in the lower lids, and only two exist in the upper lids, with the lacrimal gland assuming the lateral compartment. Fullness in the upper lateral compartment is consistent with a ptotic lacrimal gland, which should be identified to avoid the injury that can result in postoperative hemorrhage or intractable dry eye. Lacrimal-gland suspension with nonabsorbable sutures from the superior orbital rim periosteum is well described.[55]

Conservative balanced fat removal is the most appropriate strategy. Medial upper-lid fat compartments are frequently overlooked as a result of fibrous septae and vascularity. Residual fullness in an isolated compartment should be monitored for 2 to 3 months. Minor asymmetries that result from edema may resolve with a low-dose triamcinolone injection. If they are not resolved, asymmetries are likely caused by retained fat, and management requires revision transconjunctival blepharoplasty in that compartment. Alternatively, the overexcision of fat creates an undesirable hollowed-out eye that can be extremely difficult to repair. Hollow deformities have been managed with fat or fat-composite grafts with moderate success, but injectable fat may be difficult to control and can leave lumpy irregularities.

Hypesthesia

Mild diffuse hypesthesia of the orbits is common after blepharoplasty, and it usually resolves spontaneously by 6 months. It is attributed to dissection, clamping, or cauterizing the fat pads. Klatsky and Manson[56] reported numbness in the distributions of the supratrochlear and infraorbital nerves in less than 1% of patients.

Hooding or Webbing

Webbing or *hooding* refers to the band of tissue that crosses the medial punctum superiorly to the nose or inferiorly from the lateral canthus to the temple. The overexcision of skin near either canthus as well as closely spaced lateral incisions for upper and lower blepharoplasty can result in scar contracture.

To prevent hooding, upper and lower blepharoplasty incisions should be no closer than 4 mm.[57] Upper-lid incisions should be angled slightly superior,[29] whereas lower lid incisions should stop at the medial canthus and at that point be straight. Continuing into the thicker nasal or temple skin on lid incisions could cause tenting and depressions. Management includes skin grafting or Z-plasty.

Hypertrophic Scars

Surgical incisions fade over several months, but they may always be visible on close inspection. Hypertrophic scars do not usually appear in the thin eyelid skin, but they are always a possibility. Prevention involves good surgical technique, the use of 6-0 or smaller sutures (either fast absorbing or nonabsorbable) or Dermabond (Ethicon, Sommerville, NJ) and mild eversion of skin closure. Nonabsorbable sutures should be removed after 3 to 7 days to avoid suture tracks.

Milia

Milia (i.e., inclusion cysts) are caused by trapped epithelium or an obstructed glandular duct along the suture tracks of an incision line. Suture tracks, cysts, and milia can be excised with a fine blade or scissor. If necessary, substantial scars can be injected with triamcinolone or re-excised and revised.

CONCLUSION

Facial rejuvenation procedures should be undertaken by specialty-trained surgeons only after thoroughly informing the patient of the risks, benefits, alternatives, and realistic outcomes of surgery. The surgeon must screen the patient's psychologic stability and his or her ability to comply with the postoperative regimen, including dressings, activity restrictions, and follow up. A thorough knowledge of facial anatomy as well as of possible complications and their prompt management is critical. Complications should be embraced rather than avoided, with adequate time and attention given to their course and resolution. The surgeon must ensure that the patient has no medical contraindications, including hypertension, bleeding diatheses, cardiac conditions, or pulmonary problems. This is especially true for members of the older population, who typically seek facial rejuvenation.

REFERENCES

1. Baker TJ, Gordon HL, Mosienko P: Rhytidectomy: A statistical analysis. *Plast Reconstr Surg* 1977;59(1):24–30.
2. Grover R, Jones BM, Waterhouse N: The prevention of haematoma following rhytidectomy: A review of 1078 consecutive facelifts. *Br J Plast Surg* 2001;54(6):481–486.
3. Rees TD, Barone CM, Valauri FA, et al: Hematomas requiring surgical evacuation following face lift surgery. *Plast Reconstr Surg* 1994;93(6):1185–1190.
4. Perkins SW, Williams JD, Macdonald K, et al: Prevention of seromas and hematomas after face-lift surgery with the use of postoperative vacuum drains. *Arch Otolaryngol Head Neck Surg* 1997;123(7):743–745.
5. Kamer FM, Song AU: Hematoma formation in deep plane rhytidectomy. *Arch Facial Plast Surg* 2000;2(4):240–242.
6. Jones BM, Grover R: Avoiding hematoma in cervicofacial rhytidectomy: A personal 8-year quest: Reviewing 910 patients. *Plast Reconstr Surg* 2004;113(1):381–390.
7. Baker DC: Complications of cervicofacial rhytidectomy. *Clin Plast Surg* 1983;10(3):543–562.
8. Moyer JS, Baker SR: Complications of rhytidectomy. *Facial Plast Surg Clin N Am* 2005;13:469–478.
9. Straith RE, Raju DR, Hipps CJ: The study of hematomas in 500 consecutive face lifts. *Plast Reconstr Surg* 1977;59(5):694–698.
10. Berner RE, Morain WD, Noe JM: Postoperative hypertension as an etiological factor in hematoma after rhytidectomy: Prevention with chlorpromazine. *Plast Reconstr Surg* 1976;57(3):314–319.
11. Heller J, Gabbay JS, Ghadjar K, et al: Top-10 list of herbal and supplemental medicines used by cosmetic patients: What the plastic surgeon needs to know. *Plast Reconstr Surg* 2006;117(2):436–445.
12. Baker DC, Aston SJ, Guy CL, et al: The male rhytidectomy. *Plast Reconstr Surg* 1977;60(4):514–522.
13. Lawson W, Naidu RK: The male facelift: An analysis of 115 cases. *Arch Otolaryngol Head Neck Surg* 1993;119(5):535–539.
14. Grover R, Jones BM, Waterhouse N: The prevention of haematoma following rhytidectomy: A review of 1078 consecutive facelifts. *Br J Plast Surg* 2001;54(6):481–486.
15. Marchac D, Sandor G: Face lifts and sprayed fibrin glue: An outcome analysis of 200 patients. *Br J Plast Surg* 1994;47(5):306–309.

16. Fezza JP, Cartwright M, Mack W, et al: The use of aerosolized fibrin glue in face-lift surgery. *Plast Reconstr Surg* 2002;110(2):658–664.

17. MacGregor MW, Greenberg RL: Rhytidectomy. In Goldwyn RM, editor: *The unfavorable result in plastic surgery: Avoidance and treatment,* ed 1, Boston, 1972, Little, Brown.

18. Rees TD, Liverett DM, Guy CL: The effect of cigarette smoking on skin-flap survival in the face lift patient. *Plast Reconstr Surg* 1984;73(6):911–915.

19. Perkins S, Dayan S: Rhytidectomy. In Papel ID, editor: *Facial plastic and reconstructive surgery,* ed 2, New York, 2002, Thieme.

20. Baker DC, Conley J: Avoiding facial nerve injuries in rhytidectomy: Anatomical variations and pitfalls. *Plast Reconstr Surg* 1979;64(6):781–795.

21. McCollough EG, Perkins SW, Langsdon PR: SMAS suspension rhytidectomy: Rational and long term experience. *Arch Otolarygol* 1989;115:228–234.

22. Leroy IL, Rees TD, Nolan WB: Infections requiring hospital readmission following face lift surgery: Incidence, treatment, and sequelae. *Plast Reconstr Surg* 1994;93(3):533–536.

23. Goin MK, Burgoyne RW, Goin JM, et al: A prospective psychological study of 50 female facelift patients. *Plast Reconstr Surg* 1980;65(4):436–442.

24. Eremia S, Umar SH, Li CY: Prevention of temporal alopecia following rhytidectomy: The prophylactic use of minoxidil: A study of 60 patients. *Dermatol Surg* 2002;28:66–74.

25. Namazie AR, Keller GS: Current practices in endoscopic brow and temporal lifting. *Facial Plast Surg Clin North Am* 2001;9(3):439–451.

26. Elkwood A, Matarasso A, Rankin M, et al: National plastic surgery survey: Brow lifting techniques and complications. *Plast Reconstr Surg* 2001;108(7):2143–2150.

27. Mayer TG, Fleming RW: *Aesthetic and reconstructive surgery of the scalp,* St. Louis, 1992, Mosby-Year Book.

28. Isse NG: Endoscopic facial rejuvenation. *Clin Plast Surg* 1997;24(2):213–231.

29. Honrado CP, Pastorek NJ: Long-term results of lower-lid suspension blepharoplasty: A 30-year experience. *Arch Facial Plast Surg* 2004;6(3):150–154.

30. Newhouse RW, Baylis HI: Complications in lower lid blepharoplasty. In Putterman AM, editor: *Cosmetic oculoplastic surgery,* New York, 1982, Grune and Stratton.

31. Rees TD: Correction of ectropion resulting from blepharoplasty. *Plast Reconstr Surg* 1972;50(1):1–4.

32. Massry GG: Ptosis repair for the cosmetic surgeon. *Facial Plast Surg Clin North Am* 2005;13(4):533–539.

33. Iliff NT, Iwamoto M: Complications of blepharoplasty. In Eisele DW, editor: *Complications in head and neck surgery,* ed 1, St. Louis, 1993, Mosby.

34. Eliasoph I: Current techniques of entropion and ectropion correction. *Otolaryngol Clin North Am* 2005;38(5):903–919.

35. Ben Simon GJ, Lee S, Schwarcz RM, et al: Subperiosteal midface lift with or without a hard palate mucosal graft for correction of lower eyelid retraction. *Ophthalmology* 2006;113(10):1869–1873.

36. Li TG, Shorr N, Goldberg RA: Comparison of the efficacy of hard palate grafts with acellular human dermis grafts in lower eyelid surgery. *Plast Reconstr Surg* 2005;116(3):873–878.

37. Baylis HI, Wilson MC, Groth MJ: Complications of lower blepharoplasty. In Putterman AM, editor: *Cosmetic oculoplastic surgery,* ed 2, Philadelphia, 1993, WB Saunders.

38. McKinney P, Byun M: The value of tear film breakup and Schirmer's tests in preoperative blepharoplasty evaluation. *Plast Reconstr Surg* 1999;104(2):566–569.

39. De la Torre JI, Martin SA, Decordier BC: Aesthetic eyelid ptosis correction: A review of technique and cases. *Plast Reconstr Surg* 2003;112(2):655–660.

40. Baylis HI, Sutcliffe T, Fett DR: Levator injury during blepharoplasty. *Arch Ophthalmol* 1984;102(4):570–571.

41. Hayworth RS, Lisman RD, Muchnick RS: Diplopia following blepharoplasty. *Ann Ophthalmol* 1984;16(5):448–451.

42. Glavas IP: The diagnosis and management of blepharoplasty complications. *Otolaryngol Clin North Am* 2005;38:1009–1021.

43. Alfonso E, Levada AJ, Flynn JT: Inferior rectus paresis after secondary blepharoplasty. *Br J Ophthalmol* 1984;68(8):535–537.

44. Wesley RE, Pollard ZF, McCord CD: Superior oblique paresis after blepharoplasty. *Plast Reconstr Surg* 1980;66(2):283–286.

45. Syniuta LA, Goldberg RA, Thacker NM: Acquired strabismus following cosmetic blepharoplasty. *Plast Reconstr Surg* 2003;111(6):2053–2059.

46. Hass AN, Penne RB, Stefanyszyn MA: Incidence of postblepharoplasty orbital hemorrhage and associated visual loss. *Ophthal Plast Reconstr Surg* 2004;20(6):426–432.

47. Waller RR: Is blindness a realistic complication in blepharoplasty procedures? *Ophthalmology* 1978;85(7 Pt 1):730–735.

48. Teng CC, Reddy S, Wong JJ, et al: Retrobulbar hemorrhage nine days after cosmetic blepharoplasty resulting in permanent visual loss. *Ophthal Plast Reconstr Surg* 2006;22(5):388–389.

49. Mahaffery PJ, Wallace AF: Blindness following cosmetic blepharoplasty: A review. *Br J Plast Surg* 1986;39(2):213–221.

50. Anderson RL, Edwards JJ: Bilateral visual loss after blepharoplasty. *Ann Plast Surg* 1980;5(4):288–292.

51. Duke-Elder S: Orbital hemorrhage. In Duke-Elder S, editor: *System of ophthalmology: Injuries: Part 1: Mechanical injuries,* vol XIV, St. Louis, 1958 Mosby.

52. Rees TD, Craig SM, Fisher Y: Orbital abscess following blepharoplasty. *Plast Reconstr Surg* 1984;73(1):126–127.

53. Goldberg RA, Li TG: Postoperative infection with group A beta-hemolytic *Streptococcus* after blepharoplasty. *Am J Ophthalmol* 2002;134(6):908–910.

54. Morgan SC: Orbital cellulitis and blindness following a blepharoplasty. *Plast Reconstr Surg* 1979;64(6):823–826.

55. Bosniak S: Reconstructive upper lid blepharoplasty. *Ophthalmol Clin North Am* 2005;18(2):279–289.

56. Klatsky S, Manson PN: Numbness after blepharoplasty: The relation of the upper orbital fat to sensory nerves. *Plast Reconstr Surg* 1981;67(1):20–22.

57. Pastorek N: Upper lid blepharoplasty. In Papel ID, editor: *Facial plastic and reconstructive surgery,* ed 2, New York 2002, Thieme.

CHAPTER 48

Injury of the Facial Nerve

Holger G. Gassner and Kris S. Moe

Trauma is the second most common cause of facial paralysis. This includes sharp, penetrating injury, as in the case of knife or bullet wounds; blunt trauma that causes temporal bone fractures; and iatrogenic injury. Although the incidence of iatrogenic trauma is low, the number of surgical procedures performed in the area of the facial nerve and the variety of specialists operating in this region are considerable, which results in a relatively high incidence of this injury.

The magnitude of complexity involved in restoring facial-nerve function after traumatic injury is readily apparent when one considers what the process requires: the guidance of more than 11,000 nerve fibers back to their original end organs. Unfortunately, the complete restoration of function of a significantly injured facial nerve is not possible. The surgeon must therefore determine what degree of functional restoration is possible for each patient and decide which of the many reported surgical procedures is optimal.

This chapter focuses on the pathophysiology and rehabilitation of traumatic facial-nerve injury that can occur as a complication of head and neck surgery, and it provides a framework for the complex decision making that is required for the best possible care of these patients.

ANATOMIC AND PHYSIOLOGIC CONSIDERATIONS

Among the 11,000 afferent and efferent fibers of the facial nerve are 8000 myelinated motor fibers that innervate 27 muscles of the face, ear, and neck. The remaining 3000 fibers provide parasympathetic innervation to multiple salivary, mucous, and lacrimal glands; taste from the anterior tongue; and sensation from portions of the skin of the external auditory canal, the external ear, and the lateral tympanic membrane. Although on occasion autonomic and sensory dysfunction play a role in the clinical diagnosis and rehabilitation of facial-nerve injuries, the rehabilitation of these injuries focuses predominantly on motor function.

Anatomy of the Facial Nerve

The anatomy of the facial nerve is complex, with multiple branches joining and leaving the nerve along its course. Figure 48-1 depicts the multiple anatomic portions and segments of the nerve. Several anatomic characteristics render it susceptible to numerous types of injuries. The intracranial portion of the nerve lacks epineurium, and it

is particularly vulnerable to compression by tumors or surgical manipulation. The Fallopian canal is narrowest at the meatal foramen (0.7 mm), where the nerve is most susceptible to compression injury from edema. The labyrinthine segment relies solely on the internal auditory artery for perfusion; this area is therefore more susceptible to ischemic injury. Longitudinal temporal bone fractures most frequently injure the geniculate and postgeniculate tympanic segment of the facial nerve, although transection of the nerve is rare. Transverse fractures usually damage the nerve in the labyrinthine segment, with a high incidence of complete transection of the nerve when the fallopian canal is involved. The tympanic segment of the facial canal is the most frequent site of bony dehiscence, typically above the oval window. The tympanic segment also harbors the second-narrowest section of the bony canal. During tympanomastoid surgery, the tympanic and mastoid segments are at risk of injury. Some approaches to the skull base, the parotid gland, and the temporomandibular joint are associated with injuries of the extratemporal segment. In this segment, the nerve maintains its topographic orientation: isolated injuries to cephalic fibers result in deficits of the upper face and vice versa.

The facial nucleus harbors the cell bodies, which extend their axonal processes to the neuromuscular endplate at the target muscles. Each cell body innervates approximately 25 muscle fibers, which indicates the high degree of fine-motor control of the facial musculature. Schwann cells cover the axon and abut each other at the nodes of Ranvier. The myelin sheath produced by the Schwann cells greatly enhances the speed of conduction, which approximates 70 to 110 m/sec for the facial nerve. The axonal processes are surrounded by multiple membranes, which are, from the inside out, the endoneurium, the perineurium, and the epineurium. The endoneurium separates and encircles each nerve fiber. The perineurium is composed of concentric sleeves of polygonal cells; this layer acts as a diffusion barrier and lends structural strength to the fiber. The epineurium, with its loose areolar tissue, encircles the fascicles and harbors the vasa nervorum.

Pathophysiology of Acute Nerve Injury

To understand the diagnosis and treatment of traumatic facial paralysis, it is essential to understand the pathophysiology of acute nerve injury. The prolonged interruption of axoplasmic flow as a result of injury leads to the degeneration of the distal part of the fiber (i.e., Wallerian

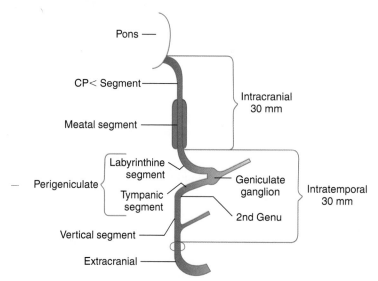

Figure 48-1. Schematic illustration of the gross anatomy of the facial nerve. *(From Adkins WY, Osguthorpe JD. Management of trauma of the facial nerve. Otolaryngol Clin North Am 1991;24:587–611.)*

degeneration). This begins within 12 hours and peaks at 72 hours. Immediately after distal injury, the proximal part of the axon begins transformation into a growth cone, enlarges considerably, and orchestrates the regeneration of sprouting axonal buds. Axonal sprouting begins at the proximal stump on the third day after injury. Concomitantly, in the distal axon stump, the myelin sheath is destroyed, and endoneurial tubules (Büngner bands) are formed from the Schwann cells. Under optimal conditions, the endoneurial tubules act as a scaffolding for the ingrowth of the sprouting axons. If successful regrowth does not occur within a critical period or if continuity between the axon stumps is lost, the endoneurial channels are eventually replaced with connective tissue, and the axons fail to reach their target organ.

In the cell body, primary reactive changes begin within hours, last for 10 to 21 days, and are characterized by the swelling of the cell body and chromatolysis with the degeneration of the Nissl bodies. The metabolic activity of the cell body increases substantially to meet the demands of the sprouting axonal fibers.

There are two main classifications of peripheral nerve injury: those of Seddon and those of Sunderland.[1,2] Seddon described three main categories of injury: neuropraxia, axonotmesis, and neurotmesis. Sunderland described five degrees of injury with increasing severity as the injury spreads from the axon to the additional encompassing layers (i.e., the endoneurium, the perineurium, and the epineurium). Table 48-1 lists the histopathologic features of these injuries and their clinical prognoses. It is helpful to consider the classifications together. The mildest form of injury—neuropraxia or first-degree injury—is a compression injury that causes a loss

of nerve conduction. This may be the result of increased intraneural pressure. The action potential may still be propagated, all layers of the nerve are intact, and axoplasmic flow is unaltered. Full recovery from this injury is expected.

Axonotmesis or second-degree injury is characterized by the disruption of the axon and its myelin sheath but with preservation of the endoneurium. Axoplasmic flow is stopped, and Wallerian degeneration occurs distal to the site of injury. As long as the endoneurium remains intact, however, the patient can expect a complete return of function.

With third-degree injury, the damage has progressed to involve the endoneurium as well. The loss of integrity of the endoneurial tubules allows the regenerating nerve fibers to escape from their original path, and incomplete recovery with synkinesis results.

When fourth-degree injury occurs, the injury has spread to include the disruption of the perineurium. This allows for the increased loss and false passage of regenerating neurites into improper tubules and fascicles, and it carries a worse prognosis.

Neurotmesis or fifth-degree injury is the most severe type. This involves total nerve disruption and includes the epineurium. When this occurs, there is very little chance of meaningful recovery without surgical intervention.

Synkinesis is a common result of abnormal axonal regeneration. The exact mechanism remains uncertain, but possible causes include axonal misdirection, faulty myelination with the shunting of electrical activity within

TABLE 48-1 The Sunderland Classification of Peripheral Nerve Injury

Type of Injury	Pattern of Injury	Clinical Prognosis
First-degree neurapraxia	• Compression injury • No histomorphologic changes • Axoplasmic flow unaltered	Full recovery
Second-degree axonotmesis	• Axon and myelin sheath disrupted • Endoneurium preserved • Axoplasmic flow stops • Wallerian degeneration occurs distal to site of injury	Fair to near-complete return of function; mild synkinesis
Third-degree injury	• Involvement of endoneurium • Loss of integrity of the endoneurial tubules allows the regenerating nerve fibers to escape from their original path	Incomplete recovery with synkinesis and mass movement
Fourth-degree injury	• Disruption of the perineurium • Increased loss and misdirection of regenerating neurites into improper tubules and fascicles	Incomplete to no recovery; synkinesis; spasm
Fifth-degree neurotmesis	• Disruption of nerve, including epineurium • Gap filled with scar tissue	Very little chance of meaningful recovery without surgical intervention

the nerve, the sprouting of multiple axons, microglial scarring in the facial nucleus, and the misdirection of regenerating axons via vertical anastomotic filaments.

It is important to note that facial-nerve damage extends proximal to the site of initial injury as well. The degree of this extension is unpredictable, but it may extend proximal to the meatal foramen into the distal intrameatal segment of the nerve. Thus acute trauma may cause direct injury to the nerve, which is then followed by delayed injury from neural edema within the confines of the Fallopian canal. This in turn results in ischemia and further damage. Delayed edema may convert an injury that is initially mild into one that is severe.

PREOPERATIVE COUNSELING AND RISK OF NERVE DAMAGE

The incidence of inadvertent iatrogenic facial nerve injury is difficult to obtain from the literature: the few reports that are available may be biased by underreporting. Furthermore, there are many types of procedures that place the nerve in jeopardy, and surgeons with varied types and degrees of training operate in this region.

The incidence of nerve damage appears to be the lowest in cosmetic procedures, and it increases with oncologic and revision surgery. The risk of damage to the facial nerve may be considerable with surgery for vestibular schwannoma, but this is an anticipated risk that is clearly explained to the patient before the decision to operate is made.

Lydiatt investigated malpractice trials involving facial-nerve paralysis.[3] In 30% of these suits, patients stated that they were unaware that facial paralysis was a potential complication of the procedure that was performed. Lydiatt also found a higher incidence of litigation after surgery for benign rather than malignant processes. He therefore stressed the importance of documenting the possibility of this complication on the consent form. He further suggested that patients with benign processes are less likely to accept a suboptimal outcome and should be counseled thoroughly.

It is helpful to some patients to give a risk estimate that based on the available literature. A search of the literature suggests an incidence of 15% to 50% temporary and up to 23% permanent facial paralysis after parotid surgery. The incidence of facial-nerve injury depends on a number of factors. Although primary lateral parotidectomy for limited benign disease should be associated with only occasional temporary and rare permanent weakness, the risk of injury increases with extensive and malignant disease, revision surgery, previous radiation therapy, deep lobe resection, and the inadequate intraoperative identification of the facial nerve.

Mastoidectomy is the most common otologic procedure that is complicated by facial-nerve injury (typically to the tympanic segment), with a reported incidence of 1% to 5%.[4] Injury to the nerve may also occur during tympanoplasty and during the removal of exostoses of the external auditory canal. Interestingly, Green and colleagues noted that, in 79% of otologic cases, the injury to the facial nerve was not noted until after surgery.[5]

For neurotologic procedures, Ryzenman reported that 45% of patients had compromised facial function after acoustic neuroma surgery and that 72% of these injuries were permanent.[6] Baumann noted that 50% of his patients had worse function after acoustic neuroma resection, but he stated that most of these were grade II on the House–Brackmann scale (HBS).[7] The incidence of facial-nerve weakness depends on the type of surgical approach and the size of tumor, and it may be higher with cystic than with solid tumors.[8]

In 96 face-lifts performed by residents, Sullivan and colleagues noted a 3% incidence of temporary facial-nerve weakness (usually of the mandibular branch) and no permanent injuries.[9] During endoscopic brow-lift, Viksraitis noted a 3% incidence of frontal-branch weakness.[10] The overall incidence of permanent paralysis of a branch of the facial nerve as a result of face-lift appears to be less than 1%.[10]

PREVENTION OF FACIAL-NERVE INJURY

Prevention of iatrogenic injury begins with the selection of the proper treatment. Nonsurgical treatment modalities should be considered, if applicable.[10] Operating in the vicinity of the facial nerve requires continuous vigilance throughout the procedure. Intricate knowledge of the surgical anatomy is necessary, including the relevant surgical landmarks and their relationship to the facial nerve. Meticulous study and thorough training by experienced surgeons is essential. Guntinas-Lichius and colleagues[11] have demonstrated in a large case series of parotidectomies that surgical teaching under expert supervision is safe and produces excellent outcomes. Surgical technique must include the meticulous maintenance of hemostasis, the use of ample lighting, and the provision of adequate exposure for optimal visualization.

Preoperative imaging will at times aid in the identification of pathology that puts the facial nerve in jeopardy. This can be invaluable during preoperative patient counseling.

Continuous intraoperative nerve monitoring with stimulation is routine during numerous procedures, including some types of otologic surgery and parotidectomy. Makeieff and colleagues[12] found that nerve monitoring decreased both the incidence and duration of paralysis after parotidectomy. Although some surgeons argue that the alarm on the monitor does not activate until the nerve has already been transected, the monitor can be extremely useful for allowing for the low-voltage stimulation of structures when searching for the nerve trunk or branches. Furthermore, excessive stretching of the nerve during dissection may also cause the alarm to trigger, which can aid in the minimization of postoperative paresis. Finally, confirming a low stimulation threshold at the end of the case reassures the surgeon that the patient will have good facial function when he or she awakens.

In some cases, sacrifice of the facial nerve is unavoidable as part of the surgical procedure. When this is anticipated, detailed preoperative counseling is essential and should include a discussion of what morbidity to expect and what subsequent treatment may or may not be possible. Educating the patient about realistic expectations and probable outcomes is critical, although fully preparing a patient emotionally for the loss of facial function is nearly impossible. Consideration should also be given to having patients begin the anticipated postoperative physical therapy before the paralysis begins. When damage of the nerve is not anticipated but is a risk of the planned surgical procedure, it is necessary to discuss the risk and its implications in detail so that the patient is fully informed.

MORBIDITY OF PARALYSIS AND ITS IMPACT ON QUALITY OF LIFE

Facial paralysis can have a severe impact on a patient's quality of life (QOL). The magnitude of this impact depends on the age of the patient. Among younger patients with higher soft-tissue elasticity, there is minimal tissue descent, and excellent resting symmetry may be maintained. Among older patients, especially smokers and those with elastosis from sun exposure, the tissue displacement can be severe. It is helpful to consider the morbidity of paralysis by facial region.

Paralysis of the Frontal Region

Paralysis of the frontal region (i.e., the temporal and zygomatic branches) leads to the descent of the forehead and eyebrow or the upper-eyelid complex. This can cause upper lateral visual field deficits as a result of ptosis of the lateral aspect of the eyebrows, and it also causes the upper-eyelid skin to descend.

Paralysis of the Periorbital Region

Paralysis of the periorbital region (i.e., the zygomatic branches) leads to an inability to actively depress the upper eyelid, which usually results in a decreased ability to close the eye. It is important to note that this effect may not become apparent until several days after the onset of paralysis and to realize that this is a cause of much of the morbidity associated with facial paralysis. Some patients benefit from a reflex superolateral excursion of the globe when attempting to close the eye (i.e., Bell reflex; Figure 48-2). This reflex has a protective effect that is analogous to blinking, and it aids in maintaining corneal moisturization. Patients who do not have this reflex are at higher risk of corneal desiccation, which is an ophthalmologic emergency. This is especially true for those patients with compromised corneal sensation (Figure 48-3).

Paralysis of the Orbicularis Oculi Muscle

Paralysis of the orbicularis oculi muscle can also lead to ectropion of the lower eyelid. In advanced stages, the inferior lacrimal punctum may roll away from the lacrimal lake. In addition, flaccidity of the orbicularis muscle may compromise the active tear-pumping mechanism. As a result, epiphora and keratoconjunctivitis sicca may be present simultaneously (Figure 48-4). In a prospective evaluation of 20 consecutive patients with complete facial paralysis, Moe and Linder[13] found that the primary ophthalmologic complaint was epiphora in 75% of cases. Other complaints, in order of descending frequency, were photophobia, a sensation of dryness, periorbital

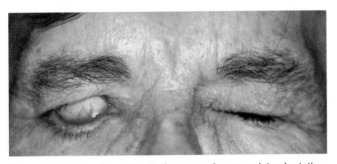

Figure 48-2. Bell reflex protects the cornea by superolateral rotation of the globe with voluntary effort at eye closure.

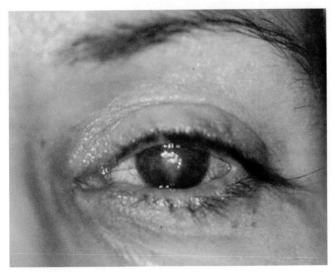

Figure 48-3. Paralytic lagophthalmos has resulted in corneal irritation.

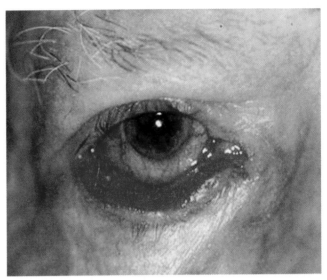

Figure 48-4. Paralytic ectropion with resulting keratoconjunctivitis sicca.

burning, and the accumulation of debris on the eyelids and eyelashes. As a result of a combination of these factors, visual acuity is often significantly compromised.

Paralysis of the Midfacial Region

Paralysis of the midfacial region (i.e., the zygomatic and buccal branches) creates a variety of disorders. Breathing is compromised because of the unopposed descent of the midfacial tissues. The musculature that elevates and lateralizes the melolabial fold, including the zygomaticus muscles, is dysfunctional, which results in an inferomedial displacement of the malar fat pad and the compression of the alar sidewall. This effect is exacerbated by the lack of an opposing force by the dilator muscles (i.e., the levator labii superioris alaeque nasi muscle and the dilator naris muscle).

Paralysis of the Lower Face

Paralysis of the lower face (i.e., the buccal and marginal mandibular nerves) results in the loss of ability to pull the corner of the mouth and the lower lid downward with dysfunction of the depressor anguli oris and depressor labii inferioris muscles, and the skin of the chin drops with the paralysis of the mentalis muscle. Asymmetry of the smile results from an impaired ability to depress the lower lip. Paralysis of the cervical branch leads to the flaccidity of the platysma muscle and the attendant inability to depress the corner of the mouth.

Paralysis of the Seventh Cranial Nerve

Paralysis of the seventh cranial nerve also affects other cranial nerves, including the first (i.e., diminished olfaction through obstruction of nasal airflow), second (i.e., impaired vision), and fifth (i.e., suboptimal mastication).

Thus any rehabilitative procedures that potentially further compromise the performance of other cranial nerves should only be performed after extensive consideration.

Unilateral Paralysis

It is also important to realize that unilateral paralysis is a bilateral problem. A phenomenon that deserves further study is one that has been referred to as *compensatory contralateral hypertonicity*. This describes the state of hypercontraction of the normal side of the face that occurs when the contralateral side becomes paralyzed (Figure 48-5). For teleologic purposes, it should be considered that the hypercontraction is the result of a subconscious effort to correct the position of the paralyzed side, thereby resulting in unintentional hypercontraction of the contralateral innervated musculature. The result is an overall "S" shape of the face, with the "S" facing away from the paralyzed side. It is interesting to note that the distortion of the innervated side of the face is arguably as great as the disfigurement of the paralyzed side. When a patient recovers from facial paralysis or undergoes the successful treatment of the paralyzed side, the normal side of the face relaxes into its premorbid position. This spontaneous repositioning of the normal side of the face is referred to as *unlocking*.

The position of midline structures with bilateral muscular insertions (e.g., the mouth and nose) can be further distorted by abnormal tension created by the hypercontraction of the innervated musculature. Thus, when evaluating a patient with facial paralysis and planning potential therapeutic interventions, it is critical to address the normal side of the face and to ascertain to what extent compensatory contralateral contraction affects the facial

distortion and to what degree this will be released when the underlying condition is relieved. The compensatory contraction can often be relieved by asking the patient to close his or her eyes and relax and then massaging the facial musculature into its native position.

Impact on the Patient's Quality of Life

A number of validated questionnaires are available to measure the impact of facial paralysis on QOL. Cross and colleagues[14] used the Derriford Appearance Scale to measure psychological distress, the COPE questionnaire to assess the patient's ability to cope with facial paralysis, and the Personal Report questionnaire to measure the self-esteem of patients with facial paralysis. These authors found a significant reduction in the QOL of these patients. The grade of motor dysfunction on the HBS did not correlate with the questionnaire scores, which is a finding that emphasizes the notion that the HBS cannot reflect the many nuances of impairment that are associated with facial paralysis. For example, nasal obstruction can have a profound impact on a patient's QOL, yet it is not included in the HBS and not consistently represented with most QOL measures. Lassaletta and colleagues[15] studied QOL with the use of the Glasgow Benefit inventory, a validated overall QOL questionnaire that takes important general, social, and physical aspects into account. These authors documented a QOL reduction in 64% of patients with an HBS grade of III or IV after surgery for vestibular schwannoma and in 100% of patients with HBS V or VI function. Patients with HBS grade of I or II reported reduced QOL in only 12% of the cases. These findings underscore the broadly accepted assumption that an outcome of an HBS grade of I or II after treatment may

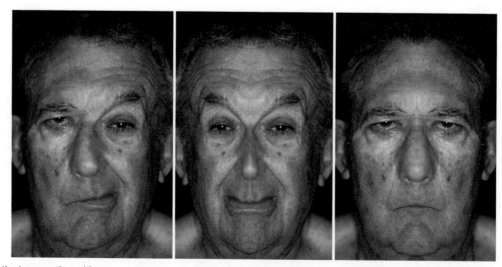

Figure 48-5. Patient presenting with compensatory contralateral (left) hypertonicity resulting from right facial paralysis. **A,** Hypertonicity of the facial musculature on the nonparalyzed side of the face contributes to an S-shaped appearance of the face. **B,** Facial image generated by mirror imaging the nonparalyzed hemiface across the midline. **C,** Facial image generated by mirror imaging the paralyzed hemiface across the midline. Hypertonicity of the forehead and perioral musculature is evident.

be regarded as successful and that the QOL of these patients is generally not impaired by their facial-nerve function.

ASSESSMENT

Before choosing a treatment option, it is critical to determine the extent and prognosis of the facial-nerve injury. The history, the physical examination, electrodiagnostic testing, and imaging studies all provide important information. The age, gender, health, life expectancy, and expectations of the patient are also important considerations. The prognosis, the previous and planned treatment of the underlying disease (e.g., radiation therapy, chemotherapy), the degree of paralysis, the compensation provided by facial tone, and the viability of the facial musculature must be well understood. The surgeon must then select the proper combination of treatment modalities and determine the timing for intervention on the basis of these data.

The HBS, which is listed in Table 48-2, is universally used because of its reproducibility and ease of use.[16] It

is a useful global scale, but it is insufficient for assessing the dysfunction of the individual branches. Functional deficits such as decreased tearing, nasal obstruction, or dysarthria are also not assessed by the HBS.

Because the patterns of facial paralysis differ substantially between primary paralysis and outcome after repair, the Repaired Facial Nerve Recovery Scale (RFNRS)[17] has been introduced to better describe and quantitate outcomes after nerve repair (Table 48-3). In clinical practice, the HBS and the RFNRS allow for the rapid classification and communication of global function. More detailed assessment typically entails description on the basis of the anatomic subsites innervated by the individual branches, as outlined later in this chapter.

FUNCTIONAL NERVE TESTING

Facial-nerve testing is indicated when the severity of injury of the nerve is unknown. Clinical topognostic tests have largely been supplanted by electrodiagnostic techniques. Limitations of topognostic tests include inaccuracies that result from the different susceptibilities

TABLE 48-2 House–Brackmann Grading System

Grade	Description	Characteristics
I	Normal	Normal facial function in all areas
II	Mild dysfunction	*Gross:* Slight weakness noticeable on close inspection; may have very slight synkinesis *At rest:* Normal symmetry and tone *Forehead:* Slight to moderate movement *Eye:* Complete closure with effort *Mouth:* Slightly weak with maximum effort
III	Moderate dysfunction	*Gross:* Obvious but not disfiguring difference between the two sides; noticeable but not severe synkinesis, contracture, and/or hemifacial spasm *At rest:* Normal symmetry and tone *Forehead:* None *Eye:* Incomplete closure *Mouth:* Asymmetric with maximum effort
IV	Moderately severe dysfunction	*Gross:* Obvious weakness and/or disfiguring asymmetry *At rest:* Normal symmetry and tone *Forehead:* None *Eye:* Incomplete closure *Mouth:* Asymmetric with maximum effort
V	Severe dysfunction	*Gross:* Only barely perceptible motion *At rest:* Asymmetry *Forehead:* None *Eye:* Incomplete closure *Mouth:* Slight movement
VI	Total paralysis	No movement

TABLE 48-3 Repaired Facial Nerve Recovery Scale

Score	Function
A	Normal facial function
B	Independent movement of eyelids and mouth; slight mass motion; slight movement of the forehead
C	Strong closure of eyelids and oral sphincter; some mass motion; no forehead movement
D	Incomplete closure of eyelids; significant mass motion; good tone
E	Minimal movement of any branch; poor tone
F	No movement

to injuries of the various types of nerve fibers (e.g., motor, sensory, visceral efferent). This often makes it difficult to pinpoint a single site of injury to the nerve.

Electrodiagnostic Tests

Electrodiagnostic tests also have important limitations. These tests can only differentiate between neuropraxia (i.e., first-degree injury) and axonotmesis (i.e., second-degree injury) in that the former will allow for the propagation of an action potential, whereas the latter will not. Hence, electrodiagnostic tests cannot differentiate between axonotmesis and neurotmesis or HBS grade II through grade V injury; this is critical information, because the prognosis for a favorable outcome is much different between these groups. In addition, the ability to stimulate neuropraxic fibers and to produce a muscle action potential does not rule out severe damage to other fibers within the nerve. In other words, the compound action potential detects fibers that have not degenerated rather than the degree of degeneration that has occurred in the nerve.[18] Furthermore, these tests are only used on the extratemporal portion of the nerve. Because conduction will continue in the distal nerve until Wallerian degeneration occurs beyond the site of stimulation, these tests are not typically useful during the first 72 hours after surgery. The condition of the intratemporal course of the nerve can only be inferred from these data, and repeat studies are often required as degeneration proceeds.

Neurodiagnostic Tests

A number of neurodiagnostic tests are available. Most of these stimulate the nerve transcutaneously with the use of an electrical pulse of chosen intensity and duration.

Minimal Nerve Excitability Test

The minimal nerve excitability test stimulates the nerve at its exit from the stylomastoid foramen with a percutaneous nerve stimulator. The current is raised until the stimulation threshold is reached, at which point the muscle contraction first becomes visible. The current required for minimal stimulation is noted for each side.

Maximal Stimulation Test

The maximal stimulation test is a modification of the minimal nerve excitability test. The threshold of excitation that results in the maximal contraction of the facial musculature is first determined on the nonparalyzed side. The nerve is then stimulated 1 mA to 2 mA above the maximal excitation threshold bilaterally. The degree of muscle contraction is then visually compared between both sides and graded.

Electroneuronography

Electroneuronography (ENoG) advances the concept of the maximal stimulation test in that it allows for the more exact measurement of the evoked contraction of the facial musculature. Needle electrodes are inserted into the stimulated muscle groups, and an evoked electromyogram (EMG) is recorded during the supramaximal percutaneous stimulation of the nerve. The amplitude of the recorded muscle compound action potential of the affected side is reported as a percentage of the response of the normal side. A 90% reduction of the compound muscle action potential on the affected side is cited as an indication for decompression surgery. The measured latency between nerve stimulation and the onset of the muscle action potential serves as an additional parameter for the assessment of nerve function.

Electromyography

EMG is performed via the intramuscular placement of a needle electrode. The electrical activity of the muscle elicited by voluntary or evoked stimulation is recorded on an oscilloscope. Physiologically, no activity is observed at rest. Within 14 to 21 days after severe nerve injury, Wallerian degeneration results in the denervation of the muscle, and fibrillation potentials are demonstrated. If the reinnervation of the motor endplates takes place, regeneration (i.e., polyphasic) potentials and spontaneous fasciculations appear before visible motion returns. EMG within the first 72 hours after injury is of limited use. Voluntary muscle action potentials will be absent, but this cannot differentiate first-degree injury from more significant injury. An evoked EMG distal to the site of injury will still demonstrate normal latency and muscle action potentials until nerve degeneration progresses.[14]

Transcranial Magnetic Stimulation

Transcranial magnetic stimulation is a technology that allows for the direct stimulation of cortical centers, and it can be applied for a variety of indications.[19] This method differs from the previously described tests in several ways. The nerve is stimulated with the use of a magnetic field produced by a coil placed on the parieto-occipital skull. This allows for the stimulation of the labyrinthine segment of the facial nerve proximal to its entrance into the Fallopian canal. The stimulator output is then increased in a stepwise fashion until a maximal response is obtained. This is performed first on the healthy nerve to determine the required stimulus intensity, and it is then performed on the affected nerve. The resulting compound muscle action potentials are then compared.[20]

Transcranial magnetic stimulation is not new technology, but the coil size has been reduced so that cortical stimulation and the stimulation of adjacent cranial nerves is less problematic. This is the only test available that allows for the determination of the condition of the nerve within the temporal bone, which is proximal to the site of most injuries. The applicability of this test is being investigated, but it seems to hold promise for increased use in the future.

MANAGEMENT OF IATROGENIC FACIAL-NERVE INJURY: SELECTION AND TIMING OF TREATMENT

The decision of how to proceed when iatrogenic damage to the facial nerve is discovered can be difficult. The realization that an injury has occurred can be emotionally devastating to the responsible surgeon, and it is often wise to obtain a second opinion from a colleague or to turn the task of reconstruction over to a colleague.

If the injury is discovered when the patient awakens in the recovery room and the surgeon was unaware of having injured the nerve, it is advisable to wait 2 to 3 hours and then reassess the patient in case the facial weakness is the result of the diffusion of local anesthetic. If function does not return, the question becomes whether or not to return to the operating room to explore the nerve. If it is noted that the facial nerve is completely paralyzed and the intraoperative site was such that it is uncertain whether the nerve has been completely preserved, reexploration of the nerve and repair as necessary are suggested. If an experienced surgeon is certain that the nerve is intact, however, it would be reasonable to perform ENoG. If the nerve degenerates during the next several days to less than 90% of the normal side, the decision should be made to explore and possibly decompress the nerve. As suggested by Fisch, the decompression is typically performed through a transcranial approach to include the internal auditory canal and the meatus.[21]

If exploration demonstrates that the nerve has been completely transected, a direct end-to-end anastomosis or an interposition nerve graft should be placed. The discovery of a partial injury to the nerve creates a more complex decision. If treatment by decompression alone is undertaken, the outcome may range from HBS grade I to grade IV. More than one third of patients will attain HBS grade I or II, which cannot be achieved by either primary anastomosis or grafting. Thus, if it appears that the nerve is less than 50% transected, decompression alone should be undertaken. If the majority of the nerve is transected, the ends should be trimmed, and a primary anastomosis should be performed, which will achieve a grade III result in most cases.

The outcomes after facial-nerve injury can be broken down as follows. If there is documented facial-nerve function after the injury and paralysis then develops or if there is paresis but not full paralysis, then the patient has a good prognosis for full recovery. If the patient does not belong to this group, the prognosis is uncertain. ENoG should be used to determine which patients develop neural degeneration of 90% or more within 14 days of injury. These patients may undergo nerve repair and decompression. Those who do not reach this degree of injury should be observed. If primary anastomosis is possible, HBS grade III (RFNRS C) function is expected. If a nerve graft is required, HBS grade IV (RFNRS D) function is realistic. Only patients who require decompression without nerve repair can obtain a grade I or II result, although most patients in this group will only achieve HBS grade III or IV.[5] The flow diagrams in Figures 48-6 and 48-7 show possible approaches to nerve injuries in uncomplicated cases. As delineated in the present discussion, a large number of factors may alter the clinical decision-making process for each individual patient.

SURGICAL

Primary Nerve Repair

The physiologic goals of facial-nerve repair are to minimize fibroblastic proliferation into the anastomosis; to maximize axonal regrowth across the anastomosis; and to minimize synkinesis. The primary reconstitution of the continuity of the facial nerve has many anatomic and physiologic advantages, and it is surgical repair that is most likely to meet these goals. Ideally performed at the time of injury, continuity from the facial motor nucleus to the neuromuscular junction is reestablished. Early repair is most promising, because a number of factors contribute to less favorable outcomes as time after injury passes: the dissection of the surgical field and the identification of the nerve endings are impeded by scar tissue; the successive degeneration of the Büngner bands reduces the ability of the axonal sprouts to regrow along the nerve; and degeneration and fibrosis reduce the contractility of the target muscle.

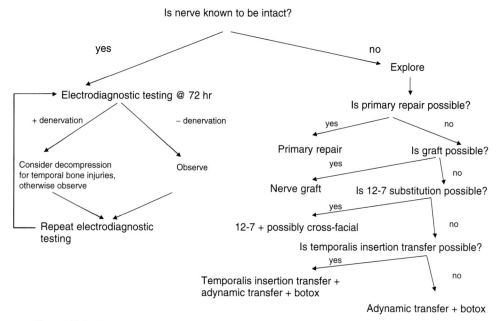

Figure 48-6. Treatment algorithm for an injury of the facial nerve proximal to the pes anserinus.

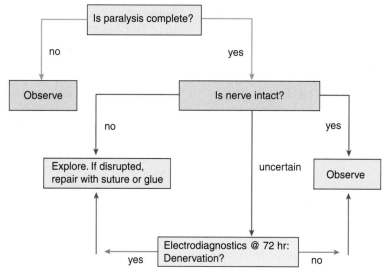

Figure 48-7. Treatment algorithm for an injury of the facial nerve distal to the pes anserinus.

Direct anastomosis will always give the best outcome, with most patients returning to HBS grade III (RFNRS C) function if there is enough laxity for coaptation. If a small gap persists, consideration should be given to mobilization so that a tension-free anastomosis can be obtained. If a larger gap is noted, an interposition nerve graft should be placed.

The historic gold standard of nerve repair has been microsurgical suture adaptation. More recently, repair proximal to the stylomastoid foramen with fibrin glue has been shown to produce equivalent results.[22] Both suture and glue repair require the atraumatic identification and dissection of the nerve ends. If tension-free reapproximation (i.e., the nerve ends should adapt without a suture) cannot be achieved, an interposition graft (most commonly

the great auricular nerve and the sural cutaneous nerve) is required. The patient should be counseled that a permanent loss of sensation of the earlobe or of the lateral aspect of the foot is expected. The great auricular nerve represents the first choice if a nonbranching interposition graft with a length of up to 7 cm to 10 cm is needed. The sural nerve may provide up to 40 cm in length, and it allows for the incorporation of a branching segment more reliably than the great auricular nerve does (Figure 48-8). Some surgeons advocate reversing the direction of the nerve graft so that regenerating neurites do not exit the nerve at graft branch points, but the importance of this maneuver has not been conclusively shown.

Under microscopic magnification, the epineurium is trimmed, and the remainder of the nerve is sharply

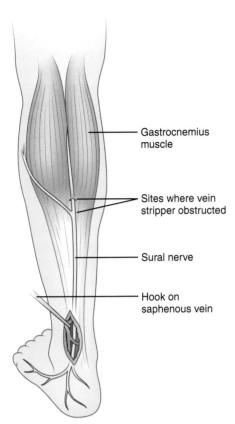

Figure 48-8. The sural nerve is harvested on the posterolateral aspect of the lower leg. The sural nerve provides for a long, branching interposition graft.

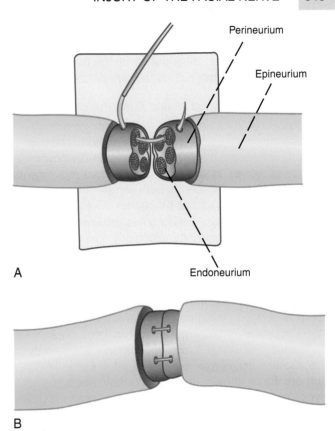

Figure 48-9. Nerve repair and the suture insertion of nerve grafts. The exact and tension-free approximation of the nerve ends is achieved with the meticulous suture of the endoneurium.

transected. Two or three 9-0 nylon sutures are used to approximate the endoneurium (Figure 48-9). Variations of the cross-sectional anatomy of the facial nerve along its course may require modifications of the suture technique. In the cerebellopontine angle, the nerve has no fascicles or epineurium, and repair with 1 or 2 stitches through the nerve using 9-0 nylon may be considered. Proximal to the geniculate ganglion, the nerve is covered only by a thin sheath of arachnoid membrane. In the perigeniculate area, the epineurium first appears, and fascicular organization is seen. Because the epineurium is still very thin, a monofascicular repair is performed. In the tympanomastoid region, the nerve contains two or three fascicles. Here the epineurium is moderately thick, and it may be incorporated in the repair. The trunk of the facial nerve as it exits the stylomastoid foramen contains multiple fascicles, and it is covered by a thick epineurium. The peripheral branches are monofascicular, and they are covered by only a thin epineurium.

Nerve repair using fibrin glue has advantages in certain situations. In general, the more proximal the injury, the more one may be inclined to prefer glue over suture. The nerve ends are carefully transected and adapted in preparation. Then 1 ml to 2 ml of fibrin glue are slowly applied to the nerve ends. The repair may be stabilized with fat grafts.

Failure to achieve the expected outcome of the repair of the facial nerve can occur for several reasons. The primary cause of delayed repair is neural fibrosis. When repairing the nerve, the distal aspect of the proximal nerve fragment should be removed where it is fibrotic. If this area is in the labyrinthine or geniculate areas, a middle cranial fossa approach may be necessary. Repair of the nerve under tension may also cause fibrosis, and the nerve should be mobilized or an interposition graft placed to avoid this complication.

Nerve Transposition and Nerve Grafts

Nerve transposition (also known as *substitution* or *crossover*) techniques rely on other cranial nerves to provide stimulation to the distal facial nerve. Hence some degree of deficit to the "donor" nerve has to be traded for the expected improvement in facial-nerve function. A number of procedures have been developed with the goal of simultaneously minimizing donor-nerve deficits and maximizing functional gain for the paralyzed face. Spinal accessory and phrenic nerve transposition grafts were used historically, and they have been replaced by facial-to-facial and hypoglossal-to-facial nerve-substitution techniques. The somewhat limited functional outcomes with these techniques are frequently accompanied by hyperkinesis, synkinesis, and morbidity related to donor-nerve deficits. Therefore the expected benefits and deficits must be well balanced and thoroughly discussed with the patient before any of the substitution techniques are performed.

Hypoglossal-to-Facial Nerve Substitution

A number of characteristics render the hypoglossal nerve advantageous for facial reanimation. There is a close functional relationship between the hypoglossal and facial nerves in the facial and lingual movements that result from connections between the two nerves at the motor cortex and the brainstem. The hypoglossal nerve courses in close topographic proximity to the facial nerve, and donor-site morbidity incurred by the sacrifice of the hypoglossal nerve is generally well compensated for, especially among younger patients. Indications for hypoglossal-to-facial nerve transposition include cases in which the proximal stump is not available for anastomosis. The distal nerve and the facial musculature must be intact. If paralysis has been present for more than 12 months, it is suggested that the viability of the facial musculature be tested with EMG. Multiple authors have shown good functional outcomes with hypoglossal-to-facial nerve transposition grafts.[23] Drawbacks associated with this technique include hemilingual atrophy as a result of the complete transection of the twelfth cranial nerve, facial hypertonia as a result of the substantial stimulatory power of the hypoglossal nerve, and synkinesis and limited voluntary animation as a result of the incomplete and nontopographic reinnervation. In an effort to reduce these side effects, various modifications to the original technique have been made. May and colleagues[24] have reported excellent results with the hypoglossal-to-facial nerve jump interposition graft. This technique involves a wedge resection of the hypoglossal nerve and the interposition of a free nerve graft. Hypoglossal nerve function is preserved, but two anastomoses have to be incorporated in the repair. With each anastomosis, regenerating axons are inevitably lost as a result of escape or the inability to locate or penetrate the tubules in the distal nerve.

To further reduce the incidence of synkinesis and mass movements with the jump anastomosis technique, selective reinnervation of only the lower facial-nerve branches has been suggested.[25] The proximal mobilization of the facial nerve and oblique end-to-side anastomosis with the hypoglossal nerve combines the advantage of the jump anastomosis (i.e., preserved functionality of the hypoglossal nerve) with that of the hypoglossal-to-facial nerve transfer (i.e., one anastomosis with the potential for better reinnervation), and it is the authors' preferred substitution technique. It must be noted that substitution techniques are typically combined with other techniques of facial reanimation and that reported results incorporate the important contributions of these ancillary techniques.

Technique

Surgical access is achieved through an anteriorly extended face-lift–parotidectomy incision. The posterior belly of the digastric muscle is located. The facial nerve is identified at the level of the stylomastoid foramen and dissected within the parotid tissue to a point just beyond the pes anserinus. The proximal stump of the facial nerve is freshened with a sharp transection. The hypoglossal nerve is then identified medial to the tendon of the digastric muscle and dissected anteriorly and posteriorly. The descendens hypoglossi branch is identified and transected. The main trunk of the hypoglossal nerve is transected distal to the descendens branch and rotated upward medial to the digastric muscle. A combined perineurial or endoneurial end-to-end anastomosis is performed under magnification with the use of 9-0 nylon sutures. If a jump graft is performed, then the distance between the branching of the descendens hypoglossi to the facial-nerve stump is measured, and a graft that is 2-cm longer than the measured distance is harvested, typically from the great auricular nerve. A wedge excision of one third of the diameter of the hypoglossal nerve is performed just distal to the descendens hypoglossi. The harvested graft is sutured end to side to the hypoglossal nerve and end to end to the facial nerve. Alternatively, a mastoidectomy may be performed and the vertical segment of the facial nerve mobilized, rotated inferiorly, and anastomosed with an oblique end-to-side technique to the partially transected hypoglossal nerve. This preferred technique eliminates the need for an interposition graft and a second anastomosis.

The best possible outcome that should be expected with hypoglossal nerve substitution techniques is HBS grade III (RFNRS C). Up to 95% of patients may obtain satisfactory facial tone and voluntary motion.[26] The initial return of function may begin as early as 3 months after surgery, and the result may continue to improve for several years.[27] The outcome diminishes with patient age and with the length of the interval between injury and repair. At least 67% of patients develop significant synkinesis.[28] Initially patients must consciously press their tongue forward and laterally to induce facial movement. With time, this appears to become spontaneous.

Cross-Facial Nerve Transposition

Cross-facial nerve transposition reroutes axons from the contralateral functional facial nerve to selected branches of the paralyzed nerve through an interposition graft. In theory, this should be the optimal solution for facial reanimation, offering the opportunity to graft between branches of like function to produce spontaneous and emotional facial function. In practice, the number of axons that can be successfully transferred to the paralyzed face without causing significant weakness of the donor nerve is limited. Furthermore, it typically requires 8 months or more for the axons to grow through the graft to the recipient nerve branch. During this time, significant fibrosis of the distal nerve and muscle atrophy may occur unless measures are taken to prevent this.

Cross-facial transposition is therefore primarily used to complement other techniques of facial reanimation. Cross-facial grafting may be performed at the time of hypoglossal-to-facial anastomosis to individual branches of the paralyzed nerve. The cross-facial grafts may initially be anastomosed to only the donor branches during the first stage of the procedure. The hypoglossal nerve provides earlier reinnervation and maintains neuromuscular integrity until the contralateral axons grow through the graft. Growth through the graft is monitored with the use of the Tinel sign, which involves a tingling sensation elicited by tapping on the graft at the distal point of nerve regrowth. Approximately 9 to 12 months later, when the donor axons have reached the end of the nerve grafts, the upper branches of the paralyzed facial nerve can be transected and anastomosed to the cross-facial grafts, thereby leaving the trunk and lower branches attached to the hypoglossal nerve. This approach provides for the separate innervation of the upper and lower face, and it reduces synkinesis.

Technique

Cross-facial nerve transposition relies on the ability to map branches of the functional nerve with intraoperative neuronography. By precisely determining the identity of each nerve branch and whether there are additional branches of strength in that muscle group, individual branches can be chosen as donors that, if sacrificed, will cause no notable weakness. Both facial nerves are approached through a face-lift incision. The donor nerve branches are located peripherally. A minimal voltage should be used for stimulation when identifying the peripheral branches to ensure that the branch does not fatigue during the procedure and to prevent postoperative facial weakness. Donor branches are selected by choosing the redundant branches that are the closest possible in function to the recipient nerves. When the recipient and donor branches have been isolated, a tunnel is dissected across the face that passes subcutaneously through the upper lip. The distance between the opposing branches is then precisely measured by passing a suture, and the appropriate length of nerve graft is harvested. The authors generally prefer the sural nerve for facial crossover anastomoses because of the redundant length and minimal morbidity associated with harvesting this graft. The medial antebrachial cutaneous nerve also provides for an excellent graft. The technique of harvesting these grafts is well described elsewhere.[29]

Cross-facial nerve grafting is generally inadequate as an isolated procedure. When used in conjunction with other techniques of facial reanimation, it is a useful adjunct to decrease synkinesis and to provide for the independent innervation of areas such as the periocular muscles.

MUSCLE REINSERTION TECHNIQUES

Technique: Muscle Insertion Transfer

Muscle insertion transfer can be an excellent technique for lower facial reanimation. These maneuvers increase facial tone and symmetry, improve mastication by obliterating the lower gingivobuccal sulcus, and re-create a voluntary partial smile. The two primary donor muscles are masticators, both of which are innervated by the trigeminal nerve: the masseter and the temporalis muscles. Temporalis muscle transfer has evolved as the gold standard technique. It was originally described by Gillies in 1934,[30] and it has evolved substantially. Attempts at re-animating the upper face with the temporalis muscle produced suboptimal results, including increased bulkiness, the risk of ectropion, and unnatural-appearing eye closure. Hence the procedure was modified to reanimate the perioral and perinasal complexes. Reported techniques have included the partial or complete elevation of the fan-shaped origin of the muscle off of the temporal bone, the reflection of the muscle over the zygoma, and attachment to the desired insertion points. Unfortunately, removing the origin of the muscle from the temporal bone and temporal fossa leaves an unsightly defect in the temporal region. Partial transfer of the muscle also leaves a defect, and it may cause the atrophy of the remaining musculature. Furthermore, reflecting the muscle over the zygoma creates a large bulge in this area, which disturbs facial symmetry. This compounds the effect of the temporal concavity. In addition, after the muscle is draped over the zygoma, it does not usually have sufficient length to reach the desired insertion point. A fascial extension must therefore be used, which adds an adynamic segment to the reconstruction with the potential for weakening or dehiscence over time.

McLaughlin[31] described a transoral approach in which the insertion of the temporalis muscle is removed from the coronoid process and, with the aid of a fascial expansion, transferred to the desired point of insertion without the translocation of the muscle. Labbé and Huault[32] used the same principle, but they elevated the origin of the muscle and mobilized the entire muscle toward the oral commissure, thereby reducing the need for a fascial extension. Sherris[33] refined the insertion technique by creating anchoring points in the midline, thus increasing lip symmetry and decreasing philtral shift. Because the ptosis of the subdermal tissues and skin laxity are substantially accentuated by facial palsy, except in the young patient population, a simultaneous face-lift procedure is often indicated and typically complemented by a staged contralateral face lift.

Technique: Temporalis Insertion Transfer

It is essential to determine preoperatively that the innervation of the donor muscle is intact, especially after skull-base surgery. The preauricular component of a face-lift incision is extended into the temporal fossa, where it is arched anteriorly to preserve the vascular supply to the temporoparietal fascia or posteriorly to respect a receding hairline. A subdermal face-lift plane is dissected past the melolabial fold and the mandibulocutaneous ligament. If a face-lift procedure is planned within the same stage, a complete face-lift incision is performed, and a postauricular and cervical flap is also dissected. The subcutaneous plane is transitioned over the zygoma to raise a skin–temporoparietal fascia flap, which is reflected anteriorly. If there is a substantial loss of tone with a resulting midfacial droop, a long sub-superficial musculo-aponeurotic system (SMAS) flap is dissected in the lower half of the face. A strip of deep temporal fascia is then harvested. The zygoma may be temporarily removed for better exposure. The coronoid process is transected beneath the insertion of the temporalis muscle and grasped. The superior aspect of the temporalis muscle is transected 5 mm to 10 mm inferior to the superior temporal line, thus preserving the anastomotic arcade between the superficial and deep vascular systems, and the entire muscle is mobilized by anterosuperior to posteroinferior subfascial dissection along the temporal bone. Care is taken to identify and preserve the deep temporal neurovascular bundle, which enters the muscle on its deep surface under the posterior aspect of the zygomatic arch. The posterior third of the muscle may be transected to facilitate mobilization. When the muscle is mobile and advanced into the face, the coronoid process is resected, and the distal periosteal extensions of the muscle are flattened and splayed out over 2 cm to 3 cm. Small incisions are made in the midline of the upper and lower lip along the vermillion border and along the melolabial fold. Tunnels are dissected that connect the lip incisions with the subdermal flap. The temporalis muscle is then suture fixated with 4-0 Prolene mattress sutures to the distal SMAS and to the perioral and paranasal muscle complexes. Strips of temporalis fascia are used to fixate the midline insertion points of the lip to the temporalis muscle. The lip should be overcorrected in such a manner that the first premolar tooth becomes visible. The origin of the muscle is then rotated slightly anteriorly and sutured to its residual cuff at the temporal line. The zygoma is returned to its original position and fixated with plates. If a face-lift is performed within the same setting, the SMAS flap is anchored to the mastoid periosteum and the posterior aspect of the deep temporal fascia. Facial skin is carefully redraped over the face, and a moderate amount of excess skin is removed. Layered closure of the face-lift incision with very little tension incorporates deep anchoring stitches around the earlobe. A fine suction drain and a bulky compression dressing complete the procedure. The patient may be discharged the same day, and he or she is seen the following morning for removal of the dressing.

In older patients, particularly after a period of muscle atrophy, the degree of laxity of the lower lip does not respond sufficiently to muscle insertion transfer. To improve the symmetry of the smile, drooling, and the pocketing of food in the gingivobuccal sulcus, a wedge resection of the lower lip may be indicated.

Temporalis insertion transfer typically results in 1 cm to 3 cm of motion at the oral commissure while at the same time improving the position of the melolabial region and decreasing the pocketing of food in the lower gingivobuccal sulcus. The overall improvement in facial appearance and motion depends to a great degree on postoperative physical therapy and the retraining of the innervated facial musculature to match the reconstructed smile.

Technique: Masseter Insertion Transfer

Masseter transfer presents an alternative for lower-face reanimation when the temporalis muscle is not available. Less overall available length, shorter excursion with contraction, and increased bulk are limiting factors that render this technique less favorable as compared with temporalis transfer.

The masseter muscle originates on the inferior and deep aspects of the zygomatic arch and inserts on the lateral surface of the angle of the mandible at the masseteric tuberosity. The motor innervation to the muscle is provided by the masseteric nerve, which reaches the medial aspect of the muscle through the sigmoid notch and runs in a superoposterior to anteroinferior direction.

The muscle can be accessed from either a lateral face-lift approach or through a transoral incision lateral and parallel to the ascending ramus of the mandible. The former approach provides greater exposure, and it is more commonly used. The lateral surface of the muscle is exposed; its insertion along the body and angle of the mandible is transected, and the muscle is elevated off of the ascending ramus, with care taken to preserve its neurovascular supply and the deep fascia. A skin incision is performed medial and parallel to the melolabial fold and along the vermillion border in the midline. The muscle is inserted in a fashion similar to that described for the temporalis muscle. Size 4-0 permanent mattress sutures should be used for fixation to prevent disinsertion. Suturing the masseter muscle to the deep aspect of the orbicularis muscle may reduce its visible bulk. Deep dermal inverted sutures tack the medial aspect of the melolabial fold to the muscle surface so that, when the muscle contracts, the fold rises and overlaps the incision site. At the conclusion of the procedure, there should be a gross overcorrection of the lateral commissure and the melolabial fold. The use of botulinum toxin (i.e., 50–100 international units) during the immediate postoperative period may help to relax the muscle and allow for significant healing before full muscular tension returns. A supporting elastic dressing should be used for the first week after surgery, during which time the patient should be kept on a liquid diet to prevent mastication and stress on the suture line.

The origin of the masseter muscle, quite lateral to the oral commissure, creates a very horizontal pull on the recipient musculature. This can help to a significant degree with obliterating the gingivobuccal pocket created by the adynamic buccinator muscle. However, the little vertical lift provided to the perioral region tends to be inadequate, particularly in patients who exhibit a "canine" smile. Significant effort to retrain the smile on the unaffected side of the face must therefore be undertaken to achieve reasonable symmetry, and the final results are often dissatisfying. However, for the patient who does not have a temporalis muscle suitable for insertion transfer, this option can create considerable improvement in the patient's QOL.

MICRONEUROVASCULAR MUSCLE TRANSPLANTATION

Microneurovascular muscle transplantation is typically the technique of last resort for unilateral dynamic facial reanimation, because these techniques are more complex and less predictable, and they address more limited areas of the paralyzed face. For congenital and bilateral facial paralysis, however, these procedures offer the patient rehabilitation options that may not otherwise be possible.

The procedure was first described for use in lower facial rehabilitation by Haarii and colleagues[34] in 1976. The original report described the transfer of the gracilis muscle from the thigh, and this remains the most common muscle transferred for this purpose, followed by the pectoralis minor and the latissimus dorsi muscle.[35]

The transplanted muscle spans from the superficial layer of the deep temporal fascia and the periosteum of the zygomatic arch to the orbicularis oris muscle. The selection of the recipient blood vessels depends on the type of muscle transferred and the condition of the recipient bed. If the patient has undergone a surgical resection in this area, the superficial temporal artery and vein may be absent or damaged, and vessels from the ipsilateral and contralateral neck may be used.

The technique of muscle reinnervation depends both on the muscle transferred and the availability of the proximal facial-nerve stump. Commonly, when this type of procedure is undertaken, the ipsilateral facial nerve is not available. For the gracilis and pectoralis minor muscle flaps, the donor nerve is usually too short, and a two-stage cross-facial interposition graft is required. Just as for cross-facial grafting, the graft is placed before the transplant is performed, and a delay of 8 to 12 months is necessary until the nerve fibers have grown across the face, as demonstrated by the Tinel sign. If the nerve transplanted with the muscle is of sufficient length, as is typically the case for the thoracodorsal nerve of the latissimus dorsi flap, a primary anastomosis to a branch of the contralateral facial nerve is performed.

Terzis and colleagues[36] reported on the outcome of 100 free-muscle transplants for facial paralysis in 1997. They reported that "a higher postoperative rating was seen in 94% of the patients, and 80% of all patients achieved a moderate or better result." They found that the functional outcome was not affected by gender, age, or ischemia time, but they emphasized the importance of the careful measurement of muscle tension before harvest so that this could be duplicated at implantation. Takushima[37] reported that 42% of patients obtained symmetry with sufficient muscle strength and natural emotional expression and that another 42% achieved a similar result but with muscle contraction that was either too strong or slightly week.

The outcomes of different series and procedures are difficult to judge as a result of the use of multiple and not easily comparable grading schemes. Studies comparing muscle insertion transfer procedures with microneurovascular muscle transplantation are lacking.

ADYNAMIC PROCEDURES FOR THE TREATMENT OF FACIAL PARALYSIS

The comprehensive management of the paralyzed face typically incorporates a combination of dynamic and static (i.e., immobile soft-tissue repositioning) procedures. The forehead, eyelid, and neck areas benefit substantially from static techniques.

As discussed previously, the phenomenon of compensatory contralateral contraction requires the surgeon to analyze both sides of the patient's face and, in some circumstances, to perform bilateral corrective procedures.

Upper Face

Forehead Lift and Blepharoplasty

The descent of the eyebrow complex frequently accentuates preexisting blepharochalasis in the patient with facial paralysis. The resulting visual-field deficits represent one of several indications to elevate the brow complex and to perform corrective upper-eyelid surgery in this patient group.

The paralyzed patient requires modifications to correct the static and dynamic asymmetries that are present with facial paralysis. The authors' observations suggest that, in the paralyzed patient, both eyebrows typically need to be treated. The eyebrow on the nonparalyzed side is frequently ptotic and exhibits marked circadian fluctuations of position. This side is corrected first, thus creating a stable mark to match on the paralyzed side. Numerous techniques have been described for the repositioning of the forehead and the eyebrow. Among other factors, the position of the hairline influences the choice of technique: coronal, trichophytic, pretrichial, mid-forehead, direct eyebrow, endoscopic, and combined endoscopic and pretrichial approaches are available. The risk of recurrence of brow ptosis after endoscopic correction of the paralyzed forehead alone is considerable, especially among older patients, unless adjunctive maneuvers are performed. The authors therefore incorporate a skin-excision technique; the trichophytic incision is well camouflaged, and it provides excellent lifting with durable results.

The endoscopic technique is excellently suited in selected patients to correct the nonparalyzed eyebrow and to elevate the paralyzed eyebrow. For a detailed review of the technique, the interested reader is referred to the pertinent literature. In short, the temporal fossae are dissected under endoscopic control in a subgaleal plane. The sentinel vein is identified and preserved or transected, and the arcus marginalis is identified. The forehead is then dissected in a subperiosteal plane through small scalp incisions at the level of the lateral canthus. The supraorbital and supratrochlear bundles are identified and preserved, and the periosteum is transected along the supraorbital rim. The deficit in frontalis muscle function on the paralyzed side can be compensated for with asymmetric endoscopic elevation and fixation. A simultaneous unilateral trichophytic or direct brow-lift is usually performed on the paralyzed side. An asymmetric subdermal trichophytic lift is preferred, because it allows for the controlled resection of the forehead skin, it hides the scar well, and it does not further lift the hairline. After subdermal undermining, the resulting defect is closed in a supragaleal plane, thus preserving the sensory innervation of the scalp.

The outcomes after forehead lifting are usually excellent. A major determinant appears to be addressing both the paralyzed and innervated sides, because the failure to do so will result in asymmetry.

Upper-Eyelid Weight Implantation

Paralysis of the facial nerve prevents the contraction of the orbicularis oculi muscle, which results in volitional and reflex lid akinesia, lagophthalmos, and, possibly, paralytic ectropion of the lower eyelid. It is still possible to raise the upper eyelid when the oculomotor nerve is functional. A sufficient blink reflex is critical for corneal nutrition and the dispersion of the normal tear film. A failure of eye closure results in corneal desiccation and exposure keratopathy, which may progress to denudement of the epithelium, ulceration, and perforation of the cornea. Lower-lid ectropion allows for the formation of a static pool of tears in the lacrimal lake, and the adynamic orbicularis oculi is unable to actively pump tears from this area. The inferior punctum may fail to contact the lacrimal lake as a result of ectropion. Thus the patient may simultaneously present with epiphora and corneal desiccation, which is a diagnostic finding that must be recognized and promptly managed. Immediate conservative management options of the dry eye include ophthalmic ointment, lubricating drops, temporary eyelid closure (e.g., tape, tarsorrhaphy suture, external weight), and a bubble dressing.

If the facial paralysis is believed to be permanent, upper-eyelid weighting may be indicated. It is necessary to consider the upper eyelid as part of the eyebrow–forehead complex, and often a brow-lift needs to be performed before upper-eyelid surgery. After the eyebrow is appropriately positioned and fixated, the placement of a lid weight allows for the counteracting and balancing of the effect of the levator muscle, and the patient is able to close the eyelid by voluntary relaxation. An implant of proper weight allows for the full closure of the vertical aperture with minimal ptosis. When the weight is tested by taping it to the eyelid, a drop of 1 mm or less in the upper-eyelid position should be observed when the eyes are fully open in neutral gaze.

Platinum implants (Figure 48-10) have an advantage over gold of being of a higher specific weight so that a smaller-volume implant can be used with the same effect. Berghaus and colleagues[38] described a platinum chain implant that flexes and conforms to the changing

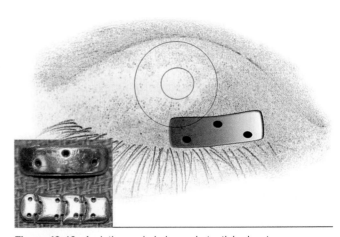

Figure 48-10. A platinum chain has substantial advantages over gold-weight implantation, because it adds less volume and is more flexible. The weight should be placed at the point of most marked lagophthalmos.

radius of the tarsus. In a prospective study of more than 60 patients, those authors found a lower rate of complications with the platinum chain implant as compared with the fixed gold weight, and they noted excellent biocompatibility.[38] The incision line along the supratarsal crease should be marked with the patient sitting upright. Lid excursion with and without the weight taped to the eyelid skin should also be carefully noted. The procedure is preferably performed with the patient under conscious sedation. A small amount of local anaesthetic is infiltrated into a supramuscular plane to minimize the diffusion of the anaesthetic to the Müller muscle. A blepharoplasty incision is placed along the supratarsal crease, the anterior aspect of the tarsal plate is dissected in a submuscular plane, and the levator aponeurosis is identified. The weight is then centered over the point of maximal lagophthalmos, typically between the mid-pupillary line and the medial limbus (Figure 48-10). The weight is attached with 6-0 Prolene sutures to the tarsal plate approximately 2 mm above the lash line. The eyelid is then everted to verify that the sutures have not perforated the tarsal plate or the conjunctiva. The levator aponeurosis is inspected for integrity, and ptosis repair is performed, if indicated. The edge of the orbicularis muscle at the inferior incision line may be fixated to the levator aponeurosis to re-create the supratarsal crease. The eyelid skin is resected as indicated. Ipsilateral or contralateral orbital fat may be harvested and positioned over the lateral and medial edge of the weight to smooth the visible contour of the implant. The incision is closed with 6-0 Prolene or 6-0 fast-absorbing gut.

The primary short-term complication of the placement of an upper-eyelid weight is the incorrect placement of the weight. If it is too high, the full weight will not be borne by the tarsus but rather in part by the globe as well. Placement too far medially or laterally will place excessive weight away from the area of greatest closure gap and fail to close the residual aperture.

Failure to choose the appropriate mass will also manifest shortly after surgery, and this can be avoided with careful preoperative evaluation. The primary long-term complication is the extrusion of the weight. The incidence of this is difficult to estimate because of the lack of appropriate prospective studies, and it quite possibly increases with the duration of implantation. The use of a flexible weight, with the techniques described previously, is a reasonable approach to mitigate this problem. The migration of the weight can also occur, but the chances of this happening can also be decreased with appropriate surgical technique.

Ectropion Repair

Dysfunction of the lower eyelid may contribute substantially to the morbidity of facial paralysis. In a prospective evaluation of ophthalmologic complaints of patients with facial paralysis, epiphora was found to be the chief ophthalmologic complaint in 75% of patients with facial paralysis, typically as a result of lower-lid ectropion.[39]

The correction of lower-eyelid malposition requires the evaluation of the entire lower-eyelid complex. With facial paralysis, the orbicularis muscle not only fails to raise the lower eyelid and maintain its resting position adjacent to the globe, but it becomes part of the problem by adding weight to the lower eyelid and its support structures. The goal of therapy, when reinnervation is not possible, is to reinforce the support structures of the lower eyelid so that they can both handle the weight of the atonic musculature and maintain the eyelid in its normal position while restoring the passive function of the lacrimal apparatus through the repositioning of the inferior punctum against the lacrimal lake. The choice of the appropriate canthopexy procedure to treat the medial and lateral canthus is based on the correct diagnosis. The authors rely on an ectropion grading scale that describes the degree and location of medial and lateral canthal pathology and that aids in the selection of the proper technique for correction[39] (Table 48-4).

TABLE 48-4 Ectropion Grading Scale

Score		Affix	
0	Normal eyelid appearance and function	L	Predominantly lateral
I	Normal appearance but symptomatic eyelid laxity present on examination	M	Predominantly medial
II	Scleral show without eversion of the lower eyelid	t	Previous tarsorrhaphy
III	Ectropion without the eversion of lacrimal punctum		
IV	Advanced ectropion with the eversion of the lacrimal punctum from the lacrimal lake		
V	Ectropion with complications (e.g., conjunctival metaplasia, retraction of anterior lamella, stenosis of lacrimal system)		

Technique: Precaruncular Medial Canthopexy

After the placement of a corneal protector and infiltration of 1% lidocaine 1:100,000 epinephrine medial to the caruncle, lacrimal probes are placed superiorly and inferiorly to reflect and protect the canaliculi. A precaruncular incision is extended into the conjunctiva, and the posterior limb of the medial canthal tendon (i.e., the Horner muscle) is used as a guide for dissection to the posterior lacrimal crest and the medial orbital wall (Figure 48-11). A CV-5 Gore-Tex suture on a TTc-13 needle (WL Gore & Associates Inc, Flagstaff, Ariz) is anchored to the periorbita or alternatively to a 4-mm titanium or resorbable screw placed at the posterosuperior lacrimal crest. The lacrimal probes and corneal shield are then removed, and the suture is anchored deeply to the medial end of the tarsal plate, close to the eyelid margin and immediately lateral to the lacrimal punctum. If the suture is placed too low, the punctum will remain everted, thereby causing epiphora. The suture is then tied on itself, which provides the appropriate tension for raising, medializing, and posteriorly tightening the medial canthus as desired. Slight overcorrection (i.e., 1 mm) is desirable. The inferior punctum should be checked for proper inversion and elevation. The incision is closed with the use of a 5-0 absorbable suture placed between the apex of the caruncle and the medial eyelid.[40]

Technique: Transorbital Lateral Canthopexy

The correction of the lateral lid is frequently required for patients with facial paralysis. Wedge resection and the tarsal strip procedure are popular, but they commonly result in asymmetry with an overriding appearance of the upper over the lower lid. Transorbital lateral canthopexy represents an alternative technique (Figure 48-12). After infiltration anesthesia of the zygomaticofrontal nerve and zygomaticofacial nerve and topical anesthesia of the conjunctiva, a 1-cm incision is placed in a crease that extends posteriorly from the lateral orbital rim at the level of the lateral canthus. Stay sutures are placed through the wound edges, the orbital aspect of the orbicularis oculi muscle is transected, and the periosteum of the arcus marginalis is incised. The insertion of the lateral canthal tendon is identified and sharply elevated off of the orbital rim in one unit, with the lateral extension of the levator aponeurosis. Size 4-0 Prolene sutures are placed through the medial aspect of the lateral canthal tendon at the canthal angle and through the lateral inferior tarsal plate. Two 1-mm bore holes are placed approximately 2 mm posterosuperior to the Whitnall tubercle in the region of the frontozygomatic suture so that the eyelid can be elevated, thus improving lacrimal drainage. The sutures are placed through the bore holes and tightened until the desired eyelid position is achieved and the lacrimal punctum is apposed to the lacrimal lake. The wound is then closed in layers.[37]

Midface

As previously mentioned, there is a dual effect of facial paralysis on the eyelids in that the orbicularis oculi muscle fails to aid in the support of the lower eyelid while also adding its mass to the structures that are already being supported by the medial and lateral canthal

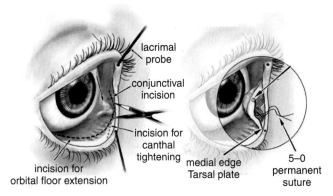

Figure 48-11. Precaruncular medial canthopexy. A conjunctival incision is extended along the Horner muscle into the precaruncular plane. The lower tarsal plate is suspended with sutures to the medial orbital wall, with a resulting posterosuperior elevation of the tarsus and apposition of the inferior lacrimal punctum.

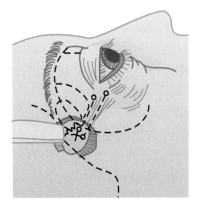
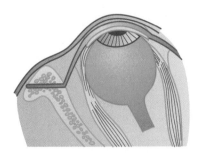

Figure 48-12. Transorbital lateral canthopexy. After the transconjunctival identification of the lateral canthal tendon, the tendon is fixated with sutures through two burr holes in the lateral orbital rim.

tendons. This phenomenon holds true for the midface as well: the musculature no longer elevates the support structures of the melolabial fold. As a result, the melolabial fold descends inferomedially together with the midfacial soft tissues that it supports.[41]

Midface Lift

The elevation of the midface is of substantial benefit to the patient with facial paralysis. The malar ptosis is not only a cosmetic issue; it may also contribute to lower-eyelid malposition as the orbitomalar ligament is stretched.[42] Elner and colleagues[43] believe that midface elevation adds significantly to the improvement gained by augmenting the tarsoligamentous support of the lower eyelid. Further studies are required to provide conclusive evidence of the clinical observation that midface elevation improves lower-eyelid function, especially when the medial and lateral canthal tendons have been properly repositioned. Midface elevation in the paralyzed face is also beneficial because of resulting improvements in nasal function and cosmesis.

The age of the patient is the most important factor for determining the surgical approach to the midface. The elderly patient who requires skin excision is best treated with a deep-plane face-lift with repositioning and the elevation of the malar fat pad. Younger patients are often good candidates for an endoscopic midface lift, which is typically combined with an endoscopic brow-lift.

Technique

An incision is placed in the gingivobuccal sulcus, and subperiosteal dissection is undertaken to elevate the soft tissues to the orbital rim and malar eminence. The infraorbital nerve is identified and preserved. An avascular plane along the deep temporal fascia is developed (as described for the endoscopic brow-lift), transitioned over the zygomatic arch into a subperiosteal plane, and followed into the midface. Two or three 3-0 polydioxanone sutures are placed in the inferior aspects of the dissected malar periosteum, pulled through the zygomatic tunnel into the temporal fossa, and fixated to the superior temporal line. Alternatively, the Coapt Endotine device (Coapt Systems, Inc., Palo Alto, CA) is used for elevation and fixation. Substantial elevation of the midface will support the lower eyelid, but this frequently results in the asymmetry of the midface. Hence consideration should be given to performing this procedure bilaterally.

Nose

The main effects of facial paralysis on nasal function are a loss of active nasal flaring and the collapse of the internal nasal valve. Kienstra and colleagues[34] have presented evidence of the important role of the nasal muscles in both actively increasing nasal airflow and maintaining resting nasal muscle tension that opens the nasal airway. Scarce data are available to quantify the effects of facial paralysis on nasal airflow and the resulting impact on the patient's QOL.

Nasal-valve collapse in the patient with facial paralysis is typically a result of the reduced dynamic resilience of the fibromuscular tissues of the ala. Inspiratory transmural pressures overcome the residual static resilience of the ala and the collapse of the internal nasal valves, the external nasal valves, or both ensues. In patients with facial paralysis, the nasal musculature with its dynamic effects on the nasal airway cannot be reliably reanimated.[44] Hence static techniques are employed to increase the resilience of the alar tissues. A face lift procedure can reposition the alar soft tissues and improve the airway. In cases of mild to moderate valve collapse the endonasal implantation of an alar batten and rim graft are sufficient to improve the airway. The authors prefer the high and vertical placement of batten grafts over the frontal process of the maxilla, because this location provides an osseous base that will project the batten graft laterally and open the airway more (Figure 48-13).

In cases of more severe valve obstruction, an open-structure rhinoplasty allows the surgeon to address various aspects of valve collapse. Senile tip ptosis is often exacerbated by facial paralysis, and it may be corrected by tip rotation through the resection of the scroll, the advancement of the columella toward the caudal septum (i.e., tongue in groove), and the mobilization and repositioning of the dorsal-skin–soft-tissue envelope (i.e., rhinolift procedure). Collapse of the fibromuscular tissues of the alar rim may result in external valve collapse, which is corrected with the placement of alar rim grafts. Collapse of the internal nasal valve may be improved with the transection of the insertion of the upper

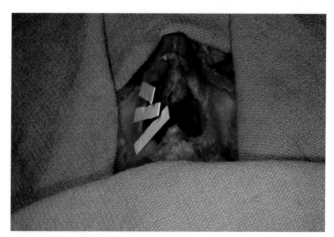

Figure 48-13. Placement of white indicators shows the effect of placement of alar batten grafts over various aspects of the piriform aperture. High placement of these grafts over the frontal process of the maxilla results in most marked lateralization of the alar sidewall.

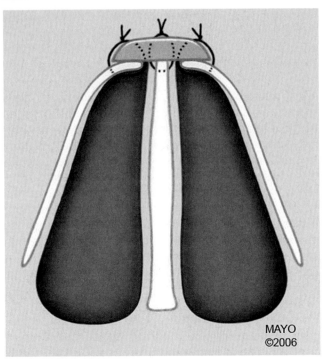

Figure 48-14. Modified dorsal onlay graft with suture fixation of the upper lateral cartilages to the graft results in opening of the nasal valve angle and lateralization of the nasal sidewall.

lateral cartilage into the septum, the placement of an onlay graft on the septum, and the suture fixation of the upper lateral cartilages to the undersurface of the onlay graft. This maneuver results in the lateral rotation of the upper lateral cartilages, and it accentuates the effects of the classic spreader grafts. The authors have found this technique to be substantially more effective than the traditional spreader-graft technique (Figure 48-14).[45]

ADJUNCTIVE PROCEDURES

Botulinum Toxin

The advent of botulinum toxin injections has contributed enormously to the adjunctive treatment of facial paralysis. Patients with facial paralysis appear to generate excessive static and to dynamically contract the nonparalyzed side of the face, which results in a shift in midline structures (e.g., nose, mouth) and an unnatural look of the nonparalyzed side. Teleologically this may be interpreted as a subconscious effort to correct the position of the paralyzed side. When comparing preoperative and postoperative photographs of patients who have recovered from facial paralysis, the improved appearance of the now relaxed nonparalyzed facial half may dramatically contribute to the overall improved appearance of the face. Treating the nonparalyzed side therefore plays an important role in the management facial paralysis. The main modalities employed for this purpose are botulinum toxin injections and retraining.

Chemodenervation with botulinum toxin is excellent for treating dynamic asymmetries of the forehead. Although a brow-lift will reposition the eyebrows symmetrically, the appearance of forehead lines and furrows remains asymmetric. The immobilization of the contralateral forehead needs to be more complete than for cosmetic purposes in nonparalyzed patients. The authors typically inject 10 to 20 units of botulinum toxin A into the frontalis, procerus, and corrugator muscles. With experience, these injections are predictable, and patients will usually require retreatment every 2 to 3 months. The treatment of the lower face is more challenging. The immobilization of the perioral musculature should be partial and allow for a better matching of the appearance of the nonparalyzed perioral and midface anatomy with the contralateral side while still preserving function. The appropriate dosage is typically found for the individual patient, with adjustments made to dosage and injection site with repeat treatments. The authors have found that the reconstitution of botulinum toxin A in 5 ml of 1% lidocaine with 1:100,000 epinephrine renders the treatment more predictable. The admixture of lidocaine results in an immediate paralysis of the injected musculature. Within the same treatment setting, additional dosages of botulinum toxin can be injected to fine tune the result.[46]

Rehabilitation

Various modalities of physical therapy are used for the adjunctive treatment of facial paralysis. One of the most important goals of rehabilitation is the retraining of the nonparalyzed side of the face to improve the overall appearance. To date there have been no trials that have demonstrated the benefit of a single type of therapy over others. However, some studies have shown a benefit for treatment groups as compared with control groups. One such study used mime therapy; a combination of massage, relaxation, and coordination; and emotional control training.[47] The basic exercises included expressing various emotions and performing tasks such as lip closure and eye closure in front of a mirror. The control group was simply placed on a waiting list for 3 months. Although the control group was not optimal and several types of therapy were included in the study group, the authors found a significant improvement with their protocol.

Electric stimulation is gaining popularity as a treatment modality for physical therapy and rehabilitation. Important goals of this therapy include the maintenance of muscle mass and assistance with retraining. To attain these goals, a visible contraction needs to be produced, typically with percutaneous stimuli of approximately 100-ms duration.[48]

The authors' present approach is to teach patients facial exercises preoperatively, when possible, including practicing the expression of all emotions and individual facial unit movements in front of a mirror. Postoperatively, the patients continue this work, spending 10 to 15 minutes at least twice a day in front of a mirror and including exercises to dampen facial expressions, such as smiling on the innervated side. Other therapies will be added as evidence of their efficacy becomes available.

REFERENCES

1. Seddon HJ: Three types of nerve injury. *Brain* 1943;66:238–283.
2. Sunderland S. The anatomy and physiology of nerve injury. *Muscle Nerve* 1990;13(9):771–784.
3. Lydiatt DD: Medical malpractice and facial nerve paralysis. *Arch Otolaryngol Head Neck Surg* 2003;129(1):50–53.
4. Long YT, bin Sabir Husin Athar PP, Mahmud R, et al: Management of iatrogenic facial nerve palsy and labyrinthine fistula in mastoid surgery. *Asian J Surg* 2004;27(3):176–179.
5. Green JD Jr, Shelton C, Brackmann DE: Surgical management of iatrogenic facial nerve injuries. *Otolaryngol Head Neck Surg* 1994;111(5):606–610.
6. Ryzenman JM, Rothholtz VS, Wiet RJ: Porencephalic cyst: a review of the literature and management of a rare cause of cerebrospinal fluid otorrhea. *Otol Neurotol* 2007;28(3):381–386.
7. Baumann I, Polligkeit J, Blumenstock G, et al: Quality of life after unilateral acoustic neuroma surgery via middle cranial fossa approach. *Acta Otolaryngol* 2005;125(6):585–591.
8. Sullivan CA, Masin J, Maniglia AJ, et al: Complications of rhytidectomy in an otolaryngology training program. *Laryngoscope* 1999;109(2 Pt 1):198–203.
9. Viksraitis S, Astrauskas T, Karbonskiene A, et al: Endoscopic aesthetic facial surgery: technique and results. *Medicina* 2004;40(2):149–155.
10. Iro H, Zenk J, Hornung J, et al: Long term results of extracorporeal piezoelectric shock wave lithotripsy of parotid stones. *Dtsch Med Wochenschr* 1998;123(40):1161–1165.
11. Guntinas-Lichius O, Klussmann JP, Wittekindt C, et al: Parotidectomy for benign parotid disease at a university teaching hospital: Outcome of 963 operations. *Laryngoscope* 2006;116(4):534–540.
12. Makeieff M, Venail F, Cartier C, et al: Continuous facial nerve monitoring during pleomorphic adenoma recurrence surgery. *Laryngoscope* 2005;115(7):1310–1314.
13. Moe KS, Linder T: The lateral transorbital canthopexy for correction and prevention of ectropion: Report of a procedure, grading system, and outcome study. *Arch Facial Plast Surg* 2000;2(1):9–15.
14. Cross T, Sheard CE, Garrud P, et al: Impact of facial paralysis on patients with acoustic neuroma. *Laryngoscope* 2000;110(9):1539–1542.
15. Lassaletta L, Alfonso C, Del Rio L, et al: Impact of facial dysfunction on quality of life after vestibular schwannoma surgery. *Ann Otol Rhinol Laryngol* 2006;115(9):694–698.
16. House JW, Brackmann DE: Facial nerve grading system. *Otolaryngol Head Neck Surg* 1985;93:146–147.
17. Gidley PW, Gantz BJ, Rubinstein JT: Facial nerve grafts: From cerebellopontine angle and beyond. *Am J Otol* 1999;20:781–788.
18. Adour KK: Facial nerve electrical testing. In Jackler RK, Brackmann DE, editors: *Neurotology*, St. Louis, 1994, Mosby.
19. Kleinjung T, Eichhammer P, Langguth B, et al: Long-term effects of repetitive transcranial magnetic stimulation (rTMS) in patients with chronic tinnitus. *Otolaryngol Head Neck Surg* 2005;132(4):566–569.
20. Nowak DA, Linder S, Topka H: Diagnostic relevance of transcranial magnetic and electric stimulation of the facial nerve in the management of facial palsy. *Clin Neurophysiol* 2005;116:2051–2057.
21. Fisch U: Surgery for Bell's palsy. *Arch Otolaryngol* 1981;107(1)1–11.
22. Greyeli AB, Mosnier I, Julien N, et al: Long-term functional outcome in facial nerve graft by fibrin glue in the temporal bone and cerebellopontine angle. *Eur Arch Otorhinolaryngol* 2005;262:404–407.
23. Hammerschlag P: Facial reanimation with jump interpositional graft hypoglossal facial anastomosis and hypoglossal facial anastomosis: Evolution in management of facial paralysis: Part 2. *Laryngoscope* 1999;109(90):1–23.
24. May M, Sobel SM, Mester SJ: Hypoglossal-facial nerve interpositional jump graft for facial reanimation without tongue atrophy. *Otolaryngol Head Neck Surg* 1991;204:818–826.
25. Kartush JM, Lundy LB: Facial nerve outcome in acoustic neuroma surgery. *Otolaryngol Clin North Am* 1992;25:623–647.
26. Gavron JP, Clemis JD: Hypoglossal-facial nerve anastomosis: A review of forty cases caused by facial nerve injuries in the posterior fossa. *Laryngoscope* 1984;94(11 Pt 1):1147–1150.
27. Malik TH, Kelly G, Ahmed A, et al: A comparison of surgical techniques used in dynamic reanimation of the paralyzed face. *Otol Neurotol* 2005;26(2):284–291.
28. Pensak ML, Jackson CG, Glasscock ME 3rd, et al: Facial reanimation with the VII-XII anastomosis: Analysis of the functional and psychologic results. *Otolaryngol Head Neck Surg* 1986;94(3):305–310.
29. May M: Nerve repair. In May M, Shaitkin B, editors: *The facial nerve,* New York, 2000, Thieme.
30. Gillies H: Experiences with fascia lata grafts in the operative treatment of facial paralysis. *Proc R Soc Med* 1934;27(10):1372–1382.
31. McLaughlin CR: Surgical report in permanent facial paralysis. *Plast Reconstr Surg* 1953;11:302–314.
32. Labbé D, Huault M: Lengthening temporalis myoplasty and lip reanimation. *Plast Reconstr Surg* 2000;105(4):1289–1297.
33. Sherris DA: Refinement in reanimation of the lower face. *Arch Facial Plast Surg* 2004;6(1):49–53.
34. Harii K, Ohmori K, Torii S: Free gracilis muscle transplantation with microneurovascular anastomoses for the treatment of facial paralysis: A preliminary report. *Plast Reconstr Surg* 1976;57(2):133–143.
35. Terzis JK: Pectoralis minor: A unique muscle for correction of facial palsy. *Plast Reconstr Surg* 1989;83(5):767–776.
36. Terzis JK, Noah ME: Analysis of 100 cases of free-muscle transplantation for facial paralysis. *Plast Reconstr Surg* 1997;99(7):1905–1921.
37. Takushima A, Harii K, Asato H, et al: Neurovascular free-muscle transfer for the treatment of established facial paralysis following ablative surgery in the parotid region. *Plast Reconstr Surg* 2004;113(6):1563–1572.
38. Berghaus A, Neumann K, Schrom T: The platinum chain. *Arch Facial Plast Surg* 2003;5(2):166–170.
39. Moe KS, Linder T: The lateral transorbital canthopexy for correction and prevention of ectropion: Report of a procedure, grading system, and outcome study. *Arch Facial Plast Surg* 2000;2(1):9–15.
40. Moe KS, Kao CH: Precaruncular medial canthopexy. *Arch Facial Plast Surg* 2005;7(4):244–250.
41. Gassner HG, Rafii A, Young A, et al: Surgical anatomy of the face: implications for modern face-lift techniques. *Arch Facial Plast Surg* 2008;10(1):9–19.
42. Kikkawa DO, Lemke BN, Dortzbach RK: Relations of the superficial musculoaponeurotic system to the orbit and characterization of the orbitomalar ligament. *Ophthal Plast Reconstr Surg* 1996;12(2):77–88.
43. Elner VM, Mauffray RO, Fante RG, et al: Comprehensive midfacial elevation for ocular complications of facial nerve palsy. *Arch Facial Plast Surg* 2003;5(5):427–433.
44. Kienstra MA, Gassner HG, Sherris DA, et al: Effects of the nasal muscles on the nasal airway. *Am J Rhinol* 2005;19(4):375–381.
45. Gassner HG, Friedman O, Sherris DA, et al: An alternative method of middle vault reconstruction. *Arch Facial Plast Surg* 2006;8(6):432–435.
46. Gassner HG, Sherris DA: Addition of an anaesthetic agent to enhance the predictability of the effects of botulinum toxin type A injections: A randomized, controlled study. *Mayo Clinic Proc* 2000;75(7):701–704.
47. Beurskens CH, Heymans PG: Mime therapy improves facial symmetry in people with long-term facial nerve paresis: A randomised controlled trial. *Aust J Physiother* 2006;52(3):177–183.
48. deLateur B: Personal communication.

CHAPTER 49

Complications of Chemical Peels, Dermabrasion, and Laser Resurfacing

F. Brian Gibson and Stephen W. Perkins

The number of aesthetic facial procedures continues to increase every year; there were a total of 11 million procedures performed in 2005, 9 million of which were nonsurgical.[1] The demand for these procedures has increased dramatically, particularly in the area of facial resurfacing, with 550,000 chemical peels, 1 million microdermabrasion procedures, and 400,000 laser resurfacing procedures carried out in 2005. Facial resurfacing is now an integral part of the aesthetic facial surgeon's palette of techniques for facial rejuvenation.

As in other areas of aesthetic surgery, patients who seek these procedures are not suffering from an illness or trauma; they are instead seeking to improvement in their physical appearance. The elective nature of these procedures imposes a different level of expectation with regard to outcomes and the avoidance of complications as compared with medically essential treatments.

Proper patient selection is paramount for the success of facial resurfacing procedures. If the surgeon has questions about the patient's likelihood of following preoperative and postprocedure care instructions and other recommendations, the best option is often to defer the performance of these procedures on that patient. For example, patients must be willing to commit to applying topical emollients or ointments after a chemical peel procedure, potentially up to 6 times a day.

Patients who are seeking aesthetic surgery should participate in a thorough process of evaluation and discussion with their surgeons. Obtaining an appropriate medical history with focused attention paid to any medications or underlying medical conditions that may affect the surgical outcome is extremely important to avoid predictable complications and to select the right procedure for the patient. The patient's habits, including sun exposure expectations, cosmetic regimen, and lifestyle, are all important factors for predicting the outcomes of their procedures. A history of abnormal scarring, collagen vascular disease, or previous surgery in the area undergoing treatment can predict possible abnormalities in postoperative healing. Previous radiation therapy may disturb the skin's architecture, reduce the number of pilosebaceous units needed to heal after resurfacing, and possibly affect recontouring efforts. The use of isotretinoin substantially increases the risk of

scarring, and it must be stopped for at least 6 months preoperatively. The assessment of the patient's psychologic stability may help to avoid performing procedures on potentially problematic individuals. At times, a preoperative psychologic consultation may be necessary. Many patients undergo resurfacing with high expectations regarding the results. Demanding or imbalanced patients may have disturbed or unrealistic expectations.

A recent study evaluated 212 patients undergoing ablative pulsed carbon-dioxide laser resurfacing. There was an 89% overall satisfaction rate (i.e., "they would do it again").[2] Predictors of patient satisfaction included expectations of mild to moderate improvement, hopes for improved appearance, and healthier-appearing skin. Correlates of dissatisfaction included preoperative expectations of improved self-esteem after therapy, a belief that the face was disfigured before treatment, and an expectation of complete or near-total improvement of the aging skin.[2]

After obtaining a thorough history, the physician must perform a thorough evaluation of the patient's physical status. For patients seeking facial resurfacing, particular attention is paid to the condition and objective qualities of the facial skin. Analyzing the degree of skin changes, assessing the skin coloration and the Fitzpatrick skin type, and determining the degree of aging changes (including assessment with the Glogau scale) are parts of this evaluation.[3] The degree of skin pigmentation is a key predictor of an uneventful outcome of particular facial resurfacing procedures and the potential need for a preprocedure regimen of topical therapy. Photographs of the patient should be obtained to document problem areas and to allow for the prospective evaluation of their improvement after the resurfacing procedure.

During their discussions about the upcoming procedure, the patient and surgeon should discuss the nature and limitations of the chosen procedure as well as the expected outcome. For example, patients with relatively fine rhytids will often do well with a variety of procedures, including medium-depth peels and other resurfacing techniques, whereas those with deeper rhytids can only achieve complete resolution with deeper resurfacing.

The normal course of healing, including that of routine symptoms (e.g., erythema, swelling, ecchymosis), should be reviewed, and this review should involve reassuring the patient that none of these symptoms represents a complication or an untoward event. As part of the consultation, some physicians recommend showing photographic examples of patients' appearance during the immediate postoperative period, patients during the course of healing, and the eventual outcome. This documentation should include outstanding results, average outcomes, and suboptimal results so that the patient has a full understanding of what can be achieved.[4] During this discussion, the patient's desired outcome (whether it can be achieved with the procedure being considered), expectations, and level of commitment to the healing process and the postoperative care regimen can be assessed.

Reviewing possible complications of the procedure, including their source, treatment, and results, is an integral part of preoperative preparation. Although uncommon, complications do occur after facial resurfacing, and they may be the result of various factors, including surgeon inexperience or inattention, inadequate postoperative care, and patient variables such as skin type and coloration, ultraviolet (UV) exposure, and compliance with care instructions.[5]

Patient satisfaction ultimately depends not only on how closely the physical result matches their expectations but also on how strong of a physician–patient relationship has developed. The process of obtaining consent is crucial to the outcome of cosmetic surgery and to the acceptance of potential complications.

RESURFACING TECHNIQUES

Chemical peels, dermabrasion, and laser resurfacing share a number of similarities, including the types of problems treated with these techniques, the histologic basis behind them, and their potential complications. In broad terms, these procedures involve mechanical, thermal, or chemical injury to the skin to produce a desired outcome through the process of healing and organized regeneration (i.e., usually a reduction in the signs of aging or sun-induced damage to the skin).[6]

Chemical Peels

Chemical peels take advantage of certain organic acids' ability to penetrate the skin and create a fairly predictable pattern of injury and subsequent repair. Modern chemical peeling includes the use of a variety of different compounds, including alpha hydroxy acids (AHAs); trichloroacetic acid (TCA); and phenol-based formulas that often incorporate phenol, croton oil (a potent vesicant), soap (e.g., Septisol), water, and vegetable oils or glycerin.

Several peel techniques are available that make use of more than one solution, such as the Jessner's TCA medium-depth peel described by Monheit.[7] These combination peels involve the use a keratolytic agent such as Jessner's solution or glycolic acid to enhance penetration by the TCA peeling solution. Reepithelialization should be complete by 5 days for superficial resurfacing, 7 to 10 days for medium-depth treatments, and nearly 10 to 14 days for deeper chemical peels.[7]

Resurfacing Procedures

Resurfacing procedures produce a level of injury to the skin that can be classified as superficial (through the epidermis to the papillary dermis), medium depth (into the upper reticular dermis), or deep (to the mid-reticular dermis). Examples of superficial treatments would include AHA or Jessner's chemical peels, light laser resurfacing, or microdermabrasion. Medium-depth treatments include combination chemical peels and many laser treatment protocols. Deep-level resurfacing includes phenol peels, more aggressive laser treatments, and most dermabrasion procedures. The body's natural process of healing produces the desired aesthetic result, and the depth of injury can be tailored on the basis of the problem to be corrected and the desired outcome.[3] In general, the reepithelialization of the skin surface occurs by the proliferation of epithelial remnants in the skin adnexa such as the hair follicles.[6,8] If these adnexa are suppressed, as in the cases of those patients taking isotretinoin or who have had radiation treatment, then care must be taken before proceeding with certain techniques of skin resurfacing. At the microscopic level, after healing, the epidermis thickens, with increased ridging at the dermal–epidermal junction. After medium and deeper resurfacing, the dermis shows increased elastin and more organized collagen formation, which is in contrast with the disorganized collagen found in sun-damaged skin.[9] Medium-depth and deep peels stimulate a new band of collagen in the dermis to further reduce the signs of aging. All of these modalities stimulate the body's natural repair processes to replace damaged, aging tissue with more organized and histologically youthful features.

The depth of injury and thus the eventual result and risk of complications depends on several factors. Patient selection, the choice of resurfacing technique including the peeling agent (e.g., TCA, Jessner's solution, phenol-based solutions, AHAs, one of numerous combination peels), the laser or dermabrasion technique, the preoperative skin preparation, the application technique, the postoperative care regimen, and compliance can all affect the patient's outcome and risk for untoward events.[10] For example, patients undergoing a Baker–Gordon phenol peel must accept certain expected results, such as some degree of persistent hypopigmentation as well as a higher risk of complications during the healing process. Similarly, if the physician chooses to use a higher concentration of TCA (i.e., ≥50%), then the patient must understand the intrinsically greater risk of postoperative scarring.

Surgeons who use these techniques must be well versed in the characteristics of the different treatment techniques, their likelihood of success for the patient's presenting clinical conditions, and their potential to cause complications. Indications for treatment include dyschromias, fine and coarse rhytids, premalignant skin lesions, and acne scars.

Laser Resurfacing

Laser resurfacing and other resurfacing techniques can be very effective for reducing the number of actinic lesions in those patients with widespread photoaging and precancerous lesions.[3] This can be a significant clinical problem because of the difficulty separating diffusely damaged skin from isolated lesions. Approximately 90% of patients may remain free of lesions for 1 year and 60% for 2 years after a single treatment. Overall 95% of actinic keratoses can be eradicated with common resurfacing techniques that allow for the removal of the lesions as well as prophylactically treating surrounding sun-damaged skin.[11] The patient must be carefully evaluated so that the depth of peeling will be appropriate for the lesion being treated. The development of more superficial treatments has expanded the range of potential patients beyond the blond, blue-eyed, fair-skinned individual originally thought to be ideal for deep peels.[12] Some physicians are now treating even Fitzpatrick types III and IV skin with medium-depth or deep peels along with very vigorous postoperative care aimed at reducing hyperpigmentation.[12]

In contrast with chemical peels and dermabrasion, laser resurfacing relies on thermal energy to wound the skin. This thermal energy has the benefit of cauterizing potential bleeding sites, but it can also damage adjacent tissue.[13] Early laser resurfacing procedures were performed with continuous-wave carbon-dioxide laser technology that led to more complications. Excessive laser energy delivery resulted in a higher incidence of scarring.[5]

After high-energy, short-pulse lasers became available during the early 1990s, controlled ablation with an acceptable incidence of complications became possible. This occurred in parallel with the development of less aggressive and safer peeling regimens. With the newer laser technologies, surgeons could deliver high-energy fluences in very short pulses, which resulted in effective cutaneous ablation with minimal collateral thermal damage. There are now a number of different

protocols for laser resurfacing that involve varying types of lasers, amounts of energy, pulse modes, and numbers of treatment passes.[13] Carbon-dioxide ablative resurfacing techniques remain the standard for laser resurfacing. Primarily absorbed by intracellular water, carbon-dioxide laser energy heats the cells to the boiling point. This results in vaporization, the removal of the surface layer of cells, the thermal coagulative necrosis of a band of cells, and the denaturation of extracellular proteins in the immediate area bordering the zone of vaporization.[14] High-energy, pulsed, carbon-dioxide lasers produce deeper penetration (i.e., 20–60 μm) with each pass and 20 μm to 150 μm of collateral thermal damage. Erbium-doped yttrium–aluminum–garnet lasers target intracellular water with a higher coefficient of absorption, and they allow for more shallow ablation in the range of 2 μm to 5 μm per pass and 20 μm to 50 μm of thermal spread.[15] With this technology, the entire epidermis and variable amounts of dermis are removed, which results in a smoother and tighter appearance of the skin as it heals as a result of the heat-induced shrinkage of extracellular collagen. The deposition of heat from the laser does cause some tightening of the tissue as well as collagen fibril shrinkage of up to 30%, which can help smooth surface skin irregularities.[4]

Reepithelialization

Reepithelialization is typically complete in 7 to 10 days for carbon-dioxide laser treatments and 5 to 7 days for erbium-doped yttrium–aluminum–garnet treatments.[5] The importance of the broader thermal spread of the carbon-dioxide laser during recovery is that more pronounced and prolonged redness will usually be seen among these patients. The other main negative effects of laser resurfacing are posttreatment edema, erythema, pruritus, and burning. Redness may last an average of 4 months. With most laser procedures today, the risk of complications depends on the number of passes performed, the energy density, the degree of pulse and scan overlap, the preoperative skin conditioning, and the relative thickness of the skin in the anatomic area being treated.[5] Other results are similar to those of similar resurfacing techniques. Overall indications for laser resurfacing include rhytides, photodamage, acne scars, actinic and seborrheic keratoses, actinic cheilitis, scar revision, and rhinophyma.

Nonablative Laser Techniques

Newer nonablative laser techniques have been developed that selectively treat the aging dermis and that increase collagen production. They also protect the epidermis through the application of cooling to the skin surface during treatment and through the use of lasers with targeted absorption at various levels of the dermis. These lasers were chosen on the basis of the principles of selective photothermolysis.[16,17] They are becoming more popular as a result of patient demand for less discomfort, reduced downtime, and a lower risk of complications along with faster recovery, and they also offer a broader range of therapies to accommodate a wider spectrum of patients. The ideal nonablative treatment protocol should involve no significant downtime, minimal discomfort, some observable improvement of the rhytids, and improvements in the skin's appearance.[18] These techniques include a number of technologies (e.g., the 585 and 595 pulsed-dye laser, the erbium-doped glass 1540-μm laser, the neodymium-doped yttrium–aluminum–garnet 1320-μm or 1450-μm diode lasers) that produce histologic effects on the dermis but that offer variable clinical improvement, as does the clinical application of intense pulsed light.[19,20] Multiple treatment sessions are most often required to effect a significant result. The best patients for these treatments probably have a mild to moderate amount of photoaging skin with fine rhytids, superficial pigmentary changes, or shallow scars.[4] Some authors report a 25% to 50% objective improvement being seen in these patients, but others report that more established techniques continue to offer greater and more predictable improvements.[18] Others have had success with extending the area of treatment to incorporate cervical rhytids. As a result of the nature of the procedures, nonablative techniques are limited to laser techniques, because chemical peels and dermabrasion procedures all require the effacement of the surface epithelium.

Dermabrasion

With the advent of other procedures, including laser resurfacing (both ablative and nonablative), chemexfoliation, and microdermabrasion, the popularity of dermabrasion has decreased.[21,22] Dermabrasion remains a valuable technique for reducing the cosmetic impact of traumatic or surgical scarring, acne, and other surface irregularities, and it is also an alternative to cosmetic facial resurfacing. It is still the best single technique for addressing deep lip and perioral rhytids. The history of dermabrasion dates into the 1930s, and Kurten wrote the first thorough review of the technique. He recommended its use for conditions including acne scars, actinic lesions, keloids, lichenoid plaques, nevi, tattoos, traumatic scars, and rhytids.[21] For scar revision, dermabrasion can reduce the contrast between the depressed scar, which lies in shadow, and the surrounding skin, possibly by beveling its edges and reducing the attention-drawing shadows cast by many scars.[23]

Dermabrasion remains much more dependent on operative technique (i.e., it requires significant manual dexterity as well as a strong and delicate touch developed through extensive training and experience) than either chemical peels or the computer-controlled laser therapies and is thus more vulnerable to operator error. Variables that affect the depth of injury during derm-

abrasion include the amount of pressure holding the instrument tip against the skin, the speed of the rotation, the coarseness of the tip chosen, and the patient's skin type and texture.[23] Full dermabrasion most often produces the removal of 350 μm of tissue into the upper reticular dermis. Avoiding complications such as the excessive removal of tissue is very dependent on training and experience. Laser techniques offer advantages with regard to predictability and accuracy, thereby reducing reliance on the surgeon's knowledge and experience as compared with dermabrasion; this contributed to their rise in popularity.[8]

Preoperative Skin Treatment Regimens

A number of different preoperative skin treatment regimens are available to help control the predicted outcome of the peeling session and to further reinvigorate the skin. Pretreating regimens are used by many resurfacing practitioners (i.e., 87% in an American Society for Aesthetic Plastic Surgery survey).[24] Tretinoin is the most common agent used preoperatively for its effects on accelerating healing, and it also improves the skin quality and its response to treatment. Glycolic acid preparations are also valuable for their exfoliating and rejuvenating effects. Some physicians prescribe a preoperative course of hydroquinones or Kligman mixture (i.e., tretinoin, hydroquinone, and hydrocortisone) to try to reduce the risk of postoperative hyperpigmentation.[25]

Wound Care After Resurfacing

Appropriate wound care after resurfacing is vital to success, and it leads to faster wound healing along with a faster resolution of minor postoperative symptoms. Most physicians rely on an open technique of treatment with the frequent application of ointments (e.g., Aquaphor [Beiersdorf AG, Hamburg, Germany], Catrix-10 [Lescarden, Inc., New York, NY], Recovery Hydra [La Roche, New York, NY]). The open technique allows for better visualization of the healing process and the better identification of problems at an earlier stage. Closed techniques of wound care involve the application of a biosynthetic dressing material such as Flexzan (UDL Laboratories, Rockford, IL), Biobrane (Smith & Nephew, Hull, UK), Silon TSR (Biomed Sciences, Allentown, PA), or Vigilon (Bard, Covington, GA). These are left in place and then removed after 2 to 7 days. Closed dressings can hide early infections and may even contribute to them as a result of wound maceration.

At some point during the postoperative period, many patients require reassurance that the sequelae they are experiencing are in fact normal processes and not complications. One example of this situation is the need to remind some patients that the improvement of—rather than the elimination of—skin problems such as scars, rhytids, and pigmentary irregularities was the expected goal. Addressing the problem of unrealistic expectations may need to be done several times during the course of evaluation and treatment.

Another example would be the postoperative pruritus experienced by up to 90% of patients who have undergone resurfacing, especially those treated with the laser.[26] In other cases, patients will need to be informed that they are experiencing an unexpected outcome and require extra care to ensure a good result.

All of these conversations during the preoperative consultation, the performance of the procedure, and the postoperative care are designed to eliminate one of the most difficult situations to manage: the dissatisfied patient. Complications of facial resurfacing include premature peeling, infection, herpetic infection or reactivation, pigmentary abnormalities, milia, prolonged erythema, phenol toxicity, and scarring.

PREMATURE EXPOSURE OF PEELED AREAS AND DELAYED HEALING

Premature Exposure of Superficial Layers

After resurfacing, at times the superficial layers of the skin will desquamate earlier than expected. After a peel, this layer of debris will usually function as a protective dressing, allowing healing to proceed predictably. The premature exposure of the fragile, partially reepithelialized areas may increase the risks of inflammation, infection, and possible scarring.

The early removal of this layer most often occurs from patients rubbing or scratching at the areas or even manually peeling off the strips of desquamating skin. If the underlying area has not yet reepithelialized, it may appear raw or moist. Intervention must be geared to reduce inflammation and to protect the area, thereby allowing normal healing to resume.

The application of topical antibiotic ointments (e.g., Bacitracin, Polysporin) 3 to 4 times a day is the best approach. Treatment with oral antibiotics that cover *Staphylococcus* and *Streptococcus* species (most often a cephalosporin) may also be indicated.

Areas that have already reepithelialized but that are not yet ready for exposure may also be uncovered by the early removal of peel debris. The risk of infection is very low, but the new skin is extremely thin and fragile. There is a high risk for increased inflammation, which may lead to hyperpigmentation or prolonged redness. The patient must be cautioned to treat the skin very carefully, with no rubbing or mechanical trauma. Reducing any inflammation is a priority, so a low-potency steroid cream or ointment (e.g., DesOwen) can be used.

Delayed Healing

Delayed healing occurs when a nonreepithelialized area within the treatment zone persists for more than 14 days. Usually laser resurfacing and chemical peel or dermabrasion patients will show complete reepithelialization within 2 weeks of the procedure, particularly if they have been treated with tretinoin preoperatively. The mainstay of treatment is to apply an occlusive dressing or ointment that protects the area and that allows for better epithelial cell migration. Care should also be taken to prevent some of the causes of delayed healing, such as infections, herpetic outbreaks, poor postoperative care, and secondary tissue injury, which may occur as a result of picking at the wound or scratching it.

INFECTION

Infection is quite uncommon after chemical peeling and dermabrasion, occurring in less than 4% to 8% of patients.[27] Facial resurfacing leads to a wound that is easily colonized with bacteria and that may become infected. Those who have an active bacterial or viral infection probably would be better managed by delaying treatment until they have recovered. Good postoperative hygiene with a reduction in the amount of surface coagulum and crusts reduces the ability of colonizing organisms to become a problem.

The removal of the epidermal barrier between the patient and the environment makes the skin more susceptible to infection. Thus care should be taken when peels or dermabrasion are performed on patients with reduced immune function (e.g., diabetic patients) or on those who are immunocompromised. Those who are unable to care for the treated area or to perform the needed cleaning and application of topical preparations are at higher risk for infection.

In many ways, facial resurfacing procedures produce an injury that mimics that of a second-degree burn.[28] Thus some basis for treatment can be found in the burn literature. Most often burn surgeons avoid systemic antibiotics unless signs of infections develop.

Prophylactic Antibiotic Therapy

Several studies have shown that, although the resurfacing wound is initially sterile, it is soon colonized with bacteria and occasionally with yeast organisms.[29,30] Prophylactic antibiotic therapy has been associated with selection for pathogenic organisms and a tendency toward higher infection rates.[30] The antibiotic must also be in the patient's bloodstream before any surgical treatment is initiated; thus any oral medication must be taken at least 1 hour before surgery.

For this reason, the Centers for Disease Control and Prevention do not recommend prophylactic antibiotics for patients with clean or clean-contaminated procedures such as facial resurfacing. Nevertheless, many surgeons still prescribe a cephalosporin or a similar antibiotic with gram-positive coverage (usually a first-generation cephalosporin) for their patients.[31]

In clinical practice, patients undergoing medium-depth or deep peels are often treated with antibiotics prophylactically (most often cephalosporins), because the most common infecting agent is *Staphylococcus aureus*. *Pseudomonas aeruginosa* and *Streptococcus* spp. are less common causes of infections. Pseudomonal infections are most commonly seen among patients who neglect to follow postoperative care instructions or who are not vigorous enough with cleaning the surface coagulum (Figure 49-1). The buildup of surface coagulum provides a medium for the more opportunistic pathogens to grow and can thereby delay the healing process. Pseudomonal infection is most commonly treated with topical acetic acid soaks and possibly with ciprofloxacin or levofloxacin orally. Topical antibiotic use after facial resurfacing is less controversial.[28] The choice of agents is wide and includes bacitracin, silver sulfadiazine, and many others.

Toxic Shock Syndrome

In rare cases, staphylococcal toxins have been reported to induce toxic shock syndrome in phenol peel patients. This is a potentially lethal condition caused by the release of toxic superantigens from *S. aureus,* which then induce cytokine release (most notably tumor necrosis factor and interleukin-1).[32] Manifestations of this problem include the acute onset of hypotension, fever, and desquamating or scarlatiniform rash along with mental confusion and, eventually, multiple-organ failure.[35]

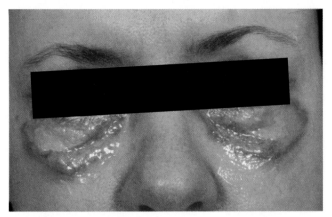

Figure 49-1. Excess surface coagulum with risk for infection.

Initial symptoms most often include fever, diarrhea, and vomiting followed by confusion and then syncopal hypotension.[32] This may be followed by acute tubular necrosis, hepatocellular inflammation, acute respiratory distress syndrome (i.e., "shock lung"), and skeletal muscle breakdown with very high creatine phosphokinase levels on laboratory evaluation. Treatment includes rapid intervention with hospital evaluation; the initiation of high-dose antistaphylococcal antibiotics; supportive care, including fluid replacement and vasopressors as needed; and appropriate consultation with infectious disease specialists and intensivists.

Bacterial Infection

Bacterial infection most often begins to appear 48 to 96 hours after a procedure. Such an infection manifests with pain and erythema at the treated areas, and it may be accompanied by some fever. Increased swelling and some crusting may also be seen, and potentially malodorous exudate may also be present. Cultures can be obtained, and they may help guide eventual therapy.

Most physicians initiate empiric treatment with topical cleaning that possibly includes 0.25% acetic acid soaks and appropriate antibiotics that cover common skin pathogens and possibly *Pseudomonas;* this usually proves to be very effective. Most patients are initially treated empirically with oral cephalexin in doses of 1000 mg to 2000 mg per day. This agent shows good activity against most gram-positive organisms and some effectiveness against gram-negative ones as well. Clindamycin can be a good substitute for a patient who is allergic to penicillin or cephalosporin. If a gram-negative infection is likely, then oral ciprofloxacin (500–1000 mg per day) must be considered. At times it can be difficult to determine what type of infection is present. Frequently these patients will be treated with both antibiotics and antiviral agents until culture results become available.[33]

Candidal Infections

Although uncommon, candidal infections can also occur. They are promoted by the use of local or systemic antibiotics, which is common with resurfacing procedures. Although not infrequently innocuous, candidal infection has been reported after all three modalities of facial resurfacing, and it can manifest up to 2 weeks after the procedure.[34,35] Signs and symptoms typically include redness and itching, significant swelling, increased exudate and crusting, and, occasionally, vesicles or pustules. The most significant manifestation may well be delayed reepithelialization. Because *Candida* prefers a warm, moist environment, exposing the wound to cool, dry air can help to reverse the infection. Topical ketoconazole or clotrimazole and oral fluconazole (150–200 mg daily for 5–7 days) or ketoconazole are frequently effective for the treatment of these infections. Most often the affected areas will clear without any sequelae after approximately 1 to 2 weeks. Acetic acid soaks may be equally as helpful for the treatment of candidal infection as they are for treating bacterial overgrowth.

Allergic Dermatitis

Allergic dermatitis can also occur after peeling or dermabrasion, and it may be confused with an infection; however, it typically develops later after the procedure than most infections. It is the most common exogenous cause of prolonged erythema.

Typically dermatitis begins about 7 to 10 days after the procedure. It is associated with intense pruritus that extends beyond the area that was treated along with copious exudate and crusting. Postoperative dermatitis is usually irritative or allergic in nature, and it can occur in up to 65% of patients.[5] It seems to occur because the newly resurfaced skin does not have a protective epithelial barrier and thus is more vulnerable to irritation. Most patients do not give a history of sensitivity to any particular topical agents and thus offer few clues regarding the source of the problem.

Choosing products for topical therapy that include few preservatives and also avoiding neomycin, which seems to affect a larger number of patients than other topical antibiotics, may help to reduce the incidence of postoperative dermatitis. Whenever patients present with an inflammatory reaction, they should be questioned about what topical agents they may be applying on their own and urged to discontinue those when appropriate. Treatment for dermatitis with mild topical steroid application and hypoallergenic soaps seems best. At times, oral antihistamines or short courses of steroids may be necessary to control the cutaneous inflammation and decrease the risk of fibrosis.

HERPETIC OUTBREAKS

Herpetic infection or reactivation is well known after chemical peels, and it may also be present after dermabrasion and laser resurfacing, occurring in up to 50% of patients with a known history of herpetic infection if no prophylaxis is given.[28,36,37] More typically, herpetic lesions may be seen in 9% to 10% of all patients undergoing facial resurfacing (Figure 49-2).

It appears that herpes virus elements latent within the trigeminal nerve ganglia are reactivated in some patients who have had either known or subclinical infections in the past. During the preoperative consultation, a

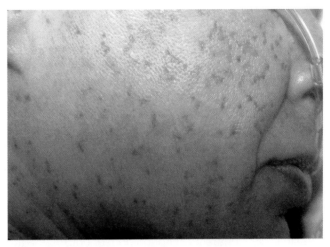

Figure 49-2. Herpetic outbreak after resurfacing.

detailed history, including a history of prior viral infections, should be obtained. At one time, previous herpes simplex virus infection was a considered to be a contraindication to facial dermabrasion or chemical peel.

With the advent of specific antivirals, these patients can now be treated effectively both on a prophylactic basis or if an infection develops. Prophylaxis for herpetic infection remains controversial, but many surgeons pretreat all patients who are undergoing skin resurfacing. The primary concern that leads to prophylactic therapy is the possibility of scarring in the areas affected by herpetic outbreaks during the healing process. The authors advocate beginning acyclovir 800 mg two times daily or valacyclovir 500 mg twice a day 3 to 4 days preoperatively. Most patients continue this regimen for 5 to 7 days postoperatively and for up to as long as 10 to 14 days.[38] McBurney and Gilbert[39] found that a regimen of 500 mg of valacyclovir begun 1 day preoperatively and continued for 14 days was 100% effective for preventing herpetic lesions in a series of 84 patients. They prefer valacyclovir (an L-val ester prodrug of acyclovir), because its oral bioavailability is 3 to 5 times as great as that of acyclovir. Their choice to treat for 14 days was based on Perkins and Sklarew's[38] finding of outbreaks as late as day 12.[36]

Reported histories of herpetic infection are given by 40% to 60% of patients, but up to 80% will have serologic evidence of prior infection.[37] These results indicate that prophylaxis on the basis of patient recollection may not be a valid approach. Beeson and Rachel compared 10- and 14-day valacyclovir regimens and found that 78% of their patients had immunoglobulin G antibodies to herpes simplex virus type 1.[37] They also found that 70% of their patients with a negative history did in fact have positive serology. They found no difference in outcome with 10- or 14-day treatment regimens.

Herpetic outbreaks typically present 4 to 5 days after peels or dermabrasion with intense, unusually severe pain and prominent redness that often includes superficial skin ulceration. Viral vesicles may not be seen as a result of the lack of complete reepithelialization, and superficial erosions may be the presenting sign.[38] If material is available, Tzanck preparations with Wright–Giemsa staining will confirm the diagnosis. Visible multinucleated giant cells confirm infection with the virus.[37] For patients who have not been undergoing prophylactic antiviral therapy, treatment should be begun immediately with acyclovir, valacyclovir, or famciclovir, usually at a dose twice that used for prophylaxis. Cultures should be obtained from the area, if possible. Fortunately, although these outbreaks are quite uncomfortable and appear to be severe, the incidences of scarring and long-term poor cosmetic outcomes are low.

PROLONGED OR PERSISTENT ERYTHEMA

Almost all patients have some degree of erythema after their procedure. Initially the treated skin may be bright red, which fairly rapidly fades to light red or pink. The length of time this takes to occur varies from 7 to 14 days for light and medium-depth peels to up to 4 to 6 weeks for phenol peels. Patients who have undergone light or medium-depth peels usually do not have any significant residual redness after about 3 weeks. After phenol-based peels, erythema may still be present up to 6 weeks after treatment (Figure 49-3). Redness may persist past these intervals without necessarily leading to any long-term problems, but a syndrome of prolonged posttreatment erythema occurring in up to 10% of phenol peel patients has been reported, with multiple causative factors being hypothesized.[39a]

The patients with this clinical syndrome also reported an increase in itching and burning in the peeled areas as well as some irregularity of skin texture and a marked prolongation of postoperative erythema. The authors of the study believe that the prolonged erythema represents a heightened inflammatory reaction that has both intrinsic and extrinsic causes,[42] including sensitivity to the peeling agent, allergic or contact dermatitis, and a preexisting clinical disorder such as lupus or rosacea that may predispose certain patients to a stronger inflammatory response.[39a] Extrinsic factors include previous skin treatments such as peels or topical agents, peeling techniques, and the use of sensitizing agents such as neomycin or certain cosmetics during the postoperative period.

As previously mentioned, the choice of agent often determines how long erythema will persist, but a genetic predisposition, factors such as sun exposure and alcohol consumption, and preoperative skin preparation may play a role.[33] Some authors report that the

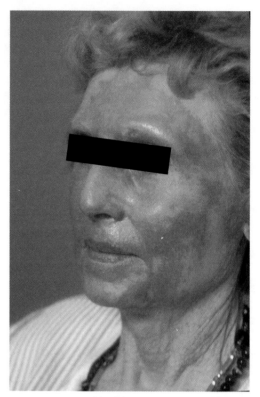

Figure 49-3. Prolonged erythema.

incidence of prolonged erythema is higher among patients undergoing laser resurfacing than among those having chemical peels or dermabrasion.[40] Prolonged erythema after laser treatment can be seen more often in patients treated with a carbon-dioxide laser as a result of its increased collateral thermal spread. Multiple laser passes, the stacking of pulses, and aggressive char removal can also contribute to a greater risk of prolonged erythema.

For all of these patients, reassurance is an integral part of their management, and education should include discussing the fact that their prolonged erythema represents a heightening of the normal repair process without long-term implications. The application of low-potency topical steroids such as 2.5% hydrocortisone, 0.25% hydrocortisone valerate (Westcort), or Elocon 0.1% (i.e., for stronger therapy) can reduce the inflammatory response, thus improving the skin's appearance. It is important to maintain good sun protection and possibly to avoid alcohol consumption to reduce additional vasodilation and further redness. Noncomedogenic cover preparations such as high-quality foundation makeup can also be helpful to reduce the apparent cosmetic deficit.

If there are still localized areas of persistent erythema after conservative treatment, these may be a precursor to scarring. Frequently these smaller areas are darker red or even purple in color rather than the color of the more uniform erythema seen immediately after the peel was performed. These localized areas should be treated topically with class I steroids topically in a way that is similar to the treatment described later in this chapter for early hypertrophic scars.[41] Topical therapy is the best choice at this juncture, and steroid injections are usually not required. The higher-potency topical steroid ointments such as betamethasone, clobetasol, and halobetasol are all worthwhile choices. They will often produce noticeable benefits within 2 weeks of initiating twice-a-day applications to the affected areas. Patients should also be cautioned to avoid rubbing or picking at these areas to reduce the possibility of creating a full-thickness injury that will lead to scarring.

PHENOL TOXICITY

TCA and glycolic acids have no known systemic effects when used as peeling agents, but phenol has possible cardiac, renal, hepatic, and neural toxicity. These toxicities have to do with the differences in metabolism between the various peeling agents. TCA and other organic acids are broken down within the skin, and they typically appear in the bloodstream as bicarbonate ions. Phenol is absorbed unchanged; 80% is excreted by the kidneys, whereas some is metabolized in the liver.[33]

The most common signs of toxicity include an initial stimulation of the central nervous system with hyperreflexia, tremors, and hypertension followed by cardiac arrhythmias; syncope; decreased respiratory function; and, rarely, coma or death. Phenol is absorbed through the skin, and the majority is excreted unchanged by the kidney, whereas some is metabolized in the liver. Patients who are to undergo phenol peels should be screened for preexisting cardiac, renal, or liver disease.

All patients who will undergo phenol peels should have cardiac monitoring performed and careful attention paid to their fluid status and hydration. Cardiac arrhythmias are by far the most common untoward occurrence, and they typically develop during phenol peels when the peeling solution is applied too rapidly, which results in the absorption of excess phenol.

Arrhythmias have been recorded in 23% of patients when full-face phenol peels were completed in 30 minutes or less as a result of the systemic accumulation of phenol.[42] To avoid this problem, each segment of the face (e.g., cheeks; forehead; and perioral, periorbital, and nasal areas) should be treated, followed by a 15-minute delay before the next segment is treated. Thus a full-face phenol peel requires approximately 90 minutes to perform, and the patient should be monitored for another 60 to 90 minutes. If an arrhythmia or another sign of complications occurs, the procedure is terminated, and the patient is treated with fluid and lidocaine.[6] Some physicians will resume the peel if the patient remains in sinus rhythm for 15 minutes, but the delay between segments will be increased to 20 to 30 minutes.

HYPERPIGMENTATION

Pigmentary changes after facial resurfacing are particularly common, with up to a third of patients having at least transient pigmentation changes that most often resolve within a few weeks to a few months[27] (Figure 49-4). This remains the most common complication after resurfacing procedures, and it can manifest as blotchy irregular areas of pigmentation or as more homogeneous dyschromia involving the entire treated areas[40] (Figure 49-5). After resurfacing, hyperpigmentation usually appears around 3 to 4 weeks after the procedure, and it may last for 2 to 3 months.[43,44] Postinflammatory hyperpigmentation is particularly common among darker-skinned patients. Those with Fitzpatrick types IV, V, and VI skin are more likely to experience prolonged and potentially permanent hyperpigmentation, particularly with deeper peels, with less but still significant risk seen in patients with type III skin.[45,46] Some authors recommend superficial peels only for those with type V and VI skin and that any more ablative procedures be avoided, whereas others have found that deeper treatments can be performed safely with aggressive intervention for any postoperative pigmentary changes.[42,45]

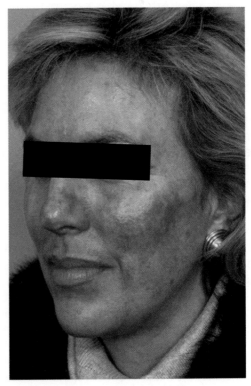

Figure 49-4. Postinflammatory hyperpigmentation.

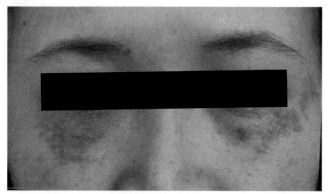

Figure 49-5. Infraorbital hyperpigmentation.

The pathogenesis of hyperpigmentation is not clear, but the culprit in these patients may be dermal injury that produces significant inflammation and leads to the activation of the dermal melanocytes.[44] Pigmentary abnormalities can also occur in all patients, particularly if postoperative instructions to avoid sun exposure are disregarded.

Good postoperative skin care and the rigorous use of sunscreen can prevent many of these patients from suffering this complication. Patients are, in general, advised to avoid sun exposure for 3 to 6 months after their peels and to use a daily moisturizer with sunscreen with a sun protection factor of at least 15 and preferably of 30 or more. The avoidance of oral contraceptives may also be suggested because of the hormonal effect on pigment production, particularly in conjunction with UV light exposure. Photosensitizing drugs, including certain antibiotics, should be avoided during this period as well.

If an early increase in pigmentation is observed, it can frequently be stopped through the application of steroid creams such as 2.5% hydrocortisone or 0.2% hydrocortisone valerate (Westcort) and possibly 4% hydroquinone cream. Fluorinated steroids have more of a tendency to cause skin atrophy, telangiectasias, and hypopigmentation, and they should be avoided in this situation. It may take several weeks or months for mild hyperpigmentation to resolve, even with appropriate therapy.

In more advanced cases, the Klingman mixture can be used: hydroquinone 4%, tretinoin 0.05%, and triamcinolone 0.1% applied twice a day to blotchy areas of hyperpigmentation. This preparation should be used for 8 to 12 weeks for optimal effectiveness. Other options include mixtures of tretinoin with hydroquinone or AHAs mixed with hydroquinone. Kojic or azelaic acid preparations can also be used, with good results. Hyperpigmented areas can be repeeled approximately 3 to 6 months after the initial treatment with the resolution of the pigmentary problems. Some authors have recommended a preoperative regimen that incorporates tretinoin, AHAs, and 4% hydroquinone to increase the rate of epithelialization and to suppress melanocyte function preoperatively.[47] This preconditioning can be particularly useful for Mediterranean skin (Fitzpatrick III or IV) by weakening the melanocytes' ability to produce pigment and by significantly reducing the likelihood of postprocedure dyspigmentation. Reported rates of postinflammatory hyperpigmentation are around 20% to 30% for Fitzpatrick type III skin and nearly 100% for Fitzpatrick type IV skin if no preoperative preparation is given.[43] However, other studies have failed to show any benefit from this regimen or from others that incorporate bleaching agents.[46] The use of a pigment-decreasing premedication regimen can help to determine which patients tolerate hydroquinones without skin reactions.

If postoperative pigmentation develops and the patient is among those who react poorly to hydroquinone, then he or she can be treated with topical azelaic or kojic acids (i.e., beta hydroxy acids) with good results. Azelaic and kojic acids along with glucosamine inhibit tyrosinase and reduce pigment production. These agents are good choices for patients who cannot tolerate hydroquinone and in cases that are not responding adequately to less aggressive therapy. Topical vitamins C and E can be employed in their capacity as free-radical scavengers, which reduce inflammation and thereby decrease melanocyte stimulation and responsiveness to UV radiation.[43]

HYPOPIGMENTATION

Hypopigmentation is very common after phenol peel and other deeper resurfacing procedures, and it should be presented to every patient as part of the expected outcome. Decreased pigmentation arises from deeper injury that results in damage to the melanocytes and a potentially permanent reduction in pigment production (Figure 49-6). Phenol is reported to be melanotoxic and thus always produces some degree of skin lightening.[40]

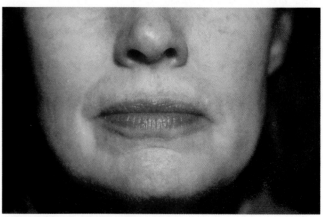

Figure 49-6. Perioral hypopigmentation.

Melanocytes are derived from the neural crest embryologically, and they are lost to some extent with all dermal resurfacing procedures.[48] They do not replicate as well as epithelial cells, through which they migrate to provide pigmentation. Deeper injury into the dermis can damage melanocytes directly, whereas the dermal fibrosis seen after deeper resurfacing adds to the hypopigmented appearance of these patients. Most cases of postresurfacing hypopigmentation develops 4 to 6 weeks after the procedure, which correlates with the maturing dermal fibrosis.[48]

Fulton and colleagues[48] have proposed a treatment plan that consists of dermabrasion or laser-assisted chemabrasion to reduce the original scar and wound healing under occlusion to allow melanocytes to migrate back into the treated areas and reduce postoperative fibrosis. The use of an occlusive dressing was critical to decrease the inflammatory response, thereby allowing for faster cell migration and reducing the unwelcome fibrotic reaction. Their postoperative care includes the use of Silon-TSR sheeting as an occlusive dressing for 5 days and then the application of petrolatum ointment 3 to 4 times a day along with use of a gentle skin cleanser (e.g., Cetaphil). After day 10, they recommend use of moisturizers with sunscreen during the day and aloe vera/hydrocortisone cream at night.

Another option is to use a pulsed topical corticosteroid treatment with clobetasol ointment for 1 week at weeks 6 and 12 postoperatively to prevent the formation of dermal fibrosis. Areas of hypopigmentation can also be treated with a combination of the topical application of 8-methoxypsoralen twice weekly with concurrent UV light application. Seventy-one percent of treated patients had clinical and histologic repigmentation with this regimen.[49]

The most common complaint about hypopigmentation is the line of demarcation between the treated and untreated areas (Figure 49-7). Feathering the margins of treatment into the hairline and into the area just below the jaw can help to reduce the cosmetic effects of this demarcation. This is accomplished by applying the peel agent with a semidry cotton applicator approximately 0.5 cm beyond the mandibular margin and into the hairline or by treating the borders of the area with lower-laser energy levels. For regional peels (e.g., the lower lids), a semidry applicator can be used to apply a small amount of the peeling agent beyond the orbital rim. Patients who have undergone deep treatment may need to wear makeup to camouflage the demarcation between the treated and untreated areas. Some surgeons recommend the use of single-pass carbon-dioxide laser in the neck to decrease the obvious demarcation at the margins of the peel.[50] In many cases, hypopigmentation may improve with time. Patients can use makeup to

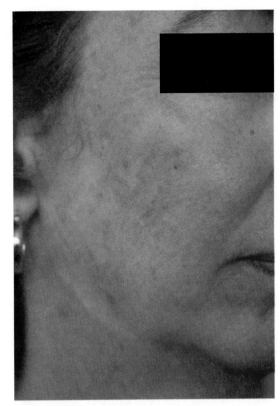

Figure 49-7. Hypopigmentation with obvious submandibular demarcation.

camouflage the area, and occasionally cosmetic tattooing may be employed.[38]

SCARRING

For most physicians and their patients, scarring represents the worst complication of chemical peels and other resurfacing procedures, although it is luckily quite uncommon. The areas around the mandible and over the bony prominences of the malar area as well as the perioral areas are most commonly affected (Figure 49-8). Certain categories of patients are at

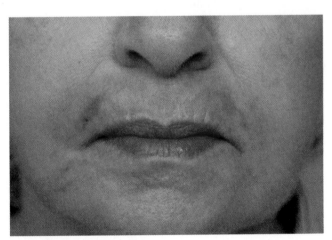

Figure 49-8. Perioral scarring.

higher-than-normal risk for scarring, even with properly applied peels or dermabrasion. These include those with a history of poor healing or keloid formation, those undergoing deep peels, those having repeated peels without allowing adequate time for full healing between peels, those who have previously been treated with isotretinoin, and those who develop an infection after the resurfacing procedure.[23]

The most significant factors relating to the potential for scarring remain the depth of injury achieved and the number and density of the skin adnexa. If the injury goes deeper than the mid reticular dermis, the risk of scarring particularly increases. Superficial peels that do not penetrate beyond the papillary dermis are not associated with scarring, and microdermabrasion is not associated with it, either. Lower-concentration (i.e., 10%–35%) TCA and other superficial and medium-depth peeling agents rarely cause scarring, because their depth of penetration (i.e., usually within the papillary dermis and not deeper than the superficial reticular dermis) does not foster scar formation to as great a degree as those treatments that produce injury to the mid reticular or deep reticular dermis.[51] Scars can be fostered by factors that promote the deeper penetration of the peel solution, such as the use of phenol-based formulas (i.e., Baker solution, which penetrates to the mid reticular dermis); differences in skin preparation and postoperative care; occlusive taping; too-frequent applications of more superficial peeling agents; and differences in technique, including the overaggressive application of peeling solutions and the use of a dermabrader or laser.

Some surgeons use the appearance of the skin during chemical peels as a guide to the depth of penetration. Although this is not universally accurate, it can serve as a guide and a warning when the appearance changes to one that indicates a deeper injury than appropriate. For example, diffuse erythema with small and scattered punctate with whitish frosting indicates an epidermal injury, whereas light-white frosting evenly over the treated area indicates injury to the epidermal or dermal junction. Dense, pure-white frosting shows that a typical medium-depth peel went into the papillary/reticular dermal junction. A grayish or yellowish frost can demonstrate injury to the deeper reticular dermis, and delayed healing with a higher risk of scarring can be anticipated.[8]

Scarring can also arise in the setting of excessive inflammation, such as keloid formation. The preoperative use of isotretinoin has been associated for years with a very high risk of postoperative scarring as a result of the reduction in skin adnexal appendages and ensuing problems with reepithelialization potential. As the use of this agent has decreased, the likelihood of this complication seems to be becoming more remote. For patients who have used isotretinoin in the past, a waiting period of at least 6 months before chemical peel or dermabrasion procedures seems prudent to allow time for the regrowth of epithelial appendages.[52] TCA concentrations of 50% or more are associated with deeper penetration and a particular increase in the risk of scarring.[47,53] Excess thermal injury from carbon-dioxide laser resurfacing can cause hypertrophic scarring in a small percentage of patients (i.e., usually <1%, which also approximates the risk after a deep chemical peel). This is most often as result of an excessive energy setting, the overlapping of pulses, or too many passes in the same area.[54] Desiccation with superficial cell death can lead to a deeper-than-expected injury, as can picking or denuding areas that have some superficial crusting. Pruritus after a peel or dermabrasion can cause intense itching that leads to the excoriation of the treated area and an increased chance of scarring.

Several different forms of scarring can occur after a chemical peel or dermabrasion. Hypopigmented, flat scars with a shiny surface and no induration are possible, as are atrophic, depressed scars with sharply defined edges. Some patients will develop thickened and elevated scars with at least some persistent erythema, but these rarely become true keloids. This last category can most vividly develop features of truly hypertrophic and cosmetically unpleasant scarring.

A special instance of scarring is lower-eyelid retraction and scleral show. Preoperative evaluation includes the assessment of lid tension or laxity, and the amount of preoperative scleral show should be recorded. In most cases, skin resurfacing can be delayed until 3 months after any procedures involving a skin flap, such as traditional lower-eyelid blepharoplasty. If there is a substantial amount of lid laxity, a pretreatment canthal reconstruction with canthoplasty or canthopexy may be helpful both for the prevention of ectropion and to prepare the patient for the resurfacing. Simultaneous resurfacing and transconjunctival blepharoplasty is a safe approach that can produce excellent results.[55] The prevention of ectropion includes using less concentrated or semidry applicators for lower-lid peeling or lower fluences for resurfacing. If some retraction begins to develop after resurfacing, massage, eyelid taping, and topical or intralesional steroids all play roles in the reduction of the problem. Mild postoperative scleral show usually resolves spontaneously.

Combined procedures that incorporate the elevation of a skin or skin–muscle flap in addition to resurfacing (especially chemical peels) have been discouraged in the past because of concerns about blood supply and flap survival.[56] Koch and Perkins[56] reviewed 30 patients who underwent simultaneous face-lift and full-face carbon-dioxide laser resurfacing, and they also performed a meta-analysis of more than 450 similar patients who had been previously described. In their own series, they found no instances of flap necrosis or other complications, no hypopigmentation, and no infection. Complications reported in their meta-analysis of other studies did not exceed those normally associated with rhytidectomy alone.[56]

The earliest signs of scarring are often persistent erythema and delayed healing. When this occurs, the affected areas should be treated with nonfluorinated steroid creams, and mechanical debridement (e.g., overaggressive cleaning) should be stopped. If a scar appears to be forming, massage and compression can help to reduce the collagen deposition and cross-linking. When overt scarring begins to develop, aggressive intervention is indicated, because early and still-developing scars are easier to manage than fully mature ones.

If persistent erythema does not resolve with less aggressive treatment, this may herald the beginning of scar formation, and a higher potency class I steroid cream such as 0.5% clobetasol, Elocon 0.1%, or Diprolene should be applied twice daily. If followed for more than 2 weeks, this regimen may lead to some skin atrophy and telangiectasia formation, but these side effects may be more desirable than the development of significant scarring.

Usually incipient scars will respond quickly, often in a week or less. However, if induration is significant, up to 3 or 4 weeks may elapse before the problem completely resolves. For this reason, a tradeoff between the side effects of the steroid cream and the future cosmetic outcome may need to be balanced.

Telangiectasias can be treated with laser therapy, and any atrophy should respond to tretinoin or AHA therapy. Steroid-impregnated tape can also be applied, as can topical silicone gel or silicone sheeting.

At times scars will not respond to topical therapy, and they will need to be treated with intralesional steroids such as 10% triamcinolone at 4-week intervals. Higher concentrations of up to 40% may be needed in some cases. Treatment with the 585-μm pulse-dye laser or the 1320-μm holmium-doped yttrium–aluminum–garnet laser also has a role in the improvement of this problem.

Laser treatments can reduce redness and soften scar tissue while reducing scar bulk and improving texture.[14] Laser treatments can be done every 6 to 8 weeks as needed, and they are performed with similar settings as those for cutaneous vascular lesions (e.g., 4–5 J/cm^2 with a 10-mm spot size). After two to four treatments, a roughly 50% improvement in scar appearance can be expected.[22,57] If atrophic scarring occurs, then the use

of soft-tissue fillers such as collagen or Restylane can sometimes reduce the soft-tissue deficit.

SKIN ATROPHY OR SKIN-TEXTURE CHANGE

Depending on the depth of injury and the process of healing, certain changes in skin quality or texture may become apparent after a chemical peel or dermabrasion. Pore size may change, and nevi may darken. Small telangiectasias can also develop or increase in number. Laser ablation remains the best treatment for these vascular lesions.

MILIA AND ACNE

Milia, which appear as small whiteheads (Figure 49-9), are tiny epidermal inclusion cysts that occur more commonly after dermabrasion than after chemical peeling or laser therapy, but they still occur in up to 15% of patients.[58] They are usually self-limited, and they clear with facial hygiene. Alternatively, they can be unroofed with an 18-gauge needle in the office if they persist.

Pretreatment with tretinoin for 2 to 3 weeks before the peel or dermabrasion and then resuming application after epithelialization is complete decreases the formation of these lesions. Acne eruptions occurred after peeling in up to 80% of resurfacing patients in some series.[58] Acne flare-ups can be treated in a routine fashion after the skin irritation from the peel resolves (i.e., with topical cleaning and other topical therapies, including clindamycin or erythromycin).[33] Oral antibiotics (e.g., minocycline) can be begun as soon as eruptions appear without having to wait for full healing to occur.

UNUSUAL REACTIONS

A case of airway obstruction related to an AHA peel has been reported.[63] No obvious mechanism of injury was obvious in this patient, although it appeared to be a

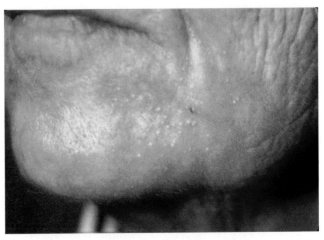

Figure 49-9. Postoperative milia of the left mental area.

direct result of deeper-than-expected burns from a citric acid peel. Clearly, if patients become tachypneic or have difficulty breathing, then airway evaluation is indicated. Previously airway edema has also been reported in a few isolated cases of phenol peels in patients who smoke.[59]

CONCLUSION

The best treatment for facial resurfacing complications is, as with most procedures, prevention. Thorough pretreatment preparation and evaluation along with the careful performance of the procedure and meticulous postoperative care and follow up are essential to achieving the best results. If untoward sequelae develop, then prompt and appropriate intervention are crucial to minimizing negative outcomes in these patients.

REFERENCES

1. American Society for Aesthetic Plastic Surgery: 2005 Cosmetic Surgery National Data Bank Statistics. *ASAPS* 2006;1–20.
2. Koch JR: Psychological predictors of patient satisfaction in laser skin resurfacing. *Arch Facial Plast Surg* 2003;5:445–446.
3. Fulton JE, Porumb S: Chemical peels: Their place within the range of resurfacing techniques. *Am J Clin Dermatol* 2004;5: 179–187.
4. Railan D, Kilmer S: Ablative treatment of photoaging. *Dermatol Ther* 2005;18:227–241.
5. Alster TS, Lupton JR: Prevention and treatment of side effects and complications of cutaneous laser resurfacing. *Plast Reconstr Surg* 2002;109:308–316.
6. Godin DA, Graham HD: Chemical peels. *J La State Med Soc* 1998;150:513–520.
7. Halas YP: Medium depth peels. *Facial Plast Surg Clin North Am* 2004;12:297–303.
8. Dinner MI, Artz JS: The art of the trichloroacetic acid peel. *Clin Plast Surg* 1998;25:53–62.
9. El-Domyati MB, Attia SK, Saleh FY, et al: Trichloroacetic acid peeling versus dermabrasion: A histometric, ultrastructural, immunohistochemical, and ultrastructural analysis. *Dermatol Surg* 2004;30:179–188.
10. Coleman WP: Dermal peels. *Dermatol Clin* 2001;19:405–411.
11. Iyer S, Friedli A, Bowes L, et al: Full face laser resurfacing: Therapy and prophylaxis for actinic keratoses and non-melanoma skin cancer. *Lasers Surg Med* 2004;34:114–119.
12. Landau M: Advances in deep chemical peels. *Dermatol Nurs* 2005;17:438–441.
13. Roy D: Ablative facial resurfacing. *Dermatol Clin* 2005;23(3): 549–559.
14. Dierickx C, Goldman MP, Fitzpatrick RE: Laser treatment of erythematous, hypertrophic and pigmented scars in 26 patients. *Plast Reconstr Surg* 1995;95:84–90.
15. Caniglia RJ: Erbium:YAG laser skin resurfacing. *Facial Plast Surg Clin North Am* 2004;12:373–377.
16. Geronemus RG: Fractional photothermolysis: Current and future applications. *Lasers Surg Med* 2006;38:169–176.
17. Doshi SN, Alster TS: 1450 nm long-pulsed diode laser for nonablative skin rejuvenation. *Dermatol Surg* 2005;31:1223–1226.
18. Carniol PJ, Farley S, Friedman A: Long-pulse 532-nm diode laser for nonablative facial skin rejuvenation. *Arch Facial Plast Surg* 2003;5:511–513.
19. Williams EF, Dahiya R: Review of nonablative laser resurfacing modalities. *Facial Plast Surg Clin North Am* 2004;12:305–310.
20. Goldman MP, Weiss RA, Weiss MA: Intense pulsed light as a nonablative approach to photoaging. *Dermatol Surg* 2005;31 (9 Pt 2):1179–1187.
21. Gold MH: Dermabrasion in dermatology. *Am J Clin Dermatol* 2003;4:467–471.
22. Grimes PE: Microdermabrasion. *Dermatol Surg* 2005;31: 1160–1164.
23. Orentreich N, Orentreich DS: Dermabrasion. *Dermatol Clin* 1995;13:313–327.
24. Apfelberg DB: Summary of ASAPS/ASPRS laser task force survey. *Plast Reconstr Surg* 1998;101:513.
25. Sensoz O, Baran CN, Alagoz MS, et al: Long-term results of ultrapulsed carbon dioxide laser resurfacing of the Mediterranean face. *Aesthetic Plast Surg* 2004;28:328–333.
26. Shook BA, Hruza GJ: Periorbital ablative and nonablative resurfacing. *Facial Plast Surg Clin North Am* 2005;13:571–582.
27. Sabini P: Classifying, diagnosing, and treating the complications of resurfacing the facial skin. *Facial Plast Surg Clin North Am* 2004;12:357–361.
28. Messingham MJ, Arpey CJ: Update on the use of antibiotics in cutaneous surgery. *Dermatol Surg* 2005;31:1068–1078.
29. Gaspar Z, Vinciullo C, Elliott T: Antibiotic prophylaxis for full-face resurfacing: Is it necessary? *Arch Dermatol* 2001;137:313–315.
30. Walia S, Alster TS: Cutaneous CO2 laser resurfacing rate with and without prophylactic antibiotics. *Dermatol Surg* 1999;25: 857–861.
31. Grunebaum LD, Reiter D: Perioperative antibiotic usage by facial plastic surgeons. *Arch Facial Plast Surg* 2006;8:88–91.
32. Garman ME, Orengo I: Unusual infectious complications of dermatologic procedures. *Dermatol Clin* 2003;21(2):321–335.
33. Resnick SS, Resnick BI: Complications of chemical peeling. *Clin Plast Surg* 2001;28:231–234.
34. Siegle RJ, Chiaramonti A, Knox DW, et al: Cutaneous candidiasis as a complication of facial dermabrasion. *J Dermatol Surg Oncol* 1984;10:891–895.
35. Nanni CA, Alster TS: Complications of carbon dioxide laser resurfacing: An evaluation of 500 patients. *Dermatol Surg* 1998;24: 315–320.
36. Perkins SW, Sklarew EC: Prevention of facial herpetic infections after chemical peel and dermabrasion: New treatment strategies in the prophylaxis of patients undergoing procedures for the perioral area. *Plast Reconstr Surg* 1996;98:427–433.
37. Beeson WH, Rachel JD: Valcyclovir prophylaxis for herpes simplex virus infection or recurrence following laser skin resurfacing. *Dermatol Surg* 2002;28:331–336.
38. Demas PN, Bridenstine JB: Diagnosis and treatment of postoperative complications after skin resurfacing. *J Oral Maxillofac Surg* 1999;57:837–841.
39. Gilbert S, McBurney E: Use of valcyclovir for herpes simplex virus-1 (HSV-1) prophylaxis after facial resurfacing: A randomized clinical trial of dosing regimens. *Dermatol Surg* 2000;26: 50–54.
39a. Maloney BP, Millman B, Monheit G, et al: The etiology of prolonged erythema after chemical peel. *Dermatol Surg* 1998;24: 337–341.
40. Ragland HP, McBurney EI: Complications of resurfacing. *Semin Cutan Med Surg* 1996;15:20–207.
41. Sadick NS: Overview of complications of nonsurgical facial rejuvenation procedures. *Clin Plast Surg* 2001;28:163–176.
42. Bernstein ER: Chemical peels. *Semin Cutan Med Surg* 2002;21: 27–45.
43. Sripracha-anunt S, Marchell NL, Fitzpatrick RE, et al: Facial resurfacing in patients with Fitzpatrick type skin type IV. *Lasers Surg Med* 2002;30:86–92.
44. Kim YJ, Lee HS, Son SW, et al: Analysis of hyperpigmentation and hypopigmentation after Er:YAG laser skin resurfacing. *Lasers Surg Med* 2005;36:47–51.
45. Briden ME: Alpha-hydroxyacid chemical peeling agents: Case studies and rationale for safe and effective use. *Cutis* 2004;73 (Suppl 2):18–24.
46. West TB, Alster TS: Effect of pretreatment on the incidence of hyperpigmentation following cutaneous carbon dioxide laser resurfacing. *Dermatol Surg* 1999;25:15–20.
47. Monheit GD: Medium-depth chemical peels. *Dermatol Clin* 2001;19: 413–425.

48. Fulton JE, Rahimi AD, Mansour S, et al: The treatment of hypopigmentation after skin resurfacing. *Dermatol Surg* 2004;30: 95–101.

49. Grimes PE, Bhawan J, Kim J, et al: Repigmentation of laser resurfacing after induced hypopigmentation: Histologic alternatives and repigmentation with topical photochemotherapy. *Dermatol Surg* 2001;27:515–22.

50. Fanous N, Prinja N, Sawaf M: Laser resurfacing of the neck: A review of 48 cases. *Aesthetic Plast Surg* 1998;22:173–179.

51. Brody HJ: Complications of chemical peeling. *J Dermatol Surg Oncol* 1989;15:1010–1019.

52. Perkins SW, Castellano R: Use of combined modality for maximal resurfacing. *Facial Plast Surg Clin North Am* 2004;12: 323–338.

53. Peters W: Full-thickness facial chemical burn from a "50% TCA" peel. *Plast Reconstr Surg* 1995;95:602–603.

54. Grossman AR, Majidian AM, Grossman PH: Thermal injuries as a result of carbon dioxide laser resurfacing. *Plast Reconstr Surg* 1998;102:1247–1252.

55. Perkins SW, Gibson FB: *Simultaneous transconjunctival blepharoplasty and phenol peel.* American Academy of Facial Plastic and Reconstructive Surgery meeting, 2002.

56. Koch BB, Perkins SW: Simultaneous rhytidectomy and full-face carbon dioxide laser resurfacing. *Arch Facial Plast Surg* 2002;4: 227–233.

57. Willey A, Anderson RA, Azpiazu JL, et al: Complications of laser dermatologic surgery. *Lasers Surg Med* 2006;38:1–15.

58. Tanzi, Alster TS: Single-pass versus multiple pass Er:YAG laser skin resurfacing: A comparison of postoperative wound healing and side effects. *Dermatol Surg* 2003;29:80–84.

59. Ghandishah D, Gorchynski J: Airway compromise after routine alpha-hydroxy facial peel administration. *J Emerg Med* 2002;22: 353–355.

CHAPTER 50

Complications of Facial Implants

Jonathan M. Sykes

During recent years, cosmetic surgery has been performed with increasing frequency and public acceptance. The greatest increase in surgical procedures is related to facial rejuvenation surgery. The pathophysiology of the aging face includes a loss of skin elasticity that results in facial sagging and soft-tissue volume depletion. Rejuvenation of the aging face includes procedures designed to lift ptotic facial soft tissue and to create structural volume in areas in which the face is volume deficient.

The recognition of the role of soft-tissue volume loss in facial aging has created many new procedures and technologies aimed at volume correction. These include injectable products and autologous fat transportation for soft-tissue augmentation and facial implants for both soft-tissue and skeletal augmentation. The decision of whether to use facial implants, fat augmentation, or injectable materials is made on the basis of the patient's specific anatomy and their acceptance of a surgical procedure. Other factors that affect procedure choice include the surgeon's comfort level and knowledge of the given procedure.

This chapter outlines the surgical complications related to the placement of facial implants. The various alloplast materials used for implantation, the surgical approaches and techniques, and the avoidance of the related complications are discussed.

CHIN IMPLANTS

Augmentation of the mentum is a commonly performed procedure designed to camouflage deficiency of the chin.[1,2] This deficiency can occur in the horizontal, vertical, or transverse dimension. Chin augmentation with an alloplast can be performed from an intraoral or submental incision, and implants can be placed in a subperiosteal or supraperiosteal plane.[3] The decision to use a camouflaging implant as compared with a horizontal osteotomy of the mentum (i.e., genioplasty) is made on the basis of the patient's specific deformity and the surgeon's experience.[4] Complications with chin implants are infrequent. Because the chin is a midline structure, asymmetry is uncommon (as opposed to paired malar, submalar, or lateral mandibular implants). If implant size is appropriate and the pocket dissection is precise, problems from implants can be minimized. A list of these complications is shown in Box 50-1.

Hypoaesthesia and Anesthesia

Minor transient sensory alterations occur frequently. These are the result of low-grade stretch injuries to the mental nerves; however, permanent changes in sensation are very uncommon with chin implants. On rare occasions, the implant can cause pressure on the mental nerve, which results in persistent postoperative pain. If a patient experiences persistent (i.e., >3 months) postoperative pain after chin augmentation, implant repositioning or surgical removal may be considered.

Bone Resorption

When facial implants are placed against bone, some degree of bone resorption over time always occurs (Figure 50-1).[5,6] The significance of this bony resorption is variable, but it is clear that resorption rarely results in clinically significant microgenia. Bone resorption is theoretically minimized when the implant is immobilized and placed in a supraperiosteal dissection plane. For this reason, many surgeons place implants in a supraperiosteal plane centrally and in a subperiosteal plane laterally (Figures 50-2 and 50-3). The supraperiosteal plane theoretically minimizes resorption centrally, whereas the subperiosteal lateral pockets facilitate implant fixation.

Another method to immobilize chin implants is to use screw fixation. The use of position screws limits implant mobility; it is the mobility of the implant and the resulting pressure on the anterior mandible that increases bone resorption.

Implant Mobility and Malposition

A potential problem with all implants is that they heal in an undesirable position (Figure 50-4). The causes for chin implant malposition are numerous, and they include the following:

- A poor choice of implant size, shape, or both
- A discrepancy in the size of the implant pocket versus the implant size
- The improper placement of the implant at the time of surgery
- The mobility of the implant after placement

Problems with implant malposition can be minimized with careful implant choice and with meticulous surgical execution.

Avoiding implant mobility begins with choosing an implant that is not too large or too small for the existing soft-tissue envelope. The implant should always be slightly smaller than an ideal chin size for the patient. Wider, more anatomically shaped implants appear to be better than smaller, button-shaped implants, and they have less chance of becoming noticed after surgery. The size of the implant pocket should be approximately 10% larger than the implant itself. If the pocket is too large, the

BOX 50-1 Complications after Chin Augmentation with an Alloplast

SENSORY NERVE INJURY
- Anesthesia
- Paresthesia

MUSCLE DYSFUNCTION (MENTALIS MUSCLE DYSKINESIS)
- Implant extrusion
- Implant malposition
- Bone resorption
- Infection
- Chin asymmetry

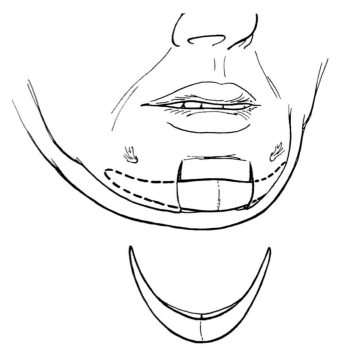

Figure 50-2. Schematic diagram of the position of a chin implant with supraperiosteal central placement and subperiosteal pockets placed laterally.

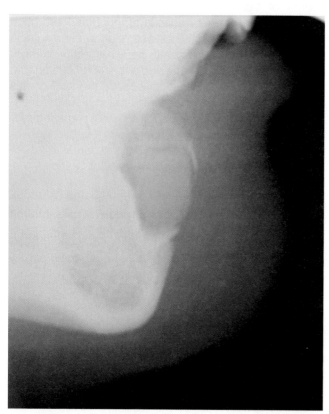

Figure 50-1. Lateral radiograph of a patient with a misplaced chin implant and obvious bone resorption above the inferior aspect of the mentum. The bone resorption is a result of pressure necrosis.

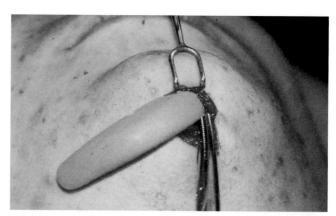

Figure 50-3. Intraoperative photograph of a submental approach to correct the placement of a chin implant with lateral subperiosteal pockets.

implant may move within the pocket and heal in an undesirable position. If the pocket is too small, the implant may be "forced" out of the pocket, thus creating distortion and a noticeable implant–host interface. The fixation of the implant is facilitated with a lateral subperiosteal pocket. If the implant is carefully selected and the procedure is carefully performed, implant malposition is very uncommon.

Infection

Infection after chin augmentation is very rare. Although it may be presumed that infections would occur more frequently with the intraoral approach, reviews of both

surgical approaches confirm the extremely low incidence of infections with either an external or an intraoral approach. The meticulous preparation of the patient, a "no-touch" technique with the implant itself, and a carefully layered closure minimize the chances of postoperative infection with chin implants. When multiple facial procedures are performed, the chin implant should be completed first, before any other procedures are initiated, to minimize bacterial contamination from other facial regions. This will decrease the incidence of implant infections.

Mentalis Muscle Dyskinesis

An unreported but commonly occurring sequela of chin implants is mentalis muscle dyskinesis. Dyskinesis of the mentalis muscle occurs as a result of the elevation

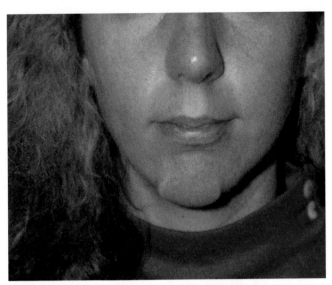

Figure 50-4. Postoperative photograph of a patient with a malpositioned alloplast chin implant.

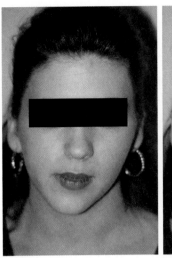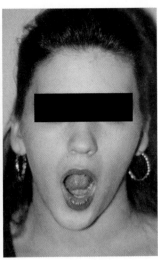

Figure 50-5. Photographs of a patient with an oculoauricular–vertebral spectrum with obvious hemifacial microsomia. This patient has a constricted right orbit, a flattened right cheek bone, and a chin that is malpositioned and asymmetric to the right side of her face.

and reattachment of the mentalis muscle during implant placement.[7] After the procedure, the mentalis muscle functions, but the muscle contraction occurs in a slightly uncoordinated fashion. This results in dimpling of the chin on the affected side and possibly a mildly altered appearance during speaking or smile animation.

The incidence of this muscle dysfunction is approximately 10% to 15%. Prevention involves the careful atraumatic dissection of the mentalis with the reapproximation of this muscle during wound closure. The treatment of mentalis muscle dyskinesis is with small amounts (i.e., 2–5 units) of botulinum toxin type A.[7,8] The treatment is effective and usually needs to be repeated only one or two times before total resolution of the problem.

Chin Asymmetry

The causes of postoperative chin asymmetry after implant placement include the following:
- Inadequate evaluation of preoperative asymmetry
- Improper operative dissection and implant placement
- Postoperative mobility of a symmetric implant

These complications can usually be avoided with thorough preoperative evaluation, meticulous surgical execution, and careful postoperative care.

Preoperative chin asymmetry is common and underdiagnosed. Many patients present with a crooked nose and request nasal straightening when they actually have mild hemifacial microsomia or some other variant of oculoauricular–vertebral spectrum (Figure 50-5). These patients usually have transverse asymmetries of the chin.[9] The placement of a symmetric chin implant will usually exacerbate the

chin asymmetry. Patients with asymmetric faces should be identified preoperatively, and the asymmetry should be discussed with the patient. Surgical treatment of the chin in a patient with existing asymmetry includes an asymmetric bony genioplasty with the rotation of the chin or the placement of a customized asymmetric chin implant.

Symmetric chin implant placement can be facilitated with the careful creation of a symmetric pocket that is the appropriate size for the given implant chosen. The implant pocket should be made and then checked with the placement of a sterile sizing implant. If the pocket is inadequate, further dissection should be accomplished. Midline fixation of the implant is performed with either suture or screw fixation. Postoperatively, the implant is immobilized with a chin-strap dressing for 3 days.

MALAR AND SUBMALAR IMPLANTS

As the face ages, two basic processes occur. First, the soft tissues of the face sag as the ligamentous supports of the face weaken. Second, volume depletion occurs as the soft tissues of the face diminish. These processes are most obvious in the midface. Treatment for midfacial aging includes the surgical lifting of the midface or the augmentation of the deficient midface with fat grafts or implants.

Malar or submalar implants can improve midfacial volume in patients with volume loss.[10] These implants also are indicated for patients with congenital malar hypoplasia and skeletal insufficiency. In general, malar or submalar implants require careful preoperative evaluation and meticulous operative execution to minimize complications. Problems with malar and submalar implants are more frequent than complications with chin implants.

The primary problems include infection, asymmetry, malposition, extrusion, eyelid malposition, and sensory abnormalities.

Surgical Approaches for Malar and Submalar Augmentation

The placement of midfacial implants can be approached through five different facial incisions:

1. Infraciliary
2. Transconjunctival (with or without lateral canthoplasty)
3. Intraoral
4. Preauricular, rhytidectomy, or both
5. Transtemporal

The most commonly used approaches are the intraoral (i.e., sublabial) and the infraorbital (i.e., either infraciliary or transconjunctival). The approach used is based on whether other simultaneous procedures are being performed and the surgeon's comfort and experience with the approach. Each approach has specific potential side effects.

Infraciliary Approach

The incision is made 2 mm to 3 mm below the eyelid margin. The preservation of the pretarsal orbicularis oculi muscle is important. Dissection is performed beneath the orbicularis oculi muscle, and a skin and muscle flap is elevated. The periosteum of the maxilla and the zygoma is incised just below the infraorbital rim. The elevation of the periosteum is achieved to create a pocket for the implant, with care taken to identify and preserve the infraorbital nerve.

Transconjunctival Approach

A transconjunctival incision is made in a standard fashion (as used during blepharoplasty or when approaching the orbital floor after trauma). The orbital rim is again exposed, and subperiosteal dissection is performed. Lateral canthotomy and cantholysis are usually necessary to provide adequate exposure for implant placement.

Intraoral Approach

The intraoral (sublabial) approach is the most commonly used approach for the placement of midfacial implants. The sublabial incision is made superior to the fixed gingiva (Figure 50-6). This incision placement creates adequate mucosa for closure and implant coverage.

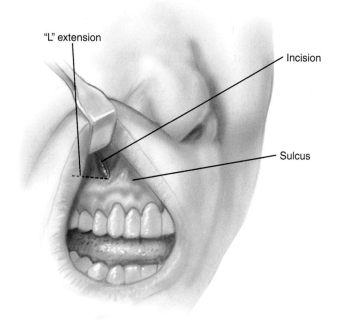

Figure 50-6. Schematic diagram of a sublabial incision radially placed to access the anterior face of the zygoma.

A subperiosteal dissection pocket is created in the predesignated area (Figure 50-7). Again, the pocket should be approximately 10% larger than the implant itself. The fixation of the implant is performed with either percutaneous bolsters or screw fixation. Meticulous layered closure is then accomplished.

Sensory Abnormalities

The infraorbital nerve supplies sensation to the skin of the cheek, the upper lip, the lateral aspect of the nose, and the ipsilateral upper teeth. This nerve is located at the mid-pupillary line approximately 7 mm below the infraorbital rim. The nerve is subject to a stretch injury (neuropraxia) during subperiosteal dissection. Complete transection of the nerve trunk or of some of the fibers can also occur. The infraorbital nerve is more at risk with the intraoral approach than it is with the infraciliary or transconjunctival approach. Careful exposure and dissection will avoid infraorbital nerve injury.

Dysesthesia or chronic pain can also occur after malar or submalar implant placement.[11] The cause of dysesthesia is either nerve regrowth after stretch injury or nerve irritation from implant mobility and pressure on the nerve. If the implant contacts and puts pressure on the infraorbital nerve, reoperation to move the implant (or to remove it) may be necessary to resolve the irritation. Chronic pain can also be the result of scar tissue adjacent to the nerve fibers. If excess scar tissue is suspected postoperatively, intralesional steroid injection (i.e., triamcinolone) may be used to lessen the discomfort.

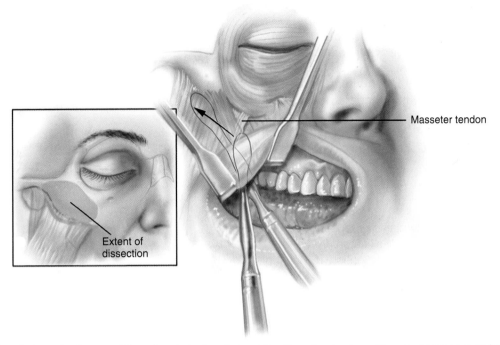

Masseter tendon

Extent of dissection

Figure 50-7. Schematic diagram of the subperiosteal pocket and the dissection to place either a submalar or a malar implant.

Infection

It is difficult to accurately quantify the incidence of infection with midfacial implants. It is clear that the intraoral approach for implant placement has an associated infection risk that warrants a discussion with and consideration by the patient. The risk of infection is related to bacterial contamination of the implant site and the colonization of the implant. Perioperative antibiotics should be used, and antibacterial mouthwash is advised postoperatively. Intraoperatively, the implant is soaked in antibiotics, and a "no-touch" technique is used when handling the implant.[12] These techniques help minimize the chance of postoperative infection.

Implant Malposition and Asymmetry

Asymmetry of the midface after malar or submalar augmentation is common. The causes of midface asymmetry include the following:
- Preoperative skeletal asymmetry
- Preoperative soft-tissue asymmetry
- The unequal creation of the implant pockets
- Implant mobility after placement

Asymmetry of the midface—either skeletal, soft tissue, or both—is common and often unnoticed preoperatively by the patient. Conditions such as hemifacial microsomia are easy to detect when the facial asymmetry is moderate to severe; however, mild facial asymmetries occur commonly and should be identified and discussed with the patient preoperatively. This will make the patient aware of the asymmetry and

will help to adjust their postoperative expectations accordingly.

Asymmetries that result from intraoperative or postoperative events should be minimized. The creation of the intraoperative dissection pocket should be performed in a meticulous fashion in the subperiosteal plane. The placement of the implant should be measured carefully and marked on the skin preoperatively. The implants are then placed and fixated in the subperiosteal pockets using the preoperative symmetric skin markings. Fixation is performed with either tie-over cutaneous bolsters or screw fixation.

Eyelid Malposition

The placement of a midfacial implant may cause or contribute to lower eyelid malposition. The condition of postoperative inferior malposition of the lower eyelid is more likely among patients who display preoperative lower eyelid laxity. Weakness or laxity of the lateral canthal tendon (LCT) of the lower eyelid may be tested preoperatively by performing the distraction test. The lower eyelid is pulled inferiorly away from the globe and allowed to "snap back" into position. If the LCT has poor tone, the lid will not return quickly to its normal anatomic position and may require a blink to regain the normal position.

The infraciliary approach to the placement of midfacial implants has a much greater chance of causing postoperative lower eyelid malposition than does the sublabial (intraoral) approach. This occurs because the suborbicularis oculi muscle dissection slightly weakens the squeezing action of the muscle. Additionally, patients with preoperative laxity of the LCT do not regain full tonicity of the tendon after it is partially detached. Among patients with preoperative LCT tendon weakness or presenile ectropion, lateral canthoplasty should be performed (with implant placement) to minimize the chance of postoperative lower eyelid malposition.

CONCLUSION

The appropriate use of facial implants produces improved balance and harmony of the facial skeleton. In the lower face, chin implants can improve projection in patients with horizontal and vertical skeletal deficiency. In the midface, malar and submalar implants can improve a deficient zygomaticomalar region and camouflage midfacial soft-tissue deficiencies. The successful placement of these implants requires careful preoperative diagnosis, precise surgical planning, and meticulous surgical execution. If these procedures are properly performed, complications are very uncommon.

REFERENCES

1. Binder WJ, Kamer FM, Parkes ML: Mentoplasty—A clinical analysis of alloplastic implants. *Laryngoscope* 1981;91:383–391.
2. Mittelman H: The anatomy of the aging mandible and its importance to facelift surgery. *Fac Plast Surg Clin North Am* 1994;2:301.
3. Sykes, JM, Tollefson TT, Frodel J: Mentoplasty and facial implants. In Cummings CM, editor: *Otolaryngology–head and neck surgery,* ed 4, Philadelphia, 2004, Mosby.
4. Sykes J, Frodel J: Genioplasty. *Op Tech Oto/HNS* Dec 1995;6(4):319–323.
5. Lilla JA, Vistnes LM, Jobe RP: The long-term effects of hard alloplastic implants when put on bone. *Plast Reconstr Surg* 1976;58:14–18.
6. Robinson M, Shuken R: Bone resorption under plastic chin implants. *J Oral Surg* 1969;27:116–118.
7. Papel ID, Capone RB: Botulinum toxin A for mentalis muscle dysfunction. *Arch Facial Plast Surg* 2001;3:268–269.
8. Blitzer A, Binder WF, Aviv JE, et al: The management of hyperfunctional facial lines with botulinum toxin: A collaborative study of 210 injection sites in 162 patients. *Arch Otolaryngol Head Neck Surg* 1997;123:389–392.
9. Gorney M, Harries T: The preoperative and postoperative consideration of natural facial asymmetry. *Plast Reconstr Surg* 1974;54:187–191.
10. Gonzalez-Ulloa M: Building out the malar prominences as an addition to rhytidectomy. *Plast Reconstr Surg* 1974;53:293–296.
11. Courtiss E: Complications in aesthetic malar augmentation-discussion. *Plast Reconstr Surg* 1983;71:648.
12. Terino EO: Complications of chin and malar augmentation. In Peck G, editor: *Complications and problems in aesthetic plastic surgery,* New York, 1991, Gower Medical Publishers.

PART 6

Skull Base and Ear

CHAPTER 51

Complications of Anterior Skull-Base Surgery

Dennis H. Kraus, Mark H. Bilsky, and Jerry Lin

The combined transcranial transfacial approach to orbital tumors was first described by Cushing[1] in 1938 and Dandy[2] in 1941. Smith and colleagues[3] and Ketchum and Van Buren[4] later expanded and applied this approach to tumors of the paranasal sinuses, thus engendering the concept of craniofacial resection and skull-base surgery. Initial attempts at craniofacial resection were limited by high morbidity rates and the inability to achieve en bloc resections of malignant tumors. Poor preoperative imaging and staging as well as limited postextirpation reconstruction methods predisposed patients to frequent cerebrospinal fluid (CSF) leak, meningitis, and surgery-related mortality.[5–7] The advent of newer radiologic techniques (e.g., computerized tomography scanning, magnetic resonance imaging) has greatly facilitated the surgeon's ability to assess the extent of tumor and to plan precise en bloc resections. Advances in reconstructive techniques, including free flap reconstruction, have significantly decreased the rates of postoperative CSF leaks and meningitis, which are two of the most common causes of morbidity and mortality from craniofacial resection. Furthermore, improvements in neuroanesthesia, brain protection, and perioperative care as well as advances in postoperative adjuvant therapy—particularly in the delivery of external-beam radiation therapy—have contributed to the ability of skull-base surgery to improve patients' long-term survival and quality of life.

Despite major innovations on multiple fronts, complication rates remain high. Mortality rates are typically reported at 5%, and overall complication rates range between 25% and 65%.[8–13] In a recent international collaborative study, complications of craniofacial resection for malignant tumors of the skull base were reviewed in 1193 patients from 17 institutions.[14] A morbidity rate of 4.7% was reported, and an overall complication rate of 36.3% was found, which was consistent with previous reports in the literature. Wound complications occurred in 19.8% of cases, central nervous system (CNS)-related complications occurred in 16.2%, systemic complications were present in 4.6%, and orbital complications occurred in 1.7%. Medical comorbidity, previous radiation therapy, dural invasion, and brain invasion were predictors of an increased incidence of postoperative complications.

This chapter describes the various complications associated with craniofacial resection and skull-base surgery.

The literature is reviewed, and the incidence of complications is discussed. Innovations in surgical technique and perioperative care that reduce morbidity and mortality are examined. Lastly, predictors of perioperative complications are identified and discussed.

SURGICAL ANATOMY

The skull base is the bony interface between the cranial cavity and the remainder of the head and neck region. Within the bony skull base lie multiple fissures and foramina that transmit nerves and blood vessels. These "natural dehiscences" of the skull base offer paths of least resistance for the spread of tumors into the neurocranium. The skull base is divided into the anterior, middle, and posterior cranial fossae. The floor of the anterior cranial fossa is formed by the crista galli, the cribriform plates, the planum sphenoidale, and the orbital roof. The majority of the paranasal sinus tumors that require craniofacial resection can be accessed through the anterior skull base. The squamous temporal bone, the greater wing of the sphenoid, and the lower part of the parietal bone compose the floor of the middle cranial fossa, and the tegmen and the petrous temporal bone are also included in the middle cranial fossa. The posterior cranial fossa consists of the posterior aspect of the temporal bone near the cerebellopontine angle, the occipital bone, and the inferior clivus.

SURGICAL TECHNIQUE

A description of the technical details regarding craniofacial resection is beyond the scope of this discussion, but the key points of the procedure will be reviewed. A spinal drain is placed before surgery to decompress the CSF and to minimize the brain retraction required for adequate exposure. Patients receive perioperative steroids and broad-spectrum antibiotics.

The intracranial aspect of the procedure is addressed using a bicoronal scalp incision. As the frontal scalp is elevated, a galeal–pericranial flap is created to facilitate skull-base reconstruction. A frontal craniotomy or a subfrontal approach with a frontal bone flap is used to gain access to the anterior skull base. At this point, if the tumor is extradural, dissection of the tumor is performed, with division of the olfactory roots at the cribriform plate and closure of the dural sleeves of the olfactory roots. If dura is involved and requires resection, which occurs in most patients, the defect is repaired with a free fascial or pericranial graft. Depending on the extent of the tumor, osteotomies are performed in the cribriform plate, the fovea ethmoidalis, the planum sphenoidale, and the orbital roof.

The transfacial aspect of the procedure is typically performed via a lateral rhinotomy incision or with the rare use of a Weber–Fergusson incision with the elevation of a cheek flap. En bloc resection incorporates the lateral nasal wall, the nasal septum, and the ethmoid contents in continuity with the bony anterior skull base. More extensive lesions may require the resection of the maxilla, the orbit, the facial skin, the infratemporal fossa, and other involved skull-base structures.

RECONSTRUCTION TECHNIQUES

Reconstructive efforts focus on four major goals:

1. Reconstructing the dura
2. Creating an effective separation between the intracranial and extracranial spaces
3. Obliterating all dead space with adequate coverage of the vital structures
4. Optimally restoring function and cosmesis

To these ends, the watertight closure of all dural defects is meticulously achieved. The frontal sinus is cranialized, and all mucosa is stripped with a diamond burr drill. The galeal–pericranial flap is used to separate the cranial cavity from the sinonasal tract, and soft-tissue transfer is then used to reconstruct the extirpated area. The bony skull base typically does not need to be reconstructed. An exception is made for cases in which a significant amount of the bony orbital roof is resected and bone reconstruction is necessary to prevent pulsatile ophthalmoplegia.

Historically, before the regular use of free-tissue transfer, skull-base defects that could not be closed primarily were reconstructed with local or regional flaps. The abundant blood supply of the head and neck region provided many choices for well-vascularized tissue that could be rotated or advanced into defects in the skull base. Local flaps came from the scalp, the galea, the pericranium, and the temporalis muscle.

Today, these local flaps are used rarely and only for smaller defects of the anterior cranial fossa that do not require the obliteration of the dead space. They are not sufficient to address larger defects that require a greater volume of tissue for reconstruction. Pedicled flaps such as the latissimus dorsi, the pectoralis major, the sternocleidomastoid, and the trapezius flaps have been considered and used for skull-base reconstruction, but their success has been limited by the distance of their vascular pedicles, which lie below the clavicle.

Free-tissue transfer is now routinely used for the closure of skull-base defects after craniofacial resection. One of the greatest advantages of free flaps is the large degree of freedom that they offer the reconstructive surgeon in terms of tissue bulk and insetting angles. Free flaps can be tailored to the defect so that all dead space is obliterated and adequate separation of the brain from the nasopharynx can be achieved. Multiple recipient vessels are available in the head and neck; the recipient vessels of choice are the superficial temporal artery and vein or the facial artery and vein. Commonly used free flaps include the radial forearm, the anterolateral thigh, the rectus abdominis, and the latissimus dorsi free flaps. Other reported flaps include the omentum, the gracilis, and the tensor fascia lata free flaps. The choice of free flap is typically based on the size and nature of the defect and the length of the pedicle that is required. Smaller defects employ radial forearm or even gracilis free flaps. The anterolateral thigh flap is becoming popular for mid-sized defects. Large defects that require a significant amount of bulk are best addressed with latissimus dorsi or rectus abdominis myocutaneous free flaps. In rare instances for extensive defects, more than one flap can be used.

COMPLICATIONS

Postoperative complications (Box 51-1) after craniofacial resection or skull-base surgery can be divided into several subtypes: intracranial or CNS-related, extracranial, systemic, and orbital. Intracranial complications include CSF leak, meningitis, subdural or intradural abscess, pneumocephalus, hematoma, delayed return of neurologic function, cerebrovascular accident, and seizure. Extradural complications include local wound infection, local wound dehiscence, and flap failure. Systemic complications can involve the respiratory, cardiovascular, hematologic, or endocrine systems. Orbital complications include corneal abrasion, epiphora, ectropion, enophthalmos, diplopia, periorbital cellulitis, and blindness.

An overview of the morbidity and mortality rates reported in several major series is shown in Table 51-1.[8–26] Operative mortality from craniofacial resection or skull-base surgery ranged from 0% to 7.6%. Meningitis and encephalitis were the most common causes of death, followed by myocardial infarction and intracranial hemorrhage. Rates of morbidity ranged from 17% to 66%. The most commonly reported complications, in descending order of frequency, were as follows: (1) wound infection; (2) CSF leak; (3) osteonecrosis of the frontal bone flap; (4) systemic complications; (5) delayed return to neurologic function; (6) meningitis; (7) ocular complications;

BOX 51-1 Complications After Skull-Base Surgery

INTRACRANIAL

- Cerebrospinal fluid leak
- Meningitis
- Subdural or intradural abscess
- Pneumocephalus
- Delayed return of neurologic function
- Cerebrovascular accident
- Seizure

EXTRACRANIAL

- Major wound infection
- Osteomyelitis of the frontal bone flap
- Delayed wound healing
- Flap failure

SYSTEMIC

- Cardiac
- Pulmonary
- Hematologic

ORBITAL

- Corneal abrasion
- Epiphora
- Ectropion
- Enophthalmos
- Diplopia
- Periorbital cellulites
- Blindness

(8) pneumocephalus; (9) delayed wound healing; (10) intracranial hematoma; and (11) intracranial abscess.

Infection

Infection remains by far the most frequently encountered complication of craniofacial resection and skull-base surgery. Dias and colleagues[17] reported that infectious complications accounted for 54.7% of all complications. Rates of wound infection range from 1.3% to 27.9%. Reported as a distinct entity, osteomyelitis of the frontal bone flap occurs in 0% to 14.8% of cases. Early reports of the craniofacial experience described intracranial infection as the most frequent complication. However, the recent literature reports a 0% to 7.7% rate of meningitis and a 0% to 11% rate of intracranial abscesses. Thus, in the more recent series of the past 15 years, the most common complication is still infectious in nature, but it has shifted to an extracranial or at least an extradural location. If wound infections and osteomyelitis of the frontal bone flap are combined into a new category of extradural infections and meningitis and intracranial abscesses are combined into a new category of intradural infections, the incidence of extradural infections nearly triples that of intradural infections. The fact that extradural infections are not spreading to the brain reflects the improved effectiveness of modern reconstructive techniques to adequately separate the intracranial space from the sinonasal tract.

Given that infectious complications comprise a significant proportion of each of the categories of wound, CNS, and systemic complications, it is not surprising that the institution of a standardized regimen of perioperative antibiotics covering key bacterial pathogens can effectively reduce both infectious and overall morbidity rates. When comparing a standardized regimen of antibiotics covering gram-positive, gram-negative, and anaerobic bacteria with nonstandardized regimens of perioperative antibiotics, Kraus and colleagues[24] reported local wound complication rates of 18% and 35%, respectively, and infectious wound complication rates of 11% and 29%, respectively. Furthermore, infectious complications that occurred with the standardized antibiotic regimen were significantly less severe and resulted in a reduction in perioperative mortality.

In addition to the standardized perioperative antibiotic regimen, several surgical techniques have been instituted to minimize postoperative infection. The neurosurgical literature recommends stripping the frontal sinuses and packing the frontal sinus ostia before entering the dura. At the conclusion of the case, the operative site is cleaned with antibiotic irrigation, and epidural and subgaleal drains are used to close the dead space. Synthetic bone products are avoided, because they often serve as a nidus for delayed infection.

Improvements in reconstruction techniques have without a doubt contributed greatly to the decrease in infection rates (particularly intradural infections) by effectively separating the intracranial space from the sinonasal tract. Kraus and colleagues[24] reported that free flap reconstruction was the sole surgical factor associated with a significant reduction in the infectious complication rate: an 8.2% complication rate was found for cases reconstructed with free flaps as compared with 27% for reconstruction methods that did not involve the use of free flaps.

Cerebrospinal Fluid Leak

Ironically, despite modern reconstruction techniques, CSF leak remains the second most common complication, with reported rates of between 0% and 13.7%. Patients with CSF leak typically complain of rhinorrhea and headaches that are worse when in an upright position. They may also suffer from nausea, tinnitus, and changes in hearing; horizontal diplopia and blurring of vision; and even facial numbness and upper limb radicular symptoms.

In and of itself, CSF leak is a clinical entity to be reckoned with. However, in addition, it suggests a connection between the intradural and extradural space that may predispose the patient to further complications such as pneumocephalus, meningitis, and intracranial

TABLE 51-1 Morbidity/Mortality of Anterior Skull-Base Surgery

Reference	Year	No. of Patients	Mortality	Morbidity	Extradural	Intradural	Ocular	Systemic
Richtsmeier et al[8]	1992	32	3.1%	—	3.1%	21.9%	—	—
Catalano et al[9]	1994	73	2.7%	63.0%	17.8%	35.6%	26.0%	—
Irish et al[10]	1994	73	—	44.0%	—	—	—	—
Janecka et al[11]	1994	183	2.0%	33.0%	2.2%	8.2%	—	—
Kraus et al[12]	1994	85	2.0%	39.0%	21.2%	11.8%	3.5%	5.9%
Clayman et al[13]	1995	39	0.0%	36.0%	—	17.9%	—	—
Bilsky et al[15]	1997	115	—	50.0%	4.3%	7.0%	—	1.7%
Shah et al[16]	1997	115	3.5%	35.0%	27.0%	5.2%	—	—
Dias et al[17]	1999	104	7.6%	48.6%	47.6%	25.0%	5.8%	10.6%
Donald[18]	1999	107	6.0%	50.5%	19.6%	15.9%	—	—
Solero et al[19]	2000	168	4.7%	34.5%	4.8%	18.5%	1.8%	—
Chang et al[20]	2001	77	—	27.0%	15.6%	10.4%	—	—
Heth et al[21]	2002	67	—	47.0%	—	—	—	19.4%
Teknos et al[22]	2002	35	5.7%	66.0%	22.9%	14.3%	25.7%	45.7%
Califano et al[23]	2003	135	3.7%	43.0%	17.8%	8.9%	—	5.9%
Kraus et al[24]	2005	211	4.3%	—	—	—	—	—
Ganly et al[14]	2005	1197	4.7%	36.3%	—	—	—	—
Newman et al[25]	2006	40	0.0%	30.0%	22.5%	—	—	10.0%
Origitano et al[26]	2006	120	0.0%	17.0%	9.2%	5.0%	—	—

abscesses. These intracranial problems could in turn exacerbate systemic issues or prolong the time that it takes to return to normal neurologic function.

Steps taken to minimize CSF leakage revolve around the meticulous watertight closure of the dura. Primary closure of the dura is performed, when possible; otherwise bovine pericardium is typically used for dural repair. Neither has been shown to be associated with higher rates of CSF leak.[20] Dural patches are typically internally overlapped with the dural edge so that the reexpansion of the CSF space serves to seal the closure. Fibrin glue can be used at the suture line to reinforce the closure. The duraplasty must be patulous to accommodate the reexpanding brain and to avoid dural banding. The avoidance of the intraoperative overdrainage of CSF can help to prevent this complication.

If a CSF leak occurs, many surgeons advocate conservative treatment with bed rest and lumbar drainage. Most of the literature reports the adequate resolution of CSF leak with this treatment. However, failing this, endoscopic reexploration can be performed with repacking via the transnasal approach. In the current era, the craniotomy rarely needs to be reexplored.

Systemic

Systemic complications comprise a significant percentage of perioperative morbidity, with rates ranging from 1.7% to 45.7%. Although they do not involve the brain, these complications should not be discounted, because they are responsible for nearly 20% of perioperative mortality. A review of the literature shows that myocardial infarction was the most common systemic cause of mortality. Other systemic complications included pneumonia, pulmonary embolism, sepsis, disseminated intravascular coagulopathy, and mesenteric artery thrombosis. As the state of the art improves, systemic complications may become more prevalent, because sicker patients with more comorbidities will be deemed appropriate candidates for craniofacial resection or skull-base surgery.

Delayed Return to Neurologic Function

Rates of delayed return to neurologic function range from 1.8% to 20.5%. Deficits in neurologic function may reflect frontal lobe edema sustained from excessive retraction or hand resting during surgery. These deficits can also be the result of other intracranial complications, such as meningitis, pneumocephalus, hematoma, or abscess. More devastatingly, they can be harbingers of acute injury to the brain, including edema, stroke, and seizure.

The key to the avoidance of brain injury is to minimize the retraction of the brain during the procedure. This can be accomplished by appropriate patient positioning, the choice of craniotomy site, and CSF decompression. Any retraction that needs to be performed should involve the use of ultrasoft blades. During the facial portion of the procedure, the brain should be protected with the replacement of the craniotomy bone flap to avoid inadvertent injury. Intraoperatively and postoperatively, brain edema can be minimized by the administration of steroids and hypertonic solutions such as mannitol.

Ocular

Ocular complication rates range from 1.8% to 26%. The most common ocular complications are corneal abrasions and the disruption of the lacrimal drainage system. In cases that do not require orbital exenteration but that do involve the resection of the orbital floor or of at least two orbital walls, rigid orbital reconstruction is necessary to avoid enophthalmos and diplopia.[27] In such cases, the medial canthal ligament must also be meticulously aligned to prevent diplopia. Nasolacrimal stents are placed to curtail postoperative stenosis and epiphora.

Blindness is the most dire ocular complication. This can occur acutely through intraoperative injury to either the optic nerve or the ophthalmic artery. Delayed blindness may also ensue from adjuvant radiation therapy to the anterior skull base that injures the optic nerve, the optic chiasm, and the optic tracts. Improvements in the delivery of radiation therapy and the advent of intensity-modulated radiation therapy in particular have reduced the incidence of radiation-induced ocular toxicity.[28]

Pneumocephalus

Reported rates of pneumocephalus range from 0% to 15.6%. As with CSF leak, pneumocephalus belies a dural defect that allows air to pass from an extradural location—most likely the sinonasal tract—into the intracranial space. If significant, pneumocephalus will certainly delay the return to neurologic function.

The avoidance of tension pneumocephalus also revolves around the achievement of a watertight dural closure. A small drain is typically placed into the epidural space at the end of the procedure. The ability of this epidural drain to hold suction is a good indication of adequate dural closure. For cases involving tension pneumocephalus, any spinal drains need to be clamped. The intracranial air can be evacuated by the placement of an intravenous catheter through an existing burr hole using meticulous antiseptic technique. Intubation or tracheostomy can be used to divert the pressure head on the closure, but this is rarely necessary. Endoscopic or open reexploration may ultimately be performed.

Delayed Wound Healing

Delayed wound healing occurs with a reported frequency of 1.8% to 15.9%. Wound complications typically arise as a result of either wound infections or reconstruction flap compromise. The administration of postoperative radiation therapy can also delay wound healing, and it has been identified in the literature as a risk factor for late wound breakdown.[8,19,23]

As previously discussed, a standardized regimen of perioperative antibiotics decreases wound complication rates. Wound complications caused by flap compromise can be minimized with meticulous surgical technique. Postoperatively, vigilant flap monitoring must be maintained. Exposed flaps can be monitored with an external Doppler probe, and buried flaps require an implantable Doppler device for monitoring. Equal in importance to the technical details of flap reconstruction is the choice of flap itself. Pedicled flaps are no longer routinely used for the reconstruction of skull-base defects. Free-tissue transfer allows for wounds to be reconstructed with tailor-made tissue that is well vascularized and appropriately sized for the defect. The incidence of free flap failure reported in the literature ranges from 0.7% to 22.9%.[17,18,20,22,23,25,26]

Emphasis on Surgical Technique

To avoid or minimize the complications of craniofacial resection and skull-base surgery, a significant emphasis is placed on surgical technique. The development of surgical technique relies heavily on experience and represents an accumulation of dynamic and often subtle alterations in practice. Many techniques that have evolved are not strictly evidence based as defined by statistical significance, because reports of surgical series have typically been underpowered. Nevertheless, the typical findings that surgical morbidity decreases with experience within reported series and that complication rates remain unchanged despite increasingly difficult cases demonstrate that the refinements in technique that come with experience have practical if not statistical significance.[9,19,23,24,26]

DISCUSSION

Need for the Standardization of Reporting

Early descriptions of craniofacial resections and skull-base surgery reported very high complication rates.[5-7] CSF leaks were expected, and resulting intracranial infectious complications were often devastating. With surgical experience and improvements in reconstruction techniques (particularly the use of galeal and pericranial flaps to reinforce dural closures), craniofacial resection has come to be considered a practical measure to address patients with skull-base neoplasms. Since the early 1990s, reported complication rates of skull-base surgery ranged from 17% to 66%. With a few exceptions, mortality rates have been less than 5%.

A systematic review of complications reported in the literature is difficult as a result of the nonstandardized methods of reporting. To date, most of the literature regarding craniofacial resection consists of retrospective reviews of a single institution's experience over a long period of time. Because of the relative infrequency of skull-base lesions, all cases are typically included in these studies, and tumor types run the gamut of histopathologies. Results for benign and malignant lesions are often reported together, without differentiation. Although most tumors are located in the anterior cranial fossa, resections of middle and posterior fossa lesions are typically included in most retrospective series. Even the approach to the skull base can be variable. In some reports (particularly those from the neurosurgical literature), cases requiring craniotomies alone were incorporated into reports of the craniofacial experience. Perioperative adjuvant therapies are not standardized, and reconstruction techniques are variable. Analyses of complications are divided into arbitrary and often inconsistently defined categories on the basis of the potential for morbidity (i.e., major vs. minor), the location (i.e., intracranial vs. extracranial or local vs. systemic), and the timing (i.e., early vs. late).

A few studies took advantage of the long reporting periods to analyze improvements in morbidity with increased surgical experience. Catalano and colleagues[9] reported a complication rate of 52.2% from 1980 to 1987 that fell to 28% from 1988 to 1994. Similarly, Solero and colleagues[19] reported a complication rate of 53% for their first 30 patients that improved to 24.6% for the subsequent 138 patients in the study. Alternatively, Califano and colleagues[23] did not report any statistically significant drops in complication rates between the time periods of 1976 to 1991 and 1992 to 1999. Kraus and colleagues[24] instituted a standardized antibiotic regimen during the course of a reported experience and used the earlier data as a retrospective control. In this manner they were able to show that the standardized antibiotic regimen decreased rates of local wound complications from 35% (i.e., prestandardized regimen) to 18% (i.e., poststandardized regimen) and that it lowered the rates of infectious wound complications from 29% (i.e., prestandardized regimen) to 11% (i.e., poststandardized regimen).

Predictors of Complications

Many reports in the literature attempted to identify predictors of increased complication rates. No consistent relationship was identified between complication rates and demographic factors such as age, sex, or medical comorbidities.[12,14,17] Heth and colleagues[21] reported the only correlation found between female gender and increased complication rate; they cited less robust reconstructive flap tissues as a possible explanation. The histopathologic type of disease, although important for survival outcomes, did not affect morbidity rates.[16]

Dias and colleagues[17] described a significant association between the extent of cranial base resection and complication rates. Patients who underwent extended cranial base resections had a 62% incidence of postoperative complications as compared with a 37% rate among those who underwent standard resections. Paradoxically, however, patients who required orbital exenteration suffered lower rates of morbidity than those with smaller resections that preserved the orbit. The resection of the orbit likely affords the surgeon better access to the skull base and therefore the improved ability to reconstruct the dura and the skull-base defect. Irish and colleagues[10] also reported a higher incidence of complications among patients who underwent skull-base resections of more than one skull-base site. Wornom and colleagues[29] described large combined defects of both the frontal and temporal regions as the most important risk factors for postoperative morbidity. Alternatively, Kraus and colleagues[24] failed to find an effect of the extent of surgery on the infectious complication rate. In an earlier study, Kraus and colleagues[12] found no effect of orbital exenteration on local wound complications.

Dural involvement of disease has been associated with significantly higher incidences of CSF leak (i.e., 25% vs. 6.5%) and meningitis (i.e., 23% vs. 4.3%) according to Dias and colleagues.[17] Kraus and colleagues[12] also observed a trend (although not a significant one) toward higher complication rates among those patients with dural invasion (i.e., 43% vs. 27%). Chang and colleagues reported no differences in postoperative morbidity associated with the type of dural repair, the type of skull-base reconstruction, or the defect location.[20] Unexpectedly, Heth and colleagues[21] described increased major wound complications with intact dural status. A closer analysis of this finding revealed that a majority of these complications occurred as a result of wound breakdown in pericranial flaps associated with high-dose radiation therapy. It was suggested that a selection bias may have resulted in this finding, because patients with an intact dural status were considered less likely to have complications and were more likely to undergo a local flap reconstruction rather than a free flap reconstruction. In turn, these local flaps, which are presumably less vascularized than free flaps, were prone to breakdown in the face of postoperative radiation therapy.

Adjuvant therapy has been scrutinized as a possible predictor of postoperative morbidity. Teknos and colleagues[22] described an association between previous irradiation and longer hospital stays (i.e., 17.7 days vs. 12.4 days), but they found no effect of previous irradiation on complication rates (i.e., 70% vs. 62.5%). Several other groups have confirmed this, failing to find any effect of previous treatment on complication rates.[17,20,21] Kraus and colleagues[12] found no relationship between morbidity and previous irradiation, orbital exenteration, or positive margin. Deschler and colleagues[30] failed to identify any effect of previous chemotherapy, previous radiation therapy, or prior craniotomy on postoperative morbidity. Alternatively, previous surgery has been shown by both Donald and colleagues[18] and Heth and colleagues[21] to significantly increase postoperative morbidity. Neither of these studies found any effect of preoperative chemotherapy or radiation therapy on postoperative complication rates. However, postoperative radiation has been associated with late wound breakdown.[8,19,23]

Interestingly, despite the evidence from individual groups refuting the relationship between either dural invasion or previous radiation therapy with increased morbidity, a multi-institutional analysis identified the extent of intracranial invasion, previous radiation therapy, and medical comorbidities as the only significant predictors of postoperative complications.[14] This same study also reported no difference in morbidity when pedicled flaps versus free flaps were employed for reconstruction.

Free Flaps Versus Local Flaps

Free-tissue transfer has become the preferred method of reconstruction after craniofacial resection or skull-base surgery. Because of its versatility, the free flap most effectively accomplishes the four major goals of reconstruction, as outlined previously. Because nearly all complications arise from a deficiency in one or more of the four major goals of reconstruction, the true usefulness of the free flap can be discerned by examining its effect on complication rates.

Califano and colleagues[23] found a complication rate of 31% for patients who were reconstructed with free-tissue transfer versus a rate of 35% for patients reconstructed with conventional pedicled flaps. Free flaps and local flaps were also comparable in terms of intracranial complication rates, mortality rates, and disease-free survival. This rate similarity existed despite a significant difference in the extent and complexity of skull-base resection: 72% of free flaps were used to reconstruct complex defects versus only 26% of local flaps. Heth and colleagues[21] also reported similar overall rates of major wound complications among patients who were reconstructed with local flaps as compared with free flaps. In this study, free flap complications typically occurred early during the postoperative period and were considered to be acute, surgery-related problems. The majority of local flap complications occurred late as a result of wound breakdown after high-dose radiation therapy. Free flaps were also associated with higher rates of systemic complications; this is possibly another example of selection bias (i.e., sicker patients with more extensive disease are offered surgery in an era when free flaps are more commonly used).

Free flaps versus local flaps are applied to the reconstruction of different kinds of cranial-base defects; thus it is unlikely that there will ever be any direct comparison between the outcomes of reconstruction for the two types of flaps. Nevertheless, the finding that free flap success rates are comparable with those of local flaps—despite the use of free flaps for more difficult cases—suggests that free flap reconstruction may be more robust.[23,25]

Free flaps and local flaps are not necessarily mutually exclusive. The use of the galeal–pericranial flap was advocated by Dias and colleagues[17] because of its ability to limit the occurrence of CSF leaks (i.e., 6.5% with its use vs. 25% without). Kraus and colleagues[12] suggested that the use of microvascular free flaps could further reinforce this closure, particularly among patients who required dural resection and repair. Califano and colleagues[23] report that they used a combination of vascularized free-tissue transfer in conjunction with pedicled flaps in nearly half of their free flap cases.

CONCLUSION

Craniofacial resection has become a relatively safe and practical surgical option for patients with tumors that involve the anterior skull base. The decision-making process for craniofacial resection no longer focuses on whether or not a resection can be performed but rather on how it will be performed and, just as importantly, on how the defect will be reconstructed. As the field continues to evolve and emphasis is placed on minimally invasive procedures, surgeons are becoming increasingly adept with intranasal endoscopic techniques. This approach is expected to be more frequently employed in the resection of skull-base tumors. With changes in surgical technique will come changes in complication profiles. Regardless of the technique used, however, repair of the dura and the prevention of CSF leak remain the greatest challenges of the reconstruction of craniofacial resections.

At this point, most of the retrospective single-institution experiences have been reported in the literature, and much information has been gleaned from these series. However, because of the relative rarity of skull-base tumors, individual studies have had to take place over protracted periods of time. Even so, many reports remain underpowered to discern the importance of demographics, tumor type, tumor locations, adjuvant therapies, and reconstruction techniques for predicting complications and outcomes. Collaborative studies performed prospectively can assemble the larger data sets that are needed to answer the questions that single-institution studies cannot. Furthermore, collaborative studies will rectify the diverse methods of reporting results, complications, and outcomes. When each institution organizes its data in a standardized fashion, that data can be compared with other data more effectively. In addition, it can be incorporated more efficiently into multi-institutional analyses that will ultimately provide the guidelines that will afford patients the best possible outcomes.

REFERENCES

1. Cushing H: *Meningiomas,* Springfield, Ill, 1938, Thomas.
2. Dandy WE: *Orbital tumors: Results following the transcranial operative attack,* New York, 1941, Oskar Priest.
3. Smith RR, Klopp CT, Williams JM: Surgical treatment of cancer of the frontal sinus and adjacent areas. *J Cancer* 1954;7:991–994.
4. Ketcham AS, Van Buren JM: Tumors of the paranasal sinuses: A therapeutic challenge. *Am J Surg* 1985;150:406–413.
5. Terz JJ, Young HF, Lawrence W Jr: Combined craniofacial resection for locally advanced carcinoma of the head and neck: I: Tumors of the skin and soft tissues. *Am J Surg* 1980;140:613–617.
6. Terz JJ, Young HF, Lawrence W Jr: Combined craniofacial resection for locally advanced carcinoma of the head and neck: II: Carcinoma of the paranasal sinuses. *Am J Surg* 1980;140:618–624.
7. Ketcham AS, Hoye RC, Van Buren JM, et al: Complications of intracranial facial resection for tumors of the paranasal sinuses. *Am J Surg* 1966;112:591–596.
8. Richtsmeier WJ, Briggs RJ, Koch WM, et al: Complications and early outcome of anterior craniofacial resection. *Arch Otolaryngol Head Neck Surg* 1992;118:913–917.
9. Catalano PJ, Hecht CS, Biller JF, et al: Craniofacial resection: An analysis of 73 cases. *Arch Otolaryngol Head Neck Surg* 1994;120:1203–1208.
10. Irish JC, Gulane PJ, Gentili F, et al: Tumors of the skull base: Outcome and survival analysis of 77 cases. *Head Neck* 1994;16:3–10.
11. Janecka IP, Sen C, Sekhar LN, et al: Cranial base surgery: Results in 183 patients. *Otolaryngol Head Neck Surg* 1994;110:539–546.
12. Kraus DH, Shah JP, Arbit E, et al: Complications of craniofacial resection for tumors involving the anterior skull base. *Head Neck* 1994;16:307–312.
13. Clayman GL, De Monte F, Jaffe DM, et al: Outcome and complications of extended cranial-base resection requiring microvascular free-tissue transfer. *Arch Otolaryngol Head Neck Surg* 1993;21:1253–1257.
14. Ganly I, Patel SG, Singh B, et al: Complications of craniofacial resection for malignant tumors of the skull base: Report of an International Collaborative Study. *Head Neck* 2005;27:445–451.
15. Bilsky MH, Kraus DH, Strong EW, et al: Extended anterior craniofacial resection for intracranial extension of malignant tumors. *Am J Surg* 1997;174:565–568.
16. Shah JP, Kraus DH, Bilsky MH, et al: Craniofacial resection for malignant tumors involving the anterior skull base. *Arch Otolaryngol Head Neck Surg* 1997;123:1312–1317.
17. Dias FL, Geraldo MS, Kligerman J, et al: Complications of anterior craniofacial resection. *Head Neck* 1999;21:12–20.
18. Donald PJ: Complications in skull base surgery for malignancy. *Laryngoscope* 1999;109(12): 1959–1966.
19. Solero CL, DiMeco F, Sampath P, et al: Combined anterior craniofacial resection for tumors involving the cribriform plate: Early postoperative complications and technical considerations. *Neurosurg* 2000;47(6):1296–1304.

20. Chang DW, Langstein HN, Gupta A: Reconstructive management of cranial base defects after tumor ablation. *Plast Reconstr Surg* 2001;107(6):1346–1355; discussion, 1356–1357.

21. Heth JA, Funk, GF, Karnell LH, et al: Free tissue transfer and local flap complications in anterior and anterolateral skull base surgery. *Head Neck* 2002;24(10):901–911; discussion, 912.

22. Teknos TN, Smith JC, Day TA, et al: Microvascular free tissue transfer in reconstructing skull base defects: Lessons learned. *Laryngoscope* 2002;112:1871–1876.

23. Califano J, Cordeiro PG, Disa JJ, et al: Anterior cranial base reconstruction using free tissue transfer: Changing trends. *Head Neck* 2003;25(2):89–96.

24. Kraus DH, Gonen J, Mener D, et al: A standardized regimen of antibiotics prevents infectious complications in skull base surgery. *Laryngoscope* 2005;115:1347–1357.

25. Newman J, O'Malley BW, Chalian A, et al: Microvascular reconstruction of cranial base defects. *Arch Otolaryngol Head Neck Surg* 2006;132:381–384.

26. Origitano TC, Petruzzelli GJ, Leonetti JP: Combined anterior and anterolateral approach to the cranial base: Complication analysis, avoidance, and management. *Operative Neurosurg* 2006;2:327–336.

27. Imola MJ, Schramm VL Jr: Orbital preservation in surgical management of sinonasal malignancy. *Laryngoscope* 2002;112:1357–1365.

28. Duthoy W, Boterberg T, Claus F, et al: Postoperative intensity-modulated radiotherapy in sinonasal carcinoma: Clinical results in 39 patients. *Cancer* 2005;104:71–82.

29. Wornom IL 3rd, Neifeld JP, Mehrhof AI Jr, et al: Closure of craniofacial defects after cancer resection. *Am J Surg* 1991;162:408–411.

30. Deschler DG, Gutin PH, Mamelak AN, et al: Complications of anterior skull base surgery. *Skull Base Surg* 1996;6:113–118.

CHAPTER 52

Complications of Lateral Skull-Base Surgery

Frank R. Lin and John K. Niparko

The lateral skull base may be defined by an arc described by the cranial nerve foramina that includes and is bounded by the sphenoid bone anteriorly and the petrous ridge posteriorly. Patients with neoplasms involving the lateral cranial base present a well-recognized therapeutic challenge. Historically access to this region via transcervical and transmaxillary approaches was often unsatisfactory, particularly when neoplasms extended beyond the palpable skull base medially to involve the dura and the brain or the infratemporal fossa inferiorly. Multidisciplinary collaboration has now expanded surgical access to the lateral cranial base, thereby presenting treatment options beyond subtotal resection and palliative radiation. The past three decades have witnessed an evolution of lateral and superior approaches that often enable the complete removal of properly selected tumors with acceptable levels of morbidity.

It is evident that no single study can provide for comprehensive surgical planning and that no single operative technique can access all lesions in this anatomically complex region. Diverse surgical approaches and techniques guided by thorough preoperative evaluation are now applicable to lateral skull-base lesions. Equally important to the success of the surgical treatment of these lesions has been progress in postoperative care for minimizing disabling and fatal complications. This chapter discusses preoperative, intraoperative, and postoperative considerations designed to optimize the management of patients with neoplasms involving the lateral skull base.

ANATOMIC AND PATHOLOGIC CONSIDERATIONS

Infratemporal Space Anatomy

The infratemporal space is formed by the greater wing of the sphenoid superomedially, the posterior wall of the maxillary sinus anteriorly, the zygomatic arch laterally, and the lateral lamina of the pterygoid fossa and the foramen magnum medially. Superiorly it is continuous with the temporal fossa medial to the zygomatic arch. The inferior and posterior boundaries of the infratemporal fossa are open (Figure 52-1).

Critical neurovascular structures course through the infratemporal fossa in intimate association with one another. The jugular bulb and vein are formed by the confluence of the inferior petrosal and sigmoid sinuses, and they are situated on the posterolateral aspect of the internal carotid artery (ICA). A bony petrous "keel" separates the jugular bulb and the carotid artery. The cervical segment of the ICA ascends to enter the tympanic bone through the posterior aperture of the carotid canal, where it then courses vertically and continues through the carotid canal anteromedially. The vertical and horizontal segments constitute the petrous segment of the ICA. At the tip of the petrous bone, the ICA exits the foramen lacerum, continuing anteriorly as the presellar and juxtasellar (cavernous) segments of the ICA.

The sympathetic plexus on the posteromedial surface of the ICA forms three cervical ganglia that supply vasomotor control via branches to the vessels of the head and neck and papillary dilation via branches from the ciliary ganglion of the orbit. Cranial nerves IX, X, and XI emanate from the pars nervosa of the jugular foramen, and cranial nerve XII comes from the hypoglossal canal. These caudal cranial nerves then descend through the infratemporal fossa in a posteroanterior direction. The facial nerve pursues a tortuous course through the petrous and mastoid portions of the temporal bone and exits from the stylomastoid foramen. Cranial nerves V2 and V3 are oriented anteriorly through the infratemporal fossa after leaving the foramina ovale and the rotundum, respectively. Refined techniques in infratemporal surgery have expanded the operability of a wide spectrum of tumors that can arise in or extend into the infratemporal fossa.

Pathology

Primary tumors of the lateral skull base may be of bony or cartilaginous origin, and they may be benign or malignant. Cranial nerve schwannomas, salivary gland neoplasms, hemangiomas, hemangiopericytomas, and fibrous dysplastic lesions may also arise primarily from infratemporal structures. Primary cholesteatomas and giant cholesterol cysts may extend inferiorly from their origin in the petrous apex or in the infralabyrinthine air cells. Chordomas, pigmented neuroectodermal neoplasms, rhabdomyosarcomas, and angiofibromas of clival and pterygopalatine origin may extend posterolaterally to involve the infratemporal fossa. Meningiomas, pituitary tumors, and craniopharyngiomas may likewise secondarily involve the infratemporal fossa.

Surgical exposure of the infratemporal fossa can also access melanomas and hematologic and metastatic

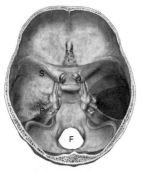
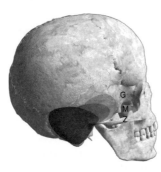

Figure 52-1. Schematic of the lateral skull base. The lateral skull base is defined broadly by the arc of the cranial nerve foramina, and it is bound anteriorly by the sphenoid bone *(S)* and posteriorly by the petrous ridge *(P)*. The infratemporal fossa lies immediately inferior to the lateral skull base, and it is bound superomedially by the greater wing of the sphenoid *(G)*, anteriorly by the posterior wall of the maxillary sinus *(M)*, laterally by the zygomatic arch *(Z)*, and medially by the foramen magnum *(F)*. Shaded areas depict the extent of temporal bone resection required for lateral skull-base tumors. More extensive resections are necessary for tumors that extend anteromedially to involve the petrous apex and the infratemporal carotid artery.

malignancies. Although the role of the surgical treatment of metastatic malignancies is often limited because of systemic involvement, patients with metastatic renal cell carcinoma (which is the most common metastatic lesion to involve the infratemporal fossa) may rarely demonstrate isolated metastasis to this region. In such cases, excision of the primary tumor and metastasis may produce a favorable clinical response.

SURGICAL APPROACHES TO THE LATERAL SKULL BASE

A thorough review of the surgical approaches to the lateral skull base has been provided in texts by Sasaki and colleagues,[1] Fisch and Mattox,[2] Jackson,[3] and Graham.[4] These approaches are described briefly to provide a foundation for the discussion of their associated complications.

Infratemporal Approach

Infratemporal approaches to the lateral skull base combine posterior and lateral access. Posterior exposure is provided by a mastoidectomy and bone removal lateral to the jugular bulb and labyrinth. Lateral and inferior access is provided by transcervical dissection and the control of the great vessels and the caudal cranial nerves. Anterior extension of lateral exposures is provided by the anterior and inferior displacement or disarticulation of the mandibular condyle. Further extension is achieved with inferior reflection of the zygoma and the lateral orbital rim.

Type A
The type A approach provides exposure of the jugular bulb, the infralabyrinthine and apical portions of the temporal bone, and the infratemporal segment of the ICA

(Figure 52-2). In combination with anterior transposition of the facial nerve, this is the procedure of choice for large glomus jugulare tumors. A canal-wall–down mastoidectomy (i.e., subtotal petrosectomy) is performed and extended anteromedially by removing petrous bone on the medial aspect of the protympanum. This exposes the proximal petrous segment of the ICA. The sigmoid sinus and the internal jugular vein are ligated, mobilized, and excised if pathologic findings and tumor location dictate. The facial nerve is displaced anteriorly from its position in the tympanic and mastoid segments of the facial canal. Transposition of the facial nerve substantially opens the angle of visualization of the infralabyrinthine compartment and the jugular bulb.

Type B
Clival lesions may arise primarily, or they may represent the anterior extension of disease of the basilar occiput. Transtemporal clival exposure can be achieved by the extension of the type A approach between the jugular foramen and the carotid canal by starting with a subtotal petrosectomy. The facial nerve is not mobilized but rather left in situ. The zygomatic arch and the temporalis muscle are reflected inferiorly to expose the pterygoid region. The mandibular condyle is dislocated and retracted anteriorly, and the glenoid fossa is drilled away. In addition to exposing and controlling its vertical segment, the genu and horizontal segments of the petrous ICA are exposed and traced anteriorly to the foramen lacerum and the cavernous sinus. The lateral clivus is exposed anterior and inferior to the ICA.

Type C
Lesions situated in the parasellar region and the lateral nasopharynx require the further extension of the type B approach anteriorly. The temporalis muscle and the zygomatic arch are reflected inferiorly, and the pterygoid plates and musculature are detached from the skull base. The maxillary nerve is divided at the foramen rotundum. The ICA is exposed and mobilized through its petrous course. Removal of the cartilaginous portion of the Eustachian tube enables the dissection of the ICA anteriorly to the presellar and juxtasellar portions of the cavernous sinus.

Craniofacial Disassembly

Enhanced exposure of the nasopharynx cavernous sinus and the middle cranial fossa structures beyond the type C approach requires transfacial and transmandibular dissections. The disassembly and translocation of the facial soft tissue can be combined with osteotomies of the orbitomaxillary skeleton and of the mandible to widely visualize the nasopharynx.[5]

When additional superior extension is required, a frontotemporal craniotomy can access the foramina spinosum,

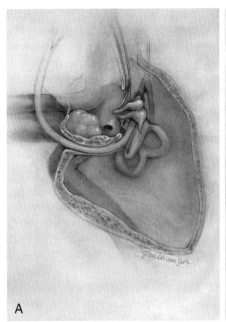 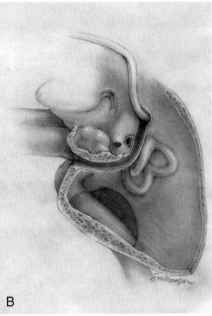 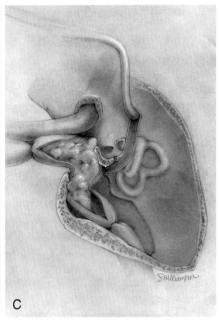

A   B   C

Figure 52-2. Approach to a glomus tumor of the jugular bulb demonstrating strategies to enhance tumor visualization and facial nerve preservation. **A,** A radical mastoidectomy (subtotal petrosectomy with tympanic membrane, ossicle, and external auditory canal removal with external auditory canal closure) is performed, and bone surrounding the intratemporal facial nerve is removed to the level of the stylomastoid foramen. The glomus jugulare tumor can be seen in the hypotympanum shielded by the facial nerve. **B,** The facial nerve is transposed and reflected laterally and anteriorly to expose the hypotympanum and the infralabyrinthine bone. The internal carotid artery is skeletonized and inspected for tumor involvement of the arterial wall. **C,** The sigmoid sinus is skeletonized from the sinodural angle to the jugular bulb with the removal of bone over the dura on each side of the sinus. The internal carotid artery and the internal jugular vein are followed from the cervical triangles to the skull base, and their bony covering is uncapped. The sigmoid sinus and the jugular vein are ligated proximally and distally for control, and the glomus tumor is exposed to enable optimal visualization and resection. Typically the superior segment of the jugular vein is resected in continuity with the glomus tumor. (Reprinted with permission from Long DM, Niparko JK, O'Malley BW Jr, et al, editors: *An atlas of skull base surgery,* London, 2003, Parthenon Publishing.)

the ovale, the rotundum, and the superior orbital fissure. Additional exposure inferiorly can be accomplished with floor-of-the-mouth incisions to expose the pharynx and the ICA in its upper cervical course.

Transcervical Approaches

Transcervical approaches to the infratemporal fossa are typically used to expose lesions that occupy the fossa and that extend into anatomic spaces adjacent to the pharynx. By virtue of transcervical dissection, the buccal, retropharyngeal, and parapharyngeal spaces can be exposed in combination with the previously described methods of exposing the infratemporal fossa.

TECHNICAL CONSIDERATIONS TO MINIMIZE THE RISK OF COMPLICATIONS

The contemporary management of lateral skull-base tumors employs many of the technical measures previously developed by neurotologic, head and neck oncologic, and neurologic surgeons. The use of microscopy with video display, constant suction, and irrigation for bony drill out as well as atraumatic, self-retaining retraction are essential for successful microsurgery of the lateral skull base. Accumulated experience with cranial

nerve[6,7] and somatosensory evoked potential monitoring[8] has demonstrated the benefits of identifying, mapping, and preserving neurologic function. Image-guided (i.e., stereotactic) computer systems have also allowed for precise intraoperative navigation,[9] thus enhancing the surgeon's ability to obtain safe and adequate margins of excision.

CAROTID ARTERY: RELATED COMPLICATIONS

The most feared complications of skull-base surgeries are hemorrhage from an inaccessible vessel on the one hand and ischemic cerebral injury on the other. In this section, the evaluation, control, and management of the ICA will be discussed.

Preoperative Radiologic Evaluation

Preoperative assessment of the carotid artery is based on detailed radiographic evaluation. Iodinated contrast-enhanced computed tomography (CT) scans of the skull base and the temporal bone can define the extent of involvement of the common carotid artery and the petrous and cavernous segments of the ICA. This evaluation can detect arterial displacement, compromise, or the invasion of the arterial lumen by tumor. Contrast-enhanced CT scans also provide a gross index of tumor vascularity and of the relationship of the tumor to the regional vessels.

Magnetic resonance (MR) scanning of the skull base has emerged as an essential study for the preoperative assessment of lateral skull-base lesions. Because MR obviates the bone artifact and can provide greater soft-tissue differentiation with the use of contrast agents (e.g., gadolinium), tumor-artery relationships can be characterized with precision. The MR scan appearance of rapid blood flow through a vessel is typically that of a "flow void" or the absence of the signal. Slow flow can produce paradoxic enhancement, and turbulence produces complex and variable patterns of enhancement.

When combined, CT and MR studies provide a comprehensive tumor map and facilitate patient education and surgical planning. Tumor–vessel relationships, however, are best delineated by angiography.[10] Four-vessel cervical–cranial angiography provides the high-resolution display of arterial involvement with tumor, tumor vascularity, and vascular supply. Angiography also determines the adequacy of posterior circulation and provides a gross measure of flow through the circle of Willis. Angiography may also detect incidental arteriovenous malformations and atheromatous stenoses that may prove problematic with skull-base dissection.

Therapeutic embolization is an extension of cervical–cranial angiography that is frequently used during the preoperative preparation of patients with highly vascular skull-base lesions. Embolization requires the initial identification of the architecture of the tumor vasculature, the tumor-feeding vessels, and both existing and potential anastomoses. The last determination is designed to minimize the risk of embolization to the intracranial circulation.

Catheterization that is selective (i.e., named vessels) or superselective (i.e., unnamed pathologic vessels) permits the injection of embolic agents or coiled springs. Polyvinyl alcohol foam and Gelfoam (i.e., absorbable gelatin sponge) offer a range of particle size and are the favored agents for vessel occlusion. When large feeding vessels render polyvinyl alcohol foam and Gelfoam inadequate for vessel occlusion, detachable balloons may achieve devascularization. These procedures are designed to facilitate tumor dissection while minimizing intraoperative blood loss.

In the past, the role of surgical management was limited in cases of lateral skull-base tumors that invaded or encased the ICA. The advisability of surgery in such cases was influenced by observations that the patency of the circle of Willis did not necessarily predict tolerance to unilateral ICA interruption. Despite the ability to bypass or reestablish flow in the ICA in some cases, the condition of the ICA adventitia after the resection of adjacent tumor often precludes revascularization, thus necessitating arterial ligation. Because of the risk of neurologic deficit associated with its ligation, a preoperative test of the ICA should be performed when extensive manipulation or ligation is anticipated.

Preoperative Evaluation of Cerebral Circulation: Assessing the Risk of Internal Carotid Artery Sacrifice

Involvement of the ICA poses an important set of clinical decisions. Sacrifice of the ICA may have the following characteristics:

1. It may be planned and performed preoperatively with angiographic techniques.

2. It may be anticipated as a possibility but not specifically planned as a part of the procedure.

3. It may be totally unplanned and unexpected.

The incidence of cerebral ischemia or stroke is greatest after unplanned carotid sacrifice, in part from the high incidence of intraoperative hemorrhage and hypotension that frequently accompany intraoperative injury to the artery. Moore and Baker[11] compared morbidity and mortality after the elective and nonelective resection of the carotid and found that the complication rate of 40% strokes and 17% mortality after elective resection rose to 88% strokes and 28% fatalities for nonelective resections. Among patients with prolonged hypotension, the mortality rate rose to 63%.

Normal cerebral blood flow is 55 ml or 100 g of brain tissue per minute. Patients usually tolerate regional blood flows of 20 ml or 100 mg of brain tissue per minute,[12] although short intervals of hypoperfusion can be tolerated by some patients.[13]

Because of the high risk associated with carotid sacrifice, a number of techniques have evolved to assess cerebral collateral blood flow. Systematic evaluation of the carotid system has been described by Valavanis.[14] Cerebral collateral flow is first assessed angiographically. The ipsilateral ICA is compressed manually while the contralateral ICA and the basilar artery are injected with contrast. The desired finding is the brisk filling of the ipsilateral middle cerebral artery. After the patency of the circle of Willis has been demonstrated, the patient is tested physiologically. The ipsilateral carotid artery is occluded with a nondetachable balloon catheter.[15] Complete obstruction of flow is demonstrated by placing contrast proximal to the balloon. Thrombosis of the vessel during the test is prevented by continuous perfusion of the vessel distal to the balloon with heparinized saline. The artery is occluded for 15 minutes, and the patient is monitored with both serial neurologic evaluations and with electroencephalography (EEG). If neurologic deficits or EEG abnormalities develop, the balloon is immediately deflated. deVries and colleagues[16] found that 11 of 136 patients developed neurologic or EEG abnormalities during temporary carotid occlusion. Intraoperative manipulation of the ICA in this group is highly risky, and 2 patients developed hemiparesis after temporary intraoperative occlusion of the ICA. Carotid stump pressures may also be measured. This is simply a reflection of the backflow pressures emanating from the collateral contralateral circulation after the occlusion of the common carotid artery. Much investigation into the use of carotid stump pressures to determine the adequacy of collateral cerebral circulation has been in the arena of carotid endarterectomy.[17,18] Such studies indicate that carotid stump pressures above 50 mm Hg suggest adequate backflow.

Although temporary balloon occlusion provides the assurance of probable safe carotid ligation, neurologic deficits have been reported in patients who maintained normal EEGs during temporary carotid occlusion.[19] Maves and colleagues[20] reported that 5 of 20 patients with normal EEGs during temporary balloon occlusion developed strokes. This suggests that, although these patients had marginal cerebral blood flow reserves, they are placed at great risk for cerebral infarction with hypotension, hypovolemia, or anemia during the procedure or the postoperative period. deVries and colleagues[16] have suggested that patients with marginal cerebral perfusion can be identified with xenon-enhanced CT blood flow measurements. Xenon is a readily absorbed radiodense gas that causes the enhancement of all tissues with high blood flow rates. With the ICA occluded, the patient breathes a mixture of 35% xenon gas and air until all tissues are saturated. Hypoperfusion of an area of the brain is demonstrated by a relative decrease in the enhancement of that area. With the use of this technique, deVries and colleagues found 13 patients who failed xenon-enhanced CT blood flow measurements out of 109 patients who passed temporary balloon occlusion. Of these 13 patients, 1 developed permanent hemiparesis after ICA resection, and 1 developed a transient hemiparesis after temporary occlusion. Conversely, of the patients who passed both temporary occlusion and the xenon study, 21 required permanent occlusion of the ligation of the carotid, and none suffered permanent sequelae directly attributable to the sacrifice of the ICA.[16]

If the patient tolerates the occlusion, the artery may be permanently occluded with detachable balloons. These balloons are filled with isotonic contrast material to allow for the easy imaging of their position postoperatively.

Balloons are usually placed in the ICA just proximal to the takeoff of the ophthalmic artery, at the carotid foramen, and just distal to the carotid bifurcation. With the use of this protocol, Andrews and colleagues[21] found no neurologic complications that were directly attributable to the preoperative balloon occlusion of the ICA in 19 patients.

Patients undergoing permanent balloon occlusion should be monitored in a neurosurgical intensive care unit for 24 hours. Particular attention must be directed to the management of hypotension, which can lead to hypoperfusion or thrombosis in the ipsilateral cerebrovascular system.

Uncontrollable intraoperative hemorrhage from the petrous or cavernous portions of the ICA presents an entirely different management problem. The immediate transfer of the patient to the angiographic suite is desirable but seldom practical. In this situation, permanent occlusion with a balloon catheter has been described.[2] A nondetachable balloon catheter is inserted into the ICA and advanced 3 cm from the carotid foramen. The balloon is not advanced further to avoid the occlusion of the ophthalmic artery. The catheter is folded on itself and ligated with strong suture to prevent deflation. If adequate soft-tissue coverage can be obtained over the catheter, it can be left permanently in place.

Delayed cerebrovascular complications can occur as a result of emboli or progressive thrombosis from the distal stump.[21] These complications are seen more commonly when the carotid artery is ligated in the neck, which leaves a large dead space distal to the ligation. An advantage of interventional neuroradiologic balloon occlusion is that the balloon can be placed immediately proximal to the ophthalmic artery, thus avoiding a large segment of the artery without flow.

Angiography itself entails significant risks. Tarr and colleagues[22] reported 11 complications of temporary balloon occlusion in 300 consecutive patients. Although 5 of these were neurologic complications, only 2 were lasting neurologic defects. The other 6 complications were asymptomatic ICA dissections. Other complications that have been reported after balloon occlusion include arrhythmias, air embolism, and intimal tear of the external iliac artery that required thrombectomy and repair.[16]

DURAL REPAIR

The maintenance of an intact dura is extremely important during the removal of extra-axial tumors. An intact dura not only protects the underlying brain, but it provides a taut plane that facilitates dissection. After the dura is torn or shredded, the surgical field is filled with cerebrospinal fluid (CSF), the likelihood of the complete removal of tumor from the dura is diminished, and wider dural resection is often required. Whenever dura is resected, attention must be given to a repair that will prevent acute CSF leak and that will also prevent long-term complications related to infection and to the formation of encephaloceles or meningoceles.

CSF leaks can occur from a number of sources, including intentional resection of the dura or from sources that are unrecognized during the procedure (Figure 52-3). Unrecognized leaks can occur as a result of small tears in the dura or openings into the pneumatic spaces of the skull base around the sphenoidal sinus and the temporal bone, particularly in the region of the petrous apex. These leaks are often difficult to identify, because the leak may have a long and circuitous path. For example, CSF leaks that originate from the temporal bone often drain through the Eustachian tube and present as rhinorrhea.

The identification of the source of a CSF leak may require high resolution thin-section CT scanning in axial and coronal planes to identify a bony defect, high-resolution CT with intrathecal contrast (metrizamide), a radioactive iodinated serum albumin study, or MR assessment. Thorough evaluation with nasal and nasopharyngeal endoscopes (occasionally with intrathecal fluorescein) can also be invaluable for the localization of CSF leaks.[23] When the rate of flow is brisk enough to allow for the capture of the fluid, analysis for β2-transferrin appears to be the most specific test to differentiate CSF from other nasopharyngeal fluids, including mucus, tears, and serum.[24] Simple testing of the fluid with a glucose dipstick fails to reliably differentiate CSF from nasal secretions.

After the site of the leak has been identified, appropriate therapy can be instituted. Leaks that occur immediately postoperatively should be treated conservatively with bed rest, the elevation of the head, and acetazolamide

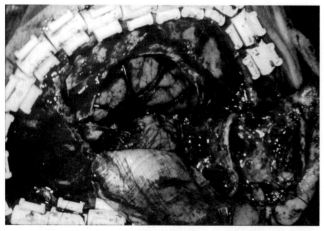

Figure 52-3. Dural defect after the resection of an ulcerative basal cell carcinoma involving the right temporal bone. The defect was repaired using a fascia lata graft covered with a superiorly based neck flap.

to decrease the production of CSF. If the leak fails to respond to these measures or is vigorous from the start, lumbar drainage can be used. A catheter is placed in the subarachnoid space of the lumbar spine. The patient is kept supine, and the drainage system is adjusted to release CSF pressure above 10 to 15 cm of water. The patient can be allowed to logroll from one side to the other, but a dangerous release of too much CSF can occur if the patient is allowed to sit up. Because of the risk of meningitis, the authors routinely use prophylactic CSF-penetrating drugs as long as the lumbar catheter is in place. To further prevent infection, the drain is removed after 5 days and replaced if needed.

It should be noted that complications associated with the use of spinal (i.e., lumbar) drains can be significant, even when procedures are properly performed.[25] The risk of complications with a CSF drainage procedure should be weighed against the risks associated with direct surgical repair; such judgments are necessarily highly individualized.

Continued CSF leakage at 5 to 10 days is considered a failure of conservative therapy, and surgical exploration and closure are needed. If the leak originates via the pneumatic system of the temporal bone, it is best approached through the mastoid. After a suboccipital craniectomy or a middle fossa procedure, it is not uncommon for a small dehiscence of the dura to leak CSF into the mastoid air-cell system. If the leak is strictly limited to the posterior mastoid, it can be repaired by the exenteration of all of the mastoid air cells and mucosa and by the obliteration of the space with a lining of the fascia and abdominal fat. It is best if the fat is packed into the wound under slight pressure. It is critically important that the connection between the mastoid antrum and the middle ear is blocked with a continuous sheet of fascia to prevent the continued leakage of the CSF through the middle ear and the Eustachian tube. This procedure does not interfere with hearing as long as the fat is kept from extending into the middle ear.

If the leak occurs in the anterior temporal bone or the pericarotid cells, then a subtotal petrosectomy (i.e., the complete obliteration of the mastoid and middle ear cleft) will be needed. The disadvantage of this procedure is that it leaves the patient with a maximal conductive hearing loss that will require a hearing aid or a semi-implantable bone oscillator for amplifications. The advantage is that the Eustachian tube can be effectively blocked, ideally with bone wax and a muscle plug, to prevent continued CSF leakage through the Eustachian tube and into the nasopharynx.[2]

CSF leaks through the anterior fossa or the sphenoid can usually be managed transnasally with nasal endoscopic techniques. The most feared leaks are those through the clivus because of the difficulty of obtaining adequate access to the defect and because of the limited local tissue available for repair. In severe cases, a microvascular free flap is brought into the defect that spans the nasopharynx to close such defects. The rectus abdominis flap is ideally suited for this situation, because it provides thin and easily harvested muscle and has a long vascular pedicle.

If dura is resected, it should be replaced with fascia lata, lyophilized dura, or another suitable substitute. It is impossible to provide an absolutely watertight closure of the dura after it is resected. However, strict attention should be paid to those factors that will promote the healing of the tissues that surround the defect. These factors include the careful suture of the dural graft without gaps or herniation of brain tissue between the graft and the dura. Moreover, the adequate reduction of CSF pressure with lumbar drainage and the adequate support of the graft with soft tissue and bone if the defect is large are critical. This support is usually provided by a myocutaneous flap (either a pedicle flap or a free microvascular flap).

The resection of many tumors leaves large intracranial and extracranial defects and little or no supporting tissue between them. If the skull base is not reconstructed, encephaloceles or pseudomeningoceles can form. Encephaloceles are herniations of the brain through the bony defect. Pseudomeningoceles are permanent accumulations of CSF in the wound or under a flap. They are distinguished from true meningoceles because they are not lined by meninges. The obliteration of the entire defect with a free revascularized tissue flap (free flap) is the best reconstructive option in these cases. The temporalis flap, although ideal for filling small dead spaces or covering small bony defects, is inadequate for both the strength and bulk needed for the repair of large defects. The failure to adequately obliterate such defects can allow for the formation of large pseudomeningoceles.

Staged Resection of Lateral Skull-Base Tumors with Intracranial Extension

Tumors of the lateral skull base that traverse the dura may require staged removal to limit complications related to CSF leakage. As mentioned, the dura should be maintained intact to protect the underlying central nervous system (CNS) and its vasculature. The CSF underlying intact dura will often push the tumor laterally, thus facilitating dissection external to the dura. This CSF pressure is particularly important for tumors that extend toward the tentorium posteriorly, which would otherwise be difficult to visualize.[2] When the dura is infiltrated by the tumor, these areas are temporarily left undissected to maintain the integrity of the dura. Residual tumor may

be removed with biopsy forceps at the end of the procedure. Fisch and Mattox[2] have emphasized the danger of widely opening the cerebellopontine angle. Disrupted venous outflow and the sacrifice of the vagus nerve that promotes coughing can combine to greatly increase the likelihood of CSF drainage. A two-stage approach to large intradural tumors can reduce unnecessary risks of morbidity and mortality.

When the tumor has substantial intradural and extradural extensions, the decision must be made whether to attempt a one-stage intracranial–extracranial resection or to perform a two-staged resection. Although single-stage resections have been reported by several authors, many others prefer a two-staged resection. Fisch[26] described a two-staged approach for removing large glomus tumors. The first stage was a lateral approach that involved removing all accessible tumor and sealing the wound, including the Eustachian tube, against CSF leak. A second-stage neurosurgical intervention can be performed without the risk of CSF leakage through a contaminated wound.

Alternatively, the order of the resections can be reversed, as described by Holliday and colleagues.[27] The first stage entails a craniotomy and the placement of fascia lata (i.e., neodura) between the brain and the tumor. After a short period of healing, a second-stage lateral approach is performed with the knowledge that the brain, the CSF, and the subarachnoid space are protected from the surgical field.

The desired effect of staging tumors in this way is to alter the tumor's location relative to the dura and brain, thus transforming the tumor from an intradural to an extradural position in preparation for the critical resection stage. In addition to the obvious advantages of reducing the likelihood of CSF leak, this approach avoids subsequent surgery on tumors found to have intracranial extension that precludes complete removal.

Drains and Retraction

Potential CSF leakage and subsequent meningitis after the removal of tumors with intradural extension can be minimized with the use of passive drains rather than suction drains. This is particularly important when dural and pharyngeal defects remain open. If suction drainage is required, the drain should be positioned away from the defects to minimize the chance of CSF leakage and the drawing of secretions into the wound.

The exposure of the lateral skull base frequently requires the sustained retraction of the temporal lobe and, when the condyle is left intact, the mandible. Specifically adapted self-retraction instruments are available.[2] CNS infarction can be avoided by adequate brain relaxation provided by intraoperative steroids, mannitol, and hyperventilation to induce mild hypocarbia. In addition, CSF diversion via a lumbar drain may be required for pronounced CSF leakage noted at the time of dura and wound closure or during the early postoperative period.[23]

TEMPOROMANDIBULAR JOINT

The anterior extension of infratemporal approaches beyond the type B approach requires either anterior or inferior displacement of the mandibular condyle after the removal of bone in the region of the glenoid fossa. This mobilization and division of the temporomandibular joint can result in functional limitations that produce impaired occlusion and diminished mandibular excursion.

The condyle is capped with a fibrous tissue layer that overlies the layers of cartilage anchored in the enchondral bone of the mandible. Although hyaline cartilage has little potential for regrowth, the dense fibrous cap of the condyle provides regenerative potential.[28] The articular disc is interposed between the condylar and glenoid articular surfaces of the temporomandibular joint. The temporomandibular joint is reinforced by the surrounding capsule and the temporomandibular (i.e., lateral) ligaments attached at the zygomatic arch above and the condylar neck below. The capsule and ligaments provide inelastic suspension of the mandible and restrain the joint from undergoing gross displacement. The full excursion of the mandible, powered by the muscles of mastication, is translated at the temporomandibular joint to a complex series of displacements of the disc–condyle complex.

The impaired function of the temporomandibular joint produces a variety of symptoms. Masticatory pain typically results from temporomandibular joint fibrosis or degeneration or the contracture and splinting of the muscles of mastication that characterizes the myofascial pain syndrome. Temporomandibular joint noises and impaired jaw mobility reflect the interruption of the rotational arc between the disc–condyle complex and the glenoid articular surface. Malocclusion may be sensed subjectively or produce discomfort when the jaw is clenched. Malocclusion may be based on the dysfunction of the muscles of mastication (particularly the lateral pterygoid) and altered relationships of the disc-condyle complex.

The clinical assessment of sites of discomfort, the degree and pattern of jaw mobility, the associated joint tenderness and sounds, and the evaluation of occlusal disharmony often indicate the source of the patient's symptoms. Standard radiographic evaluation demonstrates the subarticular bone that underlies the glenoid and condylar facets and as such does not assess the articular surfaces themselves. Panoramic projections and CT scans provide the most useful means for screening the supporting bony structures. Arthrography, which involves the injection of contrast medium into the synovial sac, images the articular disc, but it can produce artifacts and complications associated with the infusion of contrast. MR scanning of the temporomandibular joint has been used to study the articular surfaces and disc with resolution not previously achieved with conventional radiography.

Fortunately the serious impairment of joint function after infratemporal exposure is uncommon, most likely as a result of the considerable adaptive capacity of the joint. The dense fibrous tissue that lines the temporal and condylar facets maintains the capacity to regenerate and remodel as dictated by altered surface contact and functional demands.

Perioperative conditions associated with infratemporal surgery that may affect temporomandibular joint function relate to joint trauma, the division of the supporting ligaments and the muscles of mastication, and postoperative infection and immobilization. Excessive jaw manipulation can result in the stretching of the temporomandibular ligaments and the compression of the articular disc. Temporomandibular joint instability, intracapsular fibrosis, and disc deformation and displacement are potential sequelae. The derangement of the articular disc reduces the stability, flexibility, and lubrication of joint function. With the loss of the normal disc relationships, direct bony contact between condylar and glenoid facets may induce the fibrotic union of the articular surfaces. These observations suggest that the following perioperative measures can reduce temporomandibular dysfunction after infratemporal fossa surgery:

1. Intraoperative manipulation of the jaw that stretches the temporomandibular ligaments and that produces impact loading of the joint should be avoided. This may occur with excessive opening or the lateral distraction of the jaw.

2. Incision into the joint capsule should be avoided if the preservation of the joint is anticipated. An intracapsular cicatrix may exert traction on the joint capsule, the disc, or both, with resultant trismus.

3. If substantial manipulation of the temporomandibular joint is required to afford adequate exposure, the articular disc and glenoid fossa should be removed. Because the articular disc does not have the capacity to change its configuration or to undergo cellular remodeling, its removal[2] may avoid the postoperative trismus produced by ankylosis of the joint. The

removal of the bone of the glenoid fossa leads to considerable asymmetry of the resting position of the two condyles and resultant facial deformity. The problem of correcting such a deformity is difficult. Only grafts and osteotomies can be used to improve facial symmetry.[28]

4. Infection can produce ankylosis of the temporomandibular joint and should be avoided.

5. Prolonged mandibular immobilization predisposes the patient to atrophy and contracture of the muscles of mastication. When contractures involve the elevator muscles, a permanent decrease in the resting length of the muscle can produce trismus and reduced interarch opening. Patients should therefore be instructed in mouth-opening exercises to minimize muscle fibrosis. Mandibular range-of-motion exercises and prostheses to promote occlusal harmony may be required to eliminate masticatory symptoms.

CRANIAL NERVES

Infratemporal surgical approaches provide the exposure of lesions located between the jugular foramen and the parasellar–parasphenoid regions. Cranial nerves III through XII are placed at risk through such exposure, given their course through the anterolateral skull base.

Cranial Nerves III, IV, and VI

The oculomotor cranial nerves are encountered with infratemporal approaches when anterior extension involves the lateral wall of the cavernous sinus or the superior orbital fissure. Because the vast majority of lesions approached with this technique are benign, oculomotor nerve damage is often from compression, and direct nerve invasion is uncommon. Therefore surgical experience with anteriorly extending glomus tumors, for example, has shown that the oculomotor cranial nerves may be preserved in the majority of cases.[2] This stands in contrast with the postoperative results noted with regard to caudal cranial nerves IX to XII, which are directly adjacent to glomus tumors. Mild diplopia may be rehabilitated with exercise, whereas severe diplopia may require oculomotor muscle transposition or prism glasses.[29]

Cranial Nerve V

The trigeminal ganglion overlies the petrous ICA in its cavernous segment. Branches of the trigeminal ganglion are therefore encountered during approaches to the anterior clivus, the nasopharynx, and the parasellar–parasphenoid compartments. These branches are often sacrificed to expose the anterior and medial extent of tumors that extend to these regions.

Cranial Nerve V1: Ophthalmic Nerve

The ophthalmic nerve courses anteriorly from the trigeminal ganglion to enter the superior aspect of the cavernous sinus. The nerve may require division if it is involved with an intracavernous tumor or a lesion that extends to the superior orbital fissure. The division of the ophthalmic nerve produces anesthesia of the superior scalp, the forehead, and, most importantly, the anterior aspect of the globe. Unprotected by the corneal reflex, the globe is at risk for abrasion, corneal desiccation, and, ultimately, ulceration. This risk is increased by a concomitant facial paresis or paralysis. Because of this, measures to promote hydration and physical protection of the globe are needed. Ocular drops and ointments as well as protective glasses are useful adjuncts. With concomitant facial palsy, eyelid weight implantation and canthoplastic procedures may be required.

Cranial Nerve V2: Maxillary Nerve

The maxillary nerve courses straight anteriorly from the trigeminal ganglion and often shields the parasellar and parasphenoid compartments from infratemporal exposure. Sectioning of the maxillary nerve is required to adequately expose nasopharyngeal and parasellar tumors via the type C approach. Likewise, transfacial dissection typically requires V2 division peripherally to mobilize the orbitomaxillary skeleton, and this is followed by neurorrhaphy before closure.

Unilateral injury or the resection of the maxillary nerve produces midfacial and intraoral anesthesia that often recovers to some degree and that rarely produces serious sequelae.[30] A rare but notable complication of surgery proximate to the trigeminal nerve is postoperative neuralgia (i.e., anesthesia dolorosa). Although this may occur in the distribution of any cranial nerve sensory branch that is injured, in the authors' experience it is most likely to occur after the surgical manipulation of the maxillary nerve. The syndrome of anesthesia dolorosa produces dysesthesias in the distribution of the sensory branch and should be managed similarly to trigeminal neuralgia (i.e., tic douloureux). Medical therapy with analgesics is often unsatisfactory as a result of the potential for dependence on narcotics and their derivatives. Phenytoin, carbamazepine, baclofen, and other central-acting drugs may provide relief. Failing medical management, trigeminal rhizotomy proximal to the exit of the damaged branch may be indicated if trial injections of local anesthetics provide symptomatic relief.

Cranial Nerve V3: Mandibular Nerve

The mandibular branch of the trigeminal nerve is the branch that is most frequently sectioned with infratemporal exposures because of its vertical course as it descends from the middle fossa via the foramen ovale. The division of the mandibular nerve affords direct exposure of the petrous ICA from its genu forward to the foramen lacerum.

Mandibular nerve injury produces chin and intraoral anesthesia, which are unilateral and produce little disability.[30] Motor dysfunction of the muscles of mastication on one side typically produces only mild mandibular drift and trismus. Jaw-opening exercises and dental appliances may be required to strengthen those muscles of mastication that are functional to improve occlusal relationships. The importance of dental hygiene should be emphasized, because intraoral anesthesia can promote dental decay and gingival recession as a result of inconspicuous food residue. The disruption of motor innervation or of the vascular supply to the temporalis muscle may also result in temporal muscle wasting. Special care is paid to the preservation of the deep temporal artery and the motor branch of the trigeminal nerve during the lateral surgical approaches. This is especially true for the infratemporal fossa approaches to the floor of the middle cranial fossa. Temporal muscle devitalization may leave a depression (i.e., a sunken appearance) in the temporal fossa and an unsightly cosmetic defect.

In general, the sensory deficits produced by trigeminal nerve injury with infratemporal approaches are unilateral and compensated by intact sensation circumferential to the affected area.[30] In the uncommon setting of large tumors that require exposure and the possible division of trigeminal nerve branches bilaterally, sensory deficits can predispose patients to facial and oral injuries in response to extremes in temperature.

Cranial Nerve VII: Facial Nerve

The direct surgical exposure of lesions isolated to the clivus, the nasopharynx, and the parasellar–parasphenoid regions through infratemporal approaches provides a short working distance and does not require the displacement of the facial nerve.[31] Modified type C approaches that enable zygomatic arch removal and deep access to the infratemporal fossa call for the inferior displacement of the frontotemporal branches of the facial nerve without the transposition of the main trunk. However, lesions that are based in or that extend anteriorly from the jugular foramen require anterior transposition and occasionally the temporary division of the facial nerve to adequately expose the infratemporal ICA and the bony compartments medial to the artery.

Intraoperative monitoring of evoked facial nerve activity provides the ability to detect the early mechanical stimulation of the nerve.[6,7] Microphonic activity and nonrepetitive burst activity produced by drilling bone adjacent to the facial nerve epineurium may herald the exposure of the nerve.

The trauma associated with the anterior transposition of the facial nerve can be minimized by the following technical steps[2]:

1. Remove as much of the bony fallopian canal surrounding the facial nerve as possible, preferably well beyond 180 degrees.

2. Facial nerve elevation is most difficult in the region of the stylomastoid foramen, where it is tethered by periosteal and muscular attachments. Trauma to the nerve can be reduced by refraining from isolating the facial nerve trunk from these tenacious attachments and mobilizing the nerve in continuity with the adjacent periosteum and the digastric musculature.

3. Expose the superior (i.e., temporal and zygomatic) and inferior (i.e., cervical) branches of the facial nerve as far anteriorly as their initial branch points to facilitate the atraumatic elevation of the nerve.

4. The nerve should be mobilized only after complete exposure from the geniculate ganglion to the stylomastoid foramen and the sharp division of its tympanic and digastric branches.

5. Avoid dehydration, tension, and the pinching of the mobilized nerve with infratemporal retraction.

6. If tumor has invaded the fallopian canal and the facial epineurium, the epineurium should be excised only after the nerve is replaced in the mastoid. This avoids the stretch injury that is likely to occur in nerve segments that are devoid of epineurium.

Rates of preservation or recovery of facial function without transpositions are typically good. Although transposition may be associated with nerve injury and fiber degeneration, Fisch and Mattox[2] report an average recovery of 80% of facial function (i.e., House–Brackman scale grade II). The removal of tumor-involved epineurium is associated with an average return of 70% of facial function (i.e., House–Brackman scale grade III). Using a modification of the technique described by Fisch,[32] Brackmann[33] demonstrated improvements in immediate and long-term facial function without the compromise of infratemporal exposure. These modifications involve the elevation and anterior retraction of the tail and the deep lobe of the parotid gland medial to the facial nerve.

Tumors that extend to the parasellar and parasphenoid regions require anterior exposure that places excessive tension on the transposed facial nerve. In such instances, the nerve is divided, and reanastomosis is performed after tumor removal. To enhance nerve regeneration and to minimize mass movement and synkinesis, the nerve should be divided as far distally as possible, preferably beyond the pes anserinus.[3] This technique is associated with eventual excellent return of tone and good return of movement, albeit with synkinesis and occasional spasticity.

The unintentional transection of the facial nerve must be repaired immediately via primary suture neurorrhaphy repair or nerve interposition if a large segment is missing. Nerve grafts from the great auricular nerve or the sural nerve serve as good donors. Epineural repair is performed, with the maintenance of the principle of tension-free repair under magnification. The best function usually expected from such a nerve graft repair would be House–Brackmann scale grade III.[34] If facial nerve injury occurs in the cisternal or canalicular segments where an epineural layer is absent or when nerve repair is not possible, a hypoglossal–facial nerve anastomosis may be performed. These procedures may be performed with the potential for good results, the restoration of facial symmetry and muscle tone, minimal to absent synkinesis, and the restoration of a nasolabial fold.[35]

Attention to appropriate eye care should be paid anytime that facial weakness develops after surgery. This may be in the setting of paresis or paralysis. The sequelae of exposure keratitis and corneal injury may be prevented (Figure 52-4). The chances of injury are increased when there is an additional cranial nerve V deficit through a loss of corneal sensation. A combination of artificial tears and lubricating ointment are applied. In cases of incomplete eye closure, moisture chambers have been used as well. Tarsorrhaphy sutures provide more longstanding corneal protection. However, taping the eyes shut is discouraged, because this type of fixation is not absolutely secure. The lids may still open, and the adhesive side of the tape can create corneal abrasions. Surgical implantation of a gold-weight prosthesis in the upper eyelid outside of the orbital septum and under the orbicularis oculi muscle to allow the effects of gravity to aid in lid closure may be considered. This technique is particularly useful, and the gold weight may easily be removed if nerve function returns. If lower-lid ectropion is developing, a lid-tightening procedure or a lateral canthopexy may be performed.

INFECTIOUS COMPLICATIONS

Many of the precautions taken to prevent infectious complications after surgery in the lateral cranial fossa follow the same overall guidelines for clean neurosurgical procedures unless the Eustachian tube or the potentially infected mastoid–middle-ear spaces are entered. When the operation does not involve transgression into the upper aerodigestive tract, the neurosurgical literature supports the use of prophylactic perioperative antibiotics.[36] Wound infections after clean neurosurgical cases typically involve gram-positive organisms. Therefore, spectrum coverage for *Staphylococcus* spp. is necessary.

The authors routinely use intravenous prophylactic antibiotics delivered perioperatively (i.e., a preoperative dose followed by treatment for 36 hours after surgery). The selection of the antibiotic is based on the need for activity against the normal flora and expected pathogens. For cases in which preoperative radiation therapy has been delivered, antibiotic selection is further guided by the recognized higher incidence of postoperative infection with *Pseudomonas aeruginosa.*

LABYRINTHINE INJURY

Inadvertent violation into or through the bony and membranous labyrinth of the inner ear during mastoid surgery may lead to hearing loss and vestibular symptoms. However, with the translabyrinthine and transcochlear approaches, the labyrinth is purposely obliterated to

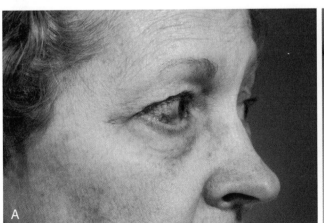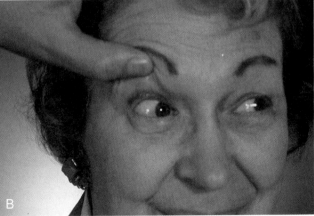

Figure 52-4. A, Early findings of conjunctival inflammation associated with reduced lacrimation and reduced strength of eye closure in a patient with clinically normal facial function after vestibular schwannoma resection. **B,** Response to topical ocular lubricant and drops.

gain access to the cerebellopontine angle and the internal auditory canal, with the expected sacrifice of hearing and balance function. With an approach such as the infratemporal fossa approach, subtotal petrosectomy is performed, which features a complete mastoidectomy with the preservation of the labyrinth. With the other approaches to the petrous apex through the mastoid or the transcanal route, care is taken to not violate the basal turn of the cochlea.

The preservation of the vestibular labyrinth is best carried out by identifying the horizontal semicircular canal, which is one of the first readily identifiable landmarks after the completion of the cortical mastoidectomy. The bone over the horizontal semicircular canal is more dense than the mastoid air-cell bone, and it is whiter in color. The horizontal semicircular canal may be found superoposterior to the body of the incus as the mastoid antrum is entered after the removal of the Koerner septum, which is a bony extension from the petrosquamous suture line. After the identification of the horizontal semicircular canal, the posterior semicircular canal may be identified posterior and inferior to it. The horizontal semicircular canal nearly bisects the arc of the posterior semicircular canal.

Any bone removal to gain access to the petrous apex via the infracochlear or infralabyrinthine approach should be performed with the identification of the basal turn of the cochlea. The bone over the promontory may be removed with the preservation of the endosteum of the inner ear so as to "blue line" the basal turn of the cochlea with the use of a diamond stone bur. Additional bone removal to gain wider access to the petrous apex through these latter approaches must then come from the bone over the jugular bulb and the petrous carotid artery.

Inadvertent entry into the labyrinth should be repaired by placing fascia over the defect immediately. Either bone wax or bone dust pate may be placed over the fascia to secure its position. Care is taken to not apply direct suction into the fistulous site to preserve the labyrinthine fluids.

SKULL-BASE SURGERY IN PREVIOUSLY RADIATED FIELDS

Preoperative radiation therapy entails inherent risks for the removal of lateral skull-base neoplasms. To minimize these risks, preoperative radiation therapy should be avoided when possible when a patient presents few risk factors for undergoing surgical resection. Postoperative radiation therapy after successful tumor removal and reconstruction with well-vascularized tissue carries far less potential for infection and necrosis. The risks of preoperative radiation therapy are related to the treatment modalities employed, including the time–dose–fraction

program, the size of the radiation ports, and the magnitude of the radiation dose.

The radiotherapy of lateral skull-base lesions is complicated by the need for the precise delivery of radiation to complex geometric figures of different sizes. Impaired CNS vasculature can predispose the patient to parenchymal injury with surgery. The concept of employing surgery for radiation failure as a salvage procedure is often difficult to justify for lateral skull-base lesions, where the incidence of major complications (e.g., osteitis, pachymeningitis, brain abscess, phlebitis, erosion of the vessel walls[1]) is greatly elevated when radiation therapy is followed by surgery.

The authors' experience with lateral skull-base surgery after radiation therapy, even when focused radiotherapy (i.e., radiosurgical) techniques are adopted, suggests that planes of cleavage between both normal and abnormal tissue are obscured.[37] Severe fibrosis of the great vessels and the cranial nerves hampers the atraumatic removal of adjacent tumor. In addition, tumors are less likely to be easily separated from the adjacent dura, which requires dural resection to provide a tumor-free margin. Preoperative radiation therapy also presents a significant risk of osteoradionecrosis, which can present years after the primary course of high-dose irradiation. The area of necrosis may be localized (i.e., only the tympanic ring is involved) or diffuse (i.e., disease has extended throughout the temporal bone, with clival involvement owing to regional vascular insufficiency). Ramsden and colleagues[38] found that approximately one third of patients with diffuse osteoradionecrosis had intracranial infections. They found temporal lobe abscesses, a cerebellar abscess, and an extradural posterior fossa abscess. The remaining patients demonstrated the exposure of the dura and lateral sinus, the erosion of the fallopian canal with facial nerve palsy, and the erosion of the horizontal semicircular canal with vertigo and deafness. The risk of future osteoradionecrosis is diminished by reconstruction with vascularized bone grafts.

As an alterative approach, when combined therapy is indicated on the basis of tumor histologic findings or distribution, postoperative radiation therapy is preferred. If postoperative radiation therapy is planned, wire sutures and osseointegrated implants should be avoided, because these can lead to the scattering of radiation.

REFERENCES

1. Sasaki C, McCabe B, Kirschner J, editors: *Surgery of the skull base,* Philadelphia, 1984, Lippincott.
2. Fisch U, Mattox D, editors: *Microsurgery of the skull base,* New York, 1988, Thieme.
3. Jackson CE: *Surgery of skull base tumors,* New York, 1991, Churchill Livingstone.
4. Graham M: Skull base surgery. *Otolaryngol Clin North Am* 1984;17:459–629.

5. Souliere CR Jr, Telian SA, Kemink JL: The infratemporal fossa approach to skull base surgery. *Ear Nose Throat J* 1991;70(9):620–636.

6. Kartush JM: Electroneurography and intraoperative facial monitoring in contemporary neurotology. *Otolaryngol Head Neck Surg* 1989;101(4):496–503.

7. Niparko JK, Kileny PR, Kemink JL, et al: Neurophysiologic intraoperative monitoring: II: Facial nerve function. *Am J Otol* 1989;10(1):55–61.

8. Aminoff MJ: The use of somatosensory evoked potentials in the evaluation of the central nervous system. *Neurol Clin* 1988;6(4):809–823.

9. Petruzzelli GJ, Origitano TC, Stankiewicz JA, et al: Frameless stereotactic localization in cranial base surgery. *Skull Base Surg* 2000;10(3):125–130.

10. Ahn HS, Sexton CS, Zinreich SJ, et al: Neuroradiologic techniques in the evaluation of lesions of the skull base. *Ear Nose Throat J* 1986;65(2):74–83.

11. Morre O, Baker HW: Carotid-artery ligation in surgery of the head and neck. *Cancer* 1955;8(4):712–726.

12. Little JR, Cook A, Lesser RP: Treatment of acute focal cerebral ischemia with dimethyl sulfoxide. *Neurosurgery* 1981;9(1):34–39.

13. Sundt TM Jr, Grant WC, Garcia JH: Restoration of middle cerebral artery flow in experimental infarction. *J Neurosurg* 1969;31(3):311–321.

14. Valavanis A: Preoperative embolization of the head and neck: Indications, patient selection, goals, and precautions. *AJNR Am J Neuroradiol* 1986;7(5):943–952.

15. Meinig G, Gunther R, Ulrich P, et al: Reduced risk of ICA ligation after balloon occlusion test. *Neurosurg Rev* 1982;5(3):95–98.

16. de Vries EJ, Sekhar LN, Horton JA, et al: A new method to predict safe resection of the internal carotid artery. *Laryngoscope* 1990;100(1):85–88.

17. Whitley D, Cherry KJ Jr: Predictive value of carotid artery stump pressures during carotid endarterectomy. *Neurosurg Clin N Am* 1996;7(4):723–732.

18. Ehrnefeld WK, Stoney RJ, Wylie EJ: Relation of carotid stump pressure to safety of carotid artery ligation. *Surgery* 1983;93(2):299–305.

19. Kwaan JH, Peterson GJ, Connolly JE: Stump pressure: An unreliable guide for shunting during carotid endarterectomy. *Arch Surg* 1980;115(9):1083–1086.

20. Maves MD, Bruns MD, Keenan MJ: Carotid artery resection for head and neck cancer. *Ann Otol Rhinol Laryngol* 1992;101(9):778–781.

21. Andrews JC, Valavanis A, Fisch U: Management of the internal carotid artery in surgery of the skull base. *Laryngoscope* 1989;99(12):1224–1229.

22. Tarr R, Jungrei C, Horton A, et al: Complications of preoperative balloon test occlusion of the internal carotid arteries: Experience in 300 cases. *Skull Base Surg* 1991;1:240–243.

23. Mattox DE, Kennedy DW: Endoscopic management of cerebrospinal fluid leaks and cephaloceles. *Laryngoscope* 1990;100(8):857–862.

24. Oberascher G, Arrer E: Efficiency of various methods of identifying cerebrospinal fluid in oto- and rhinorrhea. *ORL J Otorhinolaryngol Relat Spec* 1986;48(6):320–325.

25. Weaver KD, Wiseman DB, Farber M, et al: Complications of lumbar drainage after thoracoabdominal aortic aneurysm repair. *J Vasc Surg* 2001;34(4):623–627.

26. Fisch U: Infratemporal fossa approach for extensive tumors of the temporal bones and base of skull. In Silverstein H, Norrell H, editors: *Neurological surgery of the ear,* Birmingham, England, 1977, Aesculapius.

27. Holliday MJ, Nachlas N, Kennedy DW: Uses and modifications of the infratemporal fossa approach to skull-base tumors. *Ear Nose Throat J* 1986;65(3):101–106.

28. Sarnat BG, Laskin DM, editors: *The temporomandibular joint,* Philadelphia, 1990, WB Saunders.

29. May M: Management of cranial nerves I through VII following skull base surgery. *Otolaryngol Head Neck Surg* 1980;88(5):560–575.

30. Sataloff RT, Myers DL, Kremer FB: Management of cranial nerve injury following surgery of the skull base. *Otolaryngol Clin North Am* 1984;17(3):577–589.

31. Briggs R, Mattox DE: Management of the facial nerve in skull base surgery. *Otolaryngol Clin North Am* 1991;24(3):653–662.

32. Fisch U: Infratemporal fossa approach for glomus tumors of the temporal bone. *Ann Otol Rhinol Laryngol* 1982;91(5 Pt 1):474–479.

33. Brackmann DE: The facial nerve in the infratemporal approach. *Otolaryngol Head Neck Surg* 1987;97(1):15–17.

34. Stephanian E, Sekhar LN, Janecka IP, et al: Facial nerve repair by interposition nerve graft: Results in 22 patients. *Neurosurgery* 1992;31(1):73–76.

35. Pitty LF, Tator CH: Hypoglossal-facial nerve anastomosis for facial nerve palsy following surgery for cerebellopontine angle tumors. *J Neurosurg* 1992;77(5):724–731.

36. Dempsey R, Rapp RP, Young B, et al: Prophylactic parenteral antibiotics in clean neurosurgical procedures: A review. *J Neurosurg* 1988;69(1):52–57.

37. Limb CJ, Long DM, Niparko JK: Acoustic neuromas after failed radiation therapy: Challenges of surgical salvage. *Laryngoscope* 2005;115(1):93–98.

38. Ramsden RT, Bulman CH, Lorigan BP: Osteoradionecrosis of the temporal bone. *J Laryngol Otol* 1975;89(9):941–955.

CHAPTER 53

Complications of Acoustic Neuroma Surgery

C.Y. Joseph Chang, Brian S. Wang, and Steven W. Cheung

The rates of morbidity and mortality associated with the surgical treatment of acoustic neuromas have changed significantly during the past century. Before the early 1900s, surgical mortality rates approached 80%.[1] Harvey Cushing developed techniques to reduce the surgical mortality rate to 20% by 1917 and to an even lower level by 1931.[1–4] At that time, the preservation of hearing and facial nerve function was thought to be futile, and tumor resection was usually subtotal. There was a high rate of complications related to tumor regrowth as well.

During the 1960s, major advances in anesthesia, pharmacology, and especially surgical technique were developed, to a large extent by William House.[1] The occurrence of serious complications after acoustic tumor surgery has become uncommon, and posterior fossa surgery has become almost routine. The anatomic preservation of cranial nerves, including the facial nerve, is now routinely achievable, with the majority of patients attaining excellent functional outcomes. The preservation of serviceable hearing still remains problematic, although hearing preservation rates have been improving steadily over the past decade with the advent of improved surgical techniques and primary radiation treatments.

Serious complications still occur occasionally, and the surgeon must take all necessary precautions to avoid adverse outcomes. It is incumbent on the surgeon to diagnose and treat any complication early to provide the best possible outcome for the patient. The goals of this chapter are to discuss both the minor and major complications associated with acoustic tumor treatment as well as their timely diagnosis and the interventions used to address them.

INTRAOPERATIVE COMPLICATIONS

Many of the problems that the surgeon may encounter intraoperatively are potentially catastrophic and require immediate recognition and corrective action. The majority of these difficulties are vascular in nature and include both venous and arterial complications.

Venous Hemorrhage

Significant venous bleeding during acoustic tumor surgery can arise from the sigmoid sinus, the jugular bulb, and superior petrosal sinus. When injury to these structures occurs, it is usually during bone dissection as part of translabyrinthine, retrosigmoid, and middle fossa craniotomies. The sigmoid sinus is most commonly injured during the translabyrinthine approach, and the jugular bulb is most commonly injured during both the translabyrinthine and retrosigmoid approaches. Injury occurs during the exposure of the inferior portion of the internal auditory canal (IAC), especially if the bulb is relatively cephalad.

The superior petrosal sinus is vulnerable to injury during dural elevation off of the petrous ridge with the middle fossa approach and during petrous bone decompression with the translabyrinthine approach. In general, the violation of the dural venous sinuses occurs infrequently when diamond burrs and copious irrigation are used for dissection. In addition, during the translabyrinthine approach, the sigmoid sinus can be further protected by leaving an area of bone overlying the structure, which is often called *Bill's island.* When bleeding is encountered, expeditious management is required to control hemorrhage to proceed with the remainder of the procedure.

Because the dural sinuses are a low-pressure system, hemorrhage can usually be controlled with local pressure and the use of hemostatic agents such as oxidized cellulose (Surgicel; Ethicon, Somerville, NJ) or microfibrillar collagen (Avitene; Davol, Cranston, RI) or with bipolar electrocautery. If the laceration occurs in an area that is not fully decompressed of bone, wax can be applied to the bleeding site. An island of bone around the waxed area can be maintained for the remainder of the procedure. In some cases, repair using 6-0 or 7-0 monofilament suture can be performed, but this is rarely necessary. There are other techniques available for the control of more serious hemorrhage. Bleeding from the superior petrosal sinus that is refractory to control with bipolar electrocautery can be managed by creating dural incisions on both sides of the sinus to allow for the application of hemoclips. Large sigmoid sinus defects that are otherwise refractory can be treated with extraluminal or intraluminal packing, essentially to obliterate the sinus. Extraluminal packing can be used if there is adequate bone to pack against around the venous structure both proximal and distal to the bleeding site. When extraluminal packing is not possible, intraluminal packing can be used. The packing material used should be large enough so that a portion remains outside of the venous opening to avoid the embolization of the material to the cardiopulmonary system. When obliterating the sigmoid sinus, care must be taken to preserve the patency of the vein of Labbé to avoid temporal lobe venous infarction.

Air embolism is rarely seen today, because the sitting position, which is a significant risk factor for this complication, is rarely used for the removal of acoustic neuromas.[5,6] This complication can still occur in cases in which a large rent in a venous sinus is not closed quickly. The systemic signs of this complication include intravascular crepitation, hypotension, tachycardia, and a decline in end-expiratory partial pressure of carbon dioxide. Classically there is a mechanical-sounding heart murmur. If this complication occurs, inhalational anesthetic agents are stopped, and 100% oxygen is administered while the bleeding site is controlled as quickly as possible. To reduce airflow into the venous lumen, the local venous pressure should be increased by placing the patient in the Trendelenburg position. Other measures that can be considered include rotating the patient to the left side to trap the intravascular air within the right ventricle. In severe cases, the air can then be aspirated through a central venous catheter.[7,8]

Venous Infarction

Brain retraction during surgery can result in local venous infarctions. The cerebellum is most at risk during posterior approaches such as the retrosigmoid craniotomy, especially if the tumor is large. Direct compressive injury to the brain can cause significant edema with resulting brain dysfunction postoperatively, and this can complicate patient management. Elevated infratentorial pressure worsens the problem. Management of this condition is discussed in a later section of this chapter. Prevention is always best, so care is taken to minimize the level of brain retraction that is necessary to complete tumor resection.

A significant injury to the vein of Labbé is a rare complication of acoustic tumor surgery that can result in temporal lobe infarction with subsequent recurrent seizures. Temporal lobe infarction on the dominant side can cause language dysfunction with expressive and receptive aphasia. Again, the most common mechanism of injury during acoustic tumor surgery occurs with the middle fossa approach where temporal lobe retraction can occasionally impede venous outflow. Such venous complications can be avoided with the gentle use of temporal lobe retraction and the preservation of venous outflow from the vein of Labbé when manipulating the sigmoid and transverse sinuses. Patients who develop seizures as a result of temporal lobe infarction should be treated with antiseizure medications, and language deficits can be treated with speech and language rehabilitation.

Arterial Complications

Unless the basilar artery is involved with a large tumor, major arterial bleeding is rarely encountered during posterior fossa surgery. By contrast, injury to the anterior inferior cerebellar artery (AICA), which supplies the lateral

pontomedullary region of the brainstem, is a significant concern. This vessel is frequently encountered in association with the tumor, and it usually forms a loop within the cerebellopontine angle. It may be intermingled between cranial nerves VII and VIII, and it may form a loop within the IAC. Tumor dissection in this area must be performed with care taken to preserve the main loop of the AICA and its distal tributaries. If vasospasm occurs, papaverine should be administered to the vessel topically. The areas at risk for infarction as a result of compromise to the AICA include the vestibulocochlear nerve, the labyrinth, the nuclei of the facial and trigeminal nerves, the medial lemniscus, the lateral lemniscus, the central tegmental tract, the spinothalamic tract, and the cerebellar peduncles.[9,10] The blood flow patterns from the AICA are variable, and, therefore, the clinical symptoms can vary. The typical clinical findings include ipsilateral trigeminal nerve dysfunction, hearing loss, Horner syndrome, vertigo, cerebellar ataxia, myoclonus of the uvula and pharynx, a contralateral decrease in pain and temperature sensation, and hemiparesis.[10-12] At the present time, major deficits such as the full AICA and posterior inferior cerebellar artery syndromes are rarely encountered.[10]

The sequelae of brainstem infarction can be severe and may lead to increased intracranial pressure, autonomic dysfunction, and possible death. In these cases, supportive treatment, including the administration of corticosteroids, pharmacologic agents to support the blood pressure, mechanical ventilation, and the placement of a ventriculostomy for cerebrospinal fluid (CSF) pressure control, is provided.

POSTOPERATIVE COMPLICATIONS

Complications can be divided into emergency and nonemergency cases. Emergency cases require immediate treatment to prevent sequelae or death and include cerebral edema, intracranial hemorrhage, pneumocephalus, and bacterial meningitis. Nonemergency complications require less drastic measures and include CSF leak, cerebrovascular accident, trigeminal and lower cranial nerve dysfunction, dizziness, headache, and medical complications. Although transient facial nerve paralysis occurs frequently and is not specifically considered a complication, the management of this condition will also be discussed.

Hemorrhage

Intracranial hemorrhage after acoustic neuroma surgery occurs only rarely, but it can be catastrophic, and it can cause rapid death if it is not treated immediately. Before surgery, any clinical history of abnormal bleeding or laboratory abnormalities in platelet or coagulation function should be evaluated and treated. Aspirin, nonsteroidal anti-inflammatory agents, and other medications that can compromise hemostasis should be discontinued well in advance of surgery. Strict hemostasis should be obtained during surgery. Postoperatively, the patient should be kept on bed rest for 24 hours, and the systolic blood pressure should be maintained within 20 mm Hg of the patient's baseline blood pressure. Patients who are at risk for seizures should be treated prophylactically with phenytoin or phenobarbital.

Acute intracranial hemorrhage presents clinically with signs of acute increased intracranial pressure. The key feature is an alteration of the level of consciousness, which may be followed by acute neurologic deficits. Classic findings include hemiparalysis with obtundation, a fixed and dilated pupil, respiratory distress, bradycardia, and systolic hypertension; however, not all features may be present. A noncontrast computerized tomography (CT) scan of the head should be performed immediately for diagnosis, but, if the patient deteriorates too rapidly, immediate intracranial reexploration in the operating room is indicated. A ventriculostomy performed at the bedside can be a temporizing measure that may aid in the later management of the intracranial pressure. Treatment consists of wound reexploration, blood clot evacuation, and bleeding source control. If the patient fails to improve neurologically after the drainage of the hematoma, a magnetic resonance image (MRI) with diffusion-weighted sequences should be performed to rule out recurrent hemorrhage or other complication such as cerebrovascular accident or cerebral edema.

Cerebral Edema

Significant postoperative cerebral edema is unusual, and it is not usually observed unless the tumor is large. The removal of a large tumor may require a significant amount of cerebellar retraction. Cerebral edema can also result from ischemia or infarction. The prevention of this complication involves using the minimal amount of brain retraction to achieve the surgical objective. The degree of brain retraction can also be minimized with the use of agents such as mannitol and furosemide that reduce CSF volume as well as with the use of anesthetic techniques such as hyperventilation. An important surgical maneuver during the retrosigmoid approach is the early decompression of the medullary cistern, which allows for the relaxation of the cerebellum.

Temporal lobe edema caused by retraction can occur with the middle fossa approach. Retraction is extradural with this approach in most cases, so this complication is rare. Intraoperative somatosensory evoked potential monitoring can be used to monitor the functional status of the temporal lobe. Brain retraction can be relaxed for any change in cerebral function.

Clinical features of an acute increase in intracranial pressure include decreased level of consciousness followed by the development of progressive focal neurologic deficits such as weakness of the extremities. The differential diagnosis includes intracranial hemorrhage, acute hydrocephalus, and meningitis. A CT scan of the head should be obtained to rule out hemorrhage and acute hydrocephalus. Both MRI and CT scanning can detect the presence of cerebral edema, although the T2-weighted and fluid-attenuated inversion recovery MRI are more sensitive (Figure 53-1).

The main treatment objective is to reduce the intracranial pressure using pharmacologic, ventilatory, and surgical means. For intubated patients, hyperventilation to reduce the serum partial pressure of carbon dioxide level to 25 mm Hg to 30 mm Hg can be used over a course of 36 hours or less, after which effectiveness is reduced. To reduce CSF volume acutely, hyperosmolar agents such as mannitol can be administered intravenously (IV) in doses of 0.5 mg/kg to 2.0 mg/kg every 6 to 12 hours, and 20 mg to 60 mg of IV furosemide can be given every 4 to 6 hours. If these measures prove inadequate, a ventriculostomy can be placed to drain the CSF and to control intracranial pressure more directly. A lumbar drain is typically not used in these cases because of the risk of downward brainstem herniation. In some cases, the pressure in the posterior fossa may not be adequately reduced with supratentorial CSF drainage, in which case a surgical decompression of the posterior fossa will be needed. In a dire emergency, a

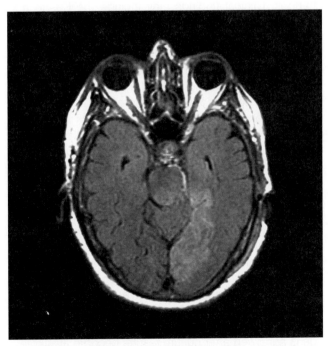

Figure 53-1. Axial fluid-attenuated inversion recovery magnetic resonance image showing cerebral edema involving the brainstem and the left calcarine cortex.

subtotal resection of the cerebellum or the temporal lobe can be undertaken as a life-saving measure.

Steroids are routinely used for the reduction of cerebral edema, but the onset of action of steroids is not immediate. Steroids are often given intraoperatively in situations involving a risk for edema, such as during the removal of large tumors. The loading dose of dexamethasone is 6 mg to 12 mg IV, whereas maintenance therapy is given in doses of 4 mg to 6 mg every 6 hours. Steroids are tapered after the risk of cerebral edema has subsided. Short-term steroid administration can be associated with gastric distress, mood changes, and hyperglycemia, especially among diabetic patients. The occurrence of other long-term sequelae with the short-term use of steroids is uncommon.

Meningitis

The risk of bacterial meningitis after acoustic tumor surgery is relatively low. It is reported to be as low as 0.14% and as high as 8.2%.[4,13–20] This complication typically occurs in the setting of CSF leakage, and, therefore, the prompt identification and treatment of the CSF leak are prudent to minimize the risk of meningitis. Despite the low incidence, the potential morbidity and mortality of bacterial meningitis is high. Those who survive can have major sequelae. Some manifestations of permanent brain damage include cognitive dysfunction, chronic seizures, motor and coordination abnormalities, and hearing loss.

Patients who develop meningitis present with headache, neck stiffness, photophobia, lethargy, and mental status changes. Clinical findings may include the Kernig and Brudzinski signs and focal neurologic deficits, although the absence of these signs does not rule out meningitis. Some of these symptoms, especially altered mental status, can also be caused by increased intracranial pressure. Head CT scanning should be performed to rule out obstructive hydrocephalus, intracranial hematoma, or other pathology that may increase the risk of cerebral herniation during lumbar puncture. If there is elevated intracranial pressure, a ventriculostomy should be performed to obtain a CSF sample. Otherwise the diagnosis of meningitis is confirmed by performing a lumbar puncture to obtain CSF for chemistries, cell counts, and cultures. Because the risk of morbidity and mortality increases significantly with a delay in therapy, antibiotics are administered soon after a CSF sample has been obtained. Antibiotics should be chosen to cover gram-positive organisms such as *Staphylococcus* and *Streptococcus* as well as gram-negative organisms such as *Klebsiella* and *Haemophilus*. Vancomycin and cefepime may be used as initial empiric therapy; antibiotic coverage is narrowed after culture results become available.

It is often difficult to differentiate bacterial meningitis from aseptic meningitis. The latter condition occurs relatively frequently after posterior fossa surgery, and it responds well to a short course of steroids. Up to 70% of such patients with CSF findings of meningitis were without clinical evidence of bacterial meningitis.[21,22] Although patients with bacterial meningitis tend to have higher fevers, a greater incidence of neurologic deficits, higher systemic white cell counts, higher CSF white cell counts, and a higher incidence of CSF leak, it is not always possible to differentiate between bacterial and aseptic meningitis on the basis of these parameters.[23,24] The diagnosis of bacterial meningitis can only be confirmed by the presence of organisms on the CSF Gram stain or with positive bacterial cultures, which may not be available for 1 to 2 days. If there is no CSF leak or implanted intracranial hardware, the continuation of antibiotics in patients with negative cultures after 2 days has not been found to be beneficial.[25] Therefore the authors use a protocol in which antibiotic coverage is continued for 2 days until the culture results are available. If the cultures are positive, the patient is treated with culture-directed antibiotics for 2 weeks. If the cultures are negative but the patient continues to have symptoms, steroids (e.g., dexamethasone 4 mg IV or by mouth every 6 hours) are given over a course of 10 days, followed by a taper. Antibiotics are not continued in cases of negative cultures unless there is a high suspicion of bacterial meningitis, as in the setting of CSF leak.

Pneumocephalus

Although intracranial air is often present after acoustic tumor surgery, it does not cause elevated intracranial pressures, and it typically resolves within 7 to 10 days. Symptomatic pneumocephalus occurs very infrequently after posterior fossa surgery. By contrast, symptomatic pneumocephalus is most often associated with craniofacial resection in which there is an interruption of the barrier between the aerodigestive tract and the intracranial space. A tissue defect that allows for communication between the subarachnoid and aerodigestive spaces can allow air to enter the intracranial space, and, if a ball–valve effect occurs, the acute elevation of intracranial pressure can occur. In suspected cases, a CT scan of the head is indicated to make the proper diagnosis and to exclude other complications (Figure 53-2). Symptomatic pneumocephalus typically responds well to conservative treatment with 100% oxygen. Generally the patient is assumed to have a CSF leak that may require closure. If the patient's neurologic status is unstable, the intracranial air should be removed percutaneously with or without CT guidance, by ventriculostomy, or with wound reexploration.

Cerebrovascular Accident

The risk of cerebrovascular accident (CVA) during or after surgery for acoustic neuroma is low. The possible causes of CVA during surgery include excessive or prolonged

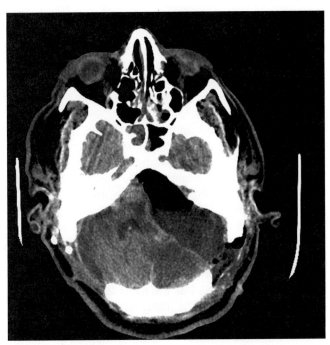

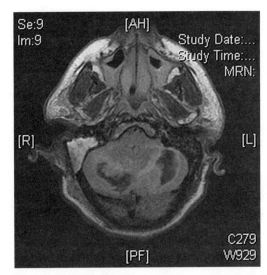

Figure 53-3. Axial fluid-attenuated inversion recovery magnetic resonance image showing bilateral cerebellar infarcts after right translabyrinthine craniectomy.

Figure 53-2. Axial noncontrast computed tomography scan showing extensive left posterior fossa pneumocephalus and fluid associated with a recent left retrosigmoid craniotomy.

brain retraction that can lead to localized ischemia and direct damage to the vessels of the posterior fossa that supply the major regions of the brainstem and the cerebellum. CT scanning and MRI are helpful for confirming the diagnosis (Figures 53-3 and 53-4). Hypotension and embolic events during or after surgery can also be contributory. The clinical presentation varies depending on the area and extent of the CVA.

Treatment for CVA is largely supportive and includes the control of intracranial pressure that can increase with cerebral edema, the spread of the infarction, and hemorrhage. The extent of ischemia may be limited by maintaining normal blood pressure and providing adequate oxygenation. Aspirin can be given as long as there is no hemorrhagic infarct, but the benefits must be weighed against the serious risk of postoperative hemorrhage. Anticoagulation therapy with heparin is controversial and not advised.

Cerebrospinal Fluid Leak

CSF leak is one of the most common complications after acoustic tumor surgery. The literature reports a range of rates from 2% to 30%; however, on average, a 10% to 12% rate is typical.[19,20,26–33] CSF leak occurs because the dural closure is rarely complete. Fat grafts and dural patches do not completely seal the intracranial space. Transtemporal procedures violate the mastoid air cells, and CSF can flow from the dural defect through the temporal bone air-cell system and exit from the wound or the Eustachian tube. When the tympanic membrane and ear-canal skin are intact, CSF otorrhea is rare. CSF leakage through the skin closure is also uncommon if the soft-tissue closure techniques are meticulously applied. CSF rhinorrhea occurs more frequently, because the pathway between the repaired dural defect and the Eustachian tube cannot be made watertight in all cases. Imaging studies such as CT scanning with the intrathecal injection of contrast (Figure 53-5) can be performed to localize the site of leakage, but they are not usually necessary in cases that occur after acoustic neuroma surgery.

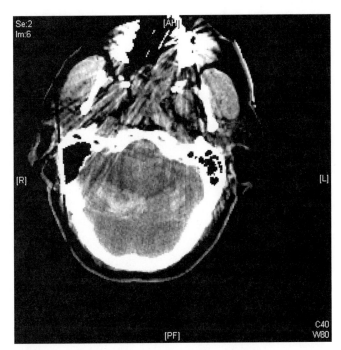

Figure 53-4. Axial noncontrast computed tomography scan showing bilateral cerebellar infarcts after right translabyrinthine craniectomy.

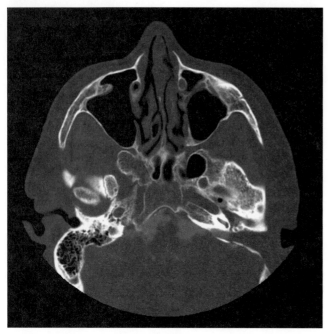

Figure 53-5. Axial computed tomography scan with intrathecal contrast showing cerebrospinal fluid leak emanating from the left posterior fossa, traversing the translabyrinthine defect into the middle ear, and exiting through the Eustachian tube.

Prevention

The key principle of the prevention of CSF leakage after acoustic tumor surgery is to provide a multilayered barrier to CSF flow. The barriers can be formed at the level of dural defects, open air cells, the middle-ear and mastoid spaces, the skin incision, and the Eustachian tube. The particular sets of barriers implemented depend on the surgical approach.

Regardless of the surgical approach, the wound closure is made watertight with multilayered tissue-closure techniques. There are reports in the literature of various

ways to create the surgical wound with staggered edges to allow for a more robust closure, but none of these techniques are proven to be more effective. The gravity-dependent portion of the wound is at greatest risk for leakage, so the inferior portion of any wound should be closed with the utmost attention.

With the retrosigmoid approach, CSF leakage through the Eustachian tube can occur with CSF traversing the retrosigmoid air cells and exiting through exposed petrous apex air cells (Figure 53-6). The first barrier to CSF leakage is a tight dural closure. Primary repair is possible in some cases, but most require a dural graft. Mastoid air cells in the craniectomy defect should be obliterated with bone wax or another suitable material to prevent CSF flow into the mastoid cavity. The dural defect in the IAC from petrosectomy cannot be closed primarily, and it represents the most vulnerable area for CSF leakage during the retrosigmoid approach. All open air cells in the IAC should be blocked by bone wax. In addition, a muscle, fascia, or fat plug should be applied to the bone defect. There have been reports of the use of angled endoscopes to visualize the air cells in the IAC defect, but their added efficacy for reducing the rate of CSF leakage has not been proven.

With the translabyrinthine approach, the potential route of CSF egress from the dural defect to the Eustachian tube can be complex and variable. CSF can trickle through any air-cell tract to the incision or the Eustachian tube. In addition, dural closure using direct suture techniques is not feasible (Figure 53-7). Some surgeons routinely remove the incus to pack the middle ear and the Eustachian tube orifice as part of surgery. CSF can also leak into the middle ear through the oval window in cases in which the stapes footplate was subluxed during incus removal. The presigmoid defect should be made just

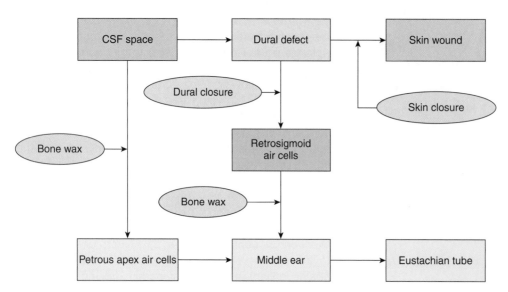

Figure 53-6. Pathways of cerebrospinal fluid leakage, retrosigmoid approach, and barriers *(oval blocks).*

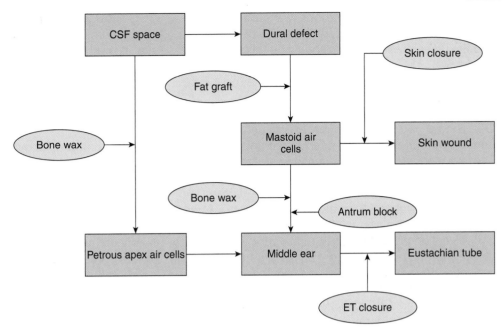

Figure 53-7. Pathways of cerebrospinal fluid leakage, translabyrinthine approach, and barriers *(oval blocks).*

large enough to allow for safe tumor removal, which leads to a smaller dural defect. The dural defect is repaired with a fat-graft plug protruding slightly into the posterior fossa. The mastoid can then be isolated from the middle ear and the Eustachian tube by the application of bone wax to all exposed mastoid air cells and by filling the mastoid defect with autologous fat graft. The aditus ad antrum is blocked with a muscle, fascia, or fat graft. Alternatively, the facial recess is opened, the incus is removed, and the middle ear and Eustachian tube are obliterated with muscle grafts. The use of a vascularized flap such as the temporalis muscle or a temporoparietal fascia flap based on the superficial temporal artery may be considered, but the use of such flaps has not been widely accepted. The use of fibrin glue or another similar material is common,

but these have not been proven to reduce the rate of CSF leakage.[27,33–36] The use of hydroxyapatite cement to improve CSF leakage rates has been attempted in the past. Recently this material has not been shown to be as good as fat grafts for controlling CSF leaks for acoustic neuroma surgery, although the combination of the cement and the fat graft may be of benefit. The cosmesis regarding the reconstruction of the bone defect is a significant benefit of the cement.[36–38]

The most common path of CSF leakage after the middle cranial fossa approach is through the dural defect in the petrous apex and the IAC. Exposed suprameatal air cells provide a conduit to the mastoid, the middle ear, and the Eustachian tube (Figure 53-8). As in the case of

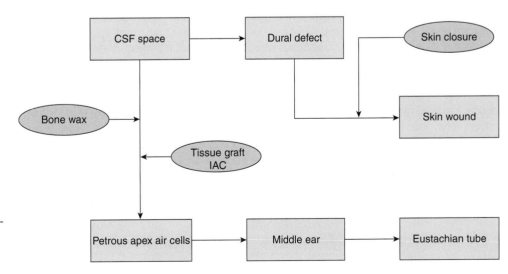

Figure 53-8. Pathways of cerebrospinal fluid leakage, middle fossa approach, and barriers *(oval blocks).*

the retrosigmoid approach, bone wax should be applied to these open air-cell tracts in the petrous apex and the IAC air cells, and this should be followed by the application of a tissue graft. The overall rate of CSF leak after the middle fossa approach is reported to be between 3.8% to 10%.[20,27,31]

One special note of caution involves patients with evidence of preoperative increased intracranial pressure. These patients may be at increased risk for CSF leakage, and they may benefit from the prophylactic placement of a CSF shunt. Patients with large tumors and chronically elevated CSF pressure as a result of tumor obstruction of the normal CSF flow may not require CSF diversion procedures, because tumor excision will relieve the obstruction. There may be a small group of patients who are prone to having elevated CSF pressures independent of the tumor size and who are at risk for postoperative CSF leakage. This group may benefit from perioperative lumbar drainage, but there is no easy way to identify these patients preoperatively.

Treatment

CSF leakage through the wound after any surgical approach for acoustic tumor surgery will typically cease after the placement of sutures to augment wound closure and the application of a pressure dressing. CSF rhinorrhea cannot be treated by any type of direct repair at the bedside. The patient should remain on bed rest as much as possible, and the head should remain elevated to at least 30 degrees. If the leakage persists despite 24 hours or more of conservative management, then a lumbar drain should be placed to remove the CSF at a rate of approximately 10 cc per hour. If the CSF leak persists after continuous lumbar drainage for 3 days, then revision surgery may be necessary.

For cases in which hearing has not been preserved, revision surgery for a CSF leak can be performed using an extradural, transmastoid procedure, regardless of the primary surgical approach. Reexploration of the primary dural defect is not usually necessary. The primary goal of revision surgery for CSF leakage is to block the Eustachian tube, because most persistent leaks exit through the nose. The most effective surgery to control the CSF leakage is to remove the ear canal, close the meatus of the ear canal, and permanently obliterate the middle ear and the Eustachian tube. Alternatively, the Eustachian tube can be temporarily obliterated through the facial recess by the application of muscle grafts to the middle ear and the Eustachian tube without damaging the mucosa. This latter technique can be used for cases in which hearing has been preserved. These materials have been shown to resorb over time, allowing for the reestablishment of a pneumatized middle-ear space.[26] The cessation of CSF flow allows for spontaneous healing at the dural defect.

For retrosigmoid cases in which the site of leakage is clearly retrosigmoid or in which posterior mastoid air cells are involved rather than the petrous apex, the easiest method of repair is to reapply bone wax to these air cells. For middle fossa cases with hearing preservation, a CSF leak repair may require reopening the craniotomy and repairing the tegmen defect.

There is compelling evidence that patients with CSF leak are at a significantly increased risk of developing bacterial meningitis.[26,27,39,40] The true efficacy of prophylactic antibiotics for preventing the bacterial meningitis that may result from CSF leaks is unknown. There is a risk that the use of antibiotics may increase the likelihood of a resistant organism causing meningitis when this complication occurs. Prophylactic antibiotics in the setting of CSF leak after acoustic neuroma surgery may be beneficial, but the best prophylaxis against the development of meningitis in the setting of CSF leakage is the prompt control of the leak.

Facial Nerve

There is a high rate of anatomic and functional facial nerve preservation with contemporary acoustic neuroma surgery.[1,15,41,42] The surgical factors that are thought to be important in facial nerve preservation include the use of the operating microscope, the application of intraoperative facial nerve monitoring, and the experience level of the surgical team. The reported overall long-term House–Brackmann scale grade I to II facial nerve function is 90% for tumors that are not larger than 2 cm in diameter.[3,28,41–45]

There is still a significant incidence of transient facial nerve dysfunction after surgery, and recovery may take weeks to several months.[1,41] These patients require eye care to prevent corneal drying and injury, especially if cranial nerve V function has also been compromised. The application of eyedrops such as carboxymethylcellulose during the day and ophthalmic ointments such as Lacri-Lube (Allergan, Irvine, CA) at night should be instituted. The use of a protective shield over the eye is useful. For prolonged or expected prolonged facial paresis, upper and lower eyelid procedures (e.g., gold-weight and spring loading) and lateral canthoplasty are effective remedies for lagophthalmos and ectropion. Older patients with diminished suspensory support of the lower eyelid as a result of aging are at increased risk for the development of ectropion. Gold-weight and spring prostheses are easily removed after facial nerve function is recovered. Lower-lid suspension procedures typically do not require reversal. If the facial nerve function fails to return after several months or is not expected to return as a result of nerve transection, a cranial nerve XII to VII cross-anastomosis may be considered.

Corneal complications are most common among patients who have facial nerve dysfunction together with corneal anesthesia and reduced tearing, which can occur after acoustic neuroma surgery. If a significant corneal complication or another ocular complication occurs, prompt consultation with an ophthalmologist is necessary.

Other Cranial Nerves

Trigeminal Nerve

It is unusual for patients to develop new facial numbness after acoustic tumor surgery unless the tumor is very large. The reported incidence of this complication is 0% to 4.7%.[13,15,19,46,47] Transient dysfunction of the trigeminal nerve often occurs together with transient facial nerve dysfunction, because both conditions are associated with the resection of large tumors. The main consideration for patients with facial numbness is corneal anesthesia, which can lead to ocular injury. It is important to provide proper postoperative eye care, as discussed previously.

Abducens Nerve

Cranial nerve VI dysfunction is rare, but it can occur during the resection of large acoustic tumors that have become adherent to this nerve. The abducens nerve may undergo mechanically induced neuropraxia. Injury to the abducens nerve results in the inability to abduct the ipsilateral eye, thus causing horizontal diplopia on lateral gaze toward the surgical side. If the diplopia is bothersome, an eye patch can be worn on the affected side until the nerve function recovers. Permanent abducens nerve dysfunction may be mitigated with extraocular muscle surgery by an ophthalmologist.

Dysphagia

There are two mechanisms of swallowing dysfunction that result from acoustic tumor surgery: acute lower cranial nerve dysfunction that causes pharyngeal and esophageal dysphagia and combined facial and trigeminal nerve dysfunction that causes oral dysphagia. The lower cranial nerves can be injured during acoustic tumor surgery. Large tumors often impinge on jugular foramen contents and on cranial nerves IX, X, and XI. It is unusual for permanent nerve injury to occur if the nerves are identified and dissected off of the tumor with the use of microsurgical techniques. Because cranial nerves IX and X control the sensory and motor function of the pharynx and larynx, acute lower cranial nerve deficits can result in dysphagia and aspiration. The patient would benefit from an evaluation by a laryngologist or a speech and swallowing pathologist. Some practitioners use a modified barium swallow study to guide therapy. If the patient is not at significant risk for aspiration, modified swallowing maneuvers may be useful during the rehabilitation period. Otherwise nutrition should be provided through a nasogastric or gastrostomy feeding tube until

the risk of aspiration has subsided. When vocal-cord paralysis causes significant vocal and swallowing dysfunction, vocal-cord injection or medialization thyroplasty can be performed.

Facial nerve and trigeminal nerve dysfunction can result in abnormalities during the oral phase of swallowing. Facial nerve dysfunction can lead to oral commissure weakness with drooling and impaired food clearance from the oral gutter. Trigeminal dysfunction can cause reduced oral sensation. In addition, tongue dysfunction as a result of cranial nerve XII injury can further compromise swallowing function. If a cranial XII to VII anastomosis for permanent facial nerve paralysis is under consideration, one must keep in mind that there is a relative contraindication to performing a XII to VII anastomosis in patients with dysphagia. The impairment of tongue function related to this procedure can result in a worsening of dysphagia. An alternative is an interposition graft from cranial nerve XII to VII with the preservation of hypoglossal function.

Vertigo and Disequilibrium

Most patients experience some degree of vertigo and disequilibrium after acoustic tumor surgery. It may be the consequence of the acute loss of residual vestibular function or transient cerebellar dysfunction. The severity of the patient's vestibular symptoms is related to the level of residual vestibular function present before surgery. Completely denervated patients experience minimal vertigo, because central compensation has already taken place. Postoperative vestibular symptoms usually subside over a period of days to weeks. Most patients recover spontaneously, but others may benefit from a short course of vestibular therapy to facilitate central compensation.

Patients who sustain significant injury to the cerebellum or brainstem, as a result of either the tumor or the surgical intervention, can develop a permanent level of balance dysfunction. Patients with other comorbidities such as advanced age, visual loss, proprioceptive dysfunction, and musculoskeletal dysfunction may be at greater risk for developing prolonged disequilibrium. The reported incidence of vertigo and disequilibrium at long-term follow up after acoustic neuroma surgery have ranged from 1% to as high as 30%.[19,46,48] Driscoll and colleagues[49] found that 31% of patients in their series had persistent disequilibrium at 3 or more months after surgery, and they identified several criteria to predict prolonged vestibular dysfunction: an age of more than 55 years, female gender, unsteadiness for 3 months before surgery, and associated central signs at vestibular testing. The vascular supply to the brainstem is better preserved with contemporary microsurgical dissection techniques for tumor removal, and cerebellar retraction is minimal with today's technique of decompressing the CSF cisternal spaces early, thus allowing for the early relaxation of the cerebellum. Prolonged disequilibrium is treated with a long course of vestibular rehabilitation therapy. Because the damage is often irreversible, it is important to use proper surgical technique to avoid brainstem and cerebellar injury.

Headache

The incidence of chronic headache after acoustic tumor surgery in the literature is widely variable, ranging from 0% to 73%, and it depends on the surgical approach, the technique, and the interval after surgery.[15,16,50–53] It is difficult to interpret these rates, because the significance, timing, and duration of headaches are not always reported. The occurrence of symptomatic headache has been attributed mainly to the retrosigmoid approach.[54] Harner and colleagues[55] reported that, after retrosigmoid surgery, significant headache occurred in 16% of patients at 1 year and in 9% of patients at 2 years. Schessel and colleagues[54] reported a chronic headache rate of 67% in suboccipital craniectomy patients, and they noted a marked reduction in postoperative pain when craniotomy with bone flap replacement was instituted.

The two main theories posited for the cause of retrosigmoid craniotomy headaches are as follows:

1. Contact between the dura and posterior neck musculature in patients whose craniectomy was not reconstructed
2. Bone dust in the CSF space from intradural drilling that causes aseptic meningitis

These theories are consistent with the relative lack of headaches in translabyrinthine and middle fossa craniotomy patients, in whom dural contact with the overlying musculature does not occur and intradural drilling is not performed. The headache problem may be alleviated by filling the craniectomy defect with bone chips, abdominal fat, methylmethacrylate, or hydroxyapatite cement and carefully irrigating the cisterns after intradural drilling.

The medical management of headaches includes the use of oral agents such as acetaminophen, aspirin, and nonsteroidal anti-inflammatory agents. Posterior fossa syndrome or aseptic meningitis patients are treated with a short course of steroid therapy. The need for long-term narcotics is uncommon. Refractory cases may require referral to a chronic pain consultant or a neurologist, who may recommend other pharmacologic agents such as antidepressants, antimigraine medications, and antiseizure medications as well as biofeedback and transcutaneous electrical nerve stimulation.

MEDICAL COMPLICATIONS

Although major morbidity after posterior fossa surgery for the removal of acoustic neuromas has become uncommon, it is still a major intracranial surgery with the potential for serious medical complications. Postoperative overnight monitoring in the intensive care unit is recommended. The duration of anesthesia can be prolonged in some cases, and significant blood loss, fluid shifts, and intracranial complications can occur. Postoperative management issues include fluid and electrolyte imbalance, cardiopulmonary stress, coagulopathy, wound infection, and aspiration pneumonia. Before surgery, significant preexisting conditions such as coronary artery disease, chronic obstructive pulmonary disease, diabetes mellitus, bleeding disorders, and malnutrition should be treated.

Pulmonary complications include atelectasis, pneumonia, and pulmonary embolus as a result of deep venous thrombosis. Prophylaxis against deep venous thrombosis may be achieved by instituting sequential compression stockings before surgery and continuing with the therapy until the patient is no longer bedridden. The patient is mobilized and encouraged to ambulate as soon as possible, and incentive spirometry is begun. Patients with acute lower cranial nerve deficits with dysphagia are at risk for aspiration, and they should be taught to clear secretions with a suction apparatus. Severely affected patients who cannot adequately handle their secretions should be fed through a nasogastric or gastrostomy tube. In addition, a tracheotomy should be considered for pulmonary toilet.

Patients with a history of or significant risk factors for coronary artery disease are at significant risk for cardiac complications. Congestive heart failure and coronary ischemia are the primary concerns. Patients should be monitored closely after surgery, with fluid and medication management shared jointly with an intensivist or a critical care specialist.

Infectious complications are especially serious with the advent of resistant organisms that are highly prevalent in hospitals and intensive care units. It is important to practice proper isolation precautions. The patients' caretakers and visitors should exercise frequent hand washing, the use of gowns, and the separation of patients. Urinary catheters, arterial lines, and central lines are potential portals of infection and should be removed as soon as they are not needed.

CONCLUSION

Acoustic tumor surgery has become relatively safe and routine, but one must keep in mind that it still represents major intracranial surgery. Although overall rates of morbidity are very low, the occurrence of a serious complication can cause significant morbidity and potential mortality. Favorable patient outcomes result from the close cooperation of all staff members, including the surgical team; anesthesia, nursing, and neuromonitoring providers; and other support staff members. All persons involved in the patient's care must work in concert to reduce factors that can lead to complications. It is imperative to diagnose and treat any complications early to minimize potential morbidity to the patient.

REFERENCES

1. Sampath P, Holliday MJ, Brem H, et al: Facial nerve injury in acoustic neuroma (vestibular schwannoma) surgery: Etiology and prevention. *J Neurosurg* 1997;87(1):60–66.
2. Ojemann RG: Management of acoustic neuromas (vestibular schwannomas) (honored guest presentation). *Clin Neurosurg* 1993;40:498–535.
3. Kaylie DM, Gilbert E, Horgan MA, et al: Acoustic neuroma surgery outcomes. *Otol Neurotol* 2001;22(5):686–689.
4. Slattery WH 3rd, Francis S, House KC: Perioperative morbidity of acoustic neuroma surgery. *Otol Neurotol* 2001;22(6):895–902.
5. Raskin JM, Benjamin E, Iberti TJ: Venous air embolism: Case report and review. *Mt Sinai J Med* 1985;52(5):367–370.
6. von Gosseln HH, Samii M, Suhr D, et al: The lounging position for posterior fossa surgery: Anesthesiological considerations regarding air embolism. *Childs Nerv Syst* 1991;7(7):368–374.
7. Kletzker GR, Smith PG, Backer RJ, et al: Complications in neurotologic surgery. In Jackler RK, Brackmann DE, editors: *Neurotology,* St. Louis, 1994, Mosby.
8. Palmon SC, Moore LE, Lundberg J, et al: Venous air embolism: A review. *J Clin Anesth* 1997;9(3):251–257.
9. Atkinson WJ: The anterior inferior cerebellar artery: Its variations, pontine distribution, and significance in the surgery of cerebello-pontine angle tumours. *J Neurol Neurosurg Psychiatry* 1949;12:137–151.
10. Hegarty JL, Jackler RK, Rigby PL, et al: Distal anterior inferior cerebellar artery syndrome after acoustic neuroma surgery. *Otol Neurotol* 2002;23(4):560–571.
11. Applebaum EL, Ferguson RJ: The latero-medial inferior pontine syndrome. *Ann Otol Rhinol Laryngol* 1975;84(3 Pt 1):379–383.
12. Perneczky A, Perneczky G, Tschabitscher M, et al: The relationship between the caudolateral pontine syndrome and the anterior inferior cerebellar artery. *Acta Neurochir (Wien)* 1981;58(3–4):245–257.
13. Wiet RJ, Kazan RP, Raslan W, et al: Complications in the approach to acoustic tumor surgery. *Ann Otol Rhinol Laryngol* 1986;95 (1 Pt 1):28–31.
14. Mangham CA: Complications of translabyrinthine vs. suboccipital approach for acoustic tumor surgery. *Otolaryngol Head Neck Surg* 1988;99(4):396–400.
15. Ebersold MJ, Harner SG, Beatty CW, et al: Current results of the retrosigmoid approach to acoustic neurinoma. *J Neurosurg* 1992;76(6):901–909.
16. Cohen NL, Lewis WS, Ransohoff J: Hearing preservation in cerebellopontine angle tumor surgery: The NYU experience 1974-1991. *Am J Otol* 1993;14(5):423–433.
17. Rodgers GK, Luxford WM: Factors affecting the development of cerebrospinal fluid leak and meningitis after translabyrinthine acoustic tumor surgery. *Laryngoscope* 1993;103(9):959–962.
18. Mamikoglu B, Wiet RJ, Esquivel CR: Translabyrinthine approach for the management of large and giant vestibular schwannomas. *Otol Neurotol* 2002;23(2):224–227.
19. Darrouzet V, Martel J, Enee V, et al: Vestibular schwannoma surgery outcomes: Our multidisciplinary experience in 400 cases over 17 years. *Laryngoscope* 2004;114(4):681–688.
20. Sanna M, Taibah A, Russo A, et al: Perioperative complications in acoustic neuroma (vestibular schwannoma) surgery. *Otol Neurotol* 2004;25(3):379–386.
21. Carmel PW, Fraser RA, Stein BM: Aseptic meningitis following posterior fossa surgery in children. *J Neurosurg* 1974;41(1):44–48.
22. Carmel PW, Greif LK: The aseptic meningitis syndrome: A complication of posterior fossa surgery. *Pediatr Neurosurg* 1993;19(5):276–280.
23. Ross D, Rosegay H, Pons V: Differentiation of aseptic and bacterial meningitis in postoperative neurosurgical patients. *J Neurosurg* 1988;69(5):669–674.
24. Negrini B, Kelleher KJ, Wald ER: Cerebrospinal fluid findings in aseptic versus bacterial meningitis. *Pediatrics* 2000;105(2):316–319.
25. Blomstedt, GC: Post-operative aseptic meningitis. *Acta Neurochir (Wien)* 1987;89(3–4):112–116.
26. Bryce GE, Nedzelski JM, Rowed DW, et al: Cerebrospinal fluid leaks and meningitis in acoustic neuroma surgery. *Otolaryngol Head Neck Surg* 1991;104(1):81–87.
27. Hoffman RA: Cerebrospinal fluid leak following acoustic neuroma removal. *Laryngoscope* 1994;104(1 Pt 1):40–58.
28. Gormley WB, Sekhar LN, Wright DC, et al: Acoustic neuromas: Results of current surgical management. *Neurosurgery* 1997;41(1):50–60.
29. Brennan JW, Rowed DW, Nedzelski JM, et al: Cerebrospinal fluid leak after acoustic neuroma surgery: Influence of tumor size and surgical approach on incidence and response to treatment. *J Neurosurg* 2001;94(2):217–223.
30. Bani A, Gilsbach JM: Incidence of cerebrospinal fluid leak after microsurgical removal of vestibular schwannomas. *Acta Neurochir (Wien)* 2002;144(10):979–982.
31. Becker SS, Jackler RK, Pitts LH: Cerebrospinal fluid leak after acoustic neuroma surgery: A comparison of the translabyrinthine, middle fossa, and retrosigmoid approaches. *Otol Neurotol* 2003;24(1):107–112.
32. Fishman AJ, Marrinan MS, Golfinos JG, et al: Prevention and management of cerebrospinal fluid leak following vestibular schwannoma surgery. *Laryngoscope* 2004;114(3):501–505.
33. Selesnick SH, Liu JC, Jen A, et al: The incidence of cerebrospinal fluid leak after vestibular schwannoma surgery. *Otol Neurotol* 2004;25(3):387–393.
34. Lebowitz RA, Hoffman RA, Roland JT Jr, et al: Autologous fibrin glue in the prevention of cerebrospinal fluid leak following acoustic neuroma surgery. *Am J Otol* 1995;16(2):172–174.
35. Sen A, Green KM, Khan MI, et al: Cerebrospinal fluid leak rate after the use of BioGlue in translabyrinthine vestibular schwannoma surgery: A prospective study. *Otol Neurotol* 2006;27(1):102–105.
36. Arriaga MA, Chen DA: Hydroxyapatite cement cranioplasty in translabyrinthine acoustic neuroma surgery. *Otolaryngol Head Neck Surg* 2002;126(5):512–517.
37. Kveton JF, Coelho DH: Hydroxyapatite cement in temporal bone surgery: A 10 year experience. *Laryngoscope* 2004;114(1):33–37.
38. Poetker DM, Pytynia KB, Meyer GA, et al: Complication rate of transtemporal hydroxyapatite cement cranioplasties: A case series review of 76 cranioplasties. *Otol Neurotol* 2004;25(4):604–609.
39. Hardy DG, Macfarlane R, Baguley D, et al: Surgery for acoustic neurinoma: An analysis of 100 translabyrinthine operations. *J Neurosurg* 1989;71(6):799–804.
40. Tos M, Thomsen J: The price of preservation of hearing in acoustic neuroma surgery. *Ann Otol Rhinol Laryngol* 1982;91(3 Pt 1): 240–245.
41. Lalwani AK, Butt FY, Jackler RK, et al: Facial nerve outcome after acoustic neuroma surgery: A study from the era of cranial nerve monitoring. *Otolaryngol Head Neck Surg* 1994;111(5): 561–570.
42. Arriaga MA, Luxford WM, Berliner KI: Facial nerve function following middle fossa and translabyrinthine acoustic tumor surgery: A comparison. *Am J Otol* 1994;15(5):620–624.
43. Silverstein H, Rosenberg SI, Flanzer J, et al: Intraoperative facial nerve monitoring in acoustic neuroma surgery. *Am J Otol* 1993;14(6):524–532.
44. Uziel A, Benezech J, Frerebeau P: Intraoperative facial nerve monitoring in posterior fossa acoustic neuroma surgery. *Otolaryngol Head Neck Surg* 1993;108(2):126–134.
45. Esses BA, LaRouere MJ, Graham MD: Facial nerve outcome in acoustic tumor surgery. *Am J Otol* 1994;15(6):810–812.

46. Harner SG, Beatty CW, Ebersold MJ: Retrosigmoid removal of acoustic neuroma: Experience 1978-1988. *Otolaryngol Head Neck Surg* July 1990;103(1):40–45.

47. Lanman TH, Brackmann DE, Hitselberger WE, et al: Report of 190 consecutive cases of large acoustic tumors (vestibular schwannoma) removed via the translabyrinthine approach. *J Neurosurg* 1999;90(4):617–623.

48. Wiegand DA, Ojemann RG, Fickel V: Surgical treatment of acoustic neuroma (vestibular schwannoma) in the United States: Report from the Acoustic Neuroma Registry. *Laryngoscope* 1996;106(1 Pt 1):58–66.

49. Driscoll CL, Lynn SG, Harner SG, et al: Preoperative identification of patients at risk of developing persistent dysequilibrium after acoustic neuroma removal. *Am J Otol* 1998;19(4):491–495.

50. Ryzenman JM, Pensak ML, Tew JM Jr: Headache: A quality of life analysis in a cohort of 1,657 patients undergoing acoustic neuroma surgery, results from the acoustic neuroma association. *Laryngoscope* 2005;115(4):703–711.

51. Wiegand DA, Fickel V: Acoustic neuroma—The patient's perspective: Subjective assessment of symptoms, diagnosis, therapy, and outcome in 541 patients. *Laryngoscope* 1989;99(2):179–187.

52. Parving A, Tos M, Thomsen J, et al: Some aspects of life quality after surgery for acoustic neuroma. *Arch Otolaryngol Head Neck Surg* 1992;118(10):1061–1064.

53. Pedrosa CA, Ahern DK, McKenna MJ, et al: Determinants and impact of headache after acoustic neuroma surgery. *Am J Otol* 1994;15(6):793–797.

54. Schessel DA, Rowed DW, Nedzelski JM, et al: Postoperative pain following excision of acoustic neuroma by the suboccipital approach: Observations on possible cause and potential amelioration. *Am J Otol* 1993;14(5):491–494.

55. Harner SG, Beatty CW, Ebersold MJ: Headache after acoustic neuroma excision. *Am J Otol* 1993;14(6):552–555.

CHAPTER 54

Complications of Surgery of the Vestibular System

Timothy E. Hullar

The diagnosis and treatment of patients with problems of balance and equilibrium has changed with the developing understanding of these conditions. In some cases, improved medical treatments have reduced the need for surgical interventions. Many otolaryngologists now use intratympanic gentamicin rather than vestibular neurectomy or labyrinthectomy to treat patients with intractable Ménière disease. Benign positional vertigo is now generally approached with a repositioning exercise such as the Epley or Semont maneuver before surgery is considered.

The most prominent adverse outcome after surgery for vestibular symptoms is the risk of continuing disequilibrium. Because many practitioners are not particularly comfortable evaluating patients with disequilibrium, the risk of an incorrect diagnosis leading to an unsuccessful surgical intervention is significant. Failed surgical treatment for Ménière disease, for example, may be the result of a missed diagnosis of vestibular migraine rather than a technical failure during the procedure itself. Soliciting a second opinion when any doubt exists regarding the diagnosis or the correct course of therapy is particularly important when contemplating surgery for imbalance.

Even when it is applied correctly, surgery for imbalance may not improve symptoms significantly. Up to 50% of patients who undergo vestibular nerve sectioning or chemical or surgical labyrinthectomy for balance symptoms will suffer from disequilibrium for at least several months after treatment.[1] This is normally addressed with the use of specialized physical therapy, which has been shown to be helpful for patients as they accommodate changes in vestibular function.[2] Adjunctive medical therapy may also be useful. Betahistine has been suggested to help compensate for vestibular loss when used in conjunction with physical therapy.[3,4] Anticonvulsants or antidepressants may also be of some use for managing the posttreatment symptoms of imbalance.[5] Vestibular suppressants such as meclizine or benzodiazepines are discouraged, particularly for use on a regular basis, because of their deleterious effect on adaptation to vestibular loss.

Another adverse outcome that must be considered for all surgeries for imbalance is sensorineural hearing loss. It has been suggested that sensorineural hearing loss after otologic procedures may be treated or prevented with high-dose steroid therapy,[6] although this remains controversial.[7] Other treatments studied in other contexts may also be effective. Antioxidants such as acetyl-L-carnitine and N-L-acetylcysteine have been suggested to reduce noise-induced hearing loss when administered before and after sound exposure.[8] Hyperbaric oxygen has been advocated for the treatment for sensorineural hearing loss caused by acoustic trauma.[9] Salicylate has been suggested as an antioxidant that may be effective against hearing loss caused by gentamicin therapy.[10] Future studies will determine whether any of these therapies are useful for treating surgery-related sensorineural hearing loss.

Other complications of surgery for imbalance are shared with other procedures that involve the ear and the skull base. Mastoid surgery risks facial nerve injury, dural injury, and venous bleeding. Complications of middle cranial fossa procedures include a risk of bleeding, particularly among older patients whose dura is more tightly adherent to the surrounding bone and whose blood vessels are more subject to tearing than younger patients. The risk of intracranial bleeding during middle cranial fossa surgery also increases with excessive anterior dissection. Neurologic deficits may result from the excessive or prolonged retraction of the temporal lobe, and they should be treated with the consultation of specialists in neurology. Optimizing exposure by careful drilling of the inferior margin of the craniotomy reduces the risks of middle cranial fossa surgery. A posterior fossa approach usually requires at least a moderate amount of retraction of the cerebellum. This may lead to complications such as cerebellar infarction or injury to the lower cranial nerves. The management of cerebellar trauma may require the partial resection of the edematous, injured cerebellum to avoid tonsillar herniation. Posterior fossa surgery leads to chronic refractory headaches in 17% of patients, but this rate can be reduced to 4% in patients if a cranioplasty is performed.[11] Presumably these headaches result from muscular adhesions to the dura.

Superior canal dehiscence, Ménière disease, vestibular schwannoma, perilymphatic fistula, and benign positional vertigo may all cause imbalance, and each may be treated surgically. For each of these conditions, observation or medical treatments must be considered carefully before surgery is recommended. Complications of surgical treatment include continuing imbalance, hearing loss, and damage to surrounding structures.

SUPERIOR CANAL DEHISCENCE

Tullio[12] described sound-induced vestibular signs among pigeons with fenestrated semicircular canals, and de Vries and Bleeker[13] showed that superior semicircular canal vestibular nerve afferents become responsive to sound after the fenestration of the canal. Minor[14] correlated Tullio's phenomenon to dehiscent superior semicircular canals in a series of patients and described surgical techniques to alleviate their symptoms of vertigo. Superior semicircular canal dehiscence has since been related to multiple otologic complaints, including vertigo, conductive hearing loss, generalized imbalance, and autophony.[15]

Diagnosis

Successful superior canal dehiscence surgery depends on an accurate diagnosis of the condition. The diagnosis of canal dehiscence requires the consideration of a constellation of factors, including the clinical history, high-resolution computed tomography (CT) scanning of the temporal bones, and other laboratory tests. The gold standard for diagnosis involves a history that is consistent with the syndrome and radiologic evidence of a dehiscence. For patients with radiologically confirmed dehiscence, loud sounds caused symptoms in 90% of patients, and the elevation of intracranial pressure (i.e., straining or coughing) caused symptoms in 73%. Sixty-seven percent of patients had symptoms induced by both sound and pressure changes, including hyperacusis in 52% of patients and autophony in 60% of patients.[15]

Ultra–high-resolution CT scans, audiograms, vestibular-evoked myogenic potentials, and other tests have been shown to help confirm the diagnosis among patients with clinical signs. Reconstructed images parallel and perpendicular to the semicircular canal (i.e., the Pöschl and Stenver views, respectively) have been advocated as being superior to standard coronal and axial images, but, given sufficiently thin slices (i.e., ≤300 μm), these oblique reconstructions may be unnecessary.[16] An air–bone gap is not uncommon among patients with superior canal dehiscence, and this sometimes manifests as a pure conductive hearing loss; however, as a result of enhanced bone conduction, it may also present with normal pure-tone air-conduction thresholds. A case series of 29 patients undergoing surgery for superior canal dehiscence reported 6 patients with a preoperative conductive hearing loss,[17] and a separate series of 10 patients with superior canal dehiscence and conductive hearing loss found 8 patients with supranormal bone lines.[18] Larger series of patients are necessary to make reliable estimates of the prevalence of these symptoms and their usefulness for the making of a correct diagnosis. Sound-evoked cervical and extraocular muscle movements have been used as diagnostic tools for superior canal dehiscence. Tests of vestibular-evoked myogenic potentials (VEMPs) generally consist of the electromyographic monitoring of sternocleidomastoid tension, which decreases when the saccule is stimulated with clicks or tones at approximately 90 dB to 100 dB. Patients with superior canal dehiscence tend to have VEMPs with a threshold that is approximately 20 dB less than normal ears, although abnormal VEMPs are not specific for superior canal dehiscence,[15] and their sensitivity and specificity have not been well documented. A promising additional diagnostic tool for superior canal dehiscence is measuring eye movements in response to clicks.[19] Intact acoustic reflex thresholds in patients with superior canal dehiscence help to differentiate them from patients with otosclerosis.

Treatment

Among patients who have been diagnosed with superior canal dehiscence, indications for the surgical repair of a superior canal dehiscence include debilitating symptoms related to vestibular function (e.g., noise- or Valsalva-induced vertigo) or to auditory function (e.g., autophony, pulsatile tinnitus).[17] Surgical techniques to correct the symptoms of superior canal dehiscence involve an extradural and intracranial approach to the floor of the middle cranial fossa (identifying the arcuate eminence and the dehiscent superior semicircular canal within it) or a transmastoid approach to the superior canal. The middle fossa approach has been shown to control vertigo in approximately 90% of patients.[15] In that report, the plugging of the defect with a piece of fascia introduced into the canal lumen resolved symptoms in 8 of 9 patients, whereas the resurfacing of the defect was successful in only 7 of 11 patients. In another series, symptoms resolved in 10 of 10 patients who were treated with canal plugging, and a single patient who underwent resurfacing did not improve.[20] Therefore canal plugging is the treatment of choice. Surgical failures for superior canal dehiscence may be related to the anatomy of the patient or to the surgical technique. Multiple dehiscences of the floor of the middle crania fossa have long been known,[21] and they may lead to difficulty with finding the proper location for repair (Figure 54-1). This problem may be particularly vexing for patients without a prominent arcuate eminence (Figure 54-2); in these cases, intraoperative guidance systems may be useful for locating the dehiscence of the canal. An unrecognized simultaneous dehiscence of the posterior semicircular canal or the contralateral semicircular canal or an ineffective repair of the defect may also contribute to the failure of the procedure to improve symptoms.[15] Material such as cortical bone used to resurface a dehiscent canal may slip out of place, thereby subjecting the patient to continuing symptoms unless the procedure is repeated. A follow-up CT examination may be helpful for determining the

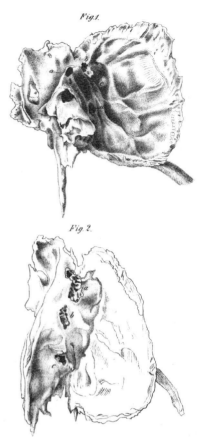

Figure 54-1. Potential anatomic source of complications during surgery for semicircular canal dehiscence: multiple tegmental dehiscences. Location *b* indicates the area of the superior semicircular canal.[21]

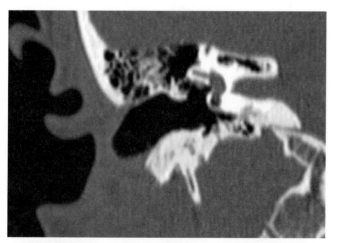

Figure 54-2. Potential anatomic source of complications during surgery for semicircular canal dehiscence: coronal computed tomography reconstruction showing semicircular canal dehiscence without a prominent arcuate eminence.

reason for surgical failure before repeat surgery is considered. If resurfacing is unsuccessful and a postoperative CT scan shows movement of the resurfacing material, reoperation is indicated.[15] A review of the rates of surgical failure described in several series of patients with superior canal dehiscence is given in Table 54-1.

TABLE 54-1 Treatment Failures for Superior Canal Dehiscence Surgery

Author	Complication	
	Continued Imbalance	Sensorineural Hearing Loss
Limb et al.[17]	Not reported	2/29
Mikulec et al.[18]	Not reported	2/8
Mikulec et al.[20]	1/11	3/11
Minor[15]	5/20	See Limb[17]
Hillman et al.[64]	1/13	1/13

Sensorineural Hearing Loss

Sensorineural hearing loss related to surgery for superior canal dehiscence has been reported in 3 of 11 patients in one series[20] and in 2 of 29 patients in another.[17] Improvement was seen in one patient who was treated with steroids after this complication.[20] A recent review of surgical outcomes showed that a history of previous middle-ear surgery was not a significant predictor for sensorineural loss, but previous middle fossa surgery for canal dehiscence was related to a poor hearing outcome in two patients in which it was performed. This review also suggested that, although canal plugging gives better control of vertigo symptoms, it may also be more prone to causing hearing loss.[17] Unfortunately, normal intraoperative auditory brainstem response recordings have not been shown to correlate with normal hearing postoperatively.[15] Hearing loss is often not immediately evident after surgery, and a prophylactic course of treatment with steroids may help to reduce the chance of this complication occurring. Given that patients with superior canal dehiscence often complain of only relatively mild symptoms and that the middle cranial fossa approach entails the risk of intracranial complications such as bleeding (especially among older patients) and stroke, many patients decide against surgery for this condition (see Table 54-1).

MÉNIÈRE DISEASE

Diagnosis

Ménière disease, which was first described by Prosper Ménière in 1861, is characterized by hearing loss, tinnitus, fullness, and vertigo, and it is correlated with the histologic finding of endolymphatic hydrops. Before embarking on a treatment course for this condition, it is wise to reconsider the diagnosis. Chiari I malformation, arachnoid cyst, vestibular schwannoma, syphilis, vestibular migraine, and other conditions may present with symptoms that are similar to those of Ménière disease but that are unlikely to improve unless addressed with therapies specific to them.[22–25] Many practitioners agree that the initial treatment of Ménière disease includes dietary modification and the use of diuretics or betahistine.[26] Despite the widespread use of these interventions among practitioners and the clinical impression that they are effective, no meta-analysis has yet shown that either is better than placebo.[27–29]

Treatment

In general, patients for whom medical treatment for Ménière disease is ineffective are offered a surgical option for treatment. Most practitioners begin with a relatively noninvasive treatment, with patients with ongoing symptoms being offered more invasive and finally ablative procedures. Management decisions for patients for whom a particular surgical intervention does not work are difficult because of limited data predicting the outcomes of each surgical option. This is a result of the intermittent nature of the disease, its tendency toward spontaneous long-term improvement, and the subjective nature of its manifestations. Treatment decisions are therefore often based on a surgeon's experience and a patient's comfort level with the potential risks of a surgery rather than a reliable prediction of the chance of an intervention being successful.

Simple nonablative surgical procedures for treating Ménière disease include the placement of a pressure equalization tube, sometimes in combination with the daily use of the Meniett low-frequency pressure device (Medtronic XOMED, Minneapolis, Minn) inserted into the external auditory canal or the intratympanic injection of steroids. Although these procedures are virtually free of risk, data do not conclusively indicate that either one of them is effective.[30,31] Persistent perforations after the placement of pressure-equalization tubes are managed expectantly or with a tympanoplasty.

Endolymphatic sac decompression or shunting is a more aggressive but no less controversial treatment for Ménière disease. The procedure involves a mastoidectomy with exposure of the endolymphatic sac by drilling away the bone that overlies the posterior fossa dura. The sac is opened, and a stent is usually placed to keep the lumen open to the mastoid cavity. Several studies have failed to show a long-term benefit of the procedure.[32,33] Quaranta and colleagues[34] showed that, 6 years after the initial evaluation, the symptoms of more than 70% of patients were well-controlled without sac surgery, whereas those who had sac decompression or shunting enjoyed no significant added benefit. Despite the ongoing question of whether the procedure improves patient outcomes and the risk of complications, many patients and practitioners are convinced of the benefit of the procedure.[35,36] The procedure has the

advantage of not being ablative, and the chance of hearing loss has been reported to be less than 5%.[37] Possible complications include damage to the posterior fossa dura that may lead to cerebrospinal fluid leak. This can be managed with a fascial patch and the application of a dural sealant such as DuraSeal (Confluent Surgical, Waltham, Mass) to the area. The posterior semicircular canal, which lies a variable distance anterior to and approximately parallel to the posterior fossa dura, may also be inadvertently entered, and it must be located positively before dural exposure proceeds (Figure 54-3). Should this canal be entered, gently placing a plug of fascial tissue into the exposed lumen may reduce the chance of hearing loss and ongoing imbalance.

Patients in whom an endolymphatic sac procedure is not performed or who do not improve after the procedure are best managed with an ablative intervention such as nerve sectioning or chemical or surgical labyrinthectomy. Intracranial sectioning of cranial nerve VIII (i.e., "vestibular neurectomy") was first proposed during the nineteenth century,[38] and it was later carefully described in a case series by Dandy.[39] A modern case series indicates that good control of symptoms can be achieved by 80% of patients who undergo a posterior fossa approach to the vestibular nerve and by 45% of patients who undergo a middle fossa approach.[40] The posterior fossa approach has the additional advantage of offering a much better chance of preserving hearing.[41] Both approaches require care with regard to the identification of

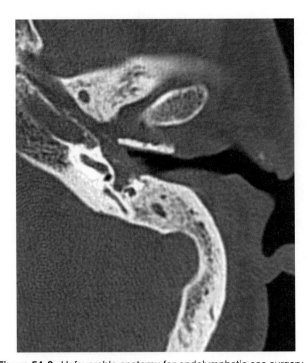

Figure 54-3. Unfavorable anatomy for endolymphatic sac surgery. The narrow space between the posterior semicircular canal and the posterior fossa dura in this patient makes for a relatively difficult approach to the endolymphatic sac, with an increased risk of violating the vestibular labyrinth.

the relevant cranial nerves. In the cerebellopontine angle, the vestibular branch of cranial nerve VIII is identified superior to the cochlear nerve (located posteroinferiorly) and the facial nerve (located anteroinferiorly). It is crucial that the surgeon recognize how this relationship changes as the nerve travels laterally (Figure 54-4). The failure to correctly identify the plane between the cochlear nerve and the vestibular nerve can result in damage to the cochlear nerve, which is an outcome that is particularly likely with medial traction. Cochlear nerve injury can be avoided by differentiating the relatively whiter auditory fibers from the grayer vestibular fibers. The presence of a small blood vessel and a sulcus between the cochlear and vestibular divisions of cranial nerve VIII can aid in defining their boundaries.

Other options that ablate labyrinthine function include a chemical labyrinthectomy via the intratympanic instillation of buffered gentamicin or a surgical labyrinthectomy. A large retrospective study that compared vestibular nerve sectioning to gentamicin therapy found greater control of vertigo and less chance of hearing loss with nerve sectioning than with gentamicin.[1] This study reported that 80% of those receiving gentamicin therapy had good control of vertigo and that 20% had hearing loss, whereas 95% of those undergoing nerve sectioning had good vertigo control and only 3% had hearing loss; however, with careful attention paid to the development of vestibular effects during a course of gentamicin therapy (using bedside and laboratory examinations to evaluate for vestibular asymmetry), gentamicin therapy may be closely titrated, and it may reduce the risk of hearing loss to approximately the 3% reported by Hillman and colleagues[42] for nerve section. Such monitoring also prevents overtreatment with gentamicin, which leads to unilateral vestibular ablation and its consequences. Gentamicin has the additional advantage of presenting none of the risks of intracranial procedures. The optimal management of hearing loss related to gentamicin or vestibular neurectomy has not been determined, but a course of high-dose steroids may be helpful.

Surgical labyrinthectomy is an appropriate approach for patients with Ménière disease who have no usable hearing and who are refractory to gentamicin treatment. A transcanal approach permits a limited labyrinthectomy to be performed. This technique requires the subluxation of the stapes, the drilling of the promontory to open the vestibule, and the removal of the vestibular neuroepithelia in the vestibule and the canal ampullae using a small right-angle hook. However, it does not allow for the sectioning of the vestibular nerve itself, which may increase the chances of this treatment being unsuccessful. A transmastoid labyrinthectomy allows for the sectioning of the vestibular nerve medial to the Scarpa ganglion within the internal auditory canal. This step may improve the control of the subjective symptoms of imbalance, probably as a result of the interruption of vestibular nerve afferents medial to the Scarpa ganglion[40,43] (Tables 54-2 and 54-3).

POSTERIOR FOSSA PATHOLOGY

Patients with vestibular schwannomas may suffer from prominent symptoms of imbalance and vertigo. Such symptoms may be constant or intermittent, and they are sometimes related to hyperventilation.[44] Although emphasis has been placed on the hearing and facial nerve outcomes of patients undergoing microsurgical or radiation treatment for vestibular schwannoma, little study has been devoted to changes in their balance. One study reported that 12 of 29 patients treated with Gamma Knife therapy for vestibular schwannoma had pretreatment imbalance. Imbalance improved in two patients, but eight patients without preoperative symptoms noted disequilibrium after the procedure.[45] Subjective symptoms of imbalance as measured by the Dizziness Handicap Inventory may be lessened after radiation therapy as compared with surgical therapy.[46]

Arnold–Chiari syndrome and vascular loops involving cranial nerve VIII may also be related to symptoms of imbalance. In a study of 27 patients operated on for Chiari I malformations, 3 of 6 who had vertigo preoperatively improved, but 1 previously asymptomatic subject developed new-onset vertigo.[47] The decompression of the vascular loops near the cranial nerve VIII complex has been reported to result in the improvement of imbalance in 80% of patients. However, symptoms of tinnitus may not be affected.[48]

PERILYMPHATIC FISTULA

The diagnosis of perilymphatic fistula is challenging. The increased recognition of disorders such as canal dehiscence and vestibular migraine, with symptoms

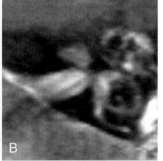

Figure 54-4. A T2-weighted magnetic resonance image showing the rotation of the contents of the internal auditory canal as seen from the standard radiologic vantage point. The failure to recognize these relationships can result in cranial nerve injury during vestibular nerve section. **A,** Right internal auditory canal. Cranial nerve VII and VIII follow a right-handed spiral. **B,** Left internal auditory canal. The contents follow a left-handed spiral.

TABLE 54-2 Failure Rates for Ménière Disease Treatments

Author	Treatment								
	Pressure Equalization Tube	Meniett Device	Diuretic	Betahistine	Intratympanic Dexamethasone Injection	Endolymphatic Sac Decompression	Chemical Labyrinthectomy	Vestibular Nerve Section	Surgical Labyrinthectomy
Gates et al.[65,66]	62/62	19/58							
Van Deelen and Huizing[26]			16/33						
Mira et al.[67]				19/71					
Silverstein et al.[68]					20/20				
Garduno-Anaya et al.[69]					2/11				
Hirvonen et al.[70]					3/17				
Telischi and Luxford[71]						87/234			
Quaranta et al.[34]						3/20			
De Beer et al.[72]							11/57		
Youssef and Poe[73]							5/37		
Hillman et al.[1]							5/25	2/39	
Thomsen et al.[74]								3/42	
De la Cruz et al.[40]						9/28		16/54	2/14

TABLE 54-3 Incidence of Sensorineural Hearing Loss After Surgical Treatment for Ménière Disease

	Endolymphatic Sac Decompression	Chemical Labyrinthectomy	Vestibular Nerve Section
Quaranta et al.[34]	1/15		
De Beer et al.[72]		9/57	
Youssef and Poe[73]		16/37	
Hillman et al.[1]		5/25	1/39
Thomsen et al.[74]			3/42

that may mimic those of perilymphatic fistula, has allowed many patients to be treated effectively without middle-ear exploration. Therefore a common "complication" related to the treatment of perilymphatic fistula is that the diagnosis was made in error. However, some patients describe a history that is convincing for fistula, such as the onset of symptoms of intermittent hearing loss, fullness, and imbalance after an episode of barotrauma. Patients with a fistula may also describe symptomatic improvement when lying on one side. Leaks are more common at the annular ligament, but careful drilling of the lip of the round-window niche allows for the complete visualization of the round window to verify that a periannular leak is not responsible for the patient's symptoms. Packing with muscle instead of fascia over the cochlear windows is standard treatment, because it is less likely to be absorbed than fat.[49] The salient complication of surgery for perilymphatic fistula is that middle-ear exploration may fail to demonstrate a fistula or that the fistula's symptoms may not be completely resolved after treatment. In a large series of pediatric patients with perilymphatic fistula, more than 90% had improvement in vertigo and no significant loss in hearing after surgery.[50] The review of a series of adults who underwent middle-ear exploration for symptoms of perilymphatic fistula revealed that 87% of patients had improvement in imbalance and that 40% had improvement in sensorineural hearing. Of note is that, although all patients were treated for fistula with packing, the level of improvement did not correlate with the demonstration of an actual leak at the time of surgery.[51] Failures of fistula surgery must be managed first and foremost by reconsidering the diagnosis, based in part on whether an actual leak was found at the time of initial surgery. If not, the diagnosis of vestibular migraine must be carefully considered, and imaging for canal dehiscence or enlarged vestibular aqueduct should be undertaken. Reoperation may clearly benefit some patients to ensure that muscle and fascia are used rather than more easily resorbable fat for sealing the leak.

BENIGN POSITIONAL VERTIGO

Treatment

Benign positional vertigo usually arises from the canalithiasis of the posterior semicircular canal. In the Dix–Hallpike position, signs include an upbeating and torsional nystagmus with the upper pole of the eyes directed toward the floor. Initial treatment consists of repositioning exercises such as the Epley maneuver,[52] with or without mastoid vibration, and the Semont maneuver.[53] Normally these maneuvers are well tolerated, although ongoing imbalance for days after even successful treatment is not uncommon. The Semont maneuver requires more rapid motion, thereby making it less feasible for some patients. The Epley and Semont maneuvers are probably equally effective, with a success rate of more than 90% after three initial treatments and a recurrence rate of approximately 15% at 6 months.[54] Treatments may need to be repeated several times to achieve these control rates.

If canalith repositioning maneuvers do not work, a reconsideration of the diagnosis is necessary. It could be that a patient has benign positional vertigo in both posterior canals or that horizontal or anterior canal variants of positional vertigo are causing symptoms. Uncomplicated horizontal canal benign positional vertigo produces horizontal nystagmus with fast phases in the geotropic direction and without a torsional component seen with the patient supine, the affected ear down, and the neck straight. All methods for treating horizontal canal canalithiasis are designed to move the otoconial debris out of the nonampullated end of the canal by rotating the head in the plane of the canal. The Vannucchi maneuver

requires the patient to roll with the affected ear up and to remain in that position for 12 hours.[55] The patient may be moved through a 360-degree rotation, starting supine with the affected ear down and rotating away from that ear.[56] The Lempert maneuver has the patient rotate the head (but not the body) 270 degrees in the same direction.[57] Such a rolling maneuver has been shown to have an efficacy of more than 90%.[54] Ageotropic horizontal nystagmus represents the cupulolithiasis of the horizontal canal with the adhesion of particles to the cupula itself, and it is much more difficult to treat.

The anterior canal variant shows torsional nystagmus similar to that seen in patients with posterior canal benign positional vertigo but with a downbeating vertical fast phase. Treatment with the patient supine and the neck flexed aggressively has been reported to have good results for clearing symptoms,[58] although many practitioners find this variant particularly resistant to treatment.

Complications

Complications related to repositioning maneuvers include the conversion of symptoms in one canal to symptoms in another canal. This has been noted to occur in 6% of patients treated for posterior canal positional vertigo, and it requires alternative repositioning maneuvers to clear the offending debris.[59] "Canalith jam" may occur when the otoconial debris exiting the posterior canal lodges in the common crus, thereby causing intense vertigo independent of the direction of the positioning of the head.[56] This requires the repositioning of the patient in the Dix–Hallpike position and then using a mastoid vibrator to loosen the wedged debris and allowing it to return to the posterior canal before reattempting the repositioning exercises.

Patients who have definite signs and symptoms of canalithiasis but for whom canal repositioning procedures are not successful may undergo surgery to plug the offending canal.[60] This procedure may be particularly useful for patients with cupulolithiasis, which is harder to clear with repositioning maneuvers. Such a surgical procedure prevents the movement of the otoconial debris from activating the canal and causing dizziness. Because it does not damage the vestibular nerve itself, it should not induce acute symptoms of unilateral vestibular loss. For the posterior canal, a transmastoid approach is used that involves blue-lining the bony canal and opening a 2 mm to 3 mm portion of the lumen to allow fascia to be introduced and to occlude the membranous duct. Fascia and fibrin glue are placed over the repair. A large study showed the relief of symptoms in all 44 subjects and only 1 case of sudden hearing loss.[61] Patients are generally imbalanced for several weeks after surgery, but careful insertion of the fascia into the lumen of the canal may

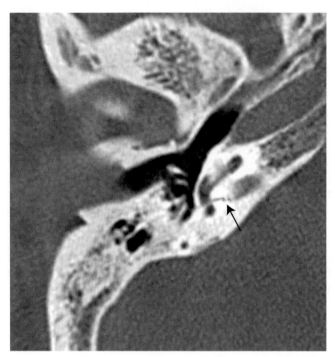

Figure 54-5. The course of a singular nerve *(arrow)*.

TABLE 54-4 Failure Rates for Benign Positional Vertigo Treatments

	Treatment			
	Epley Maneuver	**Semont Maneuver**	**Vestibular Habituation**	**Canal Plugging**
Gananca et al.[75]	2/30			
Wolf et al.[76]	2/31			
von Brevern et al.[77]	7/35			
Froehling et al.[78]	12/24			
Levrat et al.[79]		27/278		
Haynes et al.[80]		11/127		
Norre and Beckers[81]			11/40	
Brandt and Daroff[82]			1/60	
Agrawal and Parnes[61]				0/44
Walsh et al.[83]				0/13

prevent damage to the neuroepithelium and reduce recovery times.

Another surgical approach for the treatment of patients with posterior canal benign positional vertigo for whom repositioning maneuvers are ineffective is singular neurectomy.[62] The singular nerve is approached by exposing the singular canal inferior to the round window (Figure 54-5). Although this treatment has a high efficacy rate of 98%, its use is limited by a risk of sensorineural hearing loss of 4%, even in the hands of an exceptionally experienced surgeon[63] (Table 54-4).

CONCLUSION

There are many procedures available to assist in the treatment of vestibular disorders. Although these may benefit a significant number of patients, appropriate patient and procedure selection are critical. The careful explanation of the possible complications and the appropriate counseling of the patient are essential, and the vestibular surgeon must be aware of all of the potential pitfalls of these procedures to minimize their occurrence.

REFERENCES

1. Hillman TA, Chen DA, Arriaga MA: Vestibular nerve section versus intratympanic gentamicin for Ménière's disease. *Laryngoscope* 2004;114(2):216–222.
2. Herdman SJ et al: Recovery of dynamic visual acuity in unilateral vestibular hypofunction. *Arch Otolaryngol Head Neck Surg* 2003;129(8):819–824.
3. Colletti V: Medical treatment in Ménière's disease: Avoiding vestibular neurectomy and facilitating postoperative compensation. *Acta Otolaryngol Suppl* 2000;544:27–33.
4. Fujino A et al: Vestibular training for benign paroxysmal positional vertigo: Its efficacy in comparison with antivertigo drugs. *Arch Otolaryngol Head Neck Surg* 1994;120:497–504.
5. Moon IS, Hain TC: Delayed quick spins after vestibular nerve section respond to anticonvulsant therapy. *Otol Neurotol* 2005;26(1):82–85.
6. Dornhoffer JL, Milewski C: Management of the open labyrinth. *Otolaryngol Head Neck Surg* 1995;112(3):410–414.
7. Riechelmann H et al: Perioperative glucocorticoid treatment does not influence early post-laser stapedotomy hearing thresholds. *Am J Otol* 2000;21(6):809–812.
8. Kopke R et al: Prevention of impulse noise-induced hearing loss with antioxidants. *Acta Otolaryngol* 2005;125(3):235–243.
9. Lamm K, Lamm H, Arnold W: Effect of hyperbaric oxygen therapy in comparison to conventional or placebo therapy or no treatment in idiopathic sudden hearing loss, acoustic trauma, noise-induced hearing loss and tinnitus: A literature survey. *Adv Otorhinolaryngol* 1998;54:86–99.
10. Chen Y et al: Aspirin attenuates gentamicin ototoxicity: From the laboratory to the clinic. *Hear Res* 2007;226(1–2):178–182.
11. Harner SG, Beatty CW, Ebersold MJ: Impact of cranioplasty on headache after acoustic neuroma removal. *Neurosurgery* 1995;36(6):1097–1100.
12. Tullio P: *Das ohr und die entstehung der sprache und schrift,* Berlin, 1929, Urban & Schwarzenberg.
13. De Vries H, Bleeker JD: The microphonic activity of the labyrinth of the pigeon: The response of the cristae in the semicircular canals. *Acta Otolaryngol* 1949;37(4):298–306.
14. Minor LB et al: Sound- and/or pressure-induced vertigo due to bone dehiscence of the superior semicircular canal. *Arch Otolaryngol Head Neck Surg* 1998;124:249–258.
15. Minor LB: Clinical manifestations of superior semicircular canal dehiscence. *Laryngoscope* 2005;115(10):1717–1727.
16. Branstetter BF 4th et al: Superior semicircular canal dehiscence: Oblique reformatted CT images for diagnosis. *Radiology* 2006;238(3):938–942.
17. Limb CJ et al: Auditory function in patients with surgically treated superior semicircular canal dehiscence. *Otol Neurotol* 2006;27(7):969–980.
18. Mikulec AA et al: Superior semicircular canal dehiscence presenting as conductive hearing loss without vertigo. *Otol Neurotol* 2004;25(2):121–129.
19. Halmagyi GM et al: The click-evoked vestibulo-ocular reflex in superior semicircular canal dehiscence. *Neurology* 2003;60(7):1172–1175.
20. Mikulec AA, Poe DS, McKenna MJ: Operative management of superior semicircular canal dehiscence. *Laryngoscope* 2005;115(3):501–507.
21. Hyrtl J: Über spontane dehiscenz des tegmen tympani und der cellulae mastoideae. Sitzungsberichte der mathem. *Natur Classe der kais Adademie der Wissenschaften* 1858;30(16):275.
22. Milhorat TH et al: Chiari I malformation redefined: Clinical and radiographic findings for 364 symptomatic patients. *Neurosurgery* 1999;44(5):1005–1017.
23. O'Reilly RC, Hallinan EK: Posterior fossa arachnoid cysts can mimic Ménière's disease. *Am J Otolaryngol* 2003;24(6):420–425.
24. Morrison GA, Sterkers JM: Unusual presentations of acoustic tumours. *Clin Otolaryngol Allied Sci* 1996;21(1):80–83.
25. Pulec JL: Ménière's disease of syphilitic etiology. *Ear Nose Throat J* 1997;76(8):508–510, 512, 514, passim.
26. van Deelen GW, Huizing EH: Use of a diuretic (Dyazide®) in the treatment of Ménière's disease. *ORL J Otorhinolaryngol Relat Spec* 1986;48:287–292.
27. Strupp M, Brandt T: Pharmacological advances in the treatment of neuro-otological and eye movement disorders. *Curr Opin Neurol* 2006;19(1):33–40.
28. James AL, Burton MJ: Betahistine for Ménière's disease or syndrome. *Cochrane Database Syst Rev* 2001;(1):CD001873.
29. Thirlwall AS, Kundu S: Diuretics for Ménière's disease or syndrome. *Cochrane Database Syst Rev* 2006;3:CD003599.
30. Stokroos R et al: Functional outcome of treatment of Ménière's disease with the Meniett pressure generator. *Acta Otolaryngol* 2006;126(3):254–258.
31. Alles MJ, der Gaag MA, Stokroos RJ: Intratympanic steroid therapy for inner ear diseases, a review of the literature. *Eur Arch Otorhinolaryngol* 2006;263(9):791–797.
32. Jackson CG et al: Endolymphatic system shunting: A long-term profile of the Denver inner ear shunt. *Am J Otol* 1996;17:85–88.
33. Silverstein H, Smouha E, Jones R: Natural history vs. surgery for Ménière's disease. *Otolaryngol Head Neck Surg* 1989;100:6–16.
34. Quaranta A, Marini F, Sallustio V: Long-term outcome of Ménière's disease: Endolymphatic mastoid shunt versus natural history. *Audiol Neurootol* 1998;3(1):54–60.
35. Paparella MM, Fina M: Endolymphatic sac enhancement: Reversal of pathogenesis. *Otolaryngol Clin North Am* 2002;35(3):621–637.
36. Convert C et al: Outcome-based assessment of endolymphatic sac decompression for Ménière's disease using the Ménière's disease outcome questionnaire: A review of 90 patients. *Otol Neurotol* 2006;27(5):687–696.
37. Luetje CM: A critical comparison of results of endolymphatic subarachnoid shunt and endolymphatic sac incision operations. *Am J Otol* 1988;9(2):95–101.
38. Jackler RK, Whinney D: A century of eighth nerve surgery. *Otol Neurotol* 2001;22(3):401–416.
39. Dandy W: Ménière's disease, its diagnosis and a method of treatment. *Arch Surg* 1928;16:1127–1152.
40. De la Cruz A, Teufert KB, Berliner KI: Surgical treatment for vertigo: Patient survey of vertigo, imbalance, and time course for recovery. *Otolaryngol Head Neck Surg* 2006;135(4):541–548.
41. McElveen JT Jr et al: Retrolabyrinthine vestibular nerve section: A viable alternative to the middle fossa approach. *Otolaryngol Head Neck Surg* 1984;92(2):136–140.
42. Minor LB: Intratympanic gentamicin for control of vertigo in Ménière's disease: Vestibular signs that specify completion of therapy. *Am J Otol* 1999;20(2):209–212.
43. Silverstein H, Norrell H, Rosenberg S: The resurrection of vestibular neurectomy: A 10-year experience with 115 cases. *J Neurosurg* 1990;72(4):533–539.
44. Bance ML et al: Vestibular disease unmasked by hyperventilation. *Laryngoscope* 1998;108(4 Pt 1):610–614.
45. Wackym PA et al: Gamma knife radiosurgery for acoustic neuromas performed by a neurotologist: Early experiences and outcomes. *Otol Neurotol* 2004;25(5):752–761.

46. Pollock BE et al: Patient outcomes after vestibular schwannoma management: A prospective comparison of microsurgical resection and stereotactic radiosurgery. *Neurosurgery* 2006;59(1):77–85.

47. Dones J et al: Clinical outcomes in patients with Chiari I malformation: A review of 27 cases. *Surg Neurol* 2003;60(2):142–148.

48. Brackmann DE, Kesser BW, Day JD: Microvascular decompression of the vestibulocochlear nerve for disabling positional vertigo: The House Ear Clinic experience. *Otol Neurotol* 2001;22(6):882–887.

49. Suzuki M, Shigemi H, Mogi G: The leaking labyrinthine lesion resulting from direct force through the auditory canal: Report of five cases. *Auris Nasus Larynx* 1999;26(1):29–32.

50. Weber PC, Bluestone CD, Perez B: Outcome of hearing and vertigo after surgery for congenital perilymphatic fistula in children. *Am J Otolaryngol* 2003;24(3):138–142.

51. Fitzgerald D, Getson P, Brasseux C: Perilymphatic fistula: A Washington, DC experience. *Ann Otol Rhinol Laryngol* 1997;106:830–837.

52. Epley JM: The canalith repositioning procedure: For treatment of benign paroxysmal positional vertigo. *Otolaryngol Head Neck Surg* 1992;107:399–404.

53. Semont A, Freyss G, Vitte E: Curing the BPPV with a liberatory maneuver. *Adv Otorhinolaryngol* 1988;42:290–293.

54. Steenerson RL, Cronin GW, Marbach PM: Effectiveness of treatment techniques in 923 cases of benign paroxysmal positional vertigo. *Laryngoscope* 2005;115(2):226–231.

55. Vannucchi P, Giannoni B, Pagnini P: Treatment of horizontal semicircular canal benign paroxysmal positional vertigo. *J Vestib Res* 1997;7(1):1–6.

56. Epley JM: Positional vertigo related to semicircular canalithiasis. *Otolaryngol Head Neck Surg* 1995;112:154–161.

57. Lempert T, Tiel-Wilck K: A positional maneuver for treatment of horizontal-canal benign positional vertigo. *Laryngoscope* 1996;106:476–478.

58. Crevits L: Treatment of anterior canal benign paroxysmal positional vertigo by a prolonged forced position procedure. *J Neurol Neurosurg Psychiatry* 2004;75(5):779–781.

59. Herdman SJ, Tusa RJ: Complications of the canalith repositioning procedure. *Arch Otolaryngol Head Neck Surg* 1996;122:281–286.

60. Parnes LS, McClure JA: Posterior semicircular canal occlusion for intractable benign paroxysmal positional vertigo. *Ann Otol Rhinol Laryngol* 1990;99:330–334.

61. Agrawal SK, Parnes LS: Human experience with canal plugging. *Ann N Y Acad Sci* 2001;942:300–305.

62. Gacek RR: Transection of the posterior ampullary nerve for the relief of benign paroxysmal positional vertigo. *Ann Otol Rhinol Laryngol* 1974;83:596–605.

63. Gacek RR, Gacek MR: Results of singular neurectomy in the posterior ampullary recess. *ORL J Otorhinolaryngol Relat Spec* 2002;64(6):397–402.

64. Hillman TA et al: Reversible peripheral vestibulopathy: The treatment of superior canal dehiscence. *Otolaryngol Head Neck Surg* 2006;134(3):431–436.

65. Gates GA et al: The effects of transtympanic micropressure treatment in people with unilateral Ménière's disease. *Arch Otolaryngol Head Neck Surg* 2004;130(6):718–725.

66. Gates GA et al: Meniett clinical trial: Long-term follow-up. *Arch Otolaryngol Head Neck Surg* 2006;132(12):1311–1316.

67. Mira E et al: Betahistine dihydrochloride in the treatment of peripheral vestibular vertigo. *Eur Arch Otorhinolaryngol* 2003;260(2):73–77.

68. Silverstein H et al: Dexamethasone inner ear perfusion for the treatment of Ménière's disease: A prospective, randomized, double-blind, crossover trial. *Am J Otol* 1998;19:196–201.

69. Garduno-Anaya MA et al: Dexamethasone inner ear perfusion by intratympanic injection in unilateral Ménière's disease: A two-year prospective, placebo-controlled, double-blind, randomized trial. *Otolaryngol Head Neck Surg* 2005;133(2):285–294.

70. Hirvonen TP, Peltomaa M, Ylikoski J: Intratympanic and systemic dexamethasone for Ménière's disease. *ORL J Otorhinolaryngol Relat Spec* 2000;62(3):117–120.

71. Telischi F, Luxford WM: Long-term efficacy of endolymphatic sac surgery for vertigo in Ménière's disease. *Otolaryngol Head Neck Surg* 1993;109:83–87.

72. De Beer L, Stokroos R, Kingma H: Intratympanic gentamicin therapy for intractable Ménière's disease. *Acta Otolaryngol* 2007;127(6):605–612.

73. Youssef TF, Poe DS: Intratympanic gentamicin injection for the treatment of Ménière's disease. *Am J Otol* 1998;19:435–442.

74. Thomsen J, Berner B, Tos M: Vestibular neurectomy. *Auris Nasus Larynx* 2000;27(4):297–301.

75. Gananca FF et al: Is it important to restrict head movement after Epley maneuver? *Rev Bras Otorrinolaringol (Engl Ed)* 2005;71(6):764–768.

76. Wolf M et al: Epley's manoeuvre for benign paroxysmal positional vertigo: A prospective study. *Clin Otolaryngol Allied Sci* 1999;24(1):43–46.

77. von Brevern M et al: Short-term efficacy of Epley's manoeuvre: A double-blind randomised trial. *J Neurol Neurosurg Psychiatry* 2006;77(8):980–982.

78. Froehling DA et al: The canalith repositioning procedure for the treatment of benign paroxysmal positional vertigo: A randomized controlled trial. *Mayo Clin Proc* 2000;75(7):695–700.

79. Levrat E et al: Efficacy of the Semont maneuver in benign paroxysmal positional vertigo. *Arch Otolaryngol Head Neck Surg* 2003;129(6):629–633.

80. Haynes DS et al: Treatment of benign positional vertigo using the Semont maneuver: Efficacy in patients presenting without nystagmus. *Laryngoscope* 2002;112(5):796–801.

81. Norre ME, Beckers A: Vestibular habituation training for positional vertigo in elderly patients. *Arch Gerontol Geriatr* 1989;8(2):117–122.

82. Brandt T, Daroff RB: Physical therapy for benign paroxysmal positional vertigo. *Arch Otolaryngol Head Neck Surg* 1980;106:484–485.

83. Walsh RM et al: Long-term results of posterior semicircular canal occlusion for intractable benign paroxysmal positional vertigo. *Clin Otolaryngol Allied Sci* 1999;24(4):316–323.

CHAPTER 55

Complications of Tympanomastoidectomy

Ronald A. Hoffman

Complications of tympanomastoidectomy occur as result of injury to the ear or the surrounding structures, and they can be categorized as perioperative or delayed. Perioperative complications occur during, immediately after, or in near association with surgery. Delayed complications occur after months or years; there is no exact time delineation.

Excluding generic surgical complications (e.g., those associated with anesthesia and wound healing), potential complications of tympanomastoidectomy include facial nerve injury, dural injury, venous sinus injury, carotid artery injury, cochleovestibular injury, and delayed iatrogenic cholesteatoma. It is difficult to assess the true incidence of these complications, because they go largely unreported.

FACIAL NERVE INJURY

Facial nerve injury is among the most disabling to patients and the most threatening to surgeons. The incidence is understated in the literature, and it may better be determined by a review of litigation files. Greenberg and Manolides[1] reported no cases of facial paralysis in a series of 33 patients who presented with severe chronic otitis and predisposing preoperative factors such as dural dehiscence, labyrinthine fistula, facial nerve involvement by disease, and suppurative intracranial complications. Dawes[2] reported no cases of facial nerve injury in a series of 145 patients. Fayad,[3] in reporting on cochlear implantation in 705 patients, reported an incidence of delayed facial paresis of 0.71%. Although the facial nerve was routinely at risk in these cases as a result of the opening of the facial recess, gross temporal bone anatomy was otherwise normal, and the surgeons were senior and experienced.

There are three keys to avoiding facial nerve injury:

1. Preoperative high-resolution computed tomography scanning of the temporal bones in both the axial and coronal planes (Figure 55-1), thus allowing for the identification of variations in facial nerve anatomy and the extent of contiguous pathology
2. A thorough familiarity with facial nerve anatomy through surgical experience
3. The use of real-time facial nerve monitoring, including the use of a Prass probe

Although facial nerve monitoring can be an invaluable aid for avoiding facial nerve injury, it absolutely does not substitute for a thorough familiarity with facial nerve anatomy and surgical experience. The surgeon who relies inordinately on the facial nerve monitor is one who puts the patient and himself or herself at risk.

MANAGING FACIAL NERVE INJURY

The management of facial nerve injury depends on when the injury is identified. If an injury is evident intraoperatively, corrective action should be taken at that time. If the nerve is bruised or if there is an intraneural hematoma, the nerve should be decompressed for several millimeters proximal and distal to the injury. In a noninfected ear, the perineurium can be slit to allow for decompression. However, slitting the sheath is controversial, particularly in the setting of active infection, canal wall down mastoidectomy, or residual cholesteatoma. If the nerve is partially transected but more than 60% to 70% percent of the fibers are intact, decompression and a protective fascial sling are advised. If the nerve is more than 30% to 40% transected, a direct reanastomosis or nerve graft is recommended.

The facial nerve is resilient. If there is an immediate postoperative facial paralysis, the likelihood of significant injury is great. The nerve should be explored as soon as is reasonably possible, usually within 24 to 72 hours. There is no benefit to an immediate exploration if the operating surgeon is exhausted and distressed or lacks experience with managing this complication.

If facial nerve injury results in a paresis or if the facial nerve deficit is delayed, the patient should be treated with steroids, monitored with electroneuronography, and managed expectantly. Identifying the time and degree of facial nerve weakness requires an objective and honest evaluation. The status of the facial nerve should preferentially be assessed by the operating surgeon before the patient leaves the operating room. Nasal alar flare can usually be assessed as the patient is being extubated. If there is doubt, the patient must be reevaluated as soon as the state of consciousness permits. Differentiating a paresis from a complete paralysis only on the basis of eye closure is risky. The closure of the upper lid without surrounding ocularis motion is a passive activity and not indicative of cranial nerve VII function. If in doubt, explore.

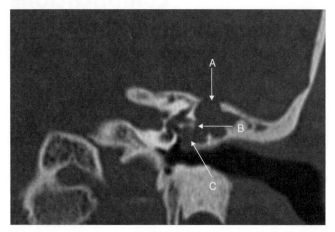

Figure 55-1. Preoperative axial computed tomography scan of the temporal bones alerting the surgeon to exposed middle fossa dura *(A)*, a horizontal canal fistula *(B)*, and an exposed facial nerve over the oval window *(C)*.

Be aware of the effects of topical anesthetics. A natural dehiscence of the bony fallopian canal has been identified in up to 55% of temporal bone specimens,[4,5] and it occurs frequently as a result of otologic pathology.[6] For example, it is not uncommon for a patient to experience a transient facial paralysis after stapedectomy performed under local anesthesia with a four-quadrant block of 1% or 2% xylocaine, with or without epinephrine. Anecdotally, the author had a patient awaken from an endolymphatic sac decompression with a complete facial paralysis. The postauricular crease had been infiltrated with 1% xylocaine with 1:100,000 epinephrine. The facial nerve was immediately explored, decompressed, and found to be completely normal. The patient emerged from anesthesia with normal facial nerve function. Such an effect of topical anesthetic would, moreover, negate the value of a facial nerve monitor. Since that experience in 1976, the author has used only epinephrine (1:200,000), mixed at the time of surgery, for local hemostasis in tympanomastoid surgery.

The chorda tympani branch of the facial nerve is routinely manipulated and sectioned during otologic surgery. Taste disturbances are common during the immediate postoperative period, and they can persist. Nin and colleagues[7] noted that 59% of patients undergoing unilateral chorda tympani section had symptoms 2 weeks after the operation. Gopalan[8] found that recovery was complete in 92% of patients at 1 one year. Taste disturbance should be a consideration in the risk–benefit analysis of elective tympanomastoid surgery, particularly if the patient's occupation involves food or wine.

DURAL INJURY

The middle cranial fossa tegmen plate and, to a lesser degree, the posterior fossa dural plate are critical anatomic landmarks of tympanomastoid surgery. The middle cranial fossa tegmen plate in particular is routinely identified during the performance of mastoid surgery. Small

areas of tegmen bone overlying the dura are often removed by the surgeon as the bone is intentionally thinned. Alternatively, dura may be exposed as a result of the disease process. Exposed intact dura rarely poses a threat of postoperative complication and merits no therapeutic intervention. Although delayed encephaloceles have been described,[9,10] they are unusual.

If the dura has been compromised with a resulting cerebrospinal fluid leak (CSF), the defect should be repaired intraoperatively. The first rule of the management of an intraoperative CSF leak is to not panic. Cover the area with gelfoam and a cottonoid to slow the leak and protect the area from further injury. Then, as best as possible, finish the indicated surgical procedure. Cholesteatoma should be removed. Decisions regarding the status of the canal wall should be skewed toward preservation, because the canal wall isolates the area of leak, protects the area postoperatively, and facilitates repair. Appropriate specimens should be taken for culture and sensitivity, and the patient should be treated postoperatively with a broad-spectrum antibiotic that crosses the blood–brain barrier.

There are many methods and approaches described for repairing CSF leaks. Some authors favor a transmastoid approach,[11] whereas others advocate a middle cranial fossa repair.[12] Tissues available for repair include fascia, local flaps, fat, bone, and bone pâte.[13] Adjunctive measures include the use of commercially available fibrin glue,[14] hydroxyapatite cement,[15] and postoperative continuous CSF drainage.[16] The method of repair and management will be dictated by each surgeon's experience.

Because the mastoid cavity has already been accessed, the initial approach to repair should be transmastoid, and the closure should be multilayered. This author prefers to initially wedge a dumbbell-shaped piece of muscle into the dural defect; this alone will usually stop the leak. A fascia graft is then tucked under the dura, above the edges of the bone defect. With larger bone defects, this can be further reinforced from below by inserting a bone plate sculpted from the occipital cortex into the defect. This is then further reinforced with a vascular flap, usually of temporalis muscle. Fibrin glue is used to seal the area. Occasionally a mini middle fossa approach can be used.[17] Foreign bodies should be avoided. The use of bone wax to repair a CSF leak is discouraged. If the surgical site becomes infected, the bone wax can act as a foreign body, develop a bacterial biofilm, and result in a persisting epidural or brain abscess.[18]

VASCULAR INJURIES

As with facial nerve injury, avoiding vascular injury is predicated on the surgeon's knowledge of anatomy and good preoperative imaging. The sigmoid sinus can be variable in location, the internal carotid artery aberrant,[19] and the dome of the jugular bulb high and potentially dehiscent in the hypotympanum.[20] The superior and inferior petrosal sinuses are also in close proximity. Moreover, otologic pathology may expose or distort these vascular structures. As with CSF leaks, the critical surgical dictum when confronted with brisk bleeding is "do not panic." Bleeding can be abated with a moist 4 × 4 or surgical Cottonoids. Assemble hemostatic aids such as Surgicel gauze or cotton (Johnson & Johnson, New Brunswick, NJ), Avitene (Davol, Inc., Cranston, RI), and thrombin. A small rent in the sigmoid or jugular bulb can usually be controlled with an Avitene, Gelfoam soaked in thrombin, or a Surgicel patch. Apply the patch, cover it with a Cottonoid, and irrigate over the Cottonoid. Reinforce the area at the termination of the procedure. Larger venous breaches may necessitate a greater amount of pressure using a larger Surgicel pack.

Mild bleeding is not unusual from the carotid adventitia, which is vascular. Techniques such as those described previously will control this bleeding. The laceration of carotid artery is a potential surgical catastrophe. Hemostasis must immediately be achieved with packing, and decisions must then made regarding possible ligation, grafting, or control with interventional radiology techniques.[21]

COCHLEOVESTIBULAR INJURY

Cochleovestibular injury results from the violation of the cochlear capsule, the semicircular canals, or the stapes footplate. The result can be tinnitus, hearing loss, or lingering vestibular symptoms. These complications most often occur because the otologic disease process creates a predisposition to them. The presence of a horizontal semicircular canal fistula can be anticipated from preoperative imaging and management strategies planned in advance.[22] Fistula of the cochlear capsule is rare.[23,24] The adherence of disease to the stapes superstructure, particularly cholesteatoma, is not unusual. When attempting to remove cholesteatoma, the stapes can be inadvertently disarticulated. If the stapes is dislocated with a perilymph leak, the safest strategy is to remove the stapes and seal the oval window. As with a stapedectomy, avoid suctioning over the oval window. Remove the stapes and the associated pathology gently, and immediately seal the oval window with a tissue graft. The author prefers fascia or perichondrium. Do not place an ossicular prosthesis on the graft, because it may prolapse into the vestibule. If stapes dislocation is recognized and managed appropriately, there will usually not be any permanent postoperative auditory or vestibular deficit. An ossiculoplasty can be performed at a subsequent sitting.

IATROGENIC CHOLESTEATOMA

Iatrogenic cholesteatoma is a delayed complication of tympanomastoidectomy that is often not recognized for years after surgery. The incidence is hard to establish, and it is often difficult to differentiate from recurrent or residual cholesteatoma. If the posterior external auditory canal wall is inadvertently violated and not repaired, a retraction cholesteatoma can occur that is indistinguishable from recurrent disease. If the skin is inadvertently seeded during the manipulation of flaps, it will appear just as the "pearl" of residual disease. The most common presentation of iatrogenic cholesteatoma are small inclusion cysts in the external auditory canal skin or on the reconstructed tympanic membrane. These will often rupture spontaneously with time, or they can be easily marsupialized in the office, often without anesthesia.

CONCLUSION

Complications of tympanomastoid surgery are unusual, but they can be serious and life-threatening. Proper preoperative planning and intraoperative management are critical to a favorable outcome. If management strategies are uncertain, the patient should be stabilized and expert consultation sought.

REFERENCES

1. Greenberg J, Manolides S: High incidence of complications encountered in chronic otitis media surgery in a U.S. metropolitan hospital. *Otolaryngol Head Neck Surg* 2001;125:623–627.
2. Dawes PJ: Early complications of surgery for chronic otitis media. *J Laryngol Otol* 1999;113(9):803–810.
3. Fayad JN, Wanna GB, Micheletto JN, et al: Facial nerve paralysis following cochlear implant surgery. *Laryngoscope* 2003;113(8):1344–1346.
4. DiMartino E, Sellhaus B, Haensel J, et al: Fallopian canal dehiscences: A survey of clinical and anatomical findings. *Eur Arch Otorhinolaryngol* 2005;262(2):120–126.
5. Baxter EH: Dehiscence of the fallopian canal: An anatomical study. *J Laryngol Otol* 1971;85:587.
6. Lin JC, Ho KY, Kuo WR, et al: Incidence of dehiscence of the facial nerve canal at surgery for middle ear cholesteatoma. *Otolaryngol Head Neck Surg* 2004;131(4):452–456.
7. Nin T, Sakagami M, Sone-Okunaka M, et al: Taste function after section of chorda tympani nerve in middle ear surgery. *Auris Nasus Larynx* 2006;33(1):13–17.
8. Gopalan P, Kumar M, Gupta D, et al: A study of chorda tympani nerve injury and related symptoms following middle-ear surgery. *J Laryngol Otol* 2005;119(3):189–192.
9. McMurphy AB, Oghalai JS: Repair of iatrogenic temporal lobe encephaloceles after canal wall down mastoidectomy in the presence of active cholesteatoma. *Otol Neurotol* 2005;26(4):587–594.
10. Wooten CT, Kaylie DM, Warren FM, et al: Management of brain herniation and cerebrospinal fluid leak in revision chronic ear surgery. *Laryngoscope* 2005;115(7):1256–1261.
11. Hoffman R: Cerebrospinal fluid leaks of temporal bone origin. In Jacker RK, Brackmann DE, editors: *Neurotology*, St Louis, 2005, Elsevier.
12. Gacek RR, Gacek MR, Tart R: Adult spontaneous cerebrospinal fluid otorrhea: Diagnosis and management. *Am J Otol* 1999;20(6):770–776.
13. Dutt SN, Mirza S, Irving RM: Middle cranial fossa approach for the repair of spontaneous cerebrospinal fluid otorrhea using autologous bone pate. *Clin Otolaryngol Allied Sci* 2001;26(2):117–123.
14. U.S. Food and Drug Administration: *FDA Talk Paper: New fibrin sealant approved to help control bleeding in surgery* (website): www.fda.gov/bbs/topics/ANSWERS/ANS00865.html. Accessed May 1, 2008.

15. Kveton JF, Goravalingappa R: Elimination of temporal bone cerebrospinal fluid otorrhea using hydroxyapatite cement. *Laryngoscope* 2000;110(Pt 1):1655–1659.

16. Fishman A, Hoffman R, Roland JT: Cerebrospinal fluid drainage in the management of CSF leak following acoustic neuroma surgery. *Laryngoscope* 1996;106(8):1002–1004.

17. Kuhweide R, Casselman JW: Spontaneous cerebrospinal fluid otorrhea from a tegmen defect: Transmastoid repair with minicraniotomy. *Ann Otol Rhinol Laryngol* 1999;108(Pt 1):653–658.

18. Unreported, personal experience of the author.

19. Sauvaget E, Paris J, Kici S, et al: Aberrant internal carotid artery in the temporal bone: Imaging findings and management. *Arch Otolaryngol Head Neck Surg* 2006;132(1):86–91.

20. Huang BR, Wang CH, Young YH: Dehiscent high jugular bulb: A pitfall in middle ear surgery. *Otol Neurotol* 2006;27(7):923–927.

21. Weber PC: Iatrogenic complications from chronic ear surgery. *Otolaryngol Clin North Am* 2005;38:711–722.

22. Soda-Mehry A, Betancourt-Suarez MA: Surgical treatment of labyrinthine fistula caused by cholesteatoma. *Otolaryngol Head Neck Surg* 2000;122(5):739–742.

23. de Zinis LO, Campovecci C, Gadola E: Fistula of the cochlear labyrinth in noncholesteatomatous chronic otitis media. *Otol Neurotol* 2005;26(5):830–833.

24. Falcioni M, Lauda L: Imaging case of the month: Cochlear fistula in recurrent cholesteatoma. *Otol Neurotol* 2006;27:284.

CHAPTER 56

Complications of Ear Surgery

Joseph G. Feghali, John T. McElveen, Jr., Bradley Thedinger,
and David Barrs

Complications are an inevitable fact of life that confronts all surgeons. The surgeon who commits to performing otologic surgery must face the particular challenges that are inherent to performing surgery in a confined space in which small errors can lead to serious complications. However, it is important to remember that all complications are not the result of errors in judgment or technique. The nature of the ear, its anatomy, its variable pneumatization, its dependence on proper Eustachian tube function, and its proximity to major vascular and neurologic structures present a unique challenge. It has been said that variation is the hallmark of otologic surgery. This variation creates an element of unpredictability that, despite every effort, can still lead to undesirable results and outcomes.

It is equally important for otologic surgeons to master techniques to avoid surgical pitfalls and methods to manage otologic complications. Avoidance is always preferred, and it is commonly achievable with the use of precise technique, sound judgment, and a realistic goal of what can be achieved in a particular situation.

The management of complications can start intraoperatively or postoperatively. During surgery, the management of complications requires experience and judgment on the part of the surgeon. During the postoperative period, it also requires the cooperation and involvement of the patient. A patient's cooperation is best secured when the patient has had adequate preoperative preparation and has appropriate expectations of the success rate—and thus the failure rate—of any procedure. Defining the success and failure of a surgical procedure is important for patients who are undergoing all types of surgery; it is of particular importance in otologic surgery, in which success may be defined differently by the patient and the surgeon. Consider the patient with a preoperative severe sensorineural loss from cholesteatoma, chronic infection, or acoustic neuroma. In such a patient, surgery is commonly indicated, but it will clearly not restore hearing. Although this fact is clear to the surgeon, it may not be clear to the patient, who might equate a successful otologic surgical result with the restoration of hearing. This is the reason that it can be useful to inform patients about the "obvious" preoperatively. This can go a long way toward adjusting expectations and improving patient satisfaction and the acceptance of imperfect function as the best expected outcome in some situations.

To organize the following discussion of the complications of otologic surgery, the authors elected to discuss complications in sections that relate to different sites and anatomic structures of the ear and the surrounding temporal bone. The sections will include discussions of complications within the ear canal, the tympanic membrane, the middle ear, the facial nerve, the labyrinth, the inner ear, and the vascular structures. The avoidance and management of these complications will be described in each of these sections.

COMPLICATIONS

Ear Canal

Complications of surgery of the external auditory canal (EAC) are surprisingly rare considering the fragile anatomic relationships of the thin skin, soft tissues, cartilage, and bone of the EAC. During various types of ear surgery, the skin of the EAC is elevated in flaps or excised and later repositioned as a free graft onto seemingly solid avascular bone. In so doing, ear surgeons are rarely concerned about the blood supply of EAC skin flaps or the vascularity of the underlying EAC bone when a free skin graft is applied directly onto that bone. The reason for this lack of concern is that experience has shown that healing is usually uneventful no matter what method or technique is used. However, when a complication does occur, the management of EAC complications tends to be difficult, slow, and frustrating to both the patient and the surgeon.

Poor healing, stenosis, web formation, inflammation, the formation of polyps, and granulation tissue in the ear canal are commonly encountered after surgery of the ear canal, such as in cases of exostosis, ear canal osteoma, or when a canalplasty is necessary during the course of a tympanoplasty.[1,2] Such complications are not uncommon, and they frequently respond to the use of antiinflammatory and antibiotic drops, recurrent cleaning, and the judicious placement of packing, as needed. In occasional cases, resultant canal stenosis, inflammation, and continuous discharge can become permanent and thus require additional surgery and reconstruction.

Tympanic Membrane

A postoperative hearing loss can result from the poor healing of the tympanic membrane. The same inflammatory processes that can afflict the external ear canal can also affect the lateral epithelial surface of the tympanic membrane and result in myringitis and polyps that are commonly associated with otorrhea and hearing loss. If this inflammatory process is new and was not present preoperatively, it tends to respond well to the same treatments as the previously described ear canal.

Thickening of the tympanic membrane is common during the immediate postoperative period, and it tends to dissipate over months. However, in rare instances, the tympanic membrane heals with a thick new membrane. Such a phenomenon has been described when dura mater is used as a graft for the repair of tympanic membrane perforation,[3] but the condition can also be seen with other methods of repair.

A tympanic membrane perforation can recur or occur de novo after ear surgery. When recurrent, this condition is considered a failure of tympanoplasty rather than a complication. In such cases, it can be the result of the technique used during surgery, postoperative infection, poor healing, and, commonly, Eustachian tube dysfunction. Forceful sneezing, flying, and wetness are also possible contributing causes.

The lateralization of the tympanic membrane is a known complication of lateral graft technique. Lateralization is the healing of a new tympanic membrane at a level that is lateral to the level of the original remnant of the tympanic membrane.[4] This lateral healing results in a lack of complete contact between the new tympanic membrane and the malleus, thereby resulting in a significant conductive hearing loss (Figure 56-1).

Blunting of the anterior sulcus is another complication of lateral graft technique tympanoplasty.[5,6] Blunting of the anterior sulcus results from the healing of the skin of the ear canal to the new tympanic membrane in such a way that the angle between the anterior wall of the ear canal and the anterior tympanic membrane is rounded rather than being sharp and well defined. This blunting reduces the effective surface of the tympanic membrane, thereby resulting in a conductive hearing loss (Figure 56-2). Although these complications may occur more frequently in the hands of inexperienced surgeons, blunting of the anterior sulcus and lateralization of the tympanic membrane occurred in 1.3% of 472 cases reported by Sheehy and Anderson.[4] Rizer[6] reported only 1 case of lateralization in a series of 158 lateral graft tympanoplasties.

Middle-Ear Space

A well-aerated middle-ear space and an intact ossicular chain are essential for the proper transmission of sound. A properly aerated middle-ear space depends on a functional Eustachian tube and, to a lesser extent, on a well-aerated mastoid air-cell system. The dependable preoperative evaluation of Eustachian tube function continues to be an elusive goal. It is common to have to proceed with tympanic membrane and middle-ear reconstructive

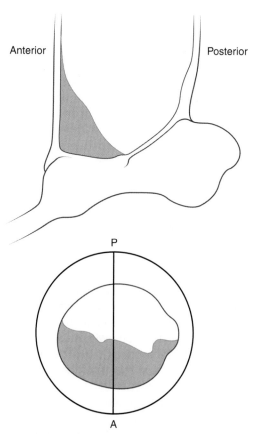

Figure 56-2. Blunting of the anterior sulcus. The shaded area shows the portion of the tympanic membrane that will not transmit sound effectively, thereby resulting in a conductive hearing loss.

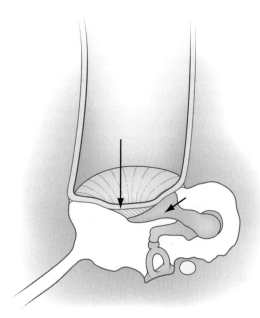

Figure 56-1. Lateralized tympanic membrane. The new membrane is lateral to the manubrium of the malleus. *Short arrow,* Lateralized tympanic membrane; *long arrow,* malleus.

surgery without a solid knowledge of the expected post-operative behavior of the Eustachian tube. In some cases, especially when Eustachian tube dysfunction is suspected preoperatively, the placement of a ventilation tube in the tympanic membrane is desirable. The aim of placing the tube would be to achieve the ventilation of the middle ear, either on a long-term basis or for a planned short postoperative duration of up to 3 months. In the latter case, the aim is to allow for the healing of the tympanic membrane, the middle ear, or a reconstructed ossicular chain without the interference of undue air pressures (either negative or positive) within the middle ear.[7–9]

Postoperative middle-ear adhesions can result in a reduction of the middle-ear space and a conductive hearing loss. In addition, middle-ear adhesions can cause a hearing loss by fixating the ossicular chain to surrounding structures. In many cases, the formation of middle-ear adhesions can be predicted and possibly prevented. Postoperative adhesions tend to recur if they were lysed during surgery. They can also develop de novo if, during surgery, denuded areas of middle-ear mucosa are created during dissection or the resection of disease (e.g., granulation tissue, cholesteatoma). For cases in which the formation of excessive adhesions is expected, the surgeon may wish to separate denuded areas by placing a sheet of Silastic or slowly absorbable material such as Gelfilm, EpiFilm, or another similar material. The placement of Silastic tends to be more effective,[10] but it has the disadvantage of requiring a second-stage procedure to remove the film. Of course, this would only be a relative disadvantage if a second-stage procedure is already planned. This is commonly the case among patients who are undergoing tympanomastoid surgery for the removal of a cholesteatoma in whom the posterior canal wall is kept intact or reconstructed during surgery.

Ossicular Chain and Conductive Mechanism

An intact ossicular chain is paramount for the proper conduction of sound. Complications relating to the disruption of the ossicular chain can be divided into planned and inadvertent disruptions of the ossicular chain.

A planned disruption or dislocation of the ossicular chain is a rare occurrence. Surgeons do intentionally disconnect the lateral chain from the stapes to reduce the transmission of vibration to the inner ear during the removal of a mass off of the lateral ossicular chain (e.g., removing glomus tympanicum tumors and cholesteatoma). A planned separation of the incudostapedial joint usually heals in such a way that hearing is preserved. Occasionally, however, the lateralization of the incus can result in a conductive hearing loss. When the incus is completely removed for access to the middle ear medial to it, it is usually not possible to reposition the incus in its original anatomic position, because that

repositioning is not always compatible with normal hearing. For cases where the incus is removed, many surgeons resort to the use of a prosthesis or to an incus interposition. The incus interposition technique requires sculpting of the incus and repositioning it between the manubrium of the malleus and the head of the stapes. This technique is commonly successful, but it can also result in a less efficient conduction of sound and a partial conductive hearing loss.[11]

The inadvertent disruption of the ossicular chain can occur during any stage of middle-ear surgery. It is most commonly associated with the use of bone curettes, angled instruments, and motorized drills. It can also occur during the elevation of the tympanomeatal flap, especially among patients with distorted anatomy of the posterior superior tympanic ring. This distortion is commonly associated with superior cholesteatoma in which the scutum is eroded and in patients who have had previous middle-ear surgery and who have undergone curetting of the scutum or atticotomy procedures. In most cases, the incus tends to be the victim of inadvertent dislocation. However, it is when the stapes is dislocated that the chances of permanent hearing loss are more likely. An inadvertent dislocation of the stapes can happen despite gentle technique in cases of cholesteatoma and glomus tumors involving the arch or footplate of the stapes. If this complication occurs, one should resort to a rapid covering of the footplate with a soft-tissue graft and avoiding the suctioning of the graft for the remainder of the procedure. Of note is that dislocations of the malleus tend to be a rare occurrence. When this dislocation occurs, it is commonly during an attempt at cutting the head of the malleus for the purpose of accessing the anterior epitympanum for the removal of anterior cholesteatoma.

Complications relating to the use of ossicular prostheses are multiple. Some complications are the result of the faulty or unstable placement of the prosthesis, whereas others relate to the biocompatibility and long-term stability of the prosthesis in its original position. During the placement of a prosthesis, the surgeon should take care to not dislocate or mobilize the remaining ossicles. Good exposure and visualization of the surgical field are essential for the safe and proper placement of a prosthesis. A good contact with the surrounding ossicles or the tympanic membrane is usually achieved with the judicious choice of a prosthesis, its shape, its size, and its adaptability to the specific hearing deficit.[12] A lack of contact with other structures such as the bony canal wall is just as important to avoid fixation of the prosthesis and interference with its function.

Despite adequate positioning during surgery, the contact of a prosthesis with the tympanic membrane can result in the extrusion of the prosthesis. Extrusion is the result of one of several factors, such as an individual patient's biologic rejection of the prosthetic material. More commonly, rejection is the result of forces that are created by poor Eustachian tube function, the flaccidity of the tympanic membrane, or both. Consider the cases of total ossicular replacement prostheses and partial ossicular replacement prostheses in that both are positioned to come in contact with the tympanic membrane. When such prostheses are positioned against the tympanic membrane, it is commonly advised to interpose a thin cartilage graft between the prosthesis and the tympanic membrane.[13] Some manufacturers maintain that such a cartilage interposition is not necessary for their type of prosthesis.[14] However, even when it is thought to be unnecessary, the placement of a graft is desirable, especially when the tympanic membrane itself is judged to be very flaccid and thin.

Inner Ear

Inner-ear complications can occur during middle-ear surgery.[15-17] These complications can result from the transmission of mechanical stimulation to the inner ear or from actual opening into the inner ear spaces.

When watching taped videos of surgeries performed by both inexperienced and skilled surgeons, one realizes that the mechanical stimulation of the inner ear is unavoidable with the current state of technology. If one watches the movement of the malleus during the elevation of a tympanomeatal flap, one becomes aware that the mechanical stimulation of the inner ear by way of the transmission of ossicular movement can occur at any stage of a middle-ear procedure. Of course, this level of transmission of mechanical energy is increased in the case of an intact and mobile ossicular chain. It is also increased in cases involving the prolonged dissection of disease off of the ossicular chain, such as is sometimes necessary during cholesteatoma surgery.

The opening of the inner ear during middle-ear and mastoid surgery is either intentional or unintentional. An intentional opening of the inner ear is typified by the case of stapes surgery for otosclerosis. During stapes surgery, most accepted techniques require opening the footplate by either creating a small or large fenestra. In rare cases, the stapes is removed, which leaves the endosteum, but this occurrence is usually the result of a desirable but unintentional event. The opening of the footplate and the inner ear in a planned manner does not usually result in a measurable hearing loss. However, the suctioning of perilymph and the manipulation of the footplate, the graft, or the prosthesis can result in some degree of hearing loss, especially in the higher frequencies. Currently there is growing evidence that a cochleostomy performed at the level of the round window for the purpose of cochlear implantation does not

always result in a sensorineural hearing loss.[18] During stapes and cochlear implant surgery, the opening of the inner ear is performed in the setting of a noninfected middle ear and in the absence of a tympanic membrane perforation.

The inadvertent, unintentional, or unplanned opening of the inner ear can result in severe sensorineural hearing loss. The presence of a fistula of the semicircular canals or the cochlea can be encountered during the removal of cholesteatoma. The stapes can be opened unexpectedly during the removal of glomus tumors in the area of the oval window. An unplanned opening into the inner ear does not always result in a partial or total sensorineural hearing loss. It is commonly thought that rapid grafting and the avoidance of the suctioning of blood or perilymph from the area of the opening or fistula is helpful to preserve inner-ear function.

Facial Nerve

Postoperative facial-nerve paralysis is a dreaded complication of ear surgery. It can occur during external-, middle-, or inner-ear surgery. Awareness of the facial-nerve anatomy (Figure 56-3) and its variants reduces but does not eliminate the chances of facial-nerve injury during ear surgery. The use of facial-nerve monitors is also helpful in many but not all situations.

In 1974, James Sheehy stated that "one of the greatest fears of the inexperienced otologic surgeon is that he may damage the facial nerve while performing mastoid surgery." This statement remains true to this day, and it does indeed apply to mastoid as well as middle-ear surgery. Green and colleagues[19,20] reviewed 22 cases of iatrogenic facial-nerve paralysis and found that

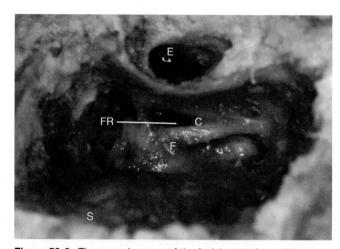

Figure 56-3. The normal course of the facial nerve (mastoid segment) as seen in a dissected cadaveric temporal bone. *C,* Corda tympani nerve; *E,* external auditory canal; *F,* mastoid segment of the facial nerve; *FR,* facial recess or posterior tympanotomy opening; *S,* sigmoid sinus.

postoperative facial paralysis can occur after stapedectomy, cochlear implant surgery, tympanoplasty, mastoidectomy, and exostosis removal. In fact, facial paralysis has been reported with all types of otologic surgery. The injury of the facial nerve can occur at any site along its long, circuitous course, depending on the type of surgery being performed.

The nerve can be injured during the performance of a postauricular incision. This is more common among very young children and infants in whom the nerve tends to reside in a more lateral position.

During outer ear canal surgery, the facial nerve is at most risk during procedures that require the drilling of the posterior aspect of the bony ear canal. The facial nerve, in its descending or mastoid portion, is in close proximity to the medial aspect of the posterior bony canal. It is a major concern during surgery for congenital atresia of the bony external auditory canal,[21] and it is of somewhat less concern for patients undergoing surgery for the removal of outer ear canal exostosis and osteoma.

Green and colleagues[19,20] found that there are predisposing factors that increase the chance of iatrogenic injury to the facial nerve during middle-ear and mastoid surgery. These factors are the presence of cholesteatoma, the findings of vascular granulation tissue, the use of a cutting burr near the course of the facial nerve, the use of a chisel, and the finding of an aberrant or anomalous course of the facial nerve.

It is of note that most facial nerve injuries are not recognized by the operating surgeon. Consequently, they are not recognized at the time of surgery (70%), and they are first noticed postoperatively. Postoperative facial paralysis is commonly immediate, but it can also be delayed in onset.

The management of postoperative facial paralysis depends on the cause and the time of onset of the paralysis. It has to be noted that postoperative facial paralysis is not necessarily always iatrogenic. Cases in point are patients who awaken after abdominal surgery with facial paralysis. One of the authors (JGF) is also aware of a patient who awakened with contralateral facial paralysis after stapes surgery. It is commonly believed that facial paralysis after nonotologic or contralateral otologic surgery is the result of a viral reactivation and should be considered and treated like Bell palsy.[22] Cases like these should also make surgeons less judgmental when facial paralysis occurs in patients with ipsilateral ear surgery when no evidence of injury is found.

The management of immediate postoperative facial paralysis requires following a few important steps. These include the proper checking of facial function and establishing whether the dysfunction is partial or complete. If paresis or paralysis is present, the surgeon should wait to make sure that the effect of any local anesthetic has worn off before proceeding to reexploration or distant referrals. If packing is present, it should be removed, and steroid treatment should be instituted. If the paralysis persists, one should make the decision to reexplore the mastoid and the middle ear or to refer the patient to another otolaryngologist or otologist for further care.

The further management of iatrogenic facial paralysis depends on the surgical findings during reexploration. The same recommendations for management apply when the facial nerve injury is recognized intraoperatively during primary ear or mastoid surgery. In both cases, the recommendations are as follows:

1. *For nerve sheath exposure:* If only the sheath of the facial nerve is exposed, no further treatment is necessary.

2. *For nerve contusion:* If the sheath and the nerve are contused without being severed, the facial nerve should be decompressed above and below the site of the contusion.

3. *For 25% or less transection:* If the nerve is transected by 25% of its diameter or less, the surgeon should decompress the nerve proximally and distally to the site of injury. In addition, the fascicles should be aligned and preferably covered by soft tissue or another suitable material.

4. *For 25% or more transection:* If the nerve is transected by 25% of its diameter or more, the surgeon should decompress the nerve proximally and distally to the site of injury. The injured segment should be resected and the nerve reconnected. If direct anastomosis is not possible, then the options of rerouting the nerve to gain length or the use of an interposition of a graft should be considered. When possible, the anastomosis should be secured with sutures or other appropriate methods (Figures 56-4 and 56-5).

As previously mentioned, these recommendations are the same whether the facial paralysis and injury are noted for the first time intraoperatively or postoperatively. However, one difference is the psychological burden that a surgeon has to carry if he or she has caused an intraoperative facial nerve injury. This is the reason, when faced with a complication, that a surgeon should try to follow certain directives:

1. Remain calm.

2. Reassess the anatomy and the surgical field by evaluating landmarks and tissue damage to achieve a good visualization of the nerve.

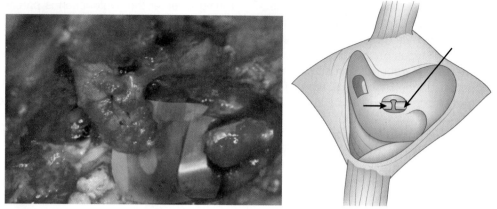

Figure 56-4. Intraoperative picture and artist's rendition of a severed facial nerve in its mastoid segment. The arrows indicate the superior *(short arrow)* and inferior *(long arrow)* segments of the facial nerve.

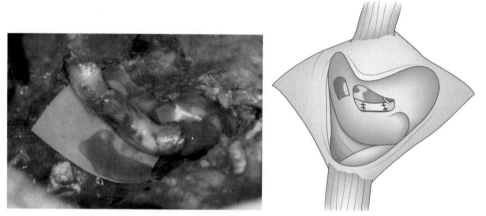

Figure 56-5. Intraoperative picture and artist's rendition of a severed facial nerve repaired with a greater auricular nerve graft.

3. Reduce losses by evaluating other possible injuries such as to the middle- or inner-ear structures.

4. Remove bone and decompress around the facial nerve course proximal and distal to the facial nerve injury site.

5. Treat with steroids.

6. Resume the operation, repair the injuries and the original pathology, or, if this cannot be done, refer the patient postoperatively to another surgeon.

7. When explaining the circumstances of the injury, maintain resolve.

8. Dictate a detailed operative report.

Labyrinthine

Labyrinthine injury can be minor or major. If the ossicular chain is intact, it is likely that the labyrinth is stimulated in every type of tympanic membrane or middle-ear surgery. This minor type of stimulation seems to leave most patients with only transient symptoms.

Operations that result in the opening of the vestibule (e.g., stapedotomy and stapedectomy operations) will likely result in an element of imbalance that can range from minimal to extreme. In these cases, too, the vast majority of patients tend to do well. This could be the result of the resiliency of the vestibular system or, more likely, of the effective mechanisms of vestibular compensation.

More severe labyrinthine surgery can be divided into two general groups. The first group consists of patients undergoing middle-ear surgery that results in an oval-window–related complication. The second group consists of patients whose surgery results in an unplanned opening into the semicircular canals, the vestibule, or the cochlea.

Oval Window

The stapes, its footplate, and the oval window can be injured during many procedures, including otosclerosis surgery, the resection of middle-ear cholesteatoma or granulation tissue, and tumor removal (e.g., glomus tympanicum tumors). As with most surgical complications, the prevention of oval-window trauma is always preferred. Minimizing the incidence of oval-window complications can be achieved by systematically identifying anatomic landmarks in the middle ear, dissecting in a posterior-to-anterior direction, and using proper instrumentation. In the particular case of otosclerosis surgery, one should avoid the application of excessive pressure when using a micro drill to create an opening in the footplate.

At times, however, and despite one's best efforts, trauma to the stapes or the oval window occurs. When footplate or oval-window complications occur, they can result in one of many scenarios. Such scenarios include oval-window fistula, footplate subluxation, or a condition known as *floating footplate* or *fragment of the footplate.*

Oval-window fistulas, such as those noted during the avulsion of the stapes, should be treated with the closure of the oval window with a soft-tissue graft such as adipose tissue, perichondrium, or temporalis fascia. After the closure of the fistula, the surgeon should avoid the manipulation and suctioning of the area of the oval window. If possible, the ossicular chain could be reconstructed, and a prosthesis can be placed over the oval-window graft if this is desired or necessary.

In the case of footplate subluxation, the stapes footplate should be elevated to its original position. A tissue graft should be used to seal the oval window, especially if the subluxation resulted in the complete exposure of the oval window (Figure 56-6).

At times, especially when the superstructure of the stapes is missing, the footplate subluxation is such that the footplate is floating within the vestibule and cannot

be retrieved easily. In such cases, one of several methods could be useful. One option would be to leave the footplate in place and to allow its refixation. This is a reasonable option when the footplate is not too deep within the vestibule and when it maintains some contact with the edges of the oval window. At times, the footplate falls more medially within the vestibule. In these cases, when feasible, a control opening can be created in the footplate using a laser. Such an opening could allow for the insertion of a hook to retrieve the footplate. Another possibility is to drill a groove adjacent to footplate within the otic capsule to allow for the insertion of proper instruments to retrieve the footplate (Figure 56-7).

One additional technique to extract a footplate fragment from the vestibule is the blood clot extraction technique described by Scheer.[23] The method of this technique includes the following steps:
- Gradually remove perilymph from the vestibule (i.e., with 24-gauge suction).
- Place 2 drops of venous blood in vestibule (i.e., tuberculin syringe and 23-gauge needle).
- Allow a clot to form (i.e., ≈10 minutes)
- Extract the clot with 22-gauge suction.
- Extract the elevated footplate fragment.

INJURY

Labyrinthine

Semicircular canal fistula is another type of labyrinthine complication that warrants discussion.[24] The inadvertent uncovering of a labyrinthine fistula during chronic ear surgery is not uncommon, especially during operations that are aimed at removing large cholesteatomas. In such cases, the cholesteatoma itself would have created a fistula into the otic capsule. The most common

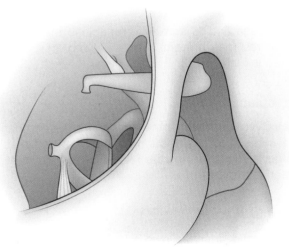
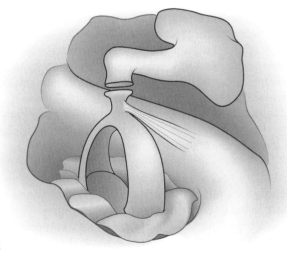

A   B

Figure 56-6. A, Subluxation of the stapes footplate. **B,** The footplate has been be elevated to its original position and placed over a temporal fascia graft.

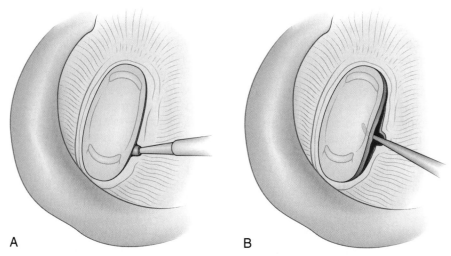

A   B

Figure 56-7. A, A micro drill is used to create an opening in the otic capsule inferior to the footplate. **B,** An angled instrument is engaged through the opening to retrieve the floating footplate.

site of such labyrinthine fistulas is the lateral portion of the arch of the lateral semicircular canal. Other areas of the otic capsule can also be involved, including any of the semicircular canals and the cochlea.

It is preferable to diagnose semicircular canal fistulas preoperatively to be better prepared to manage such fistulas in the operating room. The preoperative diagnosis of labyrinthine fistulas requires a high index of suspicion. It is also helpful to perform a fistula test preoperatively and a radiologic evaluation if the fistula test is positive. If these procedures are performed, radiologic tests should be carefully reviewed by the surgeon, because it is possible for radiologists to miss semicircular canal erosions and fistulas when they are small. Despite preoperative testing, it is still possible to miss a semicircular canal fistula, especially if it is small or in an atypical location. This is the reason that a high degree of vigilance has to be maintained for patients with larger cholesteatoma. If a fistula is diagnosed or suspected, the surgeon should, during the initial stages of the operation, excise the offending cholesteatoma while leaving the matrix in the area of the fistula, thus keeping it covered. After all disease is removed from the mastoid and the middle ear and there is no further need for drilling, cleaning, or irrigation, the area of the fistula can be uncovered and then quickly covered again. Fistulas can be covered using a variety of methods. They are commonly closed with bone wax, temporalis fascia, bone pate, perichondrium, or a combination of these.

A potentially more serious type of opening into the semicircular canals is that of iatrogenic fenestrations of the semicircular canal during mastoid surgery. If this event were to occur, the surgeon should immediately cover the defect and subsequently avoid the manipulation and suctioning of inner-ear fluids from within the defect. In addition, it is preferable to pretreat the patient

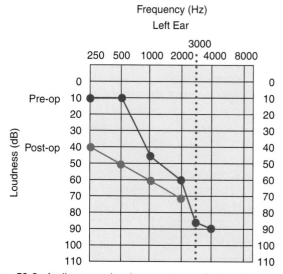

Figure 56-8. Audiograms showing a postoperative hearing loss after the inadvertent opening of the lateral semicircular canal during mastoid surgery. It is probable that the resultant hearing loss was not complete in this case, because the opening into the semicircular canal was recognized and closed immediately.

for nausea and to administer antibiotic therapy. Such measures may prevent a total hearing loss, as illustrated in Figure 56-8.

Vascular

Major vessels traverse the temporal bone and can be the subjects of injury during middle-ear and mastoid surgery. These injuries are relatively rare, but they are potentially disastrous.

Carotid Artery

The carotid artery follows a vertical course from the neck into the hypotympanic area. It then curves anteriorly and follows a horizontal course on its way to the cavernous sinus. The carotid artery is usually covered by a bony canal within its middle-ear course.[25] In the rare patient, the carotid can course in such a way that the bend at the junction of the vertical and horizontal segments is more posterior than normal. More significantly, that area can be missing its bony covering, thus rendering the carotid artery vulnerable to injuries. There are many cases (both reported and unreported) of carotid artery injuries occurring during the performance of anterosuperior myringotomies, which is a site favored by many for the placement of ventilation tubes. As infrequent as these events may be, the fact remains that the carotid artery could be just medial to the tympanic membrane. Of note is that the carotid artery in that area is whitish in color rather than red, and it is not necessarily visibly pulsatile when seen by transparency through the tympanic membrane.

In the event that the carotid artery is injured during middle-ear surgery, the surgeon should, when appropriate, pursue the following steps:

1. Pack the middle ear with oxidized cellulose (Surgicel) or other hemostatic agents that can control arterial bleeding.

2. Block the Eustachian tube orifice to prevent bleeding into the nasopharynx.

3. Return the tympanic membrane to a normal position, and pack the ear canal.

4. Prevent hypotension or hypertension.

5. Obtain a neurovascular surgery consult.

Jugular Bulb

The venous drainage of the head consists of a network of dural sinuses that converge into the sigmoid sinus. The sigmoid sinus follows an S-shaped course and curves superiorly into the jugular bulb (Figure 56-9). The jugular bulb has a dome that is occasionally dehiscent. When dehiscent, the jugular bulb can be injured during middle-ear surgery.[26,27] Bleeding from a jugular bulb injury, while dramatic, is usually less serious and less severe than carotid artery bleeding, and it can be controlled with less pressure than such bleeding.

Sigmoid Sinus

The management of venous sinus injury bleeding can be very challenging. However, it is helpful to know that venous sinus bleeding is a low-pressure bleeding that can commonly be temporized by immediate digital pressure until the area of bleeding is covered by a hemostatic pack such as Surgicel, Avitene, or Gelfoam packs. In some cases, bipolar cautery can be helpful. The use of bone wax may be helpful in cases of small

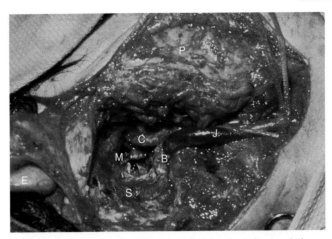

Figure 56-9. Intraoperative dissection showing the intimate relations of the vascular structures within the middle ear, the mastoid, and the upper neck. *B*, Jugular bulb; *C*, carotid artery in its middle-ear course; *E*, outer-ear lobule; *J*, jugular vein in the neck; *M*, middle-ear space; *P*, parotid gland; *S*, sigmoid sinus.

bleeders. Minimal head elevation can help reduce venous bleeding; however, additional elevation of the head could drop the venous pressure in the sigmoid sinus enough for air to be drawn into the venous system. Such air can result in an air embolism of the heart or lungs and thus be life-threatening.

In the case of a large defect, the venous sinus dura can be pushed away by extraluminal pressure. In these more complicated situations, the surgeon may have to drill out or remove surrounding bone, and he or she may very rarely have to resort to suture ligation. In all cases, the surgeon should be aware of the physiology of the venous drainage of the head. When applying a hemostatic pack to a sigmoid sinus bleeder, care should be exercised to avoid losing particles of packing material or bone wax through the defect into the lumen of the venous sinus. Such particles can easily travel distally to the right heart and become pulmonary emboli. In addition, otologic and otolaryngologic surgeons should be aware of the fact that the complete occlusion of the sigmoid sinus can result in more serious consequences than the ligation of the jugular vein in the neck. Although unilateral jugular vein ligation rarely results in significant morbidity, the ligation of the sigmoid sinus can, in some cases, result in increased intracranial pressure and venous infarction of the brain.[28]

CONCLUSION

This chapter reviewed some of the more common complications of middle-ear and mastoid surgery. Many of the complications cited in this text are commonly avoidable. However, the fact remains that surgical complications are not always preventable. The same technique, surgical move, or maneuver that has never previously failed an individual surgeon may lead to a disastrous result in one particular patient. Variations in the severity of disease, patient anatomy, postoperative physiologic function, healing ability, and a variety of factors relating to the surgeon, the patient, and the environment play very important roles in the eventual outcome of any surgical act. These factors are of utmost importance to otologic surgery.

REFERENCES

1. Fisher EW, McManus TC: Surgery for external auditory canal exostoses and osteomata. *J Laryngol Otol* 1994;108(2): 106–110.
2. Vasama JP: Surgery for external auditory canal exostoses: A report of 182 operations. *ORL J Otorhinolaryngol Relat Spec* 2003;65(4):189–192.
3. Eitschberger E, Gammert C, Pesch HH, et al: Tympanoplasty with human dura mater preserved in cialit. *Arch Otorhinolaryngol* 1978;220(1–2):141–148.
4. Sheehy JL, Anderson RG: Myringoplasty: A review of 472 cases. *Ann Otol Rhinol Laryngol* 1980;89:331–334.
5. Doyle PJ, Schleuning AJ, Echevarria J: Tympanoplasty: Should grafts be placed medial or lateral to the tympanic membrane? *Laryngoscope* 1972;82(8):1425–1430.
6. Rizer RM: Overlay versus underlay tympanoplasty: Part II: Historical review of the literature. *Laryngoscope* 1997;107(12 Suppl 84): 26–36.
7. Wehrs RE: Aeration of the middle ear and mastoid in tympanoplasty. *Laryngoscope* 1981;91(9 Pt 1):1463–1468.
8. O'Hare T, Goebel JA: Anterior subannular T-tube for long-term middle ear ventilation during tympanoplasty. *Am J Otol* 1999;20(3):304–308.
9. Gamoletti R, Lanzarini P, Sanna M, et al: Regenerated middle ear mucosa after tympanoplasty: Part II: Scanning electron microscopy. *Otolaryngol Head Neck Surg* 1986;94(4):430–434.
10. Ng M, Linthicum FH Jr: Long-term effects of Silastic sheeting in the middle ear. *Laryngoscope* 1992;102(10):1097–1102.
11. Yung M: Long-term results of ossiculoplasty: Reasons for surgical failure. *Otol Neurotol* 2006;27(1):20–26.
12. Glasscock ME: Tympanoplasty grafting and ossicular reconstruction. *J Otolaryngol* 1978;7(4):277–282.
13. Kobayashi T: Ossicular reconstruction using hydroxyapatite prostheses with interposed cartilage. *Am J Otolaryngol* 2002;23(4): 222–227.
14. Ho SY, Battista RA, Wiet RJ: Early results with titanium ossicular implants. *Otol Neurotol* 2003;24(2):149–152.
15. Bellucci RJ: Cochlear hearing loss in tympanoplasty. *Otolaryngol Head Neck Surg* 1985;93(4):482–485.
16. Strauss P, Huren H, Lobner S: The influence of tympanoplasty on bone conduction. *Laryngol Rhinol Otol (Stuttg)* 1980;59(4):244–249.
17. Smyth GD: Sensorineural hearing loss in chronic ear surgery. *Ann Otol Rhinol Laryngol* 1977;86(1 Pt 1):3–8.
18. Gantz BJ, Turner C, Gfeller KE, et al: Preservation of hearing in cochlear implant surgery: Advantages of combined electrical and acoustical speech processing. *Laryngoscope* 2005;115(5):796–802.
19. Green JD Jr, Shelton C, Brackmann DE: Iatrogenic facial nerve injury during otologic surgery. *Laryngoscope* 1994;104(8 Pt 1): 922–926.
20. Green JD Jr, Shelton C, Brackmann DE: Surgical management of iatrogenic facial nerve injuries. *Otolaryngol Head Neck Surg* 1994;111(5):606–610.
21. Jahrsdoerfer RA, Lambert PR: Facial nerve injury in congenital aural atresia surgery. *Am J Otol* 1998;19(3):283–287.
22. Gyo K, Honda N: Delayed facial palsy after middle-ear surgery due to reactivation of varicella-zoster virus. *J Laryngol Otol* 1999;113(10):914–915.
23. Scheer AA: Retrieving the lost heavy foot-plate fragment. *Arch Otolaryngol* 1970;91(5):412–413.
24. Manolidis S: Complications associated with labyrinthine fistula in surgery for chronic otitis media. *Otolaryngol Head Neck Surg* 2000;123(6):733–737.
25. Sauvaget E, Paris J, Kici S, et al: Aberrant internal carotid artery in the temporal bone. *Arch Otolaryngol Head Neck Surg* 2006;132:86–91.
26. Huang BR, Wang CH, Young YH: Dehiscent high jugular bulb: A pitfall in middle ear surgery. *Otol Neurotol* 2006;27(7):923–927.
27. Moore PJ: The high jugular bulb in ear surgery: Three case reports and a review of the literature. *J Laryngol Otol* 1994;108(9):772–775.
28. Al-Mefty O, Fox JL, Smith RR: Petrosal approach for petroclival meningiomas. *Neurosurgery* 1988;22:510–517.

CHAPTER 57

Complications of Cochlear Implantation

Lawrence R. Lustig

Since their introduction during the late 1960s, cochlear implants have allowed tens of thousands of individuals with severe to profound sensorineural hearing loss to hear, with results varying from simple environmental sound awareness to open-set speech discrimination.[1–4] As the technology has advanced, so too have the indications for implantation, which has resulted in a wider array of conditions and hearing levels suitable for a cochlear implant.[5] The success of the technology is further manifested by current research that is focused on such high-order listening tasks as music appreciation[6]; this is an unlikely achievement that was a research topic even a few years ago.

As with all surgical procedures, however, cochlear implantation is not without risk. The overall complication rate has been estimated to be approximately 2% to 6% for major complications that require intervention and up to 16% for minor complications that resolve with conservative management.[7–10] However, when one closely examines these numbers, it soon becomes obvious that any attempt to generalize these statistics toward contemporary cochlear implant surgery is problematic. There are a multitude of factors that have led to these complications, some of which are obvious and others not so obvious. These include design variations in the cochlear implant stimulator package and electrode array, historic and individual variations in the skin flap and incision employed during implantation, the use and nature of the anchoring material to secure the implant, the overall health and age of the patient, anatomic variations, expanding implant candidacy criteria over the past 20 years, and the experience of the individual surgeon as well as the cochlear implant field as a whole. Despite this variability, some general concepts learned by the field can be applied to contemporary cochlear implant surgery not only to reduce the risk of complications for this important intervention but also to properly approach complications when they do arise.

INFECTIOUS COMPLICATIONS

Meningitis

No other potential complication associated with cochlear implants has received more academic or popular press than meningitis. A headline feature in the *New York Times* in August 2002 proclaiming "Drug Agency Is Studying Ear Implants' Links to Meningitis" attests to the public interest in this issue.[11] To date a number of articles, position papers, and editorials have been published about the risk of meningitis after cochlear implants.[12–27] Despite this body of research, the precise cause of meningitis in implanted patients is still being debated, and it is likely multifactorial. Although initial studies implicated a positioning device used by one of the manufacturers to obtain a closer perimodiolar position of the electrode array as potentially causative,[21,22] additional reports and the subsequent careful analysis of the data have suggested that additional patient, surgical, and device-related factors were at play.[16,17,24]

The first detailed study of the risk of meningitis after cochlear implantation was performed by the Centers for Disease Control and Prevention.[22] In this study, 4264 children under the age of 6 years who had received cochlear implants in the United States between 1997 and 2002 were evaluated. Within this cohort, 26 children were identified as having confirmed bacterial meningitis. The calculated rate of 138.2 cases per 100,000 person-years was more than 30 times the rate found in an age-matched cohort of patients without cochlear implants. The factors that appeared to be the most predictive of the development of postimplant bacterial meningitis included the use of an implant with a perimodiolar "positioner" (i.e., a Silastic band inserted radial to the electrode array within the cochlear scala tympani to allow for the close proximity of the stimulating electrodes to the spiral ganglion neurons) and the joint presence of an inner-ear malformation and a cerebrospinal fluid leak. A study by the same group that evaluated this same cohort of children beyond 24 months after implantation identified 12 new cases of meningitis during that time period, which suggests a longer-term risk beyond the immediate postoperative period.[14] Eleven of the cases had positioners, and two children died as a result of complications related to meningitis.

Another study involved a questionnaire that was sent to all 401 cochlear implant centers in North America.[17] Although the positioner did appear to be associated with a higher risk of meningitis in this study, there were nonetheless cases of meningitis from all three implant manufacturers (the positioner was only produced by one of the three implant manufacturers), which suggests that there are additional factors at play. It was further noted that the majority of cases occurred within 1 year of surgery, that they were more common among children who were less than 5 years old, and that they were associated with inner-ear malformations. In other words, there is a patient cohort that is more prone to meningitis, regardless of the presence of a cochlear implant. The most common organisms identified were *Streptococcus pneumoniae* and *Haemophilus influenzae.* In the United Kingdom,[24] out of 1851 children with implants (including 66 patients with positioners), there were no cases of meningitis, whereas in 1779 adults (including 139 with positioners), there were 5 cases of meningitis, with 3 fatalities. It was also noted in this United Kingdom study that, of the 5 adult cases, none had a positioner, whereas 4 of the cases (including the 3 fatalities) had unrelated risk factors for the development of meningitis.

On the basis of this body of data, several important editorials and position papers emerged to provide general guidelines for cochlear implantation with respect to meningitis.[16,21] These papers noted the important fact that the incidence of meningitis in profoundly deaf patients may be greater than in the general population, thus accounting for the unusually high incidence seen in the 2003 study by Reefhuis and colleagues.[22] Furthermore, general factors that affect the likelihood of meningitis include an age of less than 5 years, impaired immune status, the presence of neurologic prostheses such as a ventricular shunt, and a history of meningitis. Additional risk factors include otitis media and inner-ear malformations.

As a result of these risk factors, some general guidelines were offered to the implant community as a whole. The positioning device was removed from the market as a result of the apparent increased incidence of meningitis associated with its use. Government agencies in the United States, the United Kingdom, and Germany have recommended universal vaccination for former and anticipated cochlear implant patients, particularly those at high risk (i.e., children <5 years old with inner-ear dysplasias and with altered immunity). It was recommended that the risk of meningitis be communicated to all patients or family members contemplating cochlear implantation as well as to those who have already undergone implantation. Patients who develop symptoms or signs of acute otitis media, meningitis, or other febrile illness should be treated as a matter of urgency by their physicians. All serious infections should be reported to the appropriate health authorities. Intraoperatively, prophylactic antibiotics should be considered. Furthermore, the cochleostomy (i.e., the surgically-created entrance to the cochlea) should be sealed with a tissue graft (e.g., fascia) to prevent the communication of the middle-ear space with the inner ear. Lastly, it is currently not recommended that positioners be surgically removed, because it is unclear whether this would lower the risk of meningitis in those patients.

There currently are four vaccines available to protect against most of the bacteria responsible for meningitis in the general population: Prevnar is a 7-valent pneumococcal conjugate; Pneumovax 23 is a 23-valent pneumococcal polysaccharide; Hib is a *Haemophilus influenzae* type b conjugate; and Menomune is a quadrivalent A,C,Y,W-135 meningococcal polysaccharide. The Center for Disease Control and Prevention has come out with the following clear guidelines for vaccination with regard to cochlear implantation (see also www.cdc.gov/nip/issues/cochlear/cochlear-gen.htm):

- Children with cochlear implants who are 2 years old or older who have completed the pneumococcal conjugate vaccine (Prevnar) series should receive one dose of the pneumococcal polysaccharide vaccine (Pneumovax 23). If they have just received the pneumococcal conjugate vaccine, they should wait at least 2 months before receiving the pneumococcal polysaccharide vaccine.
- Children with cochlear implants who are between 24 and 59 months old who have never received either pneumococcal conjugate vaccine or pneumococcal polysaccharide vaccine should receive two doses of pneumococcal conjugate vaccine 2 or more months apart and then receive one dose of pneumococcal polysaccharide vaccine at least 2 months later.
- Children 5 years old and older with cochlear implants should receive one dose of pneumococcal polysaccharide vaccine.

Several studies of the effectiveness of these vaccines for patients with cochlear implants have been carried out. Hey and colleagues[20] examined the protective effect of the 23-valent pneumococcal vaccine. In this study of 120 implant recipients who were 5 years old or older, among the patients who were less than 8 years old, only 71% of patients reached a protective antibody titer threshold. For this reason, the authors recommended a 23-valent pneumococcal vaccine booster in this younger age group. Another study by Rose and colleagues[23] prospectively evaluated 174 patients with cochlear implants and demonstrated that the 7-valent pneumococcal vaccine was significantly more immunogenic than the 23-valent vaccine for children who were less than 5 years old.

Otitis Media After Cochlear Implantation

Because one theory of the origin of meningitis after cochlear implantation is related to the direct spread of otitis media to the inner ear through the cochleostomy and array tract, the issue of otitis media after cochlear implantation is of potentially serious concern.[13] Furthermore, when one examines the causative organism identified in patients with meningitis after cochlear implantation, the most common is *Streptococcus pneumoniae,* and this is followed by *Haemophilus influenzae.* These organisms are also the two most common causes of otitis media.[14,22]

Because cochlear implants are being performed in young children, it would be obvious that this same group of patients would be at risk for otitis media simply from the standpoint of patient age. In 1996, Papsin and colleagues[28] reported that 44% of their patients with implants had peri-implant effusions, thereby attesting to the incidence of otitis media in this age group. Thus the development of otitis media is not itself considered a complication of implantation, but it could potentially lead to one. Several studies have evaluated the incidence of otitis media after cochlear implantation. In one study of 462 adults and 271 children, only 4 patients with complicated otitis media were identified, 1 of whom required surgical intervention.[29] Another study of implants in patients who were less than 2 years old showed no increase in the incidence of otitis media after cochlear implantation, and those that did get otitis media were successfully treated with standard medical therapy.[30] Another study by House and colleagues[31] demonstrated that the frequency and severity of otitis media was the same or decreased after implantation as compared with preimplantation.

An important question to ask is whether the development of otitis media places a cochlear implant recipient at any additional risk. Initial studies during the 1980s demonstrated that a cochlea with an implant is able to resist the spread of an infection nearly as well as a non-implanted ear.[32] However, these earlier studies did not take into account the younger age of the patients now being implanted, and, since that time, there have been many new iterations of electrode designs, thereby making these conclusions difficult to generalize toward contemporary implant surgery. Interestingly, one study that used a cat model of otitis media after cochlear implantation showed that the use of fascia to seal the cochleostomy (i.e., the current recommended practice) was not protective and that bioactive ceramics were better for preventing infection from spreading to the cochlea.[33]

The treatment of otitis media after cochlear implantation involves the use of antibiotics for routine infections. Antibiotics that are effective against *Staphylococcus*, *Streptococcus* and *Haemophilus* spp. should be employed. The use of ventilating tubes for otitis media after implantation is more controversial. In a study by Kennedy and Shelton,[34] a questionnaire was sent to all members of the American Neurotology Society. According to the study, 27% of surgeons would be more likely to place a tube in a child with otitis media after cochlear implantation, 27% would be less likely to place the tube, 6% would never place a tube in these patients, and 40% would treat these patients the same as they would if no implant were present. The conclusions of this study suggested that children with cochlear implants can have ventilation tubes safely placed for otitis media. Although such a retrospective questionnaire does not provide a definitive answer as to what is the most effective treatment, it nonetheless speaks to the varied attitudes and current conventional wisdom on the subject.

Postoperative Wound Infections

Wound and flap infections after cochlear implantation are potentially devastating complications. Unlike other types of implantable devices, the complete removal of a cochlear implant raises some important medical issues. If a device must be totally removed as a result of infection, the cochlear scala will likely become completely scarred, thus preventing the normal full insertion of a subsequent implant after the infection has cleared, with resulting poorer implant performance. Thus every effort must be made to salvage an infected cochlear implant, and, for cases in which the implant cannot be salvaged, an attempt must be made to leave the cochlear array in place if possible to allow for subsequent reimplantation at a later date through a preserved track. However, for life-threatening infections such as meningitis, patient safety obviously comes first, and complete removal may be necessary.

Fortunately, wound or implant infections after cochlear implantation are quite rare, and most reports consist of retrospective case studies only. In one study of 300 consecutive pediatric patients undergoing implantation, only 3 patients developed a wound infection.[7] These included a 16-month-old child with a discharging wound 1 week postoperatively as a result of *Streptococcus* and *Moraxella,* a 6-year-old child with mild but prolonged discharge from the wound that ultimately responded to both topical and oral antibiotics after 2 months, and a 5-year-old child who developed a *Pseudomonas* otitis media with a draining middle ear and a temporary facial palsy. Another study that retrospectively evaluated 290 adult cochlear implant recipients at the University of Iowa identified four patients who required revision surgery for delayed implant infections.[35] With the employment of appropriate intraoperative debridement, intravenous antibiotics, and the use of vascularized flaps, the implant was salvaged in all four of these cases.

Infections caused by *Pseudomonas* represent potentially more serious complications because of this organism's ability to form a biofilm and to evade natural host defense mechanisms and antibiotic therapy.[36,37] One retrospective review of two cases involving refractory pseudomonal infections in patients with cochlear implants highlighted the delayed nature of the presentation (i.e., 4 months and 3 years).[38] In both cases, the infection began as localized granulation tissue and progressed to the complete encasement of the implant with a poorly vascularized rubbery tissue that was resistant to antibiotics. Successful treatment in both cases required removing the infected portion of the implant (i.e., the receiver–stimulator package) while leaving the clipped array in the cochlea, employing several months of appropriate antibiotics, and then reimplanting the device through the preserved array tract.

Because of the concern regarding postoperative wound infection, the issue of antibiotic prophylaxis during cochlear implantation surgery has also been studied. A retrospective case review of 292 adults who underwent implantation evaluated the incidence of infection during the first 4 weeks after surgery.[39] The authors noted a higher rate of infection with the use of a C-shaped incision (11%) or an extended endaural incision (7.5%) and among patients with preexisting medical conditions. In addition, the infection rate was higher among patients who had received long-term antibiotics (i.e., ≤7 days) as compared with those who received a single intraoperative dose, which suggests that long-term antibiotic treatment has no advantage over a single perioperative dose.

FACIAL NERVE COMPLICATIONS

Postoperative Paresis and Paralysis

Facial nerve paralysis is a rare complication after cochlear implantation, and all reported cases have been temporary. Although all patients are counseled regarding the potential devastating risk of permanent facial nerve injury after cochlear implantation, in reality, the incidence of this complication is extraordinarily rare because of a variety of factors, including the familiarity of the surgeon with the anatomy, the use of computed tomography (CT) scans to help identify an aberrant facial nerve course preoperatively, and the widespread use of intraoperative facial nerve monitoring.

In contrast with a permanent facial nerve paralysis, temporary facial palsy after cochlear implantation is more common, although it is still extremely rare. One retrospective series of 705 patients who received implants between 1980 and 2002 identified a total of five patients who developed postoperative facial nerve weakness, for an incidence of 0.71%.[40] In all of these cases, the onset of the weakness was delayed anywhere from 18 hours to 19 days postoperatively, which is indicative of an anatomically intact facial nerve. All five patients in this study were treated with steroids with or without antiviral medication, and all recovered normal facial nerve function. A multicenter study by Hoffman and Cohen[41] also demonstrated a complete return to normal facial function in all cases of delayed facial palsy after cochlear implantation. Another study identified eight patients with facial nerve dysfunction after implantation and hypothesized that the mechanism of injury was heat transfer from the rotating shaft of the burr while transversing the facial recess.[42] Other theories of delayed facial nerve palsy include the

activation of a latent herpes virus, as has been proposed for the phenomenon of delayed facial nerve palsy seen with other types of otologic surgery.[43,44]

As with delayed facial palsy seen with other types of otologic surgery, treatment is primarily medical, with the prompt institution of steroids (i.e., prednisone 80 mg/kg/day) with or without concomitant antiviral medications (e.g., valacyclovir).[40] For patients who are unable to close the affected eye, counseling regarding appropriate eye lubrication and protection is critically important. This includes eyedrops delivered at least once every hour throughout the day and the use of a moisture eye chamber with ocular ointment (e.g., Lacri-Lube) at night while sleeping. Such measures will help protect against excessive corneal drying and the possibility of a corneal ulcer with resulting visual loss.

Facial Nerve Stimulation

In contrast with facial nerve paralysis or palsy, postoperative facial nerve stimulation is much more commonly seen, occurring in between 1% and 14% of cases.[45–51] In this scenario, electrical discharge from the activation of the cochlear implant through normal use causes twitching of the facial nerve; this symptom can range from mild irritation to an inability to use the implant entirely as a result of excessive facial pain. In the largest series reported, Kelsall and colleagues[45] reported on 14 patients with facial nerve stimulation after implantation with the Nucleus 22-channel device (Cochlear Corporation, Denver, CO) for an overall incidence of 7% of their population. In that study, the most common underlying clinical condition among patients with postoperative facial nerve stimulation was otosclerosis, and this association has been borne out by many others researchers.[52,53] Patients with otosclerosis are felt to be at risk for facial nerve stimulation as a result of changes in bone impedance associated with the underlying disease process. Anatomic analysis has suggested that it is the close proximity of the basal turn of the cochlea to the labyrinthine segment of the facial nerve that is responsible for this phenomenon.[45]

Nearly all cases of facial nerve stimulation after cochlear implantation can be controlled by reprogramming the implant. By eliminating the offending electrodes, facial nerve stimulation can often be reduced or eliminated all together.[45,49] In a smaller subset of patients, more elaborate programming strategies can be employed, such as altering stimulus or current levels or using variable programming modes.[45] For cases in which these techniques are unsuccessful for getting the facial nerve stimulation under control, revision surgery can be considered. Because some of the newer implant arrays have modiolar-facing electrodes that serve to limit the spread of current through the temporal bone, reimplantation with one of these newer devices has been successfully employed to treat intractable facial nerve stimulation.[47,54]

INTRAOPERATIVE COMPLICATIONS

Cerebrospinal Fluid Leak

Although the dura is commonly encountered during a variety of otologic surgeries, including cochlear implantation, cerebrospinal fluid (CSF) leakage is a rare complication. CSF leakage can arise intraoperatively during cochlear implantation as a result of one of several mechanisms: the middle fossa dura can be breached during the drilling of the mastoidectomy, the posterior fossa can be breached during the creation of the receiver well, or the CSF can arise from an abnormally patent communication between the cochlea and the CSF compartment, with a resultant CSF leak or "gusher" occurring during the cochleostomy.

CSF leakage as a result of a middle fossa dural breach is a rare technical error that typically occurs when encountering a low-lying middle fossa tegmen or when a drill "skips" while skeletonizing the middle fossa tegmen, thereby tearing the dura that overlies the temporal lobe. CSF leakage as a result of this mechanism is rare because of otologic surgeon familiarity with the mastoid anatomy and its relationship to the middle fossa and because of the fact that implants are typically performed in disease-free mastoids with normal bony landmarks. With the judicious drilling of the mastoid with careful tegmen identification and with the employment of commonly taught principles of mastoid surgery (e.g., saucerization), this error should be quite rare.

Another mechanism for CSF leakage comes from exposing the posterior fossa dura during the placement of the implant well or during the drilling of the holes used to secure the receiver in its well. In a review of 300 cases of pediatric cochlear implantation, CSF leakage was noted during the creation of the suture holes in 3 patients, whereas a dural tear was caused in a single case.[7] Careful attention to the underlying anatomy when drilling and the use of diamond burrs when near the dura should help to reduce the likelihood of this complication.

The treatment of such technical breaches of the dura varies depending on the location and size of the defect created. For small defects such as those created during the drill of holes for securing sutures, the leak can often be stopped using bone wax to seal the hole.[7] Large defects can be repaired with the fascia reinforcement of the defect, muscle or bone flaps, or the use of various hydroxyapatite bone substitutes or tissue glues.[55–57] Larger or brisk CSF leaks may require close observation in the hospital, lumbar drainage, the use of diuretics (e.g.,

acetazolamide), and neurosurgical consultation to control the leak and manage the complication.

The CSF gusher encountered during cochlear implantation represents a different entity, because this is not caused by a technical error; rather, a predisposition is present that is based on the patient's underlying anatomy. This finding is rare, and it occurs in approximately 1% to 2% of cases.[10,58,59] One study of 300 cases of pediatric cochlear implants identified two cases of CSF gushers after the cochleostomy.[7] These perilymphatic gushers are felt to arise from defects in the lamina cribrosa, and they are also typically seen among patients with cochlear malformations such as Mondini dysplasia.[60–62] Unfortunately preoperative scans cannot be relied on to predict this scenario, because they are predictive in only about half of cases. Intraoperative findings will include a large flow of CSF as soon as the cochleostomy is created. Abnormal and dysplastic ossicles are a frequent associated finding.[7]

When a CSF gusher is encountered, the cochlear implantation can usually be successfully completed.[59] In such cases, the surgeon will need to use one of a number of described methods for sealing the cochleostomy after the insertion of the array, including packing muscle or fascia around the array, using fibrin or tissue glue, and using additional packing in the middle ear as needed.[7,63] An alternate method has been described that employs silk suture coated with bone wax packed circumferentially around the array to stop the leak.[64] In cases of severe CSF leakage that is not controlled by these measures, more invasive measures such as lumbar drainage may need to be employed. In all cases, patients should be warned about the increased risk of meningitis associated with such conditions, although prophylaxis with antibiotics is not currently recommended.[22]

Electrode Insertion Complications

Electrode array designs have undergone a variety of updates over the past 20 years. The current aim of electrode array design is to achieve sufficient insertion depth and to allow for the proximity of the array to the cochlear modiolus in an atraumatic manner. This is achieved with some contemporary designs (Cochlear Corporation, Denver, CO, and Advanced Bionics Corporation, Valencia, CA) by using arrays with a natural curvature that mimics the cochlear spiral. To allow for insertion, the arrays come preloaded with a wire stylet, which is then removed during the placement of the implant, thus allowing the array to achieve its natural curvature within the cochlea.

As a consequence of the stiffness associated with these precurved arrays with wire stylets and the insertion technique required for their proper placement, it is possible for the implant to damage the cochlea during insertion by piercing the basilar membrane, traveling retrograde into the vestibule, or having the array itself kink or bend back on itself within the scalar lumen. In one series of temporal bone studies, even in supposedly normal implant insertions by experienced surgeons, cochlear damage from the insertion of several types of devices resulted in intracochlear damage, including the migration of the electrode into the scala tympani through the basilar membrane, damage to the spiral ligament, and damage to the Reissner membrane, particularly with deeper insertions.[65,66] Whether this actually would translate into a degradation in implant performance is not known, although prior studies have demonstrated that, where there is a fracture of the spiral lamina, there is also a focal loss of spiral ganglion neurons.[67] Because the spiral ganglion neurons are responsible for transmitting the afferent auditory signal from the cochlea, one can reasonably assume that such a loss will adversely affect implant performance.

Although such a detailed histologic analysis in human ears in not possible, electrode displacement or malpositioning can and does occur. In a review of 300 consecutive cases of pediatric cochlear implantation, 1 case was identified in which the electrode tip had curled back on itself at the junction of the middle and basal turns.[7]

The displacement of the electrode into the vestibular system has also been reported.[68,69] In such cases, the insertion of the array is uneventful, although with postoperative programming vertigo is often elicited. However, in some cases symptoms may not be readily apparent, and the problem is only noticeable on a postoperative CT scan when the patient fails to perform as expected (Figure 57-1). The more common scenario involves the electrode traveling backward through the scala tympani into the vestibule. One case has been described in which the array was ultimately identified in the superior semicircular canal.[69]

Because the cochlear modiolus is quite thin, the displacement of an array into the internal auditory canal is also possible (Figure 57-2). Cases in which patients are at risk for this complication include those with inner-ear dysplasias and in whom drilling an obliterated scala is required.

Because the potential for an aberrant array insertion into the cochlea is low, routine postoperative radiographic screening is not required. However, routine intraoperative fluoroscopy has been advocated by some as a means of identifying array kinking or displacement at the time of surgery.[70] For cases in which there is a cochlear dysplasia, a drill out is required as a result of scarring or bony overgrowth or if the insertion did not proceed smoothly. At this point, intraoperative fluoroscopy, plain radiography, or an immediate postoperative

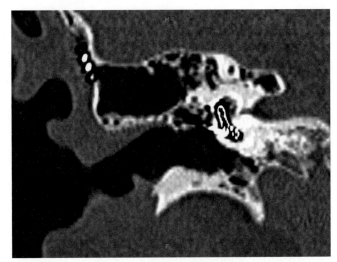

Figure 57-1. A 2-year-old child underwent an uneventful cochlear implantation. After failing to achieve expected speech and language milestones, a high-resolution computed tomography scan was obtained, which revealed that the implant array was extending into the vestibule rather than the basal turn of the cochlea. The child subsequently underwent a revision implantation with insertion into the scala tympani. At the time of the revision, it appeared that the electrode array banked off a bony ledge just anterior to the round window and traveled retrograde into the vestibule.

CT scan of the temporal bones is warranted to verify correct electrode positioning within the cochlea.[70,71]

Labyrinthine Fistula

The fenestration of the labyrinth is an uncommon complication during cochlear implant surgery. In a series of 300 pediatric implant patients, 2 cases were identified that had lateral semicircular canal fenestrations, with no postoperative sequelae noted from the violation of the labyrinth.[7] This is a technical error that can occur in the setting of abnormal anatomy and that causes the obscuration of normal bony anatomic landmarks. The treatment of this complication involves resurfacing the fistula with fascia or other connective tissue followed by bone pate and supportive vestibular care postoperatively for any associated vestibular hypofunction (e.g., vestibular therapy).

SKIN-FLAP COMPLICATIONS

Skin-flap complications are some of the most common and challenging treatment dilemmas faced by cochlear implant surgeons.[41,72–74] During the placement of the receiver–stimulator under the temporoparietal scalp, the surgeon is challenged by both the need to keep the flap thin enough to allow magnet retention for implant power and by the requirement of leaving the skin thick enough to allow adequate perfusion to maintain flap viability. There are many factors that can influence skin-flap viability, including the surgical technique used, the underlying health of the patient, comorbidities such as

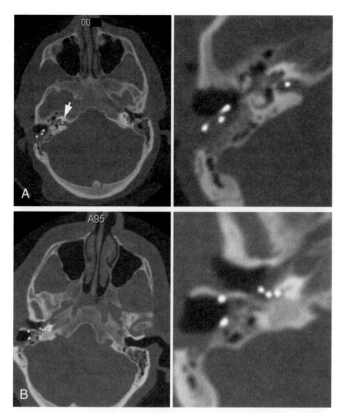

Figure 57-2. A 56-year-old woman with a history of severe cochlear otosclerosis was found to have ossification of the scala tympani at the time of implantation. A cochlear scala was identified, and an electrode array was inserted. **A,** An immediate postoperative computed tomography scan demonstrated the insertion of the array into the internal auditory canal. The patient was taken back to the operating room the following day for a revision, at which time a basal turn drill out was undertaken. **B,** The postoperative computed tomography scan for the revision is shown in which only four electrodes were placed adjacent to the cochlear nerve. The patient failed to respond to stimulation and was offered a second revision surgery with the placement of a split array but refused. The patient remains a nonuser.

the concomitant use of tobacco, associated dermatologic conditions, and the strength of the magnet used postoperatively, all of which must be taken into consideration both during and after surgery.

The overall rate of implant exposure from a skin-flap dehiscence is approximately 1%, with most reports being composed of limited case series.[7,73–77] As previously noted, the factors that lead to skin-flap breakdown and implant exposure are numerous, and they need to be addressed on a case-by-case basis. Because an exposed implant is an untenable situation, the surgeon must do everything possible to avoid this calamitous condition from the outset. Studies have shown that an extended postauricular incision is associated with fewer complications than the older C-shaped incisions.[77] The current trend toward even smaller incisions will further help promote skin-flap viability and likely lessen the incidence of skin-flap breakdown and device exposure in the future.[78] When elevating a skin flap, the surgeon should strive for

a flap thickness of at least 3 mm to 4 mm, and he or she should use bipolar rather than monopolar cautery on the skin flap itself during its elevation if any bleeding is encountered. For patients with compromised wound healing abilities, such as those taking immunosuppressive medications or who have chronic medical conditions, there does not appear to be an increased risk for postoperative infection, but close postoperative observation is warranted. However, in all other respects, these patients appear to perform as well as those with normal wound-healing capacities.[79]

After skin-flap viability becomes potentially compromised, therapy should be directed at making every attempt to save the implant and to avoid explantation and subsequent reimplantation. Interventions to consider include antibiotic therapy and the correction of thyroid hormone and blood glucose levels when indicated.[74] Hyperbaric oxygen has also been used with success in cases of a compromised skin flap.[74,76]

For cases of implant exposure, it may be advisable to reoperate in an attempt to salvage the implant (Figure 57-3). Such a surgery would involve the debridement of devitalized and infected tissue and relocating the device to a different site around the ear with healthier tissue. The use of well-vascularized rotation flaps is also advised for those with compromised wound healing or poor flap viability.[74,75] During an operation to salvage an exposed cochlear implant, it is important to avoid the use of monopolar cautery and to employ the judicious use of bipolar cautery well away from the implant, if needed. The authors have had great success with the use of the Hemostatix thermal scalpel (Hemostatix Medical Technologies, Bartlett, TN) for such cases, as described by Roland and colleagues.[80] This instrument allows for bloodless surgery without electrical current, which could damage the delicate electronics within the implant.

In some cases, the implant cannot be salvaged, and the device must be removed (Figure 57-4). In several recent articles addressing cochlear reimplantation, wound problems were the second most common cause of reimplantation after device failure.[81,82] In such a scenario, the implant is removed, with the array left within the cochlea, if possible, to maintain cochlear patency. The array can be clipped at the facial recess, which is usually free of disease in such cases. Several months after the wound has healed, one can consider the reimplantation of a new cochlear implant into a sterile wound. The use of a laser to create a circumferential cuff of charred capsule at the cochleostomy before the removal of the old array will facilitate the reintroduction of the new array through the same tract. Outcomes equivalent to prior performance scores in such cases are common, although they are by no means guaranteed.[82]

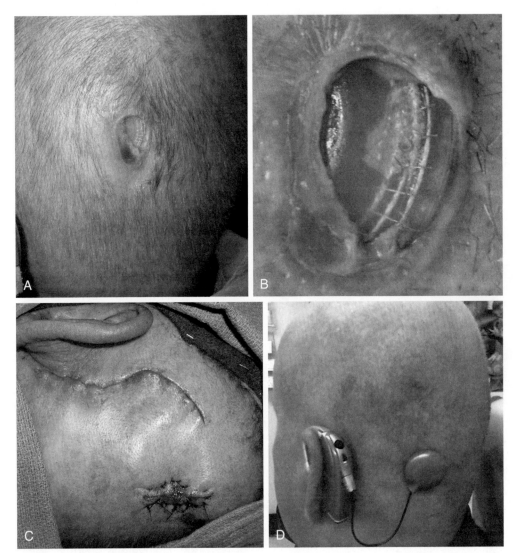

Figure 57-3. A 45-year-old immunocompromised patient underwent a routine cochlear implantation. **A** and **B,** By the second postoperative week, erythema was noted over the implanted receiver, which progressed to skin breakdown that was felt to be the result of a thermal burn while elevating the skin flap during the original implant surgery. The patient was placed on antibiotics and taken to the operating room in an attempt to salvage the implant. **C,** Intraoperatively the implant receiver was transferred inferiorly away from the region of skin breakdown, and the skin defect was closed primarily. **D,** The wounds healed well and the patient went on to achieve excellent use of the cochlear implant.

DEVICE MALFUNCTION

Hard Versus Soft Failures

There is perhaps no more frustrating complication of cochlear implantation than device failure from the standpoint of both the patient and the implant team. In most such cases, a patient's performance precipitously declines, and testing of the device demonstrates that it is no longer functioning properly; this is called a *hard failure.* In other cases, a patient's performance declines in an unexpected fashion, although all tests indicate a functioning device; this is called a *soft failure.*

In theory, it should be relatively easy to determine a cochlear implant failure rate, because this data should be available from the individual manufacturers. However, each new device iteration or change in the manufacturing

process would be expected to lead to a different failure rate, thus making generalizations difficult. Furthermore, the time course over which one measures also affects failure rates; the failure rate over a 2-year period would obviously be much different than that calculated over a 10-year period. One recent study by Maurer and colleagues[83] looked at device reliability from all manufacturers. In their 8-year retrospective study, adults had an implant failure rate of 1.7%, whereas children had a failure rate of 11.2%, for an overall failure rate of 8.3%. The primary reasons for hard failures in this group were implant design malfunctions and direct or indirect trauma to the cochlear implant receiver, particularly among children. In another retrospective review of revision cochlear implant surgeries by Buchman and colleagues,[84] 33 patients were identified. Of these patients, a total of eight operations were performed because of a failure of the external

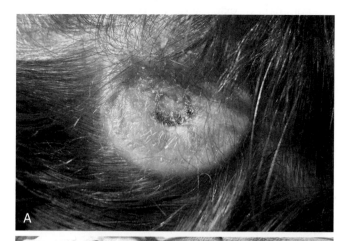

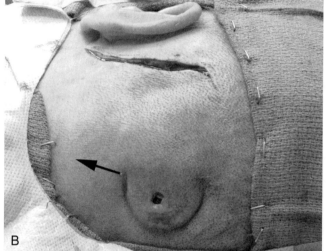

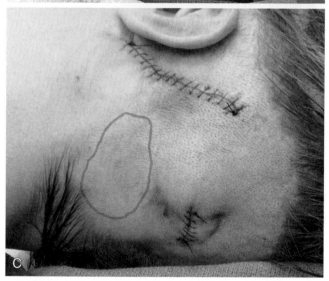

Figure 57-4. A 42-year-old woman with both deafness and blindness underwent an uneventful cochlear implantation. She developed persistent serosanguineous drainage out of her incision during the postoperative period, with edema of the skin flap. She failed to respond to a prolonged course of intravenous antibiotics for a presumed wound infection. She ultimately underwent explantation, with the clipping of the electrode at the facial recess and the array left within the cochlea, and she received 6 weeks of intravenous antibiotics. She then underwent reimplantation 3 months after the explantation, and she subsequently achieved excellent speech scores after routine activation. Two years later, she presented with pain and irritation at the receiver site overlying the magnet. **A,** Close inspection revealed an implant exposure. The patient was taken to the operating room to move the implant to a safer, more inferior location. **B,** Scar tissue and new bone formation prevented the receiver from being removed, and, as a result, the implant was removed and a new one was replaced during the same operation in a more inferior location *(arrow)*. **C,** The new location of the implant is outlined, with the primary closure of the wound breakdown site. After activation, the patient subsequently achieved similar speech scores as she had with her prior implant.

University of Michigan reported a 3.7% rate of hard failure in their population in 2005.[86] Additional reports in the literature substantiate the findings of these studies.[81,87,88]

In contrast with hard failures, which are relatively easy to identify because the receiver can no longer communicate with the external processors and the patient can no longer hear with their implant, soft failures are much more difficult to diagnose. These cases remain a diagnostic and treatment challenge, precisely because of the insidious nature of the presentation and the lack of any solid confirming evidence of device malfunction. A recent review of cochlear implant revision surgeries by Buchman and colleagues[84] noted that 25 of their 33 revision surgeries were the result of suspected soft failures. In these patients, nearly all complained of significant adverse auditory symptoms (e.g., tinnitus, hyperacusis, abnormal sounds, a noticeable drop in auditory performance) or nonauditory symptoms (e.g., pain, shock sensation, vertigo, facial stimulation), with atypical tinnitus (e.g., thumping sounds, engine-like noises) being the symptom that was most commonly reported. Although it would be straightforward to blame these symptoms on underlying physiology, subsequent reimplantation improved or abolished these symptoms in the majority of patients, which strongly suggests device malfunction as causative. Seven similar soft-failure patients were identified in a University of Michigan retrospective review with similar subjective findings, and a similar rate of symptom improvement after reimplantation was noted.[86]

As a result of reports of soft failure such as these, a Cochlear Implant Soft Failures Consensus Development Conference was held in conjunction with the Tenth Symposium on Cochlear Implantation in Children in Dallas,

processor to communicate (or "lock") with the internal device, and these were considered hard failures. In this group of hard failures, hermeticity (i.e., leak) failure was the most common reason. Another retrospective series by Balkany and colleagues[85] of 16 cochlear reimplantations also identified device failure as the most common reason for the additional surgery. A report from the

Texas, in 2005. The consensus statement[89] reaffirms that soft failures are uncommon and that they cannot be proved with the use of currently available in vivo methods. As noted from the consensus statement, the diagnosis of a soft failure is suspected in patients with declining performance or aversive symptoms such as popping or shocking sensations or intermittent function. Subsequent extensive testing, including device imaging and integrity testing, eliminates any possible role that programming or external device problems may be contributing to the problem. Lastly, the reimplantation of another device with the subsequent alleviation of symptoms lends further support to the diagnosis. In children, additional factors need to be taken into consideration, because they cannot always verbalize that a device is not functioning as expected. A suggested checklist to evaluate for soft failures that was compiled by several implant centers is shown in Table 57-1.[89]

TABLE 57-1   Soft Failure Assessment Checklist*

Young Children	B. Nonauditory
A. Behavioral	Pain over implant site
Increase in "bad" behaviors	Pain down neck
Aggressiveness	Shocking
Unwillingness to wear device	Burning
Head hitting	Itching
Inattentiveness	Facial stimulation
Regression in speech/language	**C. Performance**
B. Teacher/Therapist Concerns	Sudden drop
Intermittent responsiveness	Decrement over time
Frequent appearance of being "off task"	Failure to meet expected performance
Deterioration in grades/school performance	Intermittent performance
Plateau in performance	**D. Mapping**
Failure to meet appropriate expectations	Changes in levels over time
C. Other Factors	Changes in pulse width/duration
Educational placement	Loss of channels
Type and amount of therapy	Change in impedance
Family involvement	Shorts/open circuits
Puberty	**E. Hardware**
Adult/Older Children	Replacement of all externals
A. Auditory	**F. Objective Assessment**
Atypical tinnitus	Surface potential testing
Buzzing	Neural response measures
Roaring	Stimulus artifact
Engine-like noise	Evoked potentials
Static	
Popping	
Other	

Source: Balkany TJ et al: Cochlear reimplantation. *Laryngoscope* 1999;109:351–355

When a soft failure is suspected, treatment options will include prolonged observation, removal and reimplantation in the same ear, or implantation in the contralateral ear.[89] The individual specifics of each case will need to be taken into consideration to determine the most appropriate course of action. A decision tree regarding how to manage suspected soft failures, culled from the consensus conference, is shown in Table 57-2.[89]

To help ensure that implant failures and the reasons behind them can be tracked in the future, a European consensus statement on cochlear implant failures and explanations was put forward in 2005.[90] A summary statement by the leading European implant centers put forth the following recommendations for the times when a device failure is suspected,[90] although it is unclear whether these standards have been uniformly applied by all implant manufacturers to date:

1. All device failures must be reported to the competent authority (i.e., usually the implant manufacturer), with a calculated cumulative survival rate.

2. The manufacturer's reports of device failure should indicate the source data, sample size, and the time period over which the failure rate is being cited.

3. Reports of survival rates should provide historic data about a given device and list any technical modifications.

4. The complete data set of the manufacturer's product should be supplied when presenting data about subsequent device modifications.

5. A new device category is assigned when there has been a change in the case, the electrodes, or the electronics that has been labeled with its own CE mark.

6. Cumulative survival rates should be separated for adults and children, with 95% confidence intervals reported.

7. Device survival time should start being tracked at the closure of the cochlear implant incision.

Magnet Displacement

A potentially problematic complication after cochlear implantation is the migration or displacement of the magnet that powers the internal receiver.[91-94] For implant models in which there is a ceramic case that houses the internal receiver, this is not an issue. For some of the newer model implants (Cochlear Corporation, Denver, CO, and Advanced Bionics Corporation, Valencia, CA) that contain removable magnets, however, this is a potential complication that children seem particularly prone to developing. The advantage of having a removable magnet stems largely from the possibility of obtaining postoperative magnetic resonance imaging (MRI) scans. In a simple outpatient procedure, the internal magnet can be removed, a scan obtained, and the magnet replaced. As compared with MRI-compatible implants without a removable magnet, the quality of a head MRI in a patient with an implant with the magnet removed is far superior. However, the downside of this ability to remove the magnet

TABLE 57-2 Diagnosis of Suspected Device Malfunction in Adult Cochlear Implant Patients

Auditory	Nonauditory	Performance	Recommendation
+	+	+	Consider revision
−	+	+	Consider revision
+	−	+	Consider revision if symptoms are severe and persist
+	+	−	Consider revision
+	−	−	Monitor—noise journal, look for new symptoms over time
−	+	−	Consider revision if symptoms are severe and persist; may occur independent of device use
−	−	+	Remap, replace external hardware, re-evaluate in 1-3 months

Source: Balkany TJ et al: Cochlear implant soft failures consensus development conference statement. *Otol Neurotol* 2005;26:815–818.

is the potential displacement of the magnet from its bed within the Silastic implant receiver housing.

In the most common scenario, a child sustains some trauma to the skull overlying the receiver, thereby causing the magnet to literally pop out of its bed within the housing.[91–94] Children are likely at greater risk for this than adults as a result of their developing motor skills and associated play activities.[92] In such a scenario, the patient may notice a lack of function of the implant or a hard lump just underneath the skin adjacent to the scalp. Because of the focal nature of the magnetism between the implant and the displaced magnet just under the skin, the flap is in danger of breaking down over the displaced magnet. Thus the parents of children who have implants that contain removable magnets should be counseled to be aware of a subcutaneous hard lump adjacent to the external magnet, the focal irritation of the skin flap, or the failure of the magnet to form an effective lock on the internal receiver.

When a displaced magnet is encountered, the patient or family should be counseled to not wear the device until the magnet can be replaced as a result of the risk for injuring the skin flap. Fortunately the repair of the problem is relatively straightforward. A small incision is made just posterior to the receiver, and a skin flap is raised in continuity with the receiver. The magnet is retrieved and then replaced within its bed in the receiver. Care must be taken to ensure that the Silastic sleeve is circumferentially holding the magnet in place; otherwise the patient will be at risk for the redisplacement of the magnet. In rare cases, if the magnet becomes dislodged on multiple occasions and there is a tear in the Silastic ring holding the magnet in place, the entire implant may have to be replaced.

PERCEPTUAL COMPLICATIONS

Nonuse

Although the surgeon may perform a technically perfect operation and the implant team may flawlessly implement a programming strategy, it is possible that the patient may decide that the benefits of the implant are so minimal that it is not worth the effort to use it at all. Such a nonuse complication is a failure on many levels. This could represent an inability to correctly diagnose the patient's underlying pathophysiology to support electrical auditory stimulation, inadequate patient counseling regarding appropriate expectations, or even peer pressure among adolescents that creates a negative stigma of implant use. Because of the individual and societal costs of such an intervention, preventing a nonuse scenario is important.

Unfortunately the literature regarding the nonuse of cochlear implants is quite sparse. As was noted by Bhatt and colleagues,[95] the rate of nonuse in subjects with implants has ranged from 0.4% to 4%. In their own retrospective study, those authors identified a total of 29 adults (13.9% of their implant population) who did not use their devices for a consecutive 4-week period.[95] However, many of the patients cited in the study could not use their device as a result of the mechanical failure of the device, and they eventually went on to reuse the implant after the correction of the underlying problem. If one excludes surgical complications and device-related problems, then a total of six patients were nonusers as a result of other factors, including comorbid illness ($N = 3$) and elective nonuse ($N = 3$). The comorbid illnesses included a cerebrovascular accident that caused a decline in implant performance, an autoimmune polychondritis that caused severe malaise, and a personality disorder. A clear reason was not identified for the three patients who electively decided to not use their implants. Additional reasons cited for nonuse by other studies include depression and poor implant benefit.[9]

Although such a nonuse scenario cannot be predicted, certain measures can be taken before implantation to minimize this complication. The preoperative psychologic assessment of both children and their families is important to identify factors that could lead to nonuse after activation.[96,97] A critical factor in this assessment is to provide appropriate expectations for implant function after activation on the basis of the individual's clinical history and biology.[98] Although such a comprehensive preoperative assessment will not completely eliminate nonuse complications, it will likely greatly reduce the number of users who decline to use the implant after activation.

Tinnitus

Tinnitus after cochlear implantation has been actively studied, in part because many patients have tinnitus before receiving their implants. In fact, the majority of patients who receive cochlear implants experience an improvement in their tinnitus after cochlear implantation.[99–103] Such an effect has led to studies that have looked at high pulse train electrical stimulation as a promising potential treatment for some forms of tinnitus.[102] The precise mechanism of tinnitus suppression among patients with implants is unclear, as is the precise mechanism of tinnitus in general. Recent studies suggest that tinnitus and the residual inhibition of tinnitus with auditory stimulation are related to cortical networks of auditory higher-order processing, memory, and attention.[99]

Although a majority of patients with both implants and tinnitus do experience improvement, a small minority can develop de novo tinnitus or the exacerbation of preexisting tinnitus after the placement of the implant.[73,100,101,103] Ruckenstein and colleagues[103] demonstrated that, in a prospective series of 38 patients, 92% experienced a reduction in tinnitus intensity, whereas the remainder had no change in their underlying tinnitus; no patient experienced an increase in their tinnitus. By contrast, Webb and colleagues[73] showed that, in their series of 100 patients, a small number of patients experienced an increase in tinnitus.

The mechanism of tinnitus generation or exacerbation among patients with implants remains unclear, but it is likely related to the generation of tinnitus among individuals without implants: cochlear injury after one of a number of assaults, including noise, ototoxic medications, and age. In the case of a patient with an implant, damage to the delicate cochlear structures after the insertion of the implant may be the cause. There are no data that demonstrate that treatment strategies that have been effective for tinnitus sufferers (e.g., biofeedback, noise suppression, masking, antidepressant medications) are effective for patients with cochlear implants, in part because of the small number of patients who experience this troubling complaint after implantation. However, it is reasonable to attempt these forms of therapy for a patient with excessive tinnitus after cochlear implantation.

Vertigo

As a result of the intimate association between the cochlea and the labyrinthine structures, it may seem surprising that all patients with cochlear implants do not experience some form of dizziness. In most general retrospective series, transient vertigo has been reported in less than 10% of these patients,[9,104] although, in rare cases, it has been a cause of cochlear reimplantation.[81]

When one looks at vestibular dysfunction in greater detail after cochlear implantation, however, its incidence is probably higher than reported for these general series. For example, in a case-control prospective study of vestibular dysfunction after cochlear implantation, Fena and colleagues[105] demonstrated that 39% of patients had some degree of dizziness postoperatively. This group included 4 patients with a single, transient, acute vertigo attack within 24 hours of surgery and an additional 25 patients with delayed, episodic, positional vertigo that occurred an average 74 days after surgery. Another retrospective study by Steenerson and colleagues[106] showed that up to three fourths of their patients with implants experienced vertigo at some point after surgery. Another study by Hugyen and colleagues[107] prospectively studied patients with the use of caloric and velocity step testing before and after implantation. In four of these patients, there was significant postoperative vestibular loss, with the risk of vestibular function loss calculated at 31%. Another study that prospectively evaluated vestibular function

estimated that the risk of vestibular loss approached 60% after implantation.[108]

A majority of the cases of dizziness after cochlear implantation can be classified as episodic benign positional vertigo. In a study by Limb and colleagues,[109] 12 patients with benign positional vertigo after cochlear implantation were identified, with dizziness occurring on average 292 days after the implant surgery. In 11 of these 12 cases, the vertigo responded to traditional Epley maneuvers.

There are also rare cases of dizziness after cochlear implantation as a result of an electrode that has migrated or that has been incorrectly inserted into the labyrinth (see Electrode Insertion Complications earlier in this chapter).[68,69,110] In such cases, the activation of the electrode will often elicit vestibular rather than auditory sensations. In addition, cochlear reimplantation is required.

In most cases, vertigo after cochlear implantation is transitory and requires only supportive care or treatment for benign positional vertigo.[105,109] For cases of clear labyrinthine loss or prolonged disequilibrium after cochlear implantation, vestibular therapy is recommended to assist with compensation. Furthermore, anyone with prolonged disequilibrium or balance difficulties after surgery should undergo a CT scan to confirm that the dizziness is not a result of a misplaced electrode array.[68,69,110]

REFERENCES

1. Daya H, Ashley A, Gysin C, et al: Changes in educational placement and speech perception ability after cochlear implantation in children. *J Otolaryngol* 2000;29:224–228.
2. Fitzpatrick E, McCrae R, Schramm D: A retrospective study of cochlear implant outcomes in children with residual hearing. *BMC Ear Nose Throat Disord* 2006;6:7.
3. Nadol JB Jr, Eddington DK: Treatment of sensorineural hearing loss by cochlear implantation. *Annu Rev Med* 1988;39:491–502.
4. Rubinstein JT: Paediatric cochlear implantation: Prosthetic hearing and language development. *Lancet* 2002;360:483–485.
5. Gantz BJ: Issues of candidate selection for a cochlear implant. *Otolaryngol Clin North Am* 1989;22:239–247.
6. Limb CJ: Cochlear implant-mediated perception of music. *Curr Opin Otolaryngol Head Neck Surg* 2006;14:337–340.
7. Bhatia K, Gibbin KP, Nikolopoulos TP, et al: Surgical complications and their management in a series of 300 consecutive pediatric cochlear implantations. *Otol Neurotol* 2004;25:730–739.
8. Green KM, Bhatt YM, Saeed SR, et al: Complications following adult cochlear implantation: Experience in Manchester. *J Laryngol Otol* 2004;118:417–420.
9. Proops DW, Stoddart RL, Donaldson I: Medical, surgical and audiological complications of the first 100 adult cochlear implant patients in Birmingham. *J Laryngol Otol Suppl* 1999;24:14–17.
10. Arnoldner C, Baumgartner WD, Gstoettner W, et al: Surgical considerations in cochlear implantation in children and adults: A review of 342 cases in Vienna. *Acta Otolaryngol* 2005;125:228–234.
11. Hilts PJ: Drug agency is studying ear implants' links to meningitis. *New York Times* October 5, 2002.

12. Centers for Disease Control and Prevention: Pneumococcal vaccination for cochlear implant recipients. *MMWR Morb Mortal Wkly Rep* 2002;51:931.

13. Arnold W et al: Meningitis following cochlear implantation: Pathomechanisms, clinical symptoms, conservative and surgical treatments. *ORL J Otorhinolaryngol Relat Spec* 2002;64: 382–389.

14. Biernath KR et al: Bacterial meningitis among children with cochlear implants beyond 24 months after implantation. *Pediatrics* 2006;117:284–289.

15. Callanan V, Poje C: Cochlear implantation and meningitis. *Int J Pediatr Otorhinolaryngol* 2004;68:545–550.

16. Cohen N et al: International consensus on meningitis and cochlear implants. *Acta Otolaryngol* 2005;125:916–917.

17. Cohen NL, Roland JT Jr, Marrinan M: Meningitis in cochlear implant recipients: The North American experience. *Otol Neurotol* 2004;25:275–281.

18. Daspit CP: Meningitis as a result of a cochlear implant: Case report. *Otolaryngol Head Neck Surg* 1991;105:115–116.

19. Graveriau C, Roman S, Garrigues B, et al: Pneumococcal meningitis in an immunocompetent adult with a cochlear implant. *J Infect* 2003;46:248–249.

20. Hey C et al: Does the 23-valent pneumococcal vaccine protect cochlear implant recipients? *Laryngoscope* 2005;115:1586–1590.

21. O'Donoghue G et al: Meningitis and cochlear implantation. *Otol Neurotol* 2002;23:823–824.

22. Reefhuis J et al: Risk of bacterial meningitis in children with cochlear implants. *N Engl J Med* 2003;349:435–445.

23. Rose M et al: Immunogenicity of pneumococcal vaccination of patients with cochlear implants. *J Infect Dis* 2004;190:551–557.

24. Summerfield AQ et al: Incidence of meningitis and of death from all causes among users of cochlear implants in the United Kingdom. *J Public Health (Oxf)* 2005;27:55–61.

25. Wei BP, Shepherd RK, Robins-Browne RM, et al: Pneumococcal meningitis threshold model: A potential tool to assess infectious risk of new or existing inner ear surgical interventions. *Otol Neurotol* 2006;27:1152–1161.

26. Wilson-Clark SD, Squires S, Deeks S: Bacterial meningitis among cochlear implant recipients—Canada, 2002. *MMWR Morb Mortal Wkly Rep* 2006;55(Suppl 1):20–24.

27. Wooltorton E: Cochlear implant recipients at risk for meningitis. *CMAJ* 2002;167:670.

28. Papsin BC, Bailey CM, Albert DM, et al: Otitis media with effusion in paediatric cochlear implantees: The role of peri-implant grommet insertion. *Int J Pediatr Otorhinolaryngol* 1996;38:13–19.

29. Cunningham CD 3rd, Slattery WH 3rd, Luxford WM: Postoperative infection in cochlear implant patients. *Otolaryngol Head Neck Surg* 2004;131:109–114.

30. Lenarz T: Cochlear implantation in children under the age of two years. *Adv Otorhinolaryngol* 1997;52:204–210.

31. House WF, Luxford WM, Courtney B: Otitis media in children following the cochlear implant. *Ear Hear* 1985;6:24S–26S.

32. Webb RL, Clark GM, Shepherd RK, et al: The biologic safety of the Cochlear Corporation multiple-electrode intracochlear implant. *Am J Otol* 1988;9:8–13.

33. Jackler RK, O'Donoghue GM, Schindler RA: Cochlear implantation: Strategies to protect the implanted cochlea from middle ear infection. *Ann Otol Rhinol Laryngol* 1986;95:66–70.

34. Kennedy RJ, Shelton C: Ventilation tubes and cochlear implants: What do we do? *Otol Neurotol* 2005;26:438–441.

35. Rubinstein JT, Gantz BJ, Parkinson WS: Management of cochlear implant infections. *Am J Otol* 1999;20:46–49.

36. Calligaro KD, Veith FJ, Schwartz ML, et al: Are gram-negative bacteria a contraindication to selective preservation of infected prosthetic arterial grafts? *J Vasc Surg* 1992;16:337–346.

37. Silverstein A, Donatucci CF: Bacterial biofilms and implantable prosthetic devices. *Int J Impot Res* 2003;15(Suppl 5):S150–S154.

38. Germiller JA, El-Kashlan HK, Shah UK: Chronic *Pseudomonas* infections of cochlear implants. *Otol Neurotol* 2005;26:196–201.

39. Basavaraj S, Najaraj S, Shanks M, et al: Short-term versus long-term antibiotic prophylaxis in cochlear implant surgery. *Otol Neurotol* 2004;25:720–722.

40. Fayad JN, Wanna GB, Micheletto JN, et al: Facial nerve paralysis following cochlear implant surgery. *Laryngoscope* 2003; 113:1344–1346.

41. Hoffman RA, Cohen NL: Complications of cochlear implant surgery. *Ann Otol Rhinol Laryngol Suppl* 1995;166:420–422.

42. House JR 3rd, Luxford WM: Facial nerve injury in cochlear implantation. *Otolaryngol Head Neck Surg* 1993;109:1078–1082.

43. Gianoli GJ, Kartush JM: Delayed facial palsy after acoustic neuroma resection: The role of viral reactivation. *Am J Otol* 1996;17:625–629.

44. Vrabec JT: Delayed facial palsy after tympanomastoid surgery. *Am J Otol* 1999;20:26–30.

45. Kelsall DC, Shallop JK, Brammeier TG, et al: Facial nerve stimulation after nucleus 22-channel cochlear implantation. *Am J Otol* 1997;18:336–341.

46. Muckle RP, Levine SC: Facial nerve stimulation produced by cochlear implants in patients with cochlear otosclerosis. *Am J Otol* 1994;15:394–398.

47. Polak M, Ulubil SA, Hodges AV, et al: Revision cochlear implantation for facial nerve stimulation in otosclerosis. *Arch Otolaryngol Head Neck Surg* 2006;132:398–404.

48. Smullen JL et al: Facial nerve stimulation after cochlear implantation. *Laryngoscope* 2005;115:977–982.

49. Niparko JK et al: Facial nerve stimulation with cochlear implantation: VA cooperative study group on cochlear implantation. *Otolaryngol Head Neck Surg* 1991;104:826–830.

50. Shea JJ 3rd, Domico EH: Facial nerve stimulation after successful multichannel cochlear implantation. *Am J Otol* 1994;15:752–756.

51. Weber BP et al: Otosclerosis and facial nerve stimulation. *Ann Otol Rhinol Laryngol Suppl* 1995;166:445–447.

52. Marshall AH et al: Cochlear implantation in cochlear otosclerosis. *Laryngoscope* 2005;115:1728–1733.

53. Quaranta N et al: Cochlear implantation in otosclerosis. *Otol Neurotol* 2005;26:983–987.

54. Battmer R et al: Elimination of facial nerve stimulation by reimplantation in cochlear implant subjects. *Otol Neurotol* 2006;27: 918–922.

55. Bento RF, Padua FG: Tegmen tympani cerebrospinal fluid leak repair. *Acta Otolaryngol* 2004;124:443–448.

56. Bolger WE, McLaughlin K: Cranial bone grafts in cerebrospinal fluid leak and encephalocele repair: A preliminary report. *Am J Rhinol* 2003;17:153–158.

57. Kveton JF, Goravalingappa R: Elimination of temporal bone cerebrospinal fluid otorrhea using hydroxyapatite cement. *Laryngoscope* 2000;110:1655–1659.

58. Wootten CT, Backous DD, Haynes DS: Management of cerebrospinal fluid leakage from cochleostomy during cochlear implant surgery. *Laryngoscope* 2006;116:2055–2059.

59. Papsin BC: Cochlear implantation in children with anomalous cochleovestibular anatomy. *Laryngoscope* 2005;115:1–26.

60. Glasscock ME 3rd: The stapes gusher. *Arch Otolaryngol* 1973;98:82–91.

61. Graham JM, Ashcroft P: Direct measurement of cerebrospinal fluid pressure through the cochlea in a congenitally deaf child with Mondini dysplasia undergoing cochlear implantation. *Am J Otol* 1999;20:205–208.

62. Ito J, Sakota T, Kato H, et al: Surgical considerations regarding cochlear implantation in the congenitally malformed cochlea. *Otolaryngol Head Neck Surg* 1999;121:495–498.

63. Mylanus EA, Rotteveel LJ, Leeuw RL: Congenital malformation of the inner ear and pediatric cochlear implantation. *Otol Neurotol* 2004;25:308–317.

64. Marks HW: Simple method to control a cerebrospinal fluid gusher during cochlear implant surgery. *Otol Neurotol* 2004;25:483–484.

65. Wardrop P, Whinney D, Rebscher SJ, et al: A temporal bone study of insertion trauma and intracochlear position of cochlear implant electrodes. II: Comparison of Spiral Clarion and HiFocus II electrodes. *Hear Res* 2005;203:68–79.

66. Wardrop P et al: A temporal bone study of insertion trauma and intracochlear position of cochlear implant electrodes. I: Comparison of nucleus banded and nucleus contour electrodes. *Hear Res* 2005;203:54–67.

67. Leake PA, Hradek GT, Snyder RL: Chronic electrical stimulation by a cochlear implant promotes survival of spiral ganglion neurons after neonatal deafness. *J Comp Neurol* 1999;412:543–562.

68. Pau H, Parker A, Sanli H, et al: Displacement of electrodes of a cochlear implant into the vestibular system: Intra- and postoperative electrophysiological analyses. *Acta Otolaryngol* 2005;125:1116–1118.

69. Mecca MA, Wagle W, Lupinetti A, et al: Complication of cochlear implantation surgery. *AJNR Am J Neuroradiol* 2003;24:2089–2091.

70. Roland JT Jr, Fishman AJ, Alexiades G, et al: Electrode to modiolus proximity: A fluoroscopic and histologic analysis. *Am J Otol* 2000;21:218–225.

71. Verbist BM, Frijns JH, Geleijns J, et al: Multisection CT as a valuable tool in the postoperative assessment of cochlear implant patients. *AJNR Am J Neuroradiol* 2005;26:424–429.

72. Kempf HG, Johann K, Weber BP, et al: Complications of cochlear implant surgery in children. *Am J Otol* 1997;18:S62–S63.

73. Webb RL, et al: Surgical complications with the cochlear multiple-channel intracochlear implant: Experience at Hannover and Melbourne. *Ann Otol Rhinol Laryngol* 1991;100:131–136.

74. Leach J, Kruger P, Roland P: Rescuing the imperiled cochlear implant: A report of four cases. *Otol Neurotol* 2005;26:27–33.

75. Ito J, Taura A, Fujita S, et al: Use of rotation flap in the treatment of cutaneous ulceration after cochlear implantation. *Otolaryngol Head Neck Surg* 1999;121:830–832.

76. Schweitzer VG, Burtka MJ: Cochlear implant flap necrosis: Adjunct hyperbaric oxygen therapy for prevention of explantation. *Am J Otol* 199;12:71–75.

77. Telian SA, El-Kashlan HK, Arts HA: Minimizing wound complications in cochlear implant surgery. *Am J Otol* 1999;20:331–334.

78. O'Donoghue GM, Nikolopoulos TP: Minimal access surgery for pediatric cochlear implantation. *Otol Neurotol* 2002;23:891–894.

79. Odabasi O, Mobley SR, Bolanos RA, et al: Cochlear implantation in patients with compromised healing. *Otolaryngol Head Neck Surg* 2000;123:738–741.

80. Roland JT, Jr, Fishman AJ, Waltzman SB, et al: Shaw scalpel in revision cochlear implant surgery. *Ann Otol Rhinol Laryngol Suppl* 2000;185:23–25.

81. Migirov L, Taitelbaum-Swead R, Hildesheimer M, et al: Revision surgeries in cochlear implant patients: A review of 45 cases. *Eur Arch Otorhinolaryngol* 2007;264:3–7

82. Roland JT Jr, Huang TC, Cohen NL: Revision cochlear implantation. *Otolaryngol Clin North Am* 2006;39:viii –ix, 833–839.

83. Maurer J, Marangos N, Ziegler E: Reliability of cochlear implants. *Otolaryngol Head Neck Surg* 2005;132:746–750.

84. Buchman CA, Higgins CA, Cullen R, et al: Revision cochlear implant surgery in adult patients with suspected device malfunction. *Otol Neurotol* 2004;25:504–510.

85. Balkany TJ et al: Cochlear reimplantation. *Laryngoscope* 1999;109:351–355.

86. Lassig AA, Zwolan TA, Telian SA: Cochlear implant failures and revision. *Otol Neurotol* 2005;26:624–634.

87. Miyamoto RT, Svirsky MA, Myres WA, et al: Cochlear implant reimplantation. *Am J Otol* 1997;18:S60–S61.

88. Woolford TJ, Saeed SR, Boyd P, et al: Cochlear reimplantation. *Ann Otol Rhinol Laryngol Suppl* 1995;166:449–453.

89. Balkany TJ et al: Cochlear implant soft failures consensus development conference statement. *Otol Neurotol* 2005;26:815–818.

90. European consensus statement on cochlear implant failures and explantations. *Otol Neurotol* 2005;26:1097–1099.

91. Migirov L, Kronenberg J: Magnet displacement following cochlear implantation. *Otol Neurotol* 2005;26:646–648.

92. Weise JB et al: Impact to the head increases cochlear implant reimplantation rate in children. *Auris Nasus Larynx* 2005;32:339–343.

93. Wilkinson EP, Dogru S, Meyer TA, et al: Case report: Cochlear implant magnet migration. *Laryngoscope* 2004;114:2009–2011.

94. Yun JM, Colburn MW, Antonelli PJ: Cochlear implant magnet displacement with minor head trauma. *Otolaryngol Head Neck Surg* 2005;133:275–277.

95. Bhatt YM et al: Device nonuse among adult cochlear implant recipients. *Otol Neurotol* 2005;26:183–187.

96. Aplin DY: Psychological evaluation of adults in a cochlear implant program. *Am Ann Deaf* 1993;138:415–419.

97. Horn DL, Pisoni DB, Sanders M, et al: Behavioral assessment of prelingually deaf children before cochlear implantation. *Laryngoscope* 2005;115:1603–1611.

98. Shipp DB, Nedzelski JM: Prognostic indicators of speech recognition performance in adult cochlear implant users: A prospective analysis. *Ann Otol Rhinol Laryngol Suppl* 1995;166:194–196.

99. Osaki Y et al: Neural mechanism of residual inhibition of tinnitus in cochlear implant users. *Neuroreport* 2005;16:1625–1628.

100. Quaranta N, Wagstaff S, Baguley DM: Tinnitus and cochlear implantation. *Int J Audiol* 2004;43:245–251.

101. Miyamoto RT, Bichey BG: Cochlear implantation for tinnitus suppression. *Otolaryngol Clin North Am* 2003;36:345–352.

102. Rubinstein JT, Tyler RS, Johnson A, et al: Electrical suppression of tinnitus with high-rate pulse trains. *Otol Neurotol* 2003;24:478–485.

103. Ruckenstein MJ, Hedgepeth C, Rafter KO, et al: Tinnitus suppression in patients with cochlear implants. *Otol Neurotol* 2001;22:200–204.

104. Dutt SN et al: Medical and surgical complications of the second 100 adult cochlear implant patients in Birmingham. *J Laryngol Otol* 2005;119:759–764.

105. Fina M et al: Vestibular dysfunction after cochlear implantation. *Otol Neurotol* 2003;24:234–242.

106. Steenerson RL, Cronin GW, Gary LB: Vertigo after cochlear implantation. *Otol Neurotol* 2001;22:842–843.

107. Huygen PL et al: The risk of vestibular function loss after intracochlear implantation. *Acta Otolaryngol Suppl* 1995;520(Pt 2):270–272.

108. van den Broek P, Huygen PL, Mens LH: Vestibular function in cochlear implant patients. *Acta Otolaryngol* 1993;113:263–265.

109. Limb CJ, Francis HF, Lustig LR, et al: Benign positional vertigo after cochlear implantation. *Otolaryngol Head Neck Surg* 2005;132:741–745.

110. Tange RA, Grolman W, Maat A: Intracochlear misdirected implantation of a cochlear implant. *Acta Otolaryngol* 2006;126:650–652.

CHAPTER 58

Complications of Congenital Aural Atresia and External Auditory Canal Surgery

Paul R. Lambert

Surgery within the external auditory canal is performed routinely during the course of most middle-ear and mastoid procedures. Occasionally, the ear canal is the primary site of surgery, especially for problems of canal patency, infection, or tumor. Canal stenosis as a result of exostosis or osteomas and tumors of squamous epithelial or glandular origin are examples of primary diseases and disorders that require surgical intervention. Chronic otitis externa occasionally causes a progressive fibrosis in the medial portion of the external auditory canal that results in stenosis or the obliteration of the lumen. Trauma, including postsurgical trauma, can also cause a fibrous narrowing or closure. Finally, congenital atresia of the external auditory canal is an obvious disorder that may be amenable to surgical correction. Aural atresia repair requires an extensive procedure that encompasses the full spectrum of possible complications that are inherent to ear canal surgery and that will thus be the focus of this chapter.

A critical factor that predisposes patients to complications within the external auditory canal after surgical intervention for any reason is the loss of the normal skin lining. The approximately 2.5-cm canal is characterized by two histologically and physiologically distinct epithelia. The epithelium within the medial two thirds of the external canal (i.e., the osseous portion) rests on the periosteum and is continuous with the squamous epithelium of the tympanic membrane. The lateral one third of the canal (i.e., the cartilaginous portion) is a more complex epithelium with a subcutaneous layer that contains sebaceous and apocrine adnexa. A variety of lipid secretions from these adnexa are excreted into the hair follicle spaces and mixed with exfoliated squamous cells. This mixture forms an acidic, water-resistant coating of the external canal that is important for resisting infection.

The squamous epithelium throughout the external auditory canal is unique in its ability to self-clean. Instead of friction removing the desquamated epithelium and the keratin debris, as occurs elsewhere on the body, the ear canal is cleaned by the actual migration of squamous epithelium. Squamous epithelial cells of the tympanic membrane move radially toward the annulus and then continue in a lateral direction, from the annulus to the meatus. Any condition that disrupts this normal migration pattern or the production of the protective secretions will predispose individuals to disease. An extreme example of this is the repair of aural atresia with the creation of an ear canal lined by a split-thickness skin graft (STSG) taken from another area of the body.

CONGENITAL AURAL ATRESIA

The evaluation and treatment of atresia of the ear canal challenges the otologist's clinical acumen and surgical abilities. The improper selection of patients for surgery, an inadequate appreciation for the abnormal temporal bone development that has occurred, and a lack of attention to surgical detail can lead to diverse surgical complications, including hearing loss, facial nerve paralysis, and chronic infection. The concepts and protocols of the preoperative evaluation, the surgical procedure itself, and the postoperative care that are important for minimizing these potential problems will be reviewed.

PREOPERATIVE EVALUATION

The surgical correction of aural atresia is an elective procedure. Unilateral cases can be managed by observation alone, and bilateral cases can be rehabilitated with a bone conduction or a bone-anchored hearing aid. However, most otologic surgeons recognize the potential for a single operative procedure to restore serviceable hearing, and such a possibility is attractive to many patients. Critical to the surgeon's ability to offer predictable hearing results is proper patient selection. Only about 50% of patients with aural atresia will be surgical candidates if strict audiometric and radiographic selection criteria are followed.

Audiometric Testing

In unilateral cases, behavioral audiometry can be used, although auditory brainstem response (ABR) testing may be necessary in young infants or children who are difficult to test. Patients with bilateral atresia present the problem of a masking dilemma. Resolving this dilemma and determining the level of cochlear function in each ear is crucial to prevent operating on an only-hearing ear or on an ear with little or no potential for hearing improvement. Because most patients undergoing atresia repair will have a residual conductive hearing loss of at least 10 dB, sensorineural function should be normal in that ear to achieve binaural hearing in unilateral cases or to obviate the need for a hearing aid in bilateral cases.

Bone conduction ABR testing can be used to assess cochlear function in cases of bilateral atresia.[1] Wave I of the ABR is generated by the distal portion of the auditory nerve, and it is best measured by a recording electrode ipsilateral to the stimulated ear. Thus, when recording simultaneously from both ears with surface electrodes, the presence of wave I should represent the response only from the ear being stimulated. Although it is not possible to stimulate each ear independently with a bone-conducted signal, the wave I response is ear specific, thereby allowing for the differential assessment of cochlear function.

Computed Tomography Scanning

Computed tomography (CT) scanning of the temporal bone is necessary for all patients with congenital aural atresia. Assuming that normal sensorineural function has been confirmed audiometrically, the decision to operate will depend primarily on the degree of middle-ear development as reflected by the size of the tympanum and the status of the ossicles. The risk of surgical complications will be minimized and the chances for successful hearing results substantially increased if the middle-ear and mastoid size are at least two thirds of normal and if all three ossicles—although deformed—can be identified. Radiographic demonstration of the oval and round windows further defines the ideal surgical candidate. The inability to clearly see the course of the facial nerve is not a contraindication to surgery, assuming that the other criteria for middle-ear development are met. Proper operative technique, intraoperative facial nerve monitoring, and the expectation that the facial nerve will be anomalous, however, are critical.

CT evaluation of the architecture of the cochlea and the vestibular labyrinth is also important. Defects in the embryologic development of the first and second brachial arches and of the first branchial cleft cause congenital aural atresia. However, normal development of the labyrinth is anticipated, because it arises from the ectodermal otocyst. Nevertheless, the abnormal development of the cochlea and the semicircular canals can occur; if present, this could have an influence on the middle-ear surgery. For example, the presence of an enlarged vestibule and a horizontal semicircular canal suggests the possibility of abnormal communication between the perilymph and the cerebrospinal fluid. In such cases, manipulation of the stapes should be minimized to avoid the potential complication of a cerebrospinal fluid gusher.

INTRAOPERATIVE COMPLICATIONS

The two most serious complications of surgery for congenital aural atresia are facial nerve paralysis and sensorineural hearing loss. These concerns and the potential for the lifetime care of a mastoid cavity have prompted many surgeons to recommend delaying surgery in unilateral cases until adulthood, when the patient can make his or her own decision based on the risks and benefits. However, appropriate surgical technique and the use of facial nerve monitoring can maintain the risk of these complications and the problem of postoperative canal infection at a level comparable with that expected during surgery for chronic ear disease. Therefore surgery for unilateral atresia can be offered to carefully selected children.

The most common surgical technique for the repair of aural atresia is to expose the middle ear by drilling through the atretic bone, with limited opening into the mastoid (Figure 58-1). This "anterior approach" obviates the problem of a large mastoid cavity with its attendant problems of debris accumulation and infection. In addition, there is less surgical manipulation in the area of the mastoid segment of the facial nerve, thus minimizing trauma to that structure. The more cylindric contours of the ear canal with the anterior approach also facilitate the placement of an STSG and help to avoid postoperative healing problems such as bone exposure and the formation of granulation tissue. Facial nerve monitoring should be used.

The surgical procedure begins with a postauricular incision to expose the mastoid bone. The soft tissues are elevated anteriorly until a depression is encountered. In

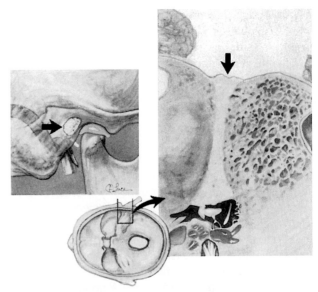

Figure 58-1. Schematic diagrams showing atretic bone *(straight arrows)* from the lateral and axial perspectives. (From Lambert PR: Major congenital ear malformations. *Ann Otol Rhinol Laryngol* 1988;97:641–649. Used with permission.)

most major malformations, this depression is the temporomandibular joint, although occasionally a stenotic bony ear canal may be encountered. Dissection within this area may be necessary to differentiate between the two, but the manipulation should be limited, because the facial nerve may exit the skull into the glenoid fossa.

Drilling is confined to an area defined by the middle cranial fossa dura superiorly, the glenoid fossa anteriorly, and the mastoid air cells posteriorly. These landmarks delimit the atretic bone lying lateral to the middle ear space. The bone that is removed is usually solid, but it may be cellular in areas. The posterior wall of the glenoid fossa (i.e., the anterior wall of the new ear canal) should be very thin to permit access to the anterior half of the middle-ear space. As the middle cranial fossa dura plate is followed medially, the epitympanum will be entered, and the fused heads of the malleus and incus will be encountered (Figure 58-2).

Fixation of the ossicular chain to the atretic bone is usually at the manubrium of the malleus. To free the ossicular chain, the atretic bone is thinned carefully with a diamond burr and completely removed with a small, right-angled instrument. Except for the fossa incudis, which may be left intact, bone should be completely removed around the ossicles, leaving at least a 2- to 3-mm space between these structures and the canal wall. The atretic bone is removed in such a way that the ossicular mass is centered in the new canal (Figure 58-3). Attention to these details will help to prevent bony refixation and permit the proper draping of the fascia and the STSG.

The stapes may be partially obscured as a result of the malformed lateral ossicular mass, the overlying facial nerve, or both. Hypoplasia of the middle-ear space, which is present to some extent in all cases of congenital atresia, can further compromise a clear view of this ossicle. Usually, however, a portion of the stapes can be seen sufficiently to assess its mobility. Abnormal development of the stapes superstructure is common, with the crura often being delicate and misshapen. It is rare to encounter a fixed stapes footplate or an absent oval window in cases of congenital aural atresia. These latter anomalies are more frequently seen among patients with congenital hearing loss who have a patent ear canal and a normal tympanic membrane.[2] The removal of the lateral ossicular mass to obtain a better view of the stapes is rarely necessary, and hearing results may be better when the ossicular chain is left intact as compared with disarticulation and the use of a prosthesis.[3]

The placement of the fascia graft in atresia cases is more problematic than in chronic ear surgery because of graft stabilization. Typically the manubrium of the malleus is either absent or represented by a short, bulbous projection from the malleus–incus complex. It is therefore difficult to anchor the graft beneath the malformed ossicular chain, and the absence of a tympanic membrane remnant or an annulus further predisposes patients to lateralization. To prevent this complication, the graft is tucked beneath the anterior and superior bony ledges of the canal wall. In addition, care is taken to smooth the canal wall so that there are no bony projections lateral to the ossicular mass. The fascia should appear to be draped over an ossicular mound centered in the exposed middle-ear space.

A STSG that is 0.009 inches thick is taken from the upper arm and used to line the ear canal. The proper dimensions of the STSG are determined by measuring the length and circumference of the canal at several levels. The resulting graft is usually shaped like a hexagon, and it measures approximately 4 cm $\times$ 6 cm. With the ear retracted forward, the STSG is positioned in the bony canal so that it overlaps the fascia graft by several millimeters. A Silastic disk contoured to the circumference of

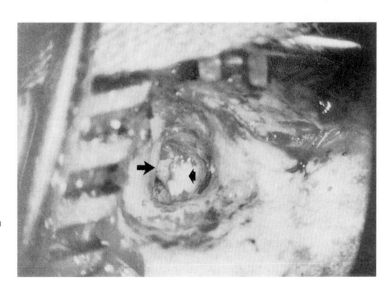

Figure 58-2. Right ear showing the fused heads of the malleus and incus that have been uncovered in the epitympanum *(arrow)*. Atretic bone covers the remainder of the middle ear *(arrowhead)*. (From Lambert PR: Major congenital ear malformations. *Ann Otol Rhinol Laryngol* 1988;97:641–649. Used with permission.)

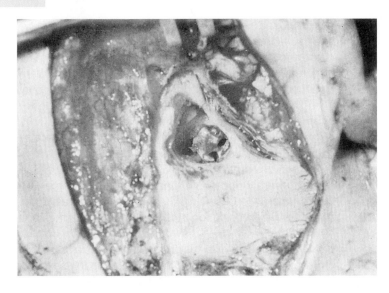

Figure 58-3. Right ear showing a fully exposed ossicular chain.

the canal is placed on top of the fascia and the overlying STSG. This helps to prevent the lateralization of the tympanic membrane and to maintain a sharp angle at the anterior sulcus. The STSG is stabilized within the canal with the placement of Merocel wicks, which are then hydrated by an antibiotic otic solution. A meatal opening about twice the normal size is made in the auricle. Working through this meatus, the lateral end of the STSG is pulled to the exterior, trimmed as necessary, and sutured to the meatal skin. The surgical procedure is completed by placing several additional Merocel wicks in the lateral or soft-tissue portion of the ear canal.

Facial Nerve Injury

Injury to the facial nerve is a potential complication with any otologic procedure, including surgery within the medial external auditory canal. The abnormal development of the temporal bone in cases of aural atresia increases the nerve's vulnerability, but injuries should still be rare if the surgeon understands the anomalies of the facial nerve that are likely to be encountered and uses facial nerve monitoring.

One should assume that the facial nerve will be anomalous in all congenital ears. Bony dehiscence of the fallopian canal is common, and the facial nerve often takes an abnormal course. In atresia cases, the facial nerve typically makes an acute (rather than obtuse) angle at the second genu, crossing the middle ear in a more anterior and lateral direction to exit near the glenoid fossa. In approximately one half of the author's major atresia cases, the facial nerve had one or more of the following abnormalities:

1. Complete dehiscence of the tympanic segment

2. Inferior displacement of the tympanic segment

3. Anterior and lateral displacement of the mastoid segment (Figure 58-4)

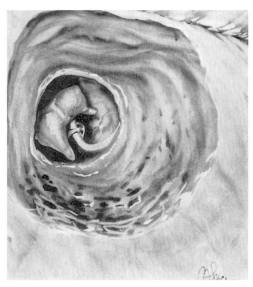

Figure 58-4. Schematic diagram showing the anterior and lateral displacement of the mastoid segment of the facial nerve.

This last abnormality may obscure the round window. The degree of external-ear deformity does provide some indication of facial nerve development in that a higher incidence of facial nerve anomalies occurs among patients with more severe microtia.[3,4]

Aberrant facial nerves can also be encountered in ears with minor malformations, such as a congenital conductive hearing loss but a normal tympanic membrane, a patent external ear canal, and little or no auricular deformity. These facial nerve abnormalities may in fact be more severe than those seen in atresia cases. Frequent findings include the dehiscence and inferior displacement of the tympanic segment of the facial nerve. In several cases, a facial nerve coursing across the mid portion of the promontory well inferior to the oval window has been noted.[2,5]

Given the abnormalities of the facial nerve anticipated in patients with aural atresia, several surgical guidelines can be set forth. First, as the atretic bone is removed, it is advisable to concentrate the drilling superiorly along the middle cranial fossa dural plate, entering the middle ear first in the epitympanum. The facial nerve is protected with this approach, because it will always lie medial to the fused heads of the malleus–incus complex in the epitympanum. Second, care should be exercised as the external canal is enlarged in the posteroinferior direction. The nerve is vulnerable to injury here because of the more anterior and lateral course of the mastoid segment.

Injury to the facial nerve can also occur in its extratemporal segment if the auricle requires undermining to better align the soft-tissue meatus and the created bony canal. Prior auricular reconstruction can cause scarring and tethering of the facial nerve in a more superficial position, thus making it vulnerable to injury. This circumstance represents the author's only case of a facial nerve weakness (i.e., temporary) in congenital ear surgery. Jahrsdoerfer and Lambert[6] have reported a 1% incidence of facial paresis or paralysis in more than 1000 patients who had undergone congenital ear surgery.

Sensorineural Hearing Loss

As previously discussed, an accurate preoperative audiometric evaluation is essential, especially in bilateral atresia cases, to prevent operating on an only-hearing ear or an ear with an existing sensorineural hearing loss and thus with little potential for gaining serviceable hearing. In an extreme case, misjudgments in patient selection or during surgery could render the patient deaf.

Postoperatively, high-frequency sensorineural hearing loss is noted in some patients, although a loss in speech frequencies is uncommon.[3,5,7–10] Because the ossicular mass is connected to the atretic bone, energy from drilling will be transmitted to the inner ear in all atresia cases, regardless of the approach. This appears to be of minor consequence, however, and most high-frequency sensorineural hearing loss is attributed to the direct manipulation of the ossicular chain by instruments or the drill. Care when removing the final portion of atretic bone from the ossicular chain is particularly important so that the incudostapedial joint is not disarticulated.

Cholesteatoma

A cholesteatoma can develop spontaneously in patients with abnormal development of the external auditory canal. The presenting symptom is usually drainage from the ear canal or from a fistulous tract postauricularly. To prevent this complication during the period of observation, it is important to have an understanding of its genesis and of the use of CT scans for its evaluation.

Embryologically, the external ear canal is derived from the first branchial groove. It is initially represented by a solid core of epithelial cells. During the fifth month of fetal life, the absorption of these epithelial cells begins, and it progresses in a medial to lateral direction. If this canalization process is arrested prematurely, it is possible for a partial tympanic membrane and a bony external ear canal to develop in association with an atretic or stenotic membranous canal. As the trapped squamous epithelium desquamates in the medial portion of the canal, a cholesteatoma forms. In a series of 50 patients with a canal diameter of 4 mm or less, a 50% incidence of cholesteatoma was noted.[11] An even higher percentage of patients developed cholesteatoma in canals of 2 mm or less in diameter. Cholesteatomas were not found in patients who were younger than 3 years old, but they were increasingly encountered as the children reached adolescence. Given these data, it is judicious to obtain a CT scan for a patient with severe stenosis of the external ear canal by the age of 5 or 6 years. If the CT findings are favorable with regard to hearing improvement, canal and middle-ear surgery are advised, even for unilateral cases. If surgery is deferred, a CT scan should be obtained every several years through adolescence. The detection of an epithelial cyst in the medial portion of the ear canal is an indication for surgery. A canaloplasty without middle-ear surgery is offered to those patients with stenosis that is sufficient to prevent the adequate cleaning of the canal but who have unfavorable middle-ear findings on a CT scan.

REVISION SURGERY

It should be recognized that revision surgery is often required after congenital aural atresia repair. In the series by Lambert[10] in which patients were followed for an average of 2.8 years, one third of the patients did require revision surgery. Stenosis of the ear canal (with or without infection), lateralization of the tympanic membrane, and persistent or recurrent conductive hearing loss were the most common problems encountered. After revision surgery, approximately half of these patients did achieve a speech reception threshold of 25 dB or better with at least 1 year of follow up.

Canal Stenosis

Some narrowing of the soft-tissue portion of the ear canal develops in as many as 25% of patients. This is of no consequence if a large meatus (i.e., approximately twice normal size) has been made. However, the development of a significant stenosis will result in chronic infection from trapped squamous epithelium and potentially cause a hearing loss. Attempts to dilate the canal with soft or hard stents are rarely effective; as a result, a meatoplasty with skin grafting will be required.

Stenosis of the ear canal can be avoided by doing the following:

1. Creating a large meatus
2. Covering all soft tissue of the lateral canal with an STSG
3. Debulking the soft tissue that is adjacent to the meatus
4. Using an anteriorly based full-thickness skin flap to line a portion of the ear canal

The ability to completely immobilize the STSG in the ear canal contributes to the extraordinary healing of these grafts that routinely occurs. However, it is important to cover all exposed soft tissue and to meticulously approximate the STSG to the meatal skin to prevent the formation of granulation tissue and subsequent stricture. The likelihood of stricture can be further diminished by generously debulking the soft tissue of the auricle in the region of the meatus. Although usually performed before the meatoplasty, the circumferential trimming of additional soft tissue from the meatus may be required. This decreases the length of the membranous canal, thereby reducing the area for stricture development. If possible, an anteriorly based full-thickness skin flap should be elevated over the area of the planned meatus. After the membranous canal has been created, the skin flap can be rotated medially to line a portion of the anterior canal, thus preventing a circumferential meatal incision and decreasing the possibility of stricture formation.

In some patients, the membranous ear canal may be narrowed by the displacement of the auricle rather than by fibrous proliferation. It is common at the time of surgery for the meatus to be offset anteriorly, inferiorly, or anteroinferiorly relative to the bony canal. In such cases, undermining the auricle is necessary so that it can be positioned without tension more posterosuperiorly. A strip of skin is usually excised from the postauricular incision to help maintain the auricle in its new location. However, because the reconstructed auricle has more mass and less muscular and soft-tissue support than a normal pinna, it can shift after surgery, thus causing a malalignment of the meatus and the bony canal. In such cases, a permanent suspension suture from the framework of the auricle to the mastoid periosteum or to a hole drilled in the mastoid cortex is necessary for the proper realignment of the soft tissue and the bony canals.

Conductive Hearing Loss

Persistent or recurrent conductive hearing loss is the most common negative outcome of aural atresia surgery. The causes of the former are varied and include the inadequate mobilization of the ossicular mass from the atretic bone, an unrecognized incudostapedial joint discontinuity, or a fixed stapes footplate. Wide exposure of the ossicular mass at surgery is necessary to ensure chain mobility and to facilitate the assessment of chain integrity. The recurrence of a conductive hearing loss after an initial satisfactory improvement in air-conduction thresholds is usually the result of the refixation of the ossicular chain or of tympanic membrane lateralization. At least a 2- to 3-mm wide area of bone removal around the ossicular mass (except at the fossa incudis) is desirable, because bony regrowth can occur, especially among children. Anchoring the fascia graft beneath a bony ledge and using a Silastic disc both help to minimize graft lateralization.

Chronic Infection

The skin-grafted ear canal lacks the normal migration of keratin debris. Protective secretions from sebaceous and apocrine glands are also absent. As a consequence, the incidence of canal infections is higher than in the normal ear. A widely patent meatus and membranous canal are obviously important for aeration and cleaning. Most postoperative patients are not restricted with regard to water activities, but an examination of the ear on a yearly basis is advised.

Otorrhea can also result from a tympanic membrane perforation. However, graft failure is uncommon, with an incidence approximating that encountered with routine tympanoplasties. Although the middle-ear and mastoid air cells in atretic ears are smaller than those seen in normal ears, no anatomic or clinical studies have demonstrated Eustachian tube dysfunction. Mucoid fluid in the middle ear has been encountered in less than 10% of the author's cases. Normal physiologic function of the Eustachian tube and of the middle-ear mucosa thus contributes to a low rate of graft failure or subsequent perforation as a result of otitis media.

REFERENCES

1. Tucci DL, Ruth RA, Lambert PR: Use of the bone, conduction ABR wave I response in determination of cochlear reserve. *Am J Otolaryngol* 1990;11:119–124.
2. Lambert PR: Congenital absence of the oval window. *Laryngoscope* 1990;100:37–40.
3. Lambert PR: Major congenital ear malformations. *Ann Otol Rhinol Laryngol* 1988;97:641–649.
4. Jahrsdoerfer RA: Congenital atresia of the ear. *Laryngoscope* 1978;88(9 Pt 3 Suppl 13):1–48.
5. Jahrsdoerfer RA: Congenital malformation of the ear. *Ann Otol Rhinol Laryngol* 1980;89:348–352.
6. Jahrsdoerfer RA, Lambert PR: Facial nerve injury in congenital aural atresia surgery. *Am J Otology* 1998;19:283–287.
7. Schuknecht HG: Congenital aural atresia. *Laryngoscope* 1989;99:908–917.
8. Molony TB, de la Cruz A: Surgical approaches to congenital atresia of the external auditory canal. *Otolaryngol Head Neck Surg* 1990;103:991–1001.
9. de la Cruz A, Teufert KB: Congenital aural atresia surgery: Long-term results. *Otolaryngol Head Neck Surg* 2003;129:121–127.
10. Lambert PR: Congenital aural atresia: Stability of surgical results. *Laryngoscope* 1998;108:1801–1805.
11. Cole RR, Jahrsdoerfer RA: The risk of cholesteatoma in congenital aural stenosis. *Laryngoscope* 1990;100:576–578.

CHAPTER 59

Complications of Otoplasty

Matthew B. Zavod, Theodore Chen, and Peter A. Adamson

It has often been stated that discussion of complications before surgery is called an explanation, and that discussion of them after surgery is called an excuse. Unexpected outcomes of facial plastic surgery can confound an otherwise satisfactory experience for a patient. Such complications can occur with otoplasty, a surgical procedure designed to correct protruding ears. The primary goal of otoplasty is to improve facial appearance, and any complication can compromise the patient's perception of having achieved this goal. Preparing patients for possible untoward outcomes serves not only to identify those possibilities but also to reinforce the surgeon's commitment to seeing the patient through to a satisfactory result. Understanding the potential complications, discussing them with patients, and taking care to avoid them as much as possible will optimize patient satisfaction.

Although credit for the original report of otoplasty for prominent ears may be under some contention,[1,2] various authors have since defined a list of predictable but infrequent complications that are encountered after this surgery. The complications have been grouped by temporal association and categorized as either early or late outcomes (Box 59-1). With the use of recent evidence, the complications are discussed, including their incidence and management. Explaining preoperatively the possible untoward outcomes as well as the frequency at which they occur can make the difference between a satisfied patient and a dissatisfied patient when a complication does occur. Only through understanding the approximate frequency of complications can a patient make an informed decision regarding surgery.

In a review of publications from the past 15 years, 14 papers were identified that described the complications of otoplasty and their incidence. The majority of the data from 11 of these studies is summarized in Table 59-1. That data and the data from the remaining three studies are discussed in the body of this chapter. The complications are discussed in relative order from highest to lowest incidence.

EARLY COMPLICATIONS

Postoperative Nausea and Vomiting

Nausea and vomiting can occur after any surgery. The risk of postoperative nausea and vomiting (PONV) may be increased after otoplasty through a postulated auriculoemetic reflex transmitted by Arnold's nerve and the auriculotemporal nerve.[3,4] Pediatric patients undergoing otoplasty have been found to have an incidence of postoperative vomiting and retching of between 15% and 40% with prophylactic antiemetics and of between 52% and 85% without prophylaxis.[3] This has led to investigations that have looked at decreasing the incidence of PONV.

In a study of 50 patients undergoing otoplasty, Honkavaara and Pyykko[3] found that patients treated with transdermal scopolamine had less PONV than their placebo cohort; the latter also received atropine as part of the study. In another study of 60 children that compared ondansetron, droperidol, and placebo for anesthetic induction, Paxton and colleagues[4] found a significant decrease in PONV only in the ondansetron group, in addition to a decrease in time to oral intake. Comparing general anesthesia with local anesthesia for pediatric outpatient otoplasty, Lancaster and colleagues[5] showed retrospectively that PONV was significantly worse among patients who received a general anesthetic. Care should be taken to minimize PONV among patients undergoing otoplasty. Vomiting will elicit a rise in blood pressure, thus increasing the risk of a hematoma. The authors administer ondansetron during induction to help prevent emesis postoperatively.

Pain

Patients are expected to have a minimal amount of pain after otoplasty. Although pain itself is generally not considered a complication, it can indicate a serious complication. A hematoma should be considered in any patient with excessive pain within the first 2 days after surgery. Malposition of the ear under the dressing can cause pain, and it is easily identified and remedied. Pain 3 to 4 days after surgery should prompt an investigation for infection, which needs to be excluded to prevent possible scarring and tissue necrosis. Pain that lasts past the first postoperative week may indicate damage to the sensory nerves that terminate in the periauricular area. This area receives sensory innervation from a host of sources, including cranial nerves V, VII, IX, and X and cervical nerves 2 and 3 from the cervical plexus. Only one study reported persistent pain.[6] This study, which mostly involved the use of a cartilage-cutting technique, reported an incidence of 5.7% at 2 years. Although one needs to be reminded that chronic pain is a potential adverse outcome, it remains an infrequent complication.

BOX 59-1 Complications of Otoplasty

EARLY COMPLICATIONS

- Postoperative nausea and vomiting
- Pain
- Allergic reactions
- Infection
- Hematoma
- Perichondritis
- Cartilage necrosis
- Atlantoaxial subluxation

LATE COMPLICATIONS

Suture Complications

- Extrusion
- Banding
- Visibility
- Granuloma
- Abscess or skin reaction

Asymmetry

Residual deformity

- Loss of correction
- Helix
- Concha
- External auditory canal distortion
- Antihelix
- Antitragus
- Lobule

Hypoesthesia/Hyperesthesia

Pathologic scarring

- Hypertrophic scar
- Keloid

Cutaneous sequelae

- Incision scar
- Dermatitis

Allergic Reactions

Skin reactions to topical antibiotic ointments occur and can irritate the skin around the incision when applied. Patients often view such a reaction as a setback. A recent study showed that positive reaction rates to topical neomycin and bacitracin were between 11.2% and 11.5% and between 8.7% and 9.2%, respectively, on patch testing.[7] The discontinued use of these ointments is usually the only treatment required. Topical steroids can be prescribed to help alleviate the symptoms. Contact reactions should be noted in the patient's chart and those medications that caused the reactions avoided in the future.

Infection

Four of the studies reported problems with postoperative infection. The range for all studies was 0% to 5.2%. The early identification of redness, pain, or discharge with rapid treatment using oral antibiotics prevented further complications in the studies by Bulstrode and colleagues,[8] Stucker and colleagues,[9] and Calder and Naasan.[10] One case of infection in which the patient was treated with intravenous antibiotics was reported by Messner and Crysdale.[11] Perioperative antibiotic prophylaxis has been shown to decrease the incidence of wound infections in clean-contaminated surgeries.[12] Its benefit in clean surgeries has not been conclusive. The authors administer a preoperative intravenous dose of clindamycin and have only needed further oral antibiotics in one recent case in which a small stitch reaction developed. If infection is suspected, drainage, culture, warm compresses, and appropriate antibiotics should be instituted.

Hematoma

The incidence of hematoma or immediate postoperative bleeding ranged from 0% to 3%. Bleeding may be caused by inadequate hemostasis, rebound from vasoconstriction, dissection outside of the appropriate surgical plane, poor wound dressing, hypertension, occult coagulopathy, trauma, and idiopathic causes.[13,14] Any early postoperative pain, especially if it is unilateral, may herald a bleed and should be investigated with the removal of the bandage. Hemostasis may require surgical intervention with the evacuation of the clot and investigation for a source. A hematoma can act as a culture medium for infection, and failure to address a hematoma can lead to a cauliflower-ear deformity as a result of cartilage necrosis. Patients should be placed on a broad-spectrum antibiotic to prevent subsequent infection and perichondritis. If the postauricular incision is initially closed with interrupted sutures, it may allow for the egress of blood and early detection, thus diminishing the chances of the development of a hematoma.

Perichondritis

No cases of perichondritis were documented in more than 2000 patients reviewed. This may reflect a move away from the use of silk suture material for antihelical definition, which may have contributed to perichondritis.[14] Although it is known to be a rare complication, rapid identification and early, aggressive treatment are important to prevent cartilage necrosis and subsequent cauliflower deformity (Figure 59-1). The authors recommend treatment with wound cultures, the debridement of compromised cartilage, and coverage with intravenous antipseudomonal and antistaphylococcal antibiotics, with close follow up.

Cartilage Necrosis

Cartilage necrosis was not encountered in any of the studies. A rare complication, necrosis of the cartilage can occur after hematoma, infection, perichondritis, dissection out of the surgical plane, excessive use of cautery, and kinking of the auricle in the dressing. The repair of defects in the skin and cartilage is difficult, and it is best avoided by judicious intraoperative and postoperative care.

Table 59-1 Comparison of Otoplasty Complications[a]

Group	Technique	Number of Patients	Residual Deformity (%)	Revision (%)	Asymmetry (%)	Suture Complication (%)	Infection (%)	Hypertrophic Scar or Keloid (%)	Hematoma or Bleeding (%)
Burstein[19]	Anterior scoring, Mustarde, Furnas	100	9	8	0	0[b]	0	2	1
Bulstrode et al[8]	Percutaneous anterior scoring, Mustarde	114	6.1	1.8	0	0[c]	3.5	1.8	0.9
Stucker et al[9]	Mustarde ± lateral conchal cartilage resection	329	0	0.6	0	0.6[d]	0.6	0.3	0.6
Epstein et al[17]	Mustarde, Furnas, cautery	60[e]	10	10	0	0[f]	0	0	0
Caouette-Laberge et al[6]	Cartilage incision and scoring ± Mustarde	500	8.4	1.2	18.4[g]	0[h]	0	0.4	3
Messner et al[11]	Mustarde, Furnas	31	6.5	6.4	6.4	8.6[i]	3.2	3.2	0
Calder et al[10]	Anterior scoring	562	8	11	11	0[j]	5.2	2.1	2
The studies below calculated percentages based on the number of ears:									
Raunig[25]	Anterior scoring	302 ears	1	0.7	0	0[k]	0	0	0
Yugueros et al[18]	Anterior scoring, Mustarde, Furnas	100 ears	3.6	3.1	0	9.8[l]	0	0	0
Erol[20]	Anterior scoring, excision, Kaye, Furnas	55 ears	3.7	1.9	0	0.9[m]	0	0	0
Adamson et al[16]	Modified Mustarde, Furnas	62 ears	5.9	5.9	0	8.4[n]	0	0.8	0.8

a Follow up is more than 12 months mean, except where indicated
b 4-0 clear nylon
c 5-0 nylon
d Non-braided
e Duration of follow-up not reported
f 4-0 clear nylon or nonabsorbable braided polyester
g Found to be secondary to a two-surgeon model
h 5-0 plain catgut
i 3-0 nonabsorbable braided polyester
j 4-0 or 5-0 polyglactin 910 (skin closure)
k 4-0 polyglactin 910 (skin closure)
l 4-0 clear nylon
m 5-0 expanded polytetrafluoroethylene
n 4-0 nonabsorbable braided polyester

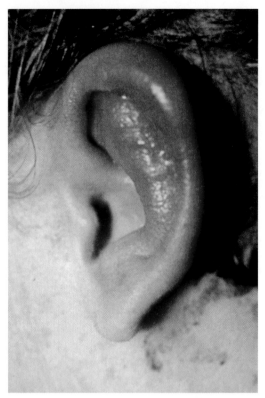

Figure 59-1. Ten days after otoplasty demonstrating perichondritis.

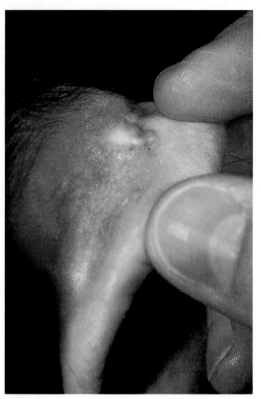

Figure 59-2. One year after otoplasty demonstrating suture banding.

Atlantoaxial Subluxation

Atlantoaxial subluxation, which is also known as *Grisel syndrome,* has been described in the literature as a result of inflammatory changes in the pharynx and the underlying fascial layers after upper aerodigestive surgery or infection. A recent report has documented atlantoaxial subluxation after otoplasty.[15] The authors of that study concluded that repeated rotation of the head during surgery may have caused the inflammation that led to subluxation. Trisomy 21 and rheumatoid arthritis may be predisposing factors in these patients. Diagnosis is made by radiography, and treatment is usually conservative if the condition is identified early during its course. Surgeons who perform otoplasty should be aware of the early signs of this process, which include severe neck pain, restricted movement of the head, and a head tilt. Although atlantoaxial subluxation can be mistaken for spasmodic torticollis, an index of suspicion should be maintained for this rare but potentially debilitating condition.

LATE COMPLICATIONS

Suture Complications

Suture extrusion, banding, visibility, granuloma formation, or skin reaction can occur with varying frequency (Figures 59-2 and 59-3). Banding occurs when the overlying skin contracts down over the suture, thereby leaving a web. This generally occurs superiorly in the

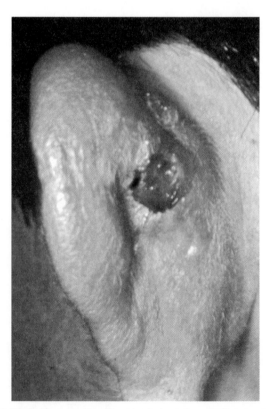

Figure 59-3. Nine months after otoplasty demonstrating a suture granuloma.

postauricular sulcus, and it is more apparent among thin-skinned individuals. Extrusion was the most common late suture complication reported in the reviewed studies. Mersilene (i.e., nonabsorbable braided polyester) was used in the studies that reported higher rates (8.4%–8.6%) of extrusion and granuloma formation,[11,16] although this was not universal.[17] Despite these higher rates, few unfavorable aesthetic outcomes were a direct result of extrusion. Interestingly, both articles that involved the use of suture-setback techniques without cartilage cutting[11,16] reported higher rates of suture complications than those studies involving the use of suture-setback techniques in combination with cartilage cutting. However, they also reported no contour irregularities to be contributing to residual deformity, which can be seen with cartilage-cutting techniques.

The risk of extrusion is neither limited to braided sutures nor avoided with the use of cartilage-cutting techniques with sutures. One study involving the use of 4-0 clear nylon for setback sutures in combination with anterior cartilage scoring also reported a high incidence (9.8%) of suture extrusion.[18] The authors of the study emphasized that high rates of extrusion may be seen in some reports and not in others, because few authors include suture extrusion as a complication in their articles.

Care for extruding sutures or granulomas requires excision and local wound care. If there is an associated loss of correction, it can be repaired at an appropriate time after the resolution of the inflammatory reaction. The choice of suture ultimately relies on the experience and preference of the surgeon. The authors have used 4-0 Mersilene for both the antihelical fold and conchal setback sutures for the past 20 years and have had excellent results with this experience. Although sutures have extruded, few patients have experienced a loss of correction as a result of extrusion if it occurs more than 6 to 8 weeks postoperatively. In addition, Mersilene is a strong suture that resists slippage. A 4-0 chromic gut suture is used for skin closure in an interrupted, inverted, and subcuticular fashion. The interrupted closure allows for the unopposed egress of any fluid that may accumulate, and it promotes the early detection of bleeding, thereby lessening the chance for hematoma formation.

Asymmetry

Three studies reported asymmetry as a late postoperative complication. The rates were between 6.4% and 18.4%. Interestingly, Caouette-Laberge and colleagues[6] initially had a rate of asymmetry of 5.6% on follow up between 0.5 and 64 months. That rate increased to 18.4% on a questionnaire that was mailed out thereafter with a much longer follow up. The authors concluded that asymmetry either increased with time or

that patients became more critical with time. Messner and Crysdale[11] found that two patients (6%) had measurable asymmetries, but only one requested revision. In the study by Calder and Naasan,[10] 11% of patients had undergone or were awaiting revision surgery to improve the symmetry of their ears.

It is important to identify preoperative asymmetries during the initial consultation. Asymmetries are commonly found in facial features, and some may not be amenable to correction with otoplasty. For example, asymmetries caused by skeletal structure may be less noticeable to patients and more difficult to correct than cartilaginous asymmetries. Human interaction is commonly performed in a face-to-face fashion in which both ears are seen simultaneously, but it only takes about 15 degrees of head rotation to obscure one ear from view. When only one ear is seen, asymmetries are impossible to see. It is interesting to note that only three studies reported problems with asymmetry, although almost every study reported problems with residual deformities, which can be appreciated from any angle. Whether asymmetries are common but just minimally noticeable, they do not appear to be consistently common complaints after otoplasty. If preoperative asymmetries are present, the authors have found that operating on the more deformed ear first allows the surgeon to attain better symmetry.

Residual Deformity

The goals of otoplasty for protruding ears are the contouring and placement of the auricles in a more natural and acceptable position. Therefore it is not surprising that one of the more common complications after surgery is a residual deformity (Figures 59-4 and 59-5). Continued prominence of the ears after surgery; loss of correction; and contour irregularities including helical, conchal, antihelical, and lobular deformities were all cited as causes of residual deformities. The incidence ranged from 0% to 10%.

Furnas[13] divided the causes of deformities into two classes: those caused by intrinsic mechanics (e.g., the strength of cartilages) and those caused by extrinsic pressures (e.g., applied dressing, the sleeping position). He warned of sutures pulling through and the buckling of cartilage. Various authors generally recommend that cartilage sutures should be placed in a broad fashion through both layers of perichondrium to prevent suture erosion through cartilage.

Certain areas may be more susceptible to postoperative deformities. Several studies advise that special effort should be directed toward the superior pole of the pinna. Both Burstein[19] and Calder[10] found that 50% of their residual deformities were the result of the

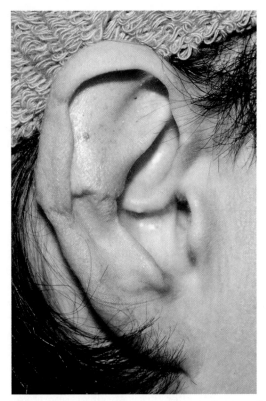

Figure 59-4. Nine years after otoplasty demonstrating an antihelical deformity after the use of a cartilage-cutting technique.

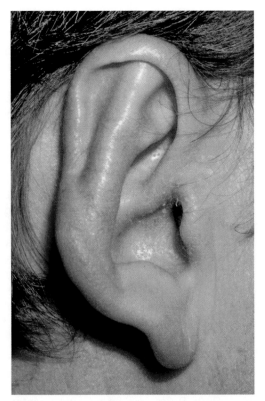

Figure 59-5. Eighteen months after otoplasty demonstrating the overcorrection of the antihelical fold.

prominence of the superior pole. Adamson and colleagues[16] and Messner and colleagues[11] reported that patients who presented with postoperative deformities had a 40% loss of correction at the superior pole. Messner and colleagues showed that this loss measured to within 3 mm of the preoperative value at the superior line. Even Caouette-Laberge and colleagues[6] found that up to one third of residual deformities were related to the prominence of the upper third of the pinna. However, Caouette-Laberge and colleagues and Messner and colleagues disagreed about the predisposition for this complication. The former group found that a short helical diameter led to a higher incidence of the loss of correction, whereas the latter investigators found that a tall vertical height led to a higher incidence of the loss of correction. Adamson and colleagues[16] recommended the placement of fossa–fascial sutures (i.e., horizontal transfixion sutures from the fossa triangularis to the temporalis fascia) to medialize the superior pole and to decrease the risk of postoperative lateralization. In addition, slight overcorrection may be necessary as a result of the frequency of some postoperative loss of correction.

The risk of deformities may be related to the experience of the surgeon. Calder and Naasan,[10] who used an anterior scoring technique, found that 73% of patients with residual deformities suffered from an error in the design of the cartilage work. They were also able to show that the only statistically significant variable for determining a postoperative deformity was the level of training of the surgeon. Training programs may take advantage of the good exposure and bilaterality of otoplasty to instruct residents. This reflects the importance of considering the supervision of trainees and one's own experience when performing otoplasty.

Conchal deformities can be avoided with the use of a cartilage-sparing technique or with the judicious use of cartilage-cutting procedures that minimize contour irregularities. For a conchal setback, enough soft tissue is excised in the area of the postauricular sulcus to accommodate the medialized concha. If a further setback is required, careful tangential shaving of the posterior surface of the concha will improve the ability to set back the concha cavum. This obviates the need to approach the cartilage anteriorly, and it minimizes the risk of scarring. The overcorrection of the concha cavum will result in the "telephone-ear" deformity. Paying close attention when setting the concha posteriorly as well as medially will decrease the risk of external auditory canal stenosis. As newer adaptations of classic techniques emerge in the literature, it is up to the surgeon to decide which methods will give the best results. On the basis of experience, the authors favor a noncutting cartilage setback technique that relies on sutures to hold the position until fibrotic tissue appears and that thus spares the anterior surface of any contour irregularities.

The antihelical edge can also pose a risk for postoperative irregularity. Folding or ridging of the antihelical surface can occur, and so can overcorrection that results in a hidden helix.[20] To avoid such deformities, the authors' preference is to secure the conchal setback sutures before placing the antihelical fold horizontal mattress sutures. Less antihelical correction may be necessary if the conchal setback is performed first. In addition, the shape of the antihelical fold can be accurately contoured, and any required changes can be made. Two to three sutures are placed along the proposed antihelical fold, and the middle sutures are tied last to avoid overcorrection in this area, which would result in the "telephone-ear" deformity. It is important to include generous amounts of cartilage in the suture and to include both layers of perichondrium to reduce the chance for erosion through cartilage. At this point, fossa–fascial sutures are placed to minimize the loss of correction, as described previously.

Antitragal and lobule deformities can occur with the excessive prominence of the cauda helicis. Treatment should focus on directing the cartilage in the proper direction rather than using the skin to pull the cartilage into the new position. In addition, it is a mistake to resect the cauda helicis, because this will prevent the ability to properly place the fibrofatty lobule. Suturing techniques, cartilage-shaping techniques, or a combination of both can be used to improve this deformity.

Hypoesthesia and Hyperesthesia

Incisions in the periauricular area and the manipulation of tissues can lead to postoperative changes in cutaneous sensation. The auricle is heavily innervated with a sensory supply from the cranial and cervical nerves, as previously described. Two studies reported complaints related to sensation postoperatively. In a patient questionnaire, Caouette-Laberge and colleagues[6] found that 3.9% of patients documented decreased sensation in the surgical area, but this was not the presenting chief complaint. Conversely, the same authors reported that 7.5% of patients noted that their ears were extremely sensitive to touch or temperature after surgery. Messner and Crysdale[11] reported that 9.7% of patients noted hyperesthesia. Again, however, this was not the presenting chief complaint. Thus changes in sensation around the operative area can occur over the long term, but patients rarely express concern about them.

Pathologic Scarring

Rates of hypertrophic scar and keloid formation varied from 0% to 3.2% in the articles reviewed (Figure 59-6). Two studies reported keloid complications,[6,16] and four

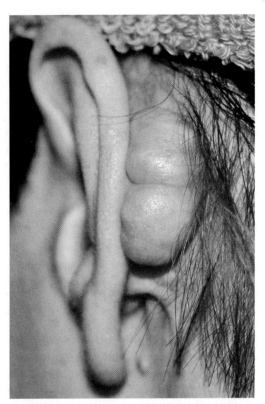

Figure 59-6. Two years after otoplasty demonstrating a keloid.

described hypertrophic scarring.[8,9,11,19] One article combined both types of scarring into one category.[10] Pediatric populations are considered to be at a higher risk for such complications, and the highest rate of hypertrophic scarring occurred in the only study that involved an entirely pediatric population.[11] However, this represented only one patient, thus highlighting the difficulty of calculating statistically meaningful conclusions with regard to scarring.

Hypertrophic scars and keloids are often lumped together in lists of complications, because they represent excessive scar formation. Although they may share certain qualities, they are inherently different, and they should be considered separate entities.[21] Hypertrophic scars tend to form within the boundary of a previous incision and to push its edges apart as they proliferate. They also can regress over time, and they rarely recur after excision if the wound is closed without tension. Alternatively, keloids proliferate outside of the confines of the incision line, they do not spontaneously diminish, and they are often recalcitrant to efforts directed at preventing their recurrence.

Although efforts are made to avoid excessive scarring by decreasing wound tension through proper closure techniques and avoiding the overresection of postauricular skin, certain populations may be at increased risk, such as young patients, patients with darker skin, and, most importantly, patients with a personal or family history of keloid formation. These scars tend to appear on the lower half of the ear. Hypertrophic scars can be monitored for regression, injected serially with 0.1 ml of triamcinolone (i.e., 10–40 mg/ml) every 2 to 3 weeks, excised, or any combination of these, sometimes with the use of silicone sheeting. The treatment for keloids may be more demanding, and it can include reexcision, steroid injection, laser treatment, and external-beam radiation therapy. No clear superior therapeutic option has emerged; therefore surgeons must preoperatively counsel their patients who may be at increased risk for excessive scar formation.

Cutaneous Sequelae

Properly executed postauricular incisions will be appreciable only on direct inspection, and they are hidden by the natural curvature of the auricle. However, the incision must be made anterior to the postauricular crease. If the incision or skin excision is made in the postauricular crease, migration of the skin postoperatively will result in a visible scar over the mastoid region. The authors use a fusiform skin excision, with 80% of the pattern anterior to the postauricular sulcus. A perpendicular limb can also be designed to aid in the placement of the antihelical sutures. In this fashion, the healing of the incision may be optimized. If the surgeon decides to use an anterior approach, the anterior incisions can be hidden under the rim of the helix or along the edge of the conchal bowl. This procedure generally heals favorably.

The ear may also be subject to occasional dermatitis. In one study, 9.8% of patients reported the intermittent appearance of "skin lesions" on the anterior and posterior surfaces of the ears within the folds on a long-term follow-up questionnaire.[6] Some of the rashes were diagnosed as eczema or intertrigo. Long-term dermatologic sequelae may be seen after otoplasty, but such occurrences have not been widely reported in the literature, either because they are rare or because they are not of sufficient severity to raise a complaint.

REVISION

Revision is one of the most important considerations of otoplasty. Revision rates were reported in every study listed, with a range of 0.6% to 11%. The importance of revision rates cannot be emphasized enough. A revision indicates that a patient or parent was dissatisfied enough to choose to undergo another procedure. Preoperative planning needs to include a discussion about the real possibility of revision surgery. Revision rates vary, and each surgeon should decide how to realistically inform patients about this possibility.

As shown in Table 59-1, the first seven studies based their data on the number of patients, whereas the last four studies reported results on the basis of the number of ears. These data cannot be directly compared, because authors who have listed complications per operated ear may have reported a lower percentage of complications than authors who have listed complications per patient, given that most otoplasty is performed bilaterally. In addition, care should be exercised when interpreting the data, because these studies are retrospective, they involve the use of different techniques, and they have not been subjected to a meta-analysis. The data should instead be used as guidelines for identifying more common or significant problems encountered by previous authors.

DISSATISFIED PATIENTS

Although complications may occur after otoplasty, it is important to ensure that patients do not feel dissatisfied with their overall experience. Although at first glance complications and dissatisfaction may seem like similar notions—and they certainly can be related—they are truly separate issues. A complication is an unexpected outcome, whereas dissatisfaction stems from failing to achieve expectations. The authors tell patients, "Ultimately, our goal is your satisfaction; it is not to perform a surgery. We could operate and get excellent results in *our* eyes, but unless the result is acceptable to *you*, we have not fulfilled our job. If we fully understand your expectations and desires and we feel that we can provide you with that result with a high degree of certainty, then the chances of your satisfaction are very high."

Patients tend to respond to this statement positively. First, they understand that the surgeons have their best interests at heart. Second, they have confirmation that the surgeons have listened to them, and this is a crucial element in the relationship. Third, they are reassured that the surgeons will do whatever is reasonable and necessary to ensure their satisfaction, even if it means revision surgery in the future. Finally, they feel less pressured knowing that the surgeons' goal is not to persuade them to have surgery, which has the added benefit of reinforcing their confidence in the surgeons. All of this together means less patient dissatisfaction and a better overall experience for both patients and surgeons.

The authors recommend that surgeons engage in a detailed preoperative discussion with the patient. During this meeting, the indications for the procedure as well as the contraindications, protocols (i.e., what the patient can expect during the surgery and the postoperative period), risks, and results are reviewed. Care is taken to address specific concerns that either commonly arise or that the surgeon has identified during the interview process as potentially problematic. The dedicated time spent for this process is the cornerstone for establishing the patient's expectations and deciding whether to proceed with surgery.

QUALITY OF LIFE

Protruding ears are a sign of good fortune in many Asian cultures; however, in Western culture, they can be the cause of ridicule. Such ridicule can lead to various behavioral and psychologic sequelae. In a young group of adolescents with behavior problems, 40% were noted to present with external-ear deformities.[22] It has been noted that those with protruding ears have almost a universal feeling of insecurity.[23] In the article by Becker,[23] it is mentioned that the insecurity may in fact be so great that it leads to an inadequacy neurosis. It has also been noted that the detrimental effects are not limited to psychologic and social problems; they may negatively affect academic performance as well.[24] All of these detrimental effects could have long-term personal and professional ramifications that could negatively affect one's quality of life.

Despite all of the potential complications and unfavorable outcomes associated with otoplasty, as previously mentioned, most patients enjoy gratifying results. A favorable result will not only alleviate the feeling of self-consciousness, but it could even help the patient become better adjusted socially, psychologically, and academically. In the authors' practice, performing otoplasty with the use of a conservative, graduated approach and employing suture techniques in combination with conchal setback provided satisfactory cosmesis for more than 95% of patients after primary or revision surgery.[16]

CONCLUSION

Otoplasty is a challenging but rewarding endeavor. Complications will arise, and steps can be taken to minimize the risk of such unexpected outcomes. Proper preoperative counseling and the proper postoperative management of complications help to ensure that otoplasty will lead to a high degree of patient satisfaction. The complications and their incidences discussed in this chapter may be used to help counsel patients and their families regarding otoplasty.

REFERENCES

1. Adamson PA, Galli SK: Otoplasty. In Cummings CW et al, editors: *Otolaryngology: Head and neck surgery,* Philadelphia, 2005, Elsevier.
2. Lam SM, Ely ET: Edward Talbot Ely: Father of aesthetic otoplasty. *Arch Facial Plast Surg* 2004;6(1):64.
3. Honkavaara P, Pyykko I: Effects of atropine and scopolamine on bradycardia and emetic symptoms in otoplasty. *Laryngoscope* 1999;109(1):108–112.
4. Paxton D, Taylor RH, Gallagher TM, et al: Postoperative emesis following otoplasty in children. *Anaesthesia* 1995;50(12):1083–1085.
5. Lancaster JL, Jones TM, Kay AR, et al: Paediatric day-case otoplasty: Local versus general anaesthetic. *Surgeon* 2003;1(2):96–98.
6. Caouette-Laberge L, Guay N, Bortoluzzi P, et al: Otoplasty: Anterior scoring technique and results in 500 cases. *Plast Reconstr Surg* 2000;105(2):504–515.
7. Wetter DA, Davis MD, Yiannias JA, et al: Patch test results from the Mayo Clinic Contact Dermatitis Group, 1998-2000. *J Am Acad Dermatol* 2005;53(3):416–421.
8. Bulstrode NW, Huang S, Martin DL: Otoplasty by percutaneous anterior scoring: Another twist to the story: A long-term study of 114 patients. *Br J Plast Surg* 2003;56(2):145–149.
9. Stucker FJ, Vora NM, Lian TS: Otoplasty: An analysis of technique over a 33-year period. *Laryngoscope* 2003;113(6):952–956.
10. Calder JC, Naasan A: Morbidity of otoplasty: A review of 562 consecutive cases. *Br J Plast Surg* 1994;47(3):170–174.
11. Messner AH, Crysdale WS: Otoplasty: Clinical protocol and long-term results. *Arch Otolaryngol Head Neck Surg* 1996;122(7):773–777.
12. Bumpous JM, Johnson JT: The infected wound and its management. *Otolaryngol Clin North Am* 1995;28(5):987–1001.
13. Furnas DW: Complications of surgery of the external ear. *Clin Plast Surg* 1990;17(2):305–318.
14. Adamson PA: Complications of otoplasty. *Ear Nose Throat J* 1985;64(12):568–574.
15. Kelly EJ, Herbert KJ, Crotty EJ, et al: Atlantoaxial subluxation after otoplasty. *Plast Reconstr Surg* 1998;102(2):543–544.
16. Adamson PA, McGraw BL, Tropper GJ: Otoplasty: Critical review of clinical results. *Laryngoscope* 1991;101(8):883–888.
17. Epstein JS, Kabaker SS, Swerdloff J: The "electric" otoplasty. *Arch Facial Plast Surg* 1999;1(3):204–207.
18. Yugueros P, Friedland JA: Otoplasty: The experience of 100 consecutive patients. *Plast Reconstr Surg* 2001;108(4):1045–1053.
19. Burstein FD: Cartilage-sparing complete otoplasty technique: A 10-year experience in 100 patients. *J Craniofac Surg* 2003;14(4):521–525.
20. Erol OO: New modification in otoplasty: Anterior approach. *Plast Reconstr Surg* 2001;107(1):193–202.
21. Atiyeh BS, Costagliola M, Hayek SN: Keloid or hypertrophic scar: The controversy: Review of the literature. *Ann Plast Surg* 2005;54(6):676–680.
22. Adamson JE, Horton CE, Crawford HH: The growth pattern of the external ear. *Plast Reconstr Surg* 1965;36(4):466–470.
23. Becker OJ: Surgical correction of the abnormally protruding ears. *Arch Otolaryngol* 1949;50(5):541–560.
24. Rhys Evans PH: Prominent ears and their surgical correction. *J Laryngol Otol* 1981;95(9):881–892.
25. Raunig H: Antihelixplasty without modeling sutures. *Arch Facial Plast Surg* 2005;7:334–341.

PART 7
Reconstructive Surgery

CHAPTER 60

Complications of Pedicled Myocutaneous Flaps

Francisco J. Civantos and James L. Netterville

A pedicled myocutaneous flap, by definition, is a muscle with an attached skin island that is transferred from an adjacent region to the area of the defect. The muscle is left hinged on a blood supply that is sufficient to nourish the entire muscle transferred, and the skin is supplied by the muscle transferred as well as by the muscle perforators that traverse the muscle and the subcutaneous tissues to reach the dermis.

Myocutaneous flaps revolutionized head and neck reconstruction 30 years ago. Surgeons now perform the single-stage reconstruction of large defects with improved cosmetic and functional results. Myocutaneous flaps offer a reliable and rich blood supply. Their distant location is usually outside of irradiated fields, and they provide bulk to protect underlying structures.

Although the subsequent development of microvascular free-tissue transfer has increased the available reconstructive options dramatically, myocutaneous pedicled flaps maintain an important role. They offer the advantages of greater technical simplicity, reduced operative time, and reduced incidence of thrombosis and complete flap loss as compared with free-tissue transfers. Alternatively, the tethering of the flap by its pedicle and the greater distance of the distal end of the flap from its blood supply may increase the potential for the geographic restriction of flap positioning, wound dehiscence, or significant partial flap necrosis relative to microvascular options. Thus the potential for complications, both minor and severe, is always present, and the appropriate reconstruction option for the specific reconstructive challenge must be selected in the context of the patient's comorbidities. Direct comparisons are difficult, because patients with severe comorbidities are less likely to be offered microvascular flaps; however, in general, the failure rates of pedicled and microvascular flaps are comparable.[1]

Strictly speaking, the midline forehead flap, which is based on the supratrochlear artery and which includes a portion of the frontalis muscle, was the first myocutaneous flap. Its use in ancient India is well documented, although the reasons for its success were probably poorly understood.[2] Similarly, during the latter half of the nineteenth century, Estlander in 1877[3] and Abbe in 1898[4] described lip transfers, which were, in fact, myocutaneous flaps based on the labial arteries and the orbicularis oris muscle. The first major myocutaneous

flap was the latissimus dorsi flap, which was described by Tansini in 1906[5] for chest wall reconstruction. Little further progress was made until the last three decades, when advances in surgical and anesthetic techniques allowed for the resection of larger tumors, thus creating a need for new reconstructive options. In 1955, Owens[6] described the use of the sternocleidomastoid flap, and McGregor[7] described the temporalis myocutaneous flap. In 1978, Futrell[8] described the platysma flap.

The pectoralis major myocutaneous flap was described by Hueston and McConchie[9] in 1968. Its use in the head and neck was reported by Ariyan[10] and also by Baek and colleagues[11] in 1979. The pectoralis major myocutaneous flap quickly became the workhorse flap of head and neck reconstruction. In 1971, Desprez and colleagues[12] described the use of a latissimus myocutaneous flap to close a lower spine defect. In 1979, Quillen[13] used the latissimus dorsi flap for head and neck reconstruction; in 1972, Dermagasse[14] reported on the trapezius myocutaneous flap. In 1979, Baek and colleagues[15] described the lower trapezius myocutaneous flap, which, in its modified form, has proved particularly useful for lateral skull-base reconstruction.[16]

Each of these flaps has specific advantages and disadvantages, but there are two overriding considerations with any myocutaneous flaps: (1) the blood supply to the muscle; and (2) the perfusion of the overlying skin. The survival of both components of the flap depends on this blood supply, which is affected by a variety of anatomic and physiologic concerns. In the next section, the present state of knowledge regarding the vascular anatomy and physiology of pedicle flaps is reviewed.

MYOCUTANEOUS FLAPS: VASCULAR ANATOMY AND PHYSIOLOGY

Not all muscles have a predominant blood supply sufficient to maintain the viability of the entire muscle, and not all areas of the skin are supplied by muscle perforators. There may be a single, a few, or multiple patterns of vascular supply to a muscle. Mathes and Nahai[17] divide these into five types that range from the completely axial to the completely segmental, with various typical variations in between. Various patterns of skin perfusion have also been described.[18-20] Musculocutaneous perforators may or may not provide sufficient vascular supply to support a particular area of skin. In addition, for any given muscle, certain areas of skin may be supplied by perforators that are derived from a minor pedicle or a segmental vessel rather than the major pedicle being preserved. Subcutaneous axial, fasciocutaneous, and random subdermal vessels also supply the skin, and they have been used for the design of flaps.[20] The relative importance of each pattern of blood supply varies among anatomic areas.

An area of skin supplied by a named artery in vivo has been described as its *angiosome.* However, the area of skin that is potentially supplied by any particular vessel is larger than that supplied by it under normal conditions. This is because of the presence of multiple subcutaneous vascular anastomoses that allow vessels from adjacent angiosomes to support the skin generally supplied by the neighboring vessel in vivo. The blood supply to the skin is best thought of as a zone of equilibrium in intravascular pressure, so that one blood supply can expand into an adjacent territory if the pressure in that territory is reduced.[21,22] The vascular supply of muscles and overlying skin areas can sometimes be explained embryologically, but rarely can flap survival be predicted theoretically. It has only been through careful anatomic dissections and trial and error that the present array of reliable myocutaneous flaps has been developed.

When a predominantly axial blood supply to a muscle exists, the vessels generally penetrate the deep muscle fascia at one end of the muscle and run longitudinally in this deep fascia, thereby creating an extensive vascular plexus. These vessels eventually perfuse the bed of arterioles, capillaries, and venules of the muscle as well as the skin via muscle perforators[23,24] (Figure 60-1). The microcirculation is sensitive to a variety of neurologic, humoral, metabolic, and physical factors. These factors vary in importance between the muscle and the skin.

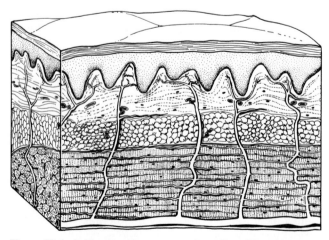

Figure 60-1. Axial myocutaneous vascular pattern. The major vessels are oriented longitudinally and run between the muscle and deep fascia, sending off perforating vessels to the muscle and skin.

Sympathetic innervation is directed at the arterioles, the precapillary sphincters, and the arteriovenous anastomoses, and it is the primary means of the regulation of blood flow to the skin under normal circumstances. Arteriovenous shunts are common in the skin, where through sympathetic innervation they can be used to alter the skin's blood flow, thus allowing for body temperature regulation. However, they are not present in muscle. Sympathetic innervation is less important in muscular blood flow, but it does provide reflex vasoconstriction in response to exercise and arterial hypertension, and acute arterial hypertension leads to vasodilation through a reflexive decrease in sympathetic tone. Humoral regulation of the microcirculation occurs in both the muscle and the skin. Norepinephrine causes vasoconstriction in muscle, and epinephrine causes vasodilation. In the skin, both substances cause vasoconstriction. Vasopressin and angiotensin cause muscular vasoconstriction, and isoproterenol and acetylcholine cause muscular vasodilation; none of these agents have significant cutaneous effects.[25,26]

Local autoregulation is also more important in muscle than in skin, although it is present in both. In neither organ are autoregulatory mechanisms as important as in the kidney, the heart, or the brain. Autoregulatory mechanisms include vasodilation in response to hypercapnia, hypoxia, acidosis, hyperosmolarity, and increased interstitial potassium. In the skin, hypothermia leads to vasoconstriction, and increased perfusion pressure leads to a myogenic reflex in the vessels as a regulatory response to maintain the capillary flow constant. Hypercapnia is the dominant autoregulatory mechanism in muscle, which is minimally responsive to temperature. Increased viscosity will decrease blood flow, but only when the viscosity is greatly increased.[25,26]

When a skin flap is raised, sympathetic innervation is lost. Humoral and autoregulatory mechanisms then take over. The physiologic mechanisms operating in fresh skin flaps have been extensively studied, but a great deal of debate persists. It is clear that a period of marked ischemia occurs initially, with a steady increase in blood flow during the first 24 hours and a gradual subsequent increase during the subsequent 2 weeks. The relative importance of arteriovenous shunting (whereby blood bypasses the skin) as compared with vasoconstriction as an explanation for this phenomenon has been debated. The latter phenomenon is the more likely mechanism during the early period. Later increases in blood flow are related to angiogenesis and the dilatation of longitudinally oriented vascular anastomosis.[27–31]

Much of the current knowledge regarding skin-flap physiology was obtained during the course of studies attempting to explain the phenomenon of flap delay, whereby a partial preliminary surgical interruption of the blood supply to a flap leads to an increased length of flap survival when the flap is raised at a later date.[32,33] Additional studies are needed to delineate the physiology of muscle flaps. Hopefully, by continuing to increase the understanding of the anatomy and physiology of myocutaneous flaps, these flaps can be optimally managed, particularly the flap with a marginal blood supply, thereby minimizing the incidence of complications.

COMPLICATIONS

Overview

In general, complications can be divided into those of the recipient site and those of the donor site (Table 60-1). In the former category, the primary complication is flap loss, either complete or partial. Complete flap necrosis occurs in less than 10% of flaps in most reports of series of major myocutaneous flaps.[34–38] Usually this is related to physical factors that cause decreased arterial flow or obstructed venous outflow (Figures 60-2 and 60-3). Either may be caused by hematoma, intraoperative kinking or stretching of the pedicle, or constriction of the pedicle by overlying skin flaps, dressings, or ties. Occasionally flaps can be saved by the early detection and correction of these factors.

Partial flap loss generally involves the loss of all or part of the skin paddle and the subcutaneous fat, with the survival of the muscle (Figure 60-4). This is more common than complete flap loss.[34,36] If significant necrosis of the skin flap occurs, prompt debridement is necessary to prevent the infection and subsequent loss of the underlying muscle. Small areas of necrosis at the edges of a flap can be treated conservatively. Skin-paddle loss can be the result of poor patient selection (e.g., a pectoralis major flap in an obese female patient). In addition, technical factors can affect the flow of blood from the muscle to the skin. Inwardly beveled skin incisions can decrease the number of perforating vessels preserved; the shearing of perforating vessels can occur

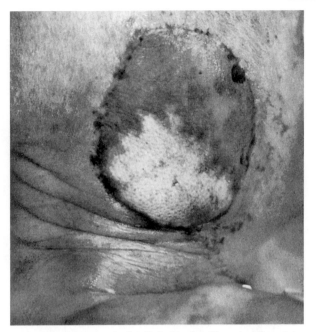

Figure 60-2. A flap that is distally ischemic with a clear line of demarcation of necrosis.

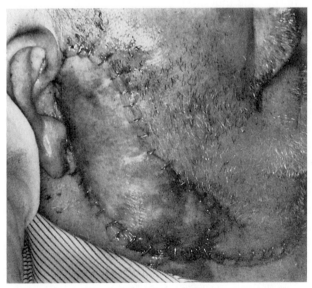

Figure 60-3. Compromised pectoralis major myocutaneous flap with moderate venous congestion. Note the ecchymosis and the mottled appearance.

TABLE 60-1 Complications of Myocutaneous Flaps

Recipient Site	Donor Site
Flap necrosis	Bleeding
Poor healing	Hematoma
Infection	Poor healing
Fistulization	Infection
Seroma	Seroma
Delayed detection of recurrence	

during the manipulation and positioning of the flap in the defect; and the ultimate position of the skin paddle can lead to skin loss if the skin is being pulled away from the muscle or excessively folded or compressed. The positioning of the flap in relation to mandibular plates and compression under tight skin flaps along any portion of the flap are additional factors of concern.

Other complications include bleeding, hematoma, seroma, infection, and fistulization. Infection and fistulization may be self-limited, but they can be quite dangerous

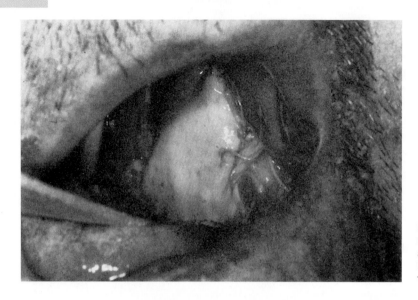

Figure 60-4. Necrotic pectoralis myocutaneous flap used to reconstruct a tonsillar defect. The flap skin and the subcutaneous tissue necrosed without muscle loss. Complete healing subsequently occurred without fistulization.

as a result of the additional risks of necrosis of the carotid or innominate arteries, with the potential for artery rupture and death. In the absence of flap necrosis, fistulization and infection related to poor healing are the complications that are most common among irradiated patients, those with poor nutritional status, and those with vascular and microcirculatory compromise as a result of smoking or medical problems. Unfortunately these factors are present in a significant portion of patients with head and neck cancer. Poor healing and the failure of the flap to adhere can ultimately lead to delayed flap necrosis. The delayed detection of tumor recurrence is an additional concern when a myocutaneous flap is used, and the awareness of this should lead to increased vigilance and the judicious use of imaging studies.

Donor-site complications also include bleeding, hematoma, seroma, poor healing, and infection. The rates of these vary among flap types. The practical necessity of working in a single operative field with certain flaps may lead to salivary contamination of the donor site with an increased risk of infection. In addition, the loss of function of the muscle being transferred can lead to functional losses at the donor site. This problem may assume greater importance in certain patients.

Leaving aside the systemic medical complications that can occur after any surgical procedure, the following is a review of the local complications of the various major myocutaneous flaps used in head and neck reconstruction.

Pectoralis Major Myocutaneous Flap

The pectoralis major myocutaneous flap has become the most popular reconstructive option available to the head and neck surgeon. Multiple large series are available that describe the results with this flap, and most of the concepts and approaches used in managing myocutaneous flaps in general are derived from these data and from experience with the pectoralis major flap.[36,39-43] The popularity of this flap is related to a number of factors, including the ease of patient positioning, the muscle bulk for carotid artery coverage, the primary closure of the donor site, and the relative technical simplicity of the procedure. However, the most important factor is its perceived reliability. Virtually all large series report an incidence of major flap necrosis of less than 5%. A great deal of variation exists in the literature regarding other complications, especially partial flap losses and wound infections. Some of this variation can be explained by differences in patient populations, including the distribution of factors such as tumor stage, previous radiation therapy, gender, age, and medical problems. Undoubtedly differences exist in the definitions of the complications, the accuracy of reporting, and the significance given to postoperative events. There may also be real differences in surgical approaches and techniques, which can affect results. These factors are difficult to qualify. In addition, the time period selected for the studies can affect results (e.g., if early patients who form a surgeon's "learning curve" are excluded). The results of the studies cited are summarized in the following paragraphs.

Partial flap losses ranged from 7% to 29%, excluding major flap necroses. Fistulas without flap necrosis occurred in 13% to 26% of patients. Purulent infections without fistulization were reported in 1% to 25% of patients, and hematoma was reported in 1% to 12% of patients. Donor-site complications, when considered separately, were described in 2% to 7% of patients. These included hematomas, seromas, and wound dehiscences. Significantly higher complication rates have been noted among patients with a history of smoking, larger tumors, previous radiation therapy, systemic diseases, lower albumin levels, and older age. Some have also found increased rates of partial flap necrosis in women and obese patients, presumably as a result of the increased amount of subcutaneous fat and breast tissue in the skin island. Decreased rates of complications have been documented in situations in which the skin island could be dispensed with, instead raising the muscle alone, possibly with skin graft placement. Unfortunately the additional length provided by the skin paddle with its random extension is essential in many situations. In fact, more distant primary site resections (e.g., anterior oral cavity) have also been associated with increased flap necrosis, possibly as a result of marginal flap reach and tension on the pedicle. Tubed pectoralis major flaps, such as those used in patients with total laryngopharyngectomies, have had a high rate of fistulization, probably as a result of flap bulk preventing a tubed closure without tension. Flaps used for skin coverage had lower complication rates because of the absence of salivary contamination. The significant prolongation of hospital stay among patients with complications is a major concern for patients with advanced disease, the majority of whom will eventually suffer tumor recurrence. Palliation with the minimization of the hospital stay is the most realistic goal for many of these patients.[36,39–43]

Additional problems with pectoralis major flaps exist that should be considered during preoperative planning, including the transfer of thick, hair-bearing skin to the upper aerodigestive tract in some men, scarring and deformity of the breast area, and the temporary deformity of the bulky pedicle in the lower neck, which resolves with subsequent atrophy of the muscle. The loss of pectoralis major function can also be important for those involved in physical labor or athletics. Rare reported complications with the pectoralis major flap have included osteomyelitis of the rib in the donor area and the metastatic spread of recurrent cancer to the base of the flap, presumably via lymphatic or intravascular seeding along the pedicle.[44,45] Patients with large skin islands taken with pectoralis major flaps have a documented increased incidence of major pulmonary atelectasis that has been attributed to the pain and restriction of chest wall motion.[46]

Overall, both Shah and colleagues[36] and Kroll and colleagues,[39] who are the authors of the two largest and most recent series, believe that the complications of pectoralis major flaps (particularly partial necrosis) are greater than generally described. Certainly both groups had referral populations with large tumors and multiple medical problems, and both groups operated on large numbers of patients with recurrent tumors after previous surgery, radiation therapy, or both. The pectoralis major flap remains one of the best options for many reconstructive problems of the head and neck. However, its limitations should be understood and its use

carefully considered, particularly for patients with the previously discussed high-risk factors.[36–39] It should be noted that, for patients with anticipated healing problems, the pectoralis major muscle is particularly suited for the protection of vascular structures in the neck on the basis of its anatomic position and its hardy muscle vascularity.[40]

Trapezius Myocutaneous Flap

Three different flaps that involve the trapezius muscle have been well described as the following[38]:

1. Superior
2. Lateral island
3. Extended island or lower trapezius flap

Each has different indications and complications. In the authors' hands, the lower or extended island flap has become the most useful of these. The superior trapezius flap is based on the occipital artery, and paraspinous perforators are necessary to ensure the adequate survival of the flap.[38,48] The flap involves the sacrifice of the upper trapezius muscle fibers that lead to winging of the scapula, which may have been avoided in patients in whom the accessory cranial nerve had not already been sacrificed. The main function of this flap is to cover cutaneous defects. Because it is not an island flap, it is less useful for internal lining reconstruction. The donor site is covered with a skin graft, thereby adding the additional risk of graft loss and leading to cosmetic deformity. In a series of 29 superior trapezius flaps, the major complication rate was 5% in nonirradiated patients and 9% in irradiated patients. Minor complications occurred in 18% of nonirradiated patients and 44% of irradiated patients. The major complications were major wound separations. The minor complications included partial flap losses (i.e., <29% of the flap), which occurred in 18% of patients, and minor wound dehiscences, which occurred in 21% of patients. Thus the superior trapezius flap is a reliable flap with usefulness that is limited by the expected loss of shoulder function, the need for a skin graft to the donor site, and the requirement of an intact skin pedicle that limits its use for internal lining reconstruction and also its arc of rotation.

The lateral island trapezius flap is based on the transverse cervical artery.[49] It also requires the sacrifice of trapezius muscle function. It is an island flap, and its thin random extension allows it to be tubed or molded to repair a variety of pharyngeal and intraoral defects. However, this flap is much less reliable than the superior or lower island flaps, with 4 (17%) major flap necroses reported in a series of 24 flaps. In addition, one major and six minor wound dehiscences, two partial flap losses, and 6 orocutaneous fistulas occurred. This questionable reliability is the major limitation of its use. Furthermore, it should not be used if the transverse cervical artery has been sacrificed during previous neck dissection. The donor site can be closed primarily in all but the largest flaps, and no donor site complications occurred in the authors' initial series.[38]

The lower or extended island trapezius flap was described in 1980 as being based on the transverse cervical artery.[14] As previously reported, the authors have found this flap to be more commonly based on the dorsal scapular artery.[16,38] Cadaver injection studies have shown the dorsal scapular artery to be the dominant blood supply in 50% of cases, and, when both vessels are preserved, the reliability of the flap is excellent. The authors have experienced only 1 partial flap loss in their first 34 cases.

Alternatively, the more proximal placement of the skin paddle may allow for adequate survival based on the transverse cervical artery, but this would decrease the arc of rotation of the flap. Previous series of lower trapezius flaps report major flap necrosis in 6% to 21% of patients and partial flap necrosis in 7% to 22% of patients.[50–52] The dorsal scapular artery can be mobilized by ligating its descending branch, and the reliable random skin extension available with this flap can reach almost any head and neck defect. It is particularly useful in the parotid and temporal regions. Other reported complications of trapezius flaps have included ulnar nerve palsy related to arm positioning and seromas in the neck, which can be managed by prolonged suction drainage.[50–52] Donor-site seromas are also quite common, and they are easily avoided by prolonged suction drainage.[50–52] Important advantages of this flap include the preservation of the upper third of the trapezius fibers, avoiding the winging of the scapula, and the primary closure of the donor site (Figure 60-5). The need for the lateral decubitus position is a disadvantage, but its low complication rate has made this flap a significant part of head and neck reconstruction in the authors' hands.

Latissimus Dorsi Myocutaneous Flap

The latissimus dorsi flap was reintroduced by Quillen[13] for head and neck reconstruction in 1979. Although slightly less reliable than the pectoralis major flap, it is a dependable source of large amounts of tissue for head and neck reconstruction. The donor site is usually outside of previously irradiated fields, and it closes primarily with minimal cosmetic or functional loss. As with the lower trapezius flap, the repositioning of the patient is required. Nevertheless, when a great deal of bulk is desirable, it may be the best alternative.

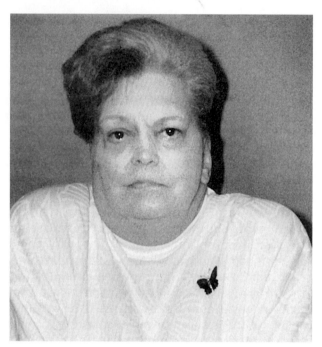

Figure 60-5. Patient with good right shoulder elevation after right trapezius flap reconstruction.

The incidences of major flap necroses in the series reported have ranged from 6.7% to 10%.[13,53,54] The major technical factor to be dealt with in the latissimus dorsi pedicle flap is the ease with which the pedicle can be kinked. The vessels are initially preserved by raising the fatty tissue between the latissimus and serratus muscles sharply off of the serratus. Superiorly the neurovascular pedicle exits the submuscular tissues to traverse the axilla. The vessels are usually identified on the axilla, and the flap is based on this area. The lack of structural support for the pedicle is in contrast with that of the pectoralis major, where intact muscle is present overlying the pedicle. Therefore great care must be taken when positioning the pedicle after flap rotation, and arm positioning during the postoperative period should be maintained in a neutral position, thereby avoiding excessive abduction or adduction. Further technical difficulty lies in the positioning of the pedicle in relation to the pectoralis major muscle. When the latissimus flap is rotated, the vessels come to lie directly over or under the muscle. To transect the pectoralis major for the ideal positioning of the pedicle would add a great deal of functional morbidity to an already weakened arm. Most authors have advised tunneling the flap through the pectoralis muscle, thus preserving as much of this muscle as possible and remaining lateral to the thoracoacromial vessels. If the technical management of the pedicle is appropriate, high success rates can be obtained with this flap.[53]

Partial flap losses have occurred in 1.6% to 40% of cases and correlate with the distal placement of the skin paddle and the harvesting of larger skin paddles.[51,52] In fact, the distal third of the latissimus dorsi cutaneous territory is primarily supplied by thoracolumbar perforators. Although the thoracodorsal system may expand to supply much of this area, the most distal areas of skin are, nevertheless, less reliably vascularized. The skin paddle must be large enough to include several perforators.

Other complications have included infection, fistulization, and failure to heal, which occurs in 10% to 30% of patients. Donor-site complications have included wound dehiscence, hypertrophic scarring, seroma formation, and brachial plexus neuropathy. Seromas, as in the lower trapezius flap, are common, and they can be avoided by prolonged suction drainage and repeated needle aspiration, if necessary. Brachial neuropathy is related to arm positioning, and it has been postulated to be related to the compression of the nerve trunks between the clavicle and the cervical vertebrae with the elevation of the arm for pedicle dissection. The incidence of this complication has ranged from 0% to 10%, and, if care is taken to avoid extremes of arm positioning, it is generally avoidable.[13,53,54]

The thoracodorsal perforator flap is a variant of the latissimus dorsi myocutaneous flap in which only principal perforators are preserved, thereby allowing for the sparing of the majority of the latissimus dorsi muscle and the minimization of donor-site morbidity. It is unclear whether the reduced muscle harvest can lead to an increase in the incidence of flap loss.[55]

The loss of latissimus dorsi function leads to mild to moderate shoulder weakness and some loss of motion, which improves gradually. It is compounded by varying degrees of loss of pectoralis major function required when positioning the pedicle as well as by losses of accessory nerve function related to neck dissection.[54] Questions regarding the reliability of the latissimus dorsi flap are probably related to the relative infrequency with which it is required by the head and neck surgeon. With proper technique, it can be used reliably, and it is very useful for those cases in which flap bulk is needed.

Other Flaps

Several other myocutaneous flaps have been described for head and neck reconstruction, but they have largely been supplanted by the flaps already described.

Sternocleidomastoid Muscle

The sternocleidomastoid muscle has been used with an overlying skin paddle for oral cavity and pharyngeal reconstruction. It is based either superiorly on the occipital and posterior auricular arteries or inferiorly on a branch of the thyrocervical trunk. Its main advantage is its regional proximity to the areas being reconstructed. It provides a non–hair-bearing skin island, and the donor site is closed primarily. However, the blood supply to the skin paddle is tenuous, with partial skin loss in more than 50% of cases.[56–59] Furthermore, if the blood supply to the flap has been interrupted during neck dissection, it cannot be used. The theoretic possibility of transplanting neck metastases is another concern. The sternocleidomastoid provides excellent carotid coverage, but it is often resected during neck dissection, and it is therefore rarely used in head and neck oncologic surgery. It probably maintains some usefulness as a muscle flap in specific situations, but the skin island is poorly vascularized. Because there is another muscle—the platysma—between the sternocleidomastoid and the overlying skin island, it is theoretically unlikely that the sternocleidomastoid perforators would be the major blood supply to this skin, and clinical experience has confirmed this.

Platysma Myocutaneous Flap

The platysma myocutaneous flap has also been used for pharyngeal and oral cavity reconstruction. Its attractiveness is the result of the thin, pliable skin island that is obtained. A high risk of major necrosis (42%) has been reported, particularly in irradiated patients. The tedious preservation of the veins and arteries to the platysma (including the facial artery and its submental branch) and the superficial branch of the transverse cervical artery increases the likelihood of success. Other complications reported with this flap include wound dehiscence in 16% of cases and injury to the marginal mandibular nerve. If carefully raised, the platysma flap can be used reliably for certain reconstructive problems of the head and neck, but it is less useful for patients with squamous cell carcinoma of the upper aerodigestive tract. In these patients, who will often receive radiation and further surgery, most surgeons would agree that the platysma is best left on the neck flaps to enhance their vascularity.[60–64]

Temporalis Muscle Flap

The temporalis muscle flap,[6] which is used for intraoral and skull-base reconstruction, provides adequate bulk but has a short pedicle.[7] The main reason that it has not been used more frequently is the donor-site deformity that it creates, with a depressed temporal fossa.

Nasolabial Island Myocutaneous Flap

The nasolabial island myocutaneous flap is a separate entity from the subdermal axial nasolabial flap. It includes the underlying facial muscles, and it is based on the facial artery. It is extremely hardy, and it can be used for intraoral reconstruction. The main complication with the use of this flap is the denervation of the upper lip, the innervation of which may return to varying degrees.[65]

AVOIDING COMPLICATIONS

The avoidance of complications in the execution of myocutaneous flaps begins long before the patient reaches the operating room. Careful planning is essential. The first step is the evaluation of the patient's risk for healing problems and poor tissue vascularity. Severe inanition, poor nutritional status, systemic disease, older age, and previous regional surgery or irradiation all decrease the likelihood of flap survival. Among certain high-risk patients, staged reconstructions, planned fistulas, prosthetic reconstructions, or simpler reconstructive options may be preferable. Of course, certain patients are best not managed by surgical resection but rather treated by nonsurgical means.

After the decision to reconstruct using a myocutaneous flap has been made, the flap to be used must be selected. Factors to consider include the size and location of the defect, the need for external or internal lining, the need for bulk, and donor-site morbidity. Function is the first consideration, but cosmesis should also be considered. The flap should fit the wound generously, without tension on the pedicle. The experienced surgeon can predict which flap is likely to achieve this for the planned resection. If a random skin extension is needed that is longer than usual, surgical delay before the reconstruction is an option to consider. To extend the random skin beyond the standard limits during a single-stage procedure is unwise. Before any incisions are made, the flap should be carefully designed with drawings on the skin and measurements made of the distance over which it must be transposed.

Attention to detail intraoperatively is the next step in the avoidance of complications. Some technical considerations have already been mentioned: inward beveling of the skin and the subcutaneous incision should be avoided, and the maximum number of cutaneous perforating vessels should be reserved; shearing of the skin from the muscle should be avoided, and, if necessary, tacking sutures placed; gentle handling of tissues and the maintenance of warmth and moisture are the rule. Above all, tension, kinking, or compression of the pedicle must be avoided. If, despite careful preoperative planning, the surgeon finds that the flap cannot be made to fully reach the defect, it is far better to exteriorize the pedicle to gain extra length and to perform a two-stage procedure rather than to suture the flap into place under tension. The meticulous positioning of the flap into the defect with a careful closure that approximates the epithelial edges as well as the deep layers is important. Insetting the flap into the defect may involve special shaping, including splitting, perforating, or enfolding the skin island. These maneuvers place additional stress on the flap and should be avoided if possible or at least minimized. Complete hemostasis must be obtained before suturing the flap in position to prevent hematoma formation. The avoidance of dead space and suction drainage also help.

The most important factor for preventing intraoperative errors is a thorough knowledge of the anatomy of the vascular pedicle and the proper tissue planes, which must be raised to protect the vessels in the submuscular space. Experience provides an understanding of the random skin extension available for each flap as well as of the optimal positioning of the pedicle. Postoperatively pressure on the pedicle or on the flap itself must be avoided. The placement of tight tracheotomy ties or wound dressings should be avoided. Drain tubing and electrocardiography monitor leads should be kept away from the flap pedicle. For each flap, optimal patient positioning to avoid pedicle compression should be explained to the nursing staff members. The patient's oxygenation status, blood pressure, and hematocrit level should be maintained within the normal limits.

If the compromise of blood flow is identified early, the situation may be correctable. Myocutaneous flaps can survive approximately 4 hours of ischemia or congestion, so immediate postoperative monitoring is crucial.[66] A variety of techniques have been used to monitor flaps. Clinical measures such as color, temperature, capillary refill after gentle compression, and dermal bleeding after a needle prick are simple and relatively accurate, but they require experienced interpretation, and they can be subjective. The use of laser Doppler velocimetry or fluorescein microfluorometry provides an objective and noninvasive means of assessing blood flow to the skin paddle. The latter is probably more accurate for assessing blood flow in the low ranges, although neither of the two methods is infallible. More recently, tissue oxygen tension monitoring using a needle probe has been used with success. In the end, a combination of clinical and objective factors will determine whether blood flow is compromised.[67–70]

If flap blood flow is clearly inadequate despite the proper execution of the flap, arterial or venous blood flow through the pedicle may be physically obstructed, and early surgical reexploration may be able to resolve the problem. If the pedicle is providing flap perfusion but the blood flow is marginal, a variety of pharmacologic means of optimizing flap survival under relatively ischemic conditions has been investigated. Guanethidine has been administered as a means of sympathetic blockade to prevent vasoconstriction during limb replantation.[71] Superoxide dismutase and topical dimethyl sulfoxide have been shown in animal studies to enhance the survival of flaps subjected to venous occlusion for 8 hours, presumably by binding oxygen free radicals and other mechanisms.[72–75] Hyperbaric oxygen therapy can also reverse arterial insufficiency.[76] Allopurinol and topical nitroglycerine have similarly proved to be beneficial after temporary venous occlusion.[76–78] Multiple stab wounds and medicinal leeches (Figure 60-6) can be used as well to relieve mild venous congestion.[79]

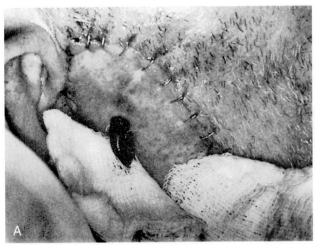 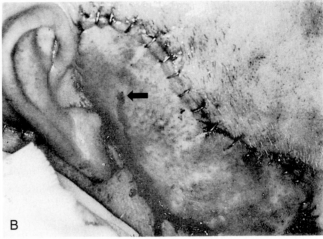

Figure 60-6. A, A medicinal leech applied to a compromised pectoralis myocutaneous flap to relieve venous congestion of the flap. **B,** Bleeding from the site of leech attachment to the flap after leech removal *(arrow).*

The exact roles of these and other agents in the postoperative management of myocutaneous flaps has yet to be delineated, although they do show promise. Nevertheless, the prevention of flap necrosis and other complications occurs primarily preoperatively and intraoperatively through careful planning, attention to detail, and good surgical technique. If the basic principles discussed in this chapter are adhered to, complications will be infrequent.

REFERENCES

1. Kroll SS, Evans GR, Goldberg D, et al: A comparison of resource costs for head and neck reconstruction with free and pectoralis flaps. *Plast Reconstr Surg* 1997;99(5):1282–1286.
2. Tiwari R, Snow GB: Role of myocutaneous flaps in reconstruction of the head and neck. *J Laryngol Otol* 1983;97:441–458.
3. Estlander JA: Methode d'autoplastie de la joue ould'une levre par un lambeau emprunte a la autre levre. *Rev Mens Med Chir* 1877;1:344–351.
4. Abbe R: A new plastic operation for the relief of deformity due to double harelip. *Med Rec* 1898;53:447–481.
5. Tansini I: Sopra il mio nuovo processo di amputazione dellia mammella. *Gaz Med Ital* 1906;57:141.
6. Owens N: A compound neck pedicle designed for the repair of massive facial defects: Formation, development, and application. *Plast Reconstr Surg* 1955;15:369–389.
7. McGregor IA: The temporal flap in intra-oral cancer: Its use in repairing the postexcisional defect. *Br J Plast Surg* 1963;16: 318–335.
8. Futrell JW: Platysma myocutaneous flap for intraoral reconstruction. *Am J Surg* 1978;136:504–507.
9. Hueston JT, McConchie JH: A compound pectoral flap. *Aust N Z J Surg* 1965;36:173–184.
10. Ariyan S: The pectoralis major myocutaneous flap. *Plast Reconstr Surg* 1979;63:73–81.
11. Baek SM, Biller HF, Krespi YP, et al: The pectoralis myocutaneous island flap for reconstruction of the head and neck. *Head Neck Surg* 1979;1:293–300.
12. Desprez JD, Kiehn CL, Eckstein W: Closure of large meningomyelocele defects by composite skin muscle flaps. *Plast Reconstr Surg* 1971;47:234–238.
13. Quillen CG: Latissimus dorsi myocutaneous flaps in head and neck reconstruction. *Plast Reconstr Surg* 1979;63:644–670.
14. Berotti J: Trapezius-musculocutaneous island flap in the repair of major head and neck cancer. *Plast Reconstr Surg* 1980;65:16–21.
15. Baek SM, Biller HF, Krespi YP, et al: The lower trapezius island flap. *Ann Plast Surg* 1980;5:108–114.
16. Netterville JL, Wood DE: The lower trapezius flap. *Arch Otolaryngol Head Neck Surg* 1991;117:73–76.
17. Mathes SJ, Nahai F: Classification of the vascular anatomy of muscles: Experimental and clinical correlation. *Plast Reconstr Surg* 1981;67:177–187.
18. Daniel RK, Williams HB: The free transfer of skin flaps by microvascular anastomoses: An experimental study and a reappraisal: Part I: The vascular supply of the skin. *Plast Reconstr Surg* 1973;52:16–31.
19. Daniel RK, Kerrigan CL: Skin flaps: An anatomical and hemodynamic approach. *Clin Plast Surg* 1979;6:181–200.
20. Taylor GI, Palmer JH: The vascular territories (angiosomes) of the body: Experimental study and clinical applications. *Br J Plast Surg* 1987;40:113–141.
21. Schafer K: Das subkutane gefasssystem (untere extremita): Mikroskoptische Untersuchungen Gegenaurs Morphal Jahrb 1975;121:492.
22. Nakajima H, Maruyama Y, Koda E: The definition of vascular skin territories with prostaglandin E1—the anterior chest, abdomen and thigh-inguinal region. *Br J Plast Surg* 1981;34:258–263.
23. McGregor IA, Morgan G: Axial and random pattern flaps. *Br J Plast Surg* 1973;26:202–213.
24. Ariyan S: Pectoralis major, sternomastoid, and other musculocutaneous flaps for head and neck reconstruction. *Clin Plast Surg* 1980;7:89–109.
25. McGraw JB, Diggell DG: Experimental definition of independent myocutaneous vascular territories. *Plast Reconstr Surg* 1977;60:212–220.
26. Hodges PL: Principles of flaps. *Setl Read Plast Surg* 1988;5:1–24.
27. Braithwaite F, Farmer FT, Edwards JRG, et al: Observations on the vascular channels of tubed pedicles using radioactive sodium: III. *Br J Plast Surg* 1951;4:38–47.
28. Hoffmeister FS: Studies on training of tissue transfer in reconstructive surgery I: Effect of delay on circulation in flaps. *Plast Reconstr Surg* 1957;19:283–298.
29. Palmer B: Sympathetic denervation and reinnervation of cutaneous blood vessels following surgery. An experimental study on rats by means of a histochemical fluorescence method. *Scand J Plast Surg* 1970;4:93–99.
30. Palmer B: Factors influencing the elimination rate of xenon injected intracutaneously. A study on rats. *Scand J Plast Reconstr Surg* 1972;6:1–5.
31. Palmer B: The influence of stress on the survival of experimental skin flaps. A study on rats. *Scand J Plast Reconstr Surg* 1972;6:110–113.
32. Reinisch JF: The pathophysiology of skin flap circulation. The delay phenomenon. *Plast Reconstr Surg* 1974;54:585–598.

33. Jonsson K, Hunt TK, Brennan SS, et al: Tissue oxygen measurements in delayed skin flaps: A reconsideration of the mechanisms of the delay phenomenon. *Plast Reconstr Surg* 1988;82:328–336.

34. Faucher A, Renaud-Salis JL, Pinsolle J, et al: Cutaneous versus myocutaneous flaps in the repair of major defects in head and neck cancer: A study of 331 flaps. *Head Neck Surg* 1984;7:104–109.

35. Biller HF, Baek SM, Lawson W, et al: Pectoralis major myocutaneous island flap in head and neck surgery. Analysis of complications in 42 cases. *Arch Otolaryngol* 1981;107:23–26.

36. Shah JP, Haribhakti V, Loree TR, et al: Complications of the pectoralis major myocutaneous flap in head and neck reconstruction. *Am J Surg* 1990;160:352–355.

37. Barton FE Jr, Spicer TE, Byrd HS: Head and neck reconstruction with tie latissimus dorsi myocutaneous flap: Anatomic observations and report of 60 cases. *Plast Reconstr Surg* 1983;71:199–204.

38. Netterville JL, Panje WR, Maves MD: The trapezius myocutaneous flap. *Arch Otolaryngol Head Neck Surg* 1987;113:271–281.

39. Kroll SS, Goepfert H, Jones M, et al: Analysis of complications in 168 pectoralis major myocutaneous flaps used for head and neck reconstruction. *Ann Plast Surg* 1990;25:93–97.

40. Zbar RI, Funk GF, McCulloch TM, et al: Pectoralis major myofascial flap: A valuable tool in contemporary head and neck reconstruction. *Head Neck* 1997;19(5):412–418.

41. Ossoff RH, Wurster CF, Berktold RE, et al: Complications after pectoralis major myocutaneous flap reconstruction of head and neck defects. *Arch Otolaryngol* 1983;109:812–814.

42. Mehrhof AI, Rosenstock A, Neifeld JP, et al: The pectoralis major myocutaneous flap in head and neck reconstruction. Analysis of complications. *Am J Surg* 1983;146:478–482.

43. Smith PG, Collins SL: Repair of head and neck defects with thin and double-lined pectoralis flaps. *Arch Otolaryngol* 1984;110:468–473.

44. Surkin MI, Lawson W, Biller HF: Analysis of the methods of pharyngoesophageal reconstruction. *Head Neck Surg* 1984;6:953–970.

45. Donegan JO, Gluckman JL: An unusual complication of the pectoralis major myocutaneous flap. *Head Neck Surg* 1984;6:982–983.

46. Ellison DE, Hoover LA, Ward PH: Tumor recurrence within myocutaneous flaps. *Ann Otolaryngol Rhinol Laryngol* 1987;96 (1 Pt 1):26–28.

47. Kuzon WM, Guilane J, Herman SJ: Pulmonary atelectasis after reconstruction with pectoralis major flaps. *Arch Otolaryngol Head Neck Surg* 1990;116:575–577.

48. Panje WR: Myocutaneous trapezius flap. *Head Neck Surg* 1980;2:206–212.

49. Tucker HM, Sobol SM, Levine H, et al: The transverse cervical trapezius myocutaneous island flap. *Arch Otolaryngol Head Neck Surg* 1981;108:194–198.

50. Cummings CW, Eisele DW, Coltrera MD: Lower trapezius myocutaneous island flap. *Arch Otolaryngol Head Neck Surg* 1989;115:1181–1185.

51. Urken ML, Naidu RK, Lawson W, et al: The lower trapezius island musculocutaneous flap revisited: Report of 45 cases and unifying concept of the vascular supply. *Arch Otolaryngol Head Neck Surg* 1991;117:502–511.

52. Chandrasekhar B, Terez JJ, Kokal WA, et al: The inferior trapezius musculocutaneous flap in head and neck surgery. *Ann Plast Surg* 1988;21:201–209.

53. Maves MD, Panje WR, Shagets FW: Extended latissimus dorsi myocutaneous flap reconstruction of flap in head and neck defects. *Otolaryngol Head Neck Surg* 1984;92:551–558.

54. Russell RC, Pribaz J, Zook EG, et al: Functional evaluation of latissimus dorsi donor site. *Plast Reconstr Surg* 1986;78:336–344.

55. Guerra AB, Metzinger SE, Lund KM, et al: The thoracodorsal artery perforator flap: Clinical experience and anatomic study with emphasis on harvest technique. *Plast Reconstr Surg* 2004;114:32–41.

56. Ariyan S: One-stage reconstruction for defects of the mouth using a sternomastoid myocutaneous flap. *Plast Reconstr Surg* 1986;78:336–344.

57. O'Brien B: A muscle-skin pedicle for total reconstruction of the lower lip. *Plast Reconstr Surg* 1970;45:395–399.

58. Ariyan S: The sternocleidomastoid myocutaneous flap. *Laryngoscope* 1980;90:676–679.

59. Larson DL, Goepfert H: Limitations of the sternocleidomastoid musculocutaneous flap in head and neck cancer reconstruction. *Plast Reconstr Surg* 1982;70:328–331.

60. Manni JJ, Bruaset I: Reconstruction of the anterior oral cavity using the platysma myocutaneous island flap. *Laryngoscope* 1986;96:564–567.

61. Coleman JJ, Jurkiewicz MJ, Nahai F, et al: The platysma musculocutaneous flap: Experience with 24 cases. *Plast Reconstr Surg* 1983;72:315–323.

62. Persky MS, Kaufman D, Cohen NL: Platysma myocutaneous flap for intraoral defects. *Arch Otolaryngol* 1983;109:463–464.

63. Conley JJ, Lanier DM, Tinsley P: Platysma myocutaneous flap revisited. *Arch Otolaryngol Head Neck Surg* 1986;112:711–713.

64. Hurwitz DJ, Rabson JA, Futrell JW: The anatomic basis for the platysma skin flap. *Plast Reconstr Surg* 1983;72:302–314.

65. Hagan WE, Walker LB: The nasolabial musculocutaneous flap: Clinical and anatomical correlations. *Laryngoscope* 1988;98:341–346.

66. Panje WR: Musculocutaneous and free flaps: Physiology and practical considerations. *Otolaryngol Clin North Am* 1984;17:401–412.

67. Cummings CW, Trachy RE, Richardson MA, et al: Prognostication of myocutaneous flap viability using laser Doppler velocimetry and fluorescein microfluorometry. *Otolaryngol Head Neck Surg* 1984;92:559–563.

68. Silverman DG, LaRossa DD, Barlow CH, et al: Quantification of tissue fluorescein delivery and prediction of flap viability with the fiberoptic dermofluorometer. *Plast Reconstr Surg* 1980;66:545–553.

69. Jones BM, Mayou BJ: The laser Doppler flowmeter for microvascular monitoring: A preliminary report. *Br J Plast Surg* 1982;35:147–149.

70. Mahoney JL, Lista FR: Variations in flap blood flow and tissue PO_2: A new technique for monitoring flap viability. *Ann Plast Surg* 1988;20:43–47.

71. Guanethidine sympathetic blockade: Its value in reimplantation surgery. *Br Med J* 1976;1:876–877.

72. Manson PN, Anthenelli RM, Im MJ, et al: The role of oxygen free radicals in ischemic tissue injury in island skin flaps. *Ann Surg* 1983;198:87–90.

73. Sagi A, Ferder M, Levens D, et al: Improved survival of island flaps after prolonged ischemia by perfusion with superoxide dismutase. *Plast Reconstr Surg* 1986;77:639–644.

74. Im MJ, Shen WH, Pak CH, et al: Effect of allopurinol on the survival of hyperemic island skin flaps. *Plast Reconstr Surg* 1984;73:276–277.

75. Rand-Luby L, Pommier RF, Williams ST, et al: Improved outcome of surgical flaps treated with topical dimethylsulfoxide. *Ann Surg* 1996;224(4):583–589.

76. McCrary BF: Hyperbaric oxygen (HBO2) treatment for a failing facial flap. *Postgrad Med J* 2007;83:e1.

77. Mes LG: Improving flap survival by sustaining cell metabolism within ischemic cells: A study using rabbits. *Plast Reconstr Surg* 1980;65:56–65.

78. Price MA, Pearl RM: Multiagent pharmacotherapy to enhance skin flap survival: Lack of additive effect of nitroglycerin and allopurinol. *Ann Plast Surg* 1994;33:52–56.

79. Hayden RE, Phillips JG, Mclear PW: Leeches: Objective monitoring of altered perfusion in congested flaps. *Arch Otolaryngol Head Neck Surg* 1988;114:1395–1399.

CHAPTER 61

Complications of Local Facial Flaps

Matthew Ashbach, Craig S. Murakami, and Mark S. Zimbler

The art of facial soft-tissue reconstruction is one that requires both forethought and the meticulous execution of a surgical plan. For the head and neck reconstructive surgeon, local facial flaps provide an excellent method of soft-tissue defect coverage with unparalleled cosmesis. The treatment of facial defects requires knowledge and experience with both facial cosmetic and head and neck reconstructive surgical techniques before the surgeon is able to achieve consistent results that are both aesthetically acceptable and anatomically functional.

Skin cancer has become the most common cancer worldwide, and it has been reported to affect one of every four Americans.[1] The reconstruction of facial skin defects, whether created by the head and neck surgeon or a Mohs dermatologic surgeon, has in recent years become the most common reason for local facial flaps. Other causes for facial flap reconstruction include traumatic injuries and scar revision surgery. However, these causes pale in number as compared with skin cancer reconstruction.

Each surgical defect is unique, and it must be placed in the context of the patient undergoing reconstruction. Factors to be considered when making decisions about reconstructive options include the location of the defect, the size of the defect, and the depth of the defect. Factors specific to the individual patient include the patient's age, the skin color and texture, the skin laxity, the facial rhytides, and the cosmetic expectations. Relative comorbidities include social habits such as smoking, medical history such as diabetes, and prior surgical reconstruction to the region or a history of radiation therapy. To further complicate the issue, in addition to the uniqueness of each defect and patient, the measurements of flap success or failure are also multifactorial and subjective. As such, a result that may be functional and cosmetically acceptable for one patient and surgeon may be completely unacceptable for another. All of the above factors coalesce to make the reconstructive surgery of facial soft-tissue defects a surgically challenging and mentally stimulating task.

The complications of local flaps are often frustrating, disheartening, and occasionally painstaking to manage for both the patient and the surgeon. In some cases, these complications could have been predicted and easily avoided if proper perioperative analysis had been performed. During this period, the surgeon should closely examine the defect as well as the surrounding tissue and systematically review the entire spectrum of reconstructive options. Relevant options should be discussed with the patient, with the benefits and risks of each reconstructive option outlined. Occasionally the patient, family, or primary care provider will request that a more simple and expeditious reconstruction be chosen despite the possibility of a less-than-perfect cosmetic result from the surgeon's perspective. The surgeon must therefore weigh economic and psychosocial issues along with the patient's reconstructive dilemma and choose the flap that is the most feasible. In certain situations, it may be perfectly appropriate to decide against using a flap altogether and to resort to using a skin graft or closure by secondary intention.

Surgeons believe that defects should be closed in a surgical manner that achieves the best cosmetic results. However, this is simply not true, and one must not forget that secondary healing also achieves excellent results if certain principles are adhered to and if the patient is meticulous with his or her wound care. Zitelli[2] has eloquently described how certain defects such as those located on concave areas of the face heal well by secondary intention. He also demonstrates nicely how convex wounds tend to heal poorly. His article includes numerous other tips for how to achieve excellent cosmetic results with secondary healing.

Most local flap complications are caused by poor flap design, ischemia, infection, bleeding, or a combination of these factors.[3] Although some of these complications are avoidable, others seem to be unfortunate outcomes of random probability. This chapter reviews the complications of local facial flaps and discusses the prevention and management of these problems. It does not address the complications of neck flaps that are used for the purpose of neck dissection.

PREOPERATIVE PLANNING

Anatomy

An integral part of designing facial flaps is acquiring knowledge of accurate surgical anatomy to avoid injury to vital anatomic structures. One should have extensive knowledge of the locations of the major nerves and vessels of the face, of the anatomic layer in which they reside, and of how to elevate a flap in these danger zones without injuring vital structures. The transection of small sensory nerves around the margins of the flap is usually unavoidable, and the mild loss in cutaneous sensation is rarely of clinical significance. One exception is the greater auricular nerve, which, when injured, can cause bothersome paresthesia or anesthesia to the affected ear. Injury to this nerve during flap elevation is avoided by remaining superficial to the fascia of the sternocleidomastoid muscle. Another exception is the infraorbital nerve, which supplies sensation to a generous portion of the midface.

Unlike sensory nerve injury, motor nerve injury (namely injury to the facial nerve) is usually a serious complication. Facial nerve injury will not only result in a devastating cosmetic deformity, but it will also create a rather dramatic functional impairment of the eyelids and the mouth. The two areas in which the facial nerve is most susceptible to surgical injury are the regions over the body of the mandible and the arch of the zygoma. In these areas, one must undermine and elevate the flaps in a subcutaneous plane and not disrupt the superficial myoaponeurotic system or the platysma.[4-6] In the forehead region, one can alternatively dissect in a subgaleal plane, which lies below the temporal branch of the facial nerve. However, special care must be taken when the dissection extends laterally over the temporal muscle and the arch of the zygoma. In this region, one must be careful to not transgress from the subgaleal plane to the subcutaneous plane, because the interposed layer of tissue contains the temporal branch of the facial nerve.

In general, the skin of the face has an excellent blood supply, and most local flaps in this region do extremely well. The microcirculatory system of the skin is comprised of two parts. First, a deep subdermal vascular plexus lies at the junction of the subcutaneous fat and the reticular dermis. A second superficial plexus lies in the superficial dermal papillae of the papillary dermis. The superficial plexus of capillaries supplies the more metabolically active epidermis via diffusion. These two plexuses are highly collateralized and lie parallel to the skin surface. They are supplied by deeper septocutaneous and musculocutaneous arteries that run perpendicular to the skin surface. Incisions at the borders of a flap interrupt these plexuses, thereby immediately decreasing perfusion. Blood supply is further diminished via norepinephrine when accompanying sympathetic nerves are severed. Fortunately the redundancy in vascular supply rarely puts a flap at risk of ischemia in the healthy patient.

It is a common misconception that the distal end of a longer flap will always survive if the width of the flap is proportionately increased. Historically the theoretic length of a flap was thought to be a function of its width, and a definitive length-to-width ratio of 2:1 to 4:1 defined flap design. The rationale was that wider flaps had more vessels available to perfuse the distal end. In reality, flap length-to-width ratios are not always reliable predictors of facial flap survival.[7] Instead, it is the length of the flap in relation to its capillary perfusion pressure and intravascular resistance that is the most critical determinant of tissue ischemia and necrosis.[8] Increasing the width of the flap does not always increase the distal capillary perfusion pressure or the intravascular resistance, unless a direct cutaneous, musculocutaneous, or large subcutaneous vessel is incorporated into the flap.[9,10] In the face, it is fortunate that there is a rich supply of sizable subcutaneous vessels; therefore, when increasing the width of a flap, one usually includes additional vessels and obtains a flap that has a greater distal blood flow.

One generally feels confident that a flap will survive when there is active bleeding present along the flap's distal margin. Because of the multiple factors that affect tissue oxygenation, however, the presence of active bleeding at the margins of a flap is not always sufficient evidence that there is adequate tissue oxygenation. The surgeon must be aware that this may not always be a reliable predictor of flap survival.[11] More extensive measures to quantify facial flap perfusion (e.g., laser Doppler, dermatofluorometry, thermocoupling, oximetry) have been suggested.[12-14] However, the use of such evaluations with local facial flaps is often time consuming, inaccurate, and rarely of clinical benefit.[15]

Patient Characteristics

The medical literature is lacking in prospective human studies comparing medical conditions with surgical technique in local facial flaps. However, considerable insight has been gained both retrospectively and through animal research. The patient who presents with compromised microvasculature (e.g., a diabetic patient or a smoker) represents an added layer of complexity to the surgeon. Microvasculature compromise limits both the length of reliable perfusion from a pedicle and wound healing. This has been exemplified in smokers undergoing rhytidectomy; these cases have demonstrated an increased risk of flap necrosis of between three- and twelvefold.[16,17] Similarly, animal models have shown a nearly 50% increase in the size of necrosis with random pattern flaps in diabetic rats[18] and a nearly twofold decrease in flap survival among island flaps.[19]

Many practitioners will give a diabetic patient or a smoker perioperative antioxidants in an effort to stop the marauding cascade of free-radical endothelial damage short. More importantly, patients are advised to stop smoking at least 2 days before surgery and for 7 days thereafter, if not indefinitely. At the time of surgery, conservative and deeper undermining of the flap is advised to preserve the more robust subdermal plexus of vessels.[20] Priority should be given to flaps of short length with abundant blood supplies. If a short flap will not suffice, one may consider using a delay technique that has been shown to be effective for increasing flap length by increasing tissue vascularity.[21,22] An alternative to the delay phenomenon is the use of a tissue expander to gain greater lengths of flap[23] (Figure 61-1). Expanded flaps have been shown to have increased flap length survival of up to 117%, which was superior to the 3% increased flap length survival with the use of the delay technique.[24]

Radiation to the skin also affects blood flow, flap survival, and soft-tissue characteristics. Tissue that has been irradiated may be atrophic, dry, scaly, fragile, and prone to even the slightest degree of injury. Both acute injury and chronic irritation to irradiated skin may result in a nonhealing ulcer or chronic dermatitis. If these lesions fail to resolve with meticulous wound care, they sometimes require surgical intervention. There is also more fibrosis in irradiated skin, and this condition tends to inhibit wound healing and to enhance tissue contracture. Histologically, previously irradiated skin displays an obliterative endarteritis that affects the subdermal plexus in addition to fibrosis.[25,26] Patients should be questioned thoroughly about any history of radiation done for facial acne or a previous malignancy, because this may affect the type of reconstruction that is recommended to the patient. In general, it is preferable to reconstruct soft-tissue defects with the use of nonirradiated flaps and to avoid the transfer of irradiated tissue, in which the circulation may be compromised. Other factors to consider include advanced age, malnutrition, immunosuppression, and actinic damage, all of which impair the healing process.

Flap Design

One of the most important aspects of facial reconstruction is to develop a systematic approach to flap design that adheres to the correct principles of

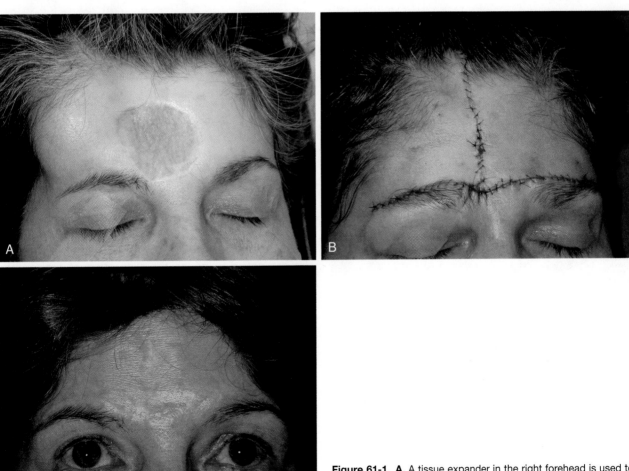

Figure 61-1. A, A tissue expander in the right forehead is used to revise a defect that was previously skin grafted. **B,** Immediate postoperative result after excision and advancement. **C,** Long-term follow-up reveals good cosmesis with minimal scarring.

soft-tissue repair. Obviously, if flaps are designed improperly, a wide spectrum of complications may subsequently arise. Some of these complications will merely result in minor and insignificant cosmetic deformities, whereas the more dramatic complications may result in deformities that become functionally and emotionally debilitating to the patient. It is essential that surgeons who are interested in facial reconstruction possess a firm grasp of head and neck anatomy, wound healing physiology, and soft-tissue dynamics.

Most errors in flap design can be avoided by adhering to the fundamental principles of relaxed skin tension lines[27,28] and lines of maximum extensibility. These principles dictate how incisions heal better when placed along, on, or within relaxed skin tension lines and how wound tension is minimized if donor tissue is transferred along lines of maximum extensibility. Similarly, the face is often described in aesthetic units, which are further categorized into subunits.[29] This schema represents a useful tool for flap planning, because the subunits are defined anatomically and with respect to the texture, contour, skin color, and thickness at subunit junctions (Figure 61-2).

These principles are especially important when designing flaps for defects around the eye, the nasal ala, and the vermilion border of the mouth, because these areas are extremely sensitive to aberrant skin tension. On the eyelid, misdirected tension will result in ectropion, epiphora, or lagophthalmos that can then lead to exposure keratitis of the cornea and possible visual impairment. Around the nose, a poorly designed flap that places excessive tension on the nasal ala will result in alar retraction (Figure 61-3), nasal obstruction (Figure 61-4), or both. In the perioral region, flaps that

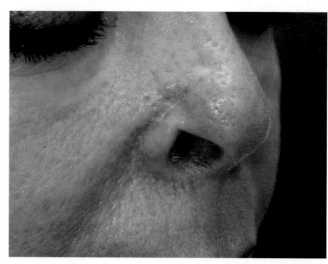

Figure 61-3. Alar retraction as a result of scar contracture from a local flap.

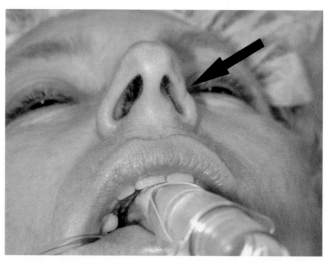

Figure 61-4. Alar collapse *(arrow)* as a result of inadequate tissue integrity.

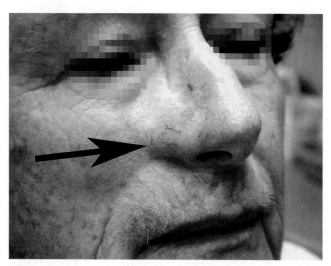

Figure 61-2. Poor cosmetic result from a flap in the superior nasolabial fold from inadequate analysis of the side and alar subunits. Telangiectasia formation has also occurred *(arrow)*.

place excessive tension on the vermilion border of the lip are prone to cause the disruption of oral competence or an aberration in speech (Figure 61-5). In addition to the functional impairment, the distortion of these anatomic areas is often difficult to correct. Therefore, at the time of operation, these anatomic structures must be examined closely after the flap has been rotated over the defect. If the flap places excessive tension on the eyelid, the nasal ala, or the lip, one should take additional measures to release the tension and rectify the situation or to perform an alternative method of defect closure.

Similarly, the type of flap affects the tension on the distal end of the flap, which is also the most common location for flap ischemia. For example, transposition flaps generally result in less distal tension than rotational or

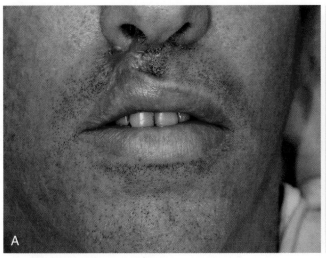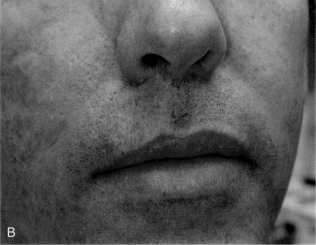

Figure 61-5. A, Lip retraction after the excision of a squamous cell carcinoma involving the vermilion border and (**B**) after full-thickness skin grafting.

advancement flaps. Flap size should also approximate the defect, because local flaps undergo minimal contracture. Lastly, the thickness should approximate that of the defect to allow for equal effacement.

There are multiple other factors (e.g., handling tissues atraumatically, minimizing wound tension, suturing tissue layers properly, reconstructing facial defects in aesthetic units) that increase the probability of achieving acceptable cosmetic results.[30,31] One can refer to numerous reference sources that review which type of local flap is the best choice for a given area of the face.[32–38] Unfortunately, there is no single book that takes into consideration all of the multiple and unique factors previously discussed. A flap that works well on an elderly patient with thin atrophic skin may not work well on a young patient with thick, sebaceous, pigmented skin. Therefore one must be extremely discriminating and cautious when selecting flaps "straight out of a textbook" if one is to avoid unnecessary complications caused by poor flap design. In general, a surgeon who is proficient with a wide variety of flap designs is able to consistently choose the best flap for any given defect on any given patient.

PERIOPERATIVE COMPLICATIONS

Ischemia

Most of the flaps created in the facial area have a random pattern of blood supply with which the distal flap is supplied by vessels in both the dermal–subdermal plexus and the subcutaneous plexus. Because the face possesses a dense subcutaneous plexus of blood vessels, these flaps do better than flaps on other regions of the body, which rely primarily on the dermal–subdermal plexus alone.[9] In addition, some flaps of the

face (e.g., the forehead flap, the dorsal nasal flap, the nasolabial flap, the various flaps of the lip) can be elevated with an axial-like or myocutaneous-like blood supply.[39–44] These particular flaps are usually based on the superficial temporal, supraorbital, supratrochlear, transverse facial, or facial–angular arteries of the face.[45] Consequently these flaps have a robust vascular supply and generally tolerate longer flap lengths than those with random patterns of blood supply alone.

The most frequent complication of local flaps is the occurrence of postoperative ischemia (Figure 61-6). Ischemia reflects an imbalance between oxygen delivery and demand. It can occur in the form of both arterial insufficiency and venous congestion. Ischemia can be detected by color changes in the flap. A pale flap with poor capillary refill and an absence of bleeding after pinprick suggests arterial insufficiency.[46] Conversely, an edematous purple- or blue-colored flap with dark-colored bleeding after pinprick suggests venous congestion.

The presence of ischemia then leads to various degrees of tissue hypoxia, and, after significant tissue hypoxia occurs, the flap becomes part of a vicious cycle of wound infection, dehiscence, the production of oxygen free radicals, and flap necrosis. The cause of flap ischemia is multifactorial and includes poor flap design (which creates excessive wound tension), bleeding, and infection. By definition, ischemia is an amount of vascular perfusion that is inadequate to support tissue oxygenation and viability. Oxygenation does not always correlate with perfusion, because tissue oxygenation is also dependent on hemoglobin saturation, oxygen binding, and pH as defined by the Bohr effect.[47] Tissue oxygenation and flap viability are also dependent on the flap's rate of oxygen consumption.

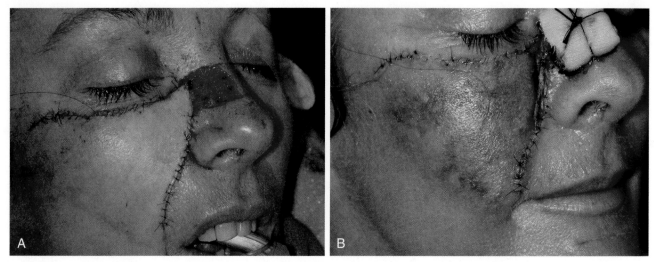

Figure 61-6. A, Flap ischemia in a smoker that became evident intraoperatively and (**B**) matured postoperatively.

Most severely, ischemia results in flap necrosis, which can be partial or full thickness. Superficial crusting and eventual reepithelialization characterize partial-thickness ischemia or epidermolysis. Full-thickness necrosis often begins at the distal end of the flap, and it may be evident as a result of pallor or vascular congestion. This is followed by mottling and, eventually, necrosis.

Undoubtedly the two most common mistakes that lead to flap ischemia are placing excessive torsion on the proximal pedicle and leaving excessive tension on the distal wound margin.[48,49] These mistakes are usually technical errors caused by improper flap design, inadequate undermining, or the inadequate redistribution of wound tension. A properly designed flap should redistribute the wound tension toward the donor site wound margin and away from the defect site. Typically the donor-site skin has a healthier blood supply than the defect site. Consequently, there is less ischemia at the donor site, and one encounters fewer problems with postoperative scar widening, tissue necrosis, and wound dehiscence.

There is an abundance of literature regarding the role of oxygen free radicals and the destruction of ischemic flaps. Ischemic tissue appears to promote the formation of oxygen free radicals[50] such as hydrogen peroxide, the superoxide radical, and the hydroxyl radical, which lead to tissue death and flap necrosis despite the presence of blood flow. The level of free radicals will also increase in infected tissues or when there is an associated wound hematoma.[51] Free-radical scavengers, such as allopurinol, superoxide dismutase, deferoxamine, ascorbic acid, mannitol, *N*-acetylcysteine, and many others have been used experimentally in animals to improve flap survival.[52-58]

Infection

Among healthy patients, the risk of infection in clean wounds is significantly low (5%),[59,60] and systemic antibiotics are rarely necessary. The necrosis of a facial flap as a result of a wound infection is even less common, and it probably occurs in only 1% of cases. Patients who are considered at higher risk for infection are those with clean-contaminated defects near oral or nasal mucosal margins, defects around the ear canal, defects with exposed cartilage, and defects that are allowed to remain open for a prolonged period before closing. In clean-contaminated wounds, the infection rate is closer to 10%, whereas, in contaminated wounds (e.g., trauma, infected cyst excision), the infection rate increases to 20%.[61] Prophylactic antibiotics are effective for clean-contaminated and contaminated wounds if the antibiotic is given preoperatively (i.e., ≥1 hour) and for a maximum 24 to 48 hours postoperatively.[62] If the antibiotics are used prophylactically, it is important to start the drugs preoperatively and to achieve adequate tissue levels of antibiotic at the time of the initial incision.

A select group of patients are at higher risk of infection as a result of compromised immune defenses (e.g., irradiated tissues, steroid therapy, cancer chemotherapy, impaired vascularity) and debility (e.g., diabetes, malnutrition).[63] Patients with human immunodeficiency virus or acquired immunodeficiency syndrome are immunocompromised and should be considered part of this infection-prone group. It is important to identify these patients with compromised immune defenses or debility and to place them on prophylactic perioperative antibiotics.

Patients with significant risk of infection are treated prophylactically with antibiotics that cover *Staphylococcus* and *Streptococcus.* Most commonly these patients are placed on a first-generation cephalosporin or dicloxacillin during the immediate perioperative period. Patients with local flaps near the mouth or nose are generally placed on a cephalosporin, although it is worth considering the use of amoxicillin–clavulanate potassium or clindamycin to increase the anaerobic coverage. On rare occasions when local flaps or skin grafts are placed over exposed cartilage or bone near the ear canal, patients may be placed on a short course of ciprofloxacin to include effective prophylaxis against *Pseudomonas.*

When insetting the flap, choosing suture material that dissolves via hydrolysis instead of via enzymatic degradation can decrease the risk of infection. Classic sutures that dissolve via hydrolysis include polyglactin (Vicryl), polyglytone (Caprosyn), polyglycolic acid (Dexon), and poliglecaprone (Monocryl), whereas plain gut and chromic suture dissolve via proteolysis. Antibiotic ointment can also be applied over suture lines, which appears to decrease infection through an improved healing environment rather than direct antibacterial action.

Bleeding

Bleeding during and after the operation is often related to poor intraoperative hemostasis, uncontrolled hypertension, poor drainage, or an occult drug or congenital coagulopathy.[64,65] Blood collecting beneath a flap invariably will elevate the flap from the surgical bed and impede the neovascularization process. Likewise, cofactors within the hematoma can cause vasospasm in the flap itself. Extreme bleeding, which occurs in approximately 4% of patients,[66] may even put the flap under significant tension and compromise blood flow from the pedicle. Evidence also supports the idea that the iron compounds of a hematoma promote local free-radical production that eventually may lead to flap necrosis. In addition, a hematoma can act as a culture medium for infection.

An inventory of the patient's medications should be taken before cutaneous surgery, with particular attention given to warfarin, nonsteroidal anti-inflammatory agents, and antiplatelet agents. The medical indication for these medications certainly needs attention before perioperative discontinuation. For example, holding coumadin in a patient with atrial fibrillation and a history of a stroke is probably unwarranted with the use of a local flap. Interestingly, the literature has actually failed to show consistent evidence that the theoretic increased risk of bleeding with these medications has had clinical significance during cutaneous surgery. For that reason, many surgeons do not insist that patients with significant comorbidities discontinue their anticoagulant medications before cutaneous surgery.

For all patients, the surgeon must pay close attention to detail at the time of operation and achieve the best hemostasis possible using electrocautery, direct pressure, and epinephrine. One must always be selective with electrocauterization to avoid excessive thermal injury to the flap, which leads to tissue necrosis or damage to the hair follicles. Tissue necrosis and the loss of hair follicles at the margins of the flap result in scarring that is more visible and less aesthetically acceptable.

Some surgeons feel that bipolar cautery is less likely to injure the flap, as it disperses a smaller amount of thermal energy than the usual monopolar cautery. A needle tip may be used rather than the usual spatulated tip, because the needle tip has pinpoint accuracy and usually requires lower power settings on the electrocautery unit. In addition, the needle tip works well for hemostasis, and it also functions well in a cutting mode as a bloodless scalpel. The one disadvantage of using needle-tip cautery is the increased risk of needle punctures for both the surgeon and the assistant. In today's environment, this is obviously not something to be taken lightly. Therefore one should take special precautions with this instrument by storing it in a protective holder when it is not in use rather than passing it on and off the field to the scrub nurse or the surgical assistant.

Occasionally the placement of some type of drain is necessary to prevent the formation of a hematoma beneath the flap. Surgical wounds should be dressed properly to provide adequate but not excessive amounts of pressure. This is generally accomplished with a bulky dressing, paper tape, and a skin adhesive. Patients should also be given proper postoperative instructions related to wound care and cautioned to avoid excessive activity that may incite bleeding.

MANAGEMENT OF COMPLICATIONS

Ischemia

Not all local flaps that become ischemic undergo flap necrosis to the degree that it becomes a clinically significant problem. It would be ideal if every surgeon possessed the ability to predict which particular ischemic flaps had "significant" amounts of ischemia so that some type of intervention could be done to prevent flap necrosis. Unfortunately, there are no easy ways of predicting local flap necrosis; for the most part, one must rely on observation, supposition, and personal experience. Flaps that are edematous, congested, or sluggish to capillary refill with digital compression are all at risk of undergoing some degree of necrosis. Preventive measures to decrease edema, increase free-radical scavenging, increase blood flow, or decrease oxygen demand can be taken at this time. Patients are instructed to keep their heads elevated and to avoid strenuous activity during the early postoperative period to keep the formation of edema to a minimum. Occasionally patients are placed on postoperative steroids (e.g., prednisone) to reduce flap edema and enhance flap survival.

The oxygen consumption of a flap can be effectively reduced by cooling the flap with an ice compress over a 48-hour period or for as long as the perfusion remains poor. Because excessive quantities of oxygen free radicals may arise in ischemic tissue and contribute to flap necrosis, patients are occasionally placed on allopurinol and ascorbic acid, which are known free-radical scavengers. Although many other free-radical scavengers exist, these particular medications have minimal adverse reactions and are tolerated well by most patients.

If significant amounts of ischemia persist, the flap will undergo various degrees of cell death that then present clinically as incremental flap loss. Mild amounts of ischemia usually result in epidermolysis alone, which presents clinically as the superficial loss of epidermis with the survival of the underlying dermis. The epithelium becomes desiccated and eventually sloughs as reepithelialization occurs. Often the epidermolysis is indistinguishable from a full-thickness tissue necrosis. Keeping the wound crust moist with an antibiotic ointment or Aquaphor will help to debride the nonviable epithelium and uncover any underlying viable tissue.

Full-thickness necrosis of small facial flaps is generally a rare occurrence in the healthy, compliant, and nonsmoking population. If the flap is small and resides in a noncritical area of the face, the ischemic area of the flap is left to necrose and clinically demarcate. After the flap demarcates, the necrotic portions of the flap can be debrided to promote reepithelialization and minimize the risk of excessive scar formation. If full-thickness crusts are not debrided, they must undergo an extensive and time-consuming autodigestion before epidermal migration can occur. If this occurs, these wounds will often form a depressed scar that is thin, fragile, and, in most cases, aesthetically unacceptable.

It is well known that the forehead, scalp, temple, and concave areas of the midface do extremely well cosmetically after healing by secondary intention.[2,67–70] In these areas, one may want to take a "wait-and-see" approach after the necrotic portions of the flap have been debrided and not aggressively attempt to reclose the defect with a second flap (Figure 61-7).

Convex areas of the face are treated more aggressively, as they are more likely to form a depressed scar from wound contraction and a bowstring effect over the convexity. Because healing by secondary intention is generally poor over convex areas of the face, surgeons may chose to reattempt the local flap closure of these defects soon after the necrotic portion of the flap demarcates. Areas such as the perioral and periocular regions, which do not tolerate contraction and distortion of the normal anatomy, should also be reconstructed as soon as possible with a flap or graft to prevent functional impairment such as oral incompetence or eyelid ectropion. If these "emergency" flaps or grafts are cosmetically unacceptable, they can be revised at a later time when there is less risk of scar contracture and functional impairment.

Infection

In most circumstances, an infected facial flap is easily identified by local erythema, edema, tenderness, and occasional drainage. For mild superficial wound infections, patients are placed on an oral antibiotic that covers *Staphylococcus* and *Streptococcus,* and the wound is treated with topical antibiotics three or four times a day. Most wound infections resolve without incident, and flap viability is not threatened.

With more severe infections, there is more edema, erythema, and tenderness. The flap begins to develop sluggish capillary refill when palpated, and signs of ischemia become apparent (i.e., if they did not precede the infection). Inflammatory cells begin to release large amounts of proteolytic enzymes that cause local cell death and vascular thrombosis. A local abscess begins to form beneath the flap, and, as it expands, it physically stretches the flap and increases wound tension. This in turn inhibits blood flow and quickly exacerbates the problem of ischemia. Abscesses must be quickly identified, drained, cultured, and copiously irrigated to rescue the portions of the flap that remain viable. Simply releasing a few of the distal flap sutures and gently probing the wound usually will accomplish drainage. This approach not only provides a route for drainage, but it also releases excessive tension on the most distal portion of the flap. It also necessitates closure with interrupted stitches rather than a running stitch. Cultures and Gram staining are performed, and the wound is packed open with gauze strips or a small Penrose drain. Although the remaining sutures theoretically create a foreign body nidus for infection, the authors are not compelled to aggressively remove all of the sutures unless the wound remains recalcitrant to systemic antibiotic therapy.

Most of the synthetic absorbable sutures are made of polyglycolic acid or polydioxanone, which are known to elicit minimal foreign body reactions. Some of the newer absorbable sutures are monofilament, and they

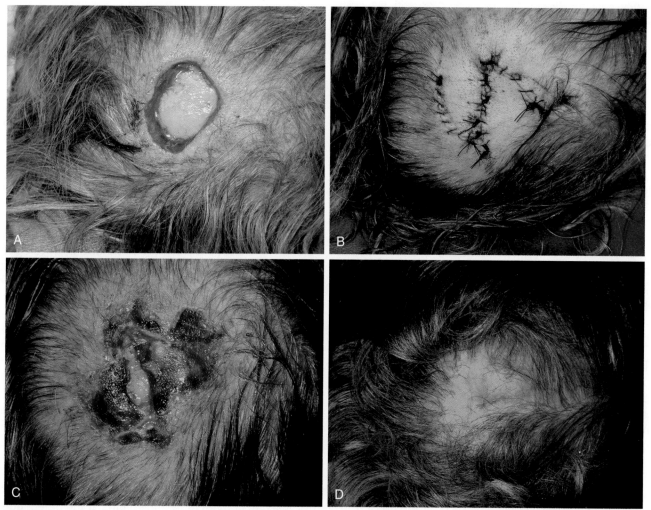

Figure 61-7. **A,** Shortly after resection and **B,** closure of a scalp squamous cell carcinoma, **C,** the flaps necrosed. **D,** Local wound care alone was able to salvage closure over the course of several weeks.

result in even less inflammation than braided sutures made of similar material. Because there is minimal foreign body reaction, synthetic sutures in the facial region generally do not act as powerful niduses for infection. Another factor to consider is that most wounds have less than 10% of their normal tensile strength at 1 week,[71] and the removal of all of the skin and subcutaneous sutures at intervals of less than 1 week may result in complete wound dehiscence and further complications.

Bleeding

Unanticipated bleeding occurs most frequently during the hours to the first couple of days after the procedure. If there is only a small amount of bleeding, the patient will suffer from greater amounts of ecchymosis and edema, but the viability of the flap is generally left unthreatened. Greater amounts of bleeding lead to hematoma formation beneath the flap; in these cases,

the viability of the flap is definitely threatened, for reasons that have already been discussed. If one is concerned at all about the contamination of the surgical site, antibiotics should promptly be started.[72,73]

A hematoma can be drained within the first 12 to 24 hours after surgery using a syringe with a 22-gauge needle or by taking out one or two sutures and applying gentle compression on the flap. Interrupted sutures make this much more feasible than a running suture, and, as such, they are the preferred method of closure if time allows. Large hematomas may necessitate the exploration of the wound to relieve the pressure on the flap and to irrigate the wound bed. This exploration will also allow the surgeon to identify and control the source of bleeding.

If the hematoma is organized or diagnosed more than 24 hours after surgery, the decision is less clear. Generally speaking, larger hematomas may require exploration and evacuation, whereas small hematomas can be observed without taking any further action. Because hematomas will liquefy in about 10 days, needle aspiration can be reconsidered at that time.

Patients who demonstrate excessive bleeding without any logical explanation should again be questioned about the recent consumption of aspirin or aspirin-containing medications. It is surprising how often one discovers that patients have taken over-the-counter medications for any number of medical problems (e.g., arthritis, colds, hay fever, headache). In addition, patients should be requestioned about any medical history of bleeding that they may have initially overshadowed. As a precautionary measure, many surgeons provide preprinted instructions about wound care to patients along with a list of over-the-counter medications that contain aspirin or other anticoagulant medications.

DELAYED COMPLICATIONS

There are a number of minor complications that may or may not be of clinical significance, and they can occur anywhere from weeks to even years after the initial procedure. These include the trapdoor deformity, pincushioning, telangiectasia formation, and suture granuloma.

The trapdoor deformity is a bulging elevation of the skin with a surrounding depressed scar that is seen after the use of transposition flaps or at the tip of rotational flaps. Several factors are likely involved in the cause of trapdoor deformity, such as lymphatic or venous obstruction, excess subcutaneous fat, redundant tissue, beveled wound edges, and excessive tension. The most widely accepted causative factor is the contraction of the scar sheet underlying the flap

toward the center of the flap.[74] The prevention or elimination of this deformity may be possible with wide undermining of the surrounding skin, because this maneuver will decrease the force of contractile vectors toward the center of the flap by increasing the area of the underlying scar sheet.

The problem of pincushioning is similar to the problem encountered with the classic trapdoor deformity (Figure 61-8). Flaps that are based superiorly will have lymphedema trapped in the dependent portion of the flap. In addition, the circular margin of the flap also undergoes contraction and a convergence of tissue, which tends to elevate the soft tissues of the flap as the scar shrinks in the length and width dimensions.[75,76] Perioperatively, the likelihood of developing pincushioning may be decreased by avoiding the beveling of the wound margin and by taking care to not harvest a flap that is too big for the given defect.

Pincushioning and trapdoor deformities can be managed similarly with steroid injections around the fourth postoperative week. It is preferable to use a 50/50 mixture of triamcinolone 10 mg/ml or 40 mg/ml with 1% plain lidocaine and to inject it subcutaneously with a 25-gauge needle. The weaker concentration is recommended for those with less experience injecting steroids, because steroids can cause excessive fat atrophy, telangiectasia, thinning of the skin, alopecia, and cutaneous hyperpigmentation. Flaps are injected with 0.3 ml to 0.6 ml of the steroid every 4 to 6 weeks for a series of three or four injections. If the defect does not appear to respond to this therapy, a higher concentration of steroid can be used, or the surgeon may elect to intervene surgically and revise the flap. Alternatively, dermabrasion may be successfully employed to resurface the elevated skin, with good results. A revision operation is considered at 3 months postoperatively,

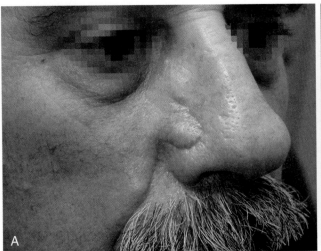 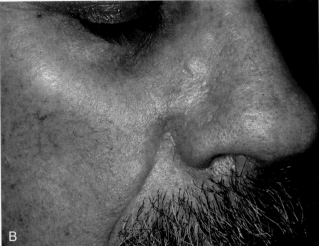

Figure 61-8. A, Pincushioning after closure with a superiorly based rotational flap that (**B**) responded well to dermabrasion.

and it usually consists of the elevation of the flap, the debulking of excess subcutaneous fat, the trimming of the excess flap margins, and the undermining of the wound edges. Occasionally, Z-plasty techniques are also necessary when the wound demonstrates excessive scar contracture.

Telangiectasias are small, enlarged blood vessels that occasionally form on patients with delicate, light-colored skin during the wound maturation period (see Figure 61-2). In most cases, they resolve spontaneously if the patient is careful to avoid excessive sun exposure. If they persist, they can be treated effectively with a laser such as the pulsed-dye laser or, alternatively, with intense pulsed light.

Suture granuloma, which is also known as a *stitch abscess,* is a benign yet bothersome complication after surgery. During facial reconstruction, it presents as a firm mass that may be tender and that is usually lying just below the level of the dermis. Occasionally it will manifest as a chronic intermittent indolent infection with or without drainage, but it should not cause a fever or show any signs of systemic infection. Suture material is a foreign body that causes local irritation and tissue necrosis. Histologically, a granulomatous tissue reaction with giant cells is diagnostic. Suture granuloma can occur many years after the primary surgical procedure, and it most commonly occurs with braided silk suture material. Fortunately monofilament and absorbable sutures carry a much lower risk of granuloma formation. Definitive treatment requires the removal of the suture material.

CONCLUSION

Although it is clear that local facial flaps can be fraught with complications, there is a good deal of satisfaction to be gained by both the patient and the reconstructive surgeon when a desired result is obtained. Successful outcomes hinge on developing plans before the operative suite is entered. These plans should consider more than just the defect and the surrounding tissue. As mentioned, patient characteristics such as tobacco use, radiation exposure, and diabetes can cause a perfectly executed local flap to fail. Furthermore, the surgeon's technique should reflect an acknowledgment of how and why failures occur. Flap characteristics such as thickness, distal tension, and pedicle torsion all affect blood supply and flap viability, and they need to be considered.

Sooner or later, all reconstructive surgeons will be faced with a flap failure. The approach to a failure requires the careful examination of the flap and the context in which it occurred. Salvage does not necessitate surgical intervention, and meticulous wound care or antibiotics may suffice. It is critical—especially early in one's career—to establish where things went wrong with the flap and to determine the least invasive technique that would rectify the situation.

REFERENCES

1. Housman TS, Feldman SR, Williford PM, et al: Skin cancer is among the most costly of all skin cancers to treat for the Medicare population. *J Am Acad Dermatol* 2003;48(3):425–429.
2. Zitelli J: Wound healing for the clinician. *Adv Dermatol* 1987; 2:243–267.
3. Vural E, Key JM: Complications, salvage, and enhancement of local flaps in facial reconstruction. *Otolaryngol Clin North Am* 2001; 34(4):739–751.
4. Loeb R: Technique for preservation of the temporal branches of the facial nerve during face-lift operations. *Br J Plast Surg* 1970; 23:390–394.
5. Robbins TH: The protection of the frontal branch of the facial nerve in face-lift surgery. *Br J Plast Surg* 1981;34:95–96.
6. Bernstein L, Nelson RH: Surgical anatomy of the extraparotid distribution of the facial nerve. *Arch Otolaryngol* 1984;110: 177–183.
7. Milton SH: Fallacy of the length-width ratio. *Br J Surg* 1970;22: 502–508.
8. Daniel RK, Williams HB: Free transfer of skin flaps by microvascular anastomosis. *Plast Reconstr Surg* 1973;52:16–31.
9. Pearl RM, Johnson D: The vascular supply to the skin: An anatomical and physiological reappraisal (Part II). *Ann Plast Surg* 1983; 11:196–205.
10. Pearl RM, Johnson D: The vascular supply to the skin: An anatomical and physiological reappraisal (Part I). *Ann Plast Surg* 1983;11:99–105.
11. Reinisch JF: The role of arteriovenous anastomoses in skin flaps. In Grabb WC, Meyers MB, editors: *Skin flaps,* Boston, 1975, Little, Brown.
12. Silverman DG, LaRossa DD, Barlow CH, et al: Quantification of tissue fluorescein delivery and prediction of flap viability with the fiberoptic dermofluorometer. *Plast Reconstr Surg* 1980;66: 545–553.
13. Marks NY, Trachy RE, Cummings CW: Dynamic variations in blood flow as measured by laser Doppler velocimetry: A study in rat skin flaps. *Plast Reconstr Surg* 1984;73:804–808.
14. Meyers B, Donovan W: An evaluation of eight methods of using fluorescein to predict the viability of skin flaps in the pig. *Plast Reconstr Surg* 1985;75:245–250.
15. Donegan JO: The assessment and enhancement of skin flap viability. *Head Neck Surg* 1980;2:470–475.
16. Goldminz D, Bennett RG: Cigarette smoking and flap and full-thickness graft necrosis. *Arch Dermatol* 1991;127(7):1012–1015.
17. Rees TD, Liverett DM, Guy CL: The effects of cigarette smoking on skin-flap survival in the face lift patient. *Plast Reconstr Surg* 1984;73(6):911–915.
18. De Carvalho EN, Ferrerira LM, de Carvalho NA, et al: Viability of a random dorsal skin flap in diabetic rats. *Acta Cir Bras* 2005; 20(3):225–228.
19. Serdaroglu I, Islamoglu K, Ozgentas E: Effects of insulin-dependent diabetes mellitus on perforator-based flaps in streptozotocin diabetic rats. *J Reconstr Microsurg* 2005;21(1):51–56.
20. Webster RC, Kazda G, Hamdan US, et al: Cigarette smoking and face lift: Conservative versus wide undermining. *Plast Reconstr Surg* 1986;77(4):596–604.
21. McFarlane RM, Heagy FC, Rodin S, et al: A study of the delay phenomenon in experimental pedicle flaps. *Plast Reconstr Surg* 1965;35:245–262.
22. Meyer MB, Cherry G: Augmentation of tissue survival by delay: An experimental study in rabbits. *Plast Reconstr Surg* 1969;39: 397–401.
23. Baker SR: Fundamentals of expanded tissue. *Head Neck Surg* 1991;2:327–333.

24. Cherry GW, Austad E, Pasyk K, et al: Increased survival and vascularity of random pattern skin flaps elevated in controlled, expanded skin. *Plast Reconstr Surg* 1983;72:680–685.

25. Stearner SP, Sanderson MH: Mechanisms of acute injury in the gamma-irradiated chicken: Effects of a protracted or split-dose exposure on the fine structure of the microvasculature. *Radiat Res* 1972;49:328.

26. Patterson TJS, Berry RJ, Hopewell JW, et al: The effect of x-radiation on the survival of experimental skin flaps. In Grabb WC, Myers MB, editors: *Skin flaps,* Boston, 1975, Little, Brown.

27. Borges AF: *Elective incisions and scar revision,* Boston, 1973, Little, Brown.

28. Borges AF, Alexander JE: Relaxed skin tension lines, Z-plasties on scars, and fusiform excision of lesions. *Br J Plast Surg* 1962;15:242–254.

29. Burget GC, Menick FJ: The subunit principle in nasal reconstruction. *Plast Reconstr Surg* 1985;76(2):239–247.

30. Menick FJ: Aesthetic refinements in use of forehead for nasal reconstruction: The paramedian forehead flap. *Clin Plast Surg* 1990;4:607–622.

31. Burgess LP, Morin BV, Rand M, et al: Wound healing: Relationship of wound closing tension to scar width in rats. *Arch Otolaryngol Head Neck Surg* 1990;116:798–802.

32. Grabb WC, Myers MB: *Skin flaps,* Boston, 1975, Little, Brown.

33. Becker FF: *Facial reconstruction with local and regional flaps,* New York, 1985, Thieme-Stratton.

34. Jackson IT: *Local flaps in head and neck reconstruction,* St. Louis, 1985, Mosby-Year Book.

35. Stauch B, Vasconez LO, Hall-Findlay EJ, editors: *Grabb's encyclopedia of flaps,* Boston, 1990, Little, Brown.

36. Thomas JR, Holt GR, editors: *Facial scars: Incision, revision, and camouflage,* St. Louis, 1989, Mosby-Year Book.

37. Tromovitch TA, Stegman S, Glogau RG: *Flaps and grafts in dermatologic surgery,* St. Louis, 1989, Mosby-Year Book.

38. Dzubow LM: *Facial flaps: Biomechanics and regional application,* Norwalk, Conn, 1990, Appleton & Lange.

39. Herbert DC, DeGeus J: Nasolabial subcutaneous pedicle flaps: II. *Br J Plast Surg* 1964;28:63.

40. Conley JC, Price JC: The midline vertical forehead flap. *Otolaryngol Head Neck Surg* 1981;89:38–44.

41. Conley JC, Donovan DT: A new technique for total reconstruction of the lower lip in a patient with malignant melanoma. *Otolaryngol Head Neck Surg* 1986;93:393–397.

42. Thomas JR, Griner N, Cook TA: The precise midline forehead flap as a musculocutaneous flap. *Arch Otolaryngol Head Neck Surg* 1988;114:79–84.

43. Ohtsuka H: Nasolabial skin flaps to the cheek. In Strauch B, Vasconez LO, Hall-Findlay EJ, editors: *Grabb's encyclopedia of flaps,* Boston, 1990, Little, Brown.

44. Burget GC: The axial paramedian forehead flap. In Strauch B, Vasconez LO, Hall-Findlay EJ, editors: *Grabb's encyclopedia of flaps,* Boston, 1990, Little, Brown.

45. Cormack GC, Lamberty BGH: *The arterial anatomy of skin flaps,* New York, 1986, Churchill Livingstone.

46. Utley DS, Koch RJ, Goode RL: The failing flap in facial plastic and reconstructive surgery: Role of the medicinal leech. *Laryngoscope* 1998;108:1129–1135.

47. Hastala MP: Gas transport and exchange. In Patton HD, Fuchs AF, Hille B, et al, editors: *Textbook of physiology,* ed 2, Philadelphia, 1989, WB Saunders.

48. Larrabee WF Jr, Holloway GA Jr, Sutton D: Wound tension and blood flow in skin flap. *Ann Otol Rhinol Laryngol* 1984;93:112–115.

49. Larrabee WF Jr, Holloway GA Jr, Trachy RE, et al: Skin flap tension and wound slough: Correlation with laser Doppler velocimetry. *Otolaryngol Head Neck Surg* 1982;90:185–187.

50. Angel MF, Ramasastry SS, Swartz WM, et al: Free radicals: Basic concepts concerning their chemistry, pathophysiology, and relevance to plastic surgery. *Plast Reconstr Surg* 1987;79:990–997.

51. Angel MF, Narayanan K, Swartz WM, et al: The etiologic role of free radicals in hematoma-induced flap necrosis. *Plast Reconstr Surg* 1986;77:795–803.

52. Angel MF, Haddadd JJ, Abramson M: A free radical scavenger reduces hematoma-induced flap necrosis in Fischer rats. *Otolaryngol Head Neck Surg* 1987;96:96–98.

53. Angel MF, Mellow CG, Knight KR, et al: The effect of deferoxamine on tolerance to secondary ischaemia caused by venous obstruction. *Br J Plast Surg* 1989;42:422–424.

54. Knight KR, MacPhadyen K, Lepore DA, et al: Enhancement of ischemic rabbit skin flap survival with the antioxidant and free-radical scavenger N-acetylcysteine. *Clin Sci* 1991;81:31–36.

55. Knight KR, Angel MF, Lepore DA, et al: Secondary ischaemia in rabbit skin flaps: The roles played by thromboxane and free radicals. *Clin Sci* 1991;80:235–240.

56. Knight KR, Mellow CG, Abbey PA, et al: Interaction between thromboxane and free radical mechanisms in experimental ischemic rabbit skin flaps. *Res Exp Med (Berl)* 1990;190:423–433.

57. Pokoryn AT, Bright DA, Cummings CW: The effects of allopurinol and superoxide dismutase in a rat model of skin flap necrosis. *Arch Otolaryngol Head Neck Surg* 1989;115:207–212.

58. Weinstein GS, Maves MD, McCormack ML: Deferoxamine decreases necrosis in dorsally based pig skin flaps. *Otolaryngol Head Neck Surg* 1989;101:559–561.

59. DiPiro JT, Record KE, Schanzenback KS, et al: Antimicrobial prophylaxis in surgery: Part I. *Am J Hosp Pharmacol* 1981;320–334.

60. Simmons BP: Guideline for the prevention of surgical wound infections. *Infect Control* 1982;3:188–196.

61. Sebben JE: Prophylactic antibiotics in cutaneous surgery. *J Dermatol Surg Oncol* 1985;11:901–906.

62. Burke JF: The effective period of preventive antibiotic protection in experimental incisions and dermal lesions. *Surgery* 1961;50:161–168.

63. Fairbanks DF: *Antimicrobial therapy in otolaryngology–head and neck surgery,* Alexandria, Va, 1991, American Academy of Otolaryngology–Head and Neck Surgery.

64. Fisher HW: Surgery on patients receiving anticoagulants. *Dermatol Surg Oncol* 1977;3:210–212.

65. Hicks PD, Stromber BV: Hemostasis in plastic surgical patients. *Clin Plast Surg* 1985;12:17–23.

66. Becker FF: *Facial reconstruction with local and regional flaps,* New York, 1985, Thieme-Stratton.

67. Tromovitch TA, Stegman S, Glogau RG: *Flaps and grafts in dermatologic surgery,* St. Louis, 1989, Mosby-Year Book.

68. Zitelli JA: Secondary intention healing: An alternative to surgical repair. *Clin Dermatol* 1984;2:92–106.

69. Burget GC: Aesthetic restoration of the nose. *Clin Plast Surg* 1985;12:463–480.

70. Becker GD, Adams LA, Levin BC: Nonsurgical repair of perinasal skin defects. *Plast Reconstr Surg* 1991;88:768–776.

71. Harris DR: Healing of the surgical wound: I: Basic considerations. *J Am Acad Dermatol* 1979;1:197–215.

72. Krizek TJ, Davis JH: The role of the red cell in subcutaneous infection. *J Trauma* 1965;5:85–89.

73. Polk HC, Miles AA: Enhancement of bacterial infection by ferric iron: Kinetics, mechanisms and surgical significance. *Surgery* 1971;70:71–77.

74. Koranda FC, Webster RC: Trapdoor effect in nasolabial flaps. *Arch Otolaryngol* 1985;111:421–424.

75. Webster RC, Benjamin RJ, Smith RC: Treatment of "trap-door" deformity. *Laryngoscope* 1978;88:707–712.

76. Holt GR: Treatment of the trapdoor scars. In Thomas JR, Holt GR, editors: *Facial scars: Incisions, revision and camouflage,* St. Louis, 1989, Mosby-Year Book.

77. Wee SS, Hruza GJ, Mustoe TA: Refinements of nasal myocutaneous flap. *Ann Plast Surg* Oct 1990;25(4):271–278.

78. Levin JM, Brauer JA, Draft K, et al: Suture granuloma following surgical neck rejuvenation procedure. *Dermatol Surg* 2006;32:768–769.

CHAPTER 62

Complications of Free-Tissue Transfer

Steven J. Wang, Theodoros N. Teknos, and Douglas B. Chepeha

The expanding application of microvascular free-tissue transfer to head and neck reconstruction during the past two decades has dramatically improved the ability to treat patients with complex head and neck defects, particularly after head and neck cancer ablative surgery. With a variety of available distant donor sites, microvascular free flaps allow for the reconstruction of virtually any type of defect in the head and neck at any location. In addition to providing better functional and cosmetic results, the placement of vascularized soft tissue or composite free flaps has also been shown to reduce complication rates as compared with other local or regional flap reconstruction techniques.[1,2] As experience among microvascular surgeons has grown, successful head and neck free flap reconstruction rates in most recent series have exceeded 95%.[3–6] However, even in the most experienced hands, complications of microvascular surgery do occur. The discussion of the factors related to the prevention and management of these complications is the subject of this chapter.

FREE FLAPS

Basic Concepts

Since successful free flap surgery was first described for the head and neck by Seldenberg[7] in 1959, this technique has become standard for the reconstruction of complex head and neck defects (Figure 62-1). In its most simplified concept, free flap reconstructive surgery refers to the harvest of a mass of tissue supplied by a single artery and drained by one or more veins that is transferred from a distant site to a recipient bed, where its vascularity is immediately reestablished through microsurgical techniques. A free flap may consist of skin, muscle, or bone tailored to what is needed for optimal reconstruction. A variety of donor sites have been described for head and neck reconstruction. For exclusively soft-tissue defects, the most commonly used donor sites include the radial forearm, the antero-lateral thigh, the rectus abdominis, the lateral arm, and the latissimus dorsi. For composite defects that require bone reconstruction, osseocutaneous flaps including the fibula, the scapula, the iliac crest, and the radius are commonly used.

Free flap reconstructive surgery begins with the harvest of the flap from its donor site. When the flap is disconnected from its native blood supply, the period of primary ischemia begins. The flap is then inset into the recipient defect, and the anastomosis of the flap vessels to recipient vessels is performed with the use of microsurgical suturing techniques. The period of primary ischemia ends when blood flow across the flap vessels is reestablished, thereby restoring normal flap physiology. Neovascularization to the new free flap occurs across the cutaneous wound edges and the recipient bed after surgery. For most soft-tissue flaps, neovascularization permits flap survival independent of what happens to the flap pedicle vessels after about 7 to 10 days.[8,9]

Physiology

Although advances in microvascular techniques have achieved a very high rate of success in free flap surgery of the head and neck, local and systemic factors do occasionally conspire to result in flap failure. An essential ingredient for flap viability is maintaining blood flow across the microvascular anastomosis. Blood flow across the microvascular anastomosis requires a favorable microenvironment. The correct interaction of the coagulation cascade, the vascular endothelium, platelet interaction, and fluid dynamics govern the fate of the flap's survival.[8–10] The tissue dissection involved with flap harvest, the division of flap pedicle vessels, and the period of primary ischemia promote factors that favor the prevention of blood flow; these factors must be minimized through meticulous surgical technique. The vascular endothelium plays a critical role, because it regulates vasomotor tone and blood flow. Although intact endothelium is nonthrombogenic, exposed subendothelium is very thrombogenic, thereby increasing platelet interaction and other events of the coagulation cascade that may result in the prevention of blood flow into the flap.[8]

Flap failures typically occur as a result of either thrombosis at the vascular anastomosis site or problems with the distal microcirculation. Thrombosis at the vascular anastomosis site may involve either the venous or arterial anastomosis or both. Studies indicate that venous thrombosis is more common.[8,11] Prolonged venous thrombosis will eventually result in arterial thrombosis. The rapid recognition of vascular anastomosis site thrombosis allows for successful salvage in about 50% of cases.[11] Problems with the distal microcirculation are more ominous, less understood, and less amenable to

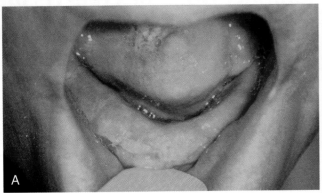

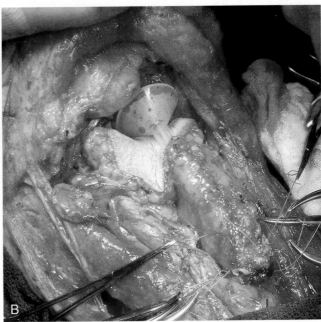

Figure 62-1. Free-tissue transfer for complex head and neck defects. **A,** A fibula free flap was used for reconstruction after the resection of a T4 squamous cell cancer of the anterior floor of the mouth, which required segmental mandibulectomy. **B,** A radial forearm free flap has been "tubed" over a salivary bypass tube for the reconstruction of a circumferential pharyngeal defect after the resection of a T4 squamous cell cancer of the hypopharynx.

salvage. Numerous factors can lead to flap failure, including the length of primary ischemia; technical factors during flap pedicle vessel dissection and microvascular anastomosis that result in intimal tears, infection, or fistula; the use of pressors; the overuse of blood products (particularly fresh frozen plasma); and the mismanagement of intravascular dynamics.[9,10] Additionally, various patient comorbidities can also contribute to flap compromise.[4,12]

Two outcomes are possible after the reperfusion of the flap after primary ischemia. In the favorable scenario, blood flow is reestablished, which brings nutrients and reverses transient physiologic derangement from ischemia. In the unfavorable scenario, there is an infusion of substrates and inflammatory mediators that results in reperfusion injury. The transition point between these two possible outcomes is poorly defined and incompletely understood. It is known that the longer the ischemia time, the more likely for irreparable damage to the microcirculation to occur.[9,10] Tolerance for ischemia varies depending on the flap tissue type. Skin flaps have the most tolerance for ischemia (5–6 hours), followed by bone, muscle, and, finally, intestinal mucosa, which has the least tolerance (1–2 hours).[9] In addition, the tolerance for secondary ischemia is less than that for primary ischemia, and the tolerance for secondary ischemia is inversely correlated with the time since primary ischemia (i.e., tolerance of >72 hours after initial surgery becomes equivalent to primary ischemia).[9]

When problems with the microcirculation occur, neutrophils, inflammatory mediators, and oxygen free radicals become activated.[9,10] There is extensive endothelial cell edema and damage, which leads to the irreversible accumulation of toxic substances in the flap. This results in the so-called *no-reflow phenomenon*. The no-reflow phenomenon exists when there is a lack of nutritive capillary perfusion despite the reperfusion of ischemic tissue. In this situation, the flap cannot be salvaged.[9,10]

Preoperative Planning and Patient Selection

Ensuring a favorable outcome of head and neck microvascular free flap surgery begins with careful preoperative planning. Consideration is made of the various reconstructive options, including both free flaps and non-free flaps, taking into account the anticipated defect and the expected functional and cosmetic goals. The patient's comorbidities and overall prognosis in the case of cancer of the head and neck are also considered. After a decision to use a free flap is made, the appropriate donor site should be selected. There are multiple factors to consider when choosing a donor site, including the size and volume of the anticipated defect, the need for bone, and pedicle length requirements. When selecting a donor site, the vascular territory (i.e., the angiosome) supplied by the flap artery limits the amount of viable tissue that may be successfully transferred. The status of the recipient site is also assessed, including the effect that any previous treatment may have on the surrounding recipient tissue, the arteries, and the veins. Consideration is made of the possible need for vein grafts, which increase the complexity and risk for complications of free flap surgery.

A number of studies have analyzed the various patient factors that may be predictive of a poor outcome after head and neck microvascular surgery.[3–6,12–15] Haughey and colleagues[3] reviewed 241 free flap reconstructive cases. In his series, the flap survival rate was 95%, and the rate of major flap complications was 29%. Multivariate analysis revealed that cigarette smoking, two or more operating surgeons, and preoperative weight loss of more than 10% correlated with major flap complications. In Classen and colleagues'[4] series of 250 free flap operations, the major flap complication rate was 17.2%, and presence of comorbid medical conditions was the only factor with a statistically significant impact on the rate of major flap complications. Singh and colleagues[5] reviewed 200 free flaps of the head and neck and found a flap survival rate of 98% and a major complication rate of 28%. In their series, multivariate analysis found that an advanced grade on the Charlson comorbidity scale correlated with complications. In a consecutive series of 400 free flaps, Suh and colleagues[6] reported a flap survival rate of 99% and a reconstruction-related complication rate of 19%. Similar to Singh and colleagues, Suh and colleagues found a significant correlation between perioperative complications and preoperative comorbidity level as indicated by American Society of Anesthesiologists status.[6]

It should be emphasized that complications of free flap surgery of the head and neck in experienced hands are a rare event, with the previously described examples showing a flap failure rate of around 1% to 2% and a major flap complication rate of 17% to 28%. Other studies have demonstrated the reliability of free flap surgery even among the characteristics common to the head and neck cancer patient population.[12–15] Choi and colleagues[13] demonstrated that radiation therapy preoperatively did not affect local complication rates of free flap reconstruction for head and neck cancer. Head and colleagues[14] and Huang and colleagues[15] reported that previous neck dissection and the development of salivary fistulas do not increase the rate of flap failure. Beausang and colleagues[12] showed that, although medical complications are more frequent among older patients who undergo the free flap reconstruction of the head and neck, the rate of surgical complications in this group was similar to that of a younger patient population.

Certain donor sites may require additional specific preoperative testing. An Allen test to confirm the ability of the hand to tolerate the sacrifice of the radial artery is mandatory for forearm flaps. Similarly, the assessment of distal lower-extremity vascular flow through conventional angiography, magnetic resonance imaging, or computed tomography angiography is necessary for the preoperative evaluation of the fibula flap[16–18] (Figure 62-2).

Surgical Technique

The vast majority of head and neck free flap reconstructive surgery is performed for head and neck cancer. Ideally head and neck free flap reconstruction is done

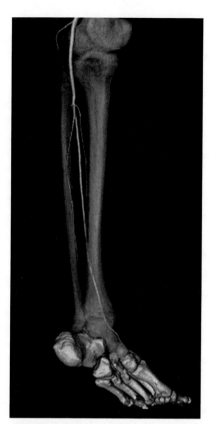

Figure 62-2. Preoperative angiography before fibula free flap harvest. Computed tomography angiography is performed to assess the adequacy of the lower-leg vasculature. It is critical that there be a sufficient vascular supply to the foot after the sacrifice of the peroneal artery during the harvest of the fibula flap.

with a two-team approach, with the reconstructive surgeon working simultaneously with the head and neck ablative team. This approach is generally more efficient and saves operative time. When the defect is known, the flap harvest is performed. The vascular pedicle is isolated but left intact to perfuse the flap. Great care is taken to avoid unnecessary stretching or otherwise traumatizing the flap pedicle vessels. The flap is allowed to perfuse along its native pedicle until the tumor resection is completed and the frozen section margin analysis is finished. The reconstructive surgeon may wish to begin preparing the recipient vessels in the neck while awaiting the frozen section results. Next, the flap pedicle is divided, and the flap is transferred to the head and neck defect. It is the authors' preference to first inset the flap, although this does lengthen the primary ischemia time. However, doing the flap inset first offers the following advantages: suturing during insetting is made easier in a nonbleeding flap; the final vessel pedicle geometry is known before the microvascular anastomosis is performed; and the movement or twisting of the vessels, which often occurs during flap inset, is avoided after microvascular anastomosis.

The preparation and suturing of the vessels are performed under the operating microscope. It is helpful when both the surgeon and the assistant are skilled with microsurgical technique. The adventitia is removed from the vessel ends, and the artery and the vein of the flap are separated from one another to allow for flexibility in the geometry of the anastomosis. The vessel lumens are instilled with heparinized saline or lactated Ringer solution. Either the artery or the vein can be anastomosed first. Sutures are meticulously placed, taking small, full-thickness bites of the vessel wall. The direct handling of the intima is avoided, and so is rough pulling or grasping of the vessel wall. An end-to-end or an end-to-side anastomosis may be performed, although the arterial anastomosis is typically end to end.

Postoperative Flap Monitoring and Management

Considerable variability exists among head and neck microvascular surgeons regarding postoperative management and free flap monitoring.[19–21] However, what all strategies share in common is an emphasis on vigilant direct clinical observation of the flap by physicians and nurses during the initial postoperative period. The ability to recognize the early signs of flap failure are critical, because a flap must be revised within hours of vascular occlusion for salvage surgery to be successful.[8,9,22]

The primary method of monitoring is through direct visual examination of the flap at the bedside. Observation is made regarding the flap's color, temperature, and capillary refill. Any changes in swelling or congestion of the flap are noted. Various additional methods of monitoring the flap are used by microvascular surgeons, including transcutaneous Doppler monitoring of the arterial flow, implantable Doppler monitoring, temperature probes, and green-light photoplethysmography.[19–21,23] Although all of these methods have some limitations, they offer the advantage of a simple tool, particularly for health personnel who are less experienced with free flap management. However, none of the currently available monitoring techniques can replace regular clinical evaluation by staff who are experienced with free flap care.

The frequency of flap monitoring is not uniformly practiced, and the optimal strategy is not definitively established.[19–21] However, most microvascular surgeons recommend that flap checks should occur at least every 1 to 2 hours for the first few postoperative days. The length of postoperative monitoring is similarly not clearly defined. The neovascularization of soft-tissue flaps certainly suggests that flap monitoring of the flap pedicle beyond 7 days is unnecessary. Furthermore, most vascular thromboses occur within the first 72 hours, and one study found that salvage surgery for flaps that develop thromboses after this time period have a very low chance for success, which suggests that frequent flap monitoring beyond postoperative day 4 may be unwarranted.[21]

Free flap failures during the initial postoperative period are primarily related to thrombosis of the arterial or venous anastomosis, and thus postoperative management specific to free flap care includes focusing on avoiding conditions known to increase the risk for vascular thrombosis. To avoid the mechanical compression of flap pedicle vessels, there is a strict avoidance of circumferential neck ties and close monitoring of the neck and neck drains for signs of hematoma or salivary leaks. Maintaining good intravascular flow dynamics with the pedicle vessels is also important. Most microvascular surgeons recommend maintaining the hematocrit level between 27% and 33% to reduce shear rate and platelet margination.[8] The use of intravascular pressors and excessive plasma-based blood products should be avoided postoperatively, if possible. Prophylactic anticoagulation is used routinely in postoperative free flap patients by most surgeons. However, there is no consensus regarding the type of anticoagulation used.[8,24] Example regimens include intravenous heparin, low-molecular-weight dextran, and aspirin. There is no evidence that clearly demonstrates the superiority of any of these methods for preventing postoperative flap vessel thrombosis.[24] However, the minimal side effects of low-dose daily aspirin have made it one of the more commonly used anticoagulation methods.

MANAGEMENT OF THE COMPROMISED FREE FLAP

Large series of head and neck free flap surgery indicate that 8% to 11% of cases require reexploration for threatened flap viability.[3–6] Venous obstruction is a more common cause of free flap compromise than arterial obstruction.[8,11] The reported salvage rate with surgical reexploration varies from 19% to 100%, with a recent analysis of 192 threatened flaps revealing a successful salvage rate of 41%.[19,22,25]

Arterial Insufficiency

The signs that are indicative of arterial insufficiency include a pale flap color, no bleeding with a pinprick of the flap, a loss of Doppler signal, and a cool temperature. However, it must be stressed that the presence of a Doppler signal does not preclude the possibility of arterial thrombosis. A pulse may be transmitted through the thrombus, the signal may be coming from a different artery (e.g., the external or internal carotid artery), or there may be problems with the vasculature distal to the location measured by the Doppler. The management of arterial insufficiency is immediate reexploration.

Venous Insufficiency

The signs that are indicative of venous insufficiency include an initial increased rubor in the flap with decreased capillary refill followed by a mottled or blue flap color. Initially there is dark and immediate bleeding with a pinprick; later, when venous insufficiency leads to arterial insufficiency, there is no bleeding with a pinprick. The Doppler signal may initially be near normal; it will then become biphasic and, later, absent. Untreated venous obstruction leads over time to arterial obstruction. The initial management of venous insufficiency is typically immediate reexploration.

Pedicle Thrombosis

In situations of threatened flap viability as a result of pedicle thrombosis, the wound is immediately reexplored. The anastomosis site is inspected visually and with a Doppler to determine whether the thrombosis is in the artery, the vein, or both. Microsurgical reanastomosis to a nonthrombosed portion of the vessel may need to be performed. It is not uncommon that the flap vessels must be cut back significantly to a point where no thrombus exists, and vein grafts may be necessary. Selective thrombolytic therapy with streptokinase, urokinase, tissue plasminogen activator, or other antithrombolytic agents may be used.

Medicinal Leech Therapy

Medicinal leech therapy is indicated in cases of surgically unsalvageable venous obstruction.[25] The *Hirudo medicinalis* species of leeches is used. The effectiveness of medicinal leech therapy for relieving venous congestion is the result of both mechanical and biologic effects. Each leech directly and indirectly extracts 25 ml to 65 ml of blood from the flap (Figure 62-3). Its saliva contains a host of coagulation and platelet aggregation inhibitors as well as histamine, collagenases,

and hyaluronidases. These facilitate the local infiltration of the leech's antithrombotic mediators into the congested tissue. Thus leech therapy addresses both the venous pedicle outflow obstruction and the microcirculation. Importantly, because the bacterium *Aeromonas hydrophila* resides in the leech gut, an infection rate of 7% to 20% is expected with leech therapy; infection related to leech therapy can also contribute to flap failure. Thus antibiotic prophylaxis for patients undergoing medicinal leech therapy is mandatory, usually with ciprofloxacin and a second-generation cephalosporin. Patients undergoing leech therapy must be kept in the intensive care unit for close hemodynamic monitoring. There is frequently a high blood transfusion requirement. All members of the health care staff, the patient, and the patient's family must be educated regarding the medical, cultural, and psychologic issues related to medicinal leech therapy.

Future Directions

Future directions in the management of the compromised flap include the potential use of free radical scavengers, antioxidant solutions, or other agents to protect against ischemia and reperfusion injury.[26–30] A few preclinical studies have demonstrated limited tissue protection from prolonged ischemia with several of these agents.[28–30] However, none to date have found widespread clinical use.

DONOR-SITE COMPLICATIONS

Additional complications after head and neck free flap surgery can occur related to the flap donor site. These complication risks may be minimized through thoughtful

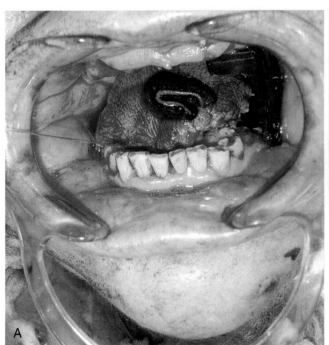

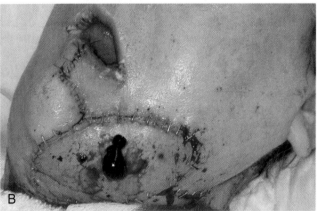

Figure 62-3. Leech therapy for free flap venous obstruction. **A,** A medicinal leech is being used to treat venous obstruction in this radial forearm flap reconstruction performed for a glossectomy defect. **B,** Medicinal leeches were applied after the skin island component of this scapula flap became congested. The main pedicle and the osseous component of the scapula flap had normal vascular flow.

patient and donor-site selection as well as careful perioperative management. Donor-site–specific complications related to the more commonly used free flaps for head and neck reconstruction are described in this section.

Radial Forearm Flaps

The radial forearm flap is one of the most common free flaps used today for head and neck reconstruction as a result of its thin, pliable nature; its long, vascular pedicle; and its ease of harvest. Sacrifice of the radial artery is generally well tolerated as long as an Allen test is performed preoperatively. Should the Allen test be abnormal or equivocal, the contralateral forearm or another donor site should be used. The forearm donor site generally requires skin grafting, which can result in wound-healing complications (Figure 62-4). Even a well-healed skin graft can be a cause of complaint because of the cosmetic appearance of this visible area of the arm. Splinting the volar surface of the forearm for a period of 1 to 4 weeks will increase the likelihood of adequate skin-graft healing. The use of compressive silicone dressings after this will maximize the cosmetic outcome of the skin graft site as well. Alternatively, the use of full-thickness skin grafts from the groin may improve the cosmetic outcome.[31] Other complications of this flap include numbness of the arm and thumb as a result of the sacrifice of the median antebrachial cutaneous nerve or unintentional injury to the superficial sensory branches of the radial nerve. Injury or paresis to the median nerve should be rare. When the harvest of the radius bone is included in this flap, the risk of pathologic fracture increases, although recent reports suggest that, with appropriate operative technique and postoperative management, this risk may be minimized.[32,33]

Anterolateral Thigh Flaps

First used widely in Asia, the anterolateral thigh flap has become increasingly popular in recent years in North America.[34–36] It is typically used as a perforator-based fasciocutaneous flap with a vascular supply that comes from the descending branch of the lateral circumflex femoral artery. Its advantages include a long

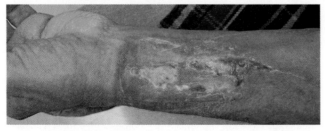

Figure 62-4. Forearm flap donor site with a partial skin graft loss. The skin-graft coverage of this radial forearm flap donor site suffered partial breakdown with tendon exposure. Immobilization of the forearm with a splint can reduce the incidence of this occurrence.

and vascular pedicle the potential for a larger skin island and more bulk than with the radial forearm flap. Usually one can close the donor site primarily without a cosmetically unsightly skin graft, and the donor site is in a less visible part of the body. The challenge of variability in the perforator vessel anatomy of this flap has become less problematic as surgeon experience with the anterolateral thigh flap increases. Because the arterial pedicle supply to this flap is not a major vessel of the lower extremity, there is little concern for vascular compromise in the donor leg postoperatively. Complications from this flap are rare.[34–36] Meticulous dissection to preserve the motor nerve to the vastus lateralis, which accompanies the main vascular pedicle to the flap, should avoid potential problems with leg motor function.

Latissimus Dorsi Flaps

Based on the thoracodorsal artery, this flap may be used as a muscle-only or a myocutaneous flap. It provides a broad, large muscle, and it is particularly useful for near-total or total scalp reconstruction.[37] The unilateral loss of latissimus dorsi muscle function is generally tolerated by most patients, although it could be problematic for individuals whose work or athletic interests require this muscle's function. During the harvest of this flap, it is important to avoid injury to surrounding neurovascular structures such as the long thoracic nerve, the brachial plexus, and the axillary vessels. Other complications that can occur with the use of latissimus dorsi flaps include the occurrence of postoperative wound seroma and lymphedema of the upper arm. Many of the complications described for the latissimus flap may be avoided by employing nerve-sparing, perforator-based flaps.[38]

Rectus Abdominis Flaps

The vascular supply of the rectus abdominis flap is the inferior epigastric artery, which can be up to 15 cm long and is of wide diameter. For this reason, this flap is frequently used for larger anterior skull-base defects.[39] The substantial volume provided by this myocutaneous flap is also frequently used for total glossectomy defects.[40] The major donor site complication that may be associated with the rectus abdominis flap is the development of ventral abdominal hernias.[39,40] The risk for this complication can be minimized with the careful closure of the abdominal wall. The posterior rectus sheath is robust above the arcuate line, and its closure should prevent ventral hernia formation. However, inferior to the arcuate line, the posterior sheath is absent, and careful reconstruction of the anterior rectus sheath inferior to the arcuate line is essential. In certain situations, the use of a synthetic mesh may be indicated. With appropriate attention given to donor-site closure, recent studies of this flap have described a very low risk for hernia formation, and this flap continues to find widespread use in head and neck reconstruction.[6,40] The ever-increasing use of perforator-based rectus free flaps has further reduced the donor-site morbidity rate, because large portions of the rectus sheath and muscle are preserved.

Fibula Flaps

The fibula flap has become one of the most popular flaps for oromandibular reconstruction that requires vascularized bone. Its advantages include a fairly long pedicle (i.e., peroneal artery) of large diameter, and an abundance of bone is available (i.e., up to 20 cm) to permit angle-to-angle mandible reconstruction. The bone may also be contoured with multiple osteotomies to precisely reconstruct the mandible profile, with adequate vascularity available for individual bone segments, because the main pedicle runs parallel to the bone itself. The major limitation of this flap is its associated skin flap, which has a variable blood supply and which may demonstrate viability issues in approximately 5% to 10% of cases.[41] The skin flap associated with the fibula may also not provide sufficient volume, area, or flexibility for more complex composite defects that require large volumes of soft tissue. The sacrifice of the peroneal artery should be well tolerated as long as the vascular anatomy and flow of the lower extremity and foot are preoperatively evaluated. The development of magnetic resonance imaging and computed tomography angiography allows for the accurate, noninvasive assessment of the lower-extremity vascular anatomy without the need for conventional angiography, and one of these tests should always be performed.[16–18] Atherosclerotic disease may be present in the lower-leg vessels. Although this is usually not problematic, severe peripheral vascular disease in combination with an overly tight wound closure or splint dressing can lead to tissue necrosis of the donor site in rare instances[42] (Figure 62-5). The segmental resection of fibula bone is also generally well tolerated, with a minimal impact on the gait. It is important to preserve about 6 cm to 7 cm of bone at both the proximal and

distal ends of the fibula to maintain the stability of the ankle and knee joints. Other reported complications of the fibula donor site include footdrop and weakness in the dorsiflexion of the great toe.[43] These problems likely occur as a result of damage to the extensor hallucis longus muscle or the peroneal nerve. When a skin island is harvested with the fibula bone, a skin graft may be required for donor-site closure, and donor-site morbidity related to skin grafting can also occur.

Scapula Flaps

Based on the circumflex scapular artery and vein, the scapula flap can be used as a soft-tissue–only flap or as an osseocutaneous flap, providing up to 10 cm of vascularized bone. Because the scapula flap contains an independent pedicle supply to its osseous and skin island component, there is great flexibility with this flap in complex composite defects, which is a major advantage for oromandibular reconstruction. However, the disadvantages of the use of this flap include difficult patient positioning for flap harvest that makes a two-team approach challenging and a thinner bone stock than the fibula flap when used for mandibular defects. In addition, shoulder dysfunction, particularly with arm abduction and external rotation, can occur after osseocutaneous scapula flaps.[44] Physical therapy should be given to limit functional morbidity related to this donor site. Pathologic fracture of the scapula after free bone harvest should be rare.

Iliac Crest Flaps

Osseous, osseocutaneous, and osseomusculocutaneous iliac crest flaps are possible for head and neck microvascular reconstruction. Iliac crest flaps are based on the deep circumflex iliac artery and vein, and the iliac crest can provide up to 14 cm of vascularized bone. The bone stock of the iliac crest is wider and thicker than fibula bone, and it is the only vascularized bone that can completely restore anterior mandibular height in the dentate patient. The internal oblique muscle and the overlying skin may be used to provide soft-tissue reconstruction. However, the main disadvantages of this flap relate to the risk of donor-site–related complications. There may be significant bleeding from the bony donor site, which can lead to postoperative hematoma formation. More long-term postoperative donor-site complications of this flap include persistent hip pain, lateral femoral cutaneous nerve hypesthesia, and ventral herniation.[44] Meticulous donor-site closure can reduce the risk for hernias, but they are still a consideration, particularly among younger patients, who will likely remain physically active, as well as among older patients, who may have weakened abdominal-wall tissues. Many surgeons routinely use synthetic mesh or other biomaterials to reinforce this closure and to decrease the risk of herniation.

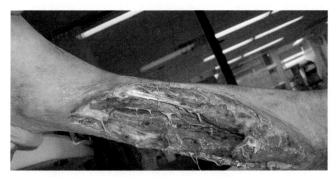

Figure 62-5. Fibula flap donor-site necrosis. Severe peripheral vascular disease in combination with an overly tight wound closure can rarely lead to extensive tissue necrosis of the fibula flap donor site. Careful patient selection, the use of skin grafts, and the avoidance of compressive splints can minimize the risk of this dreaded complication.

CONCLUSION

Free-tissue transfer techniques for head and neck reconstruction provide excellent functional and cosmetic rehabilitative outcomes for most patients who are undergoing ablative surgery for advanced head and neck cancer. A thorough understanding of the basic concepts and physiology of free flap surgery as well as appropriate preoperative planning, meticulous surgical technique, and vigilant postoperative management can minimize the risk for free flap failure and donor-site complications.

REFERENCES

1. Chepeha DB, Wang SJ, Marentette LJ, et al: Radial forearm free-tissue transfer reduces complications in salvage skull base surgery. *Otolaryngol Head Neck Surg* 2004;131(6):958–963.
2. Teknos TN, Myers LL, Bradford CR, et al: Free tissue reconstruction of the hypopharynx after organ preservation therapy: Analysis of wound complications. *Laryngoscope* 2001;111(7):1192–1196.
3. Haughey BH, Wilson E, Kluwe L, et al: Free flap reconstruction of the head and neck: Analysis of 241 cases. *Otolaryngol Head Neck Surg* 2001;125(1):10–17.
4. Classen DA, Ward H: Complications in a consecutive series of 250 free flap operations. *Ann Plast Surg* 2006;56(5):557–561.
5. Singh B, Cordeiro PG, Santamaria E, et al: Factors associated with complications in microvascular reconstruction of head and neck defects. *Plast Reconstr Surg* 1999;103(2):403–411.
6. Suh JD, Sercarz JA, Abemayor E, et al: Analysis of outcome and complications in 400 cases of microvascular head and neck reconstruction. *Arch Otolaryngol Head Neck Surg* 2004;130(8):962–966.
7. Seidenberg B: Immediate reconstruction of the cervical esophagus by a revascularized isolated jejunal segment. *Ann Surg* 1959;149(2):162–171.
8. Esclamado RM, Carroll WR: The pathogenesis of vascular thrombosis and its impact in microvascular surgery. *Head Neck* 1999;21(4):355–362.
9. Carroll WR, Esclamado RM: Ischemia/reperfusion injury in microvascular surgery. *Head Neck* 2000;22(7):700–713.
10. Siemionow M, Arslan E: Ischemia/reperfusion injury: A review in relation to free-tissue transfers. *Microsurgery* 2004;24(6):468–475.
11. Kubo T, Yano K, Hosokawa K: Management of flaps with compromised venous outflow in head and neck microsurgical reconstruction. *Microsurgery* 2002;22(8):391–395.
12. Beausang ES, Ang EE, Lipa JE, et al: Microvascular free-tissue transfer in elderly patients: The Toronto experience. *Head Neck* 2003;25(7):549–553.
13. Choi S, Schwartz DL, Farwell DG, et al: Radiation therapy does not impact local complication rates after free flap reconstruction for head and neck cancer. *Arch Otolaryngol Head Neck Surg* 2004;130(11):1308–1312.
14. Head C, Sercarz JA, Abemayor E, et al: Microvascular reconstruction after previous neck dissection. *Arch Otolaryngol Head Neck Surg* 2002;128(3):328–331.
15. Huang RY, Sercarz JA, Smith J, et al: Effect of salivary fistulas on free flap failure: A laboratory and clinical investigation. *Laryngoscope* 2005;115(3):517–521.
16. Seres L, Csaszar J, Voros E, et al: Donor site angiography before mandibular reconstruction with fibula free flap. *J Craniofac Surg* 2001;12(6):608–613.
17. Lorenz RR, Esclamado R: Preoperative magnetic resonance angiography in fibular-free flap reconstruction of head and neck defects. *Head Neck* 2001;23(10):844–850.
18. Karanas YL, Antony A, Rubin G, et al: Preoperative CT angiography for free fibula transfer. *Microsurgery* 2004;24(2):125–127.
19. Hirigoyen MB, Urken ML, Weinberg H: Free flap monitoring: a review of current practice. *Microsurgery* 1995;16(11):723–726.
20. Disa JJ, Cordeiro PG, Hidalgo DA: Efficacy of conventional monitoring techniques in free-tissue transfer: An 11-year experience in 750 consecutive cases. 1999;104(1):97–101.
21. Jallali N, Ridha H, Butler PE: Postoperative monitoring of free flaps in UK plastic surgery units. *Microsurgery* 2005;25(6):469–472.
22. Hidalgo DA, Jones CS: The role of emergent exploration in free-tissue transfer: A review of 150 consecutive cases. *Plast Reconstr Surg* 1990;86(3):492–498.
23. Futran ND, Stack BC Jr, Hollenbeak C, et al: Green light photoplethysmography monitoring of free flaps. *Arch Otolaryngol Head Neck Surg* 2000;126(5):659–662.
24. Chien W, Varvares MA, Hadlock T, et al: Effects of aspirin and low-dose heparin in head and neck reconstruction using microvascular free flaps. *Laryngoscope* 2005;115(6):973–976.
25. Chepeha DB, Nussenbaum B, Bradford CR, et al: Leech therapy for patients with surgically unsalvageable venous obstruction after revascularized free-tissue transfer. *Arch Otolaryngol Head Neck Surg* 2002;128(8):960–965.
26. Prada FS, Arrunategui G, Alves MC, et al: Effect of allopurinol, superoxide-dismutase, and hyperbaric oxygen on flap survival. *Microsurgery* 2002;22(8):352–360.
27. Kuo YR, Wang FS, Jeng SF, et al: Nitrosoglutathione promotes flap survival via suppression of reperfusion injury-induced superoxide and inducible nitric oxide synthase induction. *J Trauma* 2004;57(5):1025–1031.
28. Hom DB, Goding GS Jr, Price JA, et al: The effects of conjugated deferoxamine in porcine skin flaps. *Head Neck* 2000;22(6):579–584.
29. Hsu OK, Gabr E, Steward E, et al: Pharmacologic enhancement of rat skin flap survival with topical oleic acid. *Plast Reconstr Surg* 2004;113(7):2048–2054.
30. Tomur A, Etlik O, Gundogan NU: Hyperbaric oxygenation and antioxidant vitamin combination reduces ischemia-reperfusion injury in a rat epigastric island skin-flap model. *J Basic Clin Physiol Pharmacol* 2005;16(4):275–285.
31. Kim TB, Moe K, Eisele DW, et al: Full-thickness skin graft from the groin for coverage of the radial forearm free flap donor site. *Am J Otolaryngol* 2007;28(5):325–329.
32. Werle AH, Tsue TT, Toby EB, et al: Osteocutaneous radial forearm free flap: Its use without significant donor site morbidity. *Otolaryngol Head Neck Surg* 2000;123(6):711–717.
33. Militsakh ON, Werle A, Mohyuddin N, et al: Comparison of radial forearm with fibula and scapula osteocutaneous free flaps for oromandibular reconstruction. *Arch Otolaryngol Head Neck Surg* 2005;131(7):571–575.
34. Shieh SJ, Chiu HY, Yu JC, et al: Free anterolateral thigh flap for reconstruction of head and neck defects following cancer ablation. *Plast Reconstr Surg* 2000;105(7):2349–2357.
35. Makitie AA, Beasley NJ, Neligan PC, et al: Head and neck reconstruction with anterolateral thigh flap. *Otolaryngol Head Neck Surg* 2003;129(5):547–555.
36. Lin DT, Coppit GL, Burkey BB: Use of the anterolateral thigh flap for reconstruction of the head and neck. *Curr Opin Otolaryngol Head Neck Surg* 2004;12(4):300–304.
37. Lipa JE, Butler CE: Enhancing the outcome of free latissimus dorsi muscle flap reconstruction of scalp defects. *Head Neck* 2004;26(1):46–53.
38. Kim JT: Two options for perforator flaps in the flank donor site: Latissimus dorsi and thoracodorsal perforator flaps. *Plast Reconstr Surg* 2005;115(3):755–763.
39. Potparic Z, Starovic B: Reconstruction of extensive defects of the cranium using free-tissue transfer. *Head Neck* 1993;15(2):97–104.
40. Rosenthal E, Carroll W, Dobbs M, et al: Simplifying head and neck microvascular reconstruction. *Head Neck* 2004;26(11):930–936.
41. Schusterman MA, Reece GP, Miller MJ, et al: The osteocutaneous free fibula flap: Is the skin paddle reliable? *Plast Reconstr Surg* 1992;90(5):787–793.
42. Klein S, Hage JJ, Woerdeman LA: Donor-site necrosis following fibula free-flap transplantation: A report of three cases. *Microsurgery* 2005;25(7):538–542.
43. Zimmermann CE, Borner BI, Hasse A, et al: Donor site morbidity after microvascular fibula transfer. *Clin Oral Investig* 2001;5(4):214–219.
44. Hartman EH, Spauwen PH, Jansen JA: Donor-site complications in vascularized bone flap surgery. *J Invest Surg* 2002;15(4):185–197.

CHAPTER 63

Complications of Skin, Cartilage, and Bone Grafts

Vicente A. Resto and Daniel G. Deschler

Free grafts provide an important method for the reconstruction of head and neck defects. Their ease of harvest and inset as well as the low associated donor-site morbidity make them appealing for use. More importantly, they often provide the best structural and cosmetic tissue match for the reconstruction of facial defects. However, their successful use requires adherence to meticulous technique and exquisite donor site and tissue selection for each defect to be reconstructed. Free grafts that are available for structural defect reconstruction in the head and neck include split-thickness skin grafts, full-thickness skin grafts, fat grafts, cartilage grafts, and bone grafts. The misapplication of these will ensure poor functional and cosmetic results.

Free grafts, by definition, are avascular. As such, they require a well-vascularized and healthy recipient bed for survival. The physiology of engraftment has been best delineated for split-thickness skin grafts,[1] but its basic premise applies to all free grafts. Harvested free grafts must be maintained in a moist environment and transplanted to their recipient site as soon as possible. This ensures graft cell viability, which is critical for successful engraftment and for the integration of the transplanted tissue, which is known as *graft take.* The first 48 hours of engraftment are marked by graft swelling and fibrin deposition. The process of plasmatic imbibition supports nutrition.[2,3] Neovascularization begins approximately 48 to 72 hours after transplant. This process combines the full growth of new vessels as well as the growth of new vascular buds that connect into the established subdermal plexus of the graft, which is a process known as *inosculation.*[4,5] It is the latter process that allows for true vascular circulation with associated nutrient exchange. Thereafter healing continues with the further deposition of fibrinous matrix and the eventual maturation of graft anchorage (Figure 63-1). This process takes months to complete, and it is accompanied by wound contracture and remodeling. For this process to occur efficiently and to ensure long-term graft cell viability, several technical maneuvers must be applied. First, graft apposition to the transplant bed must be excellent.[1] Any accumulation of fluid or tenting that leads to graft–bed separation will inhibit graft–bed nutrient exchange and lead to graft necrosis. Second, graft fixation must be firm. Shear between the graft and the recipient bed will inhibit the process of vascular ingrowth, thus hampering graft viability and take.[1] Third, graft size needs to be maintained within a range that allows for adequate initial plasmatic imbibition.[1] In general, plasmatic imbibition will occur efficiently within 0.5 cm from a vascularized interphase.[3] Thus all aspects of a free graft must be within 0.5 cm from a vascularized recipient site. Deviations from these basic principles will lead to higher rates of complications and a failure of graft take (Figure 63-2).

SPLIT-THICKNESS SKIN GRAFTS

Application

Split-thickness skin grafts are composed of full-thickness epidermis and partial-thickness dermis, and they most commonly range in thickness between 0.015 inches and 0.20 inches. They provide ample donor tissue with very good pliability, thus lending themselves to cover large defects with complex topography. The thin quality of these grafts enhances imbibition and graft take, with resultant success rates of more than 90%.[6] There can be significant contracture in the long term.[7] Color match is usually adequate, but there is often a significant difference in tissue quality as compared with adjacent skin tissue. This difference is highlighted by the inherent lack of bulk associated with split-thickness skin grafts.

Harvest Sites

The most common harvest sites for use with head and neck reconstruction are the thigh and the medial aspect of the arm. Harvest is most commonly performed with a hydraulic or electric dermatome.[8] These instruments allow for the definition of size and thickness by applying the requisite blade template and setting the angle of the blade. The graft donor site heals by secondary intention, with reepithelialization occurring from residual epidermal tissue within adnexal structures left in the deep dermis. The maintenance of a moist wound enhances healing. This is most often achieved with the application of an adhesive occlusive dressing or a petrolatum-based aerated dressing.[9]

Complications

Complications associated with split-thickness graft harvest are associated with the care given to the donor site.[10] Most commonly there will be discoloration that is made worse by sun exposure. Donor-site infection can also result in poor healing and secondary scarring. If too

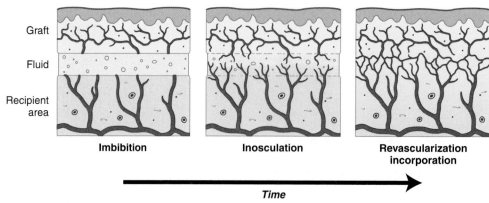

Graft		
Fluid		
Recipient area		
Imbibition	**Inosculation**	**Revascularization incorporation**

Time

Figure 63-1. Physiology of avascular donor tissue engraftment. During the early stages of graft tissue transfer, the nutrient exchange that is necessary for graft survival is primarily driven by imbibition. Inosculation, or the ingrowth of graft-bed vessels into the graft, leads to the reestablishment of early graft blood flow by connecting the native graft vasculature to the sprouting donor bed vasculature. Engraftment culminates with incorporation, which is the process of neovascularization, extracellular matrix deposition, and maturation that leads to the stable anchoring of the transplanted tissue.

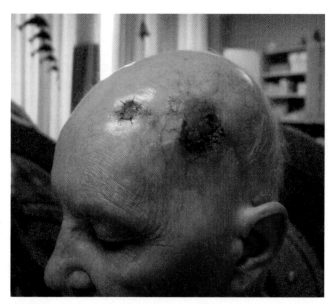

Figure 63-2. Failed skin graft. The patient was treated with split-thickness skin grafting for a moderate-sized scalp defect, with a resulting failure of the engraftment as a result of a poorly vascularized recipient bed.

thick of a graft is taken, there can be insufficient viable epidermal appendages left within the donor site wound bed to allow for rapid reepithelialization, which leads to prolonged healing and granulation tissue formation. Infection complicates the donor site in 3% of cases.[9] These problems are usually avoided by the careful selection of graft thickness, meticulous wound care, and the avoidance of sun exposure until healing is complete.[11]

Graft Take

Graft take can likewise be hampered by factors that affect the recipient site.[12] Most importantly, the wound must be clean.[13] If there has been significant granulation

over the recipient site, it must be debrided to viable healthy tissue. Active bacterial colonization will inhibit wound healing and revascularization. The transplanted split-thickness skin graft must be fully apposed to the wound bed. This is enhanced by ensuring excellent hemostasis before the application of the graft as well as adequate graft immobilization, usually by applying a bolster dressing.[14] The accumulation of fluid can be further prevented by judiciously making slits in the graft (i.e., pie-crusting) to allow for the egress of fluid and to prevent loculation. If the graft is applied over a dynamic wound bed such as a joint or an exposed muscle, the recipient site must be immobilized so as to not interfere with revascularization. This can usually be accomplished by splinting the associated area. Recently vacuum-sealed dressings have been successfully applied to promote graft immobilization as well as to enhance epithelialization.[15] Should graft take be incomplete, wound care is usually sufficient to allow for complete healing via granulation and reepithelialization (Figure 63-3). In some cases, the unhealed areas must be regrafted. The careful application of these principles allows for the use of these grafts for the reconstruction of difficult sites (e.g., the oral cavity), with great success.[16]

FULL-THICKNESS SKIN GRAFTING

Application

Full-thickness skin grafts are composed of epidermis, dermis, and subcutaneous tissue. Like split-thickness skin grafts, they provide tissue with great pliability, which is useful for the reconstruction of defects with complex contours. However, their increased thickness resists contracture and reconstructs defect volume better than split-thickness skin grafts. Full-thickness grafts also have the advantage of including epidermal appendages that further contribute to texture match.[7] These

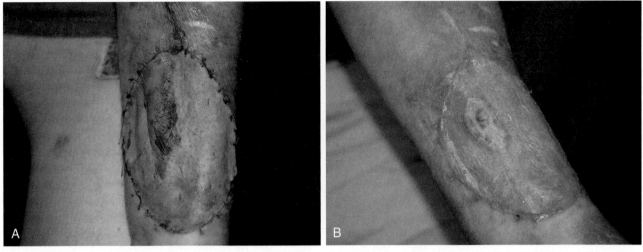

Figure 63-3. Partial split-thickness graft failure. **A,** A radial forearm free flap donor-site defect was treated with split-thickness skin grafting. Postoperative follow up at 1 week revealed a partial failure of engraftment, likely as a result of localized poor graft-to-bed approximation. **B,** The wound was treated with wet-to-dry dressings for 3 weeks, which resulted in complete healing.

qualities will afford improved contour to the reconstructed site after they have healed.[17] Donor sites can be chosen that best approximate facial skin coloration, with resulting excellent color-match results. However, their increased thickness is less conducive to the plasmatic imbibition that is critical for graft survival during the first 48 to 72 hours. For this reason, full-thickness skin grafts are generally restricted in their size. Also, because of their inclusion of full-thickness epidermis and dermis, the donor site wound will not generally heal spontaneously and thus requires primary closure. This requirement limits the available sites to those with sufficient skin laxity to allow for advancement and primary closure. This process will always result in a scar.

Full-thickness skin grafts have been found to have a great application for the reconstruction of the full-thickness facial skin defects associated with skin cancer resection. They have been particularly applied to the reconstruction of external nasal defects, because the transfer of adjacent tissues can often result in the introduction of additional highly visible scars, facial distortion, and ectropion. However, lackluster results have been reported when full-thickness skin grafts have been used for the reconstruction of intraoral defects: 23% of cases may develop graft necrosis.[18]

Harvest Sites

The most common sites of harvest are the preauricular skin, the postauricular skin, the neck, and the supraclavicular fossa. These sites provide excellent skin color matching as well as texture that closely approximates that of facial skin. In addition, these sites provide ample skin for mobilization and primary closure while also providing cosmetically tolerant sites within which to place the resultant incisions.

Complications

Complications associated with full-thickness skin grafting are very similar to those seen with split-thickness skin grafting. At the donor site, inadequate sterile technique or poor wound care can lead to infection and associated poor healing and increased scarring. These wounds can be at increased risk for this complication given the relative hypoperfusion that can result from closure under tension. It is thus critical that closure at the donor site be associated with sufficient adjacent tissue mobilization to prevent this. Should infection ensue, it should be treated with antibiotics, wound debridement, and irrigation as needed. These wounds are also at risk for hematoma formation, because vessels within the subcutaneous layer are breeched during harvest. Meticulous hemostasis is thus as important as it is for any other surgical wound. The presence of a hematoma will be associated with pain, discoloration, and fullness at the donor site. Hematoma at the donor site should be managed by drainage and irrigation. The wound should be examined for any bleeders and then reclosed. There may rarely be a need for drain placement in the wound to address potential seroma formation with larger donor sites.

Recipient-Site Complications

Recipient-site complications are generally associated with poor graft take and resulting total or partial graft necrosis. As with split-thickness skin grafts, full-thickness grafts must be inset into a clean wound. Any evidence of infection must be first treated by debridement and irrigation. In this setting, grafting ideally should be delayed. A recipient site with significant granulation should also be cleaned of any devitalized tissue. Failure to do so could lead to inefficient vascular ingrowth and graft failure. Failure can also be associated with the graft itself. As previously mentioned, graft size is important. Any portion of a full-thickness graft that is more than 0.5 cm removed from its vascularized recipient bed interface may have poor imbibition and secondary graft necrosis.[1] For this reason, it is customary to remove as much of the subcutaneous tissue as possible; this enhances dermal and epidermal proximity to the recipient bed. As for split-thickness grafts, poor graft-to-recipient contact, too much shear, or grafting onto a poorly vascularized recipient bed will be inhibitory to vascular ingrowth and thus lead to failure. Bolstering, site immobilization, and proper wound pregrafting preparation can address these factors, respectively. Partial graft failure can be managed conservatively with dressing changes and eventual healing by secondary intention. If the defect associated with the failed portion of the graft is too large, thus risking unsightly scarring, it can be regrafted. The failed take of an initial graft does not portend the failure of a second graft, as long as any identifiable factors contributing to the failure of take have been corrected.

FAT GRAFTING

Application

The dependability and versatility of free fat grafts are readily demonstrated by the wide use of these grafts for head and neck reconstruction.[19,20] As with all free grafts, success depends on the placement of the transferred adipose tissue into a stable and well-vascularized recipient bed. The tissue must undergo a similar process of revascularization for successful engraftment and long-term viability. Because free fat grafts are often designed to provide bulk, portions of the graft may be at some distance from the vascularized recipient bed. Therefore these areas are prone to cell death and resorption. For this reason, larger fat grafts are often overcorrected from 35% to 50% to account for such resorption.[21]

Large Dermal-Fat Grafts

Conley and Clairmont[22] described the use of large dermal-fat grafts for facial recontouring after tumor resection. However, success was limited by the often poor quality of radiated recipient beds. Large-volume fat grafts have also been described for recontouring after parotidectomy surgery, with good success.[21,23] Again, overcorrection is essential, and so is the presence of well-vascularized skin flaps. This technique also demonstrates success for the prevention of Frey syndrome.[21,24] Large grafts are also used extensively in otology for the obliteration of mastoid and temporal bone defects after lateral skull-base surgery.[25] Hardy and Montgomery[26] presented an extensive experience of successfully using large free fat grafts for frontal sinus obliteration. Dedo[27] described their use for pseudocord bulking in the setting of hemilaryngeal surgery.

Small Free Fat Grafts

Small free fat grafts can be injected into various sites for bulking purposes.[28] Cosmetically these have been used to plump the lips or to lessen facial creases. In laryngology, fat injections are used in the setting of vocal-fold paresis or presbylaryngis with the subsequent loss of bulk. Although smaller in size, these injected grafts are still prone to resorption.

Harvest Sites

The donor sites for free fat grafts are quite readily available. Smaller-volume grafts can be obtained with liposuction techniques, with the associated potential complications of hematoma, ecchymoses, dimpling, and anesthesia-related issues. Large grafts are often obtained from the abdominal and thigh regions. Periumbilical approaches provide excellent camouflaging of the incision, but care must be taken to avoid inadvertent entry into the umbilicus or the discovery of an associated abdominal hernia. As always, attention to hemostasis to avoid hematoma formation is critical. The main alternative abdominal site is the left lower quadrant. The left is chosen over the right so that the resultant scar is not misinterpreted as an appendectomy incision. If significant previous abdominal surgery is noted, then it may be prudent to choose an alternate site. Large dermal-fat grafts can be obtained from the groin regions with good masking of the donor-site incision. Wound drainage may be required if a significant dead space is encountered after harvest to avoid seroma or hematoma formation. Finally, some dysesthesia may be noted in the regions of larger harvests.

Recipient-Site Complications

Recipient-site complications associated with free fat grafts are primarily infectious or related to resorption and the subsequent lack of desired reconstructive effect. Although fat-grafted regions will often demonstrate some degree of erythema of the overlying skin, an infected site will be warm and ballottable with the suggestion of underlying fluid rather than the originally placed soft tissue. If purulence is noted, it is diagnostic of graft infection. In some cases, a needle aspiration is required. Although antibiotic therapy will be beneficial, wound drainage is required, and such frank infections usually result in complete liquefaction and the loss of the graft. Regrafting can be reattempted at a later date. The prevention of infection is essential. Sterile technique must be maintained, and an avoidance of placing grafts through a contaminated field (e.g., the mouth) is advised. Soaking the free fat graft in an antibiotic irrigation before placement may also be of some benefit. However, even without an infectious cause, fat grafts may undergo an aseptic liquefaction that similarly requires drainage and that will result in the loss of desired bulk.

Such events can be noted in parotid and temporal bone reconstructions.

CARTILAGE GRAFTING

Application

The primary application of cartilage grafts is to provide soft-tissue support for sites in which gravity, wound contracture, or tissue laxity may lead to undesirable cosmesis or function. In the head and neck, cartilage grafts are most often used in nasal surgery for functional conditions (e.g., nasal valve collapse) as well as for cosmetic applications (e.g., increasing tip projection in rhinoplasty).[29] Cartilage is also frequently used in microtia repair to provide the reconstructive scaffold of the new pinnae as well as for eyelid, orbital floor, skullbase, and laryngotracheal reconstruction.[30-34] The ease of harvest and handling has made cartilage grafting a mainstay of the modern facial plastic, rhinologic, and laryngologic surgeon.

Harvest Sites

The most common sites of harvest are the septum, the concha of the ear, and, in pediatric cases, the ribs.[35] These sites are similar in that they tolerate the removal of significant quantities of cartilage with minimal resulting functional or cosmetic defects. However, they differ with regard to the type of cartilage that they provide. The septum and ribs contain hyaline cartilage, whereas the ear contains elastic cartilage. They also differ with regard to their corresponding composition of type 2 collagen versus type 2 collagen with elastic fibers, respectively. Elastic cartilage is softer and more malleable than hyaline cartilage. Irrespective of type, cartilage is made up mostly of secreted extracellular matrix with a relative hypocellular component that receives its nutrients by diffusion, because cartilage is devoid of vessels. For this reason, the harvest and transplant of cartilage tissue often results in the loss of chondrocyte viability. Notwithstanding, cartilage grafts retain their structural integrity, because it is mainly derived from the acellular matrix elements.

Complications

Infection and Hematoma Formation

The most common complications associated with cartilage donor sites are related to infection and hematoma formation.[35] As for other wounds, these can result in pain and difficulty healing in the short term and worsened scarring and deformity in the long term. These infections are managed similarly to infections in donor-skin graft sites; debridement and antibiotic treatment form the mainstay of management. Additionally, the overzealous harvesting of cartilage can result in unintended donor-site disfigurement. Leaving sufficient residual cartilage for donor-site support prevents this problem. The specific amount will vary for each donor site as well as for each individual. For example, most patients require the preservation of at least a 5-mm struts of dorsal and caudal cartilage. The failure to allow for this minimal amount of septal cartilage to remain may result in a saddle-nose deformity.[36] The pinnae of the ear can tolerate the harvest of the entire concha without deformity. The harvest of cartilage from the rib is also well tolerated as long as the costosternal continuity is maintained for the same hemithorax.

Donor-Site–Specific Complications

There are additional complications associated with graft harvest that are specific to each donor site. The harvest of septal cartilage is generally performed via a standard septoplasty approach. As for septoplasty performed for nasal obstruction, there is a risk of resultant septal perforation associated with the removal of septal cartilage and bone.[37] Avoiding mucoperichondrial flap tears will prevent this complication. If tears do occur, care must be taken to prevent a tear on the contralateral flap. Opposing tears will lead to a high incidence of resultant septal perforations. Should directly opposing tears occur, these should be repaired primarily with suture. This maneuver will often enhance healing of the ipsilateral mucoperichondrial edge and not of the contralateral mucoperichondrial edge, thus preventing perforation. Should a perforation result, it can be managed in a variety of ways, including observation with nasal hygiene, delayed repair with mucosal rotation flaps, or with the insertion of a septal button.[38,39] In some cases, symptoms associated with small septal perforations can be improved by enlarging the perforation. The correct approach will vary greatly among cases and must be designed for each patient individually.

Pneumothorax Complications

Cartilage harvest from the ribs can be complicated by pneumothorax.[40] This can be life-threatening if it is not recognized and managed expeditiously, especially in children. Thus the immediate postoperative evaluation of patients with a chest x-ray film is prudent. However, in most cases, the surgeon recognizes the pleural breech intraoperatively. In these situations, the breech can be addressed primarily with the introduction of a red rubber Robinson catheter into the pleural space with the subsequent placement of a purse-string suture around it. Suction can then be applied via the catheter to evacuate any air, thus ensuring lung inflation. After this has been accomplished, the catheter is pulled out while it is still under suction as the anesthesiologist provides a Valsalva maneuver. The purse-string suture is tightened and secured simultaneously to prevent the reformation of the pneumothorax. Should this approach fail, a chest tube should be placed. During the identification and management of the pleural breech, excellent communication between the surgeon and the anesthesiologist is of paramount importance. The resolution of the pneumothorax should be documented immediately with an intraoperative chest x-ray film. Postoperatively, the patient should be observed closely and followed with serial x-ray films to ensure the stability of the repair. Thoracic surgery consultation is generally helpful in these cases.

Cartilage Graft Implantation Complications

Complications related to cartilage graft implantation sites are mostly the result of a breech in sterility, hematoma formation, or inappropriate graft fixation.[29] All three situations result in implant-site inflammation with resulting partial or total graft resorption. The loss of graft volume is permanent, because the implanted graft is acellular and thus incapable of regeneration. Infection, when present, needs to be treated aggressively. The avascular nature of cartilage makes clearing infections notoriously difficult. Management requires aggressive antibiotic therapy, with consideration given to wound exploration and irrigation. Notwithstanding these interventions, the infected graft may need to be removed in cases that prove to be unresponsive to therapy. The management of bleeding and hematoma formation within the recipient site needs to be aggressive, and it usually entails drainage with consideration for wound irrigation. Failure to do so may lead to cartilage loss as a result of the inflammatory reaction associated with the hematoma, but it may also lead to secondary wound infection. Graft resorption can also be the result of poor graft fixation. The continued graft–recipient-site shear will lead to inflammation and graft loss. This problem can be prevented by securely anchoring the graft during implantation.[41] This may be achieved by making the soft-tissue pocket only as large as needed to snugly fit the graft. Alternatively, anchoring sutures can be applied to ensure graft fixation. Improper graft fixation may also lead to graft migration and consequently to poor graft position with a concomitant poor outcome; this problem usually requires revision.

When Used as Part of a Composite Graft

Cartilage grafting can also be used as part of a composite graft, which contains cartilage, perichondrium, subcutaneous tissue, and full-thickness skin. Composite cartilage grafts are most commonly used for the reconstruction of full-thickness alar nasal defects.[35,42] The preferred donor site for these grafts is the pinnae of the ear. Their use is mostly limited by their size, because they require the ability to sustain multilayer graft cell viability during the time required for inosculation. Success is greatest when graft size is limited to less than 0.5 cm in the largest dimension. Hyperbaric oxygen therapy has been applied to help drive revascularization and thus to expand the size limitation of these

grafts, with some success.[43,44] The use of these grafts is most frequently complicated by partial or complete graft loss. This is managed by debridement and wound care, generally with consideration for alternative reconstruction. Donor-site complications and their management are the same as for the harvest of ear cartilage grafts, as previously discussed.

BONE GRAFTING

Application

Bone grafting, like cartilage grafting, is mainly used to provide soft-tissue support for sites in which gravity, wound contracture, or tissue laxity may lead to undesirable cosmesis or function. The critical difference resides in the fact that bone is best able to accomplish this within sites that are exposed to muscular stress. This technology is most frequently applied during reconstruction after head and neck cancer ablative treatment, but it also plays an important role in the management of defects associated with trauma, congenital anomalies, and the surgical treatment of infection. In the head and neck, the best example of a site that requires bone for the successful reconstitution of form and function is the mandible. At this site, the combination of the regional musculature that is active in facial mimetics, speech, and deglutition together with the prevailing forces of scar formation and gravity generally leads to extensive deformity and dysfunction unless opposed by a sufficiently strong structural framework. To a lesser extent, this phenomenon is also seen at other sites of the head and neck where muscle activity imparts load, such as the nose and the malar prominence. Free avascular bone grafts that are useful for head and neck reconstruction can be of two forms: cancellous bone or corticocancellous bone.

Harvest Sites

Cancellous bone is obtained from several sites, including cranial bone, the symphysis of the mandible, the rib, the tibial plateau, and the iliac crest.[45] The osteocompetent cells important for bony growth are the endosteal osteoblasts and the cancellous marrow stem cells that are contained within the bony marrow space. The use of cancellous bone grafts has been championed for many years because of their ease of harvest, malleability, and ease of take. They have been extensively applied for the reconstruction of intramandibular and intramaxillary defects in which alveolar height and continuity may have been lost. The reconstitution of appropriate bone height is critical for the successful placement of osseointegrated dental implants.[46] The graft is amorphous at implantation, thus necessitating a rigid and well-vascularized recipient bed initially.[47] This rigid bed can be fashioned from existing soft tissue within a recipient site or from implanted bone trays. When osteoinduction ensues, the graft acquires an independent form. Continued remodeling of the graft leads to full osteointegration with native bone.[48] The prevailing forces acting on the graft determine the resulting shape, much as normal bone morphogenesis occurs. The resultant bone stock is excellent for dental implant placement, which is currently the most advanced prosthetic rehabilitation available. Notwithstanding its versatility and success, this technique meets with lackluster success in the setting of acutely infected wounds as well as in radiated recipient beds, where vascular ingrowth from the donor site into the initially avascular graft is less efficient.[45,49] Furthermore, full osteogenesis and integration will take as long as a year, thus limiting the usefulness of these grafts for the patient with head and neck cancer. However, when applied to the appropriate patient, the technique leads to rehabilitation with bone of the highest quality.

Complications

Complications of cancellous bone grafting can be separated into donor-site complications and recipient-site complications. Cancellous bone graft harvesting requires surgical exposure through soft tissues to expose the donor bone site. As such, like most soft-tissue operations, these can be complicated by infection and hematoma formation.[50] For the case of graft harvest from the calvarial bone, the inner cortex can be breached, which leads to dural exposure with concomitant risks of cerebrospinal fluid leak, meningitis, and epidural hematoma. The management of these is stereotypical and focuses on appropriate wound care, the evacuation of any collections, and the administration of antibiotics. In addition, in the setting of dural breach, a watertight closure of the wound is important to prevent cerebrospinal fluid contamination and any risk of meningitis. Complications can also relate to site-specific anatomic structures that are at risk during graft harvest. For example, when harvesting grafts from the iliac crest, the lateral femoral cutaneous nerve can be injured, which can lead to dysesthesias and, in the worst cases, chronic pain.[45] Gait disturbance and unsightly scarring can also result from harvest in this region. When using the tibial plateau for graft harvest, care must be taken to not extend the access incision too far laterally, which places the peroneal nerve at risk for injury.[51] Lastly, when approaching the parietal skull for calvarial graft harvest, dissection within the appropriate plane must be ensured to prevent alopecia.[50,52] More specific to the actual graft harvest are complications associated with the bony donor site itself. To harvest the graft, a cortical window is generally made. The elevated plate is usually replaced and stabilized by internal fixation with

wires or plates. These sites are at risk for nonunion and possible osteomyelitis. Should these complications occur, they are managed by the debridement of the affected bone, the extraction of any infected hardware, and long-term treatment with culture-directed antibiotics.

Recipient-Site Complications

Recipient-site complications are fewer in nature and mimic those of all other free-tissue grafts: mainly failure of take. Implanting the graft into an appropriately immobilized, well-vascularized, clean bed with good apposition to native bone prevents this.[53] The failure of graft take is usually heralded by localized wound inflammation. Treatment will require debridement, wound care, and appropriate antibiotic coverage. As for most free grafts, initial failure has no impact on subsequent success as long as the factors that are identified as detrimental to take have been addressed.

Corticocancellous Grafts

Corticocancellous grafts combine the high osteointegrating potential of cancellous bone with the rigid support afforded by cortical bone. These grafts are most commonly harvested from the iliac bone, the rib, or the calvarium. Their application is most successful in the setting of the reconstruction of nasofacial defects, where they allow for the excellent reconstitution of support that is resistant to the forces of contracture and mimetic musculature. Specifically, cortical bone grafts have been successfully used for the reconstruction of nasal dorsal defects.[52] Often there is some minor cortical resorption, but, under conditions of low stress, this can be minimal and well anticipated. Corticocancellous grafts have also been used for mandibular reconstruction.[54] Here they are generally less effective at retaining their volume as a result of the increased forces inherent to this site. However, successful union can be achieved when grafting segmental mandibular defects of less than 5 cm in length in the setting of a clean, nonirradiated wound.[49] Irradiated, contaminated, or otherwise compromised wounds that are in need of segmental osseous reconstruction heal better with vascularized osseous grafts, as do wounds with segmental bone defects of more than 5 cm.

Complications of free avascular corticocancellous graft harvest are no different from those of cancellous graft harvest. Most commonly these are associated with hematoma or donor-site infections, which are treated as previously described. Specific issues may arise in relation to the lack of bone at the donor site presenting as an obvious concavity, as may occur with a calvarial bone graft. In such cases, contouring mesh plates may be placed, or the area may be resurfaced with methylmethacrylate or

TABLE 63-1. Incidence of Hematoma and Infection

Graft Tissue	Donor Site		Recipient Site	
	Hematoma (%)	Infection (%)	Hematoma (%)	Infection (%)
Split-thickness skin graft	<2	<2	<2	<2
Full-thickness skin graft	<2	<2	<2	<2
Fat	5	5	<2	5
Cartilage	<2	3	<2	5
Bone	8	5	<2	5

hydroxyapetite.[55] Complications associated with the recipient site relate mostly to a failure of graft take. Failure is usually noted as an inability to achieve bony union, obvious graft resorption, fracture of the associated fixating plate, and frank graft or hardware extrusion. These are best prevented by appropriately selecting patients with clean, well-vascularized, nonirradiated wounds in which the osseous defect is small. Importantly, the graft must be perfectly stabilized with good bone-to-bone contact to enhance the probability of take and bony union. In the case of partial graft take, there will usually be significant resorption of the cortical component of the graft. In contrast with high-stress settings, this can be well tolerated when loading stresses are low.

CONCLUSION

The field of head and neck reconstruction has enjoyed tremendous development during recent years. Advances such as free vascularized tissue transfer have greatly expanded the array of defects that can be successfully reconstructed. Notwithstanding these newer technologies, avascular tissue grafts provide important alternatives for reconstruction. When appropriately applied in isolation or in combination with other modalities of reconstruction, free avascular tissue grafts provide excellent results with low incidences of complications at both the donor and recipient sites (Table 63-1).

REFERENCES

1. Smahel J: The healing of skin grafts. *Clin Plast Surg* 1977;4(3): 409–424.
2. Clemmesen T: The early circulation in split-skin grafts: Restoration of blood supply to split-skin autografts. *Acta Chir Scand* 1964;127:1–8.
3. Converse JM, Ballantyne DL Jr, Rogers BO, et al: Plasmatic circulation in skin grafts. *Transplant Bull* 1957;4(4):154–156.
4. Converse JM, Smahel J, Ballantyne DL, Jr, et al: Inosculation of vessels of skin graft and host bed: A fortuitous encounter. *Br J Plast Surg* 1975;28(4):274–282.
5. Henry L, Marshall DC, Friedman EA, et al: A histological study of the human skin graft. *Am J Pathol* 1961;39:317–332.
6. Thourani VH, Ingram WL, Feliciano DV: Factors affecting success of split-thickness skin grafts in the modern burn unit. *J Trauma* 2003;54(3):562–658.
7. Rudolph R, Suzuki M, Guber S, et al: Control of contractile fibroblasts by skin grafts. *Surg Forum* 1977;28:524–525.
8. Bennett JE, Miller SR: Evolution of the electro-dermatome. *Plast Reconstr Surg* 1970;45(2):131–134.
9. Rakel BA, Bermel MA, Abbott LI, et al: Split-thickness skin graft donor site care: A quantitative synthesis of the research. *Appl Nurs Res* 1998;11(4):174–182.
10. Rigg BM: Importance of donor site selection in skin grafting. *Can Med Assoc J* 1977;117(9):1028–1029.
11. Tsukada S: The melanocytes and melanin in human skin autografts. *Plast Reconstr Surg* 1974;53(2):200–207.
12. Skouge JW: Techniques for split-thickness skin grafting. *J Dermatol Surg Oncol* 1987;13(8):841–849.
13. Blight A, Mountford EM, Cheshire IM, et al: Treatment of full skin thickness burn injury using cultured epithelial grafts. *Burns* 1991;17(6):495–498.
14. Hansbrough W, Dore C, Hansbrough JF: Management of skin-grafted burn wounds with Xeroform and layers of dry coarse-mesh gauze dressing results in excellent graft take and minimal nursing time. *J Burn Care Rehabil* 1995;16(5):531–534.
15. Scherer LA, Shiver S, Chang M, et al: The vacuum assisted closure device: A method of securing skin grafts and improving graft survival. *Arch Surg* 2002;137(8):930–934.
16. Alvi A, Myers EN: Skin graft reconstruction of the composite resection defect. *Head Neck* 1996;18(6):538–544.
17. Robinson JK, Dillig G: The advantages of delayed nasal full-thickness skin grafting after Mohs micrographic surgery. *Dermatol Surg* 2002;28(9):845–851.
18. Yoshimura Y, Matsuda S, Obara S: Full-thickness skin grafting of postsurgical oral defects: Short- and long-term outcomes. *J Oral Maxillofac Surg* 1995;53(9):998–1003.
19. Boyce RG, Nuss DW, Kluka EA: The use of autogenous fat, fascia, and nonvascularized muscle grafts in the head and neck. *Otolaryngol Clin North Am* 1994;27(1):39–68.
20. Davis RE, Guida RA, Cook TA: Autologous free dermal fat graft: Reconstruction of facial contour defects. *Arch Otolaryngol Head Neck Surg* 1995;121(1):95–100.
21. Deschler DG, Dileo M, Hayden RE: Free fat grafts: Do they still have a role? *J Aesthetic Derm Cosmetic Surg* 1999;3:211–216.
22. Conley JJ, Clairmont AA: Dermal-fat-fascia grafts. *Otolaryngology* 1978;86(4 Pt 1):ORL-641–649.
23. Nosan DK, Ochi JW, Davidson TM: Preservation of facial contour during parotidectomy. *Otolaryngol Head Neck Surg* 1991;104(3):293–298.
24. Harada T, Inoue T, Harashina T, et al: Dermis-fat graft after parotidectomy to prevent Frey's syndrome and the concave deformity. *Ann Plast Surg* 1993;31(5):450–452.

25. Jackler RK, Brachmann DE, editors: *Neurotology,* ed 2, St. Louis, 2005, Mosby.

26. Hardy JM, Montgomery WW: Osteoplastic frontal sinusotomy: An analysis of 250 operations. *Ann Otol Rhinol Laryngol* 1976;85 (4 Pt 1):523–532.

27. Dedo HH: *Surgery of the larynx and trachea,* Philadelphia, 1990, BC Decker.

28. Wetmore SJ: Injection of fat for soft tissue augmentation. *Laryngoscope* 1989;99(1):50–57.

29. Murrell GL: Auricular cartilage grafts and nasal surgery. *Laryngoscope* 2004;114(12):2092–2102.

30. Fayoux P, Vachin F, Merrot O, et al: Thyroid alar cartilage graft in paediatric laryngotracheal reconstruction. *Int J Pediatr Otorhinolaryngol* 2006;70(4):717–724.

31. Silva AB, Lusk RP, Muntz HR: Update on the use of auricular cartilage in laryngotracheal reconstruction. *Ann Otol Rhinol Laryngol* 2000;109(4):343–347.

32. Younis RT, Lazar RH, Astor F: Posterior cartilage graft in single-stage laryngotracheal reconstruction. *Otolaryngol Head Neck Surg* 2003;129(3):168–175.

33. Wax MK, Ramadan HH, Ortiz O, et al: Contemporary management of cerebrospinal fluid rhinorrhea. *Otolaryngol Head Neck Surg* 1997; 116(4):442–449.

34. Moon JW, Choung HK, Khwarg SI: Correction of lower lid retraction combined with entropion using an ear cartilage graft in the anophthalmic socket. *Korean J Ophthalmol* 2005;19(3):161–167.

35. Adams C, Ratner D: Composite and free cartilage grafting. *Dermatol Clin* 2005;23(1):vii, 129–140.

36. Most SP: Anterior septal reconstruction: Outcomes after a modified extracorporeal septoplasty technique. *Arch Facial Plast Surg* 2006;8(3):202–207.

37. Muhammad IA, Nabil-ur R: Complications of the surgery for deviated nasal septum. *J Coll Physicians Surg Pak* 2003;13(10):565–568.

38. Morre TD, Van Camp C, Clement PA: Results of the endonasal surgical closure of nasoseptal perforations. *Acta Otorhinolaryngol Belg* 1995;49(3):263–267.

39. Newton JR, White PS, Lee MS: Nasal septal perforation repair using open septoplasty and unilateral bipedicled flaps. *J Laryngol Otol* 2003;117(1):52–55.

40. Kawanabe Y, Nagata S: A new method of costal cartilage harvest for total auricular reconstruction: Part I: Avoidance and prevention of intraoperative and postoperative complications and problems. *Plast Reconstr Surg* 2006;117(6):2011–2018.

41. Gunter JP, Clark CP, Friedman RM: Internal stabilization of autogenous rib cartilage grafts in rhinoplasty: A barrier to cartilage warping. *Plast Reconstr Surg* 1997;100(1):161–169.

42. Friedman HI, Stonerock C, Brill A: Composite earlobe grafts to reconstruct the lateral nasal ala and sill. *Ann Plast Surg* 2003;50(3):275–281.

43. Lewis D, Goldztein H, Deschler D: Use of hyperbaric oxygen to enhance auricular composite graft survival in the rabbit model. *Arch Facial Plast Surg* 2006;8(5):310–313.

44. Li EN, Menon NG, Rodriguez ED, et al: The effect of hyperbaric oxygen therapy on composite graft survival. *Ann Plast Surg* 2004;53(2):141–145.

45. Lawson W, Biller HF: Mandibular reconstruction: Bone graft techniques. *Otolaryngol Head Neck Surg* 1982;90(5):589–594.

46. Hori M, Okaue M, Kaneko K, et al: Prosthetic restorations with osseointegrated implants after bone grafts to correct large jaw defects caused by extraction of multi-impacted teeth: A case report. *J Oral Sci* 1998;40(3):123–128.

47. Marx RE, Ehler WJ, Peleg M: "Mandibular and facial reconstruction" rehabilitation of the head and neck cancer patient. *Bone* 1996;19 (1 Suppl):59S–82S.

48. DeLacure MD: Physiology of bone healing and bone grafts. *Otolaryngol Clin North Am* 1994;27(5):859–874.

49. Pogrel MA, Podlesh S, Anthony JP, et al: A comparison of vascularized and nonvascularized bone grafts for reconstruction of mandibular continuity defects. *J Oral Maxillofac Surg* 1997; 55(11):1200–1206.

50. Sammartino G, Marenzi G, Colella G, et al: Autogenous calvarial bone graft harvest: Intraoperational complications. *J Craniofac Surg* 2005;16(2):312–319.

51. Chen YC, Chen CH, Chen PL, et al: Donor site morbidity after harvesting of proximal tibia bone. *Head Neck* 2006;28(6):496–500.

52. Cheney ML, Gliklich RE: The use of calvarial bone in nasal reconstruction. *Arch Otolaryngol Head Neck Surg* 1995;121(6): 643–648.

53. Giordano A, Brady D, Foster C, et al: Particulate cancellous marrow crib graft reconstruction of mandibular defects. *Laryngoscope* 1980;90(12):2027–2036.

54. Myoung H, Kim YY, Heo MS, et al: Comparative radiologic study of bone density and cortical thickness of donor bone used in mandibular reconstruction. *Oral Surg Oral Med Oral Pathol Oral Radiol Endod* 2001;92(1):23–29.

55. Wiltfang J, Kessler P, Buchfelder M, et al: Reconstruction of skull bone defects using the hydroxyapatite cement with calvarial split transplants. *J Oral Maxillofac Surg* 2004;62(1):29–35.

Index

Note: "b" following a page number indicates a box; "f" indicates a figure;
and "t" indicates a table.